NURSING GUIDE
TO
Physical Examination
and History Taking

BATES'
NURSING GUIDE
TO
Physical Examination
and History Taking

Beth Hogan-Quigley, MSN, RN, CRNP
Family and Community Health Department
University of Pennsylvania School of Nursing
Philadelphia, Pennsylvania

Mary Louise Palm, MS, RN
Associate Clinical Professor
University of Rhode Island College of Nursing
Kingston, Rhode Island

Lynn S. Bickley, MD
Clinical Professor of Medicine
University of New Mexico
Albuquerque, New Mexico

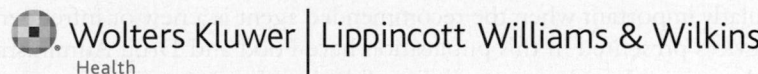
Health
Philadelphia • Baltimore • New York • London
Buenos Aires • Hong Kong • Sydney • Tokyo

Acquisitions Editor: Elizabeth Nieginski
Product Manager: Katherine Burland
Editorial Assistant: Jacalyn Clay
Design Coordinator: Holly McLaughlin
Illustration Coordinator: Brett MacNaughton
Manufacturing Coordinator: Karin Duffield
Prepress Vendor: Aptara, Inc.

9 8 7 6 5 4 3 2 1

Printed in China

Library of Congress Cataloging-in-Publication Data
Hogan-Quigley, Beth.
 Bates' nursing guide to physical examination and history taking / Beth Hogan-Quigley, Mary Louise Palm, Lynn S. Bickley.
    p. ; cm.
 Nursing guide to physical examination and history taking
 Includes bibliographical references and index.
 ISBN 978-0-7817-8069-8 (alk. paper)
 1. Physical diagnosis. 2. Medical history taking. 3. Nursing assessment. I. Palm, Mary Louise. II. Bickley, Lynn S. III. Bates, Barbara, 1928-2002. IV. Title. V. Title: Nursing guide to physical examination and history taking.
 [DNLM: 1. Nursing Assessment. 2. Medical History Taking.
3. Physical Examination. WY 100.4]
 RC76.H674 2012
 616.07'54—dc23

                                    2011027307

CCS0911

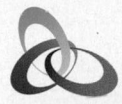

Heartfelt love and appreciation to my family:

Peter for navigating the seas with me with love and support.

Colleen and Megan for being the beams of sunlight that brighten my days.

Jim and Betty for providing me with the compass to chart my journey.

Sharon, Jim, Jan, and Laurie for "cruising" along the voyage.

And for remembering Kristin, who shines on all of us.

Beth Hogan-Quigley

With much appreciation and thanks to my family:

My husband, William J. Palm, for his support and love during this project.

My children, Aileene, Bill, and Andy, with love.

Mary Louise Palm

ACKNOWLEDGMENTS

To Lynn S. Bickley, MD and Peter G. Szilagyi, MD, MPH for creating an outstanding textbook that gave us the base to adapt the material for the undergraduate nursing student. Their thorough coverage of assessment techniques and superb writing style was a wonderful foundation for us to utilize. They set the standard for excellence in textbook writing.

We appreciate the many professionals at Lippincott, Williams and Wilkins who provided guidance throughout the creation of Bates' Nursing Guide to Physical Examination and History Taking. To Peter Darcy, Jean Rodenberger, and Renee Gagliardi, who brought us into the project. Katherine Burland, our product manager, and Mary Kinsella, who both provided day to day guidance. Our thanks to artist Anne Rains, who created drawings and altered pictures and turned our thoughts into graphics.

We would also like to thank the team at Aptara with a special thank you to Chris Miller, project manager, who was always available to answer questions at a moment's notice.

To Colleen Quigley for computer expertise and graphics.

To all our colleagues, who provided expertise and support for our endeavor and helped make this text a reality. To Patricia Burbank DNsc, RN who provided wording on sensitive topics.

To our students, past and present, who are the reason we teach and who inspire us to create and use better teaching tools.

CONTENTS

Acknowledgments   vii
Preface   xv

UNIT 1
Foundations   1

CHAPTER 1
Introduction to Health Assessment   3

HEALTH ASSESSMENT   4
Role of the Nurse in Assessment   8

CHAPTER 2
Critical Thinking in Health Assessment   11

NURSING PROCESS   14
**ASSESSMENT: THE PROCESS OF CLINICAL
REASONING   15**
Identifying Problems and Making Nursing Diagnoses:
    Steps in Clinical Reasoning   16
**RECORDING YOUR FINDINGS: THE CASE
OF MRS. N   19**
EVALUATING CLINICAL FINDINGS   30
**LIFELONG LEARNING: INTEGRATING CLINICAL
REASONING, ASSESSMENT, AND ANALYSIS OF
CLINICAL EVIDENCE   31**

CHAPTER 3
Interviewing and Communication   35

PHASES OF INTERVIEWING   36
Phase 1: Pre-interview   37
Phase 2: Introduction   39
Phase 3: Working Phase   41
Phase 4: Termination   46
THERAPEUTIC COMMUNICATION TECHNIQUES   46
**ADAPTING THE INTERVIEW FOR SPECIAL
PATIENTS   51**
ETHICS OF INTERVIEWING   58
Ethics and Professionalism   58

CHAPTER 4
The Health History   61

**THE COMPREHENSIVE ADULT HEALTH
HISTORY   63**
**SENSITIVE TOPICS THAT CALL FOR SPECIFIC
APPROACHES   72**
DOCUMENTING THE HEALTH HISTORY   76

CHAPTER 5
Cultural and Spiritual Assessment   78

CULTURAL ASSESSMENT   78
Transcultural Perspectives on the Health History   83
SPIRITUAL ASSESSMENT   85
DEATH AND THE DYING PATIENT   87

CHAPTER 6
Physical Examination   90

**THE COMPREHENSIVE ADULT PHYSICAL
EXAMINATION   91**
Beginning the Examination: Setting the Stage   91
Techniques of Examination   98
Overview—The Physical Examination   101

CHAPTER 7
Beginning the Physical Examination:
General Survey, Vital Signs, and Pain   105

General Survey   105
Vital Signs   106
Pain, the Fifth Vital Sign   106

■ **General Appearance   106**
Apparent State of Health   106
Level of Consciousness   106
Facial Expression   106
Odors of the Body and Breath   107
Posture, Gait, Motor Activity, and Speech   107
Signs of Distress   108
Skin Color and Obvious Lesions   108
Dress, Grooming, and Personal Hygiene   108

■ **The Vital Signs   109**
BLOOD PRESSURE   109
Choice of Blood Pressure Cuff (Sphygmomanometer)   109
Technique for Measuring Blood Pressure   110
Classification of Normal and Abnormal Blood
    Pressure   113
SPECIAL TECHNIQUES   114
HEART RATE AND RHYTHM   116
Heart Rate   116
Rhythm   116
RESPIRATORY RATE AND RHYTHM   116
TEMPERATURE   116
Oral Thermometers   117
Rectal Temperatures   117
Tympanic Membrane Temperatures   117
Temporal Artery Temperatures   117
Axillary Temperatures   118
Skin Temperatures   118
Fever, Chills, and Night Sweats   118

■ Acute and Chronic Pain 118

Pain 118
Understanding Acute and Chronic Pain 119
Assessing the Patient's History 119
Types of Pain 120
Pain Management 121

RECORDING YOUR FINDINGS 122
HEALTH PROMOTION 122

Temperature 122
Pulse 123
Respirations 123
Blood Pressure 123

CHAPTER 8
Nutrition 127

OVERVIEW 127

Hydration Status 128

THE HEALTH HISTORY 128

Common or Concerning Symptoms 128
Changes in Weight 129

PHYSICAL EXAMINATION 131

General Survey 131
Height Measurement 131
Weight Measurement 132
Skin, Hair, and Nails 133
Head, Ears, Eyes, Nose, and Throat (HEENT) 133
Cardiovascular and Peripheral Vascular 133
Gastrointestinal 133
Musculoskeletal 134
Neurologic 134
Calculating the BMI 134

HEALTH PROMOTION AND COUNSELING 136

Important Topics for Health Promotion and Counseling 136
Optimal Weight, Nutrition, and Diet 136
Exercise 139
Hydration 140

UNIT 2
Body Systems 151

CHAPTER 9
The Integumentary System 153

ANATOMY AND PHYSIOLOGY 154
THE HEALTH HISTORY 156

Common or Concerning Symptoms 156
Past History 157
Family History 157
Lifestyle and Personal Habits 157

PHYSICAL EXAMINATION 158

Skin 158
Hair 164
164

RECORDING YOUR FINDINGS 165
HEALTH PROMOTION AND COUNSELING 165

Important Topics for Health Promotion and Counseling 165

CHAPTER 10
The Head and Neck 189

■ The Head 189
ANATOMY AND PHYSIOLOGY OF THE HEAD 189
THE HEALTH HISTORY 190
■ The Neck 193
ANATOMY AND PHYSIOLOGY OF THE NECK 193
PHYSICAL EXAMINATION 197
RECORDING YOUR FINDINGS 202

Recording the Physical Examination—The Head and Neck 202

HEALTH PROMOTION AND COUNSELING 203

Important Topics 203

CHAPTER 11
The Eyes 211

ANATOMY AND PHYSIOLOGY 211
THE EYES 211

Eye Structures 211

THE HEALTH HISTORY 217

Eye History 219
Family History 220
Lifestyle Habits 220

PHYSICAL EXAMINATION 220

Preparation of the Patient 220
Vision Tests 221
Steps for Examining the Optic Disc 229

SPECIAL TECHNIQUES 232
RECORDING THE PHYSICAL EXAMINATION—THE EYE 234
HEALTH PROMOTION, DISEASE PREVENTION, AND EDUCATION 234

Important Topics 234
Vision Screening 234
Eye Protection 235
Care of Contact Lenses 235

CHAPTER 12
Ears, Nose, Mouth, and Throat 249

■ The Ear 250
ANATOMY AND PHYSIOLOGY 250
THE HEALTH HISTORY 252

Ear History 253
Past History 255
Family History 255
Lifestyle Habits 255

■ The Nose and Paranasal Sinuses   256
ANATOMY AND PHYSIOLOGY   256
THE HEALTH HISTORY   258

Past History   260
Family History   260
Lifestyle Habits   260

■ Mouth and Pharynx   261
ANATOMY AND PHYSIOLOGY   261
THE HEALTH HISTORY   264

Past History   266
Family History   266
Lifestyle Habits   266

PHYSICAL EXAMINATION OF THE EAR   266
PHYSICAL EXAMINATION OF THE NOSE   270
PHYSICAL EXAMINATION OF THE MOUTH AND THROAT   272
RECORDING YOUR FINDINGS   274
HEALTH PROMOTION, DISEASE PREVENTION, AND EDUCATION: EARS   274
HEALTH PROMOTION, DISEASE PREVENTION, AND EDUCATION: MOUTH AND THROAT   275

CHAPTER 13
The Respiratory System   292

ANATOMY AND PHYSIOLOGY   292
THE HEALTH HISTORY   299

Overview   299
Past History   303
Family History   304
Lifestyle and Personal Habits   304

PHYSICAL EXAMINATION   305

Overview   305

Initial Survey of Respiration and the Thorax   305
Examination of the Posterior Chest   306

Inspection   306
Palpation   307
Percussion   308
Auscultation   312

Examination of the Anterior Chest   316

Inspection   316
Palpation   316
Percussion   318
Auscultation   319

SPECIAL TECHNIQUES   320
RECORDING YOUR FINDINGS   321
HEALTH PROMOTION AND COUNSELING   321

CHAPTER 14
The Cardiovascular System   336

ANATOMY AND PHYSIOLOGY   337

Location of the Heart and Great Vessels   337
The Heart Wall   339

Cardiac Chambers, Valves, and Circulation   339
The Cardiac Cycle   340
The Splitting of Heart Sounds   342
Heart Murmurs   343
Relation of Auscultatory Findings to the Chest Wall   344
The Conduction System   345
The Heart as a Pump   347
Arterial Pulses and Blood Pressure   347
Jugular Venous Undulations   348
Jugular Venous Pressure   348

THE HEALTH HISTORY   350

Past History   354
Family History   354
Lifestyle Habits   354

PHYSICAL EXAMINATION   354

Preparation of the Patient   354
Face   355
Great Vessels of the Neck   355
The Heart   361
Peripheral Edema   376
Integrating Cardiovascular Assessment   376

RECORDING YOUR FINDINGS   376

Recording the Physical Examination—The Cardiovascular Examination   376

HEALTH PROMOTION   377

Health Promotion Topics   377
Incidence   377
Risk Reduction   379
Healthy Lifestyles   381

CHAPTER 15
The Peripheral Vascular System and Lymphatic System   398

ANATOMY AND PHYSIOLOGY   398

Arteries   399
Veins   401
The Lymphatic System and Lymph Nodes   403
Fluid Exchange and the Capillary Bed   404

THE HEALTH HISTORY   405

Past History   407
Family History   408
Lifestyle or Health Patterns   408

PHYSICAL EXAMINATION   408

Important Areas of Examination   409
Arms   409
Legs   410

RECORDING YOUR FINDINGS   416
SPECIAL TECHNIQUES   417
HEALTH PROMOTION AND COUNSELING   422

Important Topics for Health Promotion and Counseling   422

CHAPTER 16
The Gastrointestinal and Renal Systems 431

ANATOMY AND PHYSIOLOGY 431
THE HEALTH HISTORY 435
  The Gastrointestinal Tract 437
  The Urinary Tract 444
PHYSICAL EXAMINATION 447
The Abdomen 448
  Inspection 448
  Auscultation 450
  Percussion 451
  Palpation 452
  The Liver 454
  The Kidneys 457
  The Bladder 459
  The Aorta 459
SPECIAL TECHNIQUES 460
  The Spleen 460
RECORDING YOUR FINDINGS 466
  Recording the Physical Examination—The Abdomen 466
HEALTH PROMOTION 467
  Health Promotion Topics 467

CHAPTER 17
The Breasts and Axillae 490

ANATOMY AND PHYSIOLOGY 490
The Female Breast 490
The Male Breast 492
Lymphatics 493
THE HEALTH HISTORY 493
  History 495
  Family History 496
  Lifestyle Habits 497
PHYSICAL EXAMINATION 497
The Female Breast 497
  Inspection 497
  Palpation 500
The Male Breast 503
The Axillae 503
  Inspection 503
  Palpation 503
SPECIAL TECHNIQUES 504
RECORDING YOUR FINDINGS 506
  Recording the Physical Examination—Breasts and Axillae 506
HEALTH PROMOTION AND COUNSELING 506
  Important Topics for Health Promotion and Counseling 506
  Overview 506
  Selected Risk Factors That Affect Screening Decisions 509
  Recommendations for Breast Cancer Screening and Chemoprevention 510
  Counseling Women about Breast Cancer 512

CHAPTER 18
The Musculoskeletal System 517

ASSESSING THE MUSCULOSKELETAL SYSTEM 517
  Overview 517
  Joint Structure and Function 518
  Types of Joint Articulation 519
  Structure of Synovial Joints 520
THE HEALTH HISTORY 521
EXAMINATION OF JOINTS: ANATOMY AND PHYSIOLOGY AND PHYSICAL EXAMINATION 523
  Important Areas of Examination for Each of the Major Joints 523
Temporomandibular Joint 527
  Overview, Bony Structures, and Joints 527
  Muscle Groups and Additional Structures 528
  Physical Examination 528
The Shoulder 529
  Overview 529
  Bony Structures 529
  Joints 530
  Muscle Groups 531
  Additional Structures 532
  Physical Examination 533
The Elbow 538
  Overview, Bony Structures, and Joints 538
  Muscle Groups and Additional Structures 538
  Physical Examination 539
The Wrist and Hands 541
  Overview 541
  Bony Structures 541
  Joints 542
  Muscle Groups 542
  Additional Structures 543
  Physical Examination 543
The Spine 550
  Overview 550
  Bony Structures 551
  Joints 552
  Muscle Groups 553
  Physical Examination 553
The Hip 559
  Overview 559
  Bony Structures and Joints 559
  Muscle Groups 560
  Additional Structures 561
  Physical Examination 561
The Knee 566
  Overview 566
  Bony Structures 566
  Joints 567
  Muscle Groups 567
  Additional Structures 567
  Physical Examination 568

The Ankle and Foot   572
　　Overview   572
　　Bony Structures and Joints   572
　　Muscle Groups and Additional Structures   573
　　Physical Examination   574
SPECIAL TECHNIQUES   576
RECORDING YOUR FINDINGS   578
HEALTH PROMOTION   578
　　Health Promotion Topics   578

CHAPTER 19
Mental Status   595

SYMPTOMS AND BEHAVIOR   596
THE HEALTH HISTORY   597
PHYSICAL EXAMINATION   599
　　Important Areas of the Mental Status
　　　　Examination   600
　　Appearance and Behavior   601
　　Speech and Language   602
　　Mood   603
　　Thought and Perceptions   604
　　Cognitive Functions   605
　　Higher Cognitive Functions   607
SPECIAL TECHNIQUES   609
RECORDING YOUR FINDINGS   609
　　Recording Behavior and Mental Status   609
HEALTH PROMOTION AND COUNSELING   610
　　Important Topics for Health Promotion and
　　　　Counseling   610

CHAPTER 20
The Nervous System   613

ANATOMY AND PHYSIOLOGY   613
　　Central Nervous System   613
　　Peripheral Nervous System   616
　　The Peripheral Nerves   616
　　Motor Pathways   618
　　Sensory Pathways   620
　　Spinal Reflexes: The Deep Tendon Response   622
THE HEALTH HISTORY   623
PHYSICAL EXAMINATION   627
　　The Cranial Nerves   630
　　The Motor System   635
　　The Sensory System   639
　　Deep Tendon Reflexes   645
　　Cutaneous Stimulation Reflexes (Superficial Reflexes)   650
ABBREVIATED NEUROLOGIC ASSESSMENT   651
　　Assessment for Comatose Patient   651
SPECIAL TECHNIQUES   656
RECORDING YOUR FINDINGS   657
　　Recording the Examination—The Nervous System   657
HEALTH PROMOTION AND COUNSELING   658
　　Important Topics for Health Promotion and
　　　　Counseling   658

CHAPTER 21
Reproductive Systems   683

■ Female Reproductive System   684
ANATOMY AND PHYSIOLOGY   684
THE HEALTH HISTORY   686
　　Menstrual History   687
　　Obstetric History   690
PHYSICAL EXAMINATION   692
　　Important Areas of Examination   692
External Examination   694
Internal Examination   695
RECORDING YOUR FINDINGS   695
　　Recording the Pelvic Examination—Female Genitalia   695
HEALTH PROMOTION AND COUNSELING   695
　　Important Topics for Health Promotion and Counseling   695
■ Male Reproductive System   699
ANATOMY AND PHYSIOLOGY   699
THE HEALTH HISTORY   701
PHYSICAL EXAMINATION   705
The Penis   705
　　Inspection   705
The Scrotum and its Contents   706
　　Inspection   706
Hernias   706
　　Inspection   706
RECORDING YOUR FINDINGS   707
　　Recording the Physical Examination— Male Genitalia and
　　　　Hernias   707
HEALTH PROMOTION AND COUNSELING   707
　　Important Topics for Health Promotion and
　　　　Counseling   707

CHAPTER 22
Putting It All Together   720

A SAMPLE OF THE SEQUENCING FOR A HEAD-TO-TOE
ASSESSMENT   722
　　Physical Examination Overview   722

UNIT 3
Special Lifespan   729

CHAPTER 23
Assessing Children: Infancy Through Adolescence   731

■ General Principles of Child Development   733
■ Health Promotion and Counseling: Key Components   734
　　Key Components of Pediatric Health Promotion   736
■ Assessing The Infant   736

DEVELOPMENT 736
THE HEALTH HISTORY 737

Birth History 738
Past History 738
Family History 738
Health Maintenance 738
Health Patterns 739
Approaching the Infant 739
General Guidelines 740
Testing for Developmental Milestones 741

PHYSICAL EXAMINATION OF THE INFANT 744

General Survey and Vital Signs 744
The Skin 748
The Head 750
The Eyes 752
The Ears 754
The Nose and Sinuses 754
The Mouth and Pharynx 754
The Neck 755
The Thorax and Lungs 756
The Heart 759
The Breasts 763
The Abdomen 763
Male Genitalia 765
Female Genitalia 766
Rectal Examination 766
The Musculoskeletal System 767
The Nervous System 769

HEALTH PROMOTION AND COUNSELING 775

■ **Assessing Young and School-Aged Children 776**
DEVELOPMENT 776

Early Childhood: 1 to 4 Years 776
Middle Childhood: 5 to 10 Years 777

THE HEALTH HISTORY 778

Assessing Younger Children 779
Assessing Older Children 780

PHYSICAL EXAMINATION OF YOUNG AND SCHOOL-AGED CHILDREN 782

General Survey and Vital Signs 782
The Skin 785
The Head 785
The Eyes 786
The Ears 787
The Nose and Sinuses 789
The Mouth and Pharynx 790
The Neck 792
The Thorax and Lungs 793

The Heart 794
The Abdomen 796
Male Genitalia 797
Female Genitalia 798
The Rectal Examination 800
The Musculoskeletal System 800
The Nervous System 801

HEALTH PROMOTION AND COUNSELING 804

Children 1 to 4 Years 804
Children 5 to 10 Years 805

■ **Assessing Adolescents 806**
DEVELOPMENT: 11 TO 20 YEARS 806
THE HEALTH HISTORY 808
PHYSICAL EXAMINATION OF THE ADOLESCENT 810

General Survey and Vital Signs 810
The Skin 810
Head, Ears, Eyes, Throat, and Neck 811
The Heart 811
The Breasts 811
The Abdomen 813
Male Genitalia 813
Female Genitalia 815
The Musculoskeletal System 817
The Nervous System 818

HEALTH PROMOTION AND COUNSELING 818
RECORDING YOUR FINDINGS 820

CHAPTER 24
Assessing Older Adults 840

Chapter Overview: The Aging Adult 841

ANATOMY AND PHYSIOLOGY 841
THE HEALTH HISTORY 849

Approach to the Patient 849

Approach to the Older Adult Patient 849

Focus Areas When Assessing Older Adults 852

Common Concerns 852

PHYSICAL EXAMINATION OF THE OLDER ADULT 860
RECORDING YOUR FINDINGS 866
HEALTH PROMOTION AND COUNSELING 868

Important Topics for Health Promotion and Counseling in the Older Adult 868

Glossary 883
Index 887

PREFACE

Bates' Nursing Guide to Physical Assessment and History Taking is designed for undergraduate nursing students. In this ever changing and diverse health care arena, nurses are at the forefront in coordinating and providing holistic care for the patient in many venues. Assessment is a key nursing function that ensures the patient receives optimal care. The text provides assessment tools to assist the student to obtain a thorough history and perform a comprehensive physical examination of each patient. The student will learn how to ask pertinent questions and recognize verbal and nonverbal cues while eliciting information related to patient complaints in each body system. The student will then use these history findings and critical thinking skills to prioritize and guide the physical examination. The subjective and objective findings obtained during the assessment will provide the basis for the nursing diagnoses and patient plan of care. Health promotion and disease prevention are highlighted for nurses to incorporate when educating patients, families, and communities.

Bates' Nursing Guide helps students build on basic knowledge of human anatomy and physiology as the lifelong and timeless skills of patient assessment are acquired. Throughout the book, the focus and emphasis is the "normal" patient. Common or important problems are highlighted rather than the rare or obscure. Occasionally, physical signs of rare disorders are included if they hold a solid niche in classic physical assessment or represent a disorder that is critical to the life of the patient. Each chapter explicitly reflects a strong evidence based perspective, listing key citations that closely align content with new evidence from the health care literature. Color helps readers find chapter sections and tables more easily and it highlights insets of key material and special tips for challenging aspects of examination such as examining the eye or assessing the jugular venous pressure.

Bates' Nursing Guide: Highlights

The book is divided into three units: *Foundations, Body Systems,* and *Special Lifespan Considerations.*

● *Unit 1, Foundations. Chapter 1, Introduction to Health Assessment,* presents the concept of health and what defines a "healthy" individual. The indicators and purpose of Healthy People 2020 are identified, as are the components of a health assessment and the role of the nurse in assessment. *Chapter 2, Critical Thinking in Health Assessment,* focuses on how to think "like a nurse," utilizing a case study approach to implement the nursing process. *Chapter 3, Interviewing and Communication,* leads the nursing student through therapeutic communication techniques, shares mnemonics for assessment questions, and identifies strategies for handling difficult patients. *Chapter 4, The Health History,* describes the different types of health histories, the purpose for each, and the components of a comprehensive health history. *Chapter 5, Cultural and Spiritual Assessment,* explains why culture and spirituality are important in the health assessment and case studies demonstrate cultural humility. *Chapter 6, Physical Examination*, introduces a logical sequence of the physical examination with an explanation of the techniques and the equipment. *Chapter 7, Beginning the Physical Examination: General Survey, Vital Signs, and Pain, and Chapter 8, Nutrition*, continues the process of data collection and expands the process of clinical reasoning for nurses.

- *Unit 2, Body Systems.* This unit encompasses Chapters 9 through 21, which are devoted to the techniques of the regional examination of each of the body systems. These chapters are arranged in a "head-to-toe" sequence, just as the patient examination should flow. Each of the chapters contains:
  - A review of relevant anatomy and physiology
  - Key questions for a relevant nursing health history
  - Updated information for health promotion and counseling
  - Well-described and well-illustrated techniques of examination
  - Extensive citations from the clinical literature
  - Tables to assist nursing students recognize and compare normal and abnormal findings

The unit concludes with *Chapter 22, Putting It All Together*, which assists the student nurse to perform a "head to toe" examination following a sequence in which systems are integrated. Students frequently need this step-by-step guidance as they learn new skills and process how the objective data is collected in a systematic manner.

- *Unit 3, Special Lifespan Considerations.* In this unit, *Chapters 23, Assessing Children*, and *24, Assessing Older Adults*, relate to special ages in the life cycle and how the assessment techniques and physical examination findings may differ.

The first edition of this book has been written for the undergraduate student nurse. This project ensued as faculty and students requested a textbook that was geared to generalist nurses. The focus of this book is **nursing** physical examination and history taking. The health history and the physical examination are both essential for patient assessment and care.

Students are advised to return to chapters, especially in the *Foundations* unit, as they gain additional experience with patients. Each patient brings a unique background and set of abilities, ideas, issues, coping mechanisms, and family and community dynamics to the health care setting. These attributes mixed with a disease process can be confounding to even the seasoned nurse.

Students may study or review the Anatomy and Physiology sections according to their individual needs. They can study the Physical Examination sections to learn how to perform the relevant examination, practice it under faculty guidance, and review the section again afterward to consolidate their learning. Students and faculty will benefit from identifying common abnormal findings, which appear in two places. The right-hand column of the Physical Examination sections presents possible abnormal findings. These are highlighted in red and placed directly adjacent to the relevant text.

Distinguishing these findings from the normal improves learners' observations and clinical acumen. Students will learn how to clearly decipher "normal" when assessing a patient and will recognize abnormal findings. Student nurses will learn to perform inspection, palpation, percussion, and auscultation as well as to utilize the findings in the nursing plan of care.

As students progress through the body systems, they should study the write-ups of the sample patient, Mrs. N, found in Chapters 2, *Critical Thinking in Health Assessment,* and 22, *Putting It All Together.* Students should make frequent references to the sections in each of the body systems chapters titled "Recording Your Findings "that display samples of the patient record. This cross-checking will help students learn how to describe and organize information from the interview and physical examination into an understandable documentation format. Furthermore, studying Chapters 2 and 22 will help students to prioritize and analyze the data they are learning to collect.

Close scrutiny of the Tables of Abnormalities will deepen students' understanding of important clinical conditions, what they should be looking for, and why they are asking certain questions. However, they should not try to memorize all the detail that is presented. As students work to master the skills of assessment, they should return to the related signs and remember the "normal." Students should use this book to analyze the concern or finding and make use of other clinical texts or journals to pursue the patient's problems in as much depth as necessary.

Student and Instructor Resources

Student Resources
Student resources to accompany this text are available online at thePoint.lww.com.

Resources include journal articles, NCLEX-style review questions, a Spanish–English audio glossary, Watch and Learn video clips, and Concepts in Action animations.

The for-sale *Student Laboratory Manual for Bates' Nursing Guide to Physical Examination and History Taking* provides a means of student self-evaluation in a variety of formats including fill-in-the-blank, matching, sequencing, short answer and NCLEX-style questions, case studies, and sample documentation.

Instructor Resources
The instructor resource DVD available to accompany this text is a comprehensive resource that includes the following:

● Test Generator containing over 200 multiple-choice questions

● PowerPoint presentations

● Image Bank featuring all of the figures from each chapter

- Guided Lecture Notes for presenting key information to your students

- Assignments and Quizzes for gauging student understanding

- Discussion Topics to encourage critical thinking

- Case Studies providing real life application of concepts

Resources are also available online at thePoint.lww.com

Foundations

1

CHAPTER 1
Introduction to Health Assessment

CHAPTER 2
Critical Thinking in Health Assessment

CHAPTER 3
Interviewing and Communication

CHAPTER 4
The Health History

CHAPTER 5
Cultural and Spiritual Assessment

CHAPTER 6
Physical Examination

CHAPTER 7
**Beginning the Physical Examination:
General Survey, Vital Signs, and Pain**

CHAPTER 8
Nutrition

Introduction to Health Assessment

LEARNING OBJECTIVES

The student will:

1. Define health and health assessment.
2. Identify the health indicators and purpose of Healthy People 2020.
3. Explain the components of the health assessment.
4. Clarify the nurse's role in assessment.

Health is defined by the World Health Organization as being "a state of complete physical, mental, and social well-being and not merely the absence of disease or infirmity."

Health is a relative state in which a person is able to live to his or her potential and includes the "6 Facets": physical health, emotional health, social well-being, cultural influences, spiritual influences, and developmental level. Health is the sum of these facets and is not solely the absence of disease. It is influenced by a person's ability to adapt to changes in the environment. Tools for adaption include the immune system, stress reduction techniques, and support systems. Health is not a constant and is continually in a state of change. A person who feels good on all levels is a healthy person.

Nurses educate patients to think about health promotion and disease prevention. Education is paramount to assist people to make the connections between a healthy lifestyle and the prevention of disease. Health education is a vital component of nursing practice. Maintaining health is a balancing act influenced by behaviors and choices. Additional components that contribute to health include the individual's personality and attitude, resilience, family dynamics, access to health care and resources, nutrition, exercise, culture, and beliefs. The presence or absence of disease does not necessarily define health.

Healthy People 2020 is a framework that identifies risk factors, health issues, and diseases of concern in the United States. The goals and objectives serve to improve the health of individuals and communities, targeting the next ten years. Its overall goal is to increase quality of life by creating

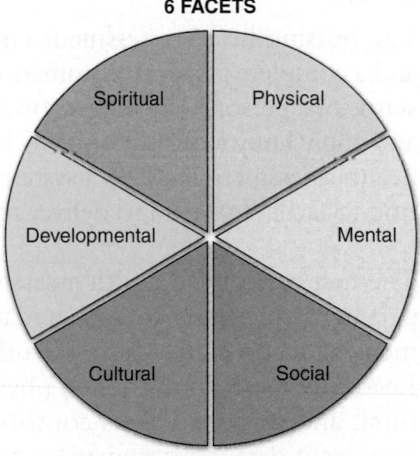

6 FACETS

guidelines for a healthy lifestyle as well as educating people and cultivating an awareness that will assist in the elimination of health disparities. Healthy People 2020 promotes health and prevents disease as it impacts the quality and length of a person's life.

The national health objectives determined by Healthy People 2020 are broad and take into consideration the results of the Healthy People 2010 outcomes of the past. These are based on current data, new developments, and challenges that are prevalent, or emerging in the United States. The U.S. Department of Health and Human Services provided this data online and invited health care leaders and the community to voice their opinions regarding the focus for this next decade.

The Healthy People 2020 indicators pertinent to each individual will be determined as the nurse completes the health assessment on each patient. Utilizing the website (http://www.healthypeople.gov), the nurse will identify appropriate interventions and resources.

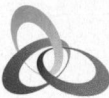 ## HEALTH ASSESSMENT

The nursing health assessment entails both a comprehensive health history and a complete physical examination, which are utilized to evaluate the health status of a person. The ability to solicit information, understand the findings, and apply knowledge can initially be daunting to the new nurse. The nursing health assessment involves a systematic data collection that provides information to facilitate a plan to deliver the best care for every patient.

The first part of the health assessment is the health history. The nurse asks pertinent questions to gather data from the patient and/or family. Past medical records may also be utilized to collect additional information. Learning about the patient's physical and psychological issues, social, cultural, and spiritual beliefs contributes to the history. The identification of important data is a systematic process.

The next component of the health assessment is the physical examination. The nurse uses a structured head-to-toe examination to identify changes in the patient's body systems. An unusual or abnormal finding may support the history data or trigger additional questions.

The information obtained throughout the health assessment should be documented in a clear, concise manner. This information is collated in the patient's medical records. The ability of the nurse to extrapolate the findings, prioritize them, and finally formulate and implement the plan of care is the overall goal. This is called "the Nursing Process."

The purpose of the nursing health assessment is to determine a patient's health status, risk factors, and need for health education as a basis for developing a nursing plan of care. The health assessment is similar to a puzzle. When the nurse meets a patient, it is like opening the puzzle box and dumping all the pieces out. Each puzzle piece represents a different aspect of the patient's life. It includes the pieces of the subjective and objective data, which form a picture of who the patient is, just like a puzzle is formed by pieces. The outside pieces and corners of the puzzle are separated into piles and pieced together first to make a frame. In the health history, the review of systems forms the frame of the assessment and outlines how to proceed with the physical examination. As each puzzle piece is inserted, the nurse is able to better see the patient as an individual. Really listening to and understanding a patient is key to having all the pieces fit. Once the frame is in place it is easier to complete the puzzle. The health assessment assists the nurse discover a patient's needs. As rapport with the patient develops, more details are acquired and more of the inside puzzle pieces are added. As the information is collated, actual health risks emerge, and eventually those last hard-to-fit puzzle pieces are found, which represent the potential health risks. This intricate puzzle is a person's life, and all the pieces need to fit correctly for the person to maintain health and quality of life. As the puzzle begins to take shape, a picture is formed. Likewise, the nurse is able to see the patient as an individual more clearly and is able to identify a specific nursing plan of care and health promotion activities.

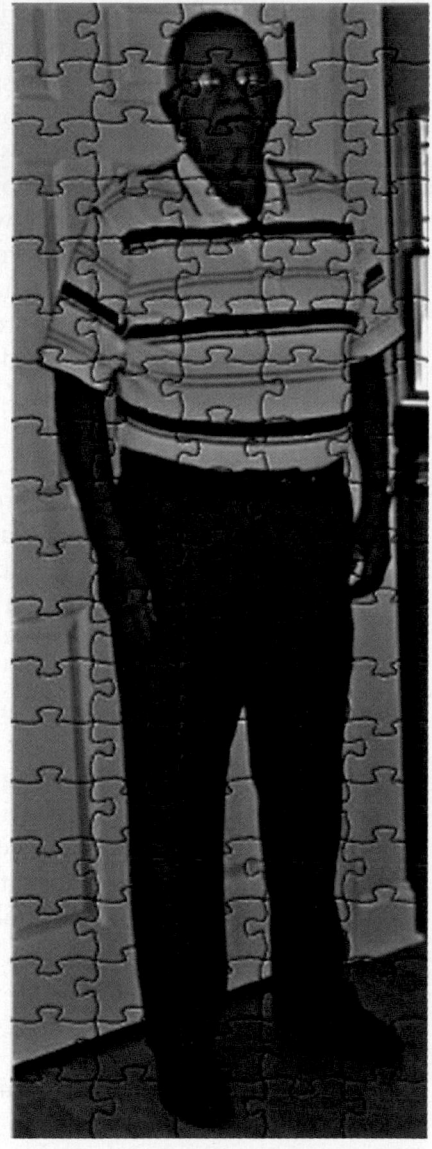

The assessment is typically performed on arrival to a health care facility. The extent of the health assessment is determined by the acuity of the patient's condition and the site of the care. For example:

● The critical patient brought into a busy emergency department would be asked basic questions revolving around the event that precipitated the admission, whether the patient is on medications, has any allergies or adverse reactions. The thorough health assessment would be completed when the patient was stable and able to answer questions.

● The patient who has a professional relationship with the nurse and had a thorough health assessment at the initial meeting does not need to have a health history repeated on each visit. Updates based on new events would be added as necessary.

● The nursing home admission of a patient with dementia may require the health assessment information be supplemented with information from the family, past health care providers, and/or medical records based on the ability of the patient to remember information.

Each person will need to have a complete health assessment. Ideally this is done on admission, but extenuating circumstances may prohibit its completion in detail at this time. The sooner the health assessment is completed fully, the better the nurse knows the patient and more holistic care can be provided to ensure health promotion and quality of life.

Nursing and medicine both perform health assessments, and although the assessment techniques may be similar, the utilization is different. The medical focus is on diagnoses and treatment of the disease, whereas the nursing focus is on diagnoses and treatment of the actual or potential human responses. The nursing assessment identifies many contributing factors to the individual's health and wellness. These include the "6 Facets" not only the physical and psychological components, but also the social, cultural, spiritual, and developmental issues. The health assessment is completed on each individual patient in order for the data collected to be specific to the patient. As the nurse spends time with the patient, he or she is able to identify concerns or changes. Any deviation is noted, as are the coping mechanisms and resources the patient has available. This information is used to determine health problems or potential problems of the patient. Development of the nursing care plan and working with the individual patient are paramount in health promotion. Once the plan is in place, evaluation continually occurs and reconfiguring may be necessary. The health care team meets to collaborate on patients and decide the best overall care. This occurs throughout the life span, from the inception of life until death. The health care team is a partnership and includes: the nurse, physician, nutritionist, social worker, physical therapist, occupational therapist, speech therapist, and/or dentist. They all work together on the same team for the benefit of the patient.

Through the health assessment nurses are able to detect areas in need of health improvement. Nurses have taken the lead in health promotion and are able to assist patients to change their behaviors and lifestyles to obtain optimal health. This enables individuals to increase control of and improve their overall health. Maintaining health is a priority in nursing and central to health care. There are three classifications of preventative health care, and assessment skills are necessary at all levels to determine what is in the best interest of the patient.

Three Levels of Preventive Care

- Primary prevention focuses on improving overall wellness and protecting from disease or disability.

- Secondary prevention focuses on early detection and treatment of a disease when it is curable or has few complications or disabilities.

- Tertiary prevention focuses on decreasing the effects of a disease or disability by preventing complications and the additional loss that happens when a defect is permanent.

Selecting the level of care and teaching is governed by the nurse as care is rendered. During the overall assessment of the patient, the nurse is able to utilize the findings and decide in which areas the patient needs the most care and which levels of prevention are necessary.

Nurses deliver care across the life span, in a variety of practice arenas, such as: pediatrics, geriatrics, medical, surgical, mental health, maternity, and community health. Nursing interventions promote health and prevent disease. Nurses educate and counsel individuals, families, groups,

● Levels of Prevention (with Examples)

Primary Prevention

- Immunizations (throughout the life span)
- Environmental measures (safe drinking water)
- Accident prevention measures (seat belts, helmets, car seats)
- Reducing risk factors (dental sealants)
- Occupational measures (hard hats, needle-free devices, sharps containers)
- Health education
- Provision of adequate housing
- Periodic selective examinations (vision, hearing, dental)
- Diet and exercise

Secondary Prevention

- Screening (blood pressure, scoliosis, mammograms, prostate-specific antigen)
- Early treatment of diseases (medications, surgery)
- Self-examination (skin lesion/mole exam, testicular self-exam)
- Communicable disease control (tuberculosis, sexually transmitted diseases)

Tertiary Prevention

- Rehabilitation programs
- Provision of hospital and community facilities
- Promotion of employing rehabilitated individuals in the workplace
- Sheltered communities
- Prevention of skin breakdown in immobile patients

and communities toward higher levels of health and wellness. Nurses view health as the focus, with the patient, the environment, and the nurse all influencing the health status of the patient. It is crucial to determine the factors that affect the patient's health as this guides the nursing plan of care. Also important is the patient's view of health and how important it is to the individual. When meeting with the patient, ask what his or her goals are:

"What do you want to get out of this visit?"
"Tell me why you are here today."

Focusing on both the answers (verbal) and the actions (nonverbal) of the patient, the nurse is constantly assessing and formulating a plan of care so that the patient can achieve the best possible health.

Health promotion goes beyond the individual patient. It also encompasses the community. Nurses are involved in the shaping of public policy and in social, economic, and workplace decisions. In order for the nurse to assist a patient with health promotion, a healthy environment must also be nurtured. The community and the environment need to be defined and realistic goals set for possible change (e.g., nurses may promote healthy diets in school cafeterias). This marks the path for prevention of illness and maintenance of health and wellness. Nurses may assess the individual, family, or community; however, the focus of this text will be the assessment of the individual.

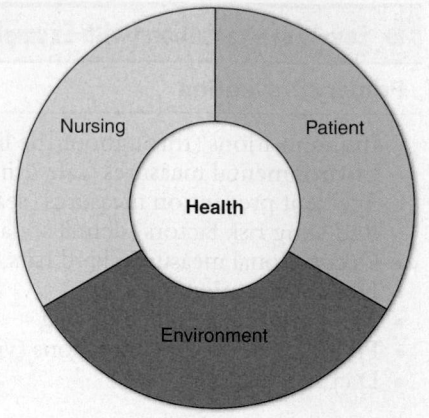

Role of the Nurse in Assessment

Nurses are instrumental in the care of patients. They oversee the holistic care of each patient. The nurse's initial role in health assessment is to collect data. Constant observation and attention to details and nuances are critical. Each person comes with a vast array of information and is influenced by his or her surroundings, including the physical, emotional, cultural, and spiritual environment. This extensive body of knowledge and the responsibility that each patient encounter requires can seem overwhelming to the new nurse. As the nurse becomes more proficient and comfortable in his or her role, accountability does not decrease, but the knowledge base and expertise increases and fosters confidence.

As a nurse, it is vital to sift through all the patient information and make judgments as to what information will impact patient safety and quality of care. The ability to identify what is important on a daily basis for each individual patient is paramount for nursing care. During the health assessment, the nurse asks questions to determine the health information that influences the day-to-day care and how it affects the person's quality of life.

This brief encounter depicts the wealth of information given by one patient. During this short interaction with Mr. P, what additional questions are you forming related to his health needs?

> Mr. P arrives at the clinic with complaints of blurred vision. During the health assessment, the patient also confides to the nurse that he has not been able to make it to the bathroom in time and has been incontinent frequently. He verbalizes that he is upset that he is unable to see well and that has slowed down his mobility. The decrease in mobility and incontinence have limited his social life with friends and he is becoming more irritable and feeling lonely. He admits to feeling like he wants to sleep all the time.

The nurse is already formulating additional questions to correlate with the standard health assessment based on what the patient has disclosed. As you read through this book, you will learn more questions to ask, those that are system specific as well as those regarding overlapping systems. How you interpret this nurse–patient interaction will be much different after learning how to do a health assessment.

As a student nurse, you might take the encounter at face value and attribute Mr. P's downward spiral to his initial blurred vision. However, after a thorough assessment, you may uncover additional issues and determine that his vision problem is not the root of his irritability and fatigue.

There is too little information available in the scenario to judge what is going on with this patient. It is important to allot a sufficient amount of time to do a detailed health assessment. Once more details are uncovered, more possibilities arise. Mr. P could potentially have multiple issues, such as: diabetes, a brain tumor, depression, blurred vision, or benign prostatic hypertrophy. However, this discovery will not be unearthed without more information.

Assessment is the foundation of nursing practice. Nurses rely heavily on their assessment skills in all aspects of nursing. The puzzle will be pieced together during the nursing assessment. For example, the patient recovering from an illness or surgery needs to be carefully assessed each shift, with changes noted that may indicate potentially dire consequences. Assessing the patient by utilizing the "6 Facets" is at the forefront of the nurse's responsibilities. Physically, the nurse may discover a change in vital signs, nausea, difficulty swallowing, or incontinence. Mentally, the patient may be experiencing changes in the level of consciousness and not know where he or she is or even who he or she is. Emotionally, is the patient more subdued, angry, or crying after a particular family member visits? The nurse will pursue the reason behind this change in the patient. Could there be abuse, money concerns, or a fear of abandonment? The nurse has developed a rapport with the patient and is now able to delve into territory that may have been off limits previously. Once these issues are acknowledged, the patient can develop a healthier life with appropriate interventions and options. Developmentally, a patient may need guidance in areas such as problem solving or moral understanding. Socially, the patient may be isolated from his or her support system in the hospital and need additional outlets. Providing information about self-help groups or health resources can provide additional avenues for people socially. Spiritually, it is best to let the patient take the lead on how he or she wants to handle spiritual care, as this dimension is very personal. If the patient wishes, connecting him or her with clergy of the same denomination while in the hospital may be welcomed, or assisting with transportation to worship services when at home may be reasonable. In all aspects it is best to work with the patient to enable partnering in choices. This allows the patient to make decisions regarding health care. The more a patient participates in these decisions, the better the outcomes are in the long term toward a healthier lifestyle.

Teaching opportunities for the patient and family present themselves during health assessments. The nurse utilizes information detected in the assessment to work with the patient to enhance quality of life. For example, the person who is overweight and has an increased body mass index (BMI) might need assistance with setting up a plan to lose weight. A plan that includes the family may be the best solution for one individual, but another may do better with an outside support group. A mutually agreed upon plan will assist the patient in maintaining autonomy and the highest level of wellness.

The nurse's ability to detect a change in a patient's physical, mental, emotional, developmental, social, or spiritual self, whether slight or significant, is instrumental in providing the best care. Just as a detective asks questions, the nurse finds clues and follows up on information in order to solve patient problems. Knowing how to facilitate the nursing health assessment by asking appropriate questions to obtain more information helps solve the mystery or create a nursing care plan. The care plan is evaluated periodically and changes made accordingly. The nurse or detective is always reassessing the patient or case for changes in order to achieve the best results. Each relies on both the science and art of their respective profession. The nursing process will be explained in detail in Chapter 2.

REFERENCES

Agency for Healthcare Research and Quality. AHRQ Quality Indicators: Guide to Patient Safety Indicators (Pub. 03-R203). Rockville, MD: Agency for Healthcare Research and Quality, 2006.

American Association of Colleges of Nursing. The Essentials of Baccalaureate Education for Professional Nursing Practice. Washington, DC: American Association of Colleges of Nursing, 1998.

American Nurses Association. Nursing: Scope and Standards of Practice. Washington, DC: American Nurses Association, 2004.

Babb M. Clinical risk assessment: identifying patients at high risk for heart failure. Assoc Periop Reg Nurse J 89(2):273–274, 277–288, 2009.

Dawood M, Gallini A. Using discovery interviews to understand the patient experience. J Nurs Manage 17(1):26–31, 2010.

Hoffman K, Aitken L, Duffield C. A comparison of novice and expert nurses' cue collection during clinical decision making: verbal protocol analysis. Int J Nurs Stud 46(10):1335–1344, 2009.

Mosby's Medical Dictionary, 8th ed. Philadelphia: Elsevier, 2009.

http://www.healthypeople.gov.

Critical Thinking in Health Assessment

LEARNING OBJECTIVES

The student will:

1. Identify the components of the nursing process.
2. Identify appropriate subjective questions based on the health assessment.
3. Categorize patient problems into a priority list.
4. Formulate a nursing diagnosis.
5. Develop a plan of care for a patient.
6. Evaluate and revise a care plan based on an individual patient.

During the time spent with the patient, you have gained your patient's trust, gathered a detailed history, and completed the requisite portions of the physical examination. You have reached the critical step of formulating your *Assessment, Nursing Diagnosis,* and *Plan.* This includes analyzing your findings, identifying the patient's problems, sharing your impressions with the patient, eliciting any concerns and coming to an agreement on the steps ahead. Finally, document the findings in the patient's record in a succinct and legible format that communicates the patient's story and your clinical reasoning and plan to other members of the health care team.

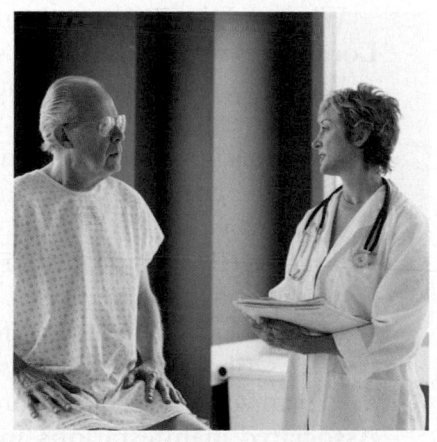

This chapter follows a step-wise approach designed to help the student acquire the important skills of clinical reasoning and critical thinking. As you listen to and examine patients, you begin to cluster information into patterns that fall into a list of problems. Each problem is listed in order of priority and clarified by an explanation of supporting findings. A nursing diagnosis is made based on the problem. Each diagnosis is followed by an individualized plan including interventions for addressing that problem. The clinical reasoning process is pivotal to determining how to interpret the patient's history and physical examination. Single out each problem listed in your assessment, and write the goals and specific nursing interventions. With experience, lifelong learning, pursuit of the clinical literature, and collaboration with colleagues, your clinical reasoning will expand and grow throughout your clinical career. The patient's record serves a dual purpose—it reflects your analysis of the patient's health status, and it documents the unique features of the patient's history, examination, laboratory and test results, assessment, and plan in a formal written format.

Critical thinking is ongoing, as is assessment of the patient. The two are intricately intertwined, and neither exists in isolation. The health assessment is the discovery and collation of facts from both the health history and physical examination. The comprehensive health history and physical assessment build the foundation of the clinical assessment.

During this collection of data, a rapport develops between the nurse and the patient and a mutual trust begins. As the fact-finding mission of the health history proceeds and data are collected, the nurse is putting pieces of the puzzle together. Through skilled interviewing, the nurse will gather the history from the patient or the family; this is the **subjective data,** which is also known as *symptoms.*

By asking questions, the nurse clarifies the most important issues that indicate areas to observe or require teaching. Each time an individual has a positive response to a question, the topic should be addressed further. As a new nurse, the questions you need to ask may seem endless, and the use of the mnemonic "OLD CART" is instrumental in assisting you to formulate the questions.

Mr. M is a 57-year-old male who presents to the clinic with complaints of a headache. During questioning you refer to "OLD CART":

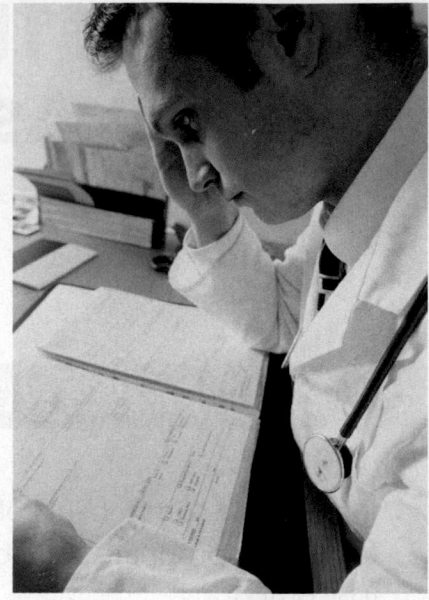

OLD CART
Onset
Location
Duration

Characteristic symptoms
Associated manifestations
Relieving factors
Treatment

Onset is when the sign or symptom began.
When did the headache begin?
Location is where the sign or symptom is located.
Where exactly is the headache? Can you point to it?
Does it radiate?
Duration is how long the sign or symptom has been going on.
Does the headache come and go? Is it nonstop? What time of day is the worst?
Characteristic symptoms are what the symptom feels like, what describes it, and its severity.
How does the headache feel? Is it throbbing? Sharp? Stabbing? Describe it. Rate it on a scale of 1 to 10, with 10 being the worst pain you have felt in your life.
Associated manifestations are what else is going on when the patient experiences the sign or symptom.
Does anything else happen when you get the headaches? Blurred vision? Nausea? Vomiting? Seizures?
Relieving factors are anything the patient has tried to relieve the headache.
Have you tried cool compresses? Rest in a dark room? Did it work?
Treatments are any interventions the patient has previously tried.
Has the patient seen a health care provider? Tried any remedies: medications (prescription, over the counter, or herbal), acupuncture to make the headache go away? Did they work?

After the interview and collection of subjective data, the nurse will perform either a head-to-toe physical examination or a systems-specific examination based on the patient's information. How to determine this will be addressed in more detail in Chapter 4, The Health History. The **objective data** is the information gathered from the physical examination and the laboratory tests. This is primarily factual and descriptive and is also known as *signs*.

As you acquire the techniques of history taking and physical examination, remember the important differences between *subjective information* and *objective information*. These distinctions are equally important for organizing written and oral presentations about patients into a logical and understandable format.

● Differences Between Subjective and Objective Data	
Subjective Data—Symptoms	**Objective Data—Signs**
What the patient tells you	What you detect during the examination
The history, from Chief Complaint through Review of Systems	All physical examination findings
Example: Mrs. G is a 54-year-old hairdresser who reports pressure over her left chest "like an elephant sitting there," which goes into her left neck and arm.	*Example:* Mrs. G is an older, overweight white female, who is pleasant and cooperative. Height 5′4″, weight 150 lbs, BMI 26, BP 160/80 right arm, sitting, HR 96 and regular, respiratory rate 24 and regular, temperature 97.5°F oral

The nurse must collect the information and synthesize it (assessment), decide what is most important (nursing diagnosis), develop a plan (goals/plan), implement the plan (interventions), and determine whether it is working for the patient (evaluation). This occurs in a multitude of sites. For example:

> At the community clinic, while assessing height and weight on an infant, you note that a 4-month-old has gained 7 lbs in the past month.
>
> At the senior center, you note that the blood pressure reading of one of the members is 192/104.
>
> Postoperatively you assess your patient and find him crying uncontrollably.

These scenarios can have different outcomes based on how the nurse and patient choose to handle the situation. As a student nurse, you may find yourself in a quandary, not certain of how to handle a situation or what to tackle first. Developing your knowledge base and diagnostic reasoning skills will assist the problem solving process. The nursing process assists you to logically and efficiently structure the patient's care.

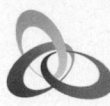 # NURSING PROCESS

The nursing process is the broad systematic framework that supplies a methodical base applicable to the practice of nursing. This problem-solving approach addresses the human responses and needs of each patient, family, and community. The nursing process has five steps: assessment, diagnosis, planning, implementation, and evaluation. The nursing process is also the scaffold that the American Nurses Association utilizes to develop the Standards of Nursing Practice.

The patient is the focus in the nursing process, with the nurse assisting the patient to achieve optimal health using individualized interventions. This is a mutually agreed upon plan of care.

ADPIE
(ASSESSMENT, DIAGNOSIS, PLANNING, IMPLEMENTATION, EVALUATION)

The five steps of the nursing process are all incorporated into the patient's plan of care and revised as the patient's health status changes.

The first step is assessment. **Assessment** is the subjective and objective data gathered during the initial health history and physical examination and collected on each patient encounter. This data is instrumental in devising a plan of care for the patient. Therapeutic communication to elicit pertinent information about the patient, the family, and the community is essential to coordinate the best care for the patient. During documentation, key points and relevant pieces of information should be clustered together, and analyzed, using the principles of: nursing, biology, psychology, sociology, and nutritional sciences. A prioritized problem list is formalized from the clustered list. The assessment phase continues throughout the entire patient encounter, which provides the potential for updates in the plan of care based on new assessments and data.

The second element is the diagnosis. **Diagnosis** has a nursing focus and is based on real or potential health problems or human responses to health problems. Diagnoses are formulated based on the assessment date. The diagnosis sets the stage for the remainder of the care plan. The diagnoses will be formulated based on the problem.

The third element is planning. **Planning** is charting the best course to address the patient's diagnoses. During planning the nurse and patient select goals for each diagnosis in order to alleviate, decrease, or prevent the problems addressed in the nursing diagnosis. There should be a short-term goal and a long-term goal with realistic time frames to be fulfilled. A successful plan requires good interpersonal skills and sensitivity to the patient's goals, economic means, competing responsibilities, and family structure and dynamics. The interventions are developed for each goal.

ADPIE
(ASSESSMENT, DIAGNOSIS, PLANNING, IMPLEMENTATION, EVALUATION) (continued)

The fourth element is the implementation of interventions. The **interventions** can be completed by the patient, the family, or members of the health care team. The interventions should clearly relate to the nursing diagnosis and the planned goals are individualized for each patient and will be modified as the patient's status or environment changes to support positive outcomes.

The fifth and final element is evaluation. **Evaluation** is a continuing process to determine if the goals have been attained. The nursing care plan is revised based on the patient's condition and whether the goals are realistic or necessary to the patient. The intervention and evaluation process is ongoing and confirms that the nursing care is relevant.

Health assessments and physical examinations are performed frequently on patients, and the information is important to document and utilize in revisions and updates of the patient's plan of care. The nursing process is ongoing. Your patient record facilitates clinical thinking, promotes communication and coordination among the many professionals caring for your patient, and documents the patient's problems and management for medical/legal purposes.

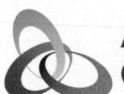

ASSESSMENT: THE PROCESS OF CLINICAL REASONING

Because assessment takes place in the nurse's mind, the process of clinical reasoning may seem inaccessible and even mysterious to beginning students. Experienced nurses often think quickly, with little overt or conscious effort. They differ widely in personal style, communication skills, clinical training, experience, and interests. Some nurses find it difficult to explain the logic behind their clinical thinking. As an active learner, it is expected that you will ask teachers and clinicians to elaborate on the fine points of their clinical reasoning and decision making.[1,2] Utilizing the nursing process and care plans as a student is instrumental in learning to think like a nurse. This framework is concrete and organized, which facilitates the learning process.

Cognitive psychologists have shown that clinicians use three types of reasoning for clinical problem solving: pattern recognition, development of schemas, and application of relevant basic and clinical science.[3-6] As you gain experience, your clinical reasoning will begin at the outset of the patient encounter, not at the end. Study the steps described below, and then apply them to the *Case of Mrs. N* that follows. Think about these steps as you see your first patients. As with all patients, focus on determining "What explains this patient's concerns?" and "What are the problems and nursing diagnoses?"[7,8]

Identifying Problems and Making Nursing Diagnoses: Steps in Clinical Reasoning

- Identify abnormal or positive findings.
- Cluster the findings.
- Interpret the findings.
- Make hypotheses about the nature of the patient's problem.
- Test the hypotheses and establish a working nursing diagnosis.
- Develop a plan agreeable to the patient.

- **Identify abnormal or positive findings.** Make a list of the patient's *symptoms,* the *signs* you observed during the physical examination, and any laboratory reports available to you. Also, identify the positive responses during the health history. For example, living in a community with a high crime level is important when organizing the issue/problem list and in plan development.

- **Cluster the findings.** This step may be easy. The symptom of a scratchy throat and the sign of an erythematous inflamed pharynx, for example, clearly localize the problem to the pharynx. A complaint of headache leads you quickly to the structures of the skull and brain. However, do not forget to include information on the patient's stress level due to being laid off work and lack of income. Other symptoms may present greater difficulty. Chest pain, for example, can originate in the coronary arteries, the stomach and esophagus, or the muscles and bones of the chest. If the pain is exertional and relieved by rest, either the heart or the musculoskeletal components of the chest wall may be involved. If the patient notes pain only when carrying groceries with the left arm, the musculoskeletal system becomes the likely culprit.

  When localizing findings, be as specific as your data allows, but bear in mind that you may have to settle for a body region, such as the chest, or a body system, such as the musculoskeletal system. On the other hand, you may be able to define the exact structure involved, such as the left pectoral muscle. Some symptoms and signs cannot be localized, such as fatigue or fever, but are useful in the next set of steps. In addition, obtaining more information regarding psychosocial issues may add more depth when trying to pinpoint the "real" problem.

- **Interpret findings in terms of probable process.** Patient problems stem from different causes, including changes: disease processes, relationships, nutritional, immunologic, infectious, congenital, traumatic, toxic, economic, or cultural causes, and many other possibilities exist.

Analyze the data to evaluate the patient's health status. It is important to differentiate a problem that should be treated by a nurse versus one that should be referred to another health discipline.

● **Make hypotheses about the nature of the patient's problem.** Draw on all the knowledge and experience you can muster, and it is here that reading is most useful for learning about patterns of abnormalities, diseases, and issues that help cluster your patient's findings. You may need to gather more data to rule in or out your hypotheses.

By consulting the clinical literature, you embark on the lifelong goal of **evidence-based decision making.**[9,10]

Until you gain broader knowledge and experience, you may not be able to develop highly specific hypotheses, but proceed as far as you can with the data and knowledge you have. The following steps should help:

CLINICAL REASONING: DEVELOPING HYPOTHESES ABOUT PATIENT PROBLEMS

The Nursing Process

1. Assessment
   Select the most specific and critical findings to support your problem list. At the community clinic while assessing height and weight on infants, you note that a 2-month-old has gained 7 pounds in the past month. The mother reports that the child does not sleep through the night and the family of seven is living in a hotel room. The baby's crying is waking everyone up, so she has started feeding him more so that he will hopefully sleep when he is full. On further questioning, you find out that the 2-month-old baby is eating rice cereal six to seven times a day. This information is critical in building a thorough assessment.

2. Diagnosis
   Use your inferences as multiple options for this child and family prevail, and the top nursing diagnosis would be:
   Ineffective infant feeding patterns related to excess food intake
   or
   Nutrition imbalance: More than body requirements
   Other choices on the list but not the best or top priority include:
   Knowledge deficit
   Risk for deficient fluid volume
   Disturbance in sleep pattern: Risk for sleep deprivation
   Potential for constipation

3. Planning
   Develop goals for the nursing diagnosis that are realistic and timely.

   (continued)

CLINICAL REASONING: DEVELOPING HYPOTHESES ABOUT PATIENT PROBLEMS (continued)

Nursing Diagnosis: Ineffective infant feeding patterns related to excess food intake

The goals for this child might be:

Short-term goal: The infant will receive adequate nutrition for growth appropriate to age within 1 day.

Long-term goal: The infant will maintain current weight over the next month.

4. Implementation/interventions:

The nursing interventions should help to achieve the goals stated.

a. Record daily weights and weekly length in a journal.

b. Educate the family regarding the importance of formula/breast milk only at this age for development and nutrition. Feeding the baby cereal at this age is not recommended as the baby's digestive tract is not ready to digest the cereal. The baby will get all the nutrients necessary for growth and development from formula/breast milk.

c. Assist the family to find alternative ways to calm the baby rather than using food. An example might be to take a walk outside as this will relax the baby and maintain quiet in the room. Another solution is to go into the bathroom and run the shower as the water may be calming to the child and separate him from the siblings so they are able to sleep, and it will limit distractions to both groups.

d. Record the sleep/wake cycle and include when and what the baby is eating. Once this is recorded, develop a schedule that will support healthy patterns for the family.

5. Evaluation

The child and family should continue to be monitored to determine if adjustments or additional teaching is necessary. Assess the child's height and weight every week and ask the family if they are obtaining more sleep.

See section on Evaluating Clinical Evidence, pp. 30–31.

Nursing diagnoses are based primarily on changes in a person's life, altered processes, and specific causes. You will frequently see patients whose complaints do not fall neatly into these categories. Some symptoms defy analysis and are medically unexplained. You may never be able to move beyond simple descriptive categories such as "fatigue" or "anorexia." Other problems relate to stressful events in the patient's life. Events such as losing a job or loved one may increase the risk for subsequent illness. Identifying these events and helping the patient develop coping strategies are as important as managing a headache or a duodenal ulcer.

Another increasingly prominent category on problem lists is *Health Maintenance*. Routinely listing Health Maintenance helps track several important health concerns more effectively: immunizations, screening measures (e.g., mammograms, prostate examinations), instructions regarding nutrition and skin or testicular self-examinations, recommendations about exercise or use of seat belts, and responses to important life events.

● **Develop a plan agreeable to the patient.** Develop and record a *Plan* for each patient problem. Your *Plan* flows logically from the problems or diagnoses you have identified. Specify which steps are needed next. These steps range from monitoring daily weights; to consultation; to timing of dressings or IVs; to arranging a family meeting. You will find that you will follow many of the same nursing diagnoses over time; however, the *Plan* is often more fluid, encompassing changes and modifications that emerge from each patient encounter. The *Plan* should reference the diagnosis, therapy, and patient education for each individual. The nursing diagnosis may be the same; however, the remainder of the care plan is much different.

Before finalizing your *Plan*, it is important to share your assessment and clinical thinking with the patient and seek out his or her opinions, concerns, and willingness to proceed with the interventions. Remember that patients may need to hear the same information multiple times and ways before they comprehend it. The patient should always be an active participant in the plan of care.

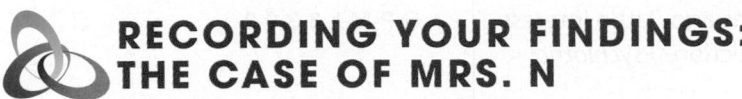

RECORDING YOUR FINDINGS: THE CASE OF MRS. N

Now turn to the case of Mrs. N and scrutinize the history, physical examination, assessment, and plan.

THE CASE OF MRS. N

1/12/11 11:00 AM
Mrs. N is a pleasant, 54-year-old widowed saleswoman residing in Amarillo, Texas.

Referral. None.
Source and Reliability. Self seems reliable.

Chief Complaint: "My head aches."

Present Illness: Mrs. N reports over the past 3 months, increasing problems with frontal headaches. These are usually bifrontal, throbbing, and mild to moderately severe. She has missed work on several occasions because of associated nausea and vomiting. Headaches average once a week, related to stress, and last 4 to 6 hours. Relieved by sleep and putting a damp towel on forehead. Little relief from aspirin. No associated visual changes, motor-sensory deficits, or paresthesias.

"Sick headaches" with nausea and vomiting began age 15, recurred through her mid-20s, decreased to one every 2 or 3 months and almost disappeared.

(continued)

THE CASE OF MRS. N (continued)

Patient reports increased pressure at work from a new and demanding boss; worried about daughter (see *Personal and Social History*). Thinks headaches may be like in the past, wants to be sure because mother died of a stroke. Concerned they interfere with work, make her irritable with family. Eats three meals a day, drinks three cups of coffee per day; cola at night.

Medications. Aspirin, 1 to 2 tablets every 4 to 6 hours as needed.
    "Water pill" in the past for ankle swelling, none recently.
Allergies. Ampicillin causes rash.
Tobacco. About 1 pack of cigarettes per day since age 18 (36 pack-years).
Alcohol/drugs. Wine rarely. No illicit drugs.

Past History

Childhood Illnesses. Measles, chickenpox. No scarlet fever or rheumatic fever.

Adult Illnesses. **Medical:** Pyelonephritis, 2001, with fever and right flank pain; treated with ampicillin; developed generalized rash with itching several days later. Reports kidney x-rays normal; no recurrence of infection. **Surgical:** Tonsillectomy, age 6; appendectomy, age 13. Sutures for laceration, 2004, after stepping on glass. **Ob/Gyn:** 3-3-0-3, normal vaginal deliveries. Menarche age 12. Last menses 6 months ago. Little interest in sex, not sexually active. No concerns about HIV infection. *Psychiatric:* None.

Gravida (G); Parity, or # deliveries (P); Miscarriages (M); Living (L), or G-P-M-L 3-3-0-3

Health Maintenance. **Immunizations:** Oral polio vaccine, year uncertain; tetanus shot, 2004; flu vaccine, 2008, no reaction; H_1N_1 vaccine, 2010.
Screening tests: Last Pap smear, 2007, normal. No mammograms to date.

Family History

The *Family History* can be recorded as a diagram or a narrative. The diagram is more helpful than the narrative for tracing genetic disorders. The negatives from the family history should follow either format.

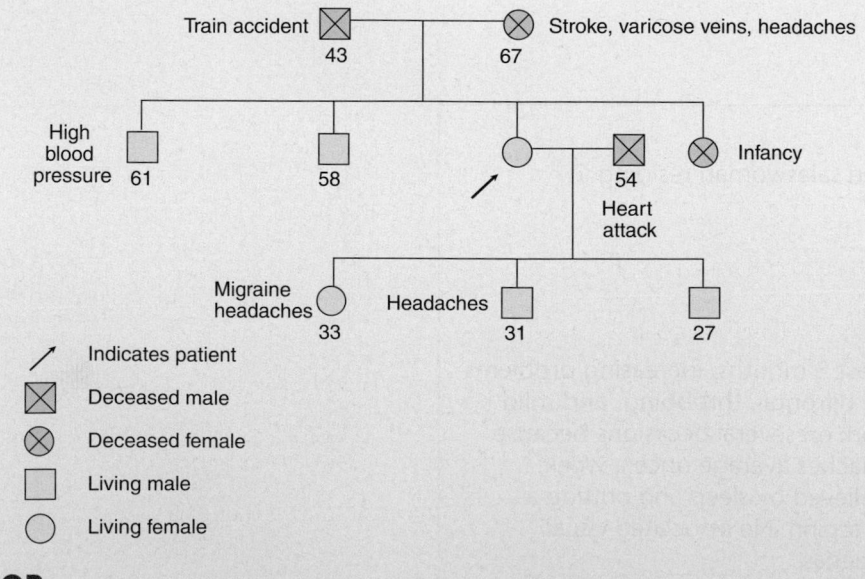

/   Indicates patient
⊠   Deceased male
⊗   Deceased female
☐   Living male
○   Living female

OR

Father died at age 43 in train accident. Mother died at age 67 from stroke; had varicose veins, headaches.

*You may wish to add an asterisk or underline important points.

Brother, 61, hypertension; brother, 58, mild arthritis; sister, died in infancy of unknown cause.

Husband died, 54 of heart attack.

Daughter, 33, with migraine headaches; son, 31, headaches; son, 27, well.

No family history of diabetes, tuberculosis, heart or kidney disease, cancer, anemia, epilepsy, or mental illness.

Personal and Social History. Born and raised in Lake City, finished high school, married at age 19. Worked as sales clerk for 2 years, moved with husband to Amarillo, had 3 children. Returned to work 15 years ago because of financial pressures. Children all married. Four years ago Mr. N died suddenly of a heart attack, leaving little savings. Mrs. N has moved to a small apartment near daughter, Dorothy. Dorothy's husband, Arthur, has an alcohol problem. Mrs. N's apartment is a haven for Dorothy and her 2 children, Kevin, 6 years, and Linda, 3 years. Mrs. N feels responsible for helping them; feels tense and nervous but denies depression. She has friends but rarely discusses family problems: "I'd rather keep them to myself. I don't like gossip." No church or other organizational support. She is typically up at 7:00 AM, works 9:00 to 5:30, eats dinner alone.

Exercise and Diet. Gets little exercise. Diet high in carbohydrates.

Safety Measures. Seat belt regularly. Sunblock SPF 15. Medications in unlocked medicine cabinet. Cleaning solutions in unlocked cabinet below sink. Shotgun and box of shells in unlocked closet.

Review of Systems

General. *Has *gained* about 10 lbs in the past 4 years.

Skin. Denies rashes or other changes.

Head, Eyes, Ears, Nose, Throat (HEENT). See *Present Illness.* Denies history of head injury. *Eyes:* Reading glasses for 5 years, last checked 1 year ago. No diplopia, blurring, halos, tearing, pain. *Ears:* Able to hear. Denies tinnitus, vertigo, infections. *Nose, sinuses:* Occasional mild cold. Denies hay fever, sinus trouble. *Throat (or mouth and pharynx):* Some bleeding of gums recently. Last dental visit 2 years ago. Occasional canker sore.

Neck. Denies lumps, goiter, pain. No swollen glands.

Breasts. Denies lumps, pain, discharge. Does breast self-examination sporadically.

Respiratory. Denies cough, wheezing, shortness of breath. Sleeps with one pillow. Last chest x-ray, 1989, St. Mary's Hospital; unremarkable.

Cardiovascular. Denies heart disease or high blood pressure; last blood pressure taken in 2006. Denies dyspnea, orthopnea, chest pain, palpitations, electrocardiogram (ECG).

Gastrointestinal. Appetite "good"; Denies nausea, vomiting, indigestion. Bowel movement about once daily, hard stools when tense; denies diarrhea, bleeding, pain, jaundice, gallbladder or liver problems.

(continued)

THE CASE OF MRS. N (continued)

Urinary. Denies frequency, dysuria, hematuria, or recent flank pain; nocturia × 1, large volume. Occasionally loses some urine when coughs hard.

Genital. Denies vaginal or pelvic infections. No dyspareunia. Last Pap smear 2007, negative results.

Peripheral Vascular. Varicose veins appeared in both legs during first pregnancy. For 10 years, has had swollen ankles after prolonged standing; wears light elastic pantyhose; tried "water pill" 5 months ago, but didn't help; denies history of phlebitis or leg pain.

Musculoskeletal. Mild, aching, low back pain, often after a long day of work; no radiation down the legs; back exercises in past, not currently. No other joint pain.

Psychiatric. Denies history of depression or treatment for psychiatric disorders. See also *Present Illness* and *Personal and Social History.*

Neurologic. Denies fainting, seizures, motor or sensory loss. Memory intact.

Hematologic. Except for bleeding gums, denies easy bleeding, anemia.

Endocrine. Denies thyroid trouble, temperature intolerance, symptoms or history of diabetes. Minimal sweating.

Physical Examination

Mrs. N is a short, overweight, middle-aged woman. Animated and responds quickly to questions. Somewhat tense, with moist, cold hands. Hair fixed neatly, clothes immaculate, color is tan, and lies flat without discomfort.

Vital Signs. Ht (without shoes) 157 cm (5'2"). Wt (dressed) 65 kg (143 lb). Body mass index (BMI) 26. Blood pressure (BP) 164/98 right arm, supine; 160/96 left arm, supine. Heart rate (HR) 88 and regular. Respiratory rate (RR) 18. Temperature (oral) 98.6°F.

Skin. Cool, moist, tan. Scattered cherry angiomas over upper trunk. Nails without clubbing, cyanosis.

Head, Eyes, Ears, Nose, Throat (HEENT). *Head:* Hair coarse, full, brown. Scalp without lesions, normocephalic/atraumatic. *Eyes:* Vision 20/30 in each eye. Visual fields full by confrontation. Conjunctiva pink; sclera white. PERRLA. EOMs intact. Disc margins sharp, without hemorrhages, exudates. No arteriolar narrowing. *Ears:* Soft, light brown cerumen partially obscures right TM; left canal clear, TM with cone of light. Acuity hears whispered voice at 1 foot BL. Weber midline. 2AC > BC. *Nose:* Mucosa pink, septum midline. No sinus tenderness or polyps. *Mouth:* Oral mucosa pink. Several interdental papillae red, slightly swollen. Dentition intact. Tongue midline, with 3 × 4-mm shallow white ulcer on red base on undersurface near tip; tender but not indurated. Tonsils absent. Pharynx without exudates.

Neck. Neck supple. Trachea midline. Thyroid isthmus barely palpable, lobes not felt.

Lymph Nodes. Small (<1 cm), soft, nontender, and mobile tonsillar and posterior cervical nodes bilaterally. No axillary or epitrochlear

PERRLA
Pupils
Equal
Round
React to
Light
Accommodate

EOM
Extra
Ocular
Movements

TM
Tympanic
Membrane

THE CASE OF MRS. N (continued)

nodes. Several 0.5-cm inguinal nodes bilaterally, soft, equal nontender, mobile.

Thorax and Lungs. Thorax symmetric with equal excursion. Lungs resonant. Breath sounds vesicular with no added sounds. Diaphragms descend 4 cm bilaterally.

Cardiovascular (CV). JVP 1 cm above the sternal angle, at 30°. Carotid upstrokes brisk, without bruits. Apical impulse discrete and tapping, barely palpable in the 5th left interspace, 8 cm lateral to the midsternal line. S_1, S_2; no S_3 or S_4. A II/VI medium-pitched midsystolic murmur at the 2nd right interspace; does not radiate to neck. No diastolic murmurs.

JVP
Jugular
Venous
Pressure

Breasts. Pendulous, left slightly larger than right. No dimpling, reactions, rashes, masses; nipples without discharge.

Abdomen. Protuberant. Well-healed 5 cm × 1 cm scar, right lower quadrant. Bowel sounds active. No tenderness or masses. Liver span 7 cm in right midclavicular line; edge smooth, palpable 1 cm below RCM. Spleen and kidneys not felt. No CVAT.

RCM
Right
Costal
Margin

CVAT
Costo
Vertebral
Angle
Tenderness

Genitalia. External genitalia without lesions. Internal exam deferred. Vaginal mucosa pink.

Rectal. Stool brown, negative for occult blood.

Extremities. Warm without edema. BL calves supple, nontender.

BL
Bi**L**ateral

Peripheral Vascular. Trace edema at both ankles. Moderate varicosities of saphenous veins, both in lower extremities. No stasis pigmentation or ulcers.

	Radial	Femoral	Popliteal	Dorsalis Pedis	Posterior Tibial
RT	2+	2+	2+	2+	2+
LT	2+	2+	2+	Absent	2+

Musculoskeletal. No joint deformities. FROM in hands, wrists, elbows, shoulders, spine, hips, knees, ankles.

FROM
Full
Range
Of
Motion

See Muscle Strength Grading, p. 527

Neurologic. *Mental Status:* Tense but alert and cooperative. Thought coherent. AA O × 3. *Cranial Nerves:* II–XII intact. *Motor:* Equal intact muscle bulk and tone. Strength 5/5 throughout. *Cerebellar:* RAMs, point-to-point movements intact. Gait stable, fluid. *Sensory:* Pinprick, light touch, position sense, vibration, and stereognosis intact. Romberg negative. *Reflexes:*

AA O × 3
Awake
Alert
Oriented (person, place, time)

RAM
Rapid
Alternating
Movements

	Biceps	Triceps	Brachio-radialis	Patellar	Achilles	Plantar
RT	2+	2+	2+	2+	1+	↓
LT	2+	2+	2+	2+	1+	↓

OR

Two methods for recording reflexes may be used: a table or a stick picture diagram; 2+ = brisk, or normal. See p. 696 for grading system.

Laboratory Data
None currently. See Plans.

Generating the Problem List. Now that you have completed your assessment and written record, you will find it helpful to generate a *Problem List* that summarizes the patient's problems. *List the most active and serious problems first, and record their date of onset.* Some nurses make separate lists for active or inactive problems; others make one list in order of priority. On follow-up visits the *Problem List* helps you remember to check the status of problems the patient may not mention. The *Problem List* also allows other members of the health care team to review the patient's health status at a glance.

A sample *Problem List* for Mrs. N is provided. You may wish to give each problem a number and use the number when referring to specific problems in subsequent notes.

● Problem List: The Case of Mrs. N From Assessment Date

Date Entered	Problem No.	Problem
1/12/11	1	Migraine headaches
	2	Elevated blood pressure
	3	Overweight
	4	Family stress
	5	Tobacco use since age 18
	6	Low back pain
	7	Health maintenance
	8	Occasional stress incontinence
	9	History of right pyelonephritis 2001
	10	Varicose veins
	11	Allergy to ampicillin

The list illustrated here includes problems that need attention now, such as Mrs. N's headaches, as well as problems that need future observation and attention, such as her blood pressure. Listing the allergy to ampicillin warns you not to distribute medications in the penicillin family. Some symptoms such as canker sores and hard stools do not appear on this list because they are minor concerns and do not require attention during this visit. Problem lists with too many relatively insignificant items diminish in value. If these symptoms increase in importance, they can always be added at a later visit.

The Challenges of Clinical Data. As you can see from the case of Mrs. N, organizing the patient's clinical data poses several challenges. The beginning student must decide whether to cluster the patient's symptoms and signs into one problem or into several problems. The amount of data may appear unmanageable. The quality of the data may be prone to error. Guidelines to help you address these challenges are provided in the following paragraphs.

● **Clustering data into single versus multiple problems.** One of the greatest difficulties facing students is how to cluster clinical data. Do selected data fit into one problem or several problems? The patient's *age* may help—young people are more likely to have a single disease, whereas older people tend to have multiple diseases. The *timing* of symptoms is often useful. For example, an episode of pharyngitis 6 weeks ago is probably unrelated to fever, chills, pleuritic chest pain, and cough that prompt a visit today. To use timing effectively, you need to know the natural history of various diseases and conditions. A yellow penile discharge followed 3 weeks later by a painless penile ulcer suggests two problems: gonorrhea and primary syphilis. In contrast, a penile ulcer followed in 6 weeks by a maculopapular skin rash and generalized lymphadenopathy suggests two stages of the same problem: primary and secondary syphilis.

Involvement of *different body systems* may help to cluster the clinical data. If symptoms and signs occur in a single system, one disease may explain them. Problems in different, apparently unrelated systems often require more than one explanation. Again, knowledge of disease patterns is necessary. You might decide, for example, to group a patient's high blood glucose and blurred vision together and place them in the Head, Eyes, Ears, Nose, and Throat system, and label the constellation "hyperglycemia." You would develop another explanation for the patient's mild fever, left lower quadrant tenderness, and diarrhea.

Some diseases involve more than one body system. As you gain knowledge and experience, you will become increasingly adept at recognizing *multisystem conditions* and building plausible explanations that link together their seemingly unrelated manifestations. To explain cough, hemoptysis, and weight loss in a 60-year-old plumber who has smoked cigarettes for 40 years, you probably even now would rank lung cancer high in the problem list. You might support your list with your observation of the patient's cyanotic fingernails. With experience and continued reading, you will recognize that his other symptoms and signs can be linked to the same diagnosis. Dysphagia would reflect extension of the cancer to the esophagus, pupillary asymmetry would suggest pressure on the cervical sympathetic chain, and jaundice could result from metastases to the liver.

● **Sifting through an extensive array of data.** It is common to confront a relatively long list of symptoms and signs and an equally long list of potential explanations. One approach is to *tease out separate clusters of observations and analyze one cluster at a time,* as just described. You can also *ask a series of key questions* that may steer your thinking in one direction and allow you to temporarily ignore the others. For example, you may ask what produces and relieves the patient's chest pain. If the answer is exercise and rest, you can focus on the cardiovascular and musculoskeletal systems and set the gastrointestinal system aside. If the pain is substernal and burning and occurs only after meals, you can logically focus on the gastrointestinal tract. A series of discriminating questions helps you form a decision tree or algorithm that is helpful in collecting and analyzing clinical data and reaching logical conclusions and explanations.

● **Assessing the quality of the data.** Almost all clinical information is subject to error. Patients forget to mention symptoms, confuse the events of their illness, avoid recounting embarrassing facts, and often slant their stories to what the nurse wants to hear. Nurses may misinterpret patient statements, overlook information, fail to ask "the one key question," jump prematurely to conclusions and diagnoses, or forget an important part of the examination, such as the funduscopic examination in a woman with headache. You can avoid some of these errors by acquiring the habits of skilled nurses, summarized below.

TIPS FOR ENSURING THE QUALITY OF PATIENT DATA

- Ask open-ended questions and listen carefully and patiently to the patient's story.
- When a patient answers "yes" to a question, continue further using "OLD CART" for additional details.
- Craft a thorough and systematic sequence to history taking and physical examination.
- Keep an open mind toward both the patient and the data.
- Always include "the worst-case scenario" in your list of possible explanations of the patient's problem, and make sure it can be safely eliminated.
- Analyze any mistakes in data collection or interpretation.
- Confer with colleagues and review the pertinent literature to clarify uncertainties.
- Apply principles of data analysis to patient information and testing.

Compose the record as soon after seeing the patient as possible, before your findings fade from memory. Record key points from each segment of the health history during the interview, leaving spaces for filling in details later.

See Table 2-1, for a Sample Progress Note for the follow-up visit of Mrs. N.

The box below details the nursing process in the case of Mrs. N. Included are the problem list, which has been developed from the assessment; the nursing diagnoses, formulated from the problem list; the plan, including the short-term goal (STG) and the long-term goal (LTG); the interventions/implementation; and the evaluation. Each of the nursing care plans would be individualized and updated for the specific patient.

NURSING PROCESS

1. **Migraine headaches**

   Assessment: A 54-year-old woman with migraine headaches since childhood, with a throbbing vascular pattern and frequent nausea and vomiting. Headaches are associated with stress and relieved by sleep and cold compresses. There is no papilledema, and there are no motor

NURSING PROCESS (continued)

or sensory deficits on the neurologic examination. The differential diagnosis includes tension headache, also associated with stress, but there is no relief with massage, and the pain is more throbbing than aching. There are no fever, stiff neck, or focal findings to suggest meningitis, and the lifelong recurrent pattern makes subarachnoid hemorrhage unlikely (usually described as "the worst headache of my life").

Nursing Diagnosis: Impaired comfort related to pain/headaches.

Plan:

STG: The patient will have decreased severity and frequency of headaches within 1 week as evidenced by journal entries.

LTG: The patient will have acceptable relief options as evidenced by her return to activities of daily living and work within 2 weeks.

Interventions:

- Log headaches—onset, location, duration, characteristic symptoms, associated manifestations, relieving factors, and treatment.
- Discuss biofeedback and stress management.
- Advise patient to avoid caffeine, including coffee, colas, and other carbonated beverages.
- Start nonsteroidal anti-inflammatory drugs (NSAIDs) for headache, as needed and prescribed.
- Follow-up appointment in 2 weeks and call doctor/nurse practitioner sooner if signs/symptoms increase.

Evaluation*:   Ideally, the patient will no longer have headaches; however, if they do persist, then the plan and goals need to be revised and/or the interventions adjusted.

2. **Elevated blood pressure**

Assessment: Systolic hypertension with wide cuff is present. May be related to obesity, also to anxiety from first visit or white coat hypertension. No evidence of end-organ damage to retina or heart.

Nursing Diagnosis: Knowledge deficit related to the relationship between increased blood pressure and increased weight and/or stress.

Plan:

STG: The patient will verbalize understanding within 5 days of importance of decreasing blood pressure and how to begin the process of diet changes, exercise, and stress reduction to assist in lowering blood pressure.

LTG: The patient will have decreased blood pressure to below 140/90 within 1 month.

Interventions:

- Discuss standards for assessing blood pressure.
- Recheck blood pressure in 2 weeks, using wide cuff.
- Check basic metabolic panel; review urinalysis.

*Evaluations will be completed for each nursing diagnosis based on the individual patient and will be updated accordingly.

(continued)

NURSING PROCESS (continued)

- Introduce weight reduction, exercise, and stress reduction techniques.
- Reduce salt intake.

3. **Overweight.**

   Assessment: Patient 5'2", weighs 143 lbs. BMI is ~26.

   Nursing Diagnosis: Ineffective health maintenance related to increased food consumption in response to stressors and insufficient energy expenditure for intake.

   Plan:

   STG: The patient will verbalize commitment to a weight loss program within 2 days.

   LTG: The patient will decrease weight by 5 lbs within 1 month (143 lbs to 138 lbs).

   Interventions:

   - Explore diet history; ask patient to keep food intake diary.
   - Explore motivation to lose weight; set target for weight loss by next visit.
   - Schedule visit with dietitian.
   - Discuss exercise program, specifically, walking 30 minutes 5–6 days a week.

4. **Family stress**

   Assessment: Son-in-law with alcohol problem; daughter and grandchildren seeking refuge in patient's apartment, leading to tension in these relationships. Patient also has financial constraints. Stress currently situational. No current evidence of major depression.

   Nursing Diagnosis: Caregiver role strain related to daughter/grandchildren situation.

   Plan:

   STG: Mrs. N will verbalize a plan to decrease strain within 5 days.

   LTG: Mrs. N will partake in the plan and have decreased signs/symptoms of stress within 1 month.

   Interventions:

   - Explore patient's views on strategies to cope with stress.
   - Explore sources of support, including Al-Anon for daughter and financial counseling for patient.
   - Continue to monitor for depression.

5. **Tobacco use**

   Assessment: 1 pack per day for 36 years.

   Nursing Diagnosis: Ineffective health maintenance related to insufficient knowledge of effects of tobacco use and resources available to quit.

   Plan:

   STG: The patient will verbalize plan to quit within 2 days.

   LTG: The patient will decrease or quit smoking within 1 month.

   Interventions:

   - Educate patient on short- and long-term effects of smoking on self and grandchildren.

NURSING PROCESS (continued)

- Identify benefits of quitting smoking (e.g., money savings, health).
- Devise strategies to decrease/eliminate smoking.
- Offer referral to tobacco cessation program.

6. **Occasional musculoskeletal low back pain**

Assessment: Usually with prolonged standing. No history of trauma or motor vehicle accident. Pain does not radiate; no tenderness or motor-sensory deficits on examination.

Nursing Diagnosis: Impaired comfort related to back pain.

Plan:

STG: The patient will demonstrate abdominal exercises that will strengthen back within 4 days.

LTG: Patient will rate back pain as 1 to 2 on pain scale within 1 month of utilizing interventions.

Interventions:

- Rate pain on scale of 1 to 10.
- Review benefits of weight loss and exercises to strengthen low back muscles.
- Continue daily exercises to strengthen abdominal muscles
- Utilize heating pad to decrease pain.

7. **Health maintenance**

Assessment: Last Pap smear 2007; has never had a mammogram.

Nursing Diagnosis:

Ineffective health maintenance related to insufficient knowledge of screening and prevention.

Plan:

STG: The patient will verbalize importance of health and prevention within 1 day.

LTG: The patient will have scheduled/completed all preventative screenings within 1 month.

Interventions:

- Teach Mrs. N breast self-examination if she would like to learn; schedule mammogram.
- Send Pap smear today.
- Provide three stool guaiac cards; discuss screening colonoscopy at next visit.
- Update immunizations.
- Suggest dental care for mild gingivitis.
- Advise patient to move medications and caustic cleaning agents to locked cabinet, if possible, above shoulder height.

8. **Occasional stress incontinence**

Assessment: Cystocele visible, probably related to bladder relaxation. Patient is perimenopausal. Incontinence reported with coughing, suggesting alteration in bladder neck anatomy. No dysuria, fever, flank pain. Not taking any contributing medications. Usually involves small amounts of urine, no dribbling, doubt urge or overflow incontinence.

(continued)

NURSING PROCESS (continued)

Nursing Diagnosis: Stress incontinence related to loss of muscle tone.

Plan:

STG: Mrs. N will verbalize understanding of stress incontinence and exercises within 2 days.

LTG: Mrs. N will report decreased or elimination of stress incontinence within 2 months.

Interventions:

- Explain cause of stress incontinence.
- Review urinalysis.
- Recommend Kegel exercises.

The remaining problems on the list do not need a care plan; they are provided as points to be aware of, such as the allergy to ampicillin, or to observe and incorporate into the patient's plan of care if they come into the forefront as more of an issue.

9. **History of right pyelonephritis, 2001**

10. **Varicose veins, lower extremities.**
    No complaints currently.

11. **Ampicillin allergy**
    Developed rash but no other allergic reaction.

 # EVALUATING CLINICAL FINDINGS

Symptoms, physical findings, tests, and x-rays should help reduce uncertainty about whether a patient does or does not have a given condition. Clinical data, including laboratory work, however, are inherently imperfect. Learn to apply the principles of *reliability, validity, sensitivity,* and *specificity* to your clinical findings.

PRINCIPLES OF TEST SELECTION AND USE

Reliability.   Indicates how well repeated measurements of the same relatively stable phenomenon will give the same result, also known as precision. Reliability may be measured for one observer or for more than one observer.

Example: If on several occasions one nurse consistently percusses the same span of a patient's liver dullness, *intraobserver reliability* is good. If, on the other hand, several observers find quite different spans of liver dullness on the same patient, *interobserver reliability* is poor.

Validity.   Indicates how closely a given observation agrees with "the true state of affairs," or the best possible measure of reality.

Example: Noninvasive blood pressure measurements by sphygmomanometers are less valid than intra-arterial pressure tracings.

PRINCIPLES OF TEST SELECTION AND USE (continued)

Sensitivity. Identifies the proportion of people who test positive in a group of people known to have the disease or condition, or the proportion of people who are *true positives* compared with the total number of people who actually have the disease. When the observation or test is negative in people with the disease, the result is termed *false negative. Good observations or tests have a sensitivity of more than 90% and help rule out disease because there are few false negatives. Such observations or tests are especially useful for screening.*

Example: The sensitivity of the Homan sign in the diagnosis of deep venous thrombosis (DVT) of the calf is 50%. In other words, compared with a group of patients with deep vein thrombosis confirmed by phlebogram, a much better test, only 50% will have a positive Homan sign, so this sign, if absent, is not helpful because 50% of patients may have a DVT.

To help remember this, experts state "when the **S**ensitivity of a symptom or sign is high, a **N**egative response rules **out** the target disorder, and the acronym for this property is "*SnNout.*"[11]

Specificity. Identifies the proportion of people who test negative in a group of people known to be *without* a given disease or condition, or the proportion of people who are *true negatives* compared with the total number of people without the disease. When the observation or test is positive in people without the disease, the result is termed *false positive. Good observations or tests have a specificity of more than 90% and help "rule in" disease because the test is rarely positive when disease is absent, and there are few false positives.*

Example: The specificity of serum amylase in patients with possible acute pancreatitis is 70%. In other words, of 100 patients without pancreatitis, 70% will have a normal serum amylase; in 30%, the serum amylase will be falsely elevated.

Likewise, when the **S**pecificity is high, a **P**ositive test result rules **in** the target disorder. The acronym is "*SpPin.*"[11]

LIFELONG LEARNING: INTEGRATING CLINICAL REASONING, ASSESSMENT, AND ANALYSIS OF CLINICAL EVIDENCE

Nurses utilize many assessment tools. These tools are used in areas of prevention such as falls, malnutrition, and skin breakdown. Screening tests for alcohol dependence (CAGE) or developmental delay (Denver II) are examples of additional tools. The concepts of sensitivity and specificity help in both the collection and the analysis of data. They even underlie some of the basic strategies of interviewing. Questions with high sensitivity, if answered in the affirmative, may be particularly useful for screening and for gathering evidence to support a hypothesis. For example, "Are you confined to bed?" is a highly sensitive question for detecting risk of skin breakdown. For patients who are immobile, there would be few false-negative responses. Thus, it is a good first screening question. However, because there are indicators other than activity and mobility that determine skin breakdown, it is not highly specific. Decreased sensory perception, friction, malnutrition, and increased moisture each are a reasonably sensitive attribute of skin breakdown and would add importantly to the growing evidence.

Data also come from the physical assessment and examination of the skin. Combining data from the history and physical examination allows screening of patients at risk for skin breakdown.

Skilled nurses use this kind of logic to generate nursing diagnoses as soon as the patient describes the *Chief Complaint,* then build evidence for one or more of these plans and discard others as they continue with the history and examination. The nurse searches explicitly for other possible manifestations of skin breakdown such as history of cerebrovascular accident or diminished lower extremity pulses of atherosclerotic peripheral vascular disease. By generating plans early and testing them sequentially, experienced nurses improve their efficiency and enhance the relevance and value of the data they collect.

This sequence of collecting data and testing hypotheses is diagrammed below.

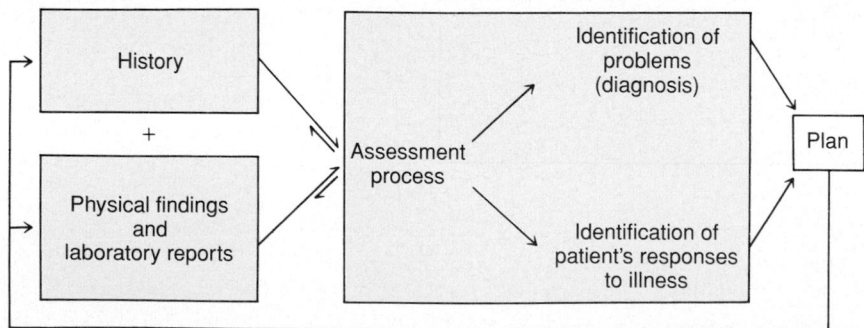

After the plan has been implemented, the process recycles. The nurse gathers more data, assesses the patient's progress, modifies the problem list if indicated, and adjusts the plan accordingly. As you gain experience, the interplay of assessment, data collection, and knowledge from the clinical literature will become increasingly familiar. You will come to value the challenges and rewards of clinical reasoning and assessment that make patient care so meaningful.

Sample Progress Note

A month later, Mrs. N returns for a follow-up visit. The format of the office progress note is quite variable, but it should meet the same standards as the initial assessment. The note should be clear, sufficiently detailed, and easy to follow. It should reflect your clinical reasoning and delineate your assessment and plan. Be sure to learn the documentation standards for billing in your institution, because this can affect the detail and type of information needed in your progress notes.

The note below follows the SOAP format: Subjective, Objective, Assessment, and Plan. You will see many other styles, some focused on the "patient-centered" record. The terms for SOAP are often not listed, but implied. Frequently nurses record the history and physical examination, then document the plan with the listing of each problem and its assessment.

2/12/11

Mrs. N returns to the clinic for follow-up of her migraine headaches. She states that she has fewer headaches since avoiding caffeinated beverages. She is now drinking decaffeinated coffee and has stopped drinking colas. She has joined a support group and started exercising to reduce stress. She is still having one to two headaches a month with some nausea, but they are less severe and generally relieved with NSAIDs. She denies any fever, stiff neck, associated visual changes, motor-sensory deficits, or paresthesias.

She has been checking her blood pressure at home. It is running about 150/90. She is walking 30 minutes three times a week in her neighborhood and has reduced her total daily calorie intake. She has been unable to stop smoking. She has been doing the Kegel exercises but still has some leakage with coughing or laughing.

Medications: Motrin 400 mg up to three times daily as needed for headache

Allergies: Ampicillin causes rash

Tobacco: 1 pack per day since age 18

Physical Examination: Pleasant, overweight, middle-aged woman, who is animated and somewhat tense. Ht 157 cm (5′2″). Wt 63 kg (140 lbs). BMI 26. BP 150/90. HR 86 and regular. RR 16. Afebrile.

Skin: No suspicious nevi. *HEENT*: Normocephalic, atraumatic. Pharynx without exudates. *Neck*: Supple, without thyromegaly. *Lymph nodes*: No lymphadenopathy. *Lungs*: Resonant and clear. *CV*: JVP 6 cm above the right atrium; carotid upstrokes brisk, no bruits. S_1, S_2. No murmurs. No S_3, S_4. *Abdomen*: Active bowel sounds. Soft, nontender, no hepatosplenomegaly. *Extremities*: Without edema.

Labs: Basic metabolic panel and urinalysis from 1/25/11 unremarkable. Pap smear normal.

Impression and Plan

1. Migraine headaches—now down to one to two per month due to reductions in caffeinated beverages and stress. Headaches are responding to NSAIDs.
   - Affirm need to stop smoking and to continue exercise program
   - Affirm patient's participation in support group to reduce stress
2. Elevated blood pressure—BP remains elevated at 150/90.
   - Educate on newly prescribed diuretic
   - Patient to take blood pressure three times a week and bring recordings to next office visit
   - Affirm need to exercise, lose weight, and stop smoking
3. Cystocele with occasional stress incontinence—stress incontinence improved with Kegel exercises but still with some urine leakage. Urinalysis from last visit no infection.
   - Educate on newly prescribed vaginal estrogen cream
   - Patient to continue Kegel exercises
4. Overweight—has lost ~3 lbs.
   - Patient to continue exercise
   - Review diet history; affirm weight reduction.
5. Family stress—patient handling this better. See Plans above.
6. Occasional low back pain—no complaints today.
7. Tobacco use—see Plans above.
8. Health maintenance—Pap smear sent last visit. Mammogram scheduled. Colonoscopy recommended.

BIBLIOGRAPHY

CITATIONS

1. Peterson MC, Holbrook JH, Von Hales DE, et al. Contributions of the history, physical examination, and laboratory investigation in making medical diagnoses. West J Med 156(2):163–165, 1992.
2. Hampton JR, Harrison MJ, Mitchell JRA, et al. Relative contributions of history-taking, physical examination, and laboratory investigation to diagnosis and management of medical outpatients. Brit Med J 2(5969):486–489, 1975.
3. Bowen J. Educational strategies to promote clinical diagnostic reasoning. New Engl J Med 355(21):2217–2225, 2006.
4. Coderre S, Mandin H, Harasym P, et al. Diagnostic reasoning strategies and diagnostic success. Med Educ 37(8):695–703, 2003.
5. Elstein A, Schwarz A. Clinical problem solving and diagnosis decision making: selective review of the cognitive literature. Brit Med J 324(7339):729–732, 2002.
6. Norman G. Research in clinical reasoning: past history and current trends. Med Educ 39(4):418–427, 2005.
7. Schneiderman H. Bedside Diagnosis. An Annotated Bibliography of Literature on Physical Examination and Interviewing, 3rd ed. Philadelphia: American College of Physicians, 1997.
8. McGee S. Evidence Based Physical Diagnosis, 2nd ed. St. Louis: Saunders/Elsevier, 2007.
9. Evidence-Based Medicine Working Group. Evidence-based medicine: a new approach to teaching the practice of medicine. JAMA 268(17):2420–2425, 1992.
10. Guyatt G. Users' Guide to the Medical Literature: A Manual for Evidence-Based Clinical Practice. New York: McGraw-Hill Medical, 2008.
11. Sackett D. A primer on the precision and accuracy of the clinical examination. JAMA 267(19):2638–2644, 1992.

ADDITIONAL REFERENCES

Alfaro-LeFevre R. Critical Thinking and Clinical Judgment: A Practical Approach to Outcome-Focused Thinking, 4th ed. St. Louis: WB Saunders–Elsevier, 2009.

Bartlett R, Bland A, Rossen E, et al. Evaluation of the outcome-present state test model as a way to teach clinical reasoning. J Nurs Educ 47(8):337–344, 2008.

Carnevali D. Diagnostic Reasoning in Nursing. Philadelphia: J. B. Lippincott Co., 2007.

Carpenito LJ. Nursing Diagnosis: Application to Clinical Practice, 12th ed. Philadelphia: Lippincott Williams & Wilkins, 2007.

Cherry B, Jacob SR. Contemporary Nursing: Issues, Trends, and Management, 4th ed. St. Louis: Mosby–Elsevier, 2008.

Cholowski K, Chan L. Diagnostic reasoning among second-year nursing students. J Adv Nurs 17(10):1171–1181, 2006.

Fletcher RH, Fletcher SW. Clinical Epidemiology: The Essentials, 4th ed. Philadelphia: Lippincott Williams & Wilkins, 2005.

Innui TS. Establishing the doctor–patient relationship: science, art, or competence? Schweiz Med Wochenschr 128:225, 1998.

Laditka JN, Laditka SB, Mastanduno MP. Hospital utilization for ambulatory care sensitive conditions: health outcome disparities associated with race and ethnicity. Soc Sci Med 57(8):1429–1441, 2003.

Lee TT. Nursing diagnoses: factors affecting their use in charting standardized care plans. J Clin Nurs 14(5):640–647, 2005.

Müller-Staub M, Needham I, Odenbreit M, et al. Implementing nursing diagnostics effectively: cluster randomized trial. J Adv Nurs 63(3):291–301, 2008.

Nettina SM. The Lippincott Manual of Nursing Practice Handbook, 3rd ed. Ambler, PA: Lippincott Williams & Wilkins, 2006.

Palese A, Saiani L, Brugnolli A, et al. The impact of tutorial strategies on student nurses' accuracy in diagnostic reasoning in different educational settings: a double pragmatic trial in Italy. Int J Nurs Stud 45(9):1285–1298, 2008.

Sackett DL. Evidence-based Medicine: How to Practice and Teach EBM, 2nd ed. New York: Churchill Livingstone, 2000.

Thompson C, Bucknall T, Estabrookes CA, et al. Nurses' critical event risk assessments: a judgement analysis. J Clin Nurs 4:601–612, 2009.

Westfall U, Tanner T, Putzier D, et al. Activating clinical inferences: a component of diagnostic reasoning in nursing. Res Nurs Health 9(4):269–277, 2009.

Interviewing and Communication

The student will:

1. Utilize therapeutic communication techniques during the patient interview.
2. Interview patients using a broad to narrow questioning technique.
3. Describe the phases of the nurse–patient interview.
4. Describe the appropriate environment to promote a successful interview.
5. Become more comfortable interviewing patients on sensitive subjects.
6. Discuss strategies for handling difficult patients.

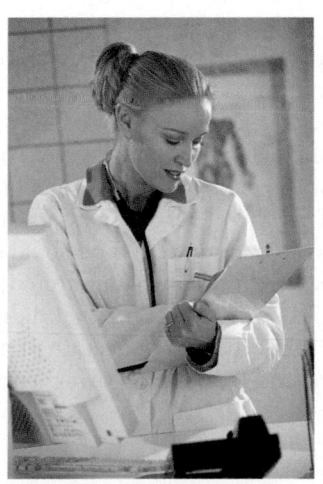

The health history interview is a conversation with a purpose. As you learn to elicit the patient's history, you will draw on many interpersonal skills that you use every day, but with important differences. Unlike social conversation, in which you can freely express your own needs and interests, the primary goal of the nurse–patient interview is to improve the well-being of the patient. At its most basic level, the purpose of conversation with a patient is threefold: to establish a trusting and supportive relationship, to gather information, and to offer information.[1-3]

Relating effectively with patients is among the most valued skills of nursing care. Using techniques that promote trust and convey respect allows the patient's story to unfold in its most full and detailed form. Establishing a supportive interaction helps the patient feel more at ease when sharing information and itself becomes the foundation for therapeutic nurse–patient relationships.[4] Illness can make patients feel discouraged and isolated. A strong nurse–patient relationship can reduce feelings of isolation and fear.[5]

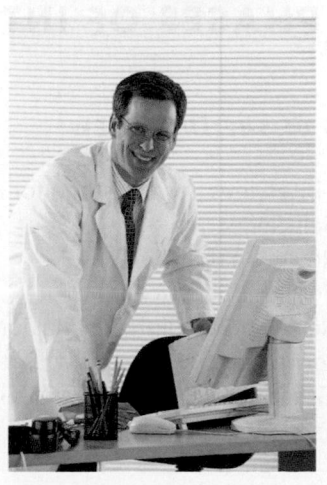

This chapter introduces the essentials of interviewing. It emphasizes interviewing techniques, but covers fundamental communication skills that will be continually used in conversations with patients. The chapter will cover the phases of interviewing, important therapeutic communication techniques and strategies for interviewing special patients.

The process of interviewing patients requires sensitivity to the patient's feelings and behavioral cues and is much more than just asking a series of questions. This process differs from the *format* of the health history as presented in Chapter 4. Both are necessary to care for patients but serve different purposes.

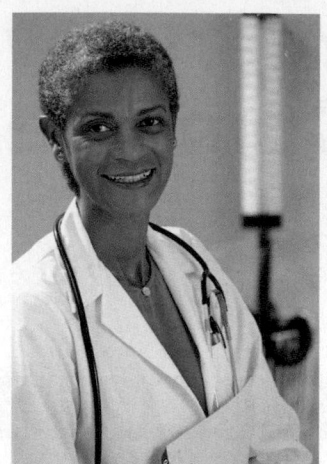

● The *health history format* is a structured framework for organizing patient information in *written or verbal form* for other health care providers; it focuses the nurse's attention on specific kinds of information that must be obtained from the patient.

● The *interviewing process* that actually generates the pieces of health information is much more fluid and demands effective communication and relational skills. It requires not only knowledge of the data needed but also the ability to elicit accurate information and the interpersonal skills that allow you to respond to the patient's feelings and concerns.

Underlying these interviewing skills is a mindset that allows the nurse to collaborate with the patient and build a healing relationship. If the patient's greatest need is for support and empathy, encouraging the patient to discuss the *experience of illness* is therapeutic, as shown by the words below from a patient with long-standing and severe arthritis:

> The patient had never talked about what the symptoms meant to her. She had never said: "This means that I can't go to the bathroom by myself, put my clothes on, even get out of bed without calling for help." When we finished the physical examination I said something like: "Rheumatoid arthritis really has not been nice to you." She burst into tears, and her daughter did also, and I sat there, very close to losing it myself. She said: "You know, no one has ever talked about it as a personal thing before. No one's ever talked to me as if this were a thing that mattered, a personal event." That was the significant thing about the encounter. I didn't really have much else to offer . . . . But something really significant had happened between us, something that she valued and would carry away with her.[6]

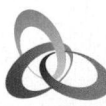

PHASES OF INTERVIEWING

PHASES OF THE INTERVIEW

> 1. Pre-interview: set the stage for a smooth interview
>   ● Self-Reflection
>   ● Review patient record
>   ● Set interview goals
>   ● Review own clinical behavior and appearance
> 2. Introduction: put the patient at ease and establish trust
>   ● Greet the patient and establish rapport
>   ● Establish the agenda for the interview

PHASES OF THE INTERVIEW (continued)

3. Working: obtain patient information
   - Invite the patient's story
   - Identify and respond to emotional clues
   - Expand and clarify the patient's story
   - Generate and test diagnostic hypotheses
   - Negotiate a plan, including further evaluation, treatment, education and self-management support and prevention
4. Termination:
   - Summarize important points
   - Discuss plan of care

Phase 1: Pre-interview

Interviewing patients requires planning. There are several preliminary steps that are crucial to success: taking time for self-reflection, reviewing the patient record, setting goals for the interview, reviewing your behavior and appearance, adjusting the environment, and being ready to take brief notes.

Take Time for Self-Reflection. As nurses, we encounter a wide variety of patients, each one unique. Establishing relationships with people from a broad spectrum of ages, social classes, races, ethnicities, and states of *health or illness* is an opportunity and privilege. Being consistently respectful and open to individual differences is one of the nurse's challenges. Because we bring our own values, assumptions, and biases to every encounter, we must look inward to clarify how our own expectations and reactions may affect

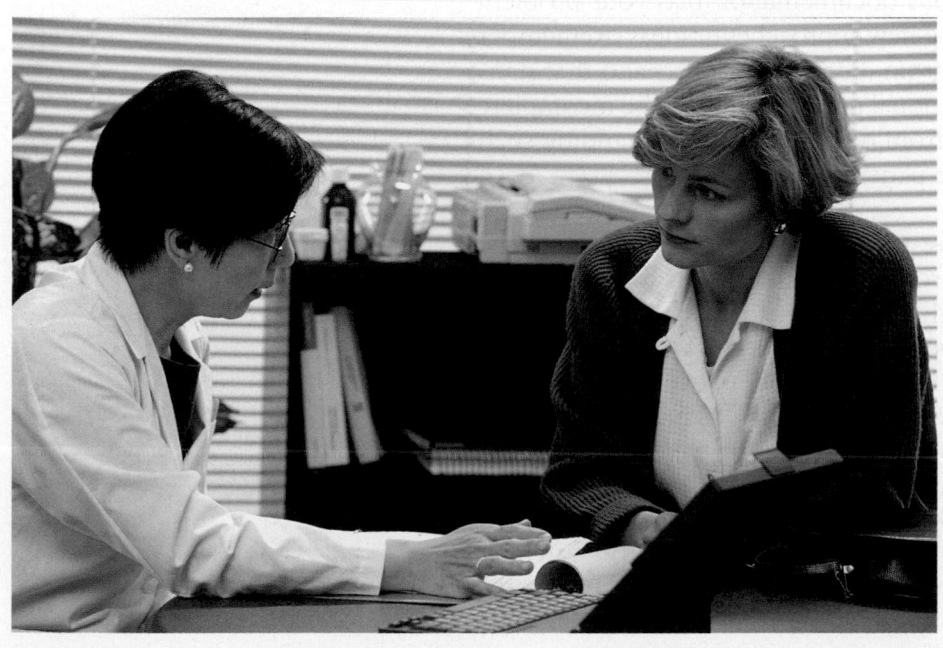

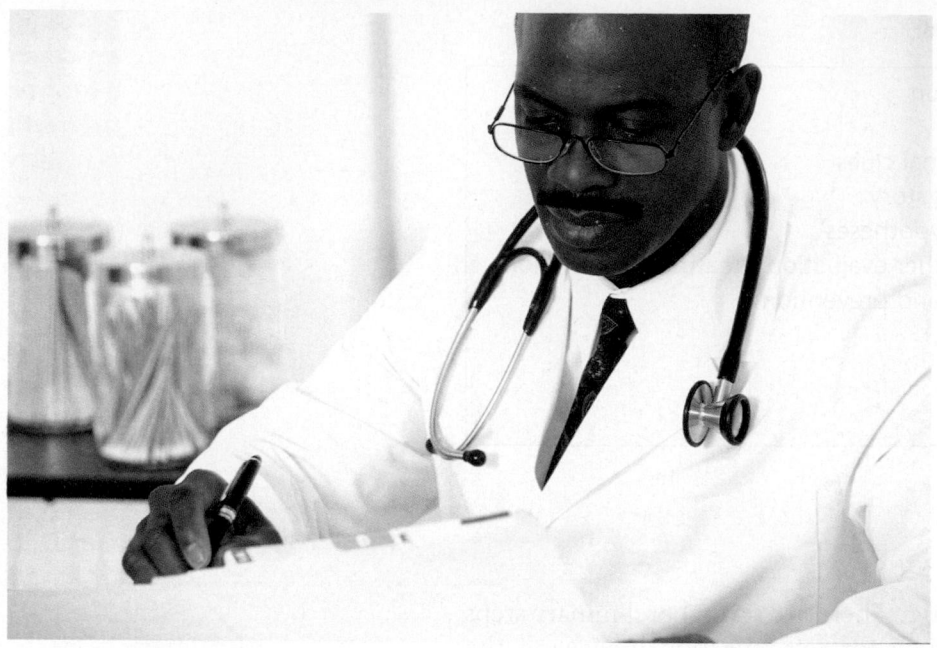

what we hear and how we behave. *Self-reflection is a continual part of professional development in clinical work. It brings a deepening personal awareness to our work with patients, which is one of the most rewarding aspects of patient care.*[7]

Review the Medical and Nursing Records.
Before seeing the patient, review the medical and nursing records. This helps gather information and plan what areas you need to explore with the patient. Look closely at identifying data such as age, gender, address, and health insurance, and peruse the problem list, the medication list, and details such as the documentation of allergies. The chart often provides valuable information about past diagnoses and treatments, but do not let previous documentation bias your problem solving or prevent you from developing new approaches or ideas. Remember that information in the record comes from different observers and that standardized forms reflect different institutional norms. Data may be incomplete or even disagree with what you learn from the patient—understanding such discrepancies may prove helpful to the patient's care.

Set Goals for the Interview.
Before talking with the patient, clarify the goals for the interview. Goals range from completing forms for health care institutions, to following up on health care issues, to obtaining a basis for developing a plan of care. *A nurse must balance these provider-centered goals with patient-centered goals.* There can be discrepancies between the needs of the nurse, the institution, and the patient and family. By taking a few minutes to think through the goals ahead of time, the interview will be smoother.

Review Clinical Behavior and Appearance.
Just as the nurse carefully observes the patient throughout the interview, the patient will be watching the nurse. Consciously or not, the nurse sends messages through both words and behavior. Posture, gestures, eye contact, and tone of voice all convey the

extent of interest, attention, acceptance, and understanding. The skilled interviewer seems calm and unhurried, even if time is limited. Reactions that betray disapproval, embarrassment, impatience, or boredom block communication, as do any behaviors that condescend, stereotype, criticize, or belittle the patient. Professionalism requires that the nurse maintain equanimity.

Personal appearance also affects the clinical relationship. Patients find cleanliness, neatness, conservative dress, and a name tag reassuring. Remember to keep *the patient's perspective* in mind in order to build the patient's trust.

Adjust the Environment. Make the interview setting as private and comfortable as possible. A proper environment improves communication, though a hospitalized patient may need to be interviewed in a two-bed room or an emergency department. If there are privacy curtains, ask permission to pull them shut. Suggest moving to an empty room instead of talking in a waiting area. Adjust the room temperature for the patient's comfort when needed. *As the nurse, it is part of your job to make adjustments to the location and seating that make the patient and you more comfortable. These efforts are always worth the time.*

Take Notes. No one can remember all the details of a comprehensive history. Jot down short phrases, specific dates, or words, but do not let note taking or written or electronic forms distract you from the patient. Maintain good eye contact, and whenever the patient is talking about sensitive or disturbing material, put down your pen or move away from the keyboard. Most patients are accustomed to note taking, but for those who find it uncomfortable, explore their concerns and explain your need to make an accurate record. When using an electronic health record, review the patient's record before entering the room; elicit the patient's story while directly facing the patient, maintaining eye contact, and observing all nonverbal behavior; and address the viewing screen only after the establishment of the relationship and with the patient included in the process.[9]

The interview moves through the introduction, working, and termination phases. *Throughout this sequence, the nurse must be attuned to the patient's feelings, help the patient express them, respond to their content, and validate their significance.*

As a beginning student, concentrate primarily on gathering the patient's story and creating a shared understanding of the problem. As you become a practicing nurse, reaching agreement on a plan for further evaluation and treatment becomes more important. Whether the interview is comprehensive or focused, you should move through this sequence with close attention to the patient's feelings and affect, always working on strengthening the relationship.

Phase 2: Introduction

Greet the Patient and Establish Rapport. The initial moments of an encounter with the patient lay the foundation for an ongoing relationship. How you greet the patient and other visitors in the room, provide for the

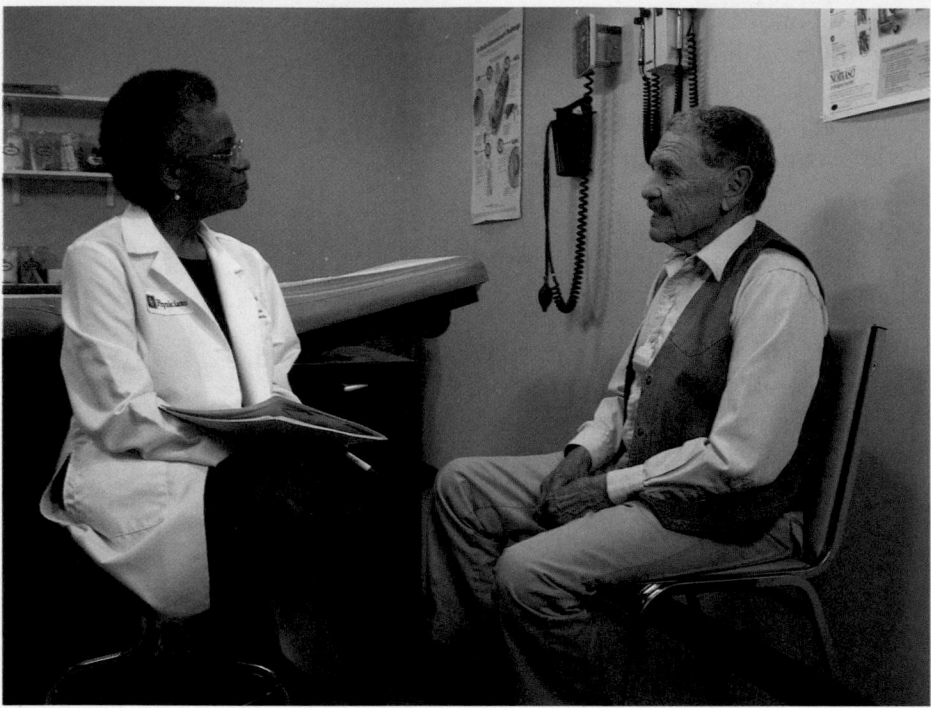

patient's comfort, and arrange the physical setting all shape the patient's first impressions.

As you begin, *greet the patient* by name and introduce yourself, giving your own name. If possible and culturally appropriate, shake hands with the patient. If this is the first contact, explain your role, including your status as a student and how you will be involved in the patient's care.

Using a formal title to address the patient—Mr. O'Neil or Ms. Washington, for example—is always best.[10,11] Except with children or adolescents, avoid first names unless you have specific permission from the patient or family. Addressing an unfamiliar adult as "granny" or "dear" can depersonalize and demean. If you are unsure how to pronounce the patient's name, do not be afraid to ask. You can say: "I am afraid of mispronouncing your name. Could you say it for me?" Then repeat it to make sure that you heard it correctly.

When visitors are in the room, be sure to acknowledge and greet each one in turn, inquiring about each person's name and relationship to the patient. Whenever visitors are present, *you are obligated to maintain the patient's confidentiality.* Let the patient decide if visitors or family members should remain in the room, and ask for the patient's permission before conducting the interview in front of them. For example, "I am comfortable with having your sister stay for the interview, Mrs. Jones, but I want to make sure that this is also what you want" or "Would you prefer if I spoke to you alone or with your sister present?"

Consider the best way to *arrange the room* and distance from the patient. Remember that cultural background and individual taste influence preferences about interpersonal space. Choose a distance that facilitates conversation and allows good eye contact, probably within several feet of the patient, close enough to be intimate but not intrusive. Pull up a chair and, if possible, sit at eye level with the patient. Move any physical barriers, such as desks or bed-side tables, out of the way. Avoid arrangements that convey disrespect or inequality of power, such as interviewing a patient on a bedpan. Such arrangements are unacceptable. Lighting also makes a difference. Sitting between a patient and a bright light or window may make the patient squint uncomfortably to see you.

Provide the patient with undivided attention. Spend enough time on small talk to put the patient at ease, and avoid looking down to take notes, read the chart, or scan a computer screen. In a first meeting, demonstrate interest in the patient as a person.[12]

Establish the Agenda.   Once rapport has been established, the nurse is ready to pursue the patient's reason for seeking health care. This reason is traditionally designated the *chief complaint,* but when there are three or four reasons for the visit, the phrase *presenting problem(s)* may be preferable.[13,14] Begin with **open-ended questions** that allow full freedom of response: "What concerns bring you here today?" or "How can I help you?" Helpful open-ended questions include "Are there specific concerns that prompted you to schedule this appointment?" and "What made you decide to come in to see us today?" Note that these questions encourage the patient to express any possible concerns and do not restrict the patient to a problem per se. Sometimes patients do not give a specific problem; they ask for "just a check-up." An important fact to remember is that the first problem the patient brings up is not necessarily the most important one. In fact, when the chief reason for coming is psychosocial, it is usually *not* the first reason the patient mentions. The order in which problems are related is not connected to their clinical importance.[15]

Identifying all the concerns at the beginning of the interview allows the patient and the nurse to negotiate which concerns are most pressing for the visit, and which can be postponed to a follow-up appointment. Questions such as "Is there anything else?" or "Have we got everything?" help elicit the patient's complete list of reasons for coming to the health care facility. The nurse may also have concerns such as blood pressure management or diabetic diet maintenance. Identifying the full agenda or even the "real reason" for the visit at the outset makes use of the time available more meaningful, facilitates time management, and reduces the short shrift given to late-emerging concerns, although negotiating the agenda at the outset still does not always avert the "hand on the doorknob syndrome"[16]—when the patient mentions a new problem as he or she is leaving.

Phase 3: Working Phase

Invite the Patient's Story.   Once the agenda has been elicited, negotiated, and prioritized, invite the patient's story by asking about the foremost concern and saying, "Tell me more about . . . ." Continue to encourage the patient to tell his or her story in his or her own words, using *a nonfocusing approach*.[17] Avoid biasing the patient's story—*inject no new information* and *do not interrupt*. Instead, use active listening skills: Lean forward as you listen; add continuers such as nodding your head and phrases like "uh huh," "go on," or "I see." Train yourself to *follow the patient's leads*. Intervening too early or asking specific questions prematurely risks trampling on the very information being sought.[13] Once interrupted, patients usually do not return to telling their stories. After the patient's initial description of each issue, use a *focusing approach to explore the patient's story in more depth*. Ask, *"How would you describe the pain?" "What happened next?" "What else did you notice?"* Using additional guided questioning helps you avoid missing any of the patient's concerns.

See p. 48 for discussions of *continuers*.

See pp. 47–49 for discussions of *guided questioning*.

Identify and Respond to the Patient's Emotional Cues. Emotional distress is frequently associated with illness.[16,18] Patients may withhold their true concerns in up to 75% of acute care visits[14] but offer various clues to their concerns that may be direct or indirect, verbal or nonverbal, and expressed as ideas or emotions.[19] Acknowledging and responding to these clues help build rapport, expand the nurse's understanding of the illness, and improve patient satisfaction.

If the patient has not mentioned his or her perspective on illness during the open-ended portion of the interview, explore this perspective prior to the directive. Probe the personal context of the illness by asking, "How has this affected you?" "What do you make of this?" or "How did you feel about that?" or stating, "Many people would be frustrated by something like this." In addition, explore the patient's ideas about the effect of the illness on his or her life.[17] See the box below for a taxonomy of the clues about the patient's perspective on illness.

Clues to the Patient's Perspective on Illness[20]

- Direct statement(s) by the patient of explanations, emotions, expectations, and effects of the illness[8]
- Expression of feelings about the illness
- Attempts to explain or understand symptoms
- Speech clues (e.g., repetition,[20] prolonged reflective pauses[21])
- Sharing a personal story
- Behavior clues indicative of unidentified concerns, dissatisfaction, or unmet needs such as reluctance to accept recommendations, seeking a second opinion, or early return appointment

Respond immediately when you hear an emotional cue. Appropriate response techniques include reflection, synonyms, and feedback indicating support and partnership. A mnemonic for responding to emotional cues is *NURS: N*aming—"That sounds like a scary experience"; *U*nderstanding or legitimization—"It's understandable that you feel that way"; and *ReS*pecting—"You've done better than most people would with this."

N – Naming
U – Understanding
ReS – Respecting

Expand and Clarify the Patient's Story. After eliciting the patient's story as fully as possible in a nondirective manner and exploring the patient's lived experience of the illness, guide the patient to elaborating on the areas of the health history that seem most significant. Clarify the attributes of each symptom, including context, associations, and chronology. For pain and many other symptoms, understanding these essential characteristics, summarized below as the seven key attributes of a symptom, is critical.

To pursue the seven attributes, two mnemonics may help:

- **OLD CART,** or **O**nset, **L**ocation, **D**uration, **C**haracteristic Symptoms, **A**ssociated Manifestations, **R**elieving/Exacerbating Factors, and **T**reatment, or

- **OPQRST,** or **O**nset, **P**alliating/**P**rovoking Factors, **Q**uality, **R**adiation, **S**ite, and **T**iming

THE SEVEN ATTRIBUTES OF A SYMPTOM

1. **O**nset. When did (does) it start? Setting in which it occurs, including environmental factors, personal activities, emotional reactions, or other circumstances that may have contributed to the illness.
2. **L**ocation. Where is it? Does it radiate?
3. **D**uration. How long does it last?
4. **C**haracteristic Symptoms. What is it like? How severe is it? (For pain, ask a rating on a scale of 1 to 10.)
5. **A**ssociated Manifestations. Have you noticed anything else that accompanies it?
6. **R**elieving/Exacerbating Factors. Is there anything that makes it better or worse?
7. **T**reatment. What have you done to treat this? Was it effective?

Whenever possible, *use the patient's words,* making sure you clarify their meaning. Do not use medical jargon, because it confuses and frustrates patients. Be aware of how quickly jargon like "take a history" and "work you up" can creep into discussions. Choose instead plain English words such as "I'd like to learn more about your illness" or "Doing these examinations can help us understand what's causing your illness."

It is important to establish *the sequence and time course* of each of the patient's symptoms if you are to arrive at accurate assessments. Encourage a chronologic account by stating, "Please describe the *symptom* from when it began to now" or "Please start at the beginning, or the last time you felt well, and go step by step" or asking such questions as "What then?" or "What happened next?" To fill in specific details, guide the patient's story by employing different types of questions and the techniques of skilled interviewing. Use focused questions to elicit information that the patient

See the Techniques of Skilled Interviewing and discussion of focused questions, pp. 47–50.

has not already offered. *In general, an interview moves back and forth from open-ended questions to increasingly focused questions and then on to another open-ended question, returning the lead in the interview to the patient.*

Generating and Testing Diagnostic Hypotheses. The skills of diagnostic reasoning are developed over time with practice. As the history is gathered, one develops and tests hypotheses about the patient problem(s). Identifying the attributes and details of the patient's symptoms is fundamental to recognizing patterns of problems and generating nursing diagnoses.

Some students visualize the process of evoking a full description of the symptom as "the cone":

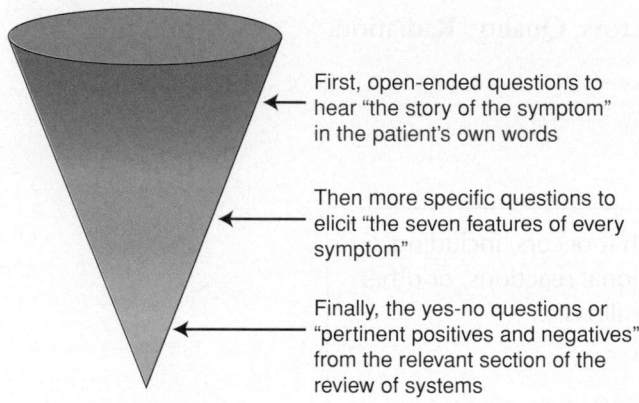

First, open-ended questions to hear "the story of the symptom" in the patient's own words

Then more specific questions to elicit "the seven features of every symptom"

Finally, the yes-no questions or "pertinent positives and negatives" from the relevant section of the review of systems

For example, in a patient with a cough, these questions would come from the Respiratory section of the Review of Systems, on pp. 21–22.

Each symptom has its own "cone," which is documented in the History of Present Illness section of the written record.

Appropriate questions about symptoms are also suggested in each of the chapters on the regional physical examinations. This is one way to build evidence for and against various diagnostic possibilities. The challenge is not letting this kind of inquiry dominate the interview and displace learning about the patient's perspective, conveying concern for the patient's well-being, and building the relationship.[5]

See also Chapter 2, Critical Thinking in Health Assessment, pp. 11–34.

Create a Shared Understanding of the Problem. Recent literature makes it clear that delivering effective health care requires exploring the deeper meanings patients attach to their symptoms. Although the "seven attributes of a symptom" add important details to the patient's history, the **disease/illness distinction model** helps to understand the full impact on the patient.[22] This model acknowledges the very different yet complementary perspectives of the nurse and the patient. *Disease* is the explanation that the *nurse* brings to the symptoms. It is the way that the nurse organizes what is learned from the patient that leads to a nursing diagnosis. *Illness* can be defined as how the *patient* experiences all aspects of the disease, including its effects on relationships, function, and sense of well-being. Many factors may shape this experience, including prior personal or family health, the effect of symptoms on everyday life, individual outlook and style of coping, and expectations about medical and nursing care. The melding of these perspectives forms the basis for planning evaluation and treatment. *The interview needs to incorporate both these views of reality.*

Even a chief complaint as straightforward as sore throat can illustrate these divergent views. The patient may be most concerned about pain and difficulty swallowing, missing time from work, or a cousin who was hospitalized with tonsillitis. The nurse, however, may focus on specific points in the history that differentiate streptococcal pharyngitis from other etiologies, or on a questionable history an allergy to penicillin. To understand the patient's expectations, the nurse needs to go beyond just the attributes of a symptom. Learning about the patient's perception of illness means asking patient-centered questions in the four domains listed below. This information is crucial to patient satisfaction, effective health care, and patient follow-through.[17,23]

A mnemonic for the patient's perspective on the illness is *FIFE—Feelings, Ideas, effect on Function, and Expectations.*

EXPLORE THE PATIENT'S PERSPECTIVE

- The patient's **F**eelings, including fears or concerns, about the problem
- The patient's **I**deas about the nature and the cause of the problem
- The effect of the problem on the patient's life and **F**unction
- The patient's **E**xpectations of the disease, of the clinician, or of health care, often based on prior personal or family experiences

To uncover the patient's feelings, the nurse might ask,

> "What concerns you most about the pain?"

> "How has this been for you?"

To explore the patient's thoughts about the cause of the problem, the nurse could say,

> "Why do you think you have this stomachache?"

Because self-treatment suggests the patient's thinking, you may ask,

> "What have you tried?"

A patient may worry that the pain is a symptom of serious disease and want reassurance. Alternatively, the patient may be less concerned about the cause of the pain and just want relief.

To determine the effect of the illness on the patient's lifestyle and function, particularly for patients with chronic illness, ask,

> "What can't you do now that you could do before?"

"How has your backache (shortness of breath, etc.) affected your ability to work? Your life at home? Your social activities? Your role as a parent? Your function in intimate relationships? The way you feel about yourself as a person?"

You need to find out what the patient expects from you, the nurse, or from health care in general . . . "I am glad that the pain is almost gone. How specifically can I help you now?" Even if the stomach pain is almost gone, the patient may need a work excuse to take to an employer.

Negotiate a Plan. Learning about the effects of the illness gives the nurse and the patient the opportunity to create a complete and congruent picture of the problem. This multifaceted picture then forms the basis for planning further evaluation (e.g., physical examination, laboratory tests, consultations) and negotiating a nursing care plan. It also plays an important role in building rapport with your patient.

See also Chapter 2, Critical Thinking in Health Assessment, for more specific techniques for negotiating a plan.

Phase 4: Termination

Summarize Important Points and Discuss Plan. Let the patient know that the end of the interview is approaching to allow time for the patient to ask any final questions. Make sure the patient understands the mutual plans you have developed. For example, before gathering your papers or standing to leave the room, you can say, "We need to stop now. Do you have any questions about what we've covered?" As you close, summarizing the patient's problems and reviewing the plan of care and follow-up are helpful. "So, you will take the medicine as we discussed, check your blood glucose daily, and make a follow-up appointment for 4 weeks. Do you have any questions about this?" Address any related concerns or questions that the patient raises.

The patient should have a chance to ask any final questions; however, the last few minutes are not the time to bring up new topics. If that happens and the concern is not life-threatening, simply assure the patient of your interest and make plans to address the problem at a future time.

THERAPEUTIC COMMUNICATION TECHNIQUES

This section describes the skills that form the basic tools of interviewing. The nurse employs these interviewing skills to achieve the tasks described in the Phases of Interviewing (see pp. 36–37) more effectively. Practice improves interviewing skills. Being observed and recorded during an interview allows for feedback from an experienced interviewer.

THE TECHNIQUES OF SKILLED INTERVIEWING

- Active listening
- Guided questioning
- Nonverbal communication
- Empathic responses
- Validation

- Reassurance
- Summarization
- Transitions
- Empowering the patient

Active Listening. Underlying all the techniques is the habit of *active listening*. Active listening is the process of closely attending to what the patient is communicating, being aware of the patient's emotional state, and using verbal and nonverbal skills to encourage the speaker to continue and expand.[24] This takes practice. It is easy to drift into thinking about the next question or the nursing diagnoses.

Guided Questioning: Options to Expand and Clarify the Patient's Story. There are several ways you can ask for more information from the patient without interfering with the flow of the patient's story. The goal is to facilitate the patient's fullest communication. Learning the following techniques encourages patient disclosures while minimizing the risk for distorting the patient's ideas or missing significant details. This is how one avoids asking a series of specific questions, which takes more time and makes the patient feel more passive.

- Moving from open-ended to focused questions
- Using questioning that elicits a graded response
- Asking a series of questions, one at a time
- Offering multiple choices for answers
- Clarifying what the patient means
- Encouraging with continuers
- Using reflection

Moving From Open-Ended to Focused Questions. Your questioning should proceed from general to specific. Think once again about the "cone," open at the top then tapering to a focal point. Start with the most general questions like "How can I help?" to still open but focused ones like "Tell me more about your experience with the medication." Then pose closed questions like "Did the new medicine cause any problems?" Begin with a truly open-ended question that does not inadvertently include an answer. A possible sequence might be

"Tell me about your chest pain." (Pause)

"What else?" (Pause)

"Where did you feel it?" (Pause) "Show me."

"Anywhere else?" (Pause) "Did it travel anywhere?" (Pause) "To which arm?"

Avoid *leading questions* that include the answer in the question or suggest a desired response: "Has your pain been improving?" or "You don't have any blood in your stools, do you?" If you ask, "Is your pain like a pressure?" and the patient answers yes, your words may turn into the patient's words. Use the more neutral "Please describe your pain." Also avoid asking the patient *why* something was not done.

Questioning That Elicits a Graded Response.   Ask questions that require a *graded response* rather than a single answer. "How many steps can you climb before you get short of breath?" is better than "Do you get short of breath climbing stairs?"

Asking a Series of Questions, One at a Time.   Be sure to *ask one question at a time*. "Any tuberculosis, pleurisy, asthma, bronchitis, pneumonia?" may lead to a negative answer out of sheer confusion. Try "Have you had any of the following problems?" Be sure to pause and establish eye contact as you list each problem.

Offering Multiple Choices for Answers.   Sometimes patients seem quite unable to describe their symptoms without help. To minimize bias, *offer multiple-choice answers:* "Which of the following words best describes your pain: aching, sharp, pressing, burning, shooting, or something else?" Almost any specific question can provide at least two possible answers. "Do you bring up any phlegm with your cough, or is it dry?"

Clarifying What the Patient Means.   At times, patients use words that are ambiguous or have unclear associations. To understand their meaning, *request clarification,* as in "Tell me exactly what you meant by 'the flu'" or "You said you were behaving just like your mother. What did you mean?"

Encouraging With Continuers.   Without specifying content, you can use posture, gestures, or words to encourage the patient to say more. Pausing with a nod of the head or remaining silent, yet attentive and relaxed, is a *cue for the patient to continue.* Leaning forward, making eye contact, and using phrases like "Mm-hmm," "Go on," or "I'm listening" all maintain the flow of the patient's story.

Reflection.   A simple repetition of the patient's last words, reflecting or echoing back the patient's words, encourages the patient to express both factual details and feelings, as in the following example:

Patient: "The pain got worse and began to spread." (Pause)

Response: "Spread?" (Pause)

Patient: "Yes, it went to my shoulder and down my left arm to the fingers. It was so bad that I thought I was going to die." (Pause)

Response: "Going to die?"

Patient: "Yes, it was just like the pain my father had when he had his heart attack, and I was afraid the same thing was happening to me."

This reflective technique has helped to reveal not only the location and severity of the pain but also its meaning to the patient. It did not bias the story or interrupt the patient's train of thought.

Nonverbal Communication. Communication that does not involve speech occurs continuously and provides important clues to feelings and emotions. Becoming sensitive to nonverbal messages allows the nurse to both "read the patient" more effectively and send messages. Pay close attention to eye contact, facial expression, posture, head position and movement such as shaking or nodding, interpersonal distance, and placement of the arms or legs—crossed, neutral, or open. Be aware that some nonverbal language is universal and some is culturally bound.

Matching your position to the patient's can signify increased rapport, just as mirroring your position can signify the patient's increasing sense of connectedness. One can also mirror the patient's *paralanguage,* or qualities of speech, such as pacing, tone, and volume, to increase rapport. Moving closer or physical contact like placing your hand on the patient's arm can convey empathy or help the patient gain control of difficult feelings. Sensitivity to the patient's culture must guide the use of nonverbal communication.

Empathic Responses. Conveying empathy greatly strengthens patient rapport. As patients talk they may express—with or without words—feelings they may or may not have consciously acknowledged. *To provide empathy, first identify the patient's feelings.* At first, this may seem unfamiliar or uncomfortable. When you sense important but unexpressed feelings from the patient's face, voice, words, or behavior, inquire about them rather than assuming that you know how the patient feels. You may simply ask, "How did you feel about that?" Unless you let patients know that you are interested in feelings as well as facts, you may miss important insights.

Once you have identified the feelings, respond with understanding and acceptance. Responses may be as simple as "I understand," "That sounds upsetting," or "You seem sad." Empathy may also be nonverbal—for example, offering a tissue to a crying patient or gently placing your hand on the patient's arm. For a response to be empathic, it must reflect a precise understanding of what the patient is feeling. If your response acknowledges how upset a patient must have been at the death of a parent when in fact the death relieved the patient of a long-standing financial and emotional burden, you have misunderstood the situation. Instead of making assumptions, you can ask directly about the patient's emotional response. "I am sorry about the death of your father. What has that been like for you?"

Validation. Another important way to make a patient feel affirmed is to validate or acknowledge the legitimacy of the emotional experience. A patient who has been in a car accident but has no physical injury may still be experiencing significant distress. Stating something like, "Being in that accident must have been very scary. Car accidents are always unsettling because they remind us of our vulnerability and mortality. That could explain why you still feel upset," reassures the patient. It helps the patient feel that such emotions are legitimate and understandable.

Reassurance.   When you are talking with patients who are anxious or upset, it is tempting to try to reassure them. Saying, "Don't worry. Everything is going to be all right" may reassure the patient about the wrong thing and provide false reassurance. Moreover, premature reassurance may block further disclosures, especially if the patient feels that the nurse is uncomfortable with the anxiety or has not appreciated the extent of the patient's distress.

The first step to effective reassurance is simply identifying and acknowledging the patient's feelings. This promotes a feeling of connection. The actual reassurance comes much later after the interview, the physical examination, and perhaps some diagnostic studies have been completed. At that point, you can interpret for the patient what you think is happening and deal openly with expressed concerns. True reassurance comes from conveying information in a competent manner, making the patient feel confident that problems have been fully understood and will be addressed.

Summarization.   Giving a capsule summary of the patient's story during the course of the interview serves several different functions. It communicates to the patient that you have been listening carefully. It identifies what you know and what you do not know. "Now, let me make sure that I have the full story. You said you've had a cough for 3 days, that it's especially bad at night, and that you have started to bring up yellow phlegm. You have not had a fever or felt short of breath, but you do feel congested, with difficulty breathing through your nose." Following with an attentive pause or asking, "Is there anything else?" lets the patient add other information and corrects any misunderstanding.

Summarization can be used at different points in the interview to structure the visit, especially at times of transition (see below). This technique also allows you to organize your clinical reasoning and to convey it to the patient, making the relationship more collaborative. *It is also a useful technique for learners when they draw a blank on what to ask the patient next.*

Transitions.   Patients have many reasons to feel vulnerable during a health care visit. To put them more at ease, tell them when you are changing directions during the interview. Just as clear signs along the highway give a sense of confidence, this "signposting" gives patients a greater sense of control. As you move from one part of the history to the next and on to the physical examination, orient the patient with brief transitional phrases like "Now I'd like to ask some questions about your past health." Make clear what the patient should expect or do next. "Before we move on to reviewing all your medications, was there anything else about past health problems?" "Now I would like to examine you. I will step out for a few minutes. Please undress and put on this gown." Specifying that the gown should close in the back protects the patient's modesty and can make examiners more comfortable.

Empowering the Patient.   Patients have many reasons to feel vulnerable. They may be in pain or worried about a symptom. They may be unfamiliar or overwhelmed with accessing the health care system. Differences of gender, ethnicity, race, or class may also contribute to power differentials. However, ultimately, patients are responsible for their own care.[25] Patients who are self-confident and understand the recommendations are most likely to adopt offered advice, make lifestyle changes, or take medications as prescribed.

Listed next are principles that help you share power with your patients. Although many of them have been discussed in other sections of this chapter, the need to reinforce patients' primary responsibility for their health is so fundamental that it is worth summarizing them here.

EMPOWERING THE PATIENT: PRINCIPLES OF SHARING POWER

- Evoke the patient's perspective.
- Convey interest in the person, not just the problem.
- Follow the patient's leads.
- Elicit and validate emotional content.
- Share information with the patient, especially at transition points during the visit.
- Make your clinical reasoning transparent to the patient.
- Reveal the limits of your knowledge.

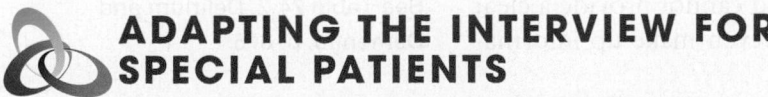

ADAPTING THE INTERVIEW FOR SPECIAL PATIENTS

Interviewing patients may precipitate behaviors and situations that seem perplexing or even vexing. Your ability to handle these situations will evolve throughout your career. *Always remember the importance of listening to the patient and clarifying the patient's concerns.*

The Silent Patient.   Novice interviewers are often uncomfortable with periods of silence and feel obligated to keep the conversation going. Silence has many meanings and many purposes. Patients frequently fall silent for short periods to collect thoughts, remember details, or decide whether you can be trusted with certain information. The period of silence usually feels much longer to the nurse than it does to the patient. The nurse should appear attentive and give brief encouragement to continue when appropriate.

During periods of silence, watch the patient closely for nonverbal cues, such as difficulty controlling emotions.

Silence may be part of the patient's culture or be the patient's response to how you are asking questions. Are you asking too many short-answer questions in rapid succession? Have you offended the patient in any way by signs of disapproval or criticism? Have you failed to recognize an overwhelming symptom such as pain, nausea, or dyspnea? If so, you may need to ask the patient directly, "You seem very quiet. Have I done something to upset you?"

Patients with depression or dementia may lose their usual spontaneity of expression, give short answers to questions, and then fall silent. If you have already tried guiding them through recent events or a typical day, try shifting your inquiry to the symptoms of depression or begin an exploratory mental status examination.

See Chapter 19, Mental Status, pp. 595–612.

The Confusing Patient.   Some patients present a confusing array of *multiple symptoms*. They seem to have every symptom that you ask about. With these patients, focus on the meaning or function of the symptom, emphasizing the patient's perspective (see p. 45), and guide the interview into a psychosocial assessment. There is little profit to exploring each symptom in detail. Although the patient may have several illnesses, a psychological disorder may be in play.

At other times, you may feel baffled, frustrated, and confused because you cannot make sense out of the patient's story. The history is vague and difficult to understand, ideas are poorly connected, and language is hard to follow. Even though you word your questions carefully, you cannot seem to get clear answers. The patient's manner of relating to you may also seem peculiar, distant, aloof, or inappropriate. Symptoms may be described in bizarre terms: "My fingernails feel too heavy" or "My stomach knots up like a snake." Perhaps there is a mental status change like psychosis or delirium, a mental illness such as schizophrenia, or a neurologic disorder. Consider delirium in acutely ill or intoxicated patients and dementia in the elderly. Such patients give histories that are inconsistent and cannot provide a clear chronology about what has happened. Some may even make up information to fill in the gaps in their memories.

See Table 24-2, Delirium and Dementia, p. 876.

When you suspect a psychiatric or neurologic disorder, do not spend too much time gathering a detailed history. Shift to the mental status examination, focusing on level of consciousness, orientation, memory, and capacity to understand. You can work in the initial questions smoothly by asking, "When was your last appointment at the clinic? Let's see . . . that was about how long ago?" "Your address now is . . . ? . . . and your phone number?" You can check these responses against the chart or seek permission to speak with family members or friends and then obtain their perspectives.

See Chapter 19, Mental Status, The Mental Status Examination, pp. 595–612.

The Patient With Altered Capacity.   Some patients cannot provide their own histories because of delirium from illness, dementia, or other health or mental health conditions. Others are unable to relate certain parts of the history, such as events related to a febrile illness or a seizure. Under these circumstances, you need to determine whether the patient has "*decision-making capacity*," or the ability to understand information related to health, to make health choices based on reason and a consistent set of values and to declare preferences about treatments. The term *capacity* is preferable to the term "*competence*," which is a legal term. You do not need to consult psychiatry to assess capacity unless mental illness impairs decision making. For many patients with psychiatric conditions or even cognitive impairments, their ability to make decisions remains intact.

For patients with capacity, obtain their consent before talking about their health with others. Even if patients communicate only with facial expressions or gestures, you must maintain confidentiality and elicit their input. Assure patients that any shared history will be kept confidential, and clarify what you can discuss with others. Your knowledge about the patient can be quite comprehensive, yet others may offer surprising and important information. A spouse, for example, may report significant family strains, depressive symptoms, or drinking habits that the patient has denied. Consider dividing the interview into two segments—one with the patient and the other with both the patient and a second informant. Each interview has its own value. Information from other sources often gives you helpful ideas for planning the patient's care, but remains confidential. Also learn the tenets of the *Health Insurance Portability and Accountability Act (HIPAA)* passed by Congress in 1996, which sets strict standards for disclosure for both institutions and providers when sharing patient information.[26]

For patients with impaired capacity, you will often need to find a *surrogate informant or decision maker* to assist with the history. Check whether the patient has a *durable power of attorney for health care* or a *health care proxy*. If not, in many cases, a spouse or family member who can represent the patient's wishes can fill this role.

Apply the basic principles of interviewing to your conversations with patients' relatives or friends. Find a private place to talk. Introduce yourself, state your purpose, inquire how they are feeling under the circumstances, and recognize and acknowledge their concerns. As you listen to their versions of the history, assess the quality of their relationship with the patient because it may color their credibility. Establish how they know the patient. For example, when a child is brought in for health care, the accompanying adult may not be the primary or even frequent caregiver, just the most available ride. Always seek the best-informed source. Occasionally, a relative or friend insists on being with the patient during your evaluation. Try to find out why, and assess the patient's wishes.

The Talkative Patient. The garrulous, rambling patient may be difficult to interview, especially when faced with limited time and the need to "get the whole story." Several techniques are helpful. Give the patient free rein for the first 5 or 10 minutes, listening closely to the conversation. Perhaps the patient simply needs a good listener and is expressing pent-up concerns, or the patient's style is to tell stories. In some cultures, social conversation of various lengths before "getting down to business" is considered polite. Does the patient seem obsessively detailed? Is the patient unduly anxious or apprehensive? Is there flight of ideas or a disorganized thought process that suggests a thought disorder?

Focus on what seems most important to the patient. Show your interest by asking questions in those areas. Interrupt only if necessary, but be courteous. Learn how to set limits when needed. Remember that part of your task is structuring the interview to gain important information about the patient's health. A brief summary may help you change the subject yet validate any concerns. "Let me make sure that I understand. You have described many concerns. In particular, I heard about two different kinds of pain, one on your left side that goes into your groin and is fairly new, and one in your upper abdomen after you eat that you have had for months. Let's focus just on the side pain first. Can you tell me what it feels like?"

See Summarization, p. 50.

Finally, do not show your impatience. If time runs out, explain the need for a second meeting. Setting a time limit for the next appointment may be helpful. "I know we have much more to talk about. We will continue after lunch. We will have a full hour then."

The Crying Patient. Crying signals strong emotions, ranging from sadness to anger or frustration. If the patient is on the verge of tears, pausing, gentle probing, or responding with empathy gives the patient permission to cry. Usually crying is therapeutic, as is your quiet acceptance of the patient's distress or pain. Offer a tissue and wait for the patient to recover. Make a supportive remark like "I am glad you were able to express your feelings." Most patients will soon compose themselves and resume their story. Aside from an acute grief or loss, it is unusual for crying to escalate and become uncontrollable.

Crying makes many people uncomfortable. If this is true for you, you need to learn how to accept displays of emotion so that as a nurse you can support patients at these moving and significant times.

The Angry or Disruptive Patient. Many patients have reasons to be angry: they are ill, they have suffered a loss, they lack their accustomed control over their own lives, and they feel powerless in the health care system.[27] They may direct this anger toward the nurse. It is possible that this hostility is justified . . . were you late for your appointment, inconsiderate, insensitive, or angry yourself? If so, acknowledge the fact and try to make amends. More often, however, patients displace their anger onto the nurse as a reflection of their frustration or pain.

Accept angry feelings from patients. Allow them to express such emotions without getting angry in return. Avoid joining such patients in their hostility toward another provider or the agency, even when privately you may feel sympathetic. You can validate their feelings without agreeing with their reasons. "I understand that you felt very frustrated by the long wait and answering the same questions over and over. Our complex health care system can seem very unsupportive when you are not feeling well." After the patient has calmed down, help find steps that will avert such situations in the future. Rational solutions to emotional problems are not always possible, however, and people need time to express and work through their angry feelings.

Some angry patients become overtly disruptive. Few people can disturb the clinic, nursing unit, or emergency department more quickly than patients who are angry, belligerent, or out of control. Before approaching such patients, alert the security staff—as a nurse, maintaining a safe environment is one of your responsibilities. Stay calm, appear accepting, and avoid being confrontational in return. Keep your posture relaxed and nonthreatening and your hands loosely open. At first, do not try to make disruptive patients lower their voices or stop if they are haranguing you or the staff. Listen carefully. Try to understand what they are saying. Once you have established rapport, gently suggest moving to a different location that is more private and will cause less disruption.

The Interview Across a Language Barrier. More than 46 million people in the United States do not speak English as their primary language, and the command of English for approximately 21 million is less than fluent.[28] Such people are less likely to have regular primary or preventive care and more likely to report problems with care or even experience medical errors. Learning to work with qualified interpreters is not only cost-effective but also important for optimal care.[28–30]

If your patient speaks a different language, make every effort to find an interpreter. A few broken words and gestures are no substitutes for the full story. The ideal interpreter is a neutral person who is familiar with both languages and cultures. Recruiting family members or friends to serve as interpreters can be hazardous—confidentiality and cultural norms may be violated, meanings may be distorted, and transmitted information may be incomplete. Untrained interpreters may try to speed up the interview by telescoping lengthy replies into a few words, losing much of what may be significant detail.

As you begin working with the interpreter, establish rapport and review what information would be most useful. Explain that you need the interpreter to translate everything, not to condense or summarize. *Make your questions clear, short, and simple.* You can also help the interpreter by outlining your goals for each segment of the history. After going over your plans, arrange the room so that you have easy eye contact and nonverbal communication with the patient. Then speak directly to the patient . . . "How long have you been sick?" rather than "How long has the patient been sick?" Having the interpreter close by the patient, or even behind you, keeps you from moving your head back and forth as though you were watching a tennis match.

When available, bilingual written questionnaires are invaluable, especially for the review of systems. First, however, be sure that patients can read in their language; otherwise, ask for help from the interpreter. In some clinical settings, there are speakerphone translators; use them if there are no better options.

GUIDELINES FOR WORKING WITH AN INTERPRETER

- Choose a trained interpreter in preference to a hospital worker, volunteer, or family member.
- Use the interpreter as a resource for cultural information.
- Orient the interpreter to the components you plan to cover in the interview; include reminders to translate everything the patient says.
- Arrange the room so that you and the patient have eye contact and can read each other's nonverbal cues. Seat the interpreter next to the patient.
- Allow the interpreter and the patient to establish rapport.
- Address the patient directly. Reinforce your questions with nonverbal behaviors.
- Keep sentences *short* and *simple*. Focus on the most important concepts to communicate.
- Verify mutual understanding by asking the patient to repeat back what was heard.
- Be patient. The interview will take more time and may provide less information.

The Patient With Low Literacy. Before giving written instructions, assess the patient's ability to read. Literacy levels are highly variable, and marginal reading skills are more prevalent than commonly believed. Explore the many reasons people do not read: language barriers, learning disorders, poor vision, or lack of education. Some patients feel uncomfortable about disclosing their reading deficits. Asking about educational level may be helpful, but practical approaches are more fruitful. Ask, "How comfortable are you with filling out medical forms?" or ask the patient to read whatever instructions you have written. (This will also address any difficulty with handwriting.) Another rapid screen is to hand the patient a written text upside down—most patients who read will turn the page around immediately. Lack of reading skill may explain why the patient has not taken medications as prescribed or adhered to recommended treatments. Respond sensitively, and do not confuse the degree of literacy with level of intelligence.

The Patient With Impaired Hearing. Communicating with the deaf presents many of the same challenges as communicating with patients who speak a different language. Even people with partial hearing may define themselves as deaf, a distinct cultural group. Find out the patient's preferred method of communicating. Patients may use American Sign Language, a unique language with its own syntax, or various other combinations of signs and speech. Thus, communication is often truly cross-cultural.

Ask when the hearing loss occurred relative to the patient's development of speech and what schools the patient attended. These questions help determine whether the patient identifies with the deaf culture or the hearing culture. If the patient prefers sign language, find an interpreter and use the principles identified earlier. Written questionnaires are also useful. Time-consuming handwritten questions and answers may be the only solution, although literacy skills may also be an issue.

Hearing deficits vary. If the patient has a hearing aid, make sure the patient is using it and it is working. For patients with unilateral hearing loss, sit on the hearing side. A person who is *hard of hearing* may not be aware of the problem, a situation you will have to tactfully address. Eliminate background noise such as television or hallway conversation as much as possible. For patients who have partial hearing or can read lips, face them directly, in good light. Patients should wear their glasses to better pick up visual cues that help them understand you.

Speak at a normal volume and rate and do not let your voice trail off at the ends of sentences. Avoid covering your mouth or looking down at papers while speaking. Remember that even the best lip readers comprehend only a percentage of what is said, so having patients repeat what you have said is important. When closing, write out any oral instructions.

The Patient With Impaired Vision. When meeting with a blind patient, shake hands to establish contact and explain who you are and why you are there. If the room is unfamiliar, orient the patient to the surroundings and report if anyone else is present. It still may be helpful to adjust the light. Encourage visually impaired patients to wear glasses whenever possible. Remember to use words because postures and gestures are unseen.

The Patient With Cognitive Disabilities. Patients with moderate cognitive disability can usually give adequate histories. In fact, you may even be able to omit their disability from their evaluations. If you suspect problems, however, pay special attention to the patient's schooling and ability to function independently. How far have such patients gone in school? If they did not finish, why not? What kinds of courses have they taken? How did they do? Have they had any testing done? Are they living alone? Do they need assistance with activities such as transportation or shopping? The sexual history is equally important and often overlooked. Find out if the patient is sexually active and provide information that may be needed about pregnancy or sexually transmitted diseases.

If you are unsure about the patient's level of disability, make a smooth transition to the mental status examination and assess simple calculations, vocabulary, memory, and abstract thinking.

See Chapter 19, Mental Status, pp. 595–612.

For patients with severe cognitive disabilities, you will have to turn to the family or caregivers to elicit the history. Identify the person who accompanies the patient, but always show interest in the patient first. Establish rapport, make eye contact, and engage in simple conversation. As with children, avoid "talking down" or using affectations of speech or condescending behavior. The patient, family members, caregivers, or friends will notice and appreciate your respect.

The Patient With Personal Problems. Patients may ask you for advice about personal problems that fall outside the range of your clinical expertise. Should the patient quit a stressful job, for example, or move out of state? Instead of responding, ask about the different approaches the patient has considered and related pros and cons, others who have provided advice, and what supports are available for different choices. Letting the patient talk through the problems is more valuable and therapeutic than any answer you could give.

Sexuality in the Nurse–Patient Relationship. Nurses of both genders occasionally find themselves physically attracted to their patients. Similarly, patients may make sexual overtures or exhibit flirtatious behavior toward nurses. The emotional and physical intimacy of the nurse–patient relationship may lend itself to these sexual feelings.

If you become aware of such feelings in yourself, accept them as a normal human response, and bring them to conscious level so they will not affect your behavior. Denying these feelings makes it more likely for you to act inappropriately. *Any* sexual contact or romantic relationship with patients is *unethical;* keep your relationship with the patient within professional bounds, and seek help if you need it.[31–33]

Sometimes nurses meet patients who are frankly seductive or make sexual advances. It is tempting to ignore this behavior because you are not sure that it really happened or are hoping it will go away. Calmly but firmly, make it clear that your relationship is professional, not personal. If unwelcome overtures continue, leave the room and find a chaperone to continue the interview. You should also reflect on your image. Has your clothing or demeanor been unconsciously seductive? Have you been overly warm with the patient? Although it is your responsibility to avoid contributing to these problems, usually you are not at fault. These problems may reflect the patient's discomfort with feeling less powerful.

 **ETHICS OF INTERVIEWING**

Ethics and Professionalism

A chapter on interviewing would not be complete without mention of the ethics related to patient information. The potential power of the nurse–patient communication calls for guidance beyond one's innate sense of morality.[34] Ethics are a set of principles crafted through reflection and discussion to define what is right and wrong. Medical ethics guide professional behavior. The principle of *confidentiality* is of paramount importance in the nurse–patient relationship. The nurse is obligated to protect patient information. Simply deleting the patient's name from a story may not be adequate protection. For example, a student may tell a friend a baby was born today with club feet at ABC hospital. If only one baby was born on this day at ABC hospital, the baby can be identified.

Information may only be shared with appropriate health care team members. At the start of the interview, the patient should be told with whom the information will be shared. Do not agree to a patient's request not to reveal a piece of information with anyone before you know what the information is. Should such a request be made, tell the patient that if information revealed is harmful to self or another person, then you are obligated to share it with the appropriate person. Confidentiality is a key quality that fosters the nurse–patient relationship.

BIBLIOGRAPHY

CITATIONS

1. Cohen-Cole SA. The Medical Interview: The Three Function Approach. St. Louis: MosbyYear Book, 1991.
2. Bird J, Cohen-Cole SA. The three function model of the medical interview. Adv Psychosom Med 20:65–88, 1990.
3. Lazare A, Putnam SM, Lipkin M Jr. Three functions of the medical interview. In: Lipkin M Jr, Putnam SM, Lazare A, et al, eds. The Medical Interview: Clinical Care, Education, and Research. New York: Springer-Verlag, 1995.
4. Novack DH. Therapeutic aspects of the clinical encounter. In Lipkin M Jr, Putnam SM, Lazare A, et al, eds. The Medical Interview: Clinical Care, Education, and Research. New York: Springer-Verlag:32, 1995.
5. Suchman AL, Matthews DA. What makes the patient-doctor relationship therapeutic? Exploring the connectional dimension of medical care. Ann Intern Med 108(1):25–130, 1988.
6. Hastings C. The lived experiences of the illness: making contact with the patient. In: Benne P, Wrubel J, eds. The Primacy of Caring: Stress and Coping in Health and Illness. Menlo Park, CA: Addison-Wesley, 1989.
7. Epstein RM. Mindful practice. JAMA 282(9):833–839, 1999.
8. Balint M. The Doctor, His Patient and the Illness, 2nd ed. New York: International Universities Press, 1964.
9. Ventres W, Kooienga S, Vuvkovic N, et al. Physicians, patients and the electronic health record: an ethnographic analysis. Ann Fam Med 4(2):124–131, 2006.
10. Conant EB. Addressing patients by their first names. N Engl J Med 308(4):226, 1998.
11. Heller ME. Addressing patients by their first names. N Engl J Med 308(18):1107, 1987.
12. Platt FW, Gaspar DL, Coulehan JL, et al. "Tell me about yourself": the patient-centered interview. Ann Int Med 134(11):1079–1085, 2001.
13. Baron RJ. An introduction to medical phenomenology: I can't hear you while I'm listening. Ann Intern Med 103(4):606–611, 1985.
14. Bass LW, Cohen RL. Ostensible versus actual reasons for seeking pediatric attention: another look at the parental ticket of admission. Pediatrics 70(6):870–874, 1982.
15. Beckman HB, Frankel RM. The effect of physician behavior on the collection of data. Ann Intern Med 101(4):692–696, 1984.
16. White J, Levinson W, Roter D. "Oh, by the way…:" the closing moments of the medical visit. J Gen Intern Med 9(1):24–28, 1994.
17. Smith RC. Patient-Centered Interviewing: An Evidence-Based Method. Philadelphia: Lippincott Williams & Wilkins, 2002.
18. Von Korff M, Shapiro S, Burke JD, et al. Anxiety and depression in a primary care clinic. Arch Gen Psychiatry 44(2):152–156, 1987.
19. Lang F, Floyd MR, Beine KL. Clues to patients' explanations and concerns about their illnesses: a call for active listening. Arch Fam Med 9(3):222–227, 2000.
20. Brown JB, Weston W, Stewart M. Patient-centered interviewing part II: finding common ground. Can Fam Physician 35:153–157, 1989.
21. Neighbour R. The Inner Consultation: How to Develop an Effective and Intuitive Consulting Style. Lancaster, England: MTP Press Ltd.:164–178, 1987.
22. Kleinman A, Eisenberg L, Good B. Culture, illness, and care: clinical lessons from anthropological and cross-cultural research. Ann Intern Med 88(2):251–258, 1978.
23. Smith RC, Lyles JS, Mettler J, et al. The effectiveness of an intensive teaching experience for residents in interviewing: a randomized controlled study. Ann Intern Med 128(2):118–126, 1998.
24. Coulehan JL, Block MR. The Medical Interview: Mastering Skills for Clinical Practice, 4th ed. Philadelphia: FA Davis Company, 2001.
25. Lipkin M Jr, Putnam SM, Lazare A, et al (eds). The Medical Interview: Clinical Care, Education, and Research. New York: Springer-Verlag, 1995.
26. Office for Civil Rights–HIPAA, U.S. Department of Health and Human Services. Available at: http://www.hhs.gov/ocr/hipaa. Accessed May 30, 2011.
27. Platt FW. Field Guide to the Difficult Patient Interview. Philadelphia: Lippincott Williams and Wilkins, 1999.
28. Jacobs EA, Shephard DS, Suya JA, et al. Overcoming language barriers in health care: costs and benefits in interpreter services. Am J Public Health 94(5):866–869, 2004.
29. Jacobs EA, Sadowski LS, Rathous PJ. The impact of enhanced interpreter service intervention on hospital costs and patient satisfaction. J Gen Intern Med 22(suppl 2):306–311, 2007.
30. Hardt E, Jacobs EA, Chen A. Insights into the problems that language barriers may pose for the medical interview. J Gen Intern Med 21(12):1357–1358, 2006.
31. Committee on Ethics, American College of Obstetricians and Gynecologists. ACOG Committee Opinion No. 373. Sexual misconduct. Obstet Gynecol 110(2 Pt 1):441–444, 2007.

32. Gabbard GO, Nadelson C. Professional boundaries in the physician-patient relationship. JAMA 273(18):1445–1449, 1995.

33. Council on Ethical and Judicial Affairs. American Medical Association: sexual misconduct in the practice of medicine. JAMA 266(19):2741–2745, 1991.

34. ABIM Foundation, American Board of Internal Medicine, ACP-ASIM Foundation, American College of Physicians-American Society of Internal Medicine, European Federation of Internal Medicine. Medical professionalism in the new millennium: a physician charter. Ann Intern Med 136(3):243–246, 2002.

ADDITIONAL REFERENCES

Building a Therapeutic Relationship: The Techniques of Skilled Interviewing

Frankel RM, Quill TE, McDanial SH. The biopsychosocial approach: past, present, and future. Rochester, NY: University of Rochester Press, 2003.

Kurtz SM, Silverman J, Draper J. Teaching and Learning Communication Skills in Medicine, 2nd ed. Oxford, San Francisco: Radcliffe Publishers, 2005.

Riley JB. Communication in Nursing. St. Louis. Mosby, 2008.

Schuster PM. Communication for Nurses: How to Prevent Harmful Events and Promote Patient Safety. Phila: F.A. Davis, 2010.

Williams C, Davis C. Therapeutic Interaction in Nursing. Boston: Jones and Bartlett, 2005.

Adapting Interviewing Techniques to Specific Situations

Agency for Healthcare Research and Quality. Health Literacy Interventions and Outcomes: An Updated Systematic Review. March 2011. Available at http://www.ahrq.gov/clinic/tp/lituptp.htm. Accessed May 30, 2011.

Americans with Disabilities Act Home Page, U.S. Department of Justice. Available at http://www.ada.gov/#Anchor-47857. Accessed May 30, 2011.

Barnett S. Cross-cultural communication with patients who use American sign language. Fam Med 34(5):376–382, 2002.

Fowler MDM. Guide to the Code of Ethics for Nurses. Silver Spring MD: American Nurses Association, 2008.

Iezzoni LI, O'Day BL, Killeen M, et al. Communicating about health care: observations from persons who are deaf or hard of hearing. Ann Intern Med 140(5):356–362, 2004.

Marcus EN. The silent epidemic—the health effects of illiteracy. N Engl J Med 355(4):339–341, 2006.

McDaniel SH, Campbell TL, Hepworth J, et al. Family-Oriented Primary Care, 2nd ed. New York: Springer, 2005.

Putsch RW. Cross-cultural communication: the special case of interpreters in health care. JAMA 254(23):3344–3348, 1985.

Rivadeneyra R, Elderkin-Thompson V, Silver RC, et al. Patient centeredness in medical encounters requiring an interpreter. Am J Med 108(6):470–474, 2000.

Schwartzberg JG, Cowett A, VanGeest J, et al. Communication techniques for patients with low health literacy: a survey of physicians, nurses, and pharmacists. Am J Health Behav 31(suppl 1): S96–104, 2007.

The Health History

LEARNING OBJECTIVES

The student will:

1. Explain the four types of histories and when they are used.
2. Describe the components of a comprehensive health history.
3. Obtain a comprehensive health history from a patient.

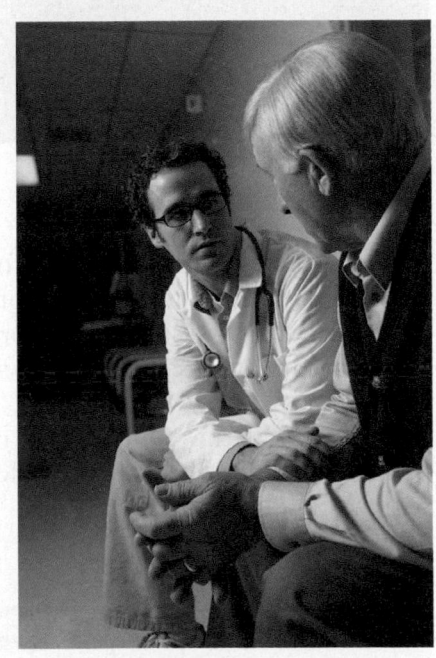

This chapter explains how to obtain a patient health history. All history information is considered subjective data. Consider the health history as a chance for the patient to tell his or her "story."

How much history to gather varies based on the purpose of the patient encounter. The admission of a new patient to a clinic, hospital, long-term care facility, or visiting nurse agency usually requires a ***comprehensive health assessment***. This allows the nurse to obtain a full picture of the patient's health status and current problems, as well as provide health promotion and risk reduction education. The comprehensive history does more than assess body systems. It is a source of personalized knowledge about the patient that strengthens the nurse–patient relationship. The comprehensive history provides a basis for assessing patient concerns, health status, risk factors and answering patient questions.

However, a ***focused or problem-oriented assessment*** is appropriate in many situations, especially when the patient is known to the nurse. Examples of such nurse–patient encounters include the patient hospitalized for surgery who develops shortness of breath or the patient presenting to an urgent care clinic. Here the nurse focuses on gathering information about the patient's problem. The patient's symptoms, age, and history will then help determine the extent of the physical examination to perform.

A ***follow-up history*** is a form of a focused assessment. The patient is returning to have a problem or treatment plan evaluated, or a second-shift nurse may be following up on a problem identified by a nurse on an earlier shift. Here the nurse gathers data to evaluate the outcomes of the plan of care.

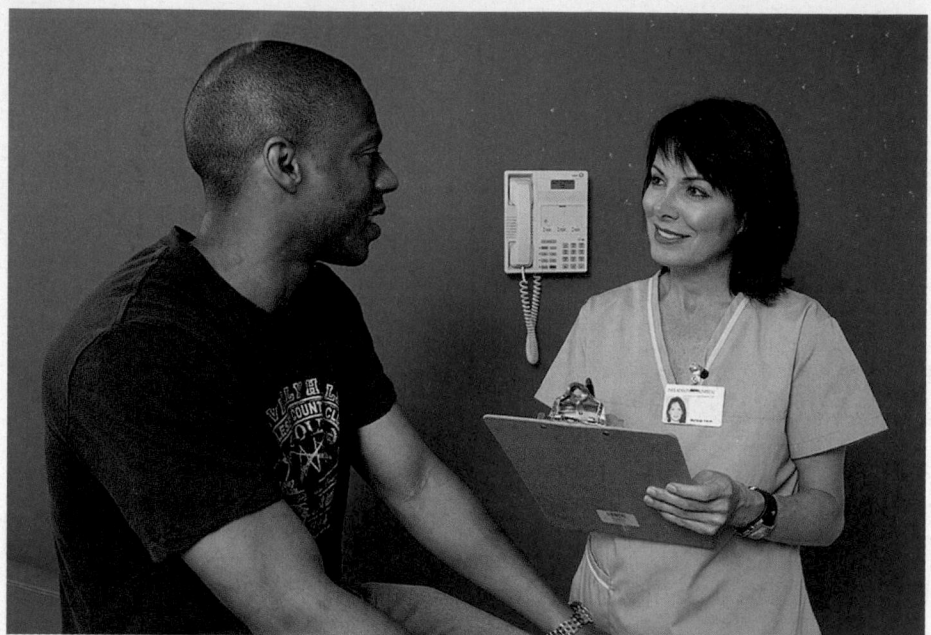

An emergency visit generates a fourth type of data collection, *the emergency history.* The data collection is focused on the patient's emergent problem with a systematic prioritization of need beginning with the ABCs of airway, breathing, and circulation.

Mastery of all the components of the comprehensive history provides proficiency and the ability to select the elements most pertinent to the patient encounter.

● The Health History: Comprehensive or Focused?

Comprehensive Assessment	Focused Assessment
• Is appropriate for new patients in all settings	• Is appropriate for established patients, especially during routine or urgent care visits
• Provides fundamental and personalized knowledge about the patient	• Addresses focused concerns or symptoms
• Strengthens the nurse–patient relationship	• Assesses symptoms restricted to a specific body system
• Provides baselines for future assessments	
• Creates a platform for health promotion through education and counseling	

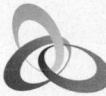

THE COMPREHENSIVE ADULT HEALTH HISTORY

Overview. The seven components of the *Comprehensive Adult Health History* are:

- Identifying Data and Source of the History

- Chief Complaint(s)

- History of Present Illness

- Past History

- Family History

- Review of Systems

- Health Patterns

See Chapter 23, Assessing Children: Infancy Through Adolescence, for *comprehensive pediatric health histories.*

As described in Chapter 3, Interviewing and Communication, the health history may not spring forth in this order! The interview is more fluid . . . follow the *patient's* cues to elicit the patient's narrative of illness, provide empathy, and strengthen rapport. For the documentation, transform the patient's language and story into the seven components of the history familiar to all members of the health care team. This restructuring can organize clinical reasoning and provide a template for identification of patient problems.

Review the features of the components of the adult health history described below; then study the more detailed explanations that follow.

● **Overview: Components of the Adult Health History**	
Identifying Data	• *Identifying data*—such as age, date of birth, gender, occupation, marital or relationship status.
	• *Source of the history*—usually the patient, but can be a family member or friend, letter of referral, or the medical record.
	• If appropriate, establish *source of referral,* because a written report may be needed.
Reliability	Varies according to the patient's memory, trust, and mood.
Chief Complaint(s)	The one or more symptoms or concerns causing the patient to seek care.
Present Illness	• Amplifies the *Chief Complaint;* describes how each symptom developed.
	• Includes patient's thoughts and feelings about the illness
	• Pulls in relevant portions of the *Review of Systems,* called "pertinent positives and negatives" (see p. 69)
	(continued)

Overview: Components of the Adult Health History (continued)

	• May include *medications, allergies,* and habits of *smoking* and *alcohol,* which are frequently pertinent to the present illness
Past History	• Lists childhood illnesses • Lists adult illnesses with dates for at least three categories: medical, surgical, and psychiatric • Includes health maintenance practices such as immunizations, screening tests, lifestyle issues, and home safety • Includes risk factors
Family History	• Outlines or diagrams age and health, or age and cause of death, of siblings, parents, and grandparents • Documents presence or absence of specific illnesses in family, such as hypertension, coronary artery disease, etc.
Review of Systems	• Documents presence or absence of common symptoms related to each major body system
Health Patterns	• Documents personal/social history

Initial Information

Date and Time of History.   The date is always important. Be sure to document the time the history was obtained.

Identifying Data.   These include age, gender, birth date, marital or relationship status, occupation, and any other biographic data appropriate to the agency. The *source of history* can be the patient (primary source) or a family member, friend, health care provider, or the medical record (secondary sources). Designating the *source* helps the nurse and reader assess the type of information provided and possible biases.

Reliability.   Document this information if relevant. For example, "The patient is vague when describing symptoms, and details are confusing" or "The patient appears reliable." This judgment reflects the quality of the information provided by the patient and is usually made at the end of the interview.

Chief Complaint(s).   *Make every attempt to quote the patient's own words.* For example, "My stomach hurts and I feel awful." Sometimes patients have no specific complaints. Report their goals instead. For example, "I have come for my regular check-up" or "I've been admitted for a thorough evaluation of my heart."

History of Present Illness (HPI).   This section of the history is a complete, clear, and chronologic account of the problems prompting the patient to seek care. The narrative should include the onset of the problem, the setting in which it has developed, its manifestations, and any treatments. The HPI should reveal the patient's responses to the symptoms and the effect the illness has had on daily living.

KEY ELEMENTS OF THE HISTORY OF PRESENT ILLNESS

- Seven attributes of each principal symptom
- Self-treatment for the symptom by the patient or family
- Past occurrences of the symptom(s)
- Pertinent positives and/or negatives from the review of systems
- Risk factors or other pertinent information related to the symptom

Seven Attributes of a Symptom

Remember the mnemonic from Chapter 3 that may help the novice history taker gather all the symptom attributes.

- **OLD CART,** or **O**nset, **L**ocation, **D**uration, **C**haracteristic Symptoms, **A**ssociated Manifestations, **R**elieving/Exacerbating Factors, and **T**reatment

1. **O**nset. When did (does) it start? Setting in which it occurs, including environmental factors, personal activities, emotional reactions, or other circumstances that may have contributed to the illness.

2. **L**ocation. Where is it? Does it radiate?

3. **D**uration. How long does it last?

4. **C**haracteristic Symptoms. What is it like? How severe is it? (For pain, ask a rating on a scale of 1 to 10.)

5. **A**ssociated Manifestations. Have you noticed anything else that accompanies it?

6. **R**elieving/Exacerbating Factors. Is there anything that makes it better or worse?

7. **T**reatment. What have you done to treat this? Was it effective?

Self-Treatment.   Be sure to ask what over-the-counter (OTC) or prescribed medication or other treatments (e.g., ice packs or alternative therapies) the patient has tried to alleviate the symptoms. If the patient has already tried the typical first course of treatment and it has failed, the provider will need to consider either more advanced treatment or an alternative diagnosis. For example, if the patient complains of heartburn that was unrelieved by an antacid, the problem may be cardiac in origin and not a gastrointestinal problem.

Past Occurrences of the Symptom. The patient may have had the same or similar problems in the past. Inquire about this and ask what treatment(s) were previously used and the results.

Pertinent Positives and/or Negatives. Pertinent positives and/or negatives from the review of systems related to the chief complaint should be sought (e.g., a history of asthma in a patient with difficulty breathing). These data may help differentiate diagnoses and individual nursing interventions.

Risk Factors or Other Pertinent Information. Risk factors or other pertinent information related to the symptom is frequently relevant, such as risk factors for coronary artery disease in a patient with chest pain, or current medications that may have side effects similar to the complaint.

Past History

KEY ELEMENTS OF THE PAST HISTORY

- *Allergies*
- *Medications*
- *Childhood illnesses*
- *Adult Illnesses*
- *Health Maintenance*

Allergies. Allergies, including specific reactions to each medication, such as rash or nausea, must be recorded. Allergies to foods, insects, or environmental factors along with the patient's reaction should also be noted.

Medications. Medications, including name, dose/route, and frequency of use, are included. Also list home remedies, nonprescription drugs, vitamins, mineral or herbal supplements, oral contraceptives, and medicines borrowed from family members or friends. If the patient is unsure, ask him or her to bring in all medications to see exactly what is taken.

Childhood illnesses. Childhood illnesses, such as measles, rubella, mumps, whooping cough, chickenpox, rheumatic fever, scarlet fever, and polio, are included in the Past History. Also included are any chronic childhood illnesses, such as asthma.

Adult Illnesses. Adult Illnesses in each of the following areas:
- *Medical:* Illnesses such as diabetes, hypertension, hepatitis, asthma, or HIV; hospitalizations
- *Surgical:* Dates, reasons for surgery, and types of operations or treatments
- *Accidents:* type, dates, treatment and residual disability of major accidents
- *Psychiatric:* Illness and time frame, hospitalizations, and treatments

Health Maintenance

- *Immunizations:* Ask whether the patient has received vaccines for tetanus, pertussis, diphtheria, polio, measles, mumps influenza, varicella, hepatitis B, *Haemophilus influenzae* type B, *Neisseria meningitides* meningitis, and *pneumococci*. Include the dates of original and booster immunizations. (The Centers for Disease Control and Prevention updates vaccine recommendations yearly for different age groups. To obtain the most current recommendations, go to the Web site: http://www.cdc.gov/vaccines/recs/schedules.)

- *Screening Tests:* Such as tuberculin tests, cholesterol tests, stool for occult blood, Pap smears, and mammograms. Include the results and the dates the tests were performed. Alternatively, screening tests may be asked about during and documented in the Review of Systems.

- *Safety Measures:* Seat belts in cars, smoke/carbon monoxide detectors, sports helmets or padding, etc.

- *Risk Factors:*

Tobacco:	Do you use or have you ever used tobacco? At what age did you start? How many packs per day (ppd) do you smoke? How many ppd in the past?
Environmental Hazards:	In home or work environment?
Substance Abuse:	Do you use or have you ever used marijuana, cocaine, heroin, or other recreational drugs?
Alcohol:	How much alcohol do you drink per sitting and per week?

Alcohol and Illicit Drugs. Many clinicians hesitate to ask patients about use of alcohol and drugs, whether prescribed or illegal. Misuse of alcohol or drugs often directly contributes to symptoms and the need for care and treatment. Despite the high lifetime prevalence of substance abuse disorders—more than 13% for alcohol and 4% for illegal drugs in the United States—they remain underdiagnosed.[1]

Avoid letting personal feelings interfere with your role. It is the nurse's job to gather data, assess the effects on the patient's health, and plan a therapeutic response. Nurses should routinely ask about current and past use of alcohol or drugs, patterns of use, and family history. Make sure to include adolescents and older adults in your questioning.[2,3]

Alcohol. Questions about alcohol and other drugs follow naturally after questions about caffeine and cigarettes. "What do you like to drink?" or "Tell me about your use of alcohol" are good opening questions that avoid the easy yes or no response. Remember to assess what the patient considers alcohol—some patients do not use this term for wine or beer. Two additional questions— "Have you ever had a drinking problem?" and "When was your last drink?"—along with a drink within 24 hours are suspicious for problem drinking.[4] To detect problem drinking, use a well-validated short screening tool that does not take much time. The most widely used screening questions are the **CAGE** questions about **C**utting down, **A**nnoyance if criticized, **G**uilty feelings, and **E**ye-openers.

THE CAGE QUESTIONNAIRE

Have you ever felt the need to **Cut down** on drinking?

Have you ever felt **Annoyed** by criticism of your drinking?

Have you ever felt **Guilty** about drinking?

Have you ever taken a drink first thing in the morning (**Eye-opener**) to steady your nerves or get rid of a hangover?

(Adapted from Mayfield D, McCleod G, Hall P. The CAGE questionnaire: validation of a new alcoholism screening instrument. Am J Psychiatry 131:1121–1123, 1974.)

Two or more affirmative answers to the CAGE questionnaire suggest alcohol misuse and have a sensitivity that ranges from 43% to 94% and a specificity that ranges from 70% to 96%.[5,6] If you detect misuse, you need to ask about blackouts (loss of memory about events during drinking), seizures, accidents or injuries while drinking, job problems, conflict in personal relationships, or legal problems. Also ask specifically about drinking while driving or operating machinery.[7,8]

Illicit Drugs. As with alcohol, questions about drugs should be more focused in order to get answers that distinguish use from misuse. A good opening question is, "Have you ever used any drugs other than those required for medical reasons?"[9] From there, either ask specifically about patterns of use (last use, how often, substances used, amount) or inquire about modes of consumption. "Have you ever injected a drug?" "Have you ever smoked or inhaled a drug?" "Have you ever taken a pill for nonmedical reasons?" As fashions in drugs of abuse change, it is important to stay up to date about the most current hazards and risks from overdose.

Another approach is to adapt the CAGE questions to screening for substance abuse by adding "or drugs" to each question. Once you identify substance abuse, continue further with questions like, "Are you always able to control your use of drugs?" "Have you had any bad reactions?" "What happened . . . Any drug-related accidents, injuries, or arrests? Job or family problems?" and "Have you ever tried to quit? Tell me about it."

Family History. Under *Family History,* outline or diagram on a genogram the age and health, or age and cause of death, of each immediate relative, including parents, grandparents, siblings, children, and grandchildren (see figure on page 69 for an example). *Review each of the following conditions and record whether they are present or absent in the family:* hypertension, coronary artery disease, elevated cholesterol levels, stroke, diabetes, thyroid or renal disease, arthritis, tuberculosis, asthma or lung disease, headache, seizure disorder, mental illness, suicide, substance abuse, and allergies, as well as symptoms reported by the patient. Ask about any history of cancer and the site. Ask about any genetically transmitted diseases.

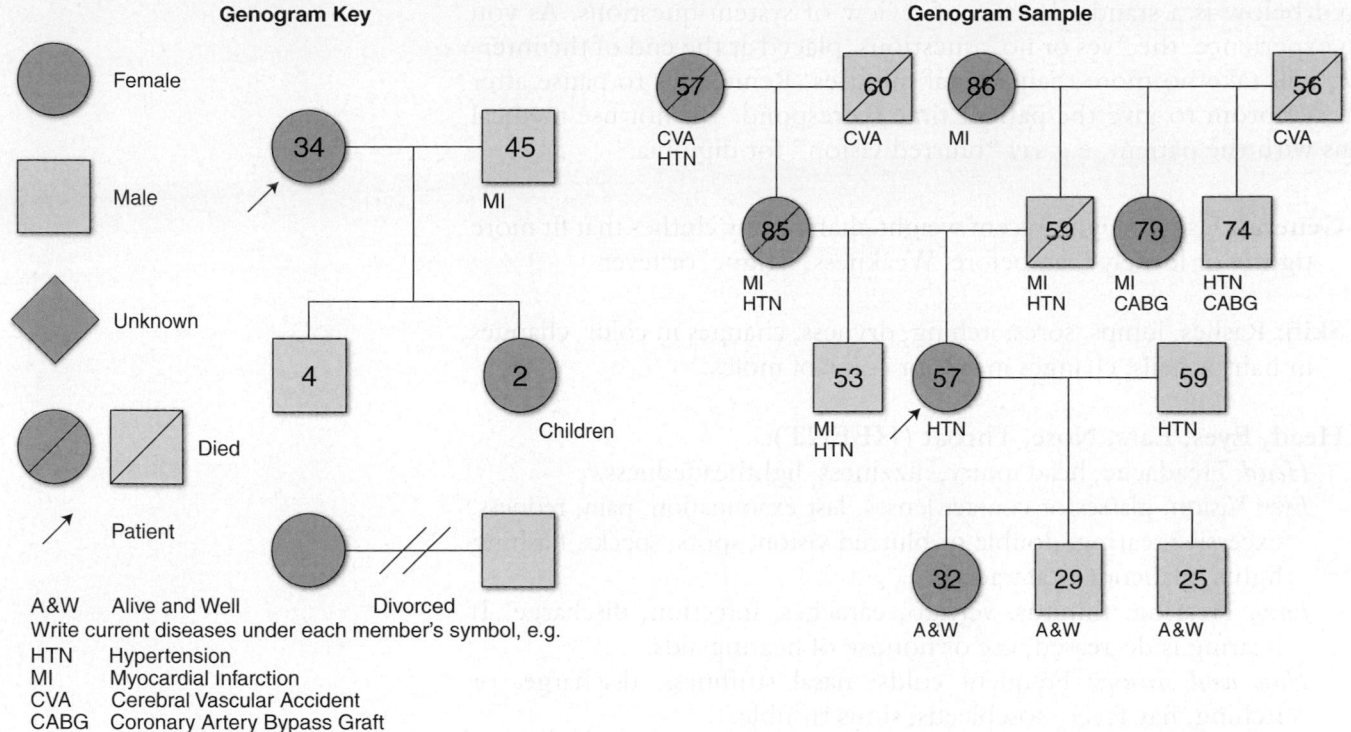

Genogram Key

Female

Male

Unknown

Died

Patient

A&W   Alive and Well   Divorced
Write current diseases under each member's symbol, e.g.
HTN   Hypertension
MI   Myocardial Infarction
CVA   Cerebral Vascular Accident
CABG   Coronary Artery Bypass Graft

Genogram Sample

Children

Review of Systems.   Understanding and using *Review of Systems* questions are often challenging for beginning students. Think about asking a series of questions going from "head to toe." It is helpful to prepare the patient for the questions to come by saying, "The next part of the history may feel like a hundred questions, but they are important and I want to be thorough." Most *Review of Systems* questions pertain to *symptoms*, but on occasion some nurses also include diseases like pneumonia or tuberculosis.

Start with a fairly general question as you address each of the different systems. This focuses the patient's attention and allows you to shift to more specific questions about systems that may be of concern. Examples of starting questions are "How are your ears and hearing?" "How about your lungs and breathing?" "Any trouble with your heart?" "How is your digestion?" "How about your bowels?" Note that you will vary the need for additional questions depending on the patient's age, complaints, and general state of health and your clinical judgment.

The *Review of Systems* questions may uncover problems that the patient has overlooked, particularly in areas unrelated to the *present illness*. Significant health events, such as a major prior illness or a parent's death, require full exploration. Remember that *major health events should be moved to the Present Illness or Past History in your write-up.* Keep your technique flexible. Interviewing the patient yields various findings that you organize into formal written format only after the interview and examination are completed.

Listed below is a standard series of review-of-system questions. As you gain experience, the "yes or no" questions, placed at the end of the interview, will take no more than several minutes. Remember to pause after each symptom to give the patient time to respond. Do not use medical terms with the patient, e.g say "blurred vision" for diplopia.

General: Usual weight, recent weight change, any clothes that fit more tightly or loosely than before. Weakness, fatigue, or fever.

Skin: Rashes, lumps, sores, itching, dryness, changes in color; changes in hair or nails; changes in size or color of moles.

Head, Eyes, Ears, Nose, Throat (HEENT):
Head: Headache, head injury, dizziness, lightheadedness.
Eyes: Vision, glasses or contact lenses, last examination, pain, redness, excessive tearing, double or blurred vision, spots, specks, flashing lights, glaucoma, cataracts.
Ears: Hearing, tinnitus, vertigo, earaches, infection, discharge. If hearing is decreased, use or nonuse of hearing aids.
Nose and sinuses: Frequent colds; nasal stuffiness, discharge, or itching; hay fever; nosebleeds; sinus trouble.
Throat (or mouth and pharynx): Condition of teeth and gums; bleeding gums; dentures, if any, and how they fit; last dental examination; sore tongue; dry mouth; frequent sore throats; hoarseness.

Neck: "Swollen glands"; goiter; lumps, pain, or stiffness in the neck.

Breasts: Lumps, pain, or discomfort; nipple discharge; self-examination practices; last mammogram.

Respiratory: Cough, sputum (color, quantity), hemoptysis, dyspnea, wheezing, pleurisy, last chest x-ray. You may include asthma, bronchitis, emphysema, pneumonia, and tuberculosis.

Cardiovascular: Heart trouble, high blood pressure, rheumatic fever, heart murmurs; chest pain or discomfort; palpitations, dyspnea, orthopnea, paroxysmal nocturnal dyspnea, edema; results of past electrocardiograms or other cardiovascular tests.

Gastrointestinal: Trouble swallowing, heartburn, appetite, nausea. Bowel movements, stool color and size, change in bowel habits, pain with defecation, rectal bleeding, black or tarry stools, hemorrhoids, constipation, diarrhea. Abdominal pain, food intolerance, excessive belching or passing of gas. Jaundice, liver, or gallbladder trouble; hepatitis.

Peripheral vascular: Intermittent claudication; leg cramps; varicose veins; past clots in the veins; swelling in calves, legs, or feet; color change in fingertips or toes during cold weather; swelling with redness or tenderness.

Urinary: Frequency of urination, polyuria, nocturia, urgency, burning or pain during urination, hematuria, urinary infections, kidney or flank pain, kidney stones, ureteral colic, suprapubic pain, incontinence; in males, reduced caliber or force of the urinary stream, hesitancy, dribbling.

Reproductive:

Male: Hernias, discharge from or sores on the penis, testicular pain or masses, scrotal pain or swelling, history of sexually transmitted diseases and their treatments.

Sexual habits, interest, function, satisfaction, birth control methods, condom use, and problems. Concerns about HIV infection. Human Papillomavirus infection or vaccine (HPV).

Female: Age at menarche; regularity, frequency, and duration of periods; amount of bleeding; bleeding between periods or after intercourse; date of last menstrual period; dysmenorrhea; premenstrual tension.

Age at menopause, menopausal symptoms, postmenopausal bleeding. Vaginal discharge, itching, sores, lumps, sexually transmitted diseases and treatments. Number of pregnancies, number and type of deliveries, number of abortions (spontaneous and induced), complications of pregnancy, birth control methods. Sexual preference, interest, function, satisfaction, any problems, including dyspareunia. Concerns about HIV infection. Human papillomavirus infection or vaccine (HPV).

If the patient was born before 1971, exposure to diethylstilbestrol (DES) from maternal use during pregnancy.

Maternal DES use during pregnancy is linked to vaginal and cervical carcinoma.

Musculoskeletal: Muscle or joint pain, stiffness, arthritis, gout, backache. If present, describe location of affected joints or muscles, any swelling, redness, pain, tenderness, stiffness, weakness, or limitation of motion or activity; include timing of symptoms (e.g., morning or evening), duration, and any history of trauma. Neck or low back pain. Joint pain with systemic features such as fever, chills, rash, anorexia, weight loss, or weakness.

Psychiatric: Nervousness; tension; mood, including depression, memory change, suicide attempts.

Neurologic: Headache, dizziness, vertigo; fainting, blackouts, seizures, weakness, paralysis, numbness or loss of sensation, tingling or "pins and needles," tremors or other involuntary movements; seizures. Changes in mood, attention, or speech; changes in orientation, memory, insight, or judgment.

Hematologic: Anemia, easy bruising or bleeding, past transfusions, transfusion reactions.

Endocrine: Thyroid issues, heat or cold intolerance, excessive sweating, excessive thirst or hunger, polyuria, change in glove or shoe size.

Health Patterns. The *Health Patterns* section provides a guide for gathering personal/social history from the patient and daily living routines that may influence health and illness.

Health Pattern	Sample Questions
Self-perception–self-concept: Describes self-concept and perceptions of self (e.g., body image, feeling state, self-esteem, personal identity, and social identity)	How would a friend describe you? How do you feel about your ability to handle ___? If you could change anything about yourself, what would you change?
Value-belief: Describes patterns of values, beliefs (including spiritual), or goals that guide choices or decisions	What is your source of strength and hope? Is religion or God significant to you? Describe how.
Activity-exercise: Describes pattern of exercise, activity, leisure, and recreation	Describe your exercise routine or activities Describe your leisure and recreation activities. Have you experienced any change in your activities due to your illness?
Sleep-rest: Describes patterns of sleep, rest, and relaxation	At what time do you usually retire and awaken? Do you feel rested?
Nutrition: Describes pattern of food and fluid consumption	Describe a typical day's diet. Are you on any special diet?
Role-relationship: Describes pattern of role interactions and relationships. Includes roles, family functioning and problems, and work and neighborhood environment *NOTE: Genogram should have provided a list of family members.*	Who lives with you? Describe the relationships you have with your family and friends. Who provides support for you? Describe your job. What is your neighborhood like?
Coping-stress-tolerance: Describes general coping pattern and its effectiveness in terms of stress tolerance	What are the current stressors in you life? What do you do to reduce stress?

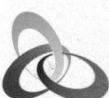

SENSITIVE TOPICS THAT CALL FOR SPECIFIC APPROACHES

Nurses talk with patients about many subjects that are emotionally charged. Even seasoned clinicians are affected by societal taboos enveloping certain subjects: abuse of alcohol or drugs, sexual practices, death and dying, financial concerns, racial and ethnic bias, family interactions, domestic violence, psychiatric illnesses, physical deformities, bowel function, and others. Many of these topics trigger strong personal responses related to family, cultural, and societal value systems. Mental illness, drug use during pregnancy, and sexual practices are examples of issues that may evoke biases that can affect the patient interview. This section explores challenges to the nurse in several of these sensitive areas.

Several basic principles can help guide your response to sensitive topics:

GUIDELINES FOR BROACHING SENSITIVE TOPICS

- *The single most important rule is to be nonjudgmental.* The nurse's role is to learn about the patient and help the patient achieve better health. Disapproval of behaviors or elements in the health history will only interfere with this goal.
- *Explain why you need to know certain information.* This makes patients less apprehensive. For example, say to patients, "Because sexual practices put people at risk for certain diseases, I ask all of my patients the following questions."
- Find opening questions for sensitive topics and learn the specific kinds of information needed for your assessments.
- Finally, consciously acknowledge whatever discomfort you are feeling. Denying your discomfort may lead you to avoid the topic altogether.

Look into strategies for becoming more comfortable with sensitive areas. Examples include reading about these topics in nursing, medical, and lay literature; talking to selected colleagues and teachers openly about your concerns; taking courses that help you explore your own feelings and reactions; and, ultimately, reflecting on your own life experience. Take advantage of all these resources. Whenever possible, listen to experienced nurses, and then practice similar discussions with your own patients.

The Sexual History. Asking questions about sexual behavior can be life-saving. Sexual behaviors determine risks for pregnancy, sexually transmitted diseases (STDs), and AIDS—good interviewing helps prevent or reduce these risks. Sexual practices may be directly related to the patient's symptoms and integral to both diagnosis and treatment. Many patients have questions or concerns about sexuality that they would discuss more freely if asked about sexual health. Finally, sexual dysfunction may result from use of medication or from misinformation that, if recognized, can be readily addressed.

You can introduce questions about sexual behavior at multiple points in an interview. If the chief complaint involves genitourinary symptoms, include questions about sexual health as part of "expanding and clarifying" the patient's story. You can ask these questions as part of the Review of Systems. You can bring them into discussions about Health Maintenance, along with diet, exercise, and screening tests, or as part of the lifestyle issues or important relationships covered in the Personal and Social History. Do not forget this area of inquiry just because the patient is elderly or has a disability or chronic illness.

An orienting sentence or two is often helpful: "To assess your risk for various diseases, I need to ask you some questions about your sexual health and practices" or "I routinely ask all patients about their sexual function." For more specific complaints you might state, "To figure out why you have this discharge and what we should do about it, I need to ask some questions about your sexual activity." Try to be matter-of-fact in your style; the patient will be likely to follow your lead. *Use specific language.* Refer to genitalia with explicit words such as penis or vagina and avoid phrases like "private parts." Choose words that the patient understands or explain what you mean. "By intercourse, I mean when a man inserts his penis into a woman's vagina."

In general, ask about both specific sexual behaviors and satisfaction with sexual function. Here are examples of questions that help patients reveal their concerns:

See specific questions in Chapter 21, The Reproductive Systems, pp. 683–719.

- "When was the last time you had intimate physical contact with someone? Did that contact include sexual intercourse?" Using the term "sexually active" can be ambiguous. Patients have been known to reply, "No, I just lie there."

- "Do you have sex with men, women, or both?" Individuals may have sex with persons of the same gender, yet not consider themselves gay, lesbian, or bisexual. Some gay and lesbian patients have had sex with the opposite gender. Your questions should always be about the behaviors.

- "How many sexual partners have you had in the last 6 months? In the last 5 years? In your lifetime?" Again, these questions give the patient an easy opportunity to acknowledge multiple partners. Ask also about routine use of condoms. "How often do you use condoms?"

- It is important to ask all patients, "Do you have any concerns about HIV infection or AIDS?" even if no explicit risk factors are evident.

Note that these questions make no assumptions about marital status, sexual preference, or attitudes toward pregnancy or contraception. Listen to each of the patient's responses, and ask additional questions as indicated.

To elicit information about sexual behaviors, you will need to ask more specific and focused questions than in other parts of the interview.

The Mental Health History. Cultural constructs of mental and physical illness vary widely, causing marked differences in acceptance and attitudes. Think how easy it is for patients to talk about diabetes and taking insulin compared with discussing schizophrenia and using psychotropic medications. Ask open-ended questions initially. "Have you ever had any problem with emotional or mental illnesses?" Then move to more specific questions such as "Have you ever visited a counselor or psychotherapist?" "Have you ever been prescribed medication for emotional issues?" "Have you or has anyone in your family ever been hospitalized for an emotional or mental health problem?"

For patients with depression or thought disorders such as schizophrenia, a careful history of their illness is in order. Depression is common world-wide but still remains underdiagnosed and undertreated. Be sensitive to reports of mood changes or symptoms such as fatigue, unusual tearfulness, appetite or weight changes, insomnia, and vague somatic complaints. Two opening screening questions are: "Over the past 2 weeks, have you felt down, depressed, or hopeless?" and "Over the past 2 weeks, have you felt little interest or pleasure in doing things?"[5] If the patient seems depressed, also ask about thoughts of suicide: "Have you ever thought about hurting yourself or ending your life?" As with chest pain, you must evaluate severity—both depression and angina are potentially lethal.

For further approaches, turn to Chapter 19, Mental Status, pp. 595–612.

Many patients with schizophrenia or other psychotic disorders can function in the community and tell you about their diagnoses, symptoms, hospitalizations, and current medications. You should investigate their symptoms and assess any effects on mood or daily activities.

Family Violence. Because of the high prevalence of physical, sexual, and emotional abuse, many authorities recommend the routine screening of all female patients for domestic violence. However men can also be victims of violence. Other patients at increased risk are children and the elderly.[10,11] As with other sensitive topics, start this part of the interview with general "normalizing" questions: "Because abuse is common in many women's lives, I've begun to ask about it routinely." "Are there times in your relationships that you feel unsafe or afraid?" "Many women tell me that someone at home is hurting them in some way. Is this true for you?" "Within the last year, have you been hit, kicked, punched, or otherwise hurt by someone you know? If so, by whom?" As with other segments of the history, use a pattern that goes from general to specific, less difficult to more difficult.

Physical abuse—often not mentioned by either victim or perpetrator—should be considered in the following situations.

- If injuries are unexplained, seem inconsistent with the patient's story, are concealed by the patient, or cause embarrassment
- If the patient has delayed getting treatment for trauma
- If there is a past history of repeated injuries or "accidents"
- If the patient or person close to the patient has a history of alcohol or drug abuse
- If the partner tries to dominate the interview, will not leave the room, or seems unusually anxious or solicitous

When abuse is suspected, it is important to spend part of the encounter alone with the patient. Use the transition to the physical examination as a reason to ask the other person to leave the room. If the patient is also resistant, do not force the situation, potentially placing the victim in jeopardy. Be attuned to diagnoses that have a higher association with abuse, such as pregnancy.

Child abuse is unfortunately also common. Asking parents about their approach to discipline is a routine part of well-child care. You can also ask parents how they cope with a baby who will not stop crying or a child who misbehaves: "Most parents get upset when their baby cries (or their child has been naughty). How do you feel when your baby cries?" "What do you do when your baby won't stop crying?" "Do you have any fears that you might hurt your child?" Find out how other caregivers or companions handle these situations as well.

DOCUMENTING THE HEALTH HISTORY

Documentation of the patient's health history is frequently computerized today. The record must be accurate and thorough no matter the type of documentation system used. A sample free form documentation of the history can be seen in Chapter 2, pp.19–23.

See Chapter 23, Assessing Children: Infancy Through Adolescence, pp. 729–839.

BIBLIOGRAPHY

CITATIONS

1. Regier DA, Farmer ME, Rae DS, et al. Comorbidity of mental disorders with alcohol and other drug abuse. Results from the Epidemiologic Catchment Area (ECA) study. JAMA 264(19):2511–2518, 1990.
2. Saitz R. Unhealthy alcohol use. N Engl J Med 352(67): 596–607, 2005.
3. Carni J, Farre M. Drug addiction. N Engl J Med 349(10): 975–986, 2003.
4. Cyr MG, Wartman SA. The effectiveness of routine screening questions in the detection of alcoholism. JAMA 259(1): 51–54, 1988.
5. Screening and Behavioral Counseling Interventions in Primary Care to Reduce Alcohol Misuse, Topic Page. April 2004. U.S. Preventive Services Task Force. http://www.uspreventiveservicestaskforce.org/uspstf/uspsdrin.htm. Accessed June 6, 2011.
6. Ewing JA. Detecting alcoholism: the CAGE questionnaire. JAMA 252(14):1905–1907, 1984.
7. National Institute on Alcohol Abuse and Alcoholism. Helping patients who drink too much. A clinician's guide. Updated 2007. Available at: http://pubs.niaaa.nih.gov/publications/Practitioner/CliniciansGuide2005/clinicians_guide.htm. Accessed June 6, 2011.
8. National Institute on Alcohol Abuse and Alcoholism. Alcohol Alert No. 62. Alcohol–an important issue in women's health. July 2004. Available at: http://pubs.niaaa.nih.gov/publications/aa62/aa62.htm. Accessed June 6, 2011.

9. Cocco KM, Carey KB. Psychometric properties of the drug abuse screening test in psychiatric outpatients. Psychol Assessment 10(4):408–414, 1998.

10. U.S. Preventive Services Task Force. Screening for family and intimate partner violence: recommendation statement. Rockville MD, Agency for Healthcare Research and Quality, March 2004. Available at: http://www.uspreventiveservicestaskforce.org/uspstf/uspsfamv.htm. Accessed June 6, 2011.

11. Rhodes KV, Frankel RM, Levinthal N, et al. "You're not the victim of domestic violence, are you?" Provider-patient communication about domestic violence. Ann Intern Med 147(9):620–627, 2007.

ADDITIONAL REFERENCES

Health Promotion and Counseling

American Public Health Association. Public Health Links (for public health professionals). Available at: http://www.apha.org/about/Public+Health+Links. Accessed March 8, 2011.

Centers for Disease Control and Prevention. Vaccines and immunizations. Available at: http://www.cdc.gov/vaccines/. Accessed March 8, 2011.

National Guideline Clearinghouse. Agency for Healthcare Research and Quality (AHRQ). Available at: http://www.ahrq.gov/clinic/ Accessed March 8, 2011.

Cultural and Spiritual Assessment

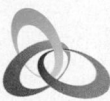 ## CULTURAL ASSESSMENT

Patients do not live in isolation; they are part of families, communities, cultures, races, and countries. In order to truly understand patients' needs, the nurse must assess them within the context of this background. Culture determines interpersonal communication style, as well as health beliefs, values, and practices. In addition, individuals from the same culture share a biologic inheritance and genetic patterns that impact health assessment, diagnoses, and medical treatment. For example, assessment of jaundice, yellowing of the skin due to excess bilirubin, requires inspection of the sclera and palate in dark-complexion patients. Certain diseases are more common in particular ethnic groups (e.g., sickle cell disease is more common in people of African origin). This chapter will discuss the importance of culture and spirituality in relation to health assessment.

There are many definitions of *culture*. Purnell and Paulanka define culture as "the totality of socially transmitted behavioral patterns, arts, beliefs, values, customs, lifeways, and all other products of human work and thought characteristic of a population of people that guide their worldview and decision making."[1] In other words, *culture* is the system of shared ideas, rules, and meanings that influences how we view the world, experience it emotionally, and behave in relation to other people.

It can be viewed as the "lens" through which we perceive and make sense of the world we inhabit. The meaning of culture is broader than the term *ethnicity*. Cultural influences are not limited to minority groups; they are relevant to everyone. Culture shapes not only the patient's beliefs, but also the nurse's.

Aspects of culture relevant to health assessment include[1,2]:

1. Communication and language

2. Kinship and social networks

3. Educational background and learning style

4. Nutrition

5. Child-bearing and child-rearing practices

6. High-risk behaviors

7. Health care beliefs and practices

8. Health care practitioners

9. Spirituality

Nursing has long recognized and practiced holistic care of the patient, and attention to culture is a part of caring for the whole patient. The nurse communicates with and cares for people of many different cultures. One does not have to be versed in every culture to provide culturally appropriate care, but one must be open and sensitive to other cultures. The term *cultural competence* recognizes the need for a set of skills necessary to care for people of different cultures. However, the concept has been difficult to define and operationalize. Too often cultural competence has been reduced to a static set of traits and beliefs for particular ethnic groups taken out of context. This can inadvertently objectify such patients as "other," implicitly reinforcing the perspectives of the dominant (often Western) culture.[3,4] In reality, "culture is ever-changing and always being revised within the dynamic context of its enactment."[5] Campinha-Bacote developed a model of cultural competence that defines culture as a process, not a state. The nurse sees herself or himself *becoming* culturally competent, not *being* culturally competent. Campinha-Bacote sees "cultural desire" as the motivation the nurse needs to "want to" and not "need to" become culturally aware, culturally knowledgeable, and culturally skillful and to seek cultural encounters. She utilizes a volcano to depict cultural competence. "When cultural desire erupts, it gives forth the desire to enter the process of becoming culturally competent by genuinely seeking cultural encounters, obtaining cultural knowledge, conducting culturally-sensitive assessments and being humble to the process of cultural awareness."[6,7]

For more information on Campinha-Bacote's model, see the Web site: http://www.transculturalcare.net/.

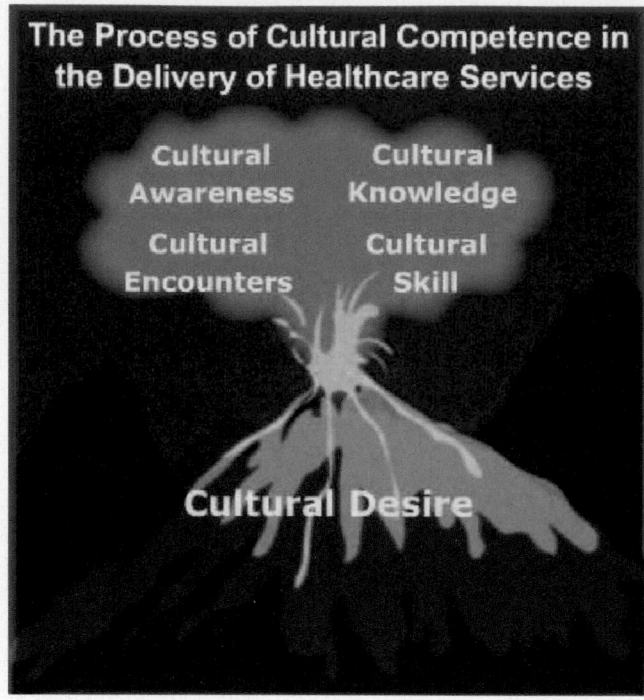

The Process of Cultural Competence in the Delivery of Healthcare Services

Cultural Awareness

Cultural Knowledge

Cultural Encounters

Cultural Skill

Cultural Desire

The concept of cultural humility is another approach for caring for patients from culturally diverse backgrounds. Cultural humility is defined as a "process that requires humility as individuals continually engage in self-reflection and self-critique as lifelong learners and reflective practitioners."[8] It is a process that includes "the difficult work of examining cultural beliefs and cultural systems of both patients and nurses to locate the points of cultural dissonance or synergy that contribute to patients' health outcomes."[9] It calls for health providers to reduce the power imbalance that exists in nurse–patient relationships and maintain mutually respectful and dynamic partnership with patients.

As you read the following vignettes, observe how cultural differences and unconscious bias can unwittingly lead to poor communication and disrupt the quality and outcomes of patient care.

CULTURAL HUMILITY: SCENARIO 1

A 28-year-old taxi driver from Ghana who has recently moved to the United States complained to a friend about U.S. medical care. He had gone to the clinic because of fever and fatigue. He described being weighed, having his temperature taken, and having a cloth wrapped tightly, to the point of pain, around his arm. The nurse, a 36-year-old woman from Washington, D.C., had asked the patient many questions, examined him, and wanted to take blood, which the patient had refused. The patient's final comment was ". . . and she didn't even give me chloroquine!"—his primary reason for seeking care. The man from Ghana was expecting few questions, no examination, and treatment for malaria, which is what fever usually means in Ghana.

In this example, cross-cultural miscommunication is understandable and thus less threatening to explore. Unconscious bias leading to miscommunication, however, occurs in many clinical interactions. Consider the next scenario, which is closer to home.

CULTURAL HUMILITY: SCENARIO 2

A 16-year-old high school student came to the local teen health center because of painful menstrual cramps that were interfering with concentrating at school. She was dressed in a tight top and short skirt and had multiple facial piercings. The 30-year-old nurse asked the following questions: "Are you passing all of your classes? What kind of job do you want after high school? What kind of birth control do you want?" The teenager felt pressured into accepting birth control pills, even though she had clearly stated she had never had intercourse and planned to postpone it until she got married. She was an honor student and planned to go to college, but the nurse did not elicit these goals. The nurse glossed over her cramps by saying, "Oh you can just take some ibuprofen. Cramps usually get better as you get older." The patient will not take the birth control pills that were prescribed, nor will she seek health care soon again. She experienced the encounter as an interrogation, therefore she failed to gain trust in her nurse. In addition, the nurse's questions made assumptions about her life and did not show respect for her health concerns. Even though the provider pursued important psychosocial domains, the patient received ineffective health care because of conflicting cultural values and nurse bias.

In both of these cases, the failure stems from mistaken assumptions or biases. In the first case, the nurse did not consider the patient's belief about his symptoms and expectations for care. In the second case, the nurse allowed stereotypes to dictate the agenda instead of listening to the patient and respecting her as an individual. Each of us has our own cultural background and biases. These do not simply fade away as we become nurses. We must continually learn about different cultures and how to therapeutically interact with each person as an individual with varying degrees of cultural influences.

Avoid allowing knowledge about specific cultural groups to turn into stereotyping rather than understanding. For example, you may have been told that Hispanic patients convey their pain more dramatically or that Asian patients are stoic. Recognize that these are stereotypes. You must evaluate each patient with pain as an individual, being aware of your reaction to the patient's communication style. Work on becoming aware of your own values and biases, developing communication skills that transcend cultural differences, and building therapeutic partnerships based on respect for each patient's life experience. The framework, described in the next section, will allow you to approach each patient as a unique individual.

THE THREE DIMENSIONS OF CULTURAL HUMILITY

- *Self-awareness.* Learn about your own biases . . . we all have them.
- *Respectful communication.* Work to eliminate assumptions about what is "normal." Learn directly from your patients—they are the experts on their culture and illness.
- *Collaborative partnerships.* Build your patient relationships on respect and mutually acceptable plans.

Self-Awareness.   Start by exploring your own cultural identity. How do you describe yourself in terms of ethnicity, class, region or country of origin, religion, and political affiliation? Don't forget the characteristics that we often take for granted—gender, life roles, sexual orientation, physical ability, and race—especially if we are in majority groups. What aspects of your family of origin do you identify with, and how are you different from your family of origin? How do these identities influence your beliefs and behaviors?

A more challenging task in learning about ourselves is to bring our own values and biases to a conscious level. *Values* are the standards we use to measure our own and others' beliefs and behaviors. These may appear to be absolutes. *Biases* are the attitudes or feelings that we attach to perceived differences. Being attuned to difference is normal; in fact, in the distant past, detecting differences may have preserved life. Intuitively knowing members of one's own group is a survival skill that we may have outgrown as a society but that is still actively at work.

Feeling guilty about our biases makes it hard to recognize and acknowledge them. Start with less threatening constructs, like the way an individual relates to time, a culturally determined phenomenon. Are you always on time—a positive value in the dominant Western culture? Or do you tend to run a little late? How do you feel about people whose habits are opposite to yours? Next time you attend a meeting or class, notice who is early, on time, or late. Is it predictable? Think about the role of physical appearance. Do you consider yourself thin, midsize, or heavy? How do you feel about your weight? What does prevailing U.S. culture teach us to value in physique? How do you feel about people who have different weights?

Respectful Communication.   Given the complexity of culture, no one can possibly know the health beliefs and practices of every culture and subculture. Let your patients be the experts on their own unique cultural perspectives. Even if patients have trouble describing their values or beliefs in the abstract, they should be able to respond to specific questions. Find out about the patient's cultural background. Use some of the same questions discussed earlier in the section Create a Shared Understanding of the Problem in Chapter 3 (see pp. 44–45). Maintain an open, respectful, and inquiring attitude. "What did you hope to get from this visit?" If you have established rapport and trust, patients will be willing to teach you. Be aware of questions that contain assumptions. And always be ready to acknowledge your areas of ignorance or bias. "I know very little about Ghana. What would have happened at a clinic there if you had these concerns?" Or, with the second patient and with much more difficulty, "I mistakenly made assumptions about you that are not right. I apologize. Would you be willing to tell me more about yourself and your future goals?"

Learning about specific cultures is valuable because it broadens what you, as a nurse, identify as areas you need to explore. Do some reading about the life experiences of individuals in ethnic or racial groups that live in your area. There may be reasons for loss of trust in nurses and health care delivery.[10] Go to movies that are filmed in different countries or explicitly present the perspective of different cultures. Learn about the concerns of different consumer groups with visible health agendas. Get to know healers of different disciplines and learn about their practices. Most importantly, be open to learning from your patients. Do not assume that what you have learned about a cultural group applies to the individual before you.

Collaborative Partnerships. Through continual work on self-awareness and seeing through the "lens" of others, the nurse lays the foundation for the collaborative relationship that best supports the patient's health. Communication based on trust, respect, and a willingness to reexamine assumptions allows patients to express concerns that may run counter to the dominant culture. These concerns may be associated with strong feelings such as anger or shame. You, the nurse, must be willing to listen to and validate these feelings, and not let your own feelings prevent you from exploring painful areas. You must also be willing to reexamine your beliefs about what is the "right approach" to clinical care in a given situation. Make every effort to be flexible and creative in your plans and respectful of patients' knowledge about their own best interests. By consciously distinguishing what is truly important to the patient's health from what is just the standard advice, you and your patients can construct the unique approach to their health care that is in concert with their beliefs and effective clinical care. Remember that if the patient stops listening, fails to follow your advice, or does not return, your health care has not been successful.

Transcultural Perspectives on the Health History

Culture impacts history taking in multiple ways. Knowledge of the cultural or minority groups in your practice region will help you better understand and interpret the patient's needs. There are some general precepts that should be noted. A patient's nonverbal communication may confuse or upset a novice nurse when it is different from the nurse's culture. Knowledge of categories of dissonance will help the novice recognize potential problems. Time in social conversation, use of silence, distance between the interviewer and client, eye contact, modesty, use of touch, and gestures vary by culture. It can be disconcerting working with a person whose culture reverses nodding the head for "yes" and shaking the head for "no," as seen in Bulgaria. Experiencing discomfort or frustration during the history may be a clue that there is cultural dissonance. It is best to stop and clarify the situation with the patient.

Cultural and racial variations are evident during the physical examination, and some of these will be noted in the text during the system examinations.

Introduction
It is generally better to begin the interview using formal titles. Ask the patient how he or she would like to be addressed. Note the specific language the patient speaks if it is not English. Some languages have different versions; for example, Chinese may be Mandarin, Cantonese, or another dialect.

Source
Note whether an interpreter was used for the history and indicate his or her relationship to the patient and a contact phone number. See Chapter 3, pp. 55–56 for more information on working with an interpreter.

Reason for Seeking Care
Patients may interpret their symptoms per their cultural view, as the man from Ghana in the example on page 80. There are also *cultural-bound syndromes*, which are "illnesses" defined by a particular culture but that have no corresponding illness in Western medicine. For example, symptoms may be attributed to actions by another individual. This may be called "evil eye," or "mal ojo" in Spanish. To the patient or parent of a child, these are very real events and must be taken seriously. Referral to a healer of the patient's culture may be the best option at times.

Self-Treatment
Be sure to ask what treatment the patient has used already and whether it helped. Traditional or alternative medicine remedies should be clarified.

Medications
When asking about medications, include herbal remedies and medicines from alternative health care providers. For example, Ayurvedic medicine is a system of traditional medicine native to India and practiced in other parts of the world as a form of alternative medicine.

Family and Social History
Family is important in all cultures, but definitions of family and who is included in the family may vary among cultures. In the history, note the family structure and who the decision makers are for the family, especially for health care issues.

Review of Systems
Ask about health promotion activities for each system as these may vary. One may also ask about symptoms of diseases commonly seen in the patient's culture or genetic background.

(Adapted from Andrews MA, Boyle JS. *Transcultural Concepts in Nursing Care,* 5th ed. Philadelphia: Lippincott Williams & Wilkins, 2008.)

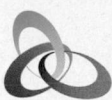

SPIRITUAL ASSESSMENT

Many definitions of spirituality have been proposed. The difficulty in defining spirituality may lie in the lack of conceptual clarity of the term.[11,12] Spirituality is a dimension of culture, and it is culture specific in how it is viewed. Nurses and researchers of Western culture have tried to separate spirituality from religion, but this may do a disservice to non-Western cultures, where spirituality rises from religious beliefs or exposure to a religious culture. An estimated 77% of the world is religious,[13] and for them religion is the basis of spirituality. Spirituality is a vital human experience shared by all humans; even atheists and nonpractitioners have a spiritual dimension. Purnell and Paulanka broadly define spirituality as "all behaviors that give meaning to life and provide strength to the individual."[1] Buck defines spirituality as "that most human of experiences that seeks to transcend self and find meaning and purpose through connection with others, nature and/or a Supreme Being, which may or may not involve religious structures or traditions."[11] Religion may be described as a system of beliefs or a practice of worship.

Spiritual distress may be a response to illness or health issues, and the North American Nursing Diagnosis Association (NANDA) recognizes Spiritual Distress as a nursing diagnosis. Therefore, nurses must be able to recognize that a patient has spiritual care needs. The generalist nurse is not prepared to provide intense spiritual counseling,[13] just as he or she does not provide intense nutrition counseling or physical therapy. However, the nurse may provide spiritual care by being present during unpleasant experiences; listening to the patient share fears, thoughts, or distress; providing opportunities for the patient to practice religious rituals; or referring the patient to a priest, minister, imam, or religious leader of the patient's choice.

The nurse approaches spiritual assessment in two tiers. Patients will not discuss deep concerns until a trusting relationship has been built with the nurse. During the first meeting, the nurse obtains a brief assessment of general information, such as the patient's religion and whether the patient would like a minister, priest, rabbi, or other religious person to be informed of the hospitalization. Does the patient have any rituals or prayers to be continued in the hospital? Nursing care schedules can be arranged to allow time for prayer during the day. Explaining to the patient that research has shown a connection between physical health and spiritual comfort will help the patient understand why questions about spirituality are being asked. The patient's diagnosis may cause fears or concerns. The nurse can ask, "Do you have any concerns or fears because of your diagnosis?" The patient may not be ready to discuss the feelings aroused by the illness. By providing an opening for discussion, the nurse communicates willingness to listen when the patient wishes to discuss spiritual concerns. Listening is an important part of being *present* with a patient. Nursing *presence* "is a holistic and reciprocal exchange between the nurse and patient that involves a sincere connection and sharing of human experience through active listening, attentiveness, intimacy and therapeutic touch, spiritual exploration, empathy, caring and compassion, and recognition of the patient's psychological, psychosocial and physiological needs."[14] Nursing presence is often what patients value most from the nurse.

Observe the patient's nonverbal cues that may indicate the patient is distressed, such as little or no affect, pitch of voice, posture, facial expression, crying, or inappropriate anger. Sitting with the patient and reflecting what the nurse sees may encourage the patient to express concerns. "I noticed that after the doctor discussed your diagnosis you have been very quiet and appear sad. Do you have any concerns?" The key nursing action here is to *listen,* not talk. Allow the patient to talk. Use the techniques discussed in Chapter 3 to encourage the patient to express feelings and concerns.

The patient may make statements that reflect spiritual distress such as "Why did I get cancer?" "I'm a burden to my family." and "I just don't know what to do." These statements should be addressed. Again, let the patient do the talking. The nurse should not offer solutions; rather, the nurse should use the interviewing techniques to help the patient identify the problem and resources utilized in the past to cope with problems: "What helps you cope?" "What is your source of strength? Source of hope?" "Who are your support persons?" If more help is needed, the nurse can refer the patient to a specialist.

Stoll's guidelines for spiritual assessment provide an outline for the novice to begin assessing a patient's spiritual needs.

STOLL'S GUIDELINES FOR SPIRITUAL ASSESSMENT

Concept of God or Deity
1. Is religion or God significant to you? If yes, can you describe how?
2. Is prayer helpful to you? What happens when you pray?
3. Does a God or deity function in your personal life? If yes, can you describe how?
4. How would you describe your God or what you worship?

Sources of Hope and Strength
1. Who is the most important person to you?
2. To whom do you turn when you need help? Are they available?
3. In what ways do they help?
4. What is your source of strength and hope?
5. What helps the most when you are afraid or need special help?

Religious Practices
1. Do you feel your faith (or religion) is helpful to you? If yes, would you tell me how?
2. Are there any religious practices that are important to you?

(continued)

STOLL'S GUIDELINES FOR SPIRITUAL ASSESSMENT (continued)

3. Has being sick (or what has happened to you) made any difference in your practice of praying or religious practices?

4. What religious books or symbols are helpful to you?

Relation Between Spiritual Beliefs and Health

1. What has bothered you most about being sick (or what is happening to you)?

2. What do you think is going to happen to you?

3. Has being sick (or what has happened to you) made any difference in your feelings about God or the practice of your faith?

4. Is there anything that is especially frightening or meaningful to you now?

(From Stoll RI. Guidelines for spiritual assessment. Am J Nurs 79(9):1574–1577, 1979.)

# DEATH AND THE DYING PATIENT

Interviewing and caring for the dying patient is challenging for a student or new nurse. Many students avoid talking about death because of their own discomfort and anxiety. It is important to work through your feelings with the help of reading and discussion. Basic concepts of care are appropriate for beginning students because you will come into contact with patients of all ages near the end of their lives.

Kubler-Ross described five stages in a person's response to loss or the anticipatory grief of impending death: denial and isolation, anger, bargaining, depression or sadness, and acceptance.[15] Later researchers discovered that these stages may occur sequentially or overlap in any order or combination. At each stage, follow the same approach. Be sensitive to the patient's feelings about dying; watch for cues that the patient is open to talking about them. Make openings for the patient to ask questions: "I wonder if you have any concerns about your illness, your treatment, and what it will be like when you go home?" Explore these concerns and provide the information the patient requests. Setting up a meeting with the physician, therapist, and other team members will help everyone understand the patient's issues and develop a cohesive plan of care. Avoid false reassurance. Accepting the patient's feelings, answering questions truthfully, and being present during difficult times will reassure the patient.

Dying patients rarely want to talk about their illnesses at each encounter, nor do they wish to confide in everyone they meet. Give them opportunities to talk, and listen, but if they choose to stay at a social level, respect their preference. Remember that illness—even a terminal one—is only a part of the total person. A smile, a touch, an inquiry about a family member, a comment on the day's events, or even some gentle humor affirms and sustains the unique individual you are caring for. Communicating effectively means getting to know the whole patient; that is part of the helping process.

Understanding the patient's wishes about treatment at the end of life is an important nursing responsibility. Failing to establish communication about end-of-life decisions is viewed as a flaw in nursing care. Even if discussions of death and dying are difficult for you, you must learn to ask specific questions. The condition of the patient and the health care setting often determine what needs to be discussed. For patients who are acutely ill and in the hospital, discussions about what the patient wants to have done in the event of a cardiac or respiratory arrest are usually mandatory. Asking about *Do Not Resuscitate (DNR) status* is difficult when you have no previous relationship with the patient or lack knowledge of the patient's values and life experience. Ask about the patient's perception of resuscitation because the media give many patients an unrealistic view of its effectiveness. "What do you know about cardiopulmonary resuscitation (CPR)?" Work with the physician to educate the patient and family about the likely success of CPR and its side effects (e.g., fractured ribs). Assure the patient that relieving pain and taking care of other spiritual and physical needs will be a priority.

Investigate hospice services in your area and be prepared to discuss how hospice can help the patient and family. Hospice care offers palliative care at the end of life. Hospice social workers and nurses help the patient and family make end-of-life decisions, complete tasks, and provide pain relief and nursing care.

BIBLIOGRAPHY

1. Purnell L, Paulanka B. Transcultural Health Care: A Culturally Competent Approach, 3rd ed. Philadelphia: F.A. Davis, 2008.
2. Andrews MA, Boyle JS. Transcultural Concepts in Nursing Care, 5th ed. Philadelphia: Lippincott Williams & Wilkins, 2008.
3. Kumas-Tan Z, Beagan B, Loppie C, et al. Measures of cultural competence: examining hidden assumptions. Acad Med 82(6):548–557, 2007.
4. Engebretson J, Mahoney J, Carlson E. Cultural competence in the era of evidence-based practice. J Prof Nurs 24(3):172–178, 2008.
5. Hunt LM. Beyond cultural competence. Park Ridge Bulletin 24:3–4, 2001. Available at: http://www.parkridgecenter.org/Page1882.html. Accessed June 7, 2011.
6. Campinha-Bacote J. The process of cultural competence in the delivery of healthcare services: a model of care. J Transcult Nurs 13(3):181–184, 2002.
7. Campinha-Bacote J. The process of cultural competence in the delivery of healthcare services, 2010. Available at: http://www.transculturalcare.net/. Accessed June 17, 2010.
8. Tervalon M, Murray-Garcia J. Cultural humility versus cultural competence: a critical distinction in defining physician training outcomes in multicultural education. J Health Care Poor Underserved 9(2):117–125, 1998.
9. Tervalon M. Components of culture in health for medical students' education. Acad Med 78(6):570–576, 2003.
10. Jacobs EA, Rolle I, Ferrans CE, et al. Understanding African Americans' views of the trustworthiness of physicians. J Gen Intern Med 21(6):642–647, 2006.
11. Buck HG. Spirituality: concept analysis and model development. Holistic Nurs Pract 20(6):288–292, 2006.
12. Sessanna L, Finnell D, Jezewski MA. Spirituality in nursing and health related literature: a concept analysis. J Holistic Nurs 25(4):252–262, 2007.
13. Fowler M. Come; give me a taste of Shalom. In: Pinch W, Haddad A, eds. Nursing and Health Care Ethics: A Legacy and a Vision. Silver Spring, MD: American Nurses Association, 2008.
14. Hessel JA. Presence in nursing practice: a concept analysis. Holistic Nurs Pract 23(5):276–281, 2009.
15. Kübler-Ross E. On Death and Dying. New York: Macmillan, 1997.

ADDITIONAL REFERENCES

Barnum BS. Spirituality in Nursing: The Challenges of Complexity, 3 ed. New York: Springer, 2011.

Kirkham S, Pesut B, Meyerhoff H, et al. Spiritual caregiving at the juncture of religion, culture and state. Can J Nurs Res 36(4): 149–169, 2004.

BIBLIOGRAPHY

Leininger M, McFarland M. Culture Care Diversity and Universality: A Worldwide Nursing Theory, 2nd ed. Boston: Jones and Bartlett Publishers, 2006.

McEvoy M. Culture and spirituality as an integrated concept in pediatric care. MCN Am J Matern/Child Nurs 25(1):39–43, 2003.

Miller S. Cultural humility is the first step to becoming global care providers. J Obstet Gynecol Neonatal Nurs 38(1):92–93, 2009.

Miner-Williams D. Putting a puzzle together: making spirituality meaningful for nursing using an evolving theoretical framework. J Clin Nurs 15:811–821, 2006.

Narayan MC. Culture's effects on pain assessment and management. Am J Nurs 110(4):38–47, 2010.

O'Brien ME. Spirituality in Nursing: Standing on Holy Ground, 3rd ed. Sudbury, MA: Jones and Bartlett, 2008.

Spector R. Cultural Diversity in Health and Illness, 7th ed. Pearson Prentice Hall, 2009.

Tarzian AJ. (2008) Exploring diversity and disparities: an evolving journey. In: Pinch W, Haddad A, eds. Nursing and Health Care Ethics: A Legacy and a Vision. Silver Spring, MD: American Nurses Association, 2008.

Taylor E. Spiritual Care: Nursing Theory, Research and Practice. Upper Saddle River, NJ: Pearson Prentice Hall, 2002.

Physical Examination

The student will:

1. Identify the components of the physical examination.
2. Recognize the best approach for physical examination based on individual needs of the patient.
3. Utilize lighting and the environment to insure an accurate physical examination.
4. Describe the equipment for performing a physical examination.
5. Demonstrate a head to toe physical examination.

Once you understand the patient's concerns and have elicited a careful history, you are ready to begin the physical examination. At first you may feel unsure of how the patient will relate to you. With practice, your skills in physical examination will grow, and you will gain confidence. Through study and repetition, the examination will flow more smoothly, and the attention will soon shift from technique and how to handle instruments to what you hear, see, and feel. Touching the patient's body will seem more natural, and you will learn to minimize any discomfort to the patient. Before long, you will gain proficiency, and what once took between 1 and 2 hours will take considerably less time.

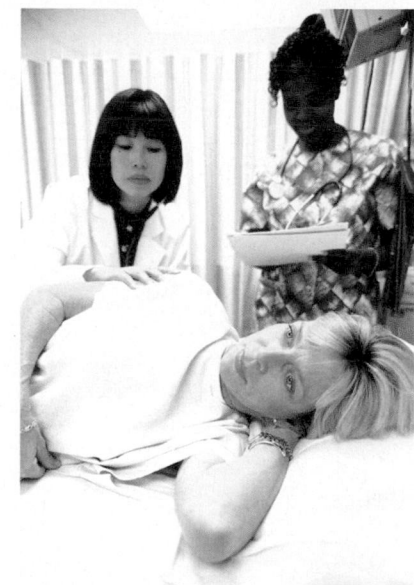

The physical examination is a process to obtain objective data from the patient. The subjective data in the health history is obtained prior to the examination and will assist the nurse to navigate through a complex examination. Each body system connects to another. A finding in one system may not be an isolated finding. For example, the patient who presents with a chief complaint of blurred vision may be having vision changes because of age, injury, a retina or macular affliction, or changes due to hyperglycemia. The purpose of the physical examination is to determine changes in a patient's health status and how to respond to a problem as well as promote healthy lifestyles and wellbeing.

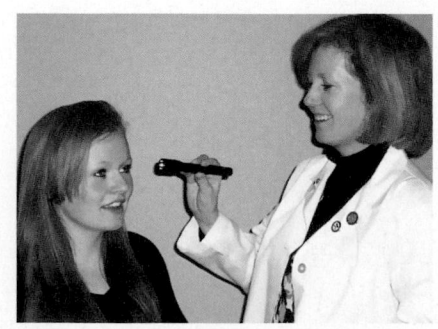

A decision to perform a complete or a focused physical assessment is made on an individual basis. A complete assessment includes: a general survey, assessment of vital signs, body measurements, and a head to toe system examination. This is performed for each patient as a baseline. A focused assessment concentrates on specific systems related to the problem or issue presented. This could be an emergent situation, follow up to a patient previously assessed, or conducted when time with the patient is brief.

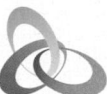

THE COMPREHENSIVE ADULT PHYSICAL EXAMINATION

Beginning the Examination: Setting the Stage

As new practitioners, the impetus is to dive in and begin the physical examination. However, as in anything worthwhile, preparation is paramount.

See Chapter 23, Assessing Children: Infancy Through Adolescence, for the comprehensive examination of infants, children, and adolescents.

Before beginning the physical examination, think through the approach to the patient, professional demeanor, and how to make the patient feel comfortable and relaxed. Review the measures that promote the patient's physical comfort and make any adjustments needed in the lighting and surrounding environment. Remember to gather the equipment and review the patient chart if available prior to entering the room.

PREPARING FOR THE PHYSICAL EXAMINATION

- Reflect on your approach to the patient.
- Adjust the lighting and the environment.
- Make the patient comfortable.
- Check your equipment.
- Choose the sequence of examination.

Reflect on Your Approach to the Patient. When first examining patients, feelings of insecurity are inevitable, but these will soon diminish with experience. Be straightforward. Identify yourself as a nursing student. Try to appear calm, organized, and competent, even when you feel differently. Forgetting part of the examination is common, especially at first! Simply examine that area out of sequence, but smoothly. It is not unusual to go back to the bedside and ask to check one or two items that might have been overlooked.

Beginners will need to spend more time than experienced nurses on selected portions of the examination, such as the ophthalmoscopic examination or cardiac auscultation. To avoid alarming the patient, warn the patient ahead of time by saying, for example, "I would like to spend extra time listening to your heart and the heart sounds, but this doesn't mean I hear anything wrong."

Most patients view the physical examination with some anxiety. They feel vulnerable, physically exposed, apprehensive about possible pain, and uneasy about what the nurse may find. At the same time, they appreciate your concern about their problems and respond to your attentiveness. With these considerations in mind, the skillful nurse is thorough without wasting time, systematic without being rigid, gentle yet not afraid to cause discomfort should this be required. The skillful nurse examines each region of the body, and at the same time senses the whole patient, notes the wince or worried glance, and shares information that calms, explains, and reassures.

Over time, you will begin sharing your findings with the patient. As a beginner, *avoid interpreting your findings.* You are not the patient's primary caregiver, and your views may be conflicting or wrong. As you grow in experience and responsibility, sharing findings will become more appropriate. If the patient has specific concerns, discuss them with your instructors before providing reassurance. At times, you may discover abnormalities such as an ominous mass or a deep oozing ulcer. Always avoid showing distaste, alarm, or other negative reactions. Keeping your verbal and nonverbal communication in check is paramount. If you find anything that is unusual or disturbing, always talk with your clinical instructor.

Adjust the Lighting and the Environment.   Surprisingly, several environmental factors affect the caliber and reliability of your physical findings. To achieve superior techniques of examination, it is important to "set the stage" so that both you and the patient are comfortable. Awkward positions may impair the quality of the examination. Take the time to adjust the bed to a convenient height (but be sure to lower it when finished!), and ask the patient to move toward you if this makes it easier to examine a region of the body more carefully.

Good lighting and a quiet environment make important contributions to what you see and hear but may be hard to arrange. Do the best you can. If a television interferes with listening to heart sounds, politely ask the nearby patient to lower the volume. Most people cooperate readily. Be courteous and remember to thank the patient as you leave.

Tangential lighting is optimal for inspecting structures such as the jugular venous pulse, the thyroid gland, and the apical impulse of the heart. It casts light across body surfaces that shows contours, elevations, and depressions, whether moving or stationary, into sharper relief.

When light is perpendicular to the surface or diffuse, shadows are reduced and subtle undulations across the surface are lost. Experiment with focused,

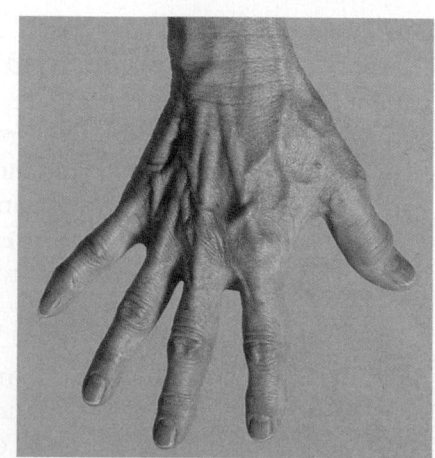

TANGENTIAL LIGHTING

tangential lighting across the tendons on the back of your hand; try to see the pulsations of the radial artery at your wrist.

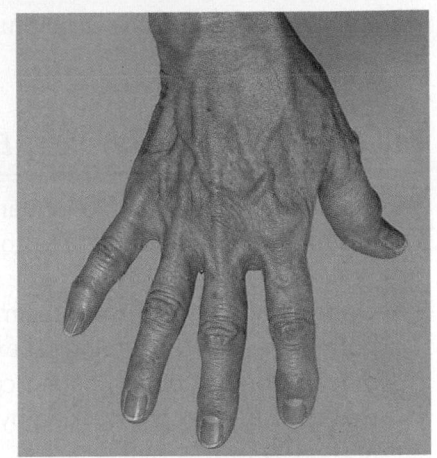

PERPENDICULAR LIGHTING

Make the Patient Comfortable.   Access to the patient's body is a unique and time-honored privilege in the role of the nurse. Showing concern for privacy and patient modesty must be ingrained in your professional behavior. These attributes help the patient feel respected and at ease. Be sure to close nearby doors and draw the curtains in the hospital or examining room before the examination begins. Also, remember to wash your hands.

You will acquire the art of *draping the patient* with the gown or draw sheet as you learn each segment of the examination in the chapters ahead. *Your goal is to visualize one area of the body at a time.* This preserves the patient's modesty but also helps focus on the area being examined. With the patient sitting, for example, untie the gown in back to better listen to the lungs. For the breast examination, uncover the right breast but keep the left chest draped. Redrape the right chest, then uncover the left chest and proceed to examine the left breast and heart. For the abdominal examination, only the abdomen should be exposed. Adjust the gown to cover the chest and place the sheet or drape at the inguinal area.

To help the patient prepare for potentially awkward segments, it is considerate to briefly describe the plan before starting. As you proceed with the examination, keep the patient informed, especially when you anticipate embarrassment or discomfort, as when checking for the femoral pulse. Also try to gauge how much the patient wants to know. Is the patient curious about the lung findings or the method for assessing the liver or spleen? Then let the patient know what you find. Also, after checking vital signs, tell the patient the results. The patient should be aware of the baseline findings.

Make sure the instructions to the patient at each step in the examination are courteous and clear. For example, "I would like to examine your lungs now, so please take a deep breath in through your nose and breathe out through your mouth."

As in the interview, be sensitive to the patient's feelings and physical comfort. Watching the patient's facial expressions and even asking "Is it okay?" as you move through the examination often reveals unexpressed worries or sources of pain. To ease patient discomfort, adjust the slant and extend the foot of the exam table. Rearranging the pillows or adding blankets for warmth shows attentiveness to the patient's well-being.

When the examination is completed, tell the patient your general impressions and what to expect next. For hospitalized patients, make sure the patient is comfortable and rearrange the immediate environment as needed. Be sure to lower the bed to avoid risk for falls and raise the bedrails if needed. As you leave, wash your hands, clean your equipment, and dispose of any waste materials.

Check Your Equipment. Equipment necessary for the physical examination includes the following:

EQUIPMENT FOR THE PHYSICAL EXAMINATION

- Stadiometer. Measures height and is attached to the wall for consistency in measurement. Ensure that this is mounted correctly and at the correct height when installed.
- Scale
- Ophthalmoscope. The ophthalmoscope requires some practice to become proficient. Utilizing the scope in both the eye and neurological exams will ease the learning process if used as often as possible. There are different brands of ophthalmoscopes however all have similar features. Before the exam, check to insure that the batteries are working by turning on the light. Re-charge if necessary.

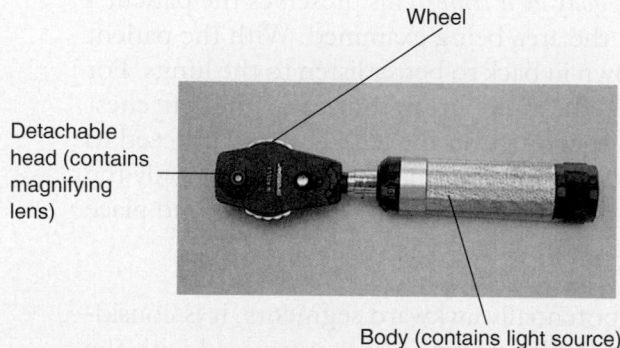

Wheel

Detachable head (contains magnifying lens)

Body (contains light source)

- Otoscope. The otoscope enables visibility of the eardrum and the external ear canal. Before the exam, check to insure that the batteries are working and do not need to be charged. Check this by turning on the light. Select the largest disposable speculum that will fit comfortably in the patient's ear.

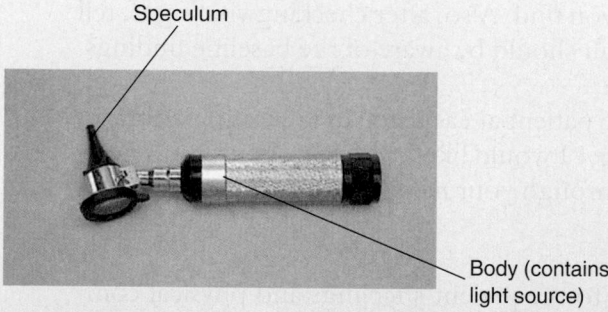

Speculum

Body (contains light source)

- Snellen chart or "E" card
- Rosenbaum or Jaegar Chart or Near vision card
- Flashlight or penlight
- Tongue depressors
- Ruler and flexible tape measure, preferably marked in centimeters
- Thermometer
- Examination gloves
- 2 × 2 gauze pads (for use during tongue examination)
- Watch with a second hand
- Sphygmomanometer. See Chapter 7.

(continued)

EQUIPMENT FOR THE PHYSICAL EXAMINATION (continued)

- Stethoscope with the following characteristics:
  - Ear tips that fit snugly and painlessly. To get this fit, choose ear tips of the proper size, align the ear pieces with the angle of the ear canals, and adjust the spring of the connecting metal band to a comfortable tightness.
  - Thick-walled tubing as short as feasible to maximize the transmission of sound: approximately 30 cm (12 inches), if possible, and no longer than 38 cm (15 inches).
  - A bell and a diaphragm.
    The disk at the end of the stethoscope is the bell and diaphragm.
    The bell is the smaller, cupped side of the stethoscope and transmits lower pitched sounds and the diaphragm is the larger, flatter side of the stethoscope and this transmits higher pitched sounds. By rotating the disk at the end of the stethoscope you can change from the bell to the diaphragm as needed. By tapping lightly on the disk you can determine which side is open for sound transmission. If you own a stethoscope that has the bell and diaphragm on the same side then you will press firmly to use the diaphragm and barely press at all to use the bell.

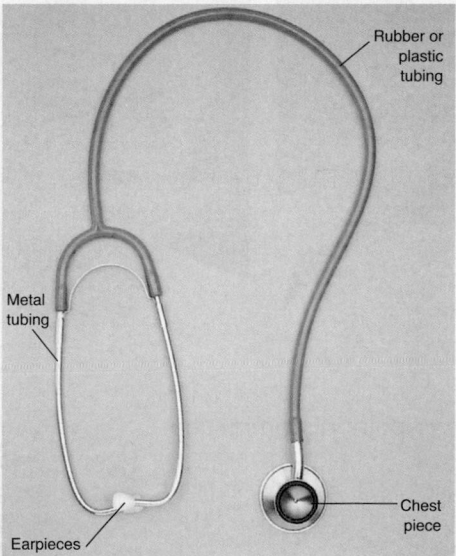

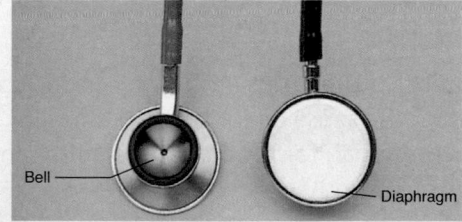

- Reflex hammer. The strength of a reflex is used to gauge central and peripheral nervous system disorders. Tapping with the head of the "hammer" will detect the reflexes. The handle of the hammer is used to detect a plantar reflex.

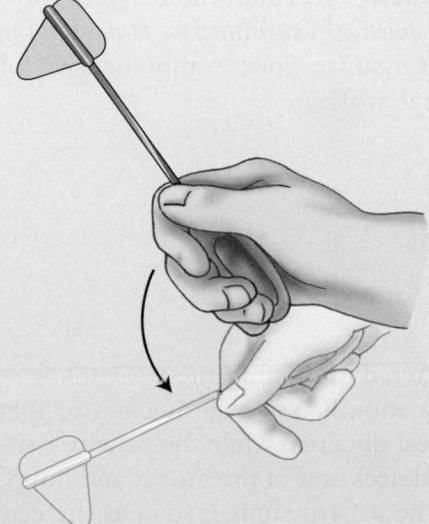

(continued)

EQUIPMENT FOR THE PHYSICAL EXAMINATION (continued)

- Tuning forks, ideally one of 128 Hz (vibration) and one of 512 Hz (sound). The tuning fork **is** a two-pronged with tines that form a U- shape. There is a constant pitch depending on which hertzog fork is vibrated. To begin the vibration the fork is hit against a surface and sound is produced. The 128 or 512 hertzog(Hz) are the frequencies of choice in physical exam. The frequency is found on the front of the tuning fork.

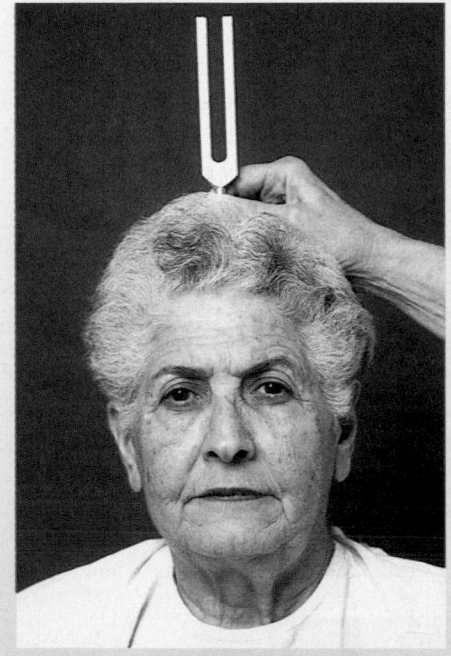
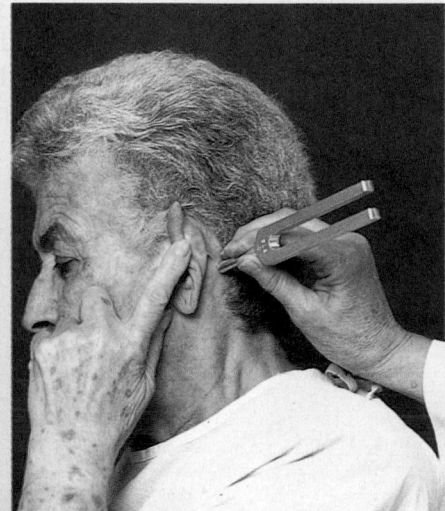
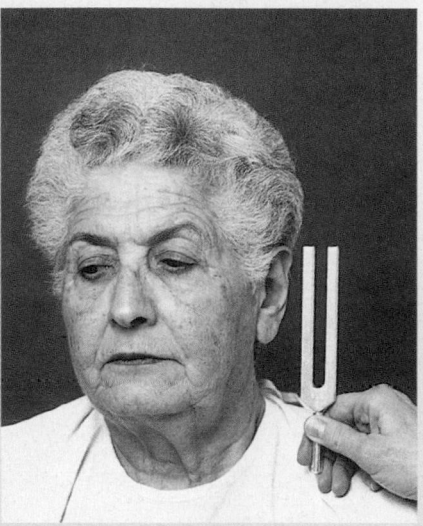

- Q-tips, paper clips, or other disposable objects for testing two-point discrimination
- Cotton for testing the sense of light touch
- Two test tubes (optional) for testing temperature sensation
- Paper and pen, or computer

Choose the Sequence of the Examination.   It is important to recognize that *the key to a thorough and accurate physical examination is developing a systematic sequence of examination.* Organize your comprehensive or focused examination around three general goals:

- Maximize the patient's comfort.

- Avoid unnecessary changes in position.

- Enhance clinical efficiency.

In general, move from "head to toe." Avoid examining the patient's feet, for example, before checking the face or mouth. You will quickly see that some segments of the examination are best obtained while the patient is sitting, such as examination of the head and neck and of the thorax and lungs, whereas others are best obtained with the patient supine, such as the cardiovascular and abdominal examinations.

You may need to examine a patient in bed, especially in the hospital. This often dictates changes in the sequence of your examination. You can examine the head, neck, and anterior chest with the patient lying supine. Then roll the patient onto each side to listen to the lungs, examine the back, and inspect the skin. Roll the patient back and finish the rest of the examination with the patient again supine.

With practice, you will develop your own sequence of examination, keeping the need for thoroughness and patient comfort in mind. At first, you may need notes to remind you what to examine in each region of the body, but with a few months of practice, you will acquire a routine of your own. This sequence will become habit, helping you to be thorough.

For an overview of the physical examination sequence, study the following outline

THE PHYSICAL EXAMINATION: SUMMARY OF SUGGESTED SEQUENCE

Patient Seated-Anterior

1. General Survey
2. VS (vital signs)
3. Skin: exam is performed throughout as you exam each part of the body
4. Head (hair, scalp, skull, nodes)
5. Face (contours, symmetry, edema, movements, sinuses, muscle strength, facial sensation, temporomandibular joint)
6. Eyes-acuity (if hand held eye chart available, otherwise do in the beginning before patient is seated or hold this part until the patient is standing for other parts of assessment), fields, position, eyebrows, lids, conjunctiva, sclera, cornea, lens, iris pupil responses, convergence, etc.
7. Ears (auricle, otoscope, auditory acuity and Weber/Rinne)
8. Nose
9. Mouth/Pharynx (tongue movement, swallow, gag-if indicated, dentition)
10. Neck (lymph nodes, trachea, thyroid exam)
11. Head and Neck range of motion
12. Spinal accessory muscles (head side to side and shrug-against resistance
13. Shoulders (ROM, inspection, palpation, muscle strength)
14. Arms (elbows, hands, wrists) (pulses, ROM, lymph nodes)
15. Chest and Thorax (ANTERIOR)- inspect, palpate percuss, diaphragmatic excursion auscultate lungs) (or may choose to do when patient is lying down)
16. Breasts (arms on hips and raised over head)
17. Axillary nodes
18. Heart sound (leaning forward) -for aortic stenosis/murmur

(continued)

THE PHYSICAL EXAMINATION: SUMMARY OF SUGGESTED SEQUENCE (continued)

Patient Seated-Posterior

19. Chest and Thorax (POSTERIOR)-inspect, palpate percuss, diaphragmatic excursion auscultate lungs)
20. Cervical Spine (inspection, palpation)
21. Costovertebral Angle (CVA tenderness)

Patient Lying Down

22. Breast exam
23. Neck (pulse, JVD, auscultate for carotid bruit)
24. Chest and thorax (anterior-inspect, palpate, percuss, auscultate breath sounds) (or may choose to do when patient is sitting up)
25. Cardiovascular-palpate for apical impulse, percuss for location/size of heart, auscultate aortic pulmonic, mitral, tricuspid areas with patient lying flat then listen over apex with patient tilted to left (listening for mitral murmur, S3, S4)
26. Abdomen (inspect, auscultate (note auscultation precedes other portions of exam . . . therefore not disturbing bowel sounds . . . then percuss, palpate, locate organs, aortic pulsation, reflex)
27. Groin, hips and knees (pulses, lymph nodes, ROM, strength)
28. Shins and ankles (soft, sharp, dull, pulses, ROM) At this time sensory assessments of trunk, arms, face, etc. can easily be incorporated

Patient Seated

29. Reflexes (knee, ankle, feet, wrists, arms)

Patient Standing

30. Spine (ROM, palpate vertebrae, alignment)
31. Romberg, gait, balance etc., other appropriate nervous system screening. Could do visual acuity here if not done previously since patient standing

Techniques of Examination

Now focus on the more detailed description of the physical examination in the section below. Review the cardinal techniques of examination, sequencing and positioning for the examination, and the need for universal precautions.

Cardinal Techniques of Examination. Note that the physical examination relies on four classic techniques: inspection, palpation, percussion, and auscultation. Later chapters show that several maneuvers are also used to amplify physical findings, such as having the patient lean forward to better detect the murmur of aortic regurgitation or bend over to assess for scoliosis.

These four techniques—inspection, palpation, percussion, and, finally, auscultation—will *always* be utilized in order in all systems with the exception of the abdomen. During the abdominal examination, the pattern will be inspection, auscultation, percussion, and palpation. Auscultation follows inspection so as not to increase bowel motility with palpation.

● Cardinal Techniques of Examination

● Inspection

Close observation of the details of the patient's appearance, behavior, and movement such as facial expression, mood, body build and conditioning, skin conditions such as petechiae or ecchymoses, eye movements, pharyngeal color, symmetry of thorax, height of jugular venous pulsations, abdominal contour, lower extremity edema, and gait.

● Palpation

Tactile pressure from the palmar fingers or fingerpads to assess areas of skin elevation, depression, warmth, or tenderness; lymph nodes; pulses; contours and sizes of organs and masses, and crepitus in the joints. Metacarpal/phalangeal joint or ulnar surface of the hand is used to detect vibration.

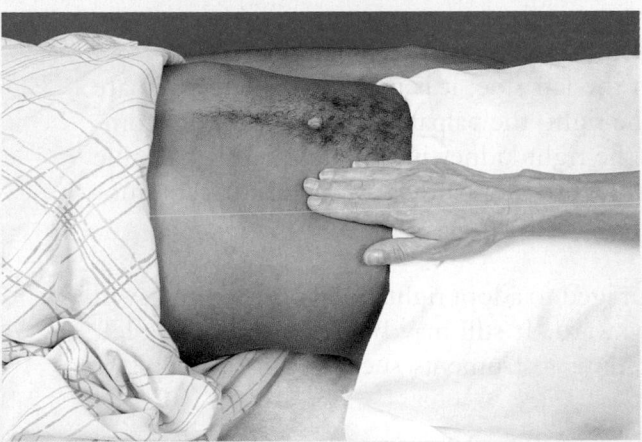

● Percussion

Use of the striking or *plexor finger*, usually the third, to deliver a rapid tap or blow against the distal *pleximeter finger*, usually the distal third finger of the left hand laid against the surface of the chest or abdomen, to evoke a sound wave such as resonance or dullness from the underlying tissue or organs. This sound wave also generates a tactile vibration against the pleximeter finger.

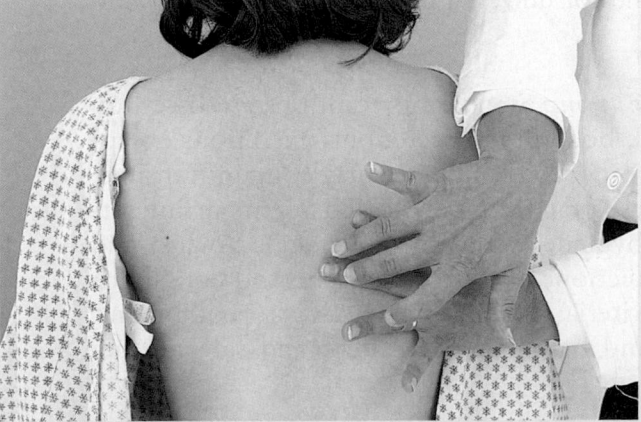

● Auscultation

Use of the diaphragm and bell of the stethoscope to detect the characteristics of heart, lung, and bowel sounds, including location, timing, duration, pitch, and intensity. For the heart this involves sounds from closing of the four valves and flow into the ventricles as well as murmurs. Auscultation also permits detection of bruits, ie, turbulence over arterial vessels.

Sequence and Positioning for the Examination. Nurses will vary in where they place different segments of the examination, especially the examinations of the musculoskeletal system and the nervous system. Some of these options are indicated in red in the right-hand column.

As you develop your own sequence of examination, *an important goal is to minimize how often you ask the patient to change position* from supine to sitting, or from standing to lying supine.

This book recommends examining the patient from the patient's **right side**, moving to the opposite side or foot of the bed or examining table as necessary. This is the standard position for the physical examination and has several advantages compared with the left side: it is more reliable to estimate jugular venous pressure from the right, the palpating hand rests more comfortably on the apical impulse, the right kidney is more frequently palpable than the left, and examining tables are frequently positioned to accommodate a right-handed approach.

Left-handed students are encouraged to adopt right-sided positioning, even though at first it may seem awkward. It still may be easier to use the left hand for percussing or for holding instruments such as the otoscope or reflex hammer.

Standard and Universal Precautions. The Centers for Disease Control and Prevention (CDC) have issued several guidelines to protect patients and examiners from the spread of infectious disease. All nurses examining patients are well advised to study and observe these precautions at the CDC Web sites. Advisories for standard and methicillin-resistant *Staphylococcus aureus* (*MRSA*) precautions and for universal precautions are briefly summarized.[10–12]

● *Standard and MRSA precautions:* Standard precautions are based on the principle that all blood, body fluids, secretions, excretions except sweat, nonintact skin, and mucous membranes may contain transmissible infectious agents. These practices apply to all patients in any setting. They include hand hygiene; when to use gloves, gowns, and mouth, nose, and eye protection; respiratory hygiene and cough etiquette; patient isolation criteria; precautions relating to equipment, toys, and solid surfaces, and handling of laundry; and safe needle-injection practices.

Be sure to wash your hands before and after examining the patient. This will show your concern for the patient's welfare and display your awareness of a critical component of patient safety. Antimicrobial fast-drying soaps are often within easy reach. Stethoscope chest pieces should be cleaned between patients. *Change your white coat frequently,* because cuffs can become damp and smudged; additional research is being done that questions whether long-sleeve lab coats should be worn into patients' rooms, and the question arises as to how often they should be laundered.

- *Universal precautions:* Universal precautions are a set of guidelines designed to prevent transmission of human immunodeficiency virus (HIV), hepatitis B virus (HBV), and other blood-borne pathogens when providing first aid or health care. The following fluids are considered potentially infectious: all blood and other body fluids containing visible blood, semen, and vaginal secretions; and cerebrospinal, synovial, pleural, peritoneal, pericardial, and amniotic fluids. Protective barriers include gloves, gowns, aprons, masks, and protective eyewear. All health care workers should *observe the important precautions for safe injections and prevention of injury from needlesticks, scalpels, and other sharp instruments and devices.* Report to your health service immediately if such injury occurs.

Overview—The Physical Examination

Read carefully this "head-to-toe" sequence, the techniques for examining each region of the body, and how to optimize patient comfort and minimize changes in the patient position.

General Survey. Observe the patient's general state of health, build, and sexual development. Note posture, motor activity, and gait; dress, grooming, and personal hygiene; and any odors of the body or breath. Watch the patient's facial expressions and note manner, affect, and reactions to people and things in the environment. Listen to the patient's manner of speaking and note the state of awareness or level of consciousness. Measure height and weight.

The survey continues throughout the history and examination.

Vital Signs. Measure the blood pressure. Count the pulse and respiratory rate. Measure the body temperature.

The **patient is sitting** on the edge of the bed or examining table. Stand in front of the patient, moving to either side as needed.

Skin. Observe the skin as you assess body parts. Assess skin moisture or dryness and temperature. Identify any lesions, noting their location, distribution, arrangement, type, and color. Inspect and palpate the hair and nails. Continue your assessment of the skin as you examine the other body regions.

Head, Eyes, Ears, Nose, Throat (HEENT). *Head:* Examine the hair, scalp, skull, face, and lymph nodes. *Eyes:* Check visual acuity and screen the visual fields. Note the position and alignment of the eyes. Observe the eyelids and inspect the sclera and conjunctiva of each eye. With oblique lighting, inspect each cornea, iris, and lens. Compare the pupils, and test their reactions to light. Assess the extraocular movements. With an ophthalmoscope, inspect the ocular fundi. *Ears:* Inspect the auricles, canals, and drums. Check auditory acuity (watch/whisper test), check lateralization (Weber test), and compare air and bone conduction (Rinne test). *Nose and sinuses:*

The room should be darkened for the ophthalmoscopic examination. This promotes pupillary dilation and visibility of the fundi.

Examine the external nose; using a light and a nasal speculum, inspect the nasal mucosa, septum, and turbinates. Palpate for tenderness of the frontal and maxillary sinuses. *Throat (mouth and pharynx):* Inspect the lips, oral mucosa, gums, teeth, tongue, palate, tonsils, uvula, and pharynx. *(You may wish to assess the cranial nerves during this portion of the examination.)*

Neck. Inspect and palpate the cervical lymph nodes. Note any masses or unusual pulsations in the neck. Feel for any deviation of the trachea. Inspect and palpate the thyroid gland.

Move behind the sitting patient to feel the thyroid gland and to examine the back, posterior thorax, and lungs.

Back. Inspect and palpate the spine and muscles of the back. Observe shoulder height for symmetry.

Posterior Thorax and Lungs. Inspect and palpate the spine and muscles of the *upper* back. Inspect, palpate, and percuss the chest. Identify the level of diaphragmatic dullness on each side. Check for respiratory expansion. Listen to the breath sounds; identify any adventitious (or added) sounds, and, if indicated, listen to the transmitted voice sounds (see p. 314). If you suspect a kidney infection, percuss posteriorly over the costovertebral angles (CVAs). Assess for CVA tenderness when the patient is standing or sitting.

A Note on the Musculoskeletal System: By this time, you have made some preliminary observations of the musculoskeletal system. Use these and subsequent observations to decide whether a full musculoskeletal examination is warranted. If indicated, *with the patient still sitting,* examine the hands, arms, shoulders, neck, and temporomandibular joints. Inspect and palpate the joints and check their range of motion. *(You may choose to examine upper extremity muscle bulk, tone, strength, and reflexes at this time, or you may wait until later.)*

Anterior Thorax and Lungs. Inspect, palpate, and percuss the chest. Assess respiratory expansion. Listen to the breath sounds, any adventitious sounds, and, if indicated, transmitted voice sounds.

Breasts, Axillae, and Epitrochlear Nodes. Inspect the breasts with arms relaxed, then elevated, and with hands pressed on the hips. Inspect the axillae and palpate the axillary nodes and epitrochlear nodes.

The patient is **still sitting**. Move to the front again.

With the Patient Supine

Cardiovascular System. Using tangential lighting, observe the jugular venous pulsations and measure the jugular venous pressure in relation to the sternal angle. Inspect and palpate the carotid pulsations. Listen for carotid bruits.

Ask the patient to lie down. The patient is supine. You should stand at the right side of the patient's bed. **Elevate the head of the bed to approximately 30°** for the cardiovascular examination, adjusting as necessary to see the jugular venous pulsations.

Inspect and palpate the precordium. Note the location, diameter, amplitude, and duration of the apical impulse. Listen at each auscultatory

Ask the patient to roll partly onto the left side while you listen at the apex area with the diaphragm of the stethoscope and then listen to each area with the bell. Listen for the first and second heart sounds and for physiologic splitting of the second heart sound. Listen for any abnormal heart sounds or murmurs.

Breasts. Palpate the breasts, while at the same time continuing inspection.

Abdomen. Inspect, auscultate, and percuss the abdomen. Palpate lightly, then deeply. Assess the liver and spleen by percussion and then palpation. Try to feel the kidneys, and palpate the aorta and its pulsations.

Lower Extremities. Examine the legs, assessing three systems while the patient is still supine. Each of these three systems can be further assessed when the patient stands.

- *Peripheral Vascular System.* Palpate the femoral pulses and, if indicated, the popliteal pulses. Palpate the inguinal lymph nodes. Inspect for lower extremity edema, discoloration, or ulcers. Palpate for pitting edema.

- *Musculoskeletal System.* Note any deformities or enlarged joints. If indicated, palpate the joints, check their range of motion, and perform any necessary maneuvers.

- *Nervous System.* Assess lower extremity muscle bulk, tone, and strength; also assess sensation and reflexes. Observe any abnormal movements.

With the Patient Sitting

Nervous System. The complete examination of the nervous system can also be done at the end of the examination. It consists of the five segments described below: *mental status, cranial nerves* (including funduscopic examination), *motor system, sensory system,* and *reflexes.*

Mental Status.   If indicated and not done during the interview, assess the patient's orientation, mood, thought process, thought content, abnormal perceptions, insight and judgment, memory and attention, information and vocabulary, calculating abilities, abstract thinking, and constructional ability.

Cranial Nerves. If not already examined, check sense of smell, strength of the temporal and masseter muscles, corneal reflexes, facial movements, gag reflex, and strength of the trapezia and sternomastoid muscles.

Motor System.   Muscle bulk, tone, and strength of major muscle groups. *Cerebellar function:* rapid alternating movements, point-to-point movements, such as finger-to-nose and heel-to-shin; gait.

Sensory System.   Pain, temperature, light touch, vibration, and discrimination. Compare right with left sides and distal with proximal areas on the limbs.

for S_3 or mitral stenosis. The patient should sit, lean forward, and exhale while you listen for the murmur of *aortic regurgitation.*

Lower the head of the bed to the flat position. **The patient should be supine.**

The patient is **sitting.**

Reflexes. Including biceps, triceps, brachioradialis, patellar, Achilles deep tendon reflexes; also plantar reflexes (see pp. 622–623).

Concluding the Examination

There are portions of the physical examination that are not possible to perform while the patient is on the examination table. For these, the patient must be standing.

With the Patient Standing

● *Peripheral Vascular System.* Inspect for varicose veins.

● *Musculoskeletal System.* Examine the alignment of the spine and its range of motion, the alignment of the legs, and the feet.

● *Nervous System.* Observe the patient's gait and ability to walk heel-to-toe, walk on the toes, walk on the heels, hop in place, and do shallow knee bends. Do a Romberg test and check for pronator drift.

As you become proficient you will develop your own style and may change the sequence for individual patients or circumstances.

The patient is **standing**. You should sit on a chair or stool.

BIBLIOGRAPHY

CITATIONS

1. U.S. Preventive Services Task Force. The guide to clinical preventive services 2007: recommendations of the U.S. Preventive Services Task Force. Washington DC: U.S. Department of Health and Human Services, Agency for Healthcare Research and Quality, September 2007. Available at: http://www.ahrq.gov/clinic/pocketgd07/pocketgd07.pdf. Accessed February 9, 2008.
2. Boulware LE, Marinopoulos S, Phillips KA, et al. Systematic review: the value of the periodic health evaluation. Ann Intern Med 146(4):289–300, 2007.
3. Oboler SK, Prochazka AV, Gonzales R, et al. Public expectations and attitudes for annual physical examinations and testing. Ann Intern Med 136(9):652–659, 2002.
4. Laine C. The annual physical examination: needless ritual or necessary routine? Ann Intern Med 136(9):701–702, 2002.
5. Culica D, Rohrer J, Ward M, et al. Medical check-ups: who does not get them? Am J Public Health 92(1):88–91, 2002.
6. Hesrud DD. Clinical preventive medicine in primary care: background and practice. Rational and current preventive practice. Mayo Clin Proc 75(4):1165–1172, 2000.

7. Simel DL, Rennie D. The clinical examination: an agenda to make it more rational. JAMA 277(7):572–574, 1997.
8. Sackett DL. A primer on the precision and accuracy of the clinical examination. JAMA 267(19):2638–2644, 1992.
9. Evidence-Based Working Group. Evidence-based medicine: a new approach to teaching the practice of medicine. JAMA 268(17):2420–2425, 1992.
10. Centers for Disease Control and Prevention (CDC). Standard precautions. Excerpt from the guidelines for isolation precautions: preventing transmission of infectious agents in healthcare settings 2007. Available at: http://www.cdc.gov/ncidod/dhqp/gl_isolation_standard.html. Accessed February 7, 2008.
11. Centers for Disease Control and Prevention. Information about MRSA for healthcare personnel. Available at: http://www.cdc.gov/ncidod/dhqp/ar_mrsa_healthcareFS.html#. Accessed February 7, 2008.
12. Centers for Disease Control and Prevention. Universal precautions for the prevention for transmission of HIV and other bloodborne infections. Updated 1996. At http://www.cdc.gov/ncidod/dhqp/bp_universal_precautions.html#. Accessed February 7, 2008.

Beginning the Physical Examination: General Survey, Vital Signs, and Pain

LEARNING OBJECTIVES

The student will:

1. Identify the components of the general survey.
2. Identify appropriate subjective questions based on initial observations.
3. Demonstrate how to measure blood pressure, pulse, respiration, and temperature.
4. Discuss variations in vital signs and the possible causes.
5. Describe the different types of pain.
6. Perform and document a pain assessment utilizing information from the health history and the physical examination.

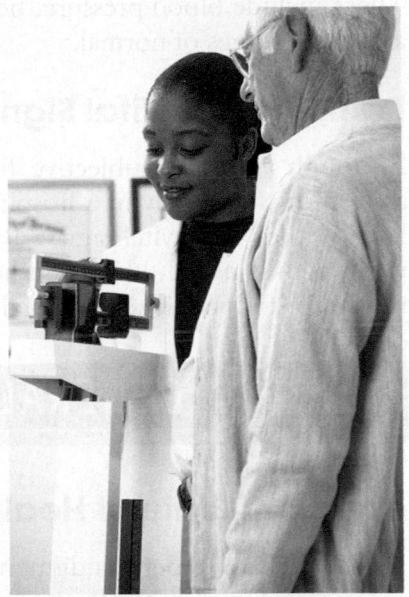

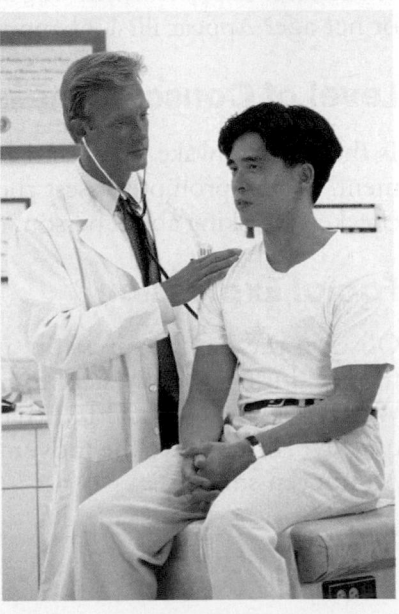

General Survey

The nurse's objective observation of the patient begins with the first moments of the encounter and continues throughout the interaction. The nonverbal cues collected during the general survey enable the nurse to select appropriate subjective questions for the individual patient to garner more information. Many factors are assessed, such as the patient's general appearance, apparent state of health, demeanor, facial affect or expression, grooming, posture, and gait. Height and weight would also be assessed at the end of the general survey and will be covered in detail in Chapter 8, Nutrition.

As the assessment skills of the nurse become more attuned to the individual patient, the distinguishing features are depicted so well in words that a colleague could envision the person.

Many factors contribute to the patient's makeup—socioeconomic status, nutrition, genetic composition, degree of fitness, mood state, early illnesses, gender, geographic location, and age cohort. Recall that the patient's status affects many of the characteristics you assess, including blood pressure, posture, mood and alertness, facial coloration, dentition, condition of the tongue and gingiva, color of the nail beds, and muscle bulk, to name a few.

Now recapture the observations you have been making since the first moments of the interaction and refine them throughout your assessment. Does the patient hear you when greeted in the waiting room or examination room? Rise with ease? Walk easily or stiffly? If hospitalized when you first meet, what is the patient doing—sitting up and enjoying television? Lying in bed? What occupies the bedside table—a magazine? A stack of "get well" cards? A Bible or a rosary? An emesis basin? Nothing at all? Each of these observations should raise one or more tentative hypotheses about the patient to consider during future assessments.

Vital Signs

These include blood pressure, heart rate, respiratory rate, and temperature and their ranges of normal.

Pain, the Fifth Vital Sign

Although pain is a subjective finding, in order to ensure frequent pain assessment, especially in a hospital or rehabilitation setting, pain has been labeled the "fifth vital sign." Pain assessment is commonly missed, and when pain is noted, it is often not effectively managed. Pain is a frequent motivator for people to seek health care.

GENERAL APPEARANCE

Apparent State of Health

Try to make a general judgment based on observations throughout the encounter. Support it with the significant details. Does the patient look his or her age? Appear ill? Unhappy? Fatigued?

Acutely or chronically ill, frail, or fit and robust.

Level of Consciousness

Is the patient awake, alert, and responsive to you and others in the environment? If not, promptly assess the level of consciousness. Orientation can be checked by asking about person, place, and time (Chapter 19, Mental Status).

Facial Expression

Observe the facial expression at rest, during conversation about specific topics, during the physical examination, and in interaction with others. Watch for eye contact. Is it natural? Sustained and unblinking? Averted quickly? Absent? Are the movements of the face symmetric? Is there ptosis? An uneven smile?

The stare of *hyperthyroidism;* the immobile face of *parkinsonism;* the flat or sad affect of *depression.* Decreased eye contact may be cultural, or may suggest anxiety, fear, or sadness. Asymmetry of the face could be a stroke, palsy, or injury to the cranial nerve.

Odors of the Body and Breath

Odors can be important diagnostic clues, such as the fruity odor of diabetes or the scent of alcohol. (For the scent of alcohol, the CAGE questions, p. 68, will help you determine possible misuse.)

Breath odors of alcohol, acetone (diabetes), pulmonary infections, uremia, or liver failure

Never assume that alcohol on a patient's breath explains changes in mental status or neurologic findings.

People with an odor of alcohol may have other serious and potentially correctable problems such as hypo-glycemia, subdural hematoma, or postictal state.

Posture, Gait, Motor Activity, and Speech

What is the patient's preferred posture? Assess the patient before calling his or her name in the waiting room. How is the patient sitting? Does that change when you are in the room with the patient?

Preference for sitting up in *left-sided heart failure,* and for leaning forward with arms braced in *chronic obstructive pulmonary disease* (COPD).

Is the patient restless or quiet? How often does the patient change position? How fast are the movements?

Fast, frequent movements of *hyperthyroidism;* slowed activity of *hypothyroidism*

Is there any apparent involuntary motor activity? Are some body parts immobile? Stiff? Jerky? Which ones?

Tremors or other involuntary movements; paralyses. See Table 20-6, Tremors and Involuntary Movements (pp. 670–671).

Does the patient walk smoothly, with comfort, self-confidence, and balance, or is there a limp or discomfort, fear of falling, loss of balance, or any movement disorder? Does the patient utilize an assistive device to ambulate? Cane? Walker? Brace?

Is the patient's speech articulate? Garbled? Rapid or slow?

See Table 20-10, Abnormalities of Gait and Posture (p. 675).

Fatigue is a nonspecific symptom with many causes. It refers to a sense of weariness or loss of energy that patients describe in various ways. "I don't feel like getting up in the morning" . . . "I don't have any energy" . . . "I just feel blah". . . "I'm all done in" . . . "I can hardly get through the day" . . . "By the time I get to the office I feel as if I've done a day's work." Because fatigue is a normal response to hard work, sustained stress, or grief, try to elicit the life circumstances in which it occurs. Fatigue unrelated to such situations requires further investigation.

Fatigue is a common symptom of depression and anxiety states, but also consider *infections* (such as hepatitis, infectious mononucleosis, and tuberculosis); *endocrine disorders* (hypothyroidism, adrenal insufficiency, diabetes mellitus, panhypopituitarism); *heart failure; chronic disease of the lungs, kidneys, or liver; electrolyte imbalance; moderate to severe anemia; malignancies; nutritional deficits;* and *medications.*

Use open-ended questions to explore the attributes of the patient's fatigue, and encourage the patient to fully describe what he or she is experiencing. Important clues about etiology often emerge from a good psychosocial history, exploration of sleep patterns, and a thorough review of systems.

Weakness is different from fatigue. It denotes a demonstrable loss of muscle power and will be discussed later with other neurologic symptoms (see p. 624).

Weakness, especially if localized in a neuroanatomic pattern, suggests possible *neuropathy* or *myopathy*.

Signs of Distress

For example, does the patient show evidence of these problems?

● Cardiac or respiratory distress

Clutching the chest, pallor, diaphoresis, labored breathing, wheezing, cough, shortness of breath, tripod position

● Pain

Facial expression, grimacing, crying, holding a body part

● Anxiety or depression

Anxious face, fidgety movements, cold and moist palms; inexpressive or flat affect, poor eye contact, psychomotor slowing. See Chapter 19 Mental Status, p. 595.

Skin Color and Obvious Lesions

See Chapter 9, Integumentary System, for details.

Pallor, cyanosis, jaundice, rashes, bruises

Dress, Grooming, and Personal Hygiene

How is the patient dressed? Is clothing appropriate to the temperature and weather? Is it clean, properly buttoned, and zipped? How does it compare with clothing worn by people of comparable age and social group?

Excess clothing may reflect the cold intolerance of *hypothyroidism* or weight loss of anorexia; hide skin rash, needle marks, or scars from self-mutilation; or signal personal lifestyle preferences.

Has the patient added additional holes on the belt to enlarge? To make smaller?

May indicate weight gain or weight loss

Glance at the patient's shoes. Have holes been cut in them? Are the laces tied? Or is the patient wearing slippers?

Cut-out holes or slippers may indicate gout, bunions, or other painful foot conditions. Untied laces or slippers also suggest edema.

Is the patient wearing any unusual jewelry? Where? Is there any body piercing? Tattoos? Where? When and where were they obtained?

Copper bracelets are sometimes worn for *arthritis*. Piercing or tattoos may appear on any part of the body.

Note the patient's hair, fingernails, and use of cosmetics. They may be clues to the patient's personality, mood, or lifestyle. Nail polish and hair coloring that have "grown out" may signify decreased interest in personal appearance.

"Grown-out" hair and nail polish can help estimate the length of an illness if the patient cannot give a history. Fingernails chewed to the quick may reflect stress.

Do personal hygiene and grooming seem appropriate to the patient's age, lifestyle, occupation, and socioeconomic group? These are norms that vary widely based on each individual.

Unkempt appearance may be seen in *depression* and *dementia,* but this appearance must be compared with the patient's probable norm.

THE VITAL SIGNS

Vital Signs are an integral part of the assessment. These include the blood pressure, heart rate, respiratory rate, and temperature. These important measurements may be completed at the start of the physical examination. If any of the vital signs are not within the normal parameters, then rechecking during the cardiovascular or respiratory system examinations would be prudent.

During the assessment, check the blood pressure and the pulse. The heart rate can be assessed by counting the radial pulse with your fingers, or the apical pulse with your stethoscope at the cardiac apex. Continue either of these techniques and count the respiratory rate without alerting the patient—breathing patterns may change if the patient knows breaths are being counted. The temperature may be taken in various anatomic sites, which depends on the patient and the equipment available. Further details on techniques for ensuring accuracy of the vital signs are provided in the following pages.

See Table 14-3, Variations and Abnormalities of the Apical Pulse (p. 386). See Table 7-1, Abnormalities in Rate and Rhythm of Breathing (p. 124).

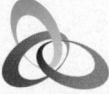 **BLOOD PRESSURE**

Choice of Blood Pressure Cuff (Sphygmomanometer)

More than 74.5 million Americans have elevated blood pressure.[1] To detect blood pressure elevations, an accurate instrument is essential. Blood pressure devices may be aneroid or electronic, and there are international protocols for evaluating their accuracy.[2–4] Some offices may continue to use mercury, although these are no longer available for sale.

Self-monitoring of blood pressure by well-instructed patients using approved devices improves blood pressure control, especially when it is done two times daily at the upper arm with automatic readouts.[5–7] Mercury products are no longer available due to possible mercury poisoning if the mercury leaks.

Take the time to choose a cuff of appropriate size for your patient's arm. Follow the guidelines listed, and advise your patients about how to choose the best cuff for home use. Urge them to have their home devices recalibrated routinely.

SELECTING THE CORRECT BLOOD PRESSURE CUFF

- Width of the inflatable bladder of the cuff should be about 40% of the limb selected (e.g., upper arm circumference [about 12–14 cm in the average adult]).
- Length of the inflatable bladder should be about 80% of upper arm circumference (almost long enough to encircle the arm).
- The standard cuff is 12 × 23 cm, appropriate for arm circumferences up to 28 cm.

If the cuff is too *small* (narrow), the blood pressure will read *high;* if the cuff is too *large* (wide), the blood pressure will read *low* on a small arm and *high* on a large arm.

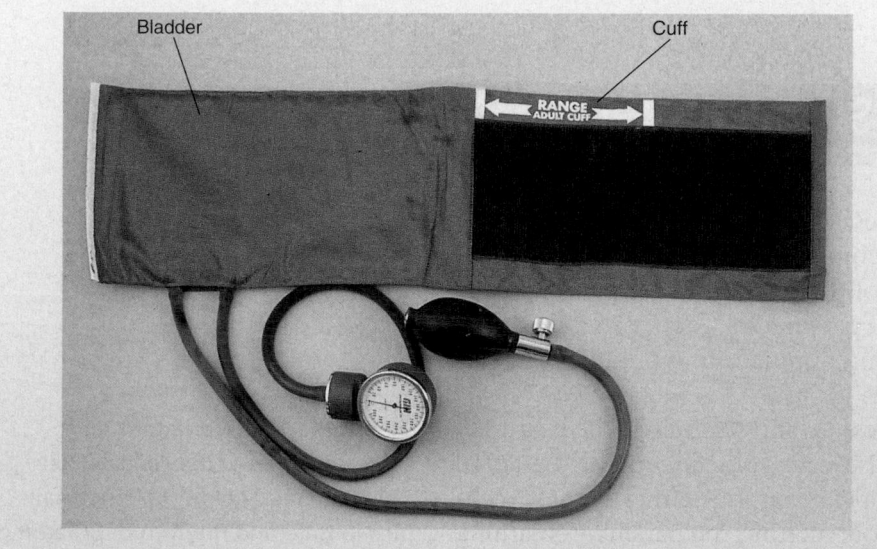

Bladder   Cuff

RANGE ADULT CUFF

Technique for Measuring Blood Pressure[8]

Before assessing the blood pressure, take several steps to make sure your measurement will be accurate. Proper technique is important and reduces the inherent variability arising from the patient or examiner, the equipment, and the procedure itself.

STEPS TO ENSURE ACCURATE BLOOD PRESSURE MEASUREMENT

- Ideally, instruct the patient to avoid smoking or drinking caffeinated beverages for 30 minutes before the blood pressure is measured.
- Check to make sure the examining room is quiet and comfortably warm.
- Ask the patient to sit quietly for at least 5 minutes in a chair, rather than on the examining table, with feet flat on the floor and legs uncrossed. The arm should be supported at heart level.

(continued)

STEPS TO ENSURE ACCURATE BLOOD PRESSURE
MEASUREMENT (continued)

- Make sure the arm selected is *free of clothing*. There should be no arterio-venous fistulas for dialysis, scarring from prior brachial artery cutdowns, or signs of lymphedema (seen after axillary node dissection or radiation therapy).
- Palpate the brachial artery to confirm that it has a viable pulse.
- Position the arm so that the brachial artery, at the antecubital crease, is *at heart level*—roughly level with the 4th interspace at its junction with the sternum.
- If the patient is seated, rest the arm on a table a little above the patient's waist; if the patient is standing, try to support the patient's arm at the midchest level.

If the brachial artery is 7 to 8 cm *below* heart level, the blood pressure will read approximately 6 cm higher; if the brachial artery is 6 to 7 cm *higher,* the blood pressure will read 5 cm lower.[9,10]

Now you are ready to measure the blood pressure.

- Center the inflatable bladder over the brachial artery. The lower border of the cuff should be about 2.5 cm above the antecubital crease. Secure the cuff snugly. Position the patient's arm so that it is slightly flexed at the elbow.

A loose cuff or a bladder that balloons outside the cuff leads to falsely high readings.

- To determine how high to raise the cuff pressure, first estimate the systolic pressure by palpation. As you feel the brachial artery with the fingers of one hand, rapidly inflate the cuff until the radial pulse disappears. Read this pressure on the manometer and add 30 mm Hg to it. Use of this sum as the target for subsequent inflations prevents discomfort from unnecessarily high cuff pressures. It also avoids the occasional error caused by an *auscultatory gap*—a silent interval that may be present between the systolic and the diastolic pressures.

An unrecognized auscultatory gap may lead to serious underestimation of systolic pressure (150/98 in the example below) or overestimation of diastolic pressure.

- Deflate the cuff promptly and completely and wait 15 to 30 seconds.

- Now place the bell or diaphragm of a stethoscope lightly over the brachial artery, taking care to make an air seal with its full rim. Do not allow the stethoscope to touch the cuff or clothing. The *Korotkoff sounds* are relatively low in pitch and are generally heard better with the bell. The diaphragm is easier to maneuver and covers a larger area. Each practitioner may choose a bell or diaphragm depending on which has clearer sounds.

If you find an auscultatory gap, record your findings completely (e.g., 200/98 with an auscultatory gap from 170 to 150).

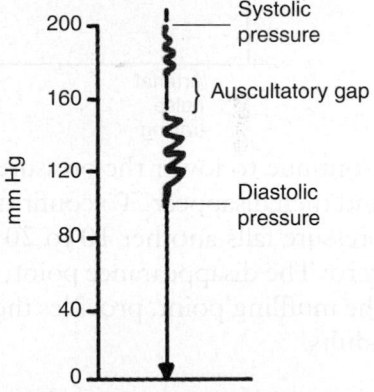

An auscultatory gap is associated with arterial stiffness, atherosclerotic disease, and wide pulse pressure.[11]

- Inflate the cuff rapidly again to the level just determined, and then deflate it slowly at a rate of about 2 to 3 mm Hg per second. Note the level at which you hear the sounds of at least two consecutive beats. This is the systolic pressure.

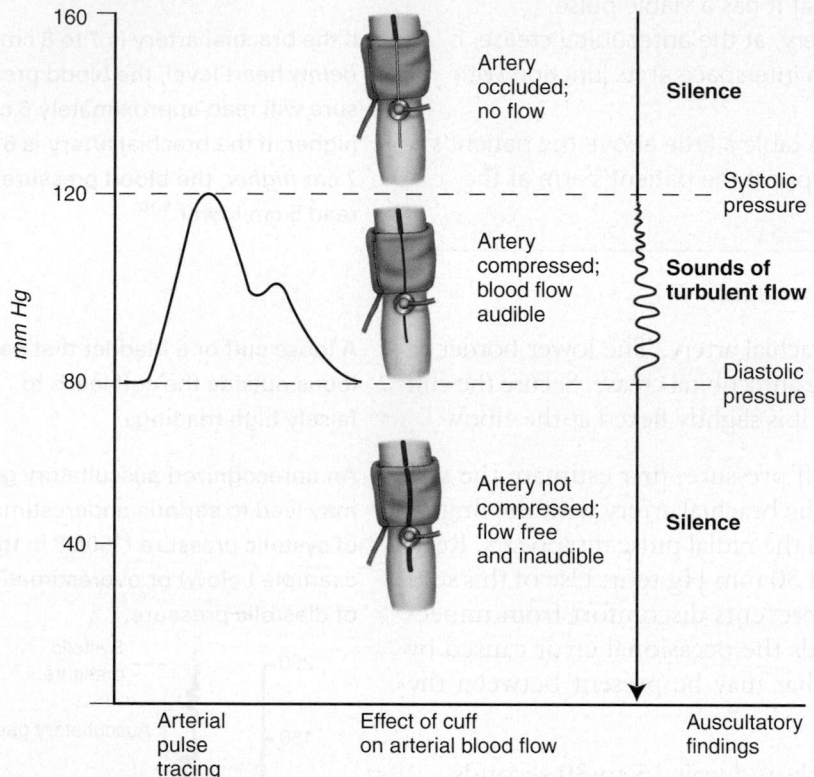

- **Continue** to lower the pressure slowly until the sounds become muffled and then disappear. To confirm the disappearance of sounds, listen as the pressure falls another 10 to 20 mm Hg. Then deflate the cuff rapidly to zero. The disappearance point, which is usually only a few mm Hg below the muffling point, provides the best estimate of true diastolic pressure in adults.

  In some people, the muffling point and the disappearance point are farther apart. Occasionally, as in aortic regurgitation, the sounds never disappear. If the difference is ≥10 mm Hg, record both figures (e.g., 154/80/68).

- Read both the systolic and the diastolic levels to the nearest 2 mm Hg.[12] Wait 2 minutes and repeat. Average your readings. If the first two readings differ by more than 5 mm Hg, take additional readings.

- When using an aneroid instrument, hold the dial so that it faces you directly. Avoid slow or repetitive inflations of the cuff, because the resulting venous congestion can cause false readings.

  By making the sounds less audible, venous congestion may produce artificially low systolic and high diastolic pressures.

- Blood pressure should be taken in both arms at least once. Normally, there may be a difference in pressure of 5 mm Hg and sometimes up to 10 mm Hg. Subsequent readings should be made on the arm with the higher pressure.

  Pressure difference of more than 10–15 mm Hg in *subclavian steal syndrome, aortic dissection.*

Blood pressure cuff selection is important:

Errors That Result in False High Readings

- Cuff too small (narrow)

- Cuff too loose or uneven

- Arm below heart level

- Arm not supported

- Inflating or deflating cuff too slowly (high diastolic)

- Deflating cuff too quickly (low systolic and high diastolic)

Errors That Result in False Low Readings

- Cuff too large (wide)

- Repeating assessments too quickly

- Inaccurate level of inflation

- Pressing stethoscope too tightly against pulse

Classification of Normal and Abnormal Blood Pressure

In its seventh report, the Joint National Committee on Prevention, Detection, Evaluation, and Treatment of High Blood Pressure recommended using the mean of two or more properly measured seated blood pressure readings, taken on two or more office visits, for diagnosis of hypertension.[8] Blood pressure measurement should be verified in the contralateral arm.

The Joint National Committee has identified four levels of systolic and diastolic hypertension. Note that either component may be high.

● JNC 7 Blood Pressure Classification — Adults Older Than 18 Years		
Category	**Systolic (mm Hg)**	**Diastolic (mm Hg)**
Normal	<120	<80
Prehypertension	120–139	80–89
Hypertension		
Stage 1	140–159	90 99
Stage 2	≥160	≥100

Note that the blood pressure goal for patients with hypertension, diabetes, or renal disease is <130/80.

Assessment of hypertension also includes its effects on target "end organs"—the eyes, heart, brain, and kidneys. Look for hypertensive retinopathy, left ventricular hypertrophy, and neurologic deficits suggesting stroke. Renal assessment requires urinalysis and blood tests of renal function.

When the systolic and diastolic levels fall in different categories, use the higher category. For example, 170/92 mm Hg is Stage 2 hypertension; 135/100 mm Hg is Stage 1 hypertension. In *isolated systolic hypertension,* systolic blood pressure is ≥140 mm Hg, and diastolic blood pressure is <90 mm Hg.

Treatment of *isolated systolic hypertension* in patients 60 years or older reduces total mortality and both mortality and complications from cardiovascular disease.[13,14]

The Hypertensive Patient with Unequal Blood Pressures in the Arms and Legs.
To detect coarctation of the aorta, make two further blood pressure measurements at least once in every hypertensive patient:

● Compare blood pressures in the arms and legs.

● Compare the volume and timing of the radial and femoral pulses. Normally, volume is equal and the pulses occur simultaneously.

Coarctation of the aorta arises from narrowing of the thoracic aorta, usually proximal but sometimes distal to the left subclavian artery.

Coarctation of the aorta and *occlusive aortic disease* are distinguished by hypertension in the upper extremities and low blood pressure in the legs and by diminished or delayed femoral pulses.[15]

To determine blood pressure in the leg, use a wide, long thigh cuff that has a bladder size of 18 × 42 cm, and apply it to the midthigh. Center the bladder over the posterior surface, wrap it securely, and listen over the popliteal artery. If possible, the patient should be prone. Alternatively, ask the supine patient to flex one leg slightly, with the heel resting on the bed. When cuffs of the proper size are used for both the leg and the arm, then the systolic blood pressure is usually 10 to 40 mm Hg higher in the leg and the diastolic blood pressure is the same in the leg and the brachial artery. (The usual arm cuff, improperly used on the leg, gives a falsely high reading.)

Relatively low levels of blood pressure should always be interpreted in light of past readings and the patient's present clinical state.

A pressure of 110/70 mm Hg would usually be normal, but could also indicate significant hypotension if past pressures have been high.

If indicated, assess *orthostatic,* or *postural, blood pressure* (see Chapter 24, Assessing Older Adults, p. 840). Measure blood pressure and heart rate in two positions—*supine* or sitting after the patient is resting up to 10 minutes, then within 3 minutes after the patient *stands up.* Normally, as the patient rises from the horizontal to the standing position, systolic pressure drops slightly or remains unchanged, while diastolic pressure rises slightly. Orthostatic hypotension is a drop in systolic blood pressure of ≥20 mm Hg or in diastolic blood pressure of ≥10 mm Hg within 3 minutes of standing.[16,17]

A fall in systolic pressure of 20 mm Hg or more, especially when accompanied by symptoms and tachycardia, indicates *orthostatic (postural) hypotension.* Causes include: drugs, moderate or severe blood loss, prolonged bed rest, and diseases of the autonomic nervous system.

SPECIAL TECHNIQUES

Weak Pulse. The Doppler ultrasound stethoscope is a device that transmits the sounds of blood flow and aids in monitoring blood pressure if the artery is unable to be palpated because of a weak pulse. The technique for auscultation of blood pressure is the same, with the change solely in the stethoscope device.

People who have a stent for dialysis or who have had breast surgery with lymph node dissection or lymphedema should not have blood pressures taken in that arm. If both arms have lymph node involvement, then the lower extremities should be used for blood pressure assessment so as not to impede blood flow, which can result in lymphedema or make it worse if it is already present.

The apical pulse should be taken (as described in Chapter 14, Cardiovascular System) instead of the radial pulse if:

● The radial pulse is difficult to find or there is an irregularity

● The patient's condition warrants a more accurate pulse reading (e.g., before administration of some medications)

Weak or Inaudible Korotkoff Sounds. Consider technical problems such as erroneous placement of your stethoscope, failure to make full skin contact with the bell, and venous engorgement of the patient's arm from repeated inflations of the cuff. Consider also the possibility of shock.

When you cannot hear Korotkoff sounds at all, you may be able to estimate the systolic pressure by palpation. Alternative methods such as Doppler techniques or direct arterial pressure tracings may be necessary.

To intensify Korotkoff sounds, one of the following methods may be helpful:

● Raise the patient's arm before and while you inflate the cuff. Then lower the arm and determine the blood pressure.

● Inflate the cuff. Ask the patient to make a fist several times, and then determine the blood pressure.

Arrhythmias. Irregular rhythms produce variations in pressure and therefore unreliable measurements. Ignore the effects of an occasional premature contraction. With frequent premature contractions or atrial fibrillation, determine the average of several observations and note the measurements are approximate. Verify the findings with an electrocardiogram.

White Coat Hypertension. "White coat hypertension" describes hypertension in people whose blood pressure measurements are higher in the office than at home or in more relaxed settings, usually >140/90. This phenomenon occurs in 10% to 25% of patients, especially women and anxious individuals, and may last for several visits. Try to relax the patient and remeasure the blood pressure later in the encounter.

Home or ambulatory hypertension, unlike "white coat" or isolated office hypertension, signals increased risk of cardiovascular disease.[18–21]

The Obese or Very Thin Patient. For the obese arm, it is important to use a wide cuff of 15 cm. If the arm circumference exceeds 41 cm, use a thigh cuff of 18 cm. For the very thin arm, a pediatric cuff may be indicated.

Using a small cuff overestimates systolic blood pressure in obese patients.[22] Palpation of an irregularly irregular rhythm reliably indicates *atrial fibrillation*. For all other irregular patterns, an electrocardiogram (ECG) is needed to identify the type of rhythm.

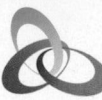 ## HEART RATE AND RHYTHM

Examine the arterial pulses, the heart rate and rhythm, and the amplitude and contour of the pulse wave.

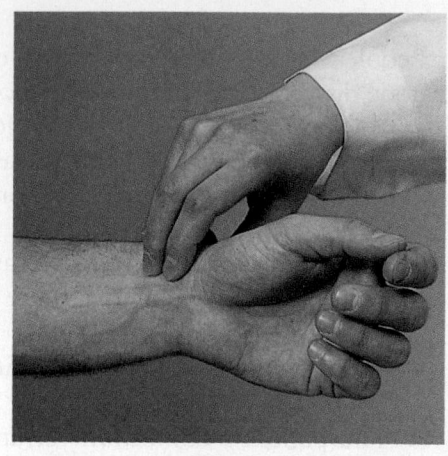

Heart Rate

The radial pulse is commonly used to assess the heart rate. With the pads of your index and middle fingers, compress the radial artery until a maximal pulsation is detected. If the rhythm is regular and the rate seems normal, count the rate for 30 seconds and multiply by 2. If the rate is unusually fast or slow, however, count it for 60 seconds. The range of normal is 60–100 beats per minute.[23]

Rhythm

To begin your assessment of rhythm, feel the radial pulse. If there are any irregularities, check the rhythm again by listening with your stethoscope at the cardiac apex. Beats that occur earlier than others may not be detected peripherally, and the heart rate can be seriously underestimated. Is the rhythm regular or irregular? If irregular, try to identify a pattern: (1) Do early beats appear in a basically regular rhythm? (2) Does the irregularity vary consistently with respiration? (3) Is the rhythm totally irregular?

See Table 14-1, Selected Heart Rates and Rhythms (p. 384), and Table 14-2, Selected Irregular Rhythms (p. 385).

If the radial pulse is irregular or the patient's condition calls for a more precise pulse rate, then an apical pulse should be assessed for 1 minute. The examiner places the stethoscope at the apex (fifth intercostal space at the midclavicular line) and auscultates the S_1 and S_2, noting the rate and rhythm.

 ## RESPIRATORY RATE AND RHYTHM

Observe the *rate, rhythm, depth,* and *effort of breathing*. Count the number of respirations (one respiration includes an inspiration and an expiration) in 1 minute either by visual inspection or by subtly listening over the patient's trachea with your stethoscope during your examination of the head and neck or chest. Normally, adults take 12–20 breaths per minute in a quiet, regular pattern. An occasional sigh is normal. Check to see if expiration is prolonged.

See Table 7-1, Abnormalities in Rate and Rhythm of Breathing (p. 124). Prolonged expiration in COPD.

 ## TEMPERATURE

The average *oral temperature,* usually quoted at 37°C (98.6°F), fluctuates considerably. In the early morning hours, it may fall as low as 35.8°C (96.4°F), and in the late afternoon or evening, it may rise as high as 37.3°C (99.1°F). *Rectal temperatures* are *higher* than oral temperatures by an average of 0.4 to 0.5°C (0.7 to 0.9°F), but this difference is also quite variable. In contrast, *axillary temperatures* are *lower* than oral temperatures by approximately 1°, but take 5 to 10 minutes to register and are generally considered less accurate than other measurements.

Fever or pyrexia refers to an elevated body temperature. *Hyperpyrexia* refers to extreme elevation in temperature, above 41.1°C (106°F), while *hypothermia* refers to an abnormally low temperature, below 35°C (95°F) rectally.

Taking oral temperatures is not recommended when patients are unconscious, restless, or unable to close their mouths. Temperature readings may be inaccurate and thermometers may be broken by unexpected movements of the patient's jaws. Options are available—rectal, tympanic, temporal artery, axilla, or skin—and should be chosen based on individual situations and availability.

Oral Thermometers

Place the disposable cover over the probe and insert the thermometer under the tongue. Ask the patient to close both lips, and then watch closely for the digital readout. An accurate temperature recording usually takes about 10 seconds. Note that hot or cold liquids, and even smoking, can alter the temperature reading. In these situations, it is best to delay measuring the temperature for 10 to 15 minutes. Due to breakage and mercury exposure, glass thermometers are giving way to electronic thermometers.

Rectal Temperatures

Select a rectal thermometer (usually red). Place the disposable cover over the probe and lubricate it. Ask the patient to lie on one side with the hip flexed and insert the thermometer about 3 to 4 cm (1.5 inches) into the anal canal, in a direction pointing to the umbilicus. Wait about 10 seconds for the digital temperature recording to appear.

Tympanic Membrane Temperatures

Another thermometer used is the *tympanic membrane thermometer*. This is an increasingly common practice and is quick, safe, and reliable if performed properly. Make sure the external auditory canal is free of cerumen, which lowers temperature readings. Place the cover on and position the probe in the canal so that the infrared beam is aimed at the tympanic membrane (otherwise the measurement will be invalid). Wait 2 to 3 seconds until the digital temperature reading appears. This method measures core body temperature, which is higher than the normal oral temperature by approximately 0.8°C (1.4°F). Tympanic measurements are more variable than oral or rectal measurements, including right and left comparisons in the same person.[24]

Temporal Artery Temperatures

A temporal artery thermometer measures the blood flow through the superficial temporal artery. There are a number of different models and the model instructions should be read prior to use. When using the Temporal Scanner model TAT 5000, place probe on the center of the forehead and depress the

Rapid respiratory rates tend to increase the discrepancy between oral and rectal temperatures. In these situations, rectal temperatures are more reliable.

Causes of *fever* include infection, trauma such as surgery or crush injuries, malignancy, blood disorders such as acute hemolytic anemia, drug reactions, and immune disorders such as collagen vascular disease.

The chief cause of *hypothermia* is exposure to cold. Other predisposing causes include reduced movement as in paralysis, interference with vasoconstriction as from sepsis or excess alcohol, starvation, hypothyroidism, or hypoglycemia. Elderly people are especially susceptible to hypothermia and also less likely to develop fever.

red button. Keeping the button depressed, slowly slide the probe midline across the forehead to the hairline. Lift the probe from the forehead and touch on the neck, just behind the earlobe. Release the button and the temperature will be visible.

Axillary Temperatures

Place a probe cover over the electronic thermometer and place the thermometer in the middle of the axilla. This technique can be used with unconscious patients. It is not recommended in patients with rapid temperature changes as it lags behind rapid core changes.

Skin Temperatures

The chemical thermometer has a sensor at the end of the thermometer. The dots change color based on the patient's temperature in about 60 seconds. Measurements can be slower to record rapid changes, and the adhesive can be lost due to diaphoresis.

Fever, Chills, and Night Sweats

Fever refers to an abnormal elevation in body temperature (see p. 116 for definitions of normal). Ask about fever if patients have an acute or chronic illness. Find out whether the patient has used a thermometer to measure the temperature. Bear in mind that errors in technique can lead to unreliable information. Has the patient felt feverish or unusually hot, noted excessive sweating, or felt chilly and cold? Try to distinguish between subjective *chilliness* and a *shaking chill* with shivering throughout the body and chattering of teeth.

Feeling cold, goosebumps, and shivering accompany a rising temperature, while feeling hot and sweating accompany a falling temperature. Normally the body temperature rises during the day and falls during the night. When fever exaggerates this swing, *night sweats* may occur. Malaise, headache, and pain in the muscles and joints often accompany fever.

Fever has many causes. Focus your questions on the timing of the illness and its associated symptoms. Become familiar with patterns of infectious diseases that may affect your patient. Inquire about travel, contact with sick people, or other unusual exposures. Be sure to inquire about medications because they may cause fever. In contrast, recent ingestion of aspirin, acetaminophen, corticosteroids, and nonsteroidal anti-inflammatory drugs may mask fever and affect the temperature recorded at the time of the physical examination.

Recurrent shaking chills suggest more extreme swings in temperature and systemic *bacteremia*.

Feelings of heat and sweating also accompany menopause. Night sweats occur in *tuberculosis* and *malignancy*.

ACUTE AND CHRONIC PAIN

Pain

Pain is one of the most common symptoms prompting office care. Each year, approximately 70 million Americans report persistent or intermittent pain, often underassessed and undertreated.[25-27] Adopt a comprehensive approach to guide your subsequent physical examination and management.

Understanding Acute and Chronic Pain

The International Association for the Study of Pain defines *pain* as "an unpleasant sensory and emotional experience". The experience of pain is complex and multifactorial. Pain involves sensory, emotional, and cognitive processing but may lack a specific physical etiology.[25]

Chronic pain is defined in several ways: pain not associated with cancer or other medical conditions that persists for more than 3 to 6 months; pain lasting more than 1 month beyond the course of an acute illness or injury; or pain recurring at intervals of months or years.[28] Chronic noncancer pain affects 5% to 33% of patients in primary care settings. More than 40% of patients report that their pain is poorly controlled.[29]

Chronic pain may be a spectrum disorder related to mental health and somatic conditions. See Chapter 19, Mental Status, "Symptoms and Behavior," pp. 596–597.

Assessing the Patient's History

Adopt a comprehensive approach to understanding the patient's pain, carefully listening to the patient's description of the many features of pain and contributing factors. Accept the patient's self-report, which experts state is the most reliable indicator of pain.[25]

Onset.   When did the pain begin? How? Does it occur at a specific time of day?

Location.   Ask the patient to point to the pain, because lay terms may not be specific enough to localize the site of origin. Also ask about radiation of pain.

Duration.   Is it constant? Does it come and go?

Characteristic Symptoms.   Assessing the severity of the pain is especially important. Use a consistent method to determine severity. Three scales are common: the Visual Analog Scale, Numeric Rating Scale and the Faces Pain Scale. Multidimensional tools like the Brief Pain Inventory are also available; these take longer to administer but address the effects of pain on the patient's activity level.[30] The Faces Pain Scale is reproduced on the next page, because it can be used by children as well as patients with language barriers or cognitive impairment.[31]

Also ask the patient the following questions:

Describe the pain. Is it sharp? Dull? Burning?
Does it follow a particular pattern?
Is it related to an injury or a particular movement? Stressful event?

Associated Manifestations.   Does anything occur when you experience the pain? Nausea? Vomiting? Headaches? Burning? Itching?

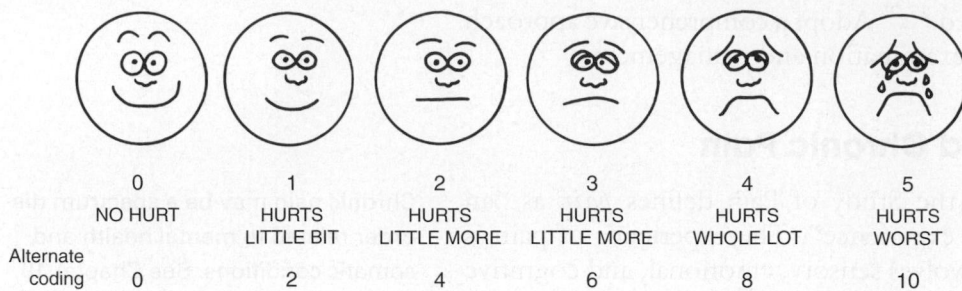

0	1	2	3	4	5
NO HURT	HURTS LITTLE BIT	HURTS LITTLE MORE	HURTS LITTLE MORE	HURTS WHOLE LOT	HURTS WORST

Alternate coding

0	2	4	6	8	10

(Adapted with permission from Hockenberry MJ, Wilson D: *Wong's essentials of pediatric nursing*, ed. 8, St. Louis, 2009, Mosby. Used with permission. Copyright Mosby).

Relieving Factors. What makes the pain better? Worse?

See Chapter 3, "The Seven Attributes of a Symptom," p. 43.

Treatments. Medications, Related Illnesses, and Impact on Daily Activities. Be sure to ask about any treatments that the patient has tried, including medications, physical therapy, and alternative medicines. A comprehensive medication history helps to identify drugs that interact with analgesics and reduce their efficacy.

Identify any comorbid conditions such as arthritis, diabetes, HIV/AIDS, substance abuse, sickle cell disease, or psychiatric disorders. These can have significant effects on the patient's experience of pain.

Chronic pain is the leading cause of disability and impaired performance at work. Inquire about the effects of pain on the patient's daily activities, mood, sleep, work, and sexual activity.

Health Disparities. Be aware of the well-documented health disparities in pain treatment and delivery of care, which range from lower use of analgesics in emergency rooms for African-American and Hispanic patients to disparities in use of analgesics for cancer, postoperative, and low back pain.[28] Studies show that clinician stereotypes, language barriers, and unconscious clinician biases in decision making all contribute to these disparities. Critique your own communication style, be aware of nonverbal cues, seek information and best practice standards, and improve your techniques of patient education and empowerment as first steps in ensuring uniform and effective pain management.

See Institute of Medicine report, *Unequal Treatment: Confronting Racial and Ethnic Disparities in Health Care*, 2002.[32]

Nonverbal cues may include: wincing, sweating, protectiveness of painful area, facial grimacing, or unusual posture favoring one limb or body area.

Types of Pain

Be familiar with recent advances in the scientific understanding of pain processes, described in several excellent modules for nurses available online.[25,28,33] Review the summary of types of pain in the following box to aid in your understanding of caring for patients in pain.

● Types of Pain[25,28,34]

Nociceptive or somatic pain	Pain related to tissue damage is termed *nociceptive*, or *somatic*. Nociceptive pain can be either acute and remitting or chronic and persistent. This form of pain is mediated by the afferent A-delta and C-fibers of the sensory system that respond to noxious stimuli and is modulated by both neurotransmitters and psychological processes. Modulating neurotransmitters include endorphins, histamines, acetylcholine, and monoamines like serotonin, norepinephrine, and dopamine. These afferent nociceptors can be sensitized by inflammatory mediators.
Neuropathic pain	Pain resulting from direct injury to the peripheral or central nervous system is termed *neuropathic*. Over time, neuropathic pain may become independent of the inciting injury, become burning, lancinating, or shock-like in quality and persisting beyond healing from the initial injury. Mechanisms postulated to evoke neuropathic pain include central nervous system brain or spinal cord injury from stroke or trauma; peripheral nervous system disorders causing entrapment or pressure on spinal nerves, plexuses, or peripheral nerves; and referred pain syndromes with increased or prolonged pain responses to inciting stimuli. These triggers appear to induce changes in pain signal processing through "neuronal plasticity," leading to pain that persists beyond healing from the initial injury.[28]
Psychogenic and idiopathic pain	*Psychogenic pain* relates to the many factors that influence the patient's report of pain—psychiatric conditions like anxiety or depression, personality and coping style, cultural norms, and social support systems. *Idiopathic pain* is pain without an identifiable etiology.

Pain Management

Treatment of pain requires sophisticated knowledge of nonopioid, opioid, and adjuvant analgesics and modalities of behavioral and physical therapy, which are beyond the scope of this book. Seek education about pain therapeutics, and turn to the literature for helpful reviews on the challenges and advances in pain management.[27,29,35] Nurses are often reluctant to administer narcotics because of fear of inducing addiction. Make use of the following definitions, and take advantage of validated screening tools for opioid assessment in patients with pain.[36,37]

Focus on the *Four A's* to monitor patient outcomes:
- *Analgesia*
- *Activities of daily living*
- *Adverse effects*
- *Aberrant drug-related behaviors*

ADDICTION, PHYSICAL DEPENDENCE, AND TOLERANCE[38]

Tolerance: A state of adaptation in which exposure to a drug induces changes that result in a diminution of one or more of the drug's effects over time.

ADDICTION, PHYSICAL DEPENDENCE, AND TOLERANCE[38] (continued)

Physical Dependence: A state of adaptation that is manifested by a drug class—specific withdrawal syndrome that can be produced by abrupt cessation, rapid dose reduction, decreasing blood level of the drug, and/or administration of an antagonist.

Addiction: A primary, chronic, neurobiologic disease, with genetic, psychosocial, and environmental factors influencing its development and manifestations. It is characterized by behaviors that include one or more of the following: impaired control over drug use, compulsive use, continued use despite harm, and craving.

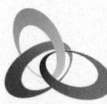

RECORDING YOUR FINDINGS

RECORDING THE PHYSICAL EXAMINATION—THE GENERAL SURVEY AND VITAL SIGNS

Choose vivid and graphic adjectives, as if you are painting a picture in words. Avoid clichés such as "well developed" or "well nourished" or "in no acute distress," because they could apply to any patient and do not convey the special features of the individual patient.

Record the vital signs taken at the time of the examination. They are preferable to those taken earlier in the day by other providers. (Common abbreviations for blood pressure, heart rate, and respiratory rate are self-explanatory.)

"Mrs. Scott is a young, healthy-appearing woman, well groomed, fit, and cheerful. 37.5°C oral, 72 regular, 16 even, 120/80 R arm sitting."

OR

"Mr. Jones is an elderly male who looks pale and chronically ill. He is alert, with eye contact but unable to speak more than two or three words at a time due to shortness of breath. He has intercostal muscle retraction when breathing and sits upright in bed. He is thin, with diffuse muscle wasting. 101.2°F tympanic, 108 irregular, 32 shallow/labored, 160/95 R arm sitting."

Suggests exacerbation of *chronic obstructive pulmonary disease.*

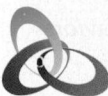

HEALTH PROMOTION

Temperature

Education of patients or parents on how to correctly take a temperature and the normal range is important. Review the various routes and instruments necessary and have them demonstrate the skill.

Patients should be aware of the risk factors for heatstroke, such as excessive exercise in hot, humid weather conditions; poor ventilation on hot days; decreased fluid intake; and sudden exposure to hot climates.

Patients also need to be aware of the risk factors for hypothermia when there is prolonged exposure to cold temperatures. Thermometers generally used to measure fevers will not register temperatures as low as hypothermia (core 95F and 35C).

Pulse

Patients taking certain cardiac medications will need to take their own pulse rate prior to taking the medication and be aware of potential side effects. They need to know at what parameters to hold the medication and when to call the health care provider. Also, patients should take a pulse rate prior to and after exercise to determine the reaction to exercise.

Teach patients how to check ONE carotid pulse by lightly placing two to three fingers on the site and counting for 1 minute. Recording the rate, rhythm, and depth is important after the assessment.

Respirations

Explain to the person assessing the respirations at home that this includes a full inspiration and a full expiration for a full minute, which is measured with a watch with a second hand. Recording the rate, rhythm, and amplitude is important after the assessment.

Blood Pressure

Monitoring a patient's blood pressure at home may be necessary, and it is important for the nurse to verify that it is correctly done. Initially, it is important to assess the environment for noise levels to ensure the reading is taken in a quiet room. Check to ensure the correct cuff size is available and the person is able to apply the cuff or has a family member who is able to correctly place the cuff. Generating a list of approved electronic instruments or sphygmomanometers for home testing is helpful, and those covered by insurance should be included. Home sphygmomanometers should be checked periodically for accuracy by simultaneously taking and comparing the readings with an office or clinic sphygmomanometer.

Everyone should be aware of his or her baseline vital signs. Notification of a health care provider of deviations is very important, especially in patients who are monitoring for a specific reason. Documentation of each vital sign should be kept in a journal with associated symptoms that are occurring at the time (e.g., shortness of breath when walking up a flight of stairs).

TABLE
7-1

Abnormalities in Rate and Rhythm of Breathing

When observing respiratory patterns, think in terms of *rate*, *depth*, and *regularity* of the patient's breathing. Describe what you see in these terms. Traditional terms, such as tachypnea, are given below so that you will understand them, but simple descriptions are recommended for use.

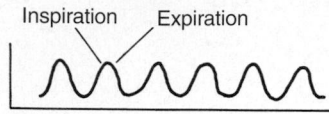

Normal

The respiratory rate is about 12–20 per minute in normal adults and up to 44 per minute in infants.

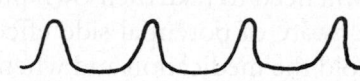

Slow Breathing (*Bradypnea*)

Slow breathing may be secondary to such causes as diabetic coma, drug-induced respiratory depression, and increased intracranial pressure.

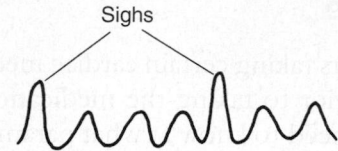

Sighing Respiration

Breathing punctuated by frequent sighs should alert you to the possibility of hyperventilation syndrome—a common cause of dyspnea and dizziness. Occasional sighs are normal.

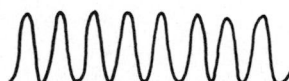

Rapid Shallow Breathing (*Tachypnea*)

Rapid shallow breathing has a number of causes, including restrictive lung disease, pleuritic chest pain, and an elevated diaphragm.

Slow, Shallow Breathing (*Hypopnea, Hypoventilation*)

Slow, shallow breathing has a number of causes, including asthma, pneumonia, pulmonary edema, shock, metabolic alkalosis, and a panic or anxiety attack.

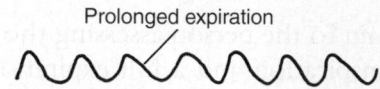

Obstructive Breathing

In obstructive lung disease, expiration is prolonged because narrowed airways increase the resistance to air flow. Causes include asthma, chronic bronchitis, and chronic obstructive pulmonary disease.

Rapid Deep Breathing (*Hyperpnea, Hyperventilation*)

Rapid deep breathing has several causes, including exercise, anxiety, and metabolic acidosis. In the comatose patient, consider infarction, hypoxia, or hypoglycemia affecting the midbrain or pons. *Kussmaul breathing* is deep breathing due to metabolic acidosis. It may be fast, normal in rate, or slow.

Ataxic Breathing (*Biot Breathing*)

Ataxic breathing is characterized by unpredictable irregularity. Breaths may be shallow or deep, and stop for short periods. Causes include respiratory depression and brain damage, typically at the medullary level.

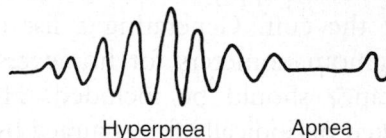

Cheyne-Stokes Breathing

Periods of deep breathing alternate with periods of apnea (no breathing). Children and aging people normally may show this pattern in sleep. Other causes include heart failure, uremia, drug-induced respiratory depression, and brain damage (typically on both sides of the cerebral hemispheres or diencephalon).

BIBLIOGRAPHY

CITATIONS

1. American Heart Association. Heart Disease and Stroke Statistics, 2010 Update. Dallas, Texas: American Heart Association; 2010. Available at: http://www.americanheart.org/downloadable/heart/1265665152970DS_3241%20HeartStrokeUpdate_2010.pdf. Accessed March 23, 2011.

2. O'Brien E, Asmar R, Beilin L, et al. European Society of Hypertension recommendations for conventional, ambulatory, and more blood pressure measurement. J Hypertens 21(5): 821–848, 2005.

3. O'Brien E, Pickering T, Asmar R, et al. International protocol for validation of blood pressure measuring devices in adults. Blood Press Monit 7(1):3–17, 2002.

4. O'Brien E, Waider B, Parati G, et al. Blood pressure measuring devices: recommendations of the European Society of Hypertension. BMJ 322(7285):531–536, 2001.

5. Verberk WJ, Kroon AA, Kessles AGH, et al. Home blood pressure measurement: a systematic review. J Am Coll Cardiol 46(5):743–751, 2005.

6. McManus RJ, Mant J, Roalfe A, et al. Targets and self monitoring in hypertension: randomized controlled trial and cost effectiveness analysis. BMJ 331(7515):493, epub 2005.

7. Bakx JC, van der Wel MC, van Weel. Self monitoring of high blood pressure. BMJ 331(7515):466–467, 2005.

8. Chobanian AV, Bakris GL, Black HR, et al. The Seventh Report of the Joint National Committee on Prevention, Detection, Evaluation, and Treatment of High Blood Pressure—The JNC 7 Report. JAMA 289(19):2560–2572, 2003. Available at: http://www.nhlbi.nih.gov/guidelines/hypertension/jnc7full.pdf. Accessed March 23, 2011.

9. McGee S. Blood pressure. In: Evidence-Based Physical Diagnosis, 2nd ed. St. Louis: Saunders, 2007:153–173.

10. Mitchell PL, Parlin RW, Blackburn H. Effect of vertical displacement of the arm on indirect blood-pressure measurements. N Engl J Med 271:72–74, 1064.

11. Cavallini MC, Roman MJ, Blank SG, et al. Association of the auscultatory gap with vascular disease in hypertensive patients. Ann Intern Med 124(10):877–883, 1996.

12. National High Blood Pressure Education Program, National Heart, Lung, and Blood Institute, National Institutes of Health. The seventh report of the Joint National Committee on Detection, Evaluation, and Treatment of High Blood Pressure. JAMA 289(19):2560, 2003.

13. Chaudhry SI, Krumholz HM, Foody JM. Systolic hypertension in older persons. JAMA 292(9):1074–1080, 2004.

14. Chobanian A. Isolated systolic hypertension in the elderly. N Engl J Med 357(8):789–796, 2007.

15. Brickner ME, Hillis LD, Lange RA. Congenital heart disease in adults: first of two parts. N Engl J Med 342(2):256–263, 2000.

16. Carslon JE. Assessment of orthostatic blood pressure: measurement technique and clinical applications. South Med J 92(2):167–173, 1999.

17. Consensus Committee of the American Autonomic Society and the American Academy of Neurology. Consensus statement on the definition of orthostatic hypotension, pure autonomic failure, and multiple system atrophy. Neurology 46(5):1470, 1996.

18. Bobrie G, Genes N, Vaur L, et al. Is "isolated home" hypertension as opposed to "isolated office" hypertension a sign of greater cardiovascular risk? Arch Int Med 161(18):2205–2211, 2001.

19. Clement DL, De Buysere ML, DeBacquer DA, et al. Prognostic value of ambulatory blood-pressure recordings in patients with treated hypertension. N Engl J Med 348(24): 2407–2415, 2003.

20. Rickerby J. The role of home blood pressure measurement in managing hypertension: an evidence-based review. J Hum Hypertens 16(7):469–472, 2002.

21. Pickering TG, Shimbo D, Hass D. Ambulatory blood pressure monitoring. N Engl J Med 354(22):2368–2374, 2006.

22. Fonseca-Reyes S, de Alba-García JG, Parra-Carrillo JZ, et al. Effect of standard cuff on blood pressure readings in patients with obese arms: how frequent are arms of a 'large circumference'? Blood Press Monit 8(3):101–106, 2003.

23. Spodick DH. Normal sinus heart rate: appropriate rate thresholds for sinus tachycardia and bradycardia. South Med J 89(7):666–667, 1996.

24. McGee S. Temperature. In: Evidence-Based Physical Diagnosis, 2nd ed. St. Louis: Saunders, 2007:174–186.

25. American Medical Association. Pain Management: The Online Series. Module 1. Pathophysiology of Pain and Pain Assessment. September 2007. Available at: http://www.ama-cmeonline.com/pain_mgmt/. Accessed March 23, 2011.

26. Epps CD, Ware LJ, Packard A. Ethnic wait time differences in analgesic administration in the emergency department. https://mail.nursing.upenn.edu/owa/redir.aspx? C=180033d1e 2f2451995f938591c198ae1&URL=http%3a%2f%2fwww. sciencedirect.com%2fscience%3f_ob%3dArticleURL%26_udi% 3dB6WP6-4SM75GH-4%26_user%3d4304014%26_ coverDate%3d06%2F30%2F2008%26_alid%3d924489990%2 6_rdoc%3d3%26_fmt%3dhigh%26_orig%3dsearch%26_cdi%3d 6982%26_sort%3dd%26_docanchor%3d%26view%3dc%26_ ct%3d14%26_acct%3dC000047720%26_version%3d1%26_url Version%3d0%26_userid%3d4304014%26md5%3dedaf86e42 0f4f892f0a2e5258c0eded7%23hit12Pain Manage Nurs 9(1): 26–32, 2008.

27. Sinatra R. Opioid analgesics in primary care: challenges and new advances in the management of noncancer pain. J Am Board Fam Med 19(2):165–167, 2006.

28. American Medical Association. Pain Management: The Online Series. Pathophysiology of Pain and Pain Assessment. Module 7—Assessing and Treating Persistent Nonmalignant Pain: An Overview. September 2007. Available at: http://www.ama-cmeonline.com/pain_mgmt/. Accessed March 23, 2011.

29. Nicholson B, Passik SD. Management of chronic noncancer pain in the primary care setting. South Med J 100(10):1028–1036, 2007.

30. Daut RL, Cleeland CS, Flanery RC. Development of the Wisconsin Brief Pain Questionnaire to assess pain in cancer and other diseases. Pain 17(2):197–210, 1983.

31. Bieri D, Reeve R, Champion GD, et al. The Faces Pain Scale for the self-assessment of the severity of pain experienced by children: development, initial validation and preliminary investigation for ratio scale properties. Pain 41(2):139–150, 1990.

32. Smedley BR, Stith AY, Nelson AR (eds). Committee on Understanding and Eliminating Racial and Ethnic Disparities in Health Care. Unequal Treatment: Confronting Racial and Ethnic Disparities in Health Care. Washington, DC: National Academies Press, 2002.

33. American Medical Association. Pain Management: The Online Series. Pathophysiology of Pain and Pain Assessment. Module 3. Pain Management: Barriers to Pain Management & Pain in Special Populations. September 2007. Available at: http://www.ama-cmeonline.com/pain_mgmt/. Accessed March 23, 2011.

34. Foley K. Opioids and chronic neuropathic pain. N Engl J Med 348(13):1279–1280, 2003.

35. Gilron I, Watson PN, Cahill CM, et al. Neuropathic pain: a practical guide for the clinician. CMAJ 175(3):256–275, 2006.

36. Butler SF, Budman SH, Fernandez K, et al. Validations of a screener and opioid assessment measure for patients with chronic pain. Pain 112(1–2):65–75, 2004.

37. Webster LR, Webster RM. Predicting aberrant behaviors in opioid-treated patients: preliminary validation of the Opioid Risk Tool. Pain Med 6(6):432–442, 2005.

38. American Pain Society. Definitions Related to the Use of Opioids for the Treatment of Pain. A consensus statement from the American Academy of Pain Medicine, the American Pain Society, and the American Society of Addiction Medicine, 2001. Available at: http://www.ampainsoc.org/advocacy/opioids2.htm. Accessed March 23, 2011.

Blood Pressure

Beevers G, Lip GY, O'Brien E. ABC of hypertension. Blood pressure measurement. Part I. Sphygmomanometry: factors common in all techniques. BMJ 322(7292):981–985, 2001.

Beevers G, Lip GY, O'Brien E. ABC of hypertension. Blood pressure measurement. Part II. Conventional sphygmomanometry: technique of auscultatory blood pressure measurement. BMJ 322(7293):1043–1047, 2001.

Bobrie G, Genes N, Vaur L, et al. Is "isolated home" hypertension as opposed to "isolated office" hypertension a sign of greater cardiovascular risk? Arch Intern Med 161(18):2205–2211, 2001.

McAlister FA, Straus SE. Evidence-based treatment of hypertension. Measurement of blood pressure: an evidence based review. BMJ 322:908–911, 2001.

Perry HM, Davis BR, Price TR, et al, for the Systolic Hypertension in the Elderly Program Cooperative Research Group. Effect of treating isolated systolic hypertension on the risk of developing various types and subtypes of stroke: the Systolic Hypertension in the Elderly Program (SHEP). JAMA 284(4):465–471, 2000.

Sacks FM, Svetkey LP, Vollmer WM, et al. Effects on blood pressure of reduced dietary sodium and the dietary approaches to stop hypertension (DASH) diet. N Engl J Med 344(1):3–10, 2001.

Tholl U, Forstner K, Anlauf M. Measuring blood pressure: pitfalls and recommendations. Nephrol Dial Transplant 19:766, 2004.

U.S. Preventive Services Task Force. Screening for High Blood Pressure: U.S. Preventive Services Task Force Reaffirmation Recommendation Statement. AHRQ Publication No. 08-05105-EF-2, December 2007; first published in Ann Intern Med 147:783–786, 2007, Rockville, MD. Available at: http://www.uspreventiveservicestaskforce.org/uspstf/uspshype.htm. Accessed March 23, 2011.

Vega CP. Wolves in sheep's clothing: don't ignore white-coat and masked hypertension. Medscape CME, July 7, 2009. Available at: http://www.medscape.org/viewarticle/705339. Accessed March 23, 2011.

Writing Group of the PREMIER Collaborative Research Group. Effects of comprehensive lifestyle modification on blood pressure control: main results of the PREMIER clinical trial. JAMA 289(16):2083–2093, 2003.

Acute and Chronic Pain

Caraceni A, Portenoy RK. An international survey of cancer pain characteristics and syndromes. IASP

Task Force on Cancer Pain. International Association for the Study of Pain. Pain 82(3):263–274, 1999.

Charlton JE (ed). Core Curriculum for Professional Education in Pain, 3rd ed. Seattle: International Association for the Study of Pain, 2005. Available at: http://www.iasp-pain.org/AM/Template.cfm?Section=Publications&Template=/CM/HTML Display.cfm&ContentID=2307#TOC. Accessed March 23, 2011.

Pellino TA, Willens J, Polomano RC, et al. The American Society of Pain Management Nurses practice analysis: role delineation study. Pain Manage Nurs 3(1):2–15, 2002.

Nutrition

8

LEARNING OBJECTIVES

The student will:

1. Assess the nutritional status of an individual through a nutrition history and physical examination.
2. Identify persons at risk for malnutrition or overnutrition.
3. Differentiate between normal and abnormal nutrition assessment findings.

 **OVERVIEW**

Nutritional status is a key element of overall health. Good nutrition is important for every body system. Poor nutrition may be a problem in itself (e.g., lack of vitamin D can cause rickets), or it may exacerbate an underlying disease, such as diabetes or cardiovascular disease. Low protein reserves will impede healing (e.g., from surgery). Poor nutrition in children may delay growth and contribute to cognitive issues in school. Problems in nutrition may be the result of many factors.

Weight gain occurs when caloric intake exceeds caloric expenditure over time and typically appears as increased body fat. Hypothyroidism may cause weight gain by reducing body metabolism. Weight gain may also reflect abnormal accumulation of body fluids. When the retention of fluid is mild, it may not be visible, but several pounds of fluid usually appear as edema.

Weight loss is an important symptom with many causes. Mechanisms include decreased intake of food for such reasons as anorexia, dysphagia, vomiting, diarrhea, inability to absorb nutrients from the gastrointestinal tract, increased metabolic needs, allergies to foods, problems with chewing, dislike of foods, and peer pressure. Poor food choices, inability to cook or poor cooking habits, inability to access food stores, or lack of financial resources may also cause nutrition problems. The nurse sorts through the data the patient provides to identify possible sources of problems and creates a plan of care. If the nurse finds the patient needs more testing or intense counseling, the patient should be referred to a nurse practitioner, physician, or registered dietician.

Causes of weight loss include *gastrointestinal diseases; endocrine disorders* (diabetes mellitus, hyperthyroidism, adrenal insufficiency); *chronic infections; malignancy; chronic cardiac, pulmonary, or renal failure; depression; and anorexia nervosa or bulimia* (see Table 8-1, Eating Disorders and Excessively Low BMI (p. 142)

Severe vitamin or mineral deficiencies or lack of protein, carbohydrates, or fats will produce characteristic signs and symptoms. However, it is preferred to recognize the potential deficiency in the patient's diet before signs and symptoms occur. For example, when a patient reports lactose intolerance, the nurse should assess the diet for adequate intake of calcium and vitamin D through nonmilk foods and supplements before signs of rickets develop.

Nutritional status is assessed at most nurse–patient encounters. A general screening assessment is done during a complete health assessment. If the patient's chief complaint involves nutrition or if the general screening finds unusual results, an in-depth nutrition assessment should be done. Patients admitted to long-term care facilities and patients with problems that require good nutrition to heal, such as pressure ulcers, should be thoroughly assessed. The U.S. Department of Agriculture's (USDA's) *Choose MyPlate* Web Site (http://www.choosemyplate.gov/) is a tool to help individuals analyze their diet and set goals for a healthier diet. The nurse can use the site with a patient to demonstrate how to perform a diet analysis and track individual progress. The ChooseMyPlate.gov web site includes nutrition tips, nutrition information for various populations, print materials, interactive tools as well as links to other nutrient and physical activity information.

> Weight loss with relatively high food intake suggests *diabetes mellitus, hyperthyroidism,* or *malabsorption.* Consider also binge eating (bulimia) with clandestine vomiting.

> Poverty, old age, social isolation, physical disability, emotional or mental impairment, lack of teeth, ill-fitting dentures, alcoholism, and drug abuse increase the likelihood of malnutrition.

> See Table 8-2, Nutrition Screening (p. 143)

Hydration Status

Hydration status is critical to a patient's health. Under or overhydration may accompany disease or medical treatment, such as intravenous fluid administration. The patient can die or suffer serious complications if alterations in hydration are not recognized immediately.

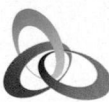

THE HEALTH HISTORY

In the general assessment the nurse assesses nutrition during the Review of Systems (ROS) and Health Patterns. Under the ROS the patient is asked about weight changes, fatigue, allergies, and problems in the gastrointestinal system, which may signal nutrition problems. Under Health Patterns the patient's nutrition and exercise patterns are elicited. These may also help the nurse identify a patient problem with nutrition. See Chapter 4, The Health History.

Common or Concerning Symptoms

- Changes in weight, usually unintended
- Anorexia
- Changes in the senses of taste or smell
- Difficulty chewing or swallowing

Changes in Weight

Changes in weight result from changes in body tissues or body fluid.

Begin with broad open-ended questions, such as "Tell me about your weight gain (loss)." Use the "OLD CART" mnemonic to ask follow-up questions.

Onset: When did you notice the change in your weight? When do you think it began?

Location: Is the weight gain (loss) distributed over your whole body or in a particular area?

Duration: Has the gain (loss) been consistent? In spurts? Have you alternated between gaining and losing weight?

Characteristic symptoms: How much weight have you gained (lost)? How does your weight compare to a year (6 months) ago? Have you experienced increased hunger (or anorexia) during this time? Do you have difficulty chewing? Has your sense of smell changed? Taste?

Assicuated manifestations: Do you tire easily? Do you often feel cold? Is your skin drier than usual? Are your ankles swollen? Have you noticed a change in the fit of your clothes? Have you changed your diet during this time? Have you changed your exercise routines or patterns of living? Who cooks for you? Who shops for you? Any change in your teeth? Dentures?

Relieving factors: Has anything helped you lose (gain) weight?

Treatment: Have you tried any diets or supplements to lose (gain) weight?

Follow up on other symptoms in a similar fashion.

Be sure to ask the patient about food allergies or intolerances, such as lactose intolerance. Ask about chronic illnesses in the patient and family, as these may be related to the nutrition problems.

If an in-depth nutrition assessment is needed, a nutrition history form is helpful. One such form is given below.

Rapid changes in weight over a few days suggest an increase or decrease in body fluids, not tissues.

Weight gain or swelling in the lower legs may indicate water retention due to peripheral vascular disease, not a nutrition problem.

● Nutrition History

Assessment Area	Sample Questions
Food pattern	How many meals/snacks are eaten a day? Which is the biggest meal?. How many meals are eaten outside the home? Where are they eaten? Is the patient on any special diet or fad diet? Are food supplements used? *(continued)*

● Nutrition History (continued)

Assessment Area	Sample Questions
Personal food preferences	Are any foods particularly liked or disliked? Are any foods the patient feels are harmful or beneficial? Are any cultural or religious preferences?
Food preparation	Who does the cooking? How are the foods prepared? What type of oil is used for frying (saturated or unsaturated)? What spices or condiments are commonly used?
Finances	Is there enough money for food? Would the patient eat any differently if more money was available? Is any supplementary financial program used?
Accessibility	Who does the shopping? When? Is there transportation to the market?
Patient health	Does the patient have any trouble with chewing or digestion? What is the bowel movement frequency? Does the patient take nutritional supplements or vitamins? What type? How much? Are there any food allergies or food intolerances? Does the patient take any medications? Does the patient drink alcohol? What type? How much? Does the patient smoke? How many packs per day? What is the patient's stress level? Does this affect appetite? Has the patient ever had hemoglobin, cholesterol, and triglyceride testing? Results? Is the patient happy with his or her health? Are there any eating disorders, heart disease, osteoporosis, diabetes, obesity, or gastrointestinal (GI) disorders?
Exercise pattern	Describe your exercise on a typical day (or week).
Body Image	Are you satisfied with your weight? What would you change about your body, if you could?
Family health	Is there any heart disease, osteoporosis, diabetes, obesity, or GI disorders in the family?
Family dietary patterns	Does anyone in the family eat a special diet? Does the family eat meals together? How often? Is mealtime a social time?

In addition to the nutrition history, the nurse should collect a sample food intake record. The nurse can ask the patient for a 24-hour recall of food and beverage intake. This is efficient if the patient can accurately remember the types and quantities of foods and beverages. If time allows, the patient can be given a sheet to record a 2-day diet intake or a weekly diary. The nurse can help the patient analyze the record at a later appointment, or if hospitalized or in a long-term care facility utilize the patient intake record.

PHYSICAL EXAMINATION

Signs of poor nutrition may occur in any body system. Usually by the time a sign appears the condition is fairly severe. See Table 8-3, Evaluating Nutritional Disorders (p. 144).

The nurse looks for signs of nutritional problems and hydration problems during the general head-to-toe physical examination. For example, assessment of the skin for nutritional deficits begins with the general survey and continues as one moves through the examination from head to toe. When a full patient examination is not necessary, the nurse can systematically look for signs of nutrition or hydration problems.

General Survey

Begin the physical examination with the patient's *height and weight* and vital signs. Note the patient's *body frame.* Is it small, medium, or large? The patient's *body mass index* (BMI) can be calculated from the height and weight. See p. 134 for how to calculate the BMI.

The proportion of weight to height can indicate whether the patient is over or underweight. Note that individuals with large muscle mass may have a falsely high calculated BMI. This must be taken into account before assuming the patient is obese or overweight.

Height Measurement

1. Have the patient remove shoes and hat.

2. Use a stadiometer attached to the wall

3. The patient should stand facing away from the wall with a straight back and the heels, hips, shoulders, and occiput aligned.

4. Record the patient's height.

5. Patients or small children who cannot stand up must be measured lying down on a firm surface, such as an examination table. Place a ruler on the crown of the head perpendicular to the bed. Use a pencil or pen to mark

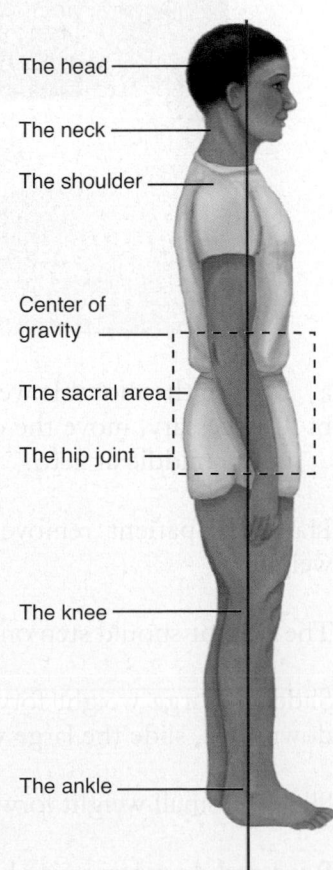

The head —
The neck —
The shoulder —
Center of gravity —
The sacral area —
The hip joint —
The knee —
The ankle —

the paper or sheet at the crown. Help the patient lay straight and mark the paper or sheet at the heel. Remove the patient or have him slide over and measure the distance between the two marks. Be sure to document that the patient's height was obtained lying down.

Weight Measurement

The balance beam scale is frequently used in health care agencies for patients who can stand up. Digital scales are used for infants and patients who cannot stand up and need chair or bed scales. Read the instructions for such scales.

Weight can vary during the day. If serial weights are needed, the patient should be weighed at the same time in the morning, on the same scale, and in the same clothing. In the hospital this is often the hospital gown.

For the balance beam scale:

1. First zero the balance beam.

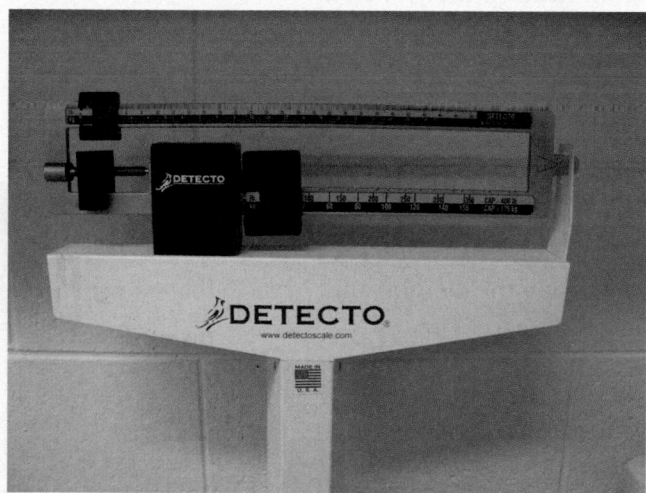

   a. Be sure the movable weights are at zero.
   b. If necessary, move the counter weights until the pointer is balanced in the middle at zero.

2. Have the patient remove shoes and outer clothing for a one-time weight.

3. The patient should step on the scale facing the balance beam.

4. Slide the large weight forward first. When the pointer is overbalanced downward, slide the large weight back to the previous notch.

5. Slide the small weight forward until the beam is balanced.

6. Read and document weight.

Skin, Hair, and Nails

Thoroughly inspect the skin for dryness, flaking, cracking, or sores that will not heal. Assess skin turgor. Inspect the hair for texture, thinning, and loss of color. Check the nails for shape and brittleness.

A pale color in fair-skinned patients or pale palms and mucous membranes in dark-skinned patients may indicate anemia.

Vitamin deficiencies may cause changes in skin, hair, and nails. See Table 8-3, Evaluating Nutrition Disorders (p. 144).

Head, Ears, Eyes, Nose, and Throat (HEENT)

Note dark circles under the eyes.

Allergies may cause circles.

Inspect the mucous membranes for dryness, color, and intactness. Note cracking at the corners of the mouth, bleeding gums, and changes in tongue color. Look for an enlarged thyroid gland.

Dry membranes indicate dehydration. Pale membranes may indicate anemia. Bleeding gums, cracking, and color changes may indicate vitamin deficiencies.

An enlarged thyroid may indicate lack of iodine or thyroid malfunction.

Cardiovascular and Peripheral Vascular

Measure pulse rate and amplitude.

Tachycardia and a weak pulse can indicate dehydration, while a bounding pulse can mean overhydration.

Inspect arms and legs for edema, petechiae, and ecchymoses.

Petechiae and ecchymoses may be due to a lack of vitamin A. Edema may be secondary to a protein deficiency or overhydration in a patient with a weak heart.

Gastrointestinal

Observe for distension and ascites. Check skin turgor on the abdomen and document findings.

Abdominal distention and ascites may be due to protein deficiency. Turgor recoil >2 seconds may indicate dehydration.

The waist circumference indicates central body fat. Waist circumference >40 inches in men and >35 inches in women is related to an increased risk for cardiovascular disease.[1]

Measure waist circumference. Place a tape measure over bare skin just above the hip bones.

Musculoskeletal

Note muscle wasting or flaccidity, bone pain, and bowing of tibia. Measure arm circumference.

Muscle wasting and flaccidity may be secondary to protein deficiency. Lack of vitamin D can cause bone pain and bowing of the legs.

Neurologic

Note changes in mental status, irritability, inability to concentrate, or paresthesias.

Dehydration and lack of vitamins may cause these symptoms.

Calculating the BMI

Use your measurements of height and weight to calculate the *Body Mass Index,* or *BMI.* Body fat consists primarily of adipose in the form of triglycerides and is stored in subcutaneous, interabdominal, and intramuscular fat deposits that are difficult to measure directly. The BMI incorporates estimated but more accurate measures of body fat than weight alone. Note that BMI criteria for overweight and obesity are not rigid cutpoints but guidelines for estimating increasing risks to patient health and well-being from both excess and low weight. For older adults, there is a disproportionate risk for undernutrition.

BMI standards are derived from two surveys: the National Health Examination Survey, consisting of three survey cycles between 1960 and 1970, and the National Health and Nutrition Examination Survey, conducted over three cycles between the 1970s and the 1990s.

There are several ways to calculate the BMI, as shown in the accompanying table. Choose the method most suited to your practice. The National Institutes of Health and the National Heart, Lung, and Blood Institute caution that people who are very muscular may have a high BMI but still be healthy.[2] Likewise, the BMI for people with low muscle mass and reduced nutrition may appear inappropriately "normal."

If the BMI is 35 or higher, measure the patient's *waist circumference.* With the patient standing, measure the waist just above the hip bones. The patient may have excess body fat if the waist measures:

- ≥35 inches for women

- ≥40 inches for men

● Methods to Calculate Body Mass Index (BMI)		
Unit of Measure	**Method of Calculation**	
Weight *in pounds,* height	(1) Body Mass Index Chart (see table on page 135)	
in inches	(2) $\left(\dfrac{\text{Weight (lbs)} \times 700*}{\text{Height (inches)}} \right)$ $\dfrac{}{\text{Height (inches)}}$	*(continued)*

● Methods to Calculate Body Mass Index (BMI) (continued)

Unit of Measure	Method of Calculation
Weight *in kilograms,* height *in meters squared*	(3) $\dfrac{\text{Weight (kg)}}{\text{Height (m}^2)}$
	(4) "BMI Calculator" at Web site www.nhlbisupport.com/bmi/bmicalc.htm

*Several organizations use 704.5, but the variation in BMI is negligible. Conversion formulas: 2.2 lbs = 1 kg; 1.0 inch = 2.54 cm; 100 cm = 1 meter.
(Source: National Institutes of Health and National Heart, Lung, and Blood Institute: Body Mass Index Calculator. Available at: http://www.nhlbisupport.com/bmi/bmicalc.htm. Accessed March 21, 2011.

● Body Mass Index Table

	Normal						Overweight						Obese							
BMI	19	20	21	22	23	24	25	26	27	28	29	30	31	32	33	34	35	36	37	38	39
Height (inches)							Body Weight (pounds)														
58	91	96	100	105	110	115	119	124	129	134	138	143	148	153	158	162	167	172	177	181	186
59	94	99	104	109	114	119	124	128	133	138	143	148	153	158	163	168	173	178	183	188	193
60	97	102	107	112	118	123	128	133	138	143	148	153	158	163	168	174	179	184	189	194	199
61	100	106	111	116	122	127	132	137	143	148	153	158	164	169	174	180	185	190	195	201	206
62	104	109	115	120	126	131	136	142	147	153	158	164	169	175	180	186	191	196	202	207	213
63	107	113	118	124	130	135	141	146	152	158	163	169	175	180	186	191	197	203	208	214	220
64	110	116	122	128	134	140	145	151	157	163	169	174	180	186	192	197	204	209	215	221	227
65	114	120	126	132	138	144	150	156	162	168	174	180	186	192	198	204	210	216	222	228	234
66	118	124	130	136	142	148	155	161	167	173	179	186	192	198	204	210	216	223	229	235	241
67	121	127	134	140	146	153	159	166	172	178	185	191	198	204	211	217	223	230	236	242	249
68	125	131	138	144	151	158	164	171	177	184	190	197	203	210	216	223	230	236	243	249	256
69	128	135	142	149	155	162	169	176	182	189	196	203	209	216	223	230	236	243	250	257	263
70	132	139	146	153	160	167	174	181	188	195	202	209	216	222	229	236	243	250	257	264	271
71	136	143	150	157	165	172	179	186	193	200	208	215	222	229	236	243	250	257	265	272	279
72	140	147	154	162	169	177	184	191	199	206	213	221	228	235	242	250	258	265	272	279	287
73	144	151	159	166	174	182	189	197	204	212	219	227	235	242	250	257	265	272	280	288	295
74	148	155	163	171	179	186	194	202	210	218	225	233	241	249	256	264	272	280	287	295	303
75	152	160	168	176	184	192	200	208	216	224	232	240	248	256	264	272	279	287	295	303	311
76	156	164	172	180	189	197	205	213	221	230	238	246	254	263	271	279	287	295	304	312	320

(Source: Adapted from National Institutes of Health and National Heart, Lung, and Blood Institute: Clinical Guidelines on the Identification, Evaluation and Treatment of Overweight and Obesity in Adults: The Evidence Report. June 1998. Available at: www.nhlbi.nih.gov/guidelines/obesity/bmi_tbl.pdf. Accessed March 20, 2011.)

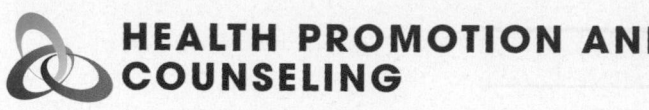

HEALTH PROMOTION AND COUNSELING

Important Topics for Health Promotion and Counseling

- Optimal weight, nutrition, and diet
- Exercise
- Hydration

Optimal Weight, Nutrition, and Diet

Fewer than half of U.S. adults maintain a healthy weight, with a BMI of 19 or above but less than 25. Obesity has increased in every segment of the U.S. population, regardless of age, gender, ethnicity, or socioeconomic status. Review the alarming statistics about the rising prevalence of obesity nationally and worldwide in the table below.

See Table 8-4, Obesity-Related Risk Factors and Diseases (p. 145).

● Obesity at a Glance

- More than 60% of U.S. adults are overweight or obese (BMI >25).
- More than 14% of U.S. children and adolescents are overweight.
- Health disparities: the prevalence of being overweight or obese is higher in selected ethnic and income groups:
  - Women: black women—69%; white women—47%
  - Women: women with an income <130% of the poverty threshold are 50% more likely to be obese than those at higher income levels
  - Men: black men—58%; white men—62%
  - Adolescents: highest prevalence in Mexican-American boys, black girls, and white boys from lower-income families
- Overweight and obesity increase risk of heart disease, numerous types of cancers, type 2 diabetes, stroke, arthritis, sleep apnea, and depression.
- More than 50% of people with non–insulin-dependent diabetes and 20% of people with hypertension or elevated cholesterol are overweight or obese.
- Obesity is increasing worldwide: although being poor in the world's poorest countries is associated with underweight and malnutrition, being poor in a middle-income country adopting a Western lifestyle is associated with increased risk of obesity.
- Only 42% of obese U.S. adults report that health care professionals have advised them to lose weight.

(Sources: Surgeon General, U.S. Department of Health and Human Services. Surgeon General's Call to Action to Prevent and Decrease Overweight and Obesity. Overweight and Obesity: At a Glance. Available at: http://www.surgeongeneral.gov/topics/obesity/calltoaction/fact_glance.html. Accessed May 19, 2011; McTigue KM, Harris R, Hemphill B, et al. Screening and interventions for obesity in adults: summary of the evidence for the U.S. Preventive Services Task Force. Ann Intern Med 139[11]:933–949, 2003; Hossain P, Kawar B, El Hahas M. Obesity and diabetes in the developing world: a growing challenge. N Engl J Med 356[3]: 213–215, 2007.)

To promote optimal patient weight and nutrition, adopt the four-pronged approach outlined below. Even reducing weight by 5% to 10% can improve blood pressure, lipid levels, and glucose tolerance and reduce the risk of diabetes or hypertension.

TIPS FOR PROMOTING OPTIMAL WEIGHT AND NUTRITION

- Measure BMI and waist circumference; identify risk of overweight and obesity.
- Establish additional risk factors for heart disease and obesity-related diseases.
- Assess dietary intake.
- Assess the patient's motivation to change; provide counseling about nutrition and exercise.

See Table 8-5, Obesity: Stages of Change Model and Assessing Readiness (p. 146).

Take advantage of the excellent resources available for patient assessment and counseling summarized in the following sections. Review the role of weight in the growing prevalence of *metabolic syndrome* in chapter 14, The Cardiovascular System.

See Table 8-4, Obesity-Related Risk Factors and Diseases (p. 145).

Responding to the BMI. Classify the BMI according to the national guidelines in the following table. If the BMI is *above 25*, assess the patient for *additional risk factors* for heart disease and other obesity-related diseases: hypertension, high low-density lipoprotein (LDL) cholesterol, low high-density lipoprotein (HDL) cholesterol, high triglycerides, high blood glucose, family history of premature heart disease, physical inactivity, and cigarette smoking. Patients with a BMI over 25 and two or more risk factors should pursue weight loss, especially if the waist circumference is elevated.

● Classification of Overweight and Obesity by BMI

	Obesity Class	BMI (kg/m²)
Underweight		<18.5
Normal		18.5–24.9
Overweight		25.0–29.9
Obesity	I	30.0–34.9
	II	35.0–39.9
Extreme obesity	III	≥40

(Source: National Institutes of Health and National Heart, Lung, and Blood Institute: Clinical Guidelines on the Identification, Evaluation, and Treatment of Overweight and Obesity in Adults: The Evidence Report. NIH Publication 98-4083. June 1998.)

Assessing Dietary Intake. Advising patients about diet and weight loss is important, especially in light of the many, often contradictory dieting options in the popular press. Review three excellent guidelines for counseling your patients:

See Table 8-6, Healthy Eating: U.S.D.A. MyPlate (p. 147).

● National Institutes of Health and National Heart, Lung, and Blood Institute. Clinical Guidelines on the Identification, Evaluation, and Treatment of Overweight and Obesity in Adults. Available at: http://www.nhlbi.nih.gov/guidelines/obesity. Accessed May 19, 2011.[2]

● U.S. Preventive Services Task Force. Screening for Obesity in Adults: Recommendations and Rationale. Rockville, MD: Agency for Healthcare Research and Quality, November 2003. Available at: http://www.uspreventiveservicestaskforce.org/uspstf/uspsobes.htm. Accessed May 19, 2011.[3]

● U.S. Department of Health and Human Services and U.S. Department of Agriculture. Dietary Guidelines for Americans 2010. Available at: http://www.health.gov/dietaryguidelines/dga2010/DietaryGuidelines 2010.pdf. Accessed May 19, 2011.[4]

Diet recommendations hinge on assessment of the patient's motivation and readiness to lose weight and individual risk factors. The *Clinical Guidelines on the Identification, Evaluation, and Treatment of Overweight and Obesity in Adults*[2] recommend the following general guidelines:

● A 10% weight reduction over 6 months, or a decrease of 300 to 500 kcal/day, for people with BMIs between 27 and 35

● A weight loss goal of ½ to 1 pound per week because more rapid weight loss does not lead to better results at 1 year.[3]

These guidelines recommend low-calorie diets of 800 to 1500 kcal per day. Interventions that combine nutrition education, diet, and moderate exercise (see Moderate and Vigorous Exercise Table on page140) with behavioral strategies are most likely to succeed. The *Clinical Guidelines* cite evidence supporting the role of moderate physical activity in weight loss and weight loss maintenance programs: it enhances and may assist with maintenance of weight; it increases cardiorespiratory fitness; and it may decrease abdominal fat.

If the BMI falls *below 18.5*, be concerned about possible anorexia nervosa, bulimia, or other medical conditions. These conditions are summarized in Table 8-1, Eating Disorders and Excessively Low BMI (p. 142).

Once you have assessed food intake, nutritional status, and motivation to adopt healthy eating behaviors or lose weight, give patients the "nine major messages" of the Dietary Guidelines for Americans 2010, as summarized and adapted on page 139.

See Table 8-6, Healthy Eating: U.S.D.A. MyPlate, p. 147.

PROMOTING PATIENT HEALTH: NINE KEY MESSAGES[4]

- Consume a variety of foods within and among the basic food groups while staying within energy needs.
- Control caloric intake and portion size to manage body weight.
- Maintain moderate physical activity for at least 30 minutes each day, for example, walking 3 to 4 miles per hour.
- Increase daily intake of fruits and vegetables, whole grains, and nonfat or low-fat milk and milk products.
- Choose fats wisely, keeping intake of saturated fat, *trans* fat found in partially hydrogenated vegetable oils, and cholesterol low.
- Choose carbohydrates—sugars, starches, and fibers—wisely for good health.
- Choose and prepare foods with little salt.
- If you drink alcoholic beverages, do so in moderation.
- Keep food safe to eat.

Be prepared to help adolescent females and women of childbearing age increase intake of iron and folic acid. Assist adults older than 50 years to identify foods rich in vitamin B_{12} and calcium. Advise older adults and those with dark skin or low exposure to sunlight to increase intake of vitamin D.

See Table 8-7, Nutrition Counseling: Sources of Nutrients (p. 148).

Blood Pressure and Diet. With respect to blood pressure, there is reliable evidence that regular and frequent exercise, decreased sodium intake, increased potassium intake, and maintenance of a healthy weight reduce the risk for developing hypertension as well as lower blood pressure in adults who are already hypertensive. Explain to patients that most dietary sodium comes from salt (sodium chloride). The recommended daily allowance (RDA) of sodium is less than 2400 mg, or 1 teaspoon, per day. However, individuals with hypertension, ≥40 years or are African-American should consume no more than 1500 mg. sodium per day.[7] Patients need to read food labels closely, especially the Nutrition Facts panel. Low-sodium foods are those with sodium listed at <5% of the RDA of 2400 mg or less. For nutritional interventions to reduce the risk for cardiac disease, refer to Chapter 14, The Cardiovascular System.

See Table 8-8, Patients With Hypertension: Recommended Changes in Diet (p. 148).

Exercise

Fitness is a key component of both weight control and weight loss. Currently, 30 minutes of moderate activity, defined as walking 2 miles in 30 minutes on most days of the week or its equivalent, is recommended. However, recent research has discovered that if a middle-aged or older woman with a normal body mass index wants to maintain her weight over an extended period, she must engage in the equivalent of 60 minutes per day of physical activity at a moderate intensity. Overweight women must restrict their caloric intake in addition to exercise to achieve weight loss.[5]

Patients can increase exercise by such simple measures as parking farther away from their place of work or using stairs instead of elevators. A safe goal for weight loss is ½ to 2 pounds per week.

● **Moderate and Vigorous Exercise**

A 154-pound man (5′10″) will use up about the number of calories listed doing each activity below. **Those who weigh more will use more calories, and those who weigh less will use fewer.** The calorie values listed include both calories used by the activity and calories used for normal body functioning.

	Approximate Calories Used by a 154-pound Man	
	In 1 hour	In 30 minutes
Moderate Physical Activities:		
Hiking	370	185
Light gardening/yard work	330	165
Dancing	330	165
Golf (walking and carrying clubs)	330	165
Bicycling (<10 miles per hour)	290	145
Walking (3½ miles per hour)	280	140
Weight training (general light workout)	220	110
Stretching	180	90
Vigorous Physical Activities:		
Running/jogging (5 miles per hour)	590	295
Bicycling (more than 10 miles per hour)	590	295
Swimming (slow freestyle laps)	510	255
Aerobics	480	240
Walking (4½ miles per hour)	460	230
Heavy yard work (chopping wood)	440	220
Weight lifting (vigorous effort)	440	220
Basketball (vigorous)	440	220

(Source: U.S. Department of Agriculture: Inside the Pyramid—Calories Used. Available at: http://www.mypyramid.gov/pyramid/calories_used_table.html. Accessed September 5, 2010.)

Hydration

According to the Report of the Dietary Guidelines Advisory Committee on the Dietary Guidelines for Americans, "In order to prevent dehydration, water must be consumed daily. Healthy individuals who have routine access to fluids and who are not exposed to heat stress consume adequate water to meet their needs. Purposeful drinking is warranted for individuals who are exposed to heat stress or who perform sustained vigorous physical activity. Although uncommon, heat waves are one setting of extreme heat stress that increases the risk of morbidity and mortality from dehydration, especially in older-aged persons. In view of the ongoing obesity epidemic, individuals are encouraged to drink water and other fluids with few or no calories.

"Based on an extensive review of evidence, an Institute Of Medicine (IOM) panel in 2004 concluded that the combination of thirst and usual drinking behavior, especially the consumption of fluids with meals, is sufficient to maintain normal hydration. However, because water needs vary considerably and because there is no evidence of chronic dehydration in the general population, a minimum intake of water cannot be set."[6]

Individuals with limited ability to obtain fluids for themselves, such as persons with disabilities, older adults in nursing homes, or persons confined to a bed, are at increased risk for dehydration. These patients' hydration status should be assessed at least daily and appropriate fluids provided.

TABLE
8-1

Eating Disorders and Excessively Low BMI

In the United States an estimated 5 to 10 million women and 1 million men suffer from eating disorders. These severe disturbances of eating behavior are often difficult to detect, especially in teens wearing baggy clothes or in individuals who binge and then induce vomiting or evacuation. Be familiar with the two principal eating disorders, anorexia nervosa and bulimia nervosa. Both conditions are characterized by distorted perceptions of body image and weight. Early detection is important, because prognosis improves when treatment occurs in the early stages of these disorders.

Clinical Features

Anorexia Nervosa

- Refusal to maintain minimally normal body weight (or BMI above 17.5 kg/m^2)
- Afraid of appearing fat
- Frequently starving but in denial; lacking insight
- Often brought in by family members
- Initial symptoms may be failure to make expected weight gains in childhood or adolescence, amenorrhea in women, loss of libido or potency in men
- Associated with depressive symptoms such as depressed mood, irritability, social withdrawal, insomnia, decreased libido
- Additional features supporting diagnosis: self-induced vomiting or purging, excessive exercise, use of appetite suppressants and/or diuretics
- Biologic complications
  - *Neuroendocrine changes:* amenorrhea, increased corticotropin-releasing factor, cortisol, growth hormone, serotonin; decreased diurnal cortisol fluctuation, luteinizing hormone, follicle-stimulating hormone, thyroid-stimulating hormone
  - *Cardiovascular disorders:* bradycardia, hypotension, arrhythmias, cardiomyopathy
  - *Metabolic disorders:* hypokalemia, hypochloremic metabolic alkalosis, increased BUN, edema
  - *Other:* dry skin, dental caries, delayed gastric emptying, constipation, anemia, osteoporosis

Bulimia Nervosa

- Repeated binge eating followed by self-induced vomiting; misuse of laxatives, diuretics, or other medications; fasting; or excessive exercise
- Often with normal weight
- Overeating at least twice a week during 3-month period; large amounts of food consumed in short period (~2 hours)
- Preoccupation with eating; craving and compulsion to eat; lack of control over eating; alternating with periods of starvation
- Dread of fatness but may be obese
- Subtypes of
  - *Purging:* bulimic episodes accompanied by self-induced vomiting or use of laxatives, diuretics, or enemas
  - *Nonpurging:* bulimic episodes accompanied by compensatory behavior such as fasting, exercise, but without purging
- Biologic complications
  See changes listed for anorexia nervosa, especially weakness, fatigue, mild cognitive disorder; also erosion of dental enamel, parotitis, pancreatic inflammation with elevated amylase, mild neuropathies, seizures, hypokalemia, hypochloremic metabolic acidosis, hypomagnesemia

(Sources: World Health Organization: The ICD-10 Classification of Mental and Behavioral Disorders: Diagnostic Criteria for Research. Geneva: World Health Organization, 1993. American Psychiatric Association: DSM-IV-TR: Diagnostic and Statistical Manual of Mental Disorders, 4th ed. Washington, DC: American Psychiatric Association, 1994. Halmi KA. Eating disorders: In: Kaplan HI, Sadock BJ, eds. Comprehensive Textbook of Psychiatry, 7th ed. Philadelphia: Lippincott Williams & Wilkins, 2000:1663–1676. Mehler PS. Bulimia nervosa. N Engl J Med 349[9]:875–880, 2003.)

Nutrition Screening

Nutrition Screening Checklist

I have an illness or condition that made me change the kind and/or amount of food I eat.	Yes (2 pts) ____
I eat fewer than 2 meals per day.	Yes (3 pts) ____
I eat few fruits or vegetables, or milk products.	Yes (2 pts) ____
I have 3 or more drinks of beer, liquor, or wine almost every day.	Yes (2 pts) ____
I have tooth or mouth problems that make it hard for me to eat.	Yes (2 pts) ____
I don't always have enough money to buy the food I need.	Yes (4 pts) ____
I eat alone most of the time.	Yes (1 pt) ____
I take 3 or more different prescribed or over-the-counter drugs each day.	Yes (1 pt) ____
Without wanting to, I have lost or gained 10 pounds in the last 6 months.	Yes (2 pts) ____
I am not always physically able to shop, cook, and/or feed myself.	Yes (2 pts) ____
	TOTAL ____

Instructions. Check "yes" for each condition that applies, then total the nutritional score. For total scores of 3–5 points (moderate risk) or ≥6 points (high risk), further evaluation is needed (especially for the elderly).

Rapid Screen for Dietary Intake

	Portions Consumed by Patient	Recommended
Grains, cereals, bread group	____	6–11
Fruit group	____	2–4
Vegetable group	____	3–5
Meat/meat substitute group	____	2–3
Dairy group	____	2–3
Sugars, fats, snack foods	____	—
Soft drinks	____	—
Alcoholic beverages	____	<2

Instructions. Ask the patient for a 24-hour dietary recall (or a 2-day diet intake) before completing the form.

(Sources: *Nutrition Screening*—American Academy of Family Physicians. Bagley, B. Editorials: Nutrition and Health. Available at: http://www.aafp.org/afp/980301ap/edits.html. Accessed May 19, 2011; *Rapid Screen for Dietary Intake*—Nestle M. Nutrition. In: Woolf SH, Jonas S, Lawrence RS, eds. Health Promotion and Disease Prevention in Clinical Practice. Baltimore: Williams & Wilkins, 1996.)

Evaluating Nutritional Disorders

This chart can help you interpret your nutritional assessment findings. Body systems are listed below with signs or symptoms and the implications for each.

Body system or region	Sign or symptom	Implications
General	• Weakness and fatigue • Weight loss	• Anemia or electrolyte imbalance • Decreased calorie intake, increased calorie use, or inadequate nutrient intake or absorption
Skin, hair, and nails	• Dry, flaky skin • Dry skin with poor turgor • Rough, scaly skin with bumps • Petechiae or ecchymoses • Sore that won't heal • Thinning, dry hair • Spoon-shaped, brittle, or ridged nails	• Vitamin A, vitamin B-complex, or linoleic acid deficiency • Dehydration • Vitamin A deficiency • Vitamin C or K deficiency • Protein, vitamin C, or zinc deficiency • Protein deficiency • Iron deficiency
Eyes	• Night blindness; corneal swelling, softening, or dryness; Bitot's spots (gray triangular patches on the conjunctiva) • Red conjunctiva	• Vitamin A deficiency • Riboflavin deficiency
Throat and mouth	• Cracks at the corner of the mouth • Magenta tongue • Beefy, red tongue • Soft, spongy, bleeding gums • Swollen neck (goiter)	• Riboflavin or niacin deficiency • Riboflavin deficiency • Vitamin B_{12} deficiency • Vitamin C deficiency • Iodine deficiency
Cardiovascular	• Edema • Tachycardia, hypotension	• Protein deficiency • Fluid volume deficit
GI	• Ascites	• Protein deficiency
Musculoskeletal	• Bone pain and bow leg • Muscle wasting	• Vitamin D or calcium deficiency • Protein, carbohydrate, and fat deficiency
Neurologic	• Altered mental status • Paresthesia	• Dehydration and thiamine or vitamin B_{12} deficiency • Vitamin B_{12}, pyridoxine, or thiamine deficiency

TABLE 8-4

Obesity-Related Risk Factors and Diseases

Cardiovascular

- Hypertension
- Congestive heart failure
- Cor pulmonale
- Varicose veins
- Pulmonary embolism
- Coronary artery disease

Endocrine

- The metabolic syndrome
- Type 2 diabetes
- Dyslipidemia
- Polycystic ovarian syndrome/androgenicity
- Amenorrhea/infertility/menstrual disorders

Gastrointestinal

- Gastroesophageal reflux disease (GERD)
- Nonalcoholic fatty liver disease (NAFLD)
- Cholelithiasis
- Hernias
- Colon cancer

Genitourinary

- Urinary stress incontinence
- Obesity-related glomerulopathy
- Hypogonadism (male)
- Breast and uterine cancers
- Pregnancy complications

Integument

- Striae distensae (stretch marks)
- Status pigmentation of legs
- Lymphedema
- Cellulitis
- Intertrigo, carbuncles
- Acanthosis nigricans/skin tags

Musculoskeletal

- Hyperuricemia and gout
- Immobility
- Osteoarthritis (knees, hips)
- Low back pain

Neurologic

- Stroke
- Idiopathic intracranial hypertension
- Meralgia paresthetica

Psychological

- Depression/low self-esteem
- Body image disturbance
- Social stigmatization

Respiratory

- Dyspnea
- Obstructive sleep apnea
- Hypoventilation syndrome
- Pickwickian syndrome
- Asthma

(Source: American Medical Association. Roadmaps for Clinical Practice—Case Studies in Disease Prevention and Health Promotion—Assessment and Management of Adult Obesity: A Primer for Physicians. Available at: http://www.ama-assn.org/ama/pub/physician-resources/public-health/general-resources-health-care-professionals/roadmaps-clinical-practice-series/assessment-management-adult-obesity.page. Accessed May 19, 2011.)

TABLE
8-5

Obesity: Stages of Change Model and Assessing Readiness

Stage	Characteristic	Patient Verbal Cue	Appropriate Intervention	Sample Dialogue
Precontemplation	Unaware of problem, no interest in change	"I'm not really interested in weight loss. It's not a problem."	Provide information about health risks and benefits of weight loss	"Would you like to read some information about the health aspects of obesity?"
Contemplation	Aware of problem, beginning to think of changing	"I know I need to lose weight, but with all that's going on in my life right now, I'm not sure I can."	Help resolve ambivalence; discuss barriers	"Let's look at the benefits of weight loss, as well as what you may need to change."
Preparation	Realizes benefits of making changes and thinking about how to change	"I have to lose weight, and I'm planning to do that."	Teach behavior modification; provide education	"Let's take a closer look at how you can reduce some of the calories you eat and how to increase your activity during the day."
Action	Actively taking steps toward change	"I'm doing my best. This is harder than I thought."	Provide support and guidance, with a focus on the long term	"It's terrific that you're working so hard. What problems have you had so far? How have you solved them?"
Maintenance	Initial treatment goals reached	"I've learned a lot through this process."	Relapse control	"What situations continue to tempt you to overeat? What can be helpful for the next time you face such a situation?"

(Sources: American Medical Association. Roadmaps for Clinical Practice—Case Studies in Disease Prevention and Health Promotion—Assessment and Management of Adult Obesity: A Primer for Physicians. Available at: http://www.ama-assn.org/ama/pub/physician-resources/public-health/general-resources-health-care-professionals/roadmaps-clinical-practice-series/assessment-management-adult-obesity.page. Accessed May 19, 2011. Adapted from Prochaska JO, DiClemente CC. Toward a comprehensive model of change. In: Miller WR, ed. Treating Addictive Behaviors. New York: Plenum, 1986:3–27.)

TABLE 8-6

Healthy Eating: U.S.D.A. MyPlate

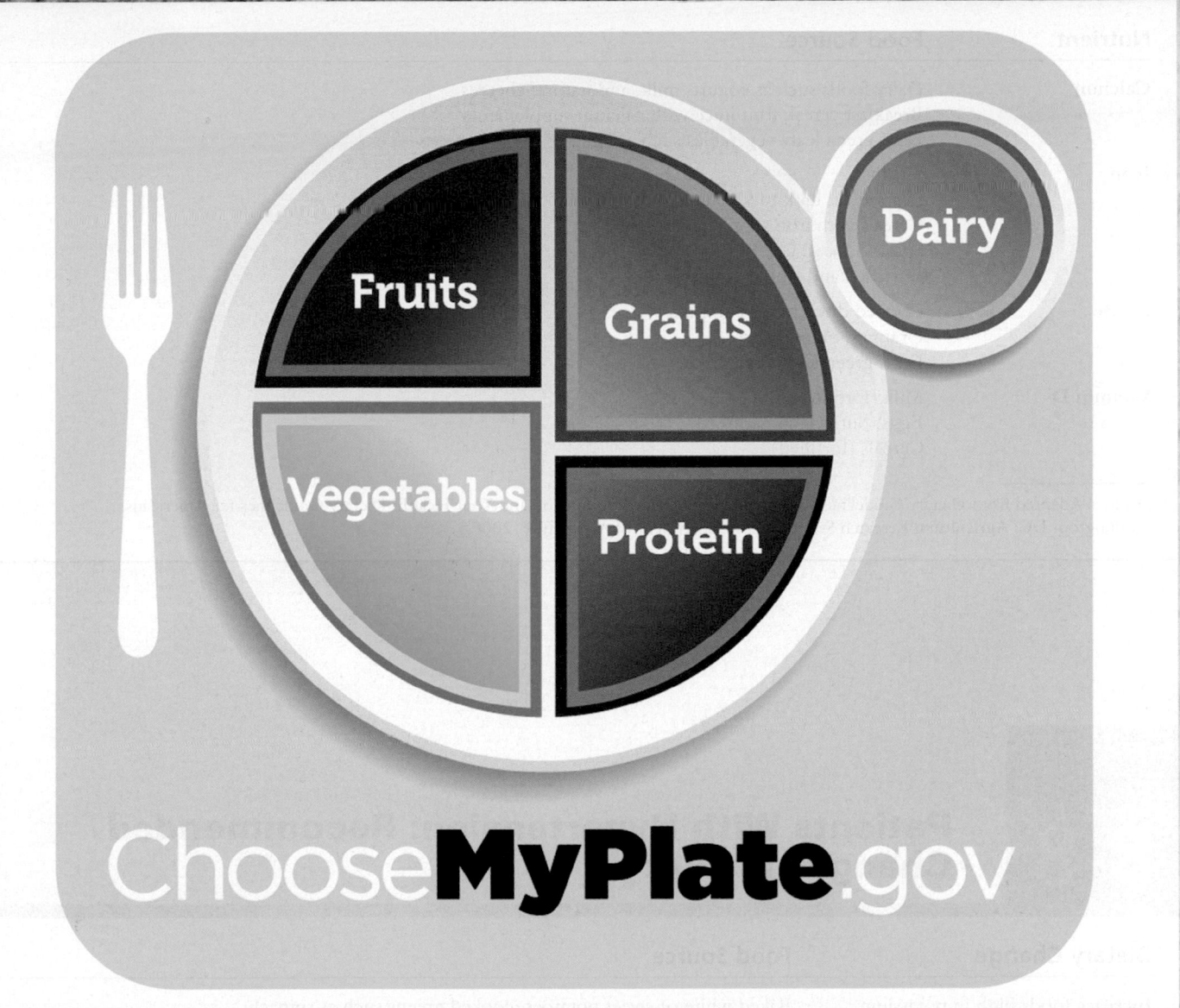

TABLE
8-7

Nutrition Counseling: Sources of Nutrients

Nutrient	Food Source
Calcium	Dairy foods such as yogurt, milk, and natural cheeses Breakfast cereal, fruit juice with calcium supplements Dark green leafy vegetables such as collards, turnip greens
Iron	Shellfish Lean meat, dark turkey meat Cereals with iron supplements Spinach, peas, lentils Enriched and whole-grain bread
Folate	Cooked dried beans and peas Oranges, orange juice Dark-green leafy vegetables
Vitamin D	Milk (fortified) Eggs, butter, margarine Cereals (fortified)

(Source: Adapted from Dietary Guidelines Committee, 2000 Report. Nutrition and Your Health: Dietary Guidelines for Americans. Washington, DC: Agricultural Research Service, U.S. Department of Agriculture, 2000.)

TABLE
8-8

Patients With Hypertension: Recommended Changes in Diet

Dietary Change	Food Source
Increase foods high in potassium	Baked white or sweet potatoes, cooked greens such as spinach Bananas, plantains, many dried fruits, orange juice
Decrease foods high in sodium	Canned foods (soups, tuna fish) Pretzels, potato chips, pickles, olives Many processed foods (frozen dinners, ketchup, mustard) Batter-fried foods Table salt, including for cooking

(Source: Adapted from Dietary Guidelines Committee, 2000 Report. Nutrition and Your Health: Dietary Guidelines for Americans. Washington, DC: Agricultural Research Service, U.S. Department of Agriculture, 2000.)

BIBLIOGRAPHY

CITATIONS

1. National Institutes of Health and National Heart, Lung, and Blood Institute. Guidelines on Overweight and Obesity: Electronic Textbook. Available at: http://www.nhlbi.nih.gov/guidelines/obesity/e_txtbk/txgd/4142.htm. Accessed March 21, 2011

2. National Institutes of Health and National Heart, Lung, and Blood Institute. Clinical Guidelines on the Identification, Evaluation, and Treatment of Overweight and Obesity in Adults. Available at: http://www.nhlbi.nih.gov/guidelines/obesity. Accessed May 19, 2011.

3. U.S. Preventive Services Task Force. Screening for Obesity in Adults: Recommendations and Rationale. Rockville, MD, Agency for Healthcare Research and Quality, November 2003. Available at: http://www.uspreventiveservicestaskforce.org/uspstf/uspsobes.htm. Accessed May 19, 2011.

4. U.S. Department of Health and Human Services and U.S. Department of Agriculture. Dietary Guidelines for Americans 2005. Available at: http://www.health.gov/dietaryguidelines/dga2010/DietaryGuidelines2010.pdf. Accessed May 19, 2011.

5. Lee I-M, Djoussé L; Sesso HD, et al. Physical activity and weight gain prevention. JAMA 303(12):1173–1179, 2010.

6. Report of the Dietary Guidelines Advisory Committee on the Dietary Guidelines for Americans, Part D, Section 6: Sodium, Potassium, and Water 2010. http://www.cnpp.usda.gov/Publications/DietaryGuidelines/2010/DGAC/Report/D-6-SodiumPotassiumWater.pdf#xml=http://65.216.150.153/texis/search/pdfhi.txt?query=water+requirement&pr=MyPyramid&rdepth=0&sufs=2&order=r&cq=&id=4c33cad817. Accessed May 19, 2011.

7. Center for Disease Control and Prevention. CDC Features: Most Americans Should Consume Less Sodium (1,500 mg./Day or Less. Available at: http://www.cdc.gov/Features/Sodium/. Accessed March 21, 2011.

ADDITIONAL REFERENCES

1. Nutrition Made Incredibly Easy, 2nd ed. Phila: Lippincott Williams & Wilkins, 2007.

2. Surgeon General, U.S. Department of Health and Human Services. Surgeon General's Call to Action to Prevent and Decrease Overweight and Obesity. Overweight and Obesity: At a Glance. Available at: http://www.surgeongeneral.gov/topics/obesity/calltoaction/fact_glance.html. Accessed May 19, 2011.

3. McTigue KM, Harris R, Hemphill B, et al. Screening and interventions for obesity in adults: summary of the evidence for the U.S. Preventive Services Task Force. Ann Intern Med 139(11): 933–949, 2003.

4. Hossain P, Kawar B, El Hahas M. Obesity and diabetes in the developing world: a growing challenge. N Engl J Med 356(3): 213–215, 2007.

5. American Heart Association. Heart Disease and Stroke Statistics, 2010 Update. Available at: http://my.americanheart.org/professional/General/Heart-Disease-and-Stroke-Statistics-2010-Update_UCM_423970_Article.jsp; and Cardiovascular Disease Statistics. Available at: http://www.americanheart.org/presenter.jhtml?identifier=4478). See also: National Center for Health Statistics. Fast Stats A to Z. Available at: http://www.cdc.gov/nchs/fastats/heart.htm. Accessed May 19, 2011.

6. Chobanian AV, Bakris GL, Black HR, et al. The Seventh Report of the Joint National Committee on Prevention, Detection, Evaluation, and Treatment of High Blood Pressure—The JNC 7 Report. JAMA 289(19):2560–2572, 2003. Available at: http://www.nhlbi.nih.gov/guidelines/hypertension/. Accessed May 19, 2011.

Body Systems

2

CHAPTER 9
The Integumentary System

CHAPTER 16
The Gastrointestinal and Renal Systems

CHAPTER 10
The Head and Neck

CHAPTER 17
The Breasts and Axillae

CHAPTER 11
The Eyes

CHAPTER 18
The Musculoskeletal System

CHAPTER 12
Ears, Nose, Mouth, and Throat

CHAPTER 19
Mental Status

CHAPTER 13
The Respiratory System

CHAPTER 20
The Nervous System

CHAPTER 14
The Cardiovascular System

CHAPTER 21
Reproductive Systems

CHAPTER 15
The Peripheral Vascular System and Lymphatic System

CHAPTER 22
Putting It All Together

CHAPTER 9

The Integumentary System

LEARNING OBJECTIVES

The student will:

1. Identify the structures of the skin, nails, and hair.
2. Explain the functions of the integumentary system.
3. Identify risk factors for pressure ulcers.
4. Identify risk factors for skin cancer.
5. Obtain an accurate history of the integumentary system.
6. Appropriately prepare and position the patient for the integumentary examination.
7. Describe the equipment necessary to perform an integumentary examination.
8. Correctly perform an integumentary examination.
9. Accurately describe primary, secondary, and vascular lesions.
10. Discuss risk reduction and health promotion strategies to reduce skin cancer.

Intact and functioning skin is essential for the life and health of the patient. The skin is the largest and heaviest organ of the body, accounting for approximately 16% of body weight and covering an area of roughly 1.2 to 2.3 m².

Nursing assessment of the integumentary system is frequently superficial, unless the patient has a significant problem, such as third-degree burns. A thorough integumentary assessment requires time; turning heavy, unconscious, or uncooperative patients in order to perform the assessment may be difficult during a busy shift. For the nurse, assessment of the skin is much more than discovering skin lesions or diseases. Examination of the skin can reveal signs of systemic diseases, medication side effects, dehydration, overhydration, or physical abuse; allow early identification of potentially cancerous lesions and risk factors for pressure ulcer formation; and identify the need for hygiene and health promotion education.

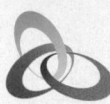 ANATOMY AND PHYSIOLOGY

The major function of the skin is to keep the body in homeostasis despite daily assaults from the environment. The skin

1. **provides a barrier** protecting the body from

    a. injury secondary to mechanical, chemical, thermal, and ultraviolet (UV) light sources.

    b. penetration by microorganisms.

    c. loss of water and electrolytes, thereby preventing dehydration.

2. **regulates body temperature** by allowing heat dissipation through sweat glands and heat storage through subcutaneous insulation.

3. **synthesizes vitamin D** from cholesterol by the action of UV light.

4. has end sensory organs for touch, pain, temperature, and pressure allowing **sensory perception.**

5. **provides nonverbal communication,** such as posture, facial movements, or vasomotor responses such as blushing.

6. **provides identity** through skin color and facial features.

7. **allows wound repair** through cell replacement of surface injuries.

8. **allows excretion of metabolic wastes,** such as electrolytes, minerals, sugar, or uric acid.

Hair, nails, and sebaceous and sweat glands are considered appendages of the skin. The skin and its appendages undergo many changes during aging. Turn to Chapter 24, Assessing Older Adults (pp. 895–896), to review normal and abnormal changes of the skin with aging.

Skin. The skin contains three layers: the epidermis, the dermis, and the subcutaneous tissues.

The most superficial layer, the *epidermis,* is thin, devoid of blood vessels, and itself divided into two layers: an outer horny layer of dead keratinized cells and

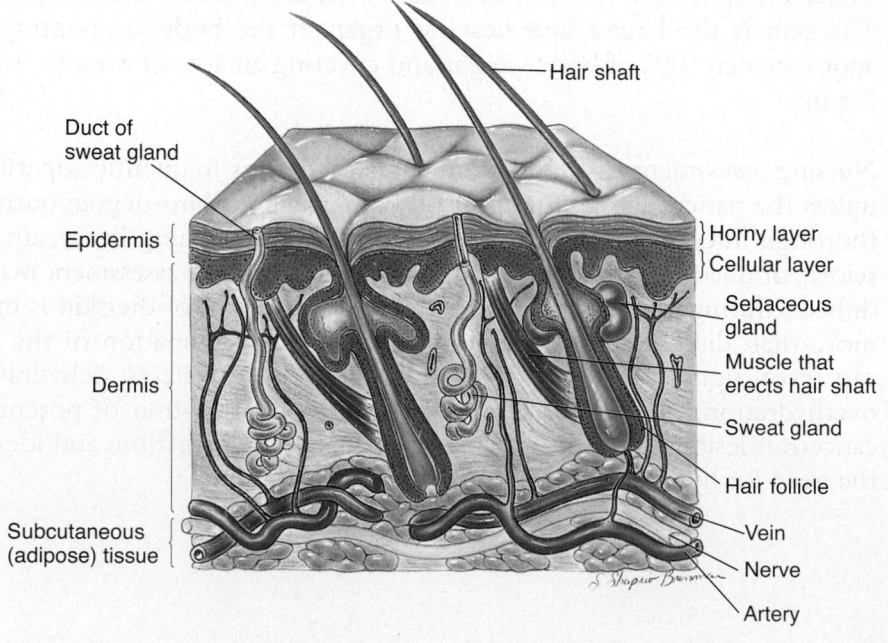

Duct of sweat gland

Hair shaft

Epidermis

Horny layer
Cellular layer

Sebaceous gland

Muscle that erects hair shaft

Dermis

Sweat gland

Hair follicle

Subcutaneous (adipose) tissue

Vein

Nerve

Artery

an inner cellular layer where both melanin and keratin are formed. Migration from the inner layer to the top layer takes approximately 1 month.

The epidermis depends on the underlying *dermis* for its nutrition. The dermis is well supplied with blood. It contains connective tissue, sebaceous glands, sweat glands, and hair follicles. It merges below with *subcutaneous*, or *adipose, tissue*, also known as fat.

The color of normal skin depends primarily on four pigments: melanin, carotene, oxyhemoglobin, and deoxyhemoglobin. The amount of *melanin*, the brownish pigment of the skin, is genetically determined and is increased by exposure to sunlight. *Carotene* is a golden yellow pigment that exists in subcutaneous fat and in heavily keratinized areas such as the palms and soles.

Another yellow color in the skin may be jaundice, due to deposition of bilirubin in the skin. Liver disease, biliary duct obstruction, or increased destruction of red blood cells increases serum bilirubin, which is then deposited in the skin. It is easiest to observe in the sclera, nails, palms, and soles. See Chapter 16, Gastrointestinal and Renal Systems, for further discussion of jaundice.

Hemoglobin, which circulates in the red cells and carries most of the oxygen of the blood, exists in two forms. *Oxyhemoglobin,* a bright red pigment, predominates in the arteries and capillaries. An increase in blood flow through the arteries to the capillaries causes a reddening of the skin (e.g., with blushing), whereas the opposite change usually produces pallor. The skin of light-colored people is normally redder on the palms, soles, face, neck, and upper chest.

As blood passes through the capillary bed, oxyhemoglobin loses its oxygen to the tissues and changes to *deoxyhemoglobin*—a darker and somewhat bluer pigment. An increased concentration of deoxyhemoglobin in cutaneous blood vessels gives the skin a bluish cast known as *cyanosis.*

Cyanosis is of two kinds. If the oxygen level in the arterial blood is low, cyanosis is *central* and indicates decreased oxygenation in the patient. If the oxygen level is normal, cyanosis is *peripheral*. Peripheral cyanosis occurs when cutaneous blood flow decreases and slows, and tissues extract more oxygen than usual from the blood. Peripheral cyanosis may be a normal response to anxiety or a cold environment.

Skin color is also affected by the scattering of light reflected back through the cloudy superficial layers of the skin or vessel walls. This scattering makes the color look more blue and less red. The bluish color of a subcutaneous vein results from this effect; it appears much bluer than the venous blood obtained on venipuncture.

Hair.   Adults have two types of hair: *vellus hair,* which is short, fine, inconspicuous, and relatively unpigmented; and *terminal hair,* which is coarser, thicker, more conspicuous, and usually pigmented. Scalp hair and eyebrows are examples of terminal hair.

Nails. Nails protect the distal ends of the fingers and toes. The firm, rectangular, and usually curving *nail plate* gets its pink color from the vascular *nail bed* to which the plate is firmly attached. Note the white moon, or *lunula,* and the white free edge of the nail plate. Roughly one fourth of the nail plate (the *nail root*) is covered by the proximal nail fold. The *cuticle* extends from the fold and, functioning as a seal, protects the space between the fold and the plate from external moisture. *Lateral nail folds* cover the sides of the nail plate. Note that the angle between the proximal nail fold and nail plate is normally less than 180°.

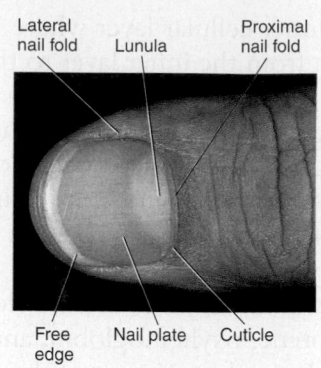

Fingernails grow approximately 0.1 mm daily; toenails grow more slowly.

Sebaceous Glands and Sweat Glands. *Sebaceous glands* produce sebum, a fatty substance secreted onto the skin surface through the hair follicles. These glands are present on all skin surfaces except the palms and soles. The sebum lubricates hair and skin and reduces water loss through the skin.

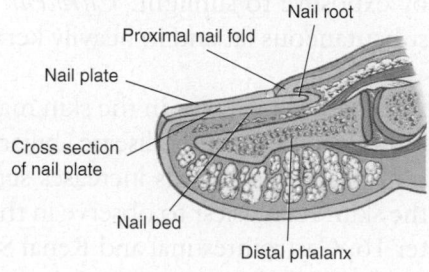

Sweat glands are of two types: eccrine and apocrine. The *eccrine glands* are widely distributed, open directly onto the skin surface, and by their sweat production help to control body temperature. In contrast, the *apocrine glands* are found chiefly in the axillary and genital regions, usually open into hair follicles, and are stimulated by emotional stress. Bacterial decomposition of apocrine sweat is responsible for adult body odor.

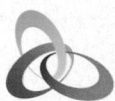

THE HEALTH HISTORY

The purpose of the integumentary history is to identify the following:

Diseases of the skin
Systemic diseases that have skin manifestations
Physical abuse
Risk for pressure ulcer formation
Risk for skin cancer
Need for health promotion education regarding the skin

Common or Concerning Symptoms

Rash	Lesions
Nonhealing lesions	Bruising (ecchymosis)
Moles	Hair loss

The patient with an integumentary issue will frequently state the problem when asked the purpose of the visit. The nurse can use the OLD CART mnemonic to ask follow-up questions in order to obtain a full description of the condition. For example, if the patient reports a rash, ask:

Onset: When did it start?
  Have you started any new medications or changed existing medications?

Have you been out of the country recently?
Have you ever had similar symptoms in the past?
Location: Where is it located?
Has it changed size or spread to another part of your body?
Duration: How long have you had it?
Does it come and go?
Characteristic symptoms: Describe your rash.
What did it first look like?
Has it changed?
Associated manifestations: Does it itch?
Is there any discharge?
Relieving/exacerbating factors: Have you used or done anything that
seems to make it better?
Treatment: Have you put anything on it to treat it?

If the patient does not offer a specific complaint, be sure to ask about each of the symptoms above. Start with broad open-ended questions:

"Have you noticed any changes in your skin? Your hair? Your nails?"
"Have you had any rashes? Sores? Lumps? Itching?"

Even subtle changes in moles or skin lesions may indicate cancerous changes and need follow-up. Ask, "Have you noticed any moles you are concerned about or that have changed at all?" "Any new moles?" If the patient reports such moles, ask how they have changed and pursue any personal or family history of melanoma or skin cancer.

Past History

Do you have any skin diseases such as melanoma, eczema, or psoriasis?
Do you have diabetes or peripheral vascular disease?
Do you have any allergies or food sensitivities?
Have you ever had a severe sunburn? How many second-degree sunburns have you experienced?
Have you ever been on corticosteroid medications for more than 2 weeks?
What prescribed or over-the-counter medications do you take?
What immunizations have you had?

Family History

Do any family members have the same or similar symptoms?
Has anyone in your family had melanoma, eczema, or psoriasis or skin biopsies?
Does anyone have allergies?

Lifestyle and Personal Habits

Describe your bathing and shampooing routines. Have you changed product brands recently?
Do you wear false nails or wigs?

Do you go to a nail salon or gym?

How much sun exposure do you receive daily?

How often do you use sunscreen? What SPF value of sunscreen do you use?

Do you perform skin self-examinations? How often?

Are you exposed to any chemicals or radiation at home or work?

What are your hobbies?

Describe a typical day's diet.

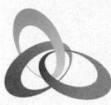 **PHYSICAL EXAMINATION**

The examination of the skin, hair, and nails begins with the General Survey and continues throughout the physical examination. Take time, however, to ensure that the patient wears a gown and is draped to facilitate close inspection of the hair, anterior and posterior surfaces of the body, palms, soles, and web spaces between the fingers and toes.

Inspect the entire skin surface in good light, preferably natural light or artificial light that resembles it. Correlate your findings with observations of the mucous membranes, especially when assessing skin color, because diseases may appear in both areas. Techniques for examining these membranes are described in Chapter 11, The Eyes and Chapter 12, Ears, Nose, Mouth and Throat.

Artificial light often distorts colors and masks jaundice.

To sharpen your observations, Turn to the tables at the end of the chapter to better identify skin colors and patterns and types of lesions that you may encounter during the examination.

SKIN

Inspect and palpate the skin. Note these characteristics:

1. *Color.* Skin color will vary according to genetic background and may have fair, olive, tan, brown, or golden hues. Patients may notice a change in their skin color before the nurse does. Ask about it.

   a. Look for increased pigmentation (brownness), loss of pigmentation, or redness of the skin.

   See Table 9-1, pp. 169–170, Skin Color Changes

   b. Assess for cyanosis or pallor. Note the red color of oxyhemoglobin and the pallor in its absence where the horny layer of the epidermis is thinnest and causes the least scatter: the fingernails, the lips, and the mucous membranes, particularly those of the mouth and the palpebral conjunctiva. In dark-skinned people, inspecting the palms and soles may also be useful.

   Pallor results from decreased redness in *anemia* and decreased blood flow, as occurs in fainting or arterial insufficiency.

Central cyanosis is best identified in the lips, oral mucosa, and tongue. The lips, however, may turn blue in the cold, and melanin in the lips may simulate cyanosis in darker-skinned people.

Cyanosis of the nails, hands, and feet may be central or peripheral in origin. Anxiety or a cold examining room may cause peripheral cyanosis.

Causes of *central cyanosis* include advanced lung disease, congenital heart disease, and hemoglobinopathies.

Cyanosis in *congestive heart failure* is usually peripheral, reflecting decreased blood flow, but in *pulmonary edema*, it may also be central. *Venous obstruction* may cause peripheral cyanosis.

c. Look for the yellow color of jaundice in the sclera. Do not confuse a normal scleral yellow pigmentation in dark-skinned individuals with jaundice. Rather, observe the hard palate with a bright light for jaundice. Jaundice may also appear in the palpebral conjunctiva, lips, hard palate, undersurface of the tongue, tympanic membrane, and skin. Press the skin over a bony prominence and observe the color when your finger is removed.

Jaundice suggests liver disease or excessive hemolysis of red blood cells.

d. For the yellow color that accompanies high levels of carotene, look at the palms, soles, and face. See Table 9-1, pp. 169–170, Skin Color Changes.

Carotenemia

2. *Moisture.* Note excessive dryness, sweating, and oiliness. Skin should be dry to touch without flaking or cracking. Perspiration may appear on the face, hands, axillae, or skin folds in response to a warm environment; increased metabolic activity, such as fever or exercise; and anxiety or pain. Excessive dryness, often accompanied by flaking, or excessive sweating (diaphoresis) may indicate a problem. Carefully inspect skin folds where moisture may cause skin breakdown.

Dryness in hypothyroidism; oiliness in acne. Dry skin with parched cracked lips, dry mucous membranes, and lack of tears indicate dehydration.

3. *Temperature.* Use the backs of your hands to make this assessment. In addition to identifying generalized warmth or coolness of the skin, note the temperature of any areas with increased pigmentation or erythema.

Generalized warmth in fever, *hyperthyroidism;* coolness in *hypothyroidism.* Local warmth of inflammation or cellulitis.

4. *Texture.* Note the roughness or smoothness of the skin. Normal skin feels smooth and firm with an even surface.

Roughness in *hypothyroidism;* velvety texture in *hyperthyroidism*

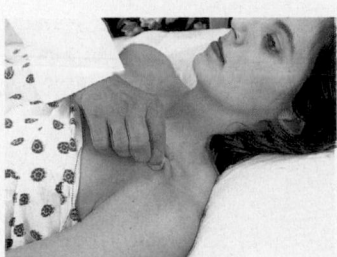

5. *Mobility and Turgor.* Lift a fold of skin and note the ease with which it lifts up (mobility) and the speed with which it returns into place (turgor). Normally the skin promptly returns into place.

Decreased mobility in edema, *scleroderma;* decreased turgor in dehydration.

6. **Edema.** The presence of excess fluid in the interstitial spaces is edema. It may be localized due to an injury or may be the result of a systemic problem (e.g., heart failure). Systemic edema most often occurs in the dependent portions of the body, the feet, legs, and sacral area. The skin appears puffy and feels tight. Mobility is decreased and cyanosis or jaundice in the skin is obscured.

Edema may be pitting or nonpitting. In pitting edema the interstitial water is mobile and can be translocated with the pressure exerted by a finger. A "pit" or depression is left for 5 to 30 seconds. The degree of pitting is measured on a 1 to 4 scale.

See Chapter 15, Peripheral Vascular System, for a further discussion of edema.

Scale	Depression
1+	2 mm
2+	4 mm
3+	6 mm
4+	8 mm

Nonpitting edema reflects a condition in which serum proteins have accumulated in the interstitial space with the water and coagulated. This is frequently seen with local infection or trauma and is called brawny edema.

7. **Lesions.** Observe any lesions of the skin, noting their characteristics:

   a. Their *anatomic location and distribution* over the body. Are they generalized or localized? Do they, for example, involve the exposed surfaces, the intertriginous or skin-fold areas, extensor or flexor areas, or acral (peripheral) areas? Do they involve areas exposed to specific allergens or irritants, such as wrist bands, rings, or industrial chemicals?

   Many skin diseases have typical distributions. *Acne* affects the face, upper chest, and back; *psoriasis*, the knees and elbows (among other areas); and *Candida* infections, the intertriginous areas. See patterns in Table 9-2, p. 171, Skin Lesions—Anatomic Location and Distribution.

   b. Their *patterns and shapes*. For example, are they linear, clustered, annular (in a ring), arciform (in an arc), geographic, or serpiginous (serpent- or worm-like)? Are they dermatomal, covering a skin band that corresponds to a sensory nerve root (see pp. 632–633)?

   Vesicles in a unilateral dermatomal pattern are typical of herpes zoster.[1] See patterns in Table 9-3, p. 172, Skin Lesions—Patterns and Shapes.

   c. The *types of skin lesions* (e.g., macules, papules, vesicles, nevi). If possible, find representative and recent lesions that have not been traumatized by scratching or otherwise altered. Inspect them carefully and feel them.

   See Table 9-4, pp. 173–175, Primary Skin Lesions; Table 9-5, p. 176, Secondary Skin Lesions; Table 9-6, p. 177, Secondary Skin Lesions—Depressed; Table 9-7, p. 178, Acne Vulgaris—Primary and Secondary Lesions; Table 9-8, p. 179, Vascular and Purpuric Lesions of the Skin; Table 9-9, p. 180, Skin Tumors; and Table 9-10, p. 181, Benign and Malignant Nevi.

d. Their *color*.

e. Their *elevation*. For example, are they flat, raised, or pedunculated (attached to a stalk, as a skin tag)?

See Table 9-4, pp. 173–175, Primary Skin; Table 9-7, p. 178, Acne Vulgaris—Primary and Secondary Lesions; Table 9-9, p. 180, Skin Tumors; Table 9-10, p. 181, Benign and Malignant Nevi; Table 9-11, p. 182, Skin Lesions in Context.

Evaluating the Patient With Decreased Mobility. People with decreased mobility or who are hospitalized, especially when they are emaciated, elderly, or neurologically impaired, are particularly susceptible to skin damage and ulceration. *Pressure sores* result when sustained compression obliterates arteriolar and capillary blood flow to the skin. Sores may also result from the shearing forces created by bodily movements. When a person slides down in bed from a partially sitting position or is dragged rather than lifted up from a supine position, for example, the movements may distort the soft tissues of the buttocks and close off the arteries and arterioles. Friction and moisture further increase the risk.

See Table 9-12, p. 183, Pressure Ulcers.

Assess every patient by carefully inspecting the skin that overlies the sacrum, buttocks, greater trochanters, knees, and heels. Roll the patient onto one side to see the sacrum and buttocks. Inspect the skin folds where moisture promotes maceration and skin breakdown.

It is easier to prevent pressure ulcers than heal them. Every patient with decreased mobility and all hospitalized patients should be assessed for the risk factors that lead to pressure ulcers. The risk factors may then be mitigated to prevent pressure ulcers. The Braden Scale is a simple effective tool that evaluates levels of risk for ulcer development in the patient. With its high reliability, predictive validity, and ease of use, the Braden Scale can be used to assess patients as often as every shift if needed.[2,3] Six factors are rated using a matrix scoring system: sensory perception, moisture, activity, mobility, nutrition, and friction and shear. A lower score indicates that the patient has a lower functional level and is at higher risk for ulcer formation. Levels of risk for developing pressure ulcers are rated according to the following scores:

See Table 9-12, p, 183, Pressure Ulcers.

Local redness of the skin warns of impending necrosis, although some deep pressure sores develop without antecedent redness. Ulcers may be seen.

- 19 to 23: not at risk

- 15 to 18: mild risk

- 13 to 14: moderate risk

- 10 to 12: high risk

- 9 or lower: very high risk

● Braden Scale for Predicting Pressure Sore Risk

Patient's Name _____ Evaluator's Name _____ Date of Assessment _____

	1	2	3	4
SENSORY PERCEPTION Ability to respond meaningfully to pressure-related discomfort	**1. Completely Limited** Unresponsive (does not moan, flinch, or grasp) to painful stimuli, due to diminished level of consciousness or sedation OR limited ability to feel pain over most of body.	**2. Very Limited** Responds only to painful stimuli. Cannot communicate discomfort except by moaning or restlessness OR has a sensory impairment which limits the ability to feel pain or discomfort over half of body.	**3. Slightly Limited** Responds to verbal commands, but cannot always communicate discomfort of the need to be turned. OR has some sensory impairment which limits ability to feel pain or discomfort in 1 or 2 extremities.	**4. No Impairment** Responds to verbal commands. Has no sensory deficit which would limit ability to feel or voice pain or discomfort.
MOISTURE Degree to which skin is exposed to moisture	**1. Constantly Moist** Skin is kept moist almost constantly by perspiration, urine, etc. Dampness is detected every time patient is moved or turned.	**2. Very Moist** Skin is often, but not always moist. Linen must be changed at least once a shift.	**3. Occasionally Moist** Skin is occasionally moist, requiring an extra linen change approximately once a day.	**4. Rarely Moist** Skin is usually dry. Linen only requires changing at routine intervals.
ACTIVITY Degree of physical activity	**1. Bedfast** Confined to bed.	**2. Chairfast** Ability to walk severely limited or non-existent. Cannot bear own weight and/or must be assisted into chair or wheelchair.	**3. Walks Occasionally** Walks occasionally during day, but for very short distances, with or without assistance. Spends majority of each shift in bed or chair.	**4. Walks Frequently** Walks outside room at least twice a day and inside room at least once every two hours during waking hours.
MOBILITY Ability to change and control body position	**1. Completely Immobile** Does not make even slight changes in body or extremity position without assistance.	**2. Very Limited** Makes occasional slight changes in body or extremity position but unable to make frequent or significant changes independently.	**3. Slightly Limited** Makes frequent though slight changes in body or extremity position independently.	**4. No Limitation** Makes major and frequent changes in position without assistance.

	1. Very Poor	2. Probably Inadequate	3. Adequate	4. Excellent	
NUTRITION Usual food intake pattern	Never eats a complete meal. Rarely eats more than half of any food offered. Eats 2 servings or less of protein (meat or dairy products) per day. Takes fluids poorly. Does not take a liquid dietary supplement OR Is NPO and/or maintained on clear liquids or IVs for more than 5 days.	Rarely eats a complete meal and generally eats only about half of any food offered. Protein intake includes only 3 servings of meat or dairy products per day. Occasionally will take a dietary supplement. OR Receives less than optimum amount of liquid diet or tube feeding.	Eats over half of most meals. Eats a total of 4 servings of protein (meat, dairy products) per day. Occasionally will refuse a meal, but will usually take a supplement when offered OR Is on a tube feeding or TPN regimen which probably meets most nutritional needs.	Eats most of every meal. Never refuses a meal. Usually eats a total of 4 or more servings of meat and dairy products. Occasionally eats between meals. Does not require supplementation.	
FRICTION AND SHEAR	**1. Problem** Requires moderate to maximum assistance in moving. Complete lifting without sliding against sheets is impossible. Frequently slides down in bed or chair, requiring frequent repositioning with maximum assistance. Spasticity, contractures, or agitation leads to almost constant friction.	**2. Potential Problem** Moves feebly or requires minimum assistance. During a move skin probably slides to some extent against sheets, chair, restraints, or other devices. Maintains relatively good position in chair or bed most of the time but occasionally slides down.	**3. No Apparent Problem** Moves in bed and in chair independently and has sufficient muscle strength to lift up completely during move. Maintains good position in bed or chair.		Total Score

(Copyright: Barbara Braden and Nancy Bergstrom, 1988. Reprinted with permission.)

HAIR

Inspect and palpate the hair. Note its quantity, distribution, and texture.

Alopecia refers to hair loss—diffuse, patchy, or total. Sparse hair is seen in *hypothyroidism*; fine, silky hair in *hyperthyroidism*. See Table 9-13, p. 184, Hair Loss.

The color of hair depends on the amount of melanin present and varies from pale blond to black. Graying occurs with aging and may begin in the 20s. Texture varies from silky fine to coarse and thick, straight to varying degrees of curly. As people age, hair tends to feel coarser and drier. However, if such changes occur over a few weeks or months, it may indicate a systemic disease or poor nutrition.

The amount of hair tends to decrease with aging in both men and women. Male pattern baldness is considered a normal change. See Table 9-13, p. 184, Hair Loss.

Inspect the scalp for lesions, flaking, and parasites by separating the hair at 1- to 2-inch intervals.

Inspect the body, axillae, and pubic hair for amount and distribution as well as parasites. Loss of hair on the legs may indicate peripheral artery disease, while changes in pubic or axilla hair may indicate hormonal problems.

NAILS

Inspect and palpate the fingernails and toenails. Note their color and shape and any lesions. Nails should be pink with white lunulae; smooth and firm in texture; rounded in shape with a 160° angle between the nail base and skin; and firmly attached to the nail bed. Longitudinal bands of pigment may be seen in the nails of people who have darker skin.

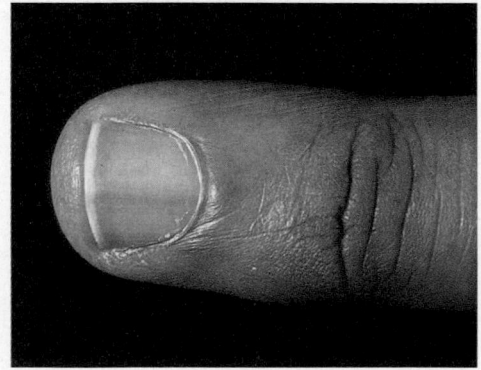

See Table 9-14, pp. 185–186, Findings in or Near the Nails.

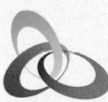

RECORDING YOUR FINDINGS

Note that initially you may use sentences to describe your findings; later you will use phrases. The style below contains phrases appropriate for most write-ups.

RECORDING THE PHYSICAL EXAMINATION—THE SKIN

> "Color pink. Skin warm and moist. Nails without clubbing or cyanosis. No suspicious nevi. No rash, petechiae, or ecchymoses."
>
> **OR**
>
> "Marked facial pallor, with circumoral cyanosis. Palms cold and moist. Cyanosis in nailbeds of fingers and toes. One raised blue-black nevus, 1 × 2 cm, with irregular border on right forearm. No rash."
>
> **OR**
>
> "Facial ruddiness. Skin icteric. 3 spider angiomas over anterior torso. Palmar erythema. Single pearly papule with depressed center and telangiectasias, 1 × 1 cm, on posterior neck above collarline. No suspicious nevi. Nails with clubbing but no cyanosis."

Suggests central cyanosis and possible melanoma

Suggests possible liver disease and basal cell carcinoma

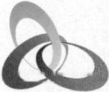

HEALTH PROMOTION AND COUNSELING

Important Topics for Health Promotion and Counseling

- Risk factors for skin cancers
- Avoidance of excessive sun exposure and artificial tanning lamps

Nurses play an important role in educating patients about early detection of suspicious moles, protective measures for skin care, and the hazards of excessive sun exposure. Skin cancers are the most common cancers in the United States and usually arise on sun-exposed areas, particularly the head, neck, and hands. Almost all skin cancers are of three types[4]:

- *Basal cell carcinoma,* arising in the lowest, or basal, level of the epidermis, accounts for approximately 80% of skin cancers. These cancers arise in sun-exposed areas, usually on the head and neck. They are pearly white and translucent, tend to grow slowly, and rarely metastasize.

- *Squamous cell carcinoma,* in the upper layer of the epidermis, accounts for approximately 16% of skin cancers. These cancers are often crusted and scaly with a red inflamed or ulcerated appearance; they can metastasize.

- *Melanoma,* arising from the pigment-producing melanocytes in the epidermis that give the skin its color, accounts for approximately 4% of skin cancers and is the most lethal type. Although rare, melanomas are the most rapidly increasing U.S. malignancy. Lifetime risk for melanoma in men is 1 in 37, and in women is 1 in 56.[5] Melanomas can spread rapidly to the lymph system and internal organs, and they cause 75% of deaths from skin cancer.[6] Mortality rates are highest in white men possibly because of lower "skin awareness" and lower rates of self-examination.[7]

Risk Factors for Melanoma. Educate patients about *risk factors for melanoma*. Early detection of melanoma, when 3 mm or less, significantly improves prognosis.

RISK FACTORS FOR MELANOMA

- History of previous melanoma
- Age over 50
- Regular dermatologist absent
- Mole changing
- Male gender
- 50 or more common moles
- One to four atypical or unusual moles, especially if dysplastic (abnormal skin change)[8,9]
- Red or light hair
- Actinic keratoses, lentigines, or macular brown or tanned spots usually on sun-exposed areas, such as freckles
- Ultraviolet radiation from heavy sun exposure, sunlamps, or tanning booths
- Light eye or skin color, especially skin that freckles or burns easily
- Severe blistering sunburns in childhood
- Immunosuppression from HIV or chemotherapy
- Family history of melanoma[7,10]

The most commonly recommended screening measure for skin cancer is *total-body skin examination*, although data on the utility of this method for nondermatologists are limited. Although the U.S. Preventive Services Task Force has found insufficient evidence to recommend inspection for routine screening, the American Cancer Society recommends skin examination as part of a routine cancer-related check-up.[11,12] Only a few studies have shown that *skin self-examination* enhances detection,[13–15] but this low-cost method of patient education can promote health awareness in at-risk patients.

Instructions for the Skin Self-Examination. The American Academy of Dermatology recommends regular self-examination of the skin using the following techniques. The patient will need a full-length mirror, a hand-held mirror, and a well-lit room that provides privacy. Teach the patient the **ABCDE** method for assessing moles, and show the patient the photos of benign and malignant nevi in Table 9-10, p. 181, Benign.

PATIENT INSTRUCTIONS FOR THE SKIN SELF-EXAMINATION

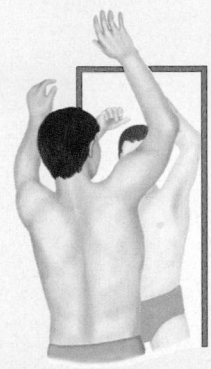

Examine your body front and back in the mirror, then right and left sides with arms raised.

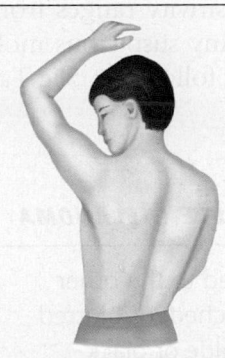

Bend elbows and look carefully at forearms, upper underarms, and palms.

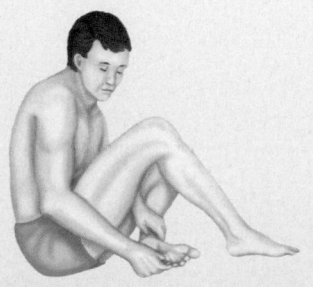

Look at the backs of your legs and feet, the spaces between your toes, and the sole.

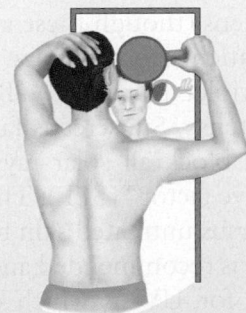

Examine the back of your neck and scalp with a hand mirror. Part hair for a closer look.

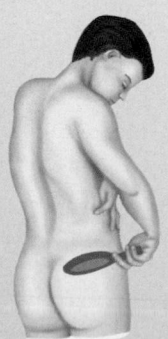

Finally, check your back and buttocks with a hand mirror.

(Source: Adapted from American Academy of Dermatology. SkinCancerNet. Available at: http://www.skincarephysicians.com/skincancernet; and from American Academy of Dermatology. How to perform a self-examination. Available at: http://www.aad.org/skin-conditions/skin-cancer-detection/about-skin-self-exams/how-to-examine-your-skin. Accessed March 24, 2011.)

Detecting Moles. Patients and clinicians who find moles should apply the *ABCDE method* to screen for melanoma. Sensitivity ranges from 50% to 97%, and specificity from 96% to 99%.[12,16,17] Any suspicious mole or skin lesion should be referred to a dermatologist for follow-up. See Table 9-10, p. 181, Benign and Malignant Nevi.

ABCDEs OF EXAMINING MOLES FOR POSSIBLE MELANOMA

- **A** for asymmetry of one side of mole compared to the other
- **B** for irregular borders, especially ragged, notched, or blurred
- **C** for variation or change in color, especially blue or black
- **D** for diameter ≥6 mm or different from others, especially if changing, itching, or bleeding
- **E** for evolving, a mole or skin lesion that looks different from the rest or is changing in size, shape, or color[18]

Preventing Skin Cancer. Counsel patients about preventive strategies such as reducing sun exposure and using sunscreens (though these are not conclusively validated as effective).[13] Caution patients to minimize direct sun exposure, especially at midday, when ultraviolet B rays (UV-B), the most common cause of skin cancer, are most intense. Sunscreens fall into two categories: thick, paste-like ointments that block all solar rays, and light-absorbing sunscreens rated by "sun protective factor" (SPF). The SPF is a ratio of the number of minutes for treated versus untreated skin to redden with exposure to UV-B. An SPF of at least 15 is recommended and protects against 93% of UV-B. (There is no scale for UV-A, which causes photoaging, or UV-C, the most carcinogenic ray but blocked in the atmosphere by ozone.) Water-resistant sunscreens that remain on the skin for prolonged periods are preferable. Be aware, however, that use of sunscreens may give patients a false sense of security and increase sun exposure.

TABLE
9-1

Skin Color Changes

Changes in Pigmentation

Cyanosis

Cyanosis is the somewhat bluish color that is visible in these toenails and toes. Compare this color with the normally pink fingernails and fingers of the same patient. Impaired venous return in the leg caused this example of peripheral cyanosis. Cyanosis, especially when slight, may be hard to distinguish from normal skin color.

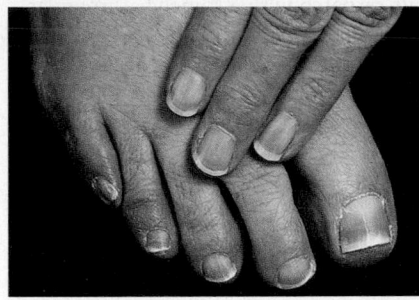

Erythema

Red hue, increased blood flow, seen here as the "slapped cheeks" of *erythema infectiosum* ("fifth disease").

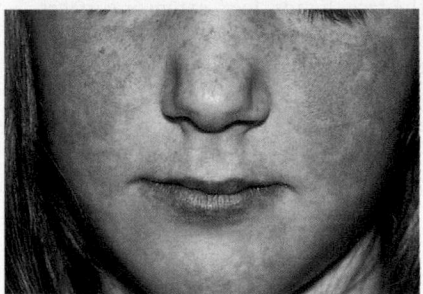

Carotenemia

The yellowish palm of carotenemia is compared with a normally pink palm, sometimes a subtle finding. Unlike jaundice, carotenemia does not affect the sclera, which remains white. The cause is a diet high in carrots and other yellow vegetables or fruits. Carotenemia is not harmful but indicates the need for assessing dietary intake.

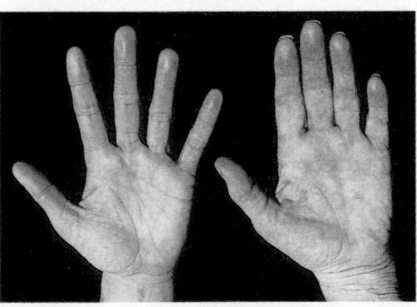

Jaundice

Jaundice makes the skin diffusely yellow. Contrast this patient's skin color with the examiner's hand. Jaundice is seen most easily and reliably in the sclera, as shown here. It may also be visible in mucous membranes. Causes include *liver disease* and *hemolysis of red blood cells*.

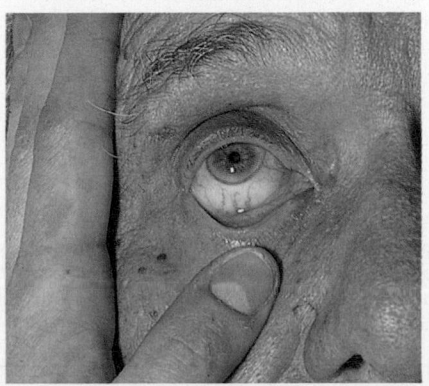

(table continues on page 170)

TABLE 9-1
Skin Color Changes (continued)

Café-Au-Lait Spot

A slightly but uniformly pigmented macule or patch with a somewhat irregular border, usually 0.5 to 1.5 cm in diameter; benign. Six or more such spots, each with a diameter of >1.5 cm, however, suggest neurofibromatosis (p. 188). (The small, darker macules are unrelated.)

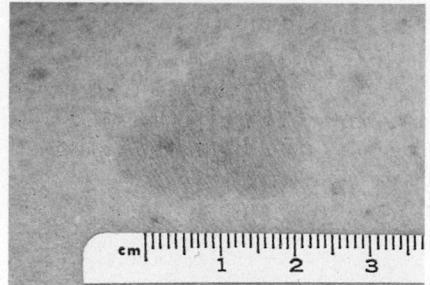

Vitiligo

In vitiligo, depigmented macules appear on the face, hands, feet, extensor surfaces, and other regions and may coalesce into extensive areas that lack melanin. The brown pigment is normal skin color; the pale areas are vitiligo. The condition may be hereditary. These changes may be distressing to the patient.

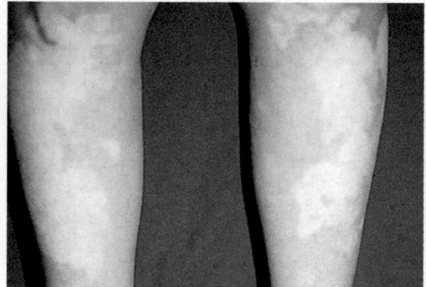 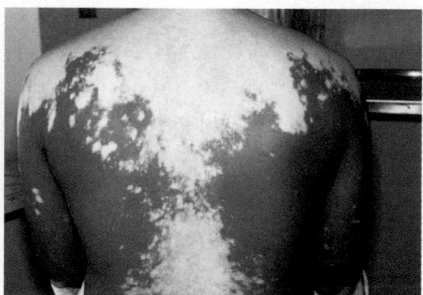

Tinea Versicolor

Common superficial fungal infection of the skin, causing hypopigmented, slightly scaly macules on the trunk, neck, and upper arms (short-sleeved shirt distribution). They are easier to see in darker skin and in some are more obvious after tanning. In lighter skin, macules may look reddish or tan instead of pale.

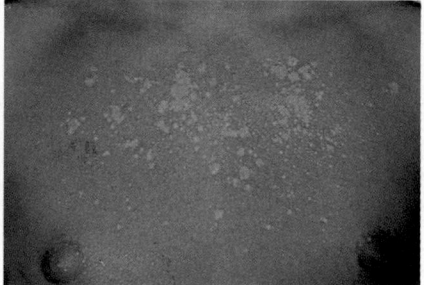 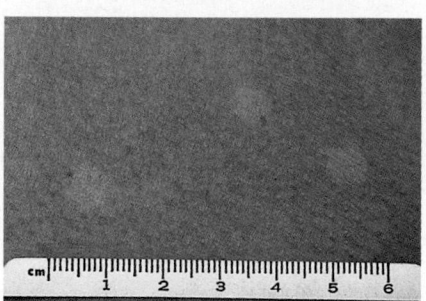

Acanthosis Nigricans

Violaceous eruption over the eyelids in the collagen vascular disease *dermatomyositis.*

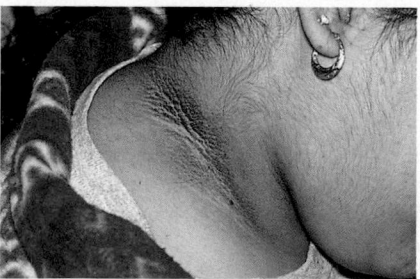

(Sources of photos: *Tinea Versicolor*—Ostler HB, Mailbach HI, Hoke AW, et al. Diseases of the Eye and Skin: A Color Atlas. Philadelphia: Lippincott Williams & Wilkins, 2004; *Vitiligo, Erythema*—Goodheart HP. Goodheart's Photoguide of Common Skin Disorders: Diagnosis and Management, 2nd ed. Philadelphia: Lippincott Williams & Wilkins, 2003; *Heliotrope*—Hall JC. Sauer's Manual of Skin Diseases, 8th ed. Philadelphia: Lippincott Williams & Wilkins, 2000.)

TABLE
9-2

Skin Lesions—Anatomic Location and Distribution

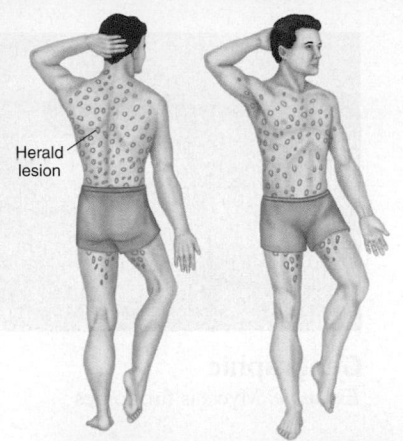

Herald lesion

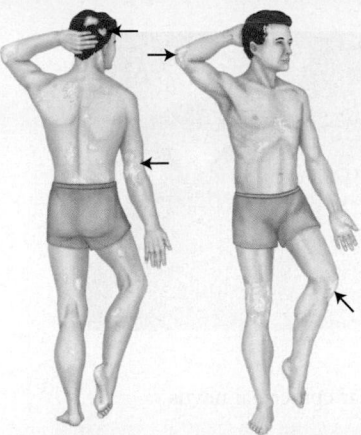

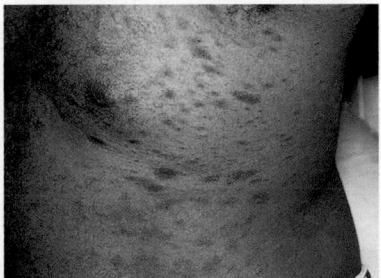

Pityriasis Rosea
Reddish oval ringworm-like lesions

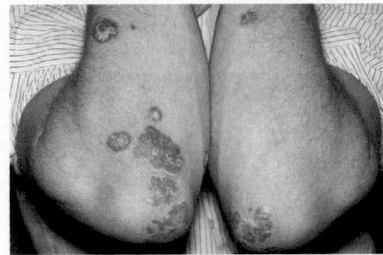

Psoriasis
Silvery scaly lesions, mainly on the extensor surfaces

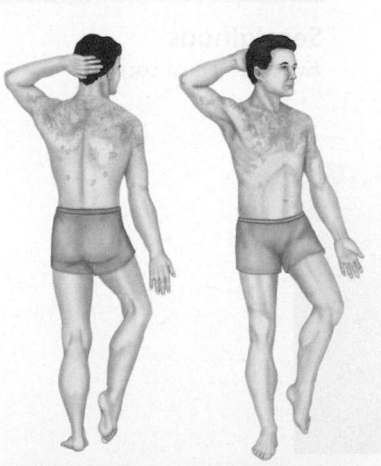

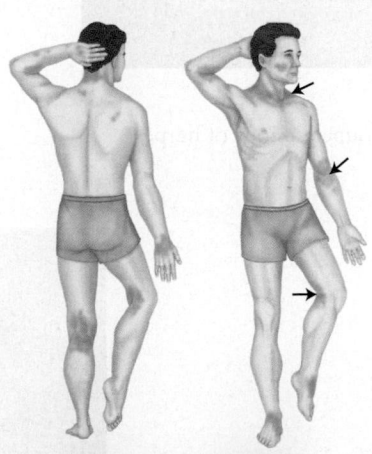

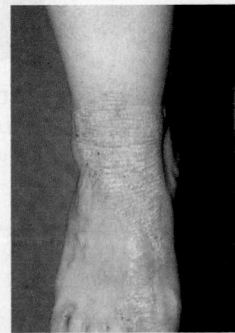

Tinea Versicolor
Tan, flat, scaly lesions

Atopic Eczema
(adult form)
Appears mainly on flexor surfaces

(Source: Hall JC. *Sauer's Manual of Skin Diseases*, 8th ed. Philadelphia: Lippincott Williams & Wilkins, 2000; Photos from: Goodheart HP. *Goodheart's Photoguide of Common Skin Disorders: Diagnosis and Management*, 2nd ed. Philadelphia: Lippincott Williams & Wilkins, 2003.)

Skin Lesions—Patterns and Shapes

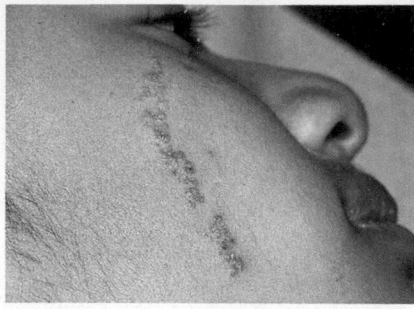

Linear

Example: Linear epidermal nevus

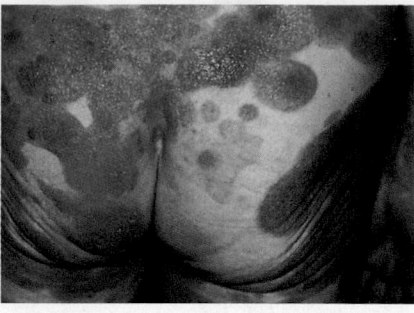

Geographic

Example: Mycosis fungoides

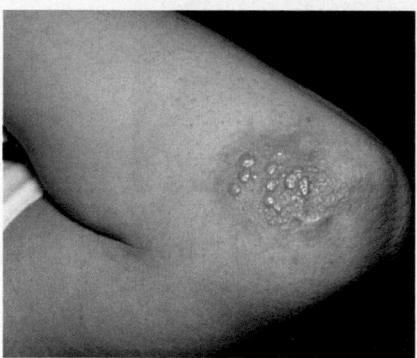

Clustered

Example: Grouped lesions of herpes simplex

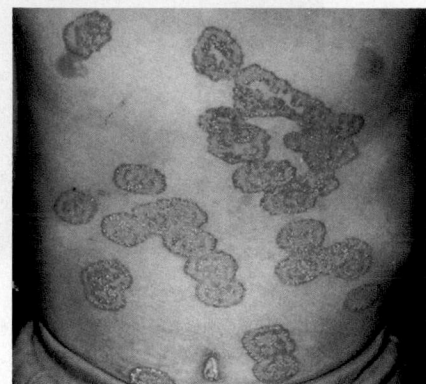

Serpiginous

Example: Tinea corporis

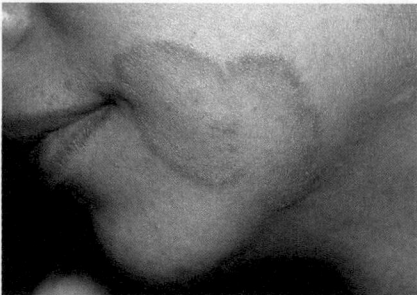

Annular, arciform

Example: Annular lesion of tinea faciale (ringworm)

(Sources of photos: *Linear Epidermal Nevus, Herpes Simplex, Tinea Faciale*—Goodheart HP. Goodheart's Photoguide of Common Skin Disorders: Diagnosis and Management, 2nd ed. Philadelphia: Lippincott Williams & Wilkins, 2003; *Mycosis Fungoides, Tinea Corporis*—Hall JC. Sauer's Manual of Skin Diseases, 8th ed. Philadelphia: Lippincott Williams & Wilkins, 2000.)

TABLE
9-4

Primary Skin Lesions (*initial presentation*)

Flat, Nonpalpable Lesions With Changes in Skin Color

Macule—Small flat spot, up to 1.0 cm

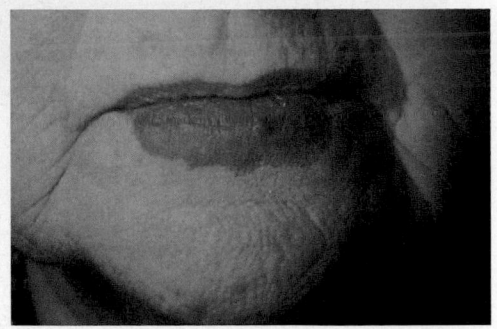

HEMANGIOMA

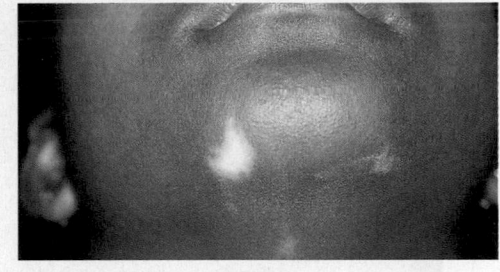

VITILIGO

Patch—Flat spot, 1.0 cm or larger

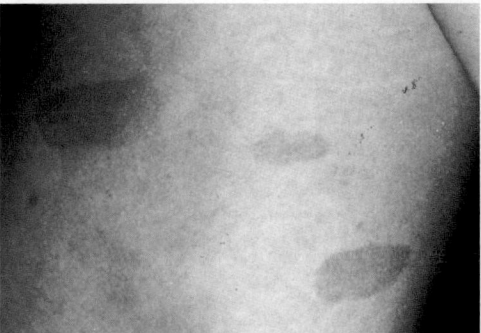

CAFÉ-AU-LAIT SPOT

Palpable Elevations: Solid Masses

Plaque—Elevated superficial lesion 1.0 cm or larger, often formed by coalescence of papules

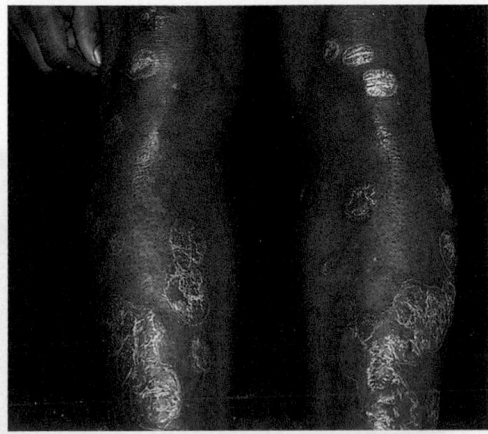

PSORIASIS

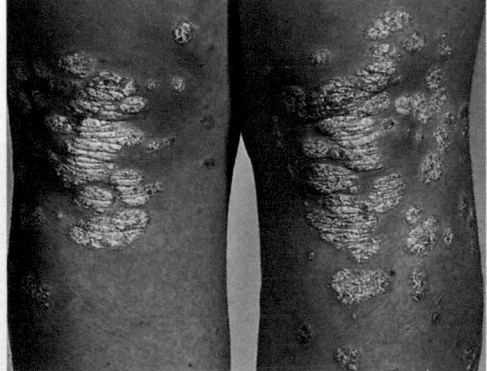

PSORIASIS

(table continues on page 174)

TABLE 9-4

Primary Skin Lesions
(*initial presentation*) (continued)

Papule—Up to 1.0 cm

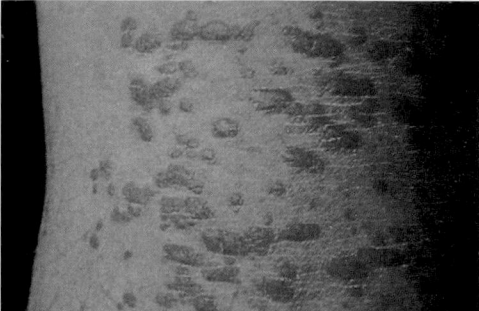

PSORIASIS

Nodule—Marble-like lesion larger than 0.5 cm, often deeper and firmer than a papule

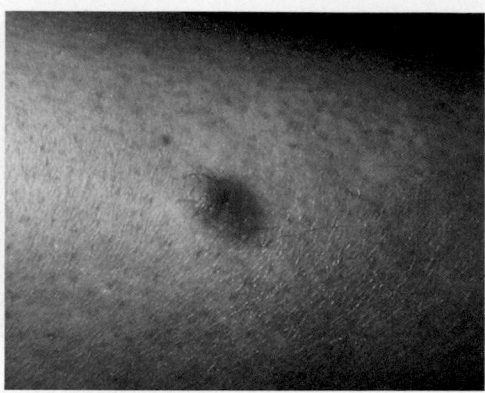

DERMATOFIBROMA

Cyst—Nodule filled with expressible material, either liquid or semisolid

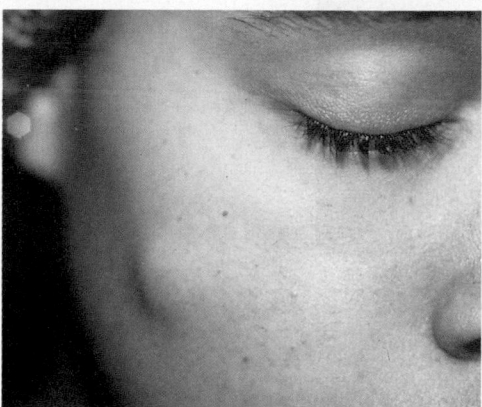

EPIDERMAL INCLUSION CYST

Wheal—A somewhat irregular, relatively transient, superficial area of localized skin edema

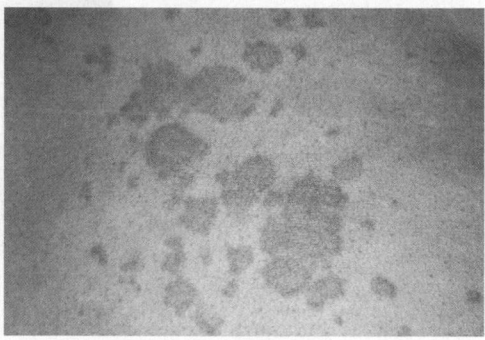

URTICARIA

Palpable Elevations With Fluid-Filled Cavities
Vesicle—Up to 1.0 cm; filled with serous fluid

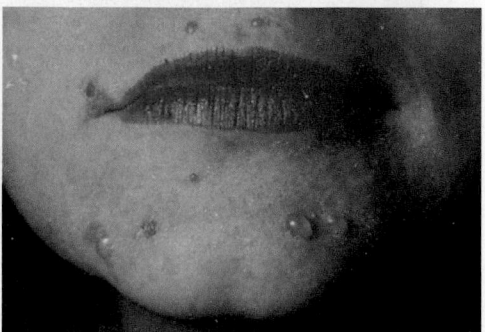

HERPES SIMPLEX

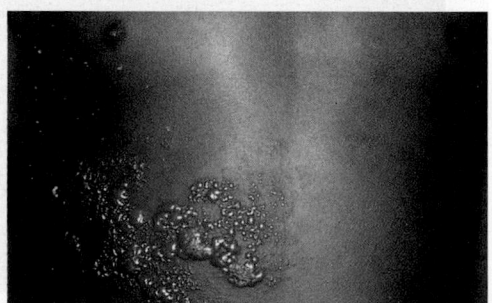

HERPES ZOSTER

Bulla—1.0 cm or larger; filled with serous fluid

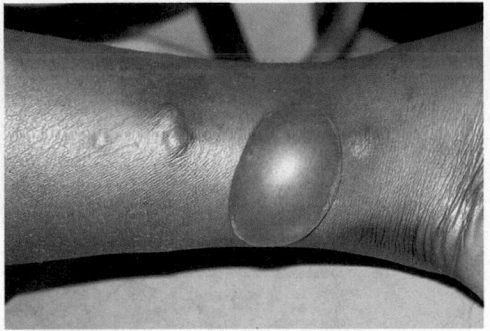

INSECT BITE

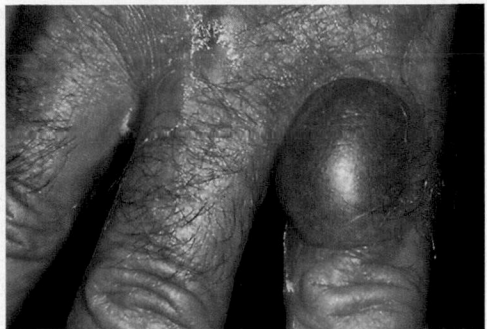

INSECT BITE

Pustule—Filled with pus

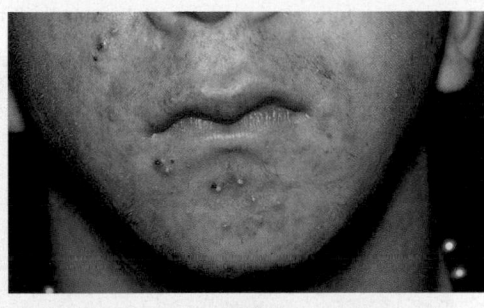

ACNE

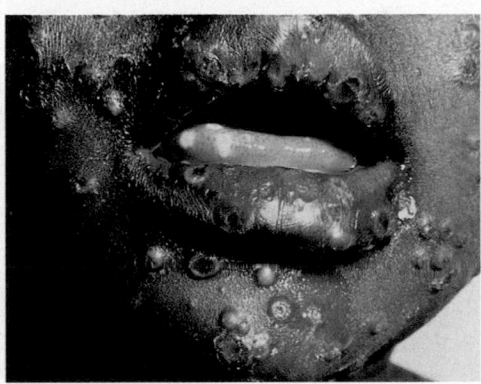

SMALL POX

Burrow (scabies)—A minute, slightly raised tunnel in the epidermis, commonly found on the finger webs and on the sides of the fingers. It looks like a short (5–15 mm), linear or curved gray line and may end in a tiny vesicle. Skin lesions include small papules, pustules, lichenified areas, and excoriations. With a magnifying lens, look for the *burrow* of the mite that causes scabies.

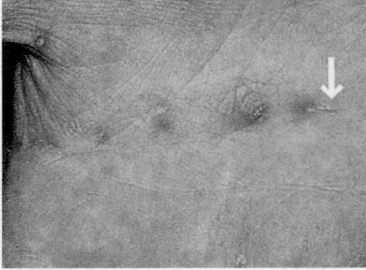

SCABIES

(Sources of photos: *Hemangioma, Café-au-Lait Spot, Psoriasis* [bottom], *Dermatofibroma, Herpes Simplex, Herpes Zoster, Insect Bite* [right]—Hall JC. Sauer's Manual of Skin Diseases, 9th ed. Philadelphia: Lippincott Williams & Wilkins, 2006; *Vitiligo, Psoriasis* [top], *Epidermal Inclusion Cyst, Urticaria, Insect Bite* [left], *Acne, Scabies*—Goodheart HP. Goodheart's Photoguide of Common Skin Disorders: Diagnosis and Management, 2nd ed. Philadelphia: Lippincott Williams & Wilkins, 2003; *Small Pox*—Ostler, HB, Mailbach HI, Hoke AW, et al. Diseases of the Eye and Skin: A Color Atlas. Philadelphia: Lippincott Williams & Wilkins, 2004.)

TABLE
9-5

Secondary Skin Lesions (*seen in overtreatment, excess scratching, infection of primary lesions*)

Scale—A thin flake of dead exfoliated epidermis.

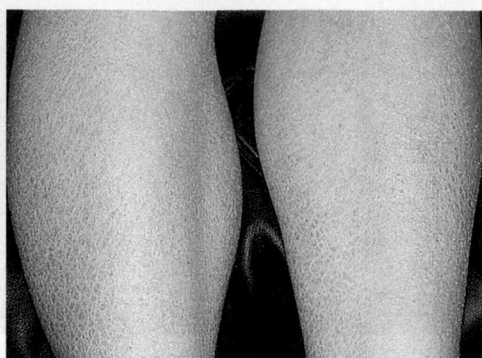

ICHTHYOSIS VULGARIS

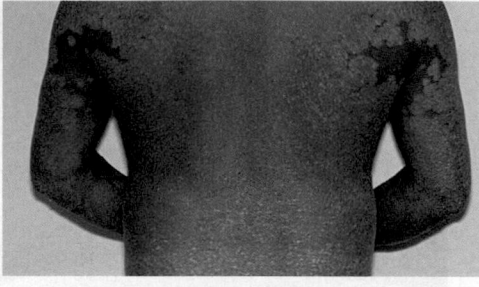

DRY SKIN

Crust—The dried residue of skin exudates such as serum, pus, or blood

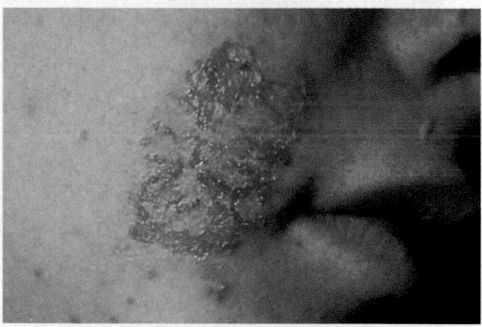

IMPETIGO

Lichenification—Visible and palpable thickening of the epidermis and roughening of the skin with increased visibility of the normal skin furrows (often from chronic rubbing)

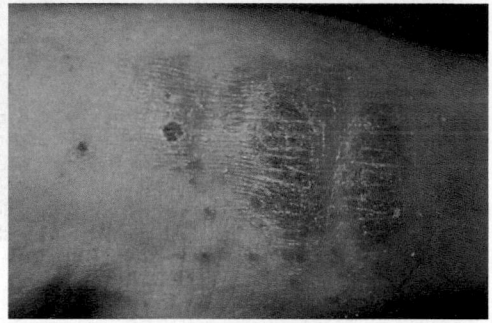

NEURODERMATITIS

Scars—Connective tissue that arises from injury or disease

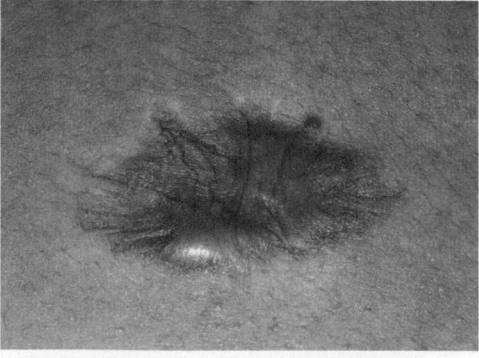

HYPERTROPHIC SCAR FROM STEROID INJECTIONS

Keloids—Hypertrophic scarring that extends beyond the borders of the initiating injury

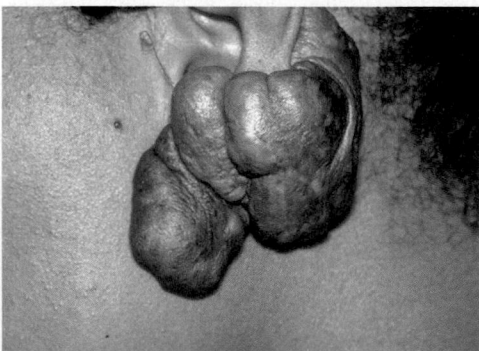

KELOID—EAR LOBE

(Sources of photos: *Lichenification*—Hall JC. Sauer's Manual of Skin Diseases, 9th ed. Philadelphia, Lippincott Williams & Wilkins, 2006; *Ichthyosis, Dry Skin, Hypertrophic Scar, Keloids*—Goodheart HP. Goodheart's Photoguide of Common Skin Disorders: Diagnosis and Management, 2nd ed. Philadelphia, Lippincott Williams & Wilkins, 2003.)

TABLE
9-6

Secondary Skin Lesions—Depressed

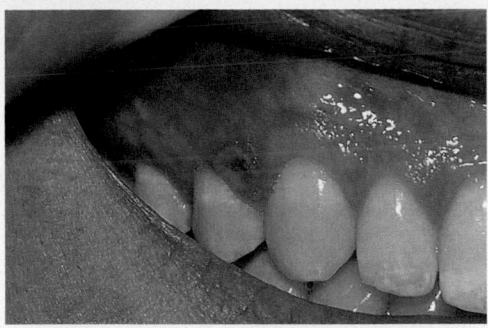

Erosion—Nonscarring loss of the superficial epidermis; surface is moist but does not bleed

Example: Aphthous stomatitis, moist area after the rupture of a vesicle, as in chickenpox

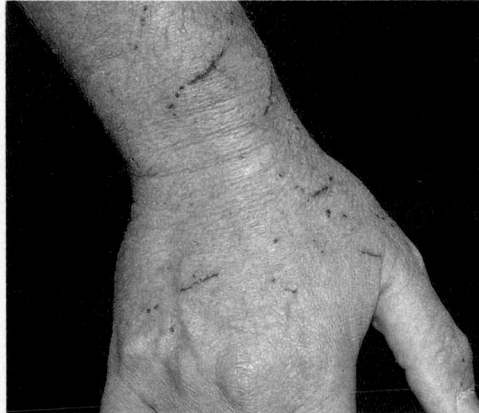

Excoriation—Linear or punctate erosions caused by scratching

Example: Cat scratches

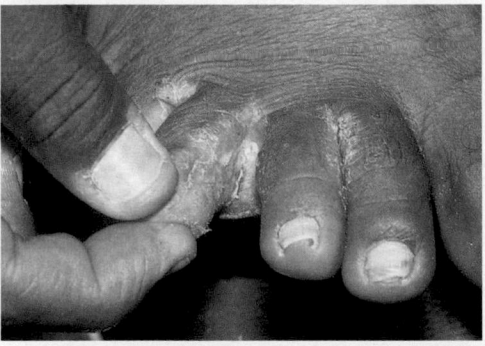

Fissure—A linear crack in the skin, often resulting from excessive dryness

Example: Athlete's foot

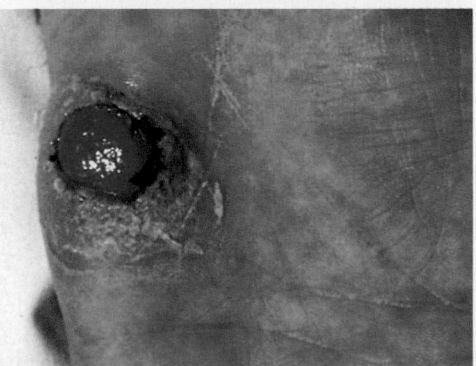

Ulcer—A deeper loss of epidermis and dermis; may bleed and scar

Examples: Stasis ulcer of venous insufficiency, syphilitic chancre

(Sources of photos: *Erosion, Excoriation, Fissure*—Goodheart HP. Goodheart's Photoguide of Common Skin Disorders: Diagnosis and Management, 2nd ed. Philadelphia: Lippincott Williams & Wilkins, 2003; *Ulcer*—Hall JC. Sauer's Manual of Skin Diseases, 8th ed. Philadelphia: Lippincott Williams & Wilkins, 2000)

TABLE 9-7

Acne Vulgaris—Primary and Secondary Lesions

Acne vulgaris is the most common cutaneous disorder in the United States, affecting more than 85% of adolescents.[19] Acne is a disorder of the pilosebaceous follicle that involves proliferation of the keratinocytes at the opening of the follicle; increased production of sebum, stimulated by androgens, which combines with keratinocytes to plug the follicular opening; growth of *Propionibacterium acnes,* an anaerobic diphtheroid normally found on the skin; and inflammation from bacterial activity and release of free fatty acids and enzymes from activated neutrophils.[19] Cosmetics, humidity, heavy sweating, and stress are contributing factors.

Lesions appear in areas with the greatest number of sebaceous glands, namely, the face, neck, chest, upper back, and upper arms. They may be primary, secondary, or mixed.

Primary Lesions

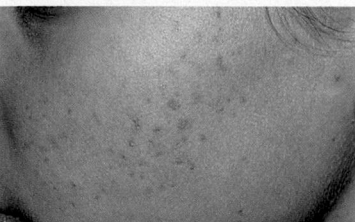

Mild Acne
Open and closed comedones, occasional papules

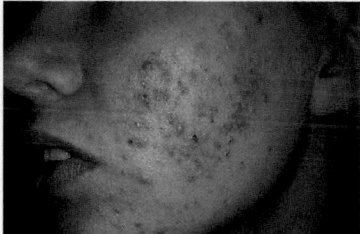

Moderate Acne
Comedones, papules, pustules

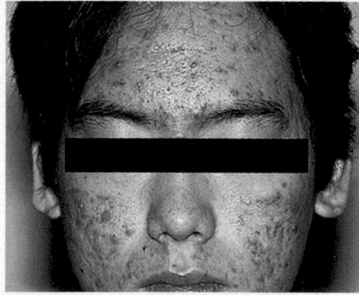

Severe Cystic Acne

Secondary Lesions

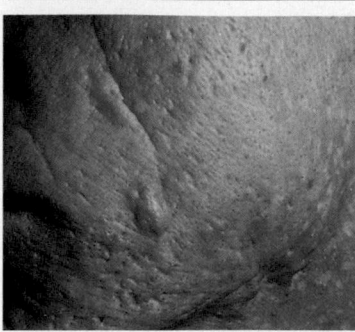

Acne With Pitting and Scars

TABLE 9-8

Vascular and Purpuric Lesions of the Skin

Vascular Lesions

	*Spider Angioma**	*Spider Vein**	*Cherry Angioma*
	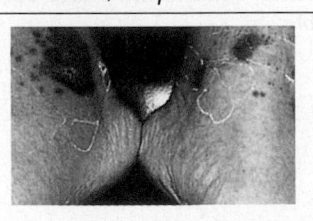		
Color and Size	Fiery red. From very small to 2 cm	Bluish. Size variable, from very small to several inches	Bright or ruby red; may become brownish with age. 1–3 mm
Shape	Central body, sometimes raised, surrounded by erythema and radiating legs	Variable. May resemble a spider or be linear, irregular, cascading	Round, flat or sometimes raised, may be surrounded by a pale halo
Pulsatility and Effect of Pressure	Often seen in center of the spider, when pressure with a glass slide is applied. Pressure on the body causes blanching of the spider.	Absent. Pressure over the center does not cause blanching, but diffuse pressure blanches the veins.	Absent. May show partial blanching, especially if pressure applied with edge of a pinpoint
Distribution	Face, neck, arms, and upper trunk; almost never below the waist	Most often on the legs, near veins; also on the anterior chest	Trunk; also extremities
Significance	Liver disease, pregnancy, vitamin B deficiency; also occurs normally in some people	Often accompanies increased pressure in the superficial veins, as in varicose veins	None; increases in size and numbers with aging

Purpuric Lesions

	Petechia/Purpura	*Ecchymosis*
	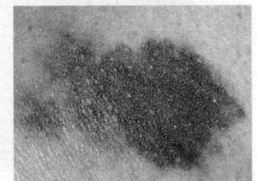	
Color and Size	Deep red or reddish purple, fading away over time. Petechia, 1–3 mm; purpura, larger	Purple or purplish blue, fading to green, yellow, and brown with time. Variable size, larger than petechiae, >3 mm
Shape	Rounded, sometimes irregular; flat	Rounded, oval, or irregular; may have a central subcutaneous flat nodule (a hematoma)
Pulsatility and Effect of Pressure	Absent. No effect from pressure	Absent. No effect from pressure
Distribution	Variable	Variable
Significance	Blood outside the vessels; may suggest a bleeding disorder or, if petechiae, emboli to skin, palpable purpura in *vasculitis*	Blood outside the vessels; often secondary to bruising or trauma; also seen in bleeding disorders

*These are telangiectasias, or dilated small vessels that look red or bluish.
(Sources of photos: *Spider Angioma*—Marks R. Skin Disease in Old Age. Philadelphia: JB Lippincott, 1987; *Petechia/Purpura*—Kelley WN. Textbook of Internal Medicine. Philadelphia: JB Lippincott, 1989.)

TABLE
9-9 **Skin Tumors**

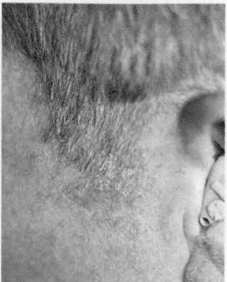 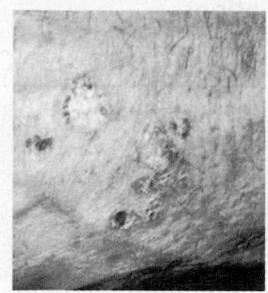

Actinic Keratosis

Superficial, flattened papules covered by a dry scale. Often multiple; can be round or irregular; pink, tan, or grayish. Appear on sun-exposed skin of older, fair-skinned people. Though benign, 1 of every 1000 per year develops into squamous cell carcinoma (suggested by rapid growth, induration, redness at the base, and ulceration). Keratoses on face and hand, typical locations, are shown.

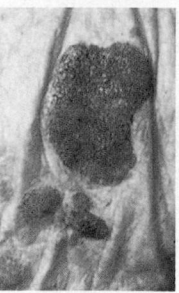 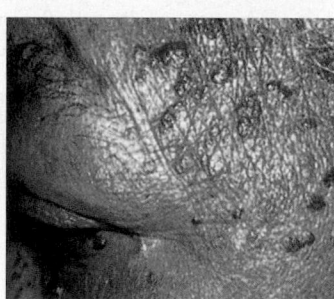

Seborrheic Keratosis

Common, benign, yellowish to brown raised lesions that feel slightly greasy and velvety or warty and have a "stuck on" appearance. Typically multiple and symmetrically distributed on the trunk of older people, but may also appear on the face and elsewhere. In black people, often younger women, may appear as small, deeply pigmented papules on the cheeks and temples (dermatosis papulosa nigra).

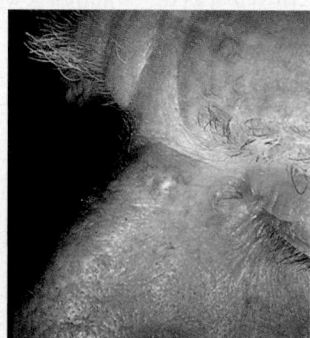

Basal Cell Carcinoma

A basal cell carcinoma, though malignant, grows slowly and seldom metastasizes. It is most common in fair-skinned adults 40 years or older, and usually appears on the face. An initial translucent nodule spreads, leaving a depressed center and a firm, elevated border. Telangiectatic vessels are often visible.

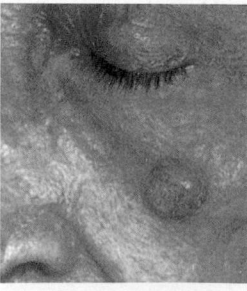 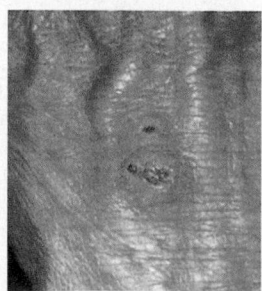

Squamous Cell Carcinoma

Usually appears on sun-exposed skin of fair-skinned adults older than 60 years. May develop in an actinic keratosis. Usually grows more quickly than a basal cell carcinoma, is firmer, and looks redder. The face and the back of the hand are often affected, as shown here.

(Sources of photos: *Basal Cell Carcinoma*—Rapini R. *Squamous Cell Carcinoma, Actinic Keratosis, Seborrheic Keratosis*—Hall JC. Sauer's Manual of Skin Diseases, 9th ed. Philadelphia, Lippincott, Williams & Wilkins, 2006.)

TABLE
9-10

Benign and Malignant Nevi

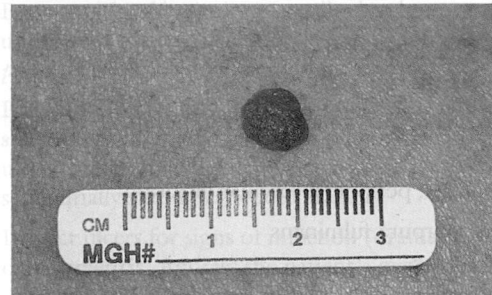

Benign Nevus

The *benign nevus,* or common mole, usually appears in the first few decades. Several nevi may arise at the same time, but their appearance usually remains unchanged. Note the following typical features and contrast them with those of atypical nevi and melanoma:

- Round or oval shape
- Sharply defined borders
- Uniform color, especially tan or brown
- Diameter <6 mm
- Flat or raised surface

Changes in these features raise the specter of *atypical (dysplastic) nevi,* or melanoma. Atypical nevi are varied in color but often dark and larger than 6 mm, with irregular borders that fade into the surrounding skin. Look for atypical nevi primarily on the trunk. They may number more than 50 to 100.

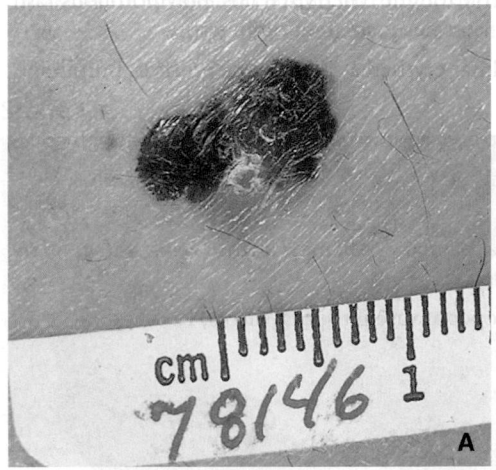

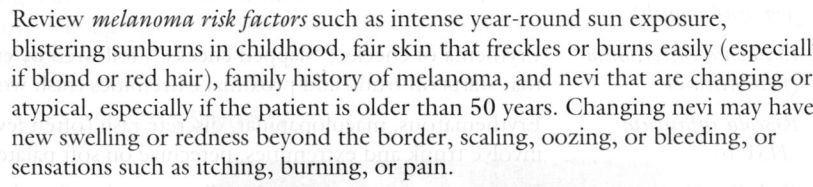

A

Malignant Melanoma

Learn the **ABCDEs** of melanoma from these reference standard photographs from the American Cancer Society:

- *Asymmetry* (Fig. A)
- Irregular *Borders,* especially notching (Fig. B)
- Variation in *Color,* especially mixtures of black, blue, and red (Figs. B, C)
- *Diameter* >6 mm (Fig. C)
- *Evolving,* a mole changing in size, shape or color.

Review *melanoma risk factors* such as intense year-round sun exposure, blistering sunburns in childhood, fair skin that freckles or burns easily (especially if blond or red hair), family history of melanoma, and nevi that are changing or atypical, especially if the patient is older than 50 years. Changing nevi may have new swelling or redness beyond the border, scaling, oozing, or bleeding, or sensations such as itching, burning, or pain.

On darker skin, look for melanomas under the nails, on the hands, or on the soles of the feet.

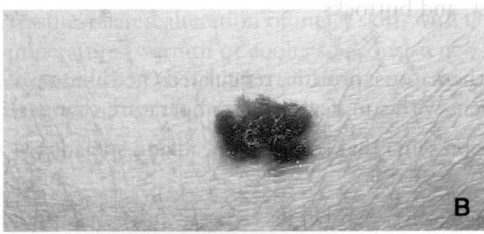

B

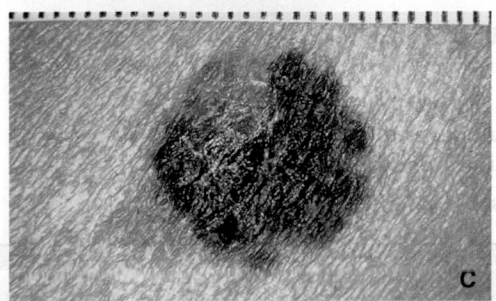

C

(Source: Courtesy of American Cancer Society; American Academy of Dermatology.

TABLE
9-13

Hair Loss

Alopecia Areata

Clearly demarcated round or oval patches of hair loss, usually affecting young adults and children. There is no visible scaling or inflammation.

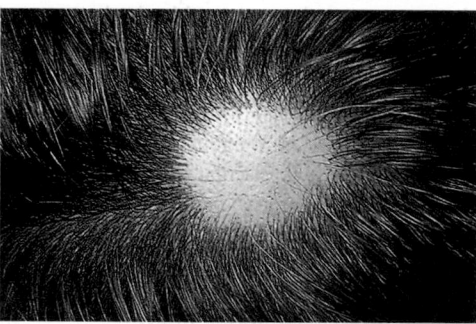 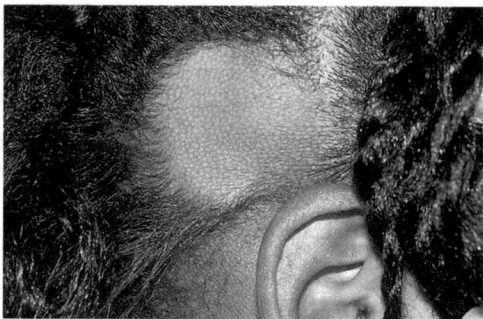

Trichotillomania

Hair loss from pulling, plucking, or twisting hair. Hair shafts are broken and of varying lengths. More common in children, often in settings of family or psychosocial stress.

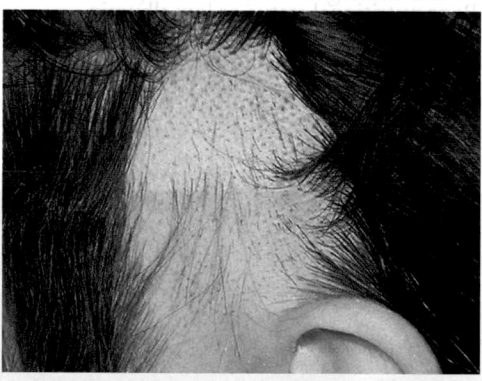 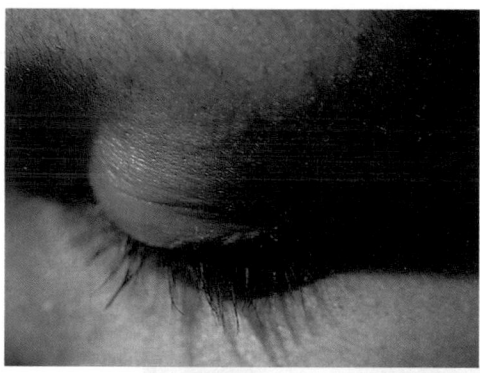

Tinea Capitis ("Ringworm")

Round scaling patches of alopecia. Hairs are broken off close to the surface of the scalp. Usually caused by fungal infection from *tinea tonsurans*. Mimics seborrheic dermatitis.

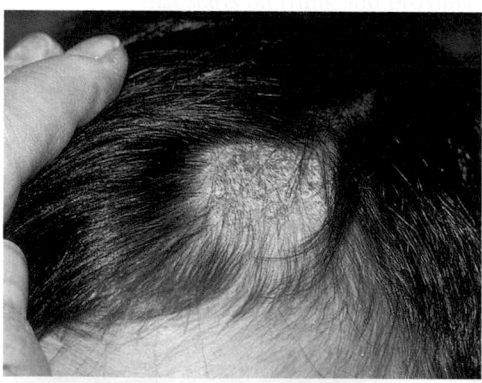 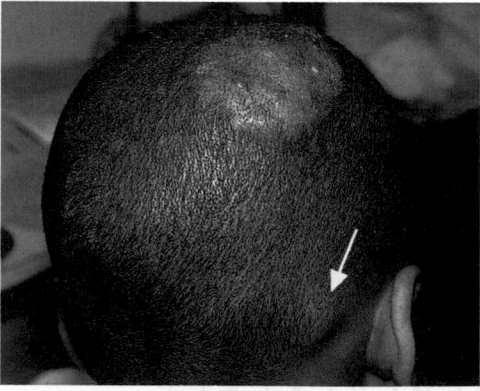

(Sources of photos: *Alopecia Areata [left]*, *Trichotillomania [top]*—Hall JC. Sauer's Manual of Skin Diseases, 9th ed. Philadelphia: Lippincott Williams & Wilkins, 2006; *Alopecia Areata [bottom]*, *Tinea Capitis*—Goodheart HP. Goodheart's Photoguide of Common Skin Disorders: Diagnosis and Management, 2nd ed. Philadelphia: Lippincott Williams & Wilkins, 2003; *Trichotillomania [bottom]*—Ostler HB, Mailbach HI, Hoke AW, et al. Diseases of the Eye and Skin: A Color Atlas. Philadelphia: Lippincott Williams & Wilkins, 2004.)

TABLE	
9-14	**Findings in or Near the Nails**

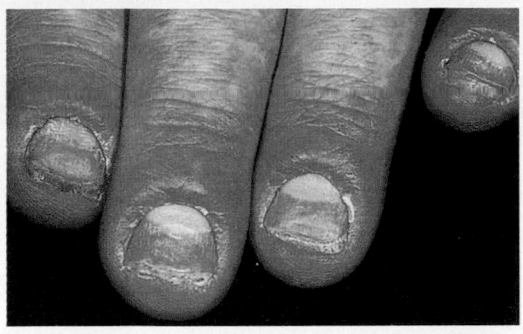

Paronychia

A superficial infection of the proximal and lateral nail folds adjacent to the nail plate. The nail folds are often red, swollen, and tender. Represents the most common infection of the hand, usually from *Staphylococcus aureus* or *Streptococcus* species, and may spread until it completely surrounds the nail plate. Creates a felon if it extends into the pulp space of the finger. Arises from local trauma due to nail biting, manicuring, or frequent hand immersion in water.

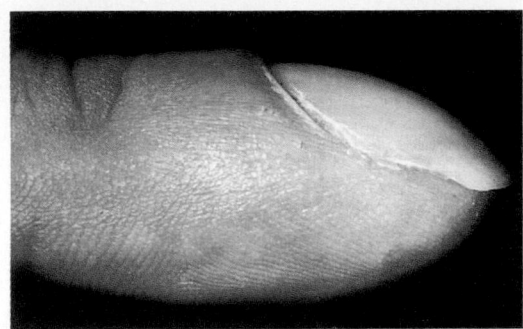

Clubbing of the Fingers

Clinically a bulbous swelling of the soft tissue at the nail base, with loss of the normal angle between the nail and the proximal nail fold. The angle increases to 180° or more, and the nail bed feels spongy or floating. The mechanism is still unknown but involves vasodilatation with increased blood flow to the distal portion of the digits and changes in connective tissue, possibly from hypoxia, changes in innervation, genetics, or a platelet-derived growth factor from fragments of platelet clumps. Seen in congenital heart disease, interstitial lung disease and lung cancer, inflammatory bowel diseases, and malignancies.[20]

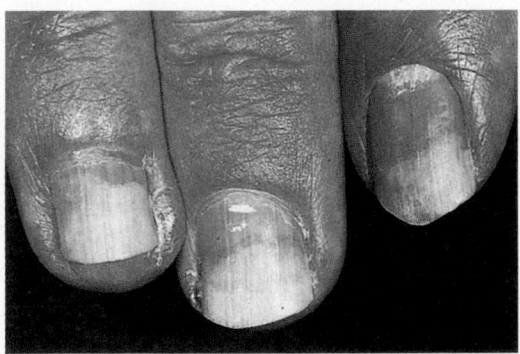

Onycholysis

A painless separation of the whitened opaque nail plate from the pinker translucent nail bed. Starts distally and progresses proximally, enlarging the free edge of the nail. Local causes include trauma from excess manicuring, psoriasis, fungal infection, and allergic reactions to nail cosmetics. Systemic causes include diabetes, anemia, photosensitive drug reactions, hyperthyroidism, peripheral ischemia, bronchiectasis, and syphilis.

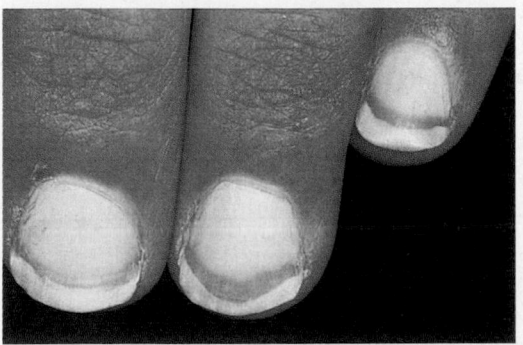

Terry Nails

Nail plate turns white with a ground-glass appearance, a distal band of reddish brown, and obliteration of the lunula. Commonly affects all fingers, although may appear in only one finger. Seen in liver disease, usually cirrhosis, congestive heart failure, and diabetes. May arise from decreased vascularity and increased connective tissue in nail bed.

(table continues on page 186)

TABLE
9-14 **Findings in or Near the Nails** (continued)

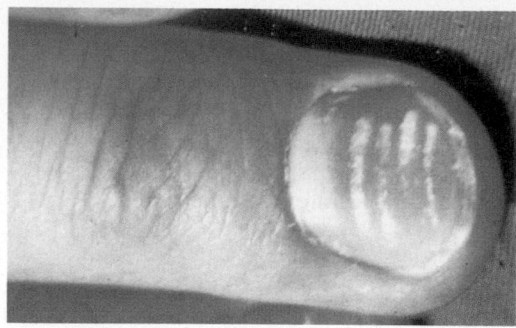

White Spots (*Leukonychia*)

Trauma to the nails is commonly followed by nonuniform white spots that grow slowly out with the nail. Spots in the pattern illustrated are typical of overly vigorous and repeated manicuring. The curves in this example resemble the curve of the cuticle and proximal nail fold.

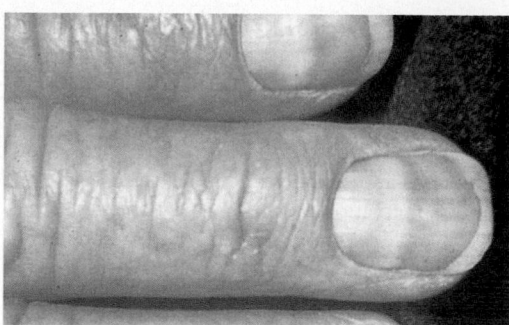

Transverse White Bands (*Mees Lines*)

Curving transverse white bands that cross the nail parallel to the lunula. Arising from the disrupted matrix of the proximal nail, they vary in width and move distally as the nail grows out. Seen in arsenic poisoning, heart failure, Hodgkin disease, chemotherapy, carbon monoxide poisoning, and leprosy.[21]

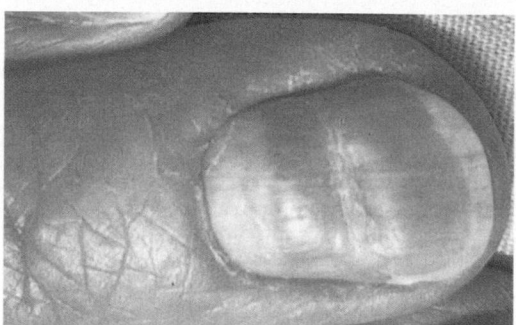

Transverse Linear Depressions (*Beau Lines*)

Transverse depressions of the nail plates, usually bilateral, resulting from temporary disruption of proximal nail growth from systemic illness. As with Mees lines, timing of the illness may be estimated by measuring the distance from the line to the nail bed (nails grow approximately 1 mm every 6 to 10 days). Seen in severe illness, trauma, and cold exposure if Raynaud disease is present.[21,22]

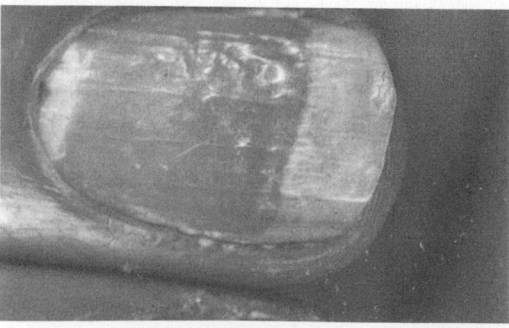

Pitting

Punctate depressions of the nail plate caused by defective layering of the superficial nail plate by the proximal nail matrix. Usually associated with psoriasis but also seen in Reiter syndrome, sarcoidosis, alopecia areata, and localized atopic or chemical dermatitis.[21]

(Sources of photos: *Clubbing of the Fingers, Paronychia, Onycholysis, Terry Nails*—Habif TP. Clinical Dermatology: A Color Guide to Diagnosis and Therapy, 2nd ed. St. Louis: CV Mosby, 1990; *White Spots, Transverse White Lines, Psoriasis, Beau Lines*—Sams WM Jr, Lynch PJ. Principles and Practice of Dermatology. New York: Churchill Livingstone, 1990.)

BIBLIOGRAPHY

CITATIONS

1. Hall, JC. Sauer's Manual of Skin Diseases, 9th ed. Philadelphia: Lippincott Williams & Wilkins, 2006.

2. Braden B, Maklebust J. Preventing pressure ulcers with the braden scale. Am J Nurs 105(6):70–72, 2005.

3. Bergstrom N, Braden B, Kemp M, Champagne M, & Ruby E. (1998). Predicting pressure ulcer risk: a multisite study of the predictive validity of the Braden Scale. *Nursing Research,* 1998 Sep–Oct, 47(5), 261–269.

4. American Academy of Dermatology. What is skin cancer? Skincare.net. Available at: http://www.skincarephysicians.com/ skincancernet/whatis.html. Accessed April 8, 2011.

5. American Cancer Society, Cancer Facts & Figures 2010. Available at: http://www.cancer.org/Research/CancerFacts Figures/CancerFactsFigures/cancer-facts-and-figures-2010. Accessed April 8, 2011.

6. American Academy of Dermatology, Melanoma Fact Sheet, 2011. Available at: http://www.aad.org/media-resources/stats-and-facts/conditions/melanoma/melanoma. Accessed April 8, 2011.

7. Wolff T, Tai E, Miller T. Screening for Skin Cancer: An Update of the Evidence for the U.S. Preventive Services Task Force: Rockville, MD: Available at: http://www.ncbi.nlm.nih.gov/books/NBK34051/. Accessed March 29, 2011.

8 Naeyaert JM, Broches L. Dysplastic nevi. N Engl J Med 349(23):2233–2240, 2003.

9. Tucker MA, Halpern A, Holly EA, et al. Clinically recognized dysplastic nevi: a central risk factor for cutaneous melanoma. JAMA 277(18):1439–1444, 1997.

10. National Cancer Institute. Melanoma & Other Skin Cancers: Risk Factors. Available at: http://www.cancer.gov/cancer-topics/wyntk/melanoma/page5. Accessed April 8, 2011.

11. U.S. Preventive Services Task Force. Screening for Skin Cancer: Recommendations Statement. [Article originally published in *Ann Intern Med* 2009;150:188-93.] Rockville, MD: Agency for Healthcare Research and Quality. Available at: http://www.uspreventiveservicestaskforce.org/uspstf09/skincancer/skincanrs.htm. Accessed March 29, 2011.

12. American Cancer Society. Skin cancer Prevention and Early Detection, 2010. Available at: http://www.cancer. org/acs/groups/cid/documents/webcontent/003184-pdf.pdf. Accessed March 29, 2011.

13. U.S. Preventive Services Task Force: Counseling to Prevent Skin Cancer: Recommendations and Rationale. Rockville, MD: Agency for Healthcare Research and Quality, 2003. Available at: http://www.uspreventiveservicestaskforce.org/3rduspstf/skcacoun/skcarr.htm. Accessed March 29, 2011.

14. Berwick M, Begg CB, Fine JA, et al. Screening for cutaneous melanoma by skin self-examination. J Natl Cancer Inst 88:17–23, 1996.

15. Robinson JK, Fisher SG, Turrisi RJ. Predictors of skin self-examination performance. Cancer 95(1):135–146, 2002.

16. Whited JD, Grichnik JM. Does this patient have a mole or a melanoma? The rational clinical examination. JAMA 279(9): 696–701, 1998.

17. American Academy of Dermatology. SkinCancerNet. Skin Examinations. Available at: http://www.skincarephysicians.com/skincancernet/skin_examinations.html#Examination% 20by%20a%20Dermatologist. Accessed March 29, 2011.

18. American Academy of Dermatology. ABCDEs of melanoma detection. Available at: http://www.aad.org/skin-conditions/skin-cancer-detection/about-skin-self-exams/how-to-examine-your-skin. Accessed March 29, 2011.

19. Goodheart HP. Goodheart's Photoguide of Common Skin Disorders: Diagnosis and Management, 2nd ed. Philadelphia: Lippincott Williams & Wilkins, 2003.

20. Spicknall KE, Zirwas MJ, English JC 3rd. Clubbing: an update on diagnosis, differential diagnosis, pathophysiology, and clinical relevance. J Am Acad Dermatol 52(6): 1020–1028, 2005.

21. Fawcett RS, Hart TM, Lindford S, et al. Nail abnormalities: clues to systemic diseases. Am Fam Phys 69(6):1418–1425, 2004.

22. Hanford RR, Cobb MW, Banner NT. Unilateral Beau's lines associated with a fractured and immobilized wrist. Cutis 56(5):263–264, 1995.

ADDITIONAL READINGS

Alam M, Ratner D. Cutaneous squamous cell carcinoma. N Engl J Med 344(13):975–983, 2001.

American Academy of Dermatology. Malignant Melanoma. Available at: http://www.aad.org/public/Publications/pamphlets/MalignantMelanoma.htm. Accessed April 9, 2011.

Anderson J, Langemo D, Hanson D, et al. Wound & skin care. What you can learn from a comprehensive skin assessment. Nursing 37(4):65–66, 2007.

Barr J. Nursing assessment of the integumentary system. Ostomy Wound Manag 52(6):20–22, 2006.

Boulton AJM, Kirsner RS, Vileikyte L. Neuropathic diabetic foot ulcers. N Engl J Med 351(1):48–55, 2004.

Fitzpatrick TB, Wolff K, Johnson RA, et al. Fitzpatrick's Color Atlas and Synopsis of Clinical Dermatology, 5th ed. New York: McGraw-Hill, 2005.

Fitzpatrick TB, Wolff K. Fitzpatrick's Dermatology in General Medicine, 7th ed. New York: McGraw-Hill, 2008.

Gnann JW, Whitley RJ. Herpes zoster. N Engl J Med 347(5):340–346, 2002.

Habif TP. Clinical Dermatology: A Color Guide to Diagnosis and Therapy, 4th ed. New York: Mosby, 2004.

Habif TP. Skin Disease: Diagnosis and Treatment, 2nd ed. Philadelphia: Elsevier–Mosby, 2005.

Hess C. Performing a skin assessment. Adv Skin Wound Care 21(8):392, 2008.

Hordinsky M, Sawaya M, Roberts JL. Hirsutism and hair loss in the elderly. Clin Geriatr Med 18(1):121–133, 2002.

Johannsen L. Skin assessment. Dermatol Nurs 17(2):165–166, 2005.

Joint Commission on Accreditation of Healthcare Organizations. Assessing a patients' risk for pressure ulcers: compliance tips for national patient safety goal 14. Joint Commission Perspectives on Patient Safety 8(10):9–11, October 2008.

Massey D. The value and role of skin and nail assessment in the critically ill. Nurs Crit Care 11(2):80–85, 2006.

Miller AJ, Mihm MC. Melanoma. N Engl J Med 355(1):51–65, 2006.

Myers KA, Farquhar DRE. Does this patient have clubbing? JAMA 286(3):341–347, 2001.

Rubin A, Elbert HC, Ratner D. Basal-cell carcinoma. N Engl J Med 353(21):2262–2269, 2005.

Scanlon E, Stubbs N. Pressure ulcer risk assessment in patients with darkly pigmented skin. Professional Nurse 19(6):339–341, 2004.

Schon MP, Henning-Boehncke W. Psoriasis. N Engl J Med 352(18): 1899–1912, 2005.

Singer AJ, Clark RAF. Cutaneous wound healing. N Engl J Med 341(10):738–746, 1999.

Singh N, Armstrong DG, Lipsky BA. Preventing foot ulcers in patients with diabetes. JAMA 293(2):217–228, 2005.

Swartz MN. Cellulitis. N Engl J Med 350(9):904–912, 2004.

U.S. Preventive Services Task Force. Counseling to prevent skin cancer: recommendations and rationale. Am J Nurs 104(4): 87–91, 2004.

CHAPTER 10

The Head and Neck

10

LEARNING OBJECTIVES

The student will:

1. Identify the structures and function of the head and neck and the purpose of each.
2. Collect an accurate health history of the head and neck.
3. Perform the physical examination techniques to evaluate the head and neck.
4. Document the physical examination results.
5. Identify the measures for prevention of traumatic brain injury.

The head and neck system contains the cranium, face, neck, thyroid gland, and lymph nodes.

THE HEAD

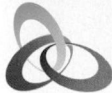

ANATOMY AND PHYSIOLOGY OF THE HEAD

Regions of the head take their names from the underlying bones of the skull, the frontal, parietal, temporal, and occipital areas. Knowing this anatomy helps locate and describe physical findings.

Two paired salivary glands lie near the mandible: the *parotid gland,* superficial to and behind the mandible (both visible and palpable when enlarged), and the *submandibular gland,* located deep to the mandible. Feel for the latter as you bow and press your tongue against your lower incisors. Its lobular surface can often be felt against the tightened muscle. The openings of the parotid and submandibular ducts are visible within the oral cavity (see p. 263).

The *superficial temporal artery* passes upward just in front of the ear, where it is readily palpable. The twisting path of one of its branches can be traced across the forehead in many people, especially in those who are thin or elderly.

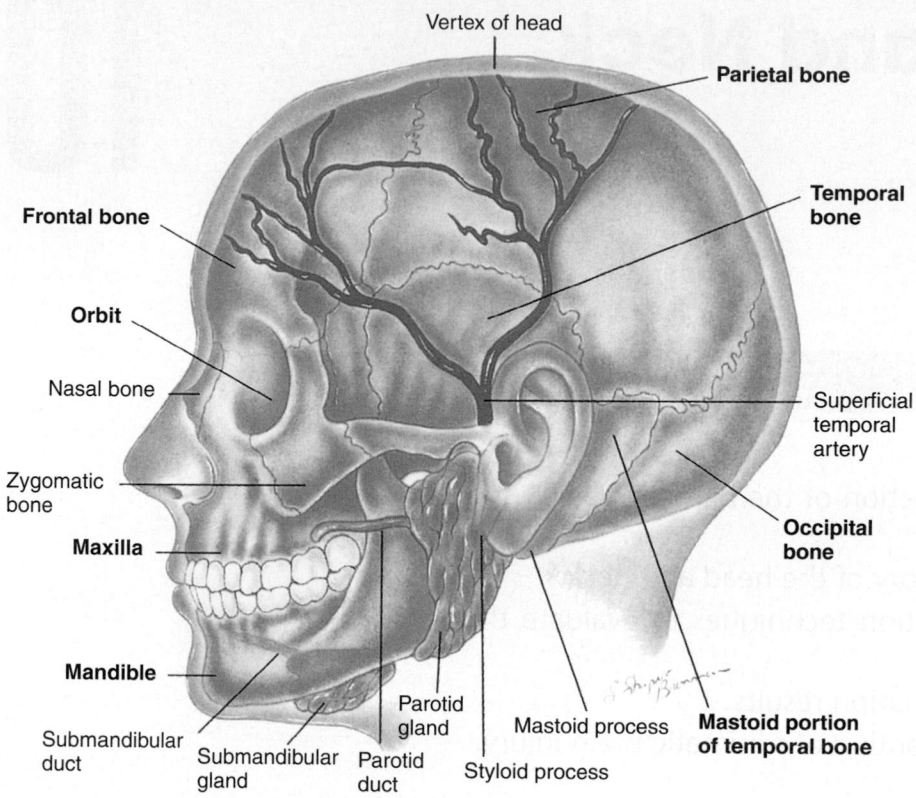

Vertex of head

Parietal bone

Frontal bone

Temporal bone

Orbit

Nasal bone

Superficial temporal artery

Zygomatic bone

Occipital bone

Maxilla

Mandible

Submandibular duct

Submandibular gland

Parotid gland

Parotid duct

Styloid process

Mastoid process

Mastoid portion of temporal bone

THE HEALTH HISTORY

COMMON OR CONCERNING SYMPTOMS OF THE HEAD

- Headache
- Head injury
- Head or neck surgery
- Traumatic brain injury

Headache. *Headache* is one of the most common symptoms in clinical practice, with a lifetime prevalence of 30% in the general population.[1,2] Migraine headaches are by far the most frequent cause of headaches seen in office practice, approaching 80% with careful diagnosis. Nevertheless, every headache warrants careful evaluation for life-threatening causes such as meningitis, subdural or intracranial hemorrhage, or tumor. It is important to elicit a full description of the headache and all seven attributes of the patient's pain (see p. 12). Is the headache one-sided or bilateral? Severe with sudden onset? Steady or throbbing? Continuous or intermittent (comes and goes)?

Look for "red flags" that raise suspicion of worrisome secondary causes: recent onset (less than 6 months); onset after 50 years; acute onset like a

See Table 10-1, Primary Headaches, p. 205, and Table 10-2, Secondary Headaches; Cranial Neuralgias pp. 206–207.

Primary headaches have no identifiable underlying cause. *Secondary headaches* arise from other conditions—some of these may endanger the patient's life.[3]

"thunderclap," or "the worst headache of my life"; markedly elevated blood pressure; presence of rash or signs of infection; presence of cancer, HIV, or pregnancy; vomiting; recent head trauma; or persisting neurologic deficits.

The subjective section of the physical examination is critical in determining the focus of the objective examination. Utilizing "OLD CART," ask the patient specifically about symptoms related to each system.

The opening questions are:

"Have you experienced unusually severe headaches?"
"Have you experienced unusually frequent headaches?"

If the patient noticed unusually severe or frequent headaches, then further assessment is helpful.

The most important attributes are the headaches' severity and chronologic patterns. If a headache is severe and of sudden onset, consider subarachnoid hemorrhage related to head injury, meningitis, or stroke.

Onset: When did you first notice the headache?

Migraine and *tension headaches* are episodic and tend to peak over several hours. New and persisting, progressively severe headaches raise concerns of *tumor, abscess,* or *mass.* Unilateral headache is seen in *migraine and cluster headaches.*[1,3] Tension headaches often arise in the temporal areas; cluster headaches may be retro-orbital.

Location: Where do you feel the headache? Can you point to the area(s)?
Duration: How long has this been going on?
  Did the headache begin suddenly (in a few minutes or less than an hour) or gradually (over a few hours or days)?
  Is it temporary or constant?
  When does the pain begin (morning, evening)? Does it wake you at night?
  How long do the headaches last?
  Are they recurring?
  Is there a pattern?
Characteristic Symptoms: Describe what it feels like (throbbing, hammering, squeezing).
  Describe the pain on a scale of 1 to 10 with 1 being minimal pain and 10 being the worst pain you ever felt.

Associated Manifestations: Do you notice any other symptoms when this occurs? Blurred vision? Nausea? Vomiting? Dizziness?

Nausea and vomiting are common with *migraine* but also occur with *brain tumors* and *subarachnoid hemorrhage.*

What happened prior to the headache? Did anything precipitate the pain?

Is there a prodrome of unusual feelings such as euphoria, craving for food, fatigue, or dizziness? Is there an aura with neurologic symptoms, such as change in vision or numbness or weakness in an arm or leg?

Approximately 60% to 70% of patients with migraine have a prodrome prior to onset; 20% experience an aura, including photophobia, scintillating scotomata, or reversible visual and sensory symptoms.

What brings the headache on (specific foods or drinks, exercise, stress, work, environment, menstruation)?

Is there a history of overuse of analgesics (for eg. NSAIDS), ergotamine, or triptans?

Consider medication overuse in patients with chronic daily headache taking symptomatic medications more than 2 days a week.[1,3]

Do you have a family or personal history of headaches?

Family history may be positive in patients with migraines.

Did you experience a head injury or brain trauma in the past? When?

Relieving Factors: What have you tried to make the headache go away? (for eg. Sleep? Dark room? Cool compresses? Relaxation techniques?)

Ask whether coughing, sneezing, or changing the position of the head has any effect (better, worse, or none) on the headache. Such maneuvers may increase pain from a brain tumor and acute sinusitis.

What has worked the best? What has not worked at all?
Does anything make it worse?
How have the headaches affected your daily life and activities?
Treatment:
Has anyone treated you for headaches in the past? (eg. physician, nurse practitioner, or massage therapist).
Have you used any medication? If yes, then the name of the medication, dosage, and affect?

Traumatic Brain Injury

Traumatic brain injury (TBI) is a blow to the head or a piercing head injury that interferes with the function of the brain. Not all injuries to the head result in a TBI, and those that do occur span from mild to severe. There are 1.7 million people who sustain a TBI each year in the United States[4]

Head Trauma or Brain Injury

Have you experienced head trauma or brain injury in the past?

Onset: When did this occur? Can you describe what happened?

Do you remember when you hurt your head?

Precipitating Factors: What happened to cause the traumatic brain injury? (eg. Lack of protective equipment or helmet? Environmental)?

Location: Can you show me where you hurt your head?

Duration: Did you lose consciousness? If yes, for how long? Did you fall first or lose consciousness first?

Characteristic Symptoms: Did you experience any symptoms prior to the head injury (headache, shortness of breath, chest pain, numbness, or tingling)?

Do you have any medical issues (cardiac history, diabetes, seizures)?

Associated Manifestations: Do you experience vision changes; nausea or vomiting; attention span deficits; drainage from the ears, nose, eyes, or mouth; tremors; seizures; or gait changes?

Relieving Factors/Strategies: Prevention of further injury (p. 203)

THE NECK

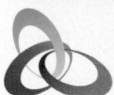

ANATOMY AND PHYSIOLOGY OF THE NECK

For descriptive purposes, divide each side of the neck into two triangles bounded by the sternomastoid muscle. Visualize the borders of the two triangles as follows:

- For the *anterior triangle:* the mandible above, the sternomastoid laterally, and the midline of the neck medially

- For the *posterior triangle:* the sternomastoid muscle, the trapezius, and the clavicle. Note that a portion of the omohyoid muscle crosses the lower portion of this triangle and can be mistaken for a lymph node or mass.

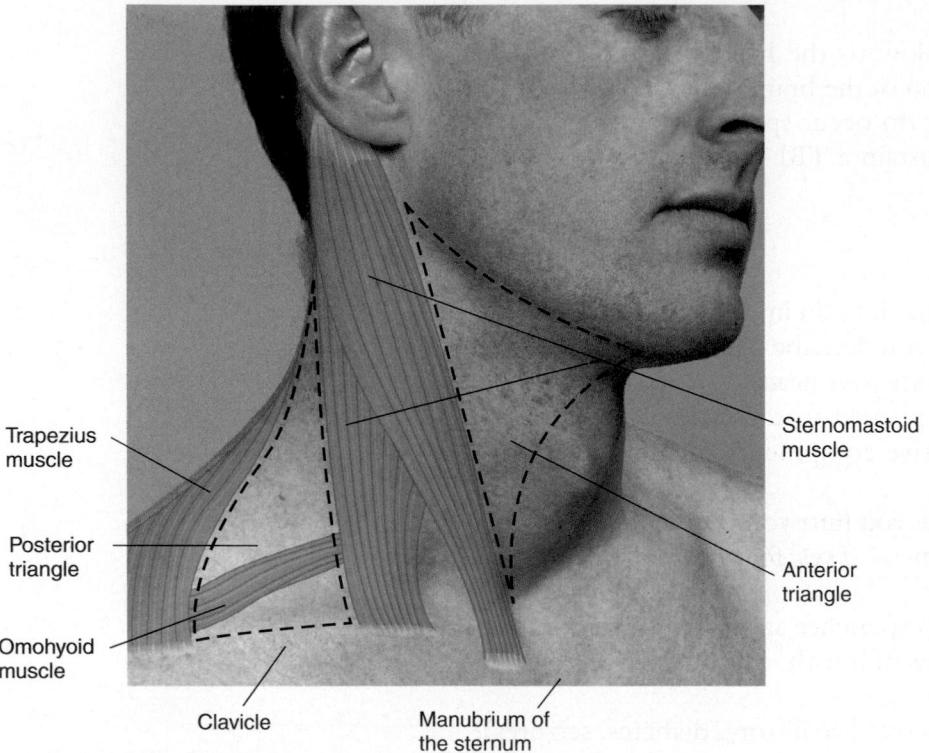

Trapezius muscle

Posterior triangle

Omohyoid muscle

Clavicle

Sternomastoid muscle

Anterior triangle

Manubrium of the sternum

Great Vessels. Under the sternomastoids run the great vessels of the neck: the *carotid artery* and the *internal jugular vein*. The *external jugular vein* passes diagonally over the surface of the sternomastoid and may be helpful when trying to identify the jugular venous pressure (see pp. 348–350).

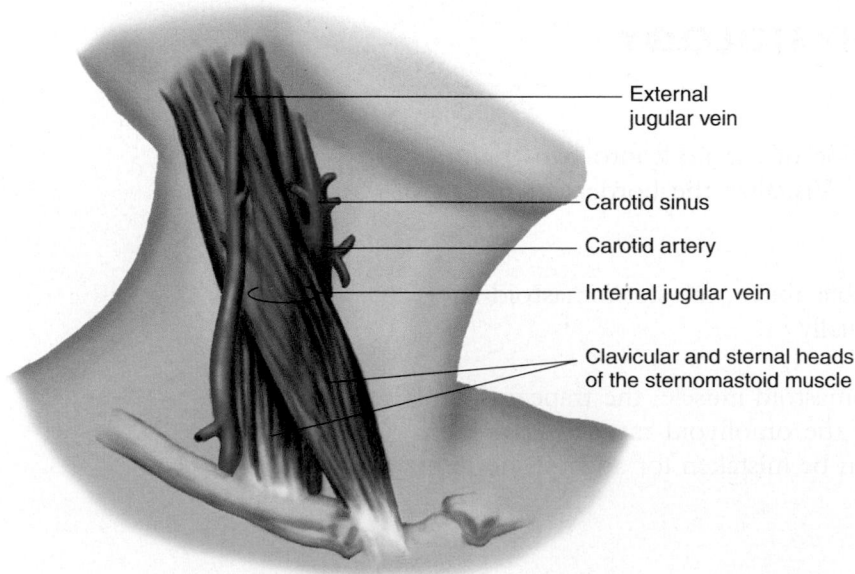

External jugular vein

Carotid sinus

Carotid artery

Internal jugular vein

Clavicular and sternal heads of the sternomastoid muscle

Midline Structures and Thyroid Gland. Now identify the following midline structures: (1) the mobile *hyoid bone* just below the mandible, (2) the *thyroid cartilage*, readily identified by the notch on its superior edge, (3) the *cricoid cartilage*, (4) the *tracheal rings*, and (5) the *thyroid gland*.

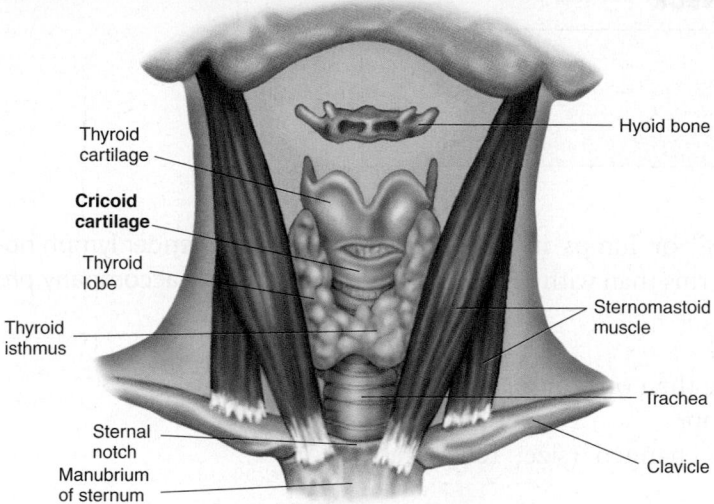

The isthmus of the thyroid gland lies across the trachea below the cricoid cartilage. The lateral lobes of this gland curve posteriorly around the sides of the trachea and the esophagus. Except in the midline, the thyroid gland is covered by thin strap-like muscles. Of these, only the sternomastoids are visible. Women have larger and more easily palpable glands than men.

Lymph Nodes. The lymphatic system is a part of the immune system. Its function is to detect and eliminate foreign substances. One part of the lymph system is in the head and neck. The nurse needs to be aware of the drainage pattern.

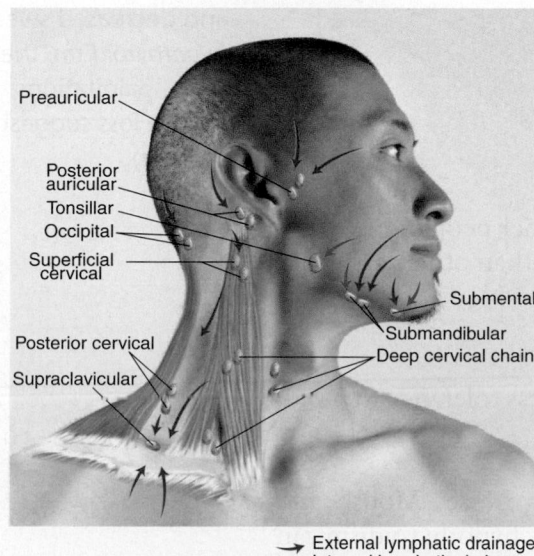

Knowledge of the lymphatic system is important to a thorough assessment: whenever a malignant or inflammatory lesion is observed, look for involvement of the regional lymph nodes that drain it; whenever a node is enlarged or tender, look for a source such as infection in the area that it drains.

Common or Concerning Symptoms of the Neck

- Swollen lymph nodes or neck lumps
- Enlarged thyroid gland
- Hoarseness

Ask, "Have you noticed any swollen "glands" or lumps in your neck?" because patients are more familiar with the lay terms than with "*lymph nodes.*"

Enlarged tender lymph nodes commonly accompany *pharyngitis*.

Onset: When did you first notice the lump?
Location: Where is the lump? Is there more than one lump?
Duration: How long have you had the lump?
Characteristic Symptoms: Has the lump changed (size, tenderness, drainage, shape, consistency)?
Associated Manifestations: Do you have difficulty swallowing? Have you had any recent infections? Trauma? Radiation? Surgery? History of smoking? Drinking alcohol? Chewing tobacco?
Relieving Factors: Does anything make the lump smaller? Less tender? Have you tried compresses on the site?
Treatment: Have you been to a health care provider?

Assess thyroid function and ask about any evidence of an enlarged thyroid gland or *goiter*. To evaluate thyroid function, ask about *temperature intolerance* and *sweating*. Opening questions include:

With *goiter*, thyroid function may be increased, decreased, or normal.

Do you prefer hot or cold weather?

Intolerance to cold, preference for warm clothing and many blankets, and decreased sweating suggest *hypothyroidism*; the opposite symptoms, palpitations, and involuntary weight loss suggest *hyperthyroidism* (p. 209).

Do you dress more warmly or less warmly than other people?
What about blankets . . . do you use more or fewer than others at home?
Do you perspire more or less than others?
Any new palpitations or change in weight?

Note that as people grow older, they sweat less, have less tolerance for cold, and tend to prefer warmer environments.

Hoarseness, which is addressed in Chapter 12, Ear, Nose, Mouth and Throat, will frequently arise from the larynx. However, hypothyroidism can cause chronic hoarseness.

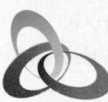

PHYSICAL EXAMINATION

EQUIPMENT

- Tangential light
- Cup of water
- Stethoscope

Abnormalities covered by the hair are easily missed, so ask if the patient has noticed anything wrong with the scalp or hair. Ask the patient to remove any hair pieces, hair adornments, scarves, or rubber bands. Take into consideration a cultural view when examining patients.

The Hair. Note its quantity, distribution, texture, and pattern of loss, if any. You may see loose flakes of dandruff.

Fine hair accompanies *hyperthyroidism*; coarse hair is found with *hypothyroidism*.

Tiny white ovoid granules that adhere to hairs may be nits (eggs of lice).

The Scalp. Part the hair in several places and look for scaliness, lumps, nevi, or other lesions.

Redness and scaling may indicate *seborrheic dermatitis, psoriasis*; soft lumps of *pilar cysts*; or pigmented nevi.

The Skull. Observe the general size and contour of the skull. Note any deformities, depressions, lumps, or tenderness. Learn to recognize the irregularities in a normal skull, such as those near the suture lines between the parietal and occipital bones.

Microcephaly is an anomaly characterized by a small head in proportion to the body and an underdeveloped brain. The circumference of the head is more than two standard deviations below average for the person's age and sex.

Macrocephaly is an anomaly characterized by a large head in proportion to the body and an underdeveloped brain. The circumference of the head is more than two standard deviations above average for the person's age and sex.

The Face. Note the patient's facial expression and contours. Observe for asymmetry, involuntary movements, edema, and masses.

See Table 10-3, Selected Facies (p. 208).

The Skin. Observe the skin, noting its color, pigmentation, texture, thickness, hair distribution, and any lesions.

Acne is found in many adolescents. *Hirsutism* (excessive facial hair) occurs in some women with *polycystic ovary syndrome*.

The Neck. Observe the skin, noting its color, pigmentation, texture, thickness, hair distribution, and any lesions. *Inspect the neck,* noting its symmetry and any masses or scars. Look for enlargement of the parotid or submandibular glands, and note any visible lymph nodes.

The Lymph Nodes. *Palpate the lymph nodes.* Using the pads of your index and middle fingers, move the skin over the underlying tissues in each area in a circular motion. The patient should be relaxed, with neck flexed slightly forward and, if needed, slightly toward the side being examined. You can usually examine both sides at once. For the submental node, however, it is helpful to feel with one hand while bracing the top of the head with the other.

Feel in sequence for the following nodes:

1. *Preauricular*—in front of the ear

2. *Posterior auricular*—superficial to the mastoid process

3. *Occipital*—at the base of the skull posteriorly

4. *Tonsillar*—at the angle of the mandible

5. *Submandibular*—midway between the angle and the tip of the mandible. These nodes are usually smaller and smoother than the lobulated submandibular gland against which they lie.

6. *Submental*—in the midline a few centimeters behind the tip of the mandible

7. *Superficial cervical*—superficial to the sternomastoid

8. *Posterior cervical*—along the anterior edge of the trapezius

9. *Deep cervical chain*—deep to the sternomastoid and often inaccessible to examination. Hook your thumb and fingers around either side of the sternomastoid muscle to find them.

10. *Supraclavicular*—deep in the angle formed by the clavicle and the sternomastoid

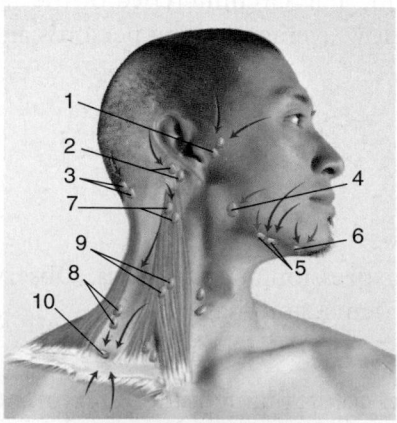

→ External lymphatic drainage
→ Internal lymphatic drainage
  (e.g., from mouth and throat)

A scar of past thyroid surgery is often a clue to unsuspected thyroid disease.

A "tonsillar node" that pulsates is really the carotid artery. A small, hard, tender "tonsillar node" high and deep between the mandible and the sternomastoid is probably a styloid process.

Enlargement of a supraclavicular node, especially on the left, suggests possible metastasis from a thoracic or an abdominal malignancy.

Begin palpation using the pads of the second and third fingers, and palpate the *preauricular nodes* with a gentle rotary motion. Then examine the *posterior auricular* and *occipital* lymph nodes and follow sequentially to *tonsillar,* then *submandibular.* The *submental* is palpated with one hand.

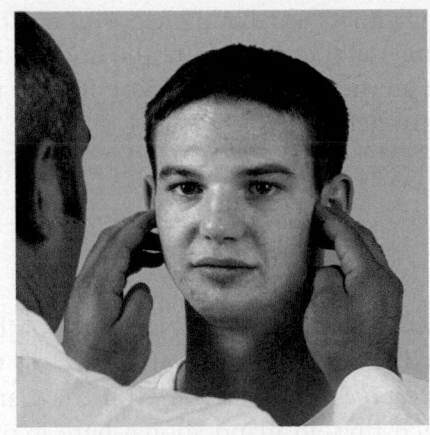

The last lymph nodes in the neck to be palpated are the *superficial cervical* and the *deep cervical chains,* located anterior and superficial to the sternomastoid. Then palpate the *posterior cervical chain* along the trapezius (anterior edge) and along the sternomastoid (posterior edge). Flex the patient's neck slightly forward toward the side being examined. Examine the *supraclavicular* nodes in the angle between the clavicle and the sternomastoid.

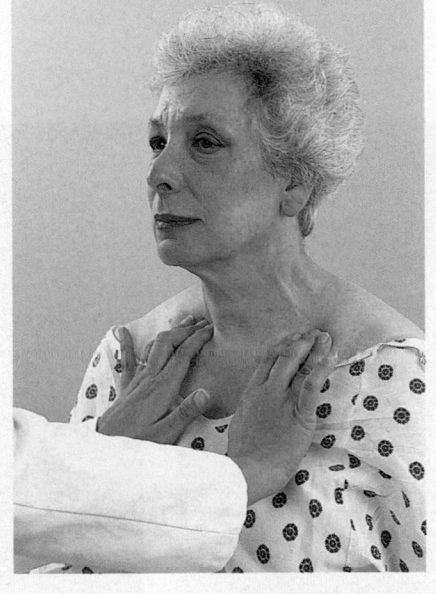

Oftentimes a lymph node is unable to be palpated. When a node is palpated, note its size, shape, delimitation (discrete or matted together), mobility, consistency, and any tenderness. Small, mobile, discrete, nontender nodes, sometimes termed "shotty," can frequently be found, especially in children.

Tender nodes suggest inflammation; hard or fixed nodes suggest malignancy.

Enlarged or tender nodes, if unexplained, call for (1) reexamination of the regions they drain and (2) careful assessment of lymph nodes elsewhere so that you can distinguish between regional and generalized lymphadenopathy.

Diffuse lymphadenopathy raises the suspicion of HIV or AIDS.

Occasionally you may mistake a band of muscle or an artery for a lymph node. You should be able to roll a node in two directions: up and down, and side to side. Neither a muscle nor an artery will pass this test.

The Trachea and the Thyroid Gland. To orient yourself to the neck, identify the thyroid and cricoid cartilages and the trachea below them.

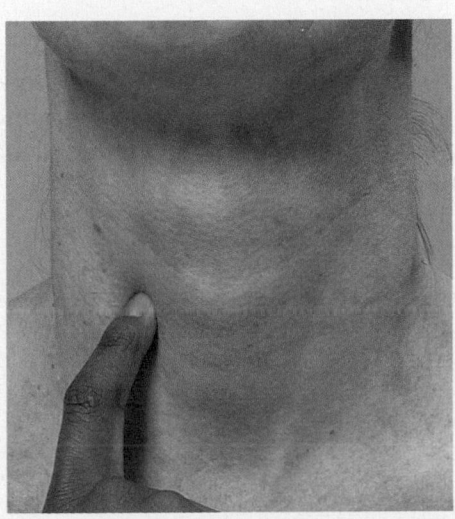

- *Inspect the trachea* for any deviation from its usual midline position. Then *feel for any deviation*. Place your finger along one side of the trachea and note the space between it and the sternomastoid. Compare it with the other side. The spaces should be symmetric.

Masses in the neck may push the trachea to one side. Tracheal deviation may also signify important problems in the thorax, such as a mediastinal mass, atelectasis, or a large pneumothorax (see Table 13-7, p. 332–333).

- *Inspect the neck for the thyroid gland*. Tip the patient's head back a bit. Using tangential lighting directed downward from the tip of the patient's chin, *inspect the region below the cricoid cartilage* for the gland. The lower shadowed border of each thyroid gland shown here is outlined by arrows.

The lower border of this large thyroid gland is outlined by tangential lighting. *Goiter* is a general term for an enlarged thyroid gland.[5,6]

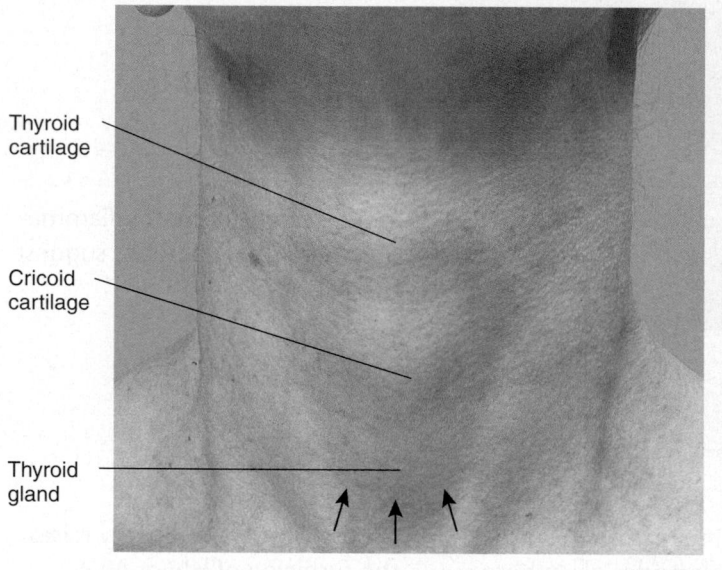

Thyroid cartilage

Cricoid cartilage

Thyroid gland

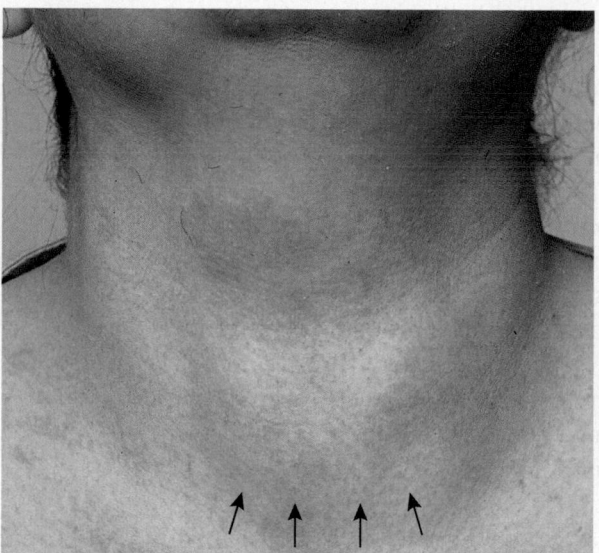

AT REST

Ask the patient to sip some water and to extend the neck again and swallow. Watch for upward movement of the thyroid gland, noting its contour and symmetry. The thyroid cartilage, the cricoid cartilage, and the thyroid gland all rise with swallowing and then fall to their resting positions.

With swallowing, the lower border of this large gland rises and looks less symmetric.

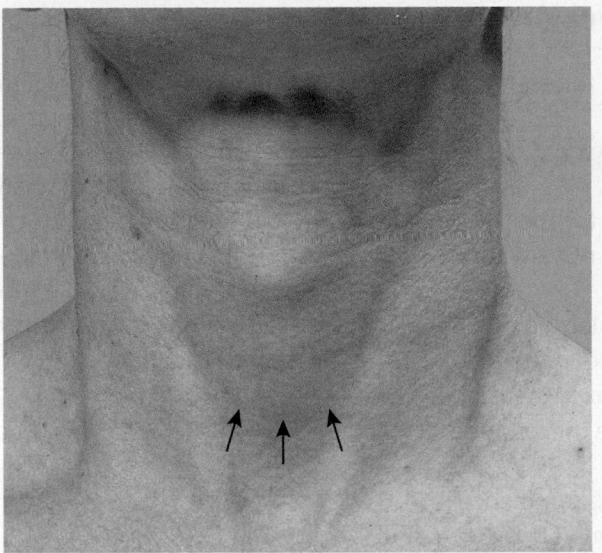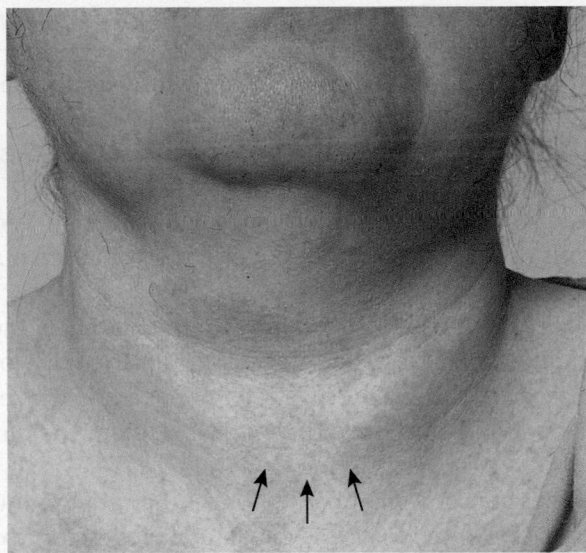

SWALLOWING

Until you become familiar with this examination, check your visual observations with your fingers from in front of the patient. This will orient you to the next step.

You are now ready to *palpate the thyroid gland*. This may seem difficult at first. Use the cues from visual inspection. Find your landmarks—the notched thyroid cartilage and the cricoid cartilage below it. Locate the *thyroid isthmus*, usually overlying the second, third, and fourth tracheal rings.

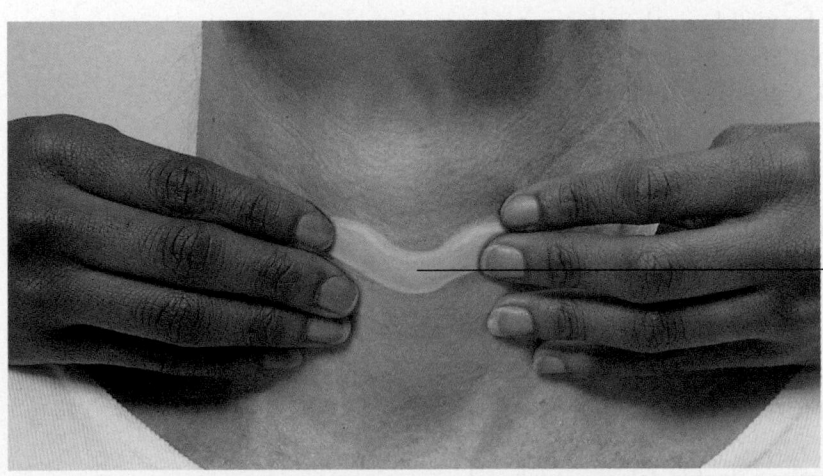

Cricoid cartilage

Adopt good technique, and follow the steps below, which outline the posterior approach (technique for the anterior approach is similar). With experience you will become more adept. The thyroid gland is usually easier to feel in a long slender neck than in a short stocky one. In shorter necks, added extension of the neck may help. In some people, however, the thyroid gland is partially or wholly substernal and not amenable to physical examination.

STEPS FOR PALPATING THE THYROID GLAND (POSTERIOR APPROACH)

- Ask the patient to flex the neck slightly forward to relax the sternomastoid muscles.
- Place the fingers of both hands on the patient's neck so that your index fingers are just below the cricoid cartilage.
- Ask the patient to sip and swallow water as before. Feel for the thyroid isthmus rising up under your finger pads. It is often but not always palpable.
- Displace the trachea to the right with the fingers of the left hand; with the right-hand fingers, palpate laterally for the right lobe of the thyroid in the space between the displaced trachea and the relaxed sternomastoid. Find the lateral margin. In similar fashion, examine the left lobe.

  The lobes are somewhat harder to feel than the isthmus, so practice is needed. The anterior surface of a lateral lobe is approximately the size of the distal phalanx of the thumb and feels somewhat rubbery.
- Note the *size, shape,* and *consistency* of the gland and identify any *nodules* or *tenderness.*

  > Soft in *Graves disease;* firm in *Hashimoto thyroiditis,* malignancy. Benign and malignant nodules,[8,9] tenderness in thyroiditis

  If the thyroid gland is enlarged, listen over the lateral lobes with a stethoscope to detect a *bruit,* a sound similar to a cardiac murmur but of noncardiac origin.

  > A localized systolic or continuous bruit may be heard in *hyperthyroidism.*

Although physical characteristics of the thyroid gland, such as size, shape, and consistency, are diagnostically important, assessment of thyroid function depends on symptoms, signs elsewhere in the body, and laboratory tests.[7] See Table 10-4, Thyroid Enlargement and Function (p. 209).

The Carotid Arteries and Jugular Veins. Defer a detailed examination of these vessels until the patient lies down for the cardiovascular examination. Jugular venous distention, however, may be visible in the sitting position and should not be overlooked. You should also be alert to unusually prominent arterial pulsations. See Chapter 14 Cardiovascular System, for further discussion.

RECORDING YOUR FINDINGS

Recording the Physical Examination— The Head and Neck

Head—The skull is normocephalic/atraumatic (NC/AT). Hair straight, brown, and soft.
Neck—Trachea midline. Neck supple; thyroid isthmus palpable, lobes not felt.
Lymph Nodes—No head or neck adenopathy.

OR

Head—The skull is normocephalic/atraumatic. Frontal balding; thin, brown.
Neck—Trachea midline. Neck supple; thyroid isthmus midline, lobes palpable but not enlarged.
Lymph Nodes—R submandibular and R occipital lymph nodes tender, 1×1 cm, rubbery, non tender and mobile.

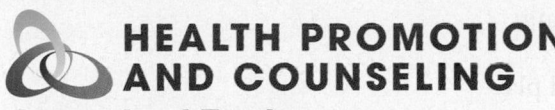

HEALTH PROMOTION AND COUNSELING

Important Topics

Prevention of Traumatic Brain Injury

The Centers for Disease Control and Prevention note the age groups at highest risk for TBI injury are children 0- to 4-years-old, adolescents 15- to 19-year-olds, and adults 65 years and older. The adults over 75 years old have higher rates of hospitalization and death. In every age group, TBI rates are higher for males.[4]

The leading causes of traumatic brain injury are falls, motor vehicle accidents, and being hit or struck by an object. Teaching patients about prevention of head injuries is paramount.

To decrease the likelihood of falls, suggest the following:

- Install safety features in the home such as grab bars in the bathroom and nonslip mats in the bathtub.

- Avoid the use of throw rugs.

- Remove extension or phone cords from high-traffic areas.

- Use rails on stairs.

- Wear nonslip, well-fitting shoes.

- Install gates on stairs.

- Install window guards.

- Do not use walkers for babies.

To prevent head injuries in motor vehicle accidents, recommend the following:

- Always use seat belts.

- Ensure small children are using car seats or booster seats appropriate for their size and weight.

- Small children should sit in the back seat especially if the car has a passenger airbag.

- Never drive under the influence of alcohol or drugs, including over-the-counter medications that cause drowsiness.

- Wear a helmet when riding motorcycles, all-terrain vehicles, motorized scooters, bicycles, horses or snowmobiles.

To avert injuries from being hit by an object, recommend the following:

- Wear helmets when skiing, snowboarding, skating, batting, and playing all contact sports.

- Place heavy objects on shelves at eye level or lower.

- Avoid dangerous situations or fights.

- Lock firearms and store bullets in a separate area.

Safety and prevention are ongoing, and every possible situation is not addressed. This is an awareness issue that each individual needs to account for in his or her own surroundings.

TABLE
10-1

Primary Headaches[1,3,10]

	Migraines	Tension	Cluster
	• With aura • Without aura • Variants		
Process	Primary neuronal dysfunction, possibly of brainstem origin, causing imbalance of excitatory and inhibitory neurotransmitters and affecting craniovascular modulation	Unclear—muscle contraction or vasoconstriction unlikely	Unclear—possibly extracranial vasodilation from neural dysfunction with trigeminovascular pain
Location	Unilateral in ~70%; bifrontal or global in ~30%	Usually bilateral; may be generalized or localized to the back of the head and upper neck or to the frontotemporal area	Unilateral, usually behind or around the eye
Quality and Severity	Throbbing or aching, variable in severity	Pressing or tightening pain; mild to moderate intensity	Deep, continuous, severe
Timing			
Onset	Fairly rapid, reaching a peak in 1–2 hours	Gradual	Abrupt; peaks within minutes
Duration	4–72 hours	Minutes to days	Up to 3 hours
Course	Peak incidence early to midadolescence; prevalence is ~6% in men and ~15% in women. Recurrent—usually monthly, but weekly in ~10%	Often recurrent or persistent over long periods; annual prevalence ~40%	Episodic, clustered in time, with several each day for 4–8 weeks and then relief for 6–12 months; prevalence <1%, more common in men
Associated Factors	Nausea, vomiting, photophobia, phonophobia, visual auras (flickering, zigzagging lines), motor auras affecting hand or arm, sensory auras (numbness, tingling usually precede attack)	Sometimes photophobia, phonophobia; nausea absent	Lacrimation, rhinorrhea, miosis, ptosis, eyelid edema, conjunctival infection
Factors That Aggravate or Provoke	Alcohol, certain foods, or tension may provoke; more common premenstrually; aggravated by noise and bright light	Sustained muscle tension, as in driving or typing	During attack, sensitivity to alcohol may increase
Factors That Relieve	Quiet, dark room; sleep; sometimes transient relief from pressure on the involved artery, if early in the course	Possibly massage, relaxation	

TABLE
10-2

Secondary Headaches[3]; Cranial Neuralgias

Type	Process	Location	Quality and Severity	Onset
Secondary Headaches				
Analgesic Rebound	Withdrawal of medication	Previous headache pattern	Variable	Variable
Headaches From Eye Disorders				
Errors of Refraction (farsightedness and astigmatism, but not nearsightedness)	Probably the sustained contraction of the extraocular muscles, and possibly of the frontal, temporal, and occipital muscles	Around and over the eyes; may radiate to the occipital area	Steady, aching, dull	Gradual
Acute Glaucoma	Sudden increase in intraocular pressure (see p. 238)	In and around one eye	Steady, aching, often severe	Often rapid
Headache From Sinusitis	Mucosal inflammation of the paranasal sinuses	Usually above the eye (frontal sinus) or over the maxillary sinus	Aching or throbbing, variable in severity; consider possible migraine	Variable
Meningitis	Infection of the meninges surrounding the brain	Generalized	Steady or throbbing, very severe	Fairly rapid
Subarachnoid Hemorrhage	Bleeding, most often from a ruptured intracranial aneurysm	Generalized	Very severe, "the worst of my life"	Usually abrupt, severe; prodromal symptoms may occur
Brain Tumor	Displacement of or traction on pain-sensitive arteries and veins or pressure on nerves	Varies with the location of the tumor	Aching, steady, variable in intensity	Variable
Giant Cell (Temporal) Arteritis[11]	Vasculitis from cell-mediated immune response to elastic lamina of artery	Localized near the involved artery, most often the temporal, but also the occipital; age related	Throbbing, generalized, persistent; often severe	Gradual or rapid
Posttraumatic Headache	Mechanism unclear; episodes similar to tension-type and migraine without aura headaches[6]	May be localized to the injured area, but not necessarily	Generalized, dull, aching, constant	Within hours to 1–2 days of the injury
Cranial Neuralgias				
Trigeminal Neuralgia (CN V)	Compression of CN V, often by aberrant loop or artery of vein	Cheek, jaws, lips, or gums; trigeminal nerve divisions 2 and 3 > 1	Shock-like, stabbing, burning; severe	Abrupt, paroxysmal

Note: Blanks appear in this table when the categories are not applicable or not usually helpful in assessing the problem.

Timing		Associated Factors	Factors That Aggravate or Provoke	Factors That Relieve
Duration	*Course*			
Depends on prior headache pattern	Depends on frequency of "mini-withdrawals"	Depends on prior headache pattern	Fever, carbon monoxide, hypoxia, withdrawal of caffeine, other headache triggers	Depends on cause
Variable	Variable	Eye fatigue, "sandy" sensations in the eyes, redness of the conjunctiva	Prolonged use of the eyes, particularly for close work	Rest of the eyes
Variable, may depend on treatment	Variable, may depend on treatment	Diminished vision, sometimes nausea and vomiting	Sometimes provoked by drops that dilate the pupils	
Often several hours at a time, recurring over days or longer	Often recurrent in a repetitive daily pattern	Local tenderness, nasal congestion, discharge, and fever	May be aggravated by coughing, sneezing, or jarring the head	Nasal decongestants, antibiotics
Variable, usually days	A persistent headache in an acute illness	Fever, stiff neck		
Variable, usually days	A persistent headache in an acute illness	Nausea, vomiting, possibly loss of consciousness, neck pain		
Often brief	Often intermittent but progressive	May be aggravated by coughing, sneezing, or sudden movements of the head		
Variable	Recurrent or persistent over weeks to months	Tenderness of the adjacent scalp; fever (in ~50%), fatigue, weight loss; new headache (~60%), jaw claudication (~50%), visual loss or blindness (~15%–20%), polymyalgia rheumatica (~50%)	Movement of neck and shoulders	
Weeks, months, or even years	Tends to diminish over time	Poor concentration, problems with memory, vertigo, irritability, restlessness, fatigue	Mental and physical exertion, straining, stooping, emotional excitement, alcohol	Rest
Each jab lasts seconds but recurs at intervals of seconds or minutes	May last for months, then disappear for months, but often recurs. It is uncommon at night.	Exhaustion from recurrent pain	Touching certain areas of the lower face or mouth; chewing, talking, brushing teeth	

TABLE
10-3

Selected Facies

Facial Swelling

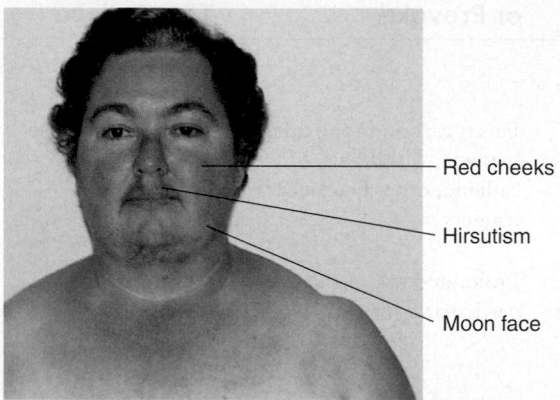

Red cheeks

Hirsutism

Moon face

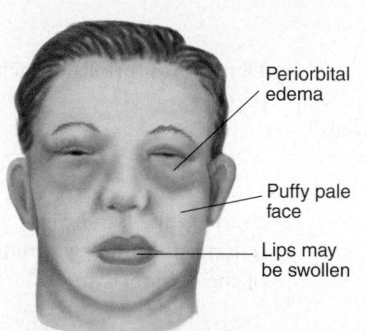

Periorbital edema

Puffy pale face

Lips may be swollen

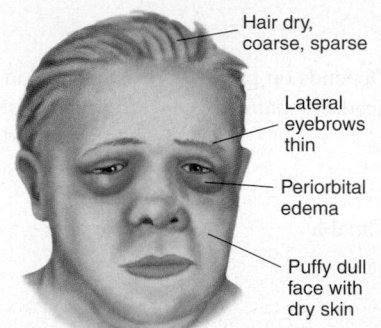

Hair dry, coarse, sparse

Lateral eyebrows thin

Periorbital edema

Puffy dull face with dry skin

Cushing Syndrome

The increased adrenal cortisol production of Cushing syndrome produces a round or "moon" face with red cheeks. Excessive hair growth may be present in the mustache and sideburn areas and on the chin.

Nephrotic Syndrome

The face is edematous and often pale. Swelling usually appears first around the eyes and in the morning. The eyes may become slitlike when edema is severe.

Myxedema

The patient with severe hypothyroidism (myxedema) has a dull, puffy facies. The edema, often pronounced around the eyes, does not pit with pressure. The hair and eyebrows are dry, coarse, and thinned. The skin is dry.

Other Facies

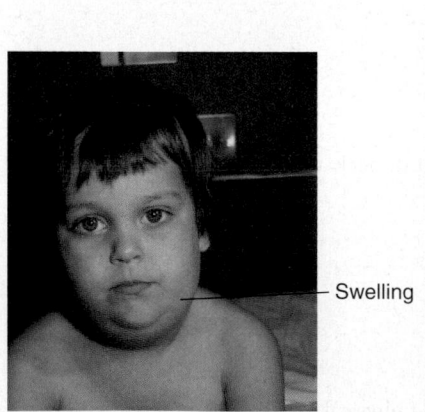

Swelling

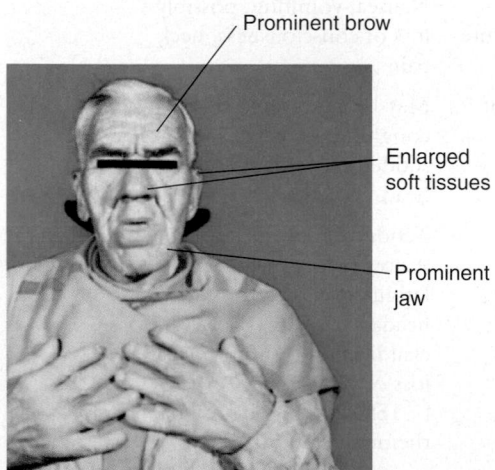

Prominent brow

Enlarged soft tissues

Prominent jaw

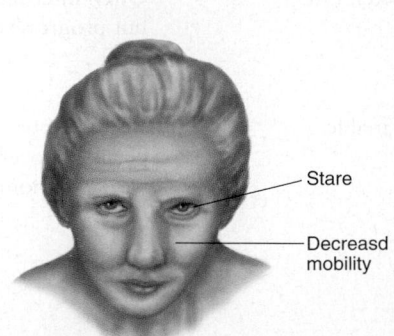

Stare

Decreasd mobility

Parotid Gland Enlargement

Chronic bilateral asymptomatic parotid gland enlargement may be associated with obesity, diabetes, cirrhosis, and other conditions. Note the swellings anterior to the ear lobes and above the angles of the jaw. Gradual unilateral enlargement suggests neoplasm. Acute enlargement is seen in mumps.

Acromegaly

The increased growth hormone of acromegaly produces enlargement of both bone and soft tissues. The head is elongated, with bony prominence of the forehead, nose, and lower jaw. Soft tissues of the nose, lips, and ears also enlarge. The facial features appear generally coarsened.

Parkinson Disease

Decreased facial mobility blunts expression. A masklike face may result, with decreased blinking and a characteristic stare. Since the neck and upper trunk tend to flex forward, the patient seems to peer upward toward the observer. Facial skin becomes oily, and drooling may occur.

TABLE
10-4

Thyroid Enlargement and Function

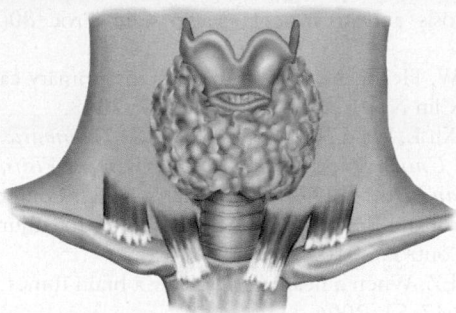

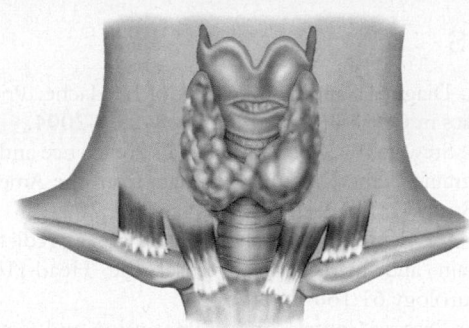

Diffuse Enlargement. Includes the isthmus and lateral lobes; there are no discretely palpable nodules. Causes include Graves disease, Hashimoto thyroiditis, and endemic goiter.

Single Nodule. May be a cyst, a benign tumor, or one nodule within a multinodular gland. It raises the question of malignancy. Risk factors are prior irradiation, hardness, rapid growth, fixation to surrounding tissues, enlarged cervical nodes, and occurrence in males.[8]

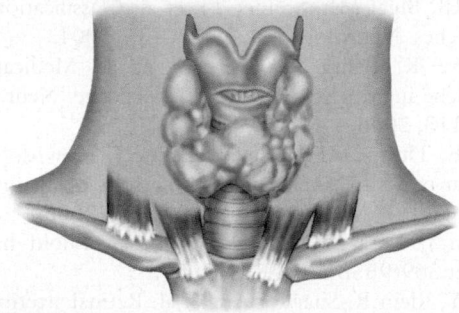

Multinodular Goiter. An enlarged thyroid gland with two or more nodules suggests a metabolic rather than a neoplastic process. Positive family history and continuing nodular enlargement are additional risk factors for malignancy.

TABLE
10-5

Symptoms and Signs of Thyroid Dysfunction[7,12–14]

	Hyperthyroidism	Hypothyroidism
Symptoms	Nervousness	Fatigue, lethargy
	Weight loss despite increased appetite	Modest weight gain with anorexia
	Excessive sweating and heat intolerance	Dry, coarse skin and cold intolerance
	Palpitations	Swelling of face, hands, and legs
	Frequent bowel movements	Constipation
	Muscular weakness of the proximal type and tremor	Weakness, muscle cramps, arthralgias, paresthesias, impaired memory and hearing
Signs	Warm, smooth, moist skin	Dry, coarse, cool skin, sometimes yellowish from carotene, with nonpitting edema and loss of hair
	With Graves disease, eye signs such as stare, lid lag, and exophthalmos	Periorbital puffiness
	Increased systolic and decreased diastolic blood pressures	Decreased systolic and increased diastolic blood pressures
	Tachycardia or atrial fibrillation	Bradycardia and, in late stages, hypothermia
	Hyperdynamic cardiac pulsations with an accentuated S_1	Intensity of heart sounds sometimes decreased
	Tremor and proximal muscle weakness	Impaired memory, mixed hearing loss, somnolence, peripheral neuropathy, carpal tunnel syndrome

BIBLIOGRAPHY

CITATIONS

1. Taylor FR. Diagnosis and classification of headache. Primary Care: Clinics in Office Practice 31(2):243–259, 2004.
2. Lipton RB, Stewart WF, Seymour D, et al. Prevalence and burden of migraine in the United States: data from the American Migraine Study II. Headache 41(7):646–657, 2001.
3. Zwart JA, Dyb G, Hagen K, et al. Analgesic use: a predictor of chronic pain and medication overuse: the Head-HUNT Study. Neurology 61:160–164, 2003.
4. Centers for Disease Control. Injury Prevention and Control: Traumatic Brain Injury. Available at: http://www.cdc.gov/traumaticbraininjury/statistics.html. Accessed April 1, 2011.
5. McGuirt WF. The neck mass. Med Clin N Am 83:219–234, 1989.
6. Siminoski K. Does this patient have a goiter? JAMA 273(10):813–817, 1995.
7. Surks MI, Ortiz E, Daniels GH, et al. Subclinical thyroid disease: scientific review and guidelines for diagnosis and management. JAMA 291(2):228–238, 2004.
8. Hegedus L. The thyroid nodule. N Engl J Med 351(17):1764–1771, 2004.
9. Castro MR, Gharib H. Controversies in the management of thyroid nodules. Ann Intern Med 142(11):926–931, 2005.
10. Goadsby PJ, Lipton RB, Ferrari MD. Migraine: current understanding and treatment. N Engl J Med 346(4):257–270, 2002.
11. Smetana GW, Shmerling RH. Does this patient have temporal arteritis? JAMA 287(1):92–101, 2002.
12. Gladstone GJ. Ophthalmologic aspects of thyroid-related orbitopathy. Endocrinol Metab Clin North Am 27:91–100, 1998.
13. Bartley GB, Fatourechi V, Kadrmas EF, et al. Clinical features of Graves' ophthalmopathy in an incidence cohort. Am J Ophthalmol 121:284–290, 1996.
14. Hallin ES, Feldon SE. Graves' ophthalmopathy. II. Correlation of clinical signs with measures derived from computed tomography. Br J Ophthalmol 72:678–682, 1988.

ADDITIONAL REFERENCES

The Head

Bahra A, May A. Cluster headache: a prospective clinical study with diagnostic implications. Neurology 58(3):354–361, 2002.

Cady RK, Dodick DW, Levine HL, et al. Sinus headache: a neurology, otolaryngology, allergy, and primary care consensus on diagnosis and treatment. Mayo Clin Proc 80(7):908–916, 2005.

Evans RW. Headache case studies for the primary care physician. Med Clin North Am 87(3):589–607, 2003.

Faul M, Xu L, Wald MM, Coronado VG. *Traumatic Brain Injury in the United States: Emergency Department Visits, Hospitalizations and Deaths 2002–2006.* Atlanta (GA): Centers for Disease Control and Prevention, National Center for Injury Prevention and Control; 2010.

Franges EZ. When a headache is really a brain tumor. Nurse Pract 31(4):47–51, 2006.

Langlois JA, Rutland-Brown W, Thomas KE. Traumatic Brain Injury in the United States: Emergency Department Visits, Hospitalizations, and Deaths. Atlanta, GA: Centers for Disease Control and Prevention, National Center for Injury Prevention and Control, 2006.

Lipton RB, Bigal ME, Steiner TJ, et al. Classification of primary headaches. Neurology 63(3):427–435, 2004.

Paemeleire K, Bahra A, Evers S, et al. Medication-overuse headache in patients with cluster headache. Neurology 67(1):109–113, 2006.

Straus SE, Thorpe KE, Holroyd-Leduc J. How do I perform a lumbar puncture and analyze the results to diagnose bacterial meningitis? JAMA 296(16):2012–2022, 2006.

Van Gijn J, Kerr RS, Rinkel GJ. Subarachnoid haemorrhage Lancet 369(9558):306–318, 2007.

Wong TY, Klein R, Sharrett AR, et al. Retinal arteriolar diameter and risk for hypertension. Ann Intern Med 140(4):248–255, 2004.

The Neck

Bliss SJ, Flanders SA, Saint S. A pain in the neck. N Engl J Med 350(10):1037–1042, 2004.

Dorshimer GW, Kelly M. Cervical pain in the athlete: common conditions and treatment. Prim Care 32(1):231–243, 2005.

Henry PH, Long DL. Enlargement of the lymph nodes and spleen. In: Kasper DL, Fauci AS, Longo DL, et al., eds. Harrison's Principles of Internal Medicine, 16th ed. New York: McGraw-Hill, 2005:343–348.

Prisco MK. Evaluating neck masses. Nurse Pract 25(4):30–32, 35–36, 38, 2000.

Schwetschenau E, Kelley DJ. The adult neck mass. Am Fam Phys 67(6):1190, 1192, 1195, 2003.

The Eyes

LEARNING OBJECTIVES

The student will:

1. Identify the components and function of the eye.
2. Collect an accurate health history of the eye.
3. Describe the physical examination techniques performed to evaluate the eye.
4. Demonstrate how to use the ophthalmoscope.
5. Identify the measures for prevention or early detection of eye disease, infections, or vision loss.
6. Perform a complete eye examination.
7. Document a complete eye assessment utilizing information from the health history and physical examination.

 ## ANATOMY AND PHYSIOLOGY

The eye is the sensory organ of vision and has many critical components, including the cranial nerves. During the assessment various signs and symptoms signal changes in the eyes. The nurse's role is to detect these changes and work with the health care team to prevent injury or loss of vision.

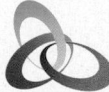 ## THE EYES

Eye Structures

The structures of the eye are identified on this page. Note that the upper eyelid covers a portion of the iris but does not touch the pupil. The opening between the eyelids is called the *palpebral fissure*. The white sclera may look somewhat darker at its periphery. The *conjunctiva* is a clear mucous membrane with two easily visible components. The *bulbar conjunctiva*, also known as the sclera covers most of the anterior eyeball, adhering loosely to the underlying tissue. The *palpebral conjunctiva* lines the eyelids. The two parts of the conjunctiva merge in a folded recess that permits movement of the eyeball.

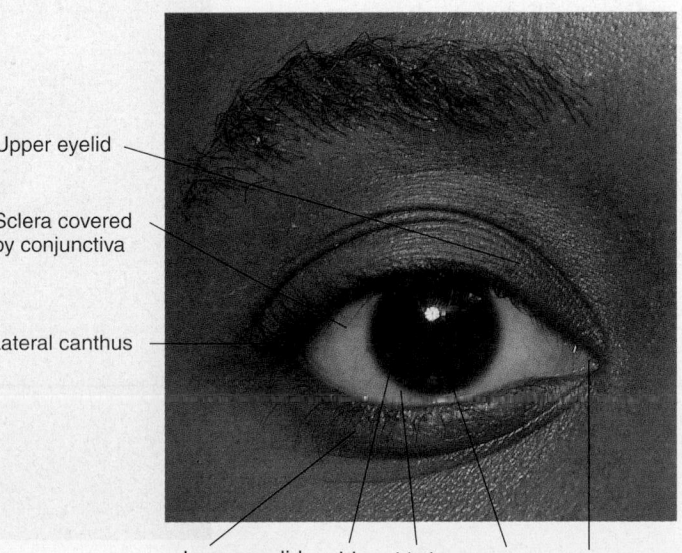

Upper eyelid

Sclera covered by conjunctiva

Lateral canthus

Lower eyelid   Iris   Limbus   Pupil   Medial canthus

Within the eyelids lie firm strips of connective tissue called *tarsal plates.* Each plate contains a parallel row of *meibomian glands,* which open on the lid margin. The *levator palpebrae,* the muscle that raises the upper eyelid, is innervated by the oculomotor nerve, cranial nerve (CN) III. Smooth muscle, innervated by the sympathetic nervous system, also contributes to lid elevation.

A film of tear fluid protects the conjunctiva and cornea from drying, inhibits microbial growth, and gives a smooth optical surface to the cornea. This fluid comes from the meibomian glands, conjunctival glands, and lacrimal gland. The *lacrimal gland* lies mostly within the bony orbit, above and lateral to the eyeball. The tear fluid spreads across the eye and drains medially through two tiny holes called *lacrimal puncta.* The tears then pass into the *lacrimal sac* and into the nose through the *nasolacrimal duct.* You can easily find a *punctum* atop the small elevation of the lower lid medially. The lacrimal sac rests in a small depression inside the bony orbit and is not visible.

The eyeball is a spherical structure that focuses light on the neurosensory elements within the retina. The muscles of the iris control pupillary size, constricting in bright light and dilating in the dark. Muscles of the *ciliary body* control the thickness of the lens, allowing the eye to focus on near or distant objects.

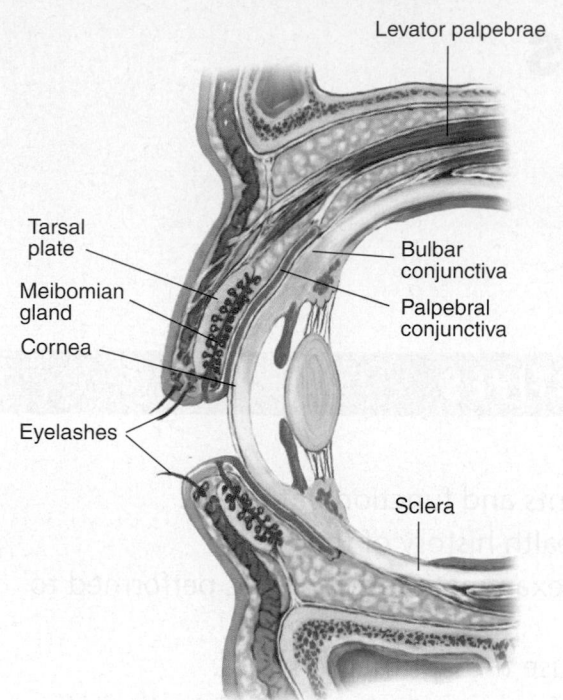

SAGITTAL SECTION OF ANTERIOR EYE WITH LIDS CLOSED

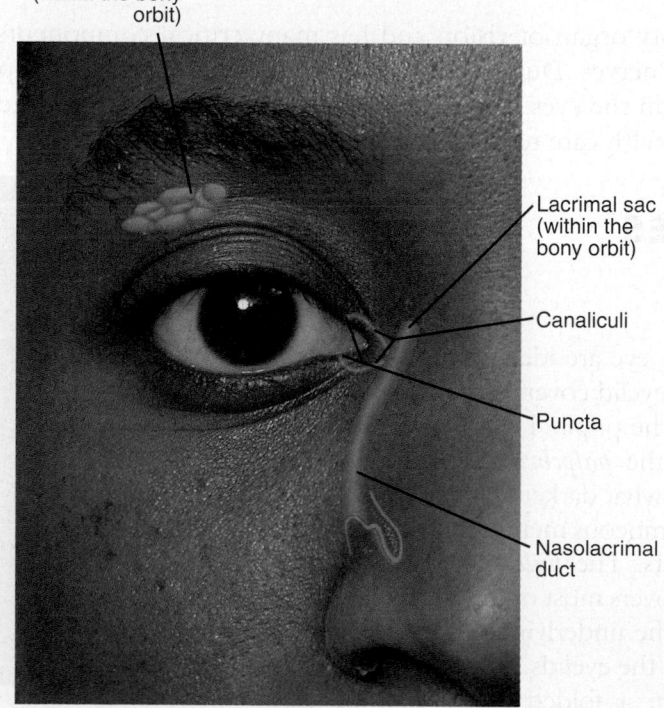

Vitreous humor is the clear gel that fills the space between the lens and the retina. The aqueous humor is a clear liquid that fills the anterior and posterior chambers of the eye, circulating between the cornea and the lens. Aqueous humor is produced by the *ciliary body,* circulates from the posterior chamber through the pupil into the anterior chamber, and drains out through the *canal of Schlemm.* This circulatory system helps to control the pressure inside the eye.

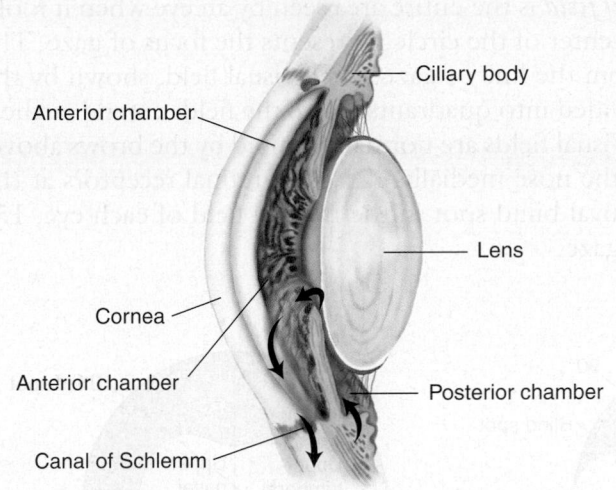

CIRCULATION OF AQUEOUS HUMOR

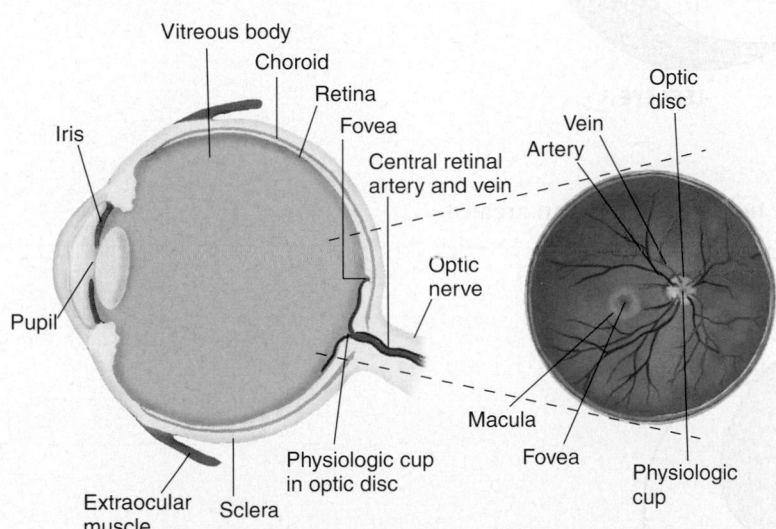

CROSS SECTION OF THE RIGHT EYE SHOWING A PORTION OF THE FUNDUS COMMONLY SEEN WITH THE OPHTHALMOSCOPE

The posterior part of the eye seen through an ophthalmoscope is often called the *fundus* of the eye. Structures here include the retina, choroid, fovea, macula, optic disc, and retinal vessels. The eye is not visible at once and as the ophthalmoscope is adjusted sections of the eye appear. The optic nerve with its retinal vessels enters the eyeball posteriorly. You can find it with an ophthalmoscope at the *optic disc.* When looking into the eye with the ophthalmoscope, it is best to locate the optic disc medially and utilize this as your landmark. Note the margins of the disc and then locate the arteries and veins. Lateral and slightly inferior to the disc, there is a small depression in the retinal surface that marks the point of central vision. Around it is a darkened circular area called the *fovea.* The roughly circular *macula* (named for a microscopic yellow spot) surrounds the fovea but has no discernible margins. It is unusual to see the normal *vitreous body,* a transparent mass of gelatinous material that fills the eyeball behind the lens. It helps to maintain the shape of the eye.

ANATOMY AND PHYSIOLOGY

Visual Fields. A *visual field* is the entire area seen by an eye when it looks at a central point. The center of the circle represents the focus of gaze. The circumference is 90° from the line of gaze. Each visual field, shown by the white areas below, is divided into quadrants. Note the fields extend farthest on the temporal sides. Visual fields are normally limited by the brows above, the cheeks below, and the nose medially. A lack of retinal receptors at the optic disc produces an oval blind spot in the normal field of each eye, 15° temporal to the line of gaze.

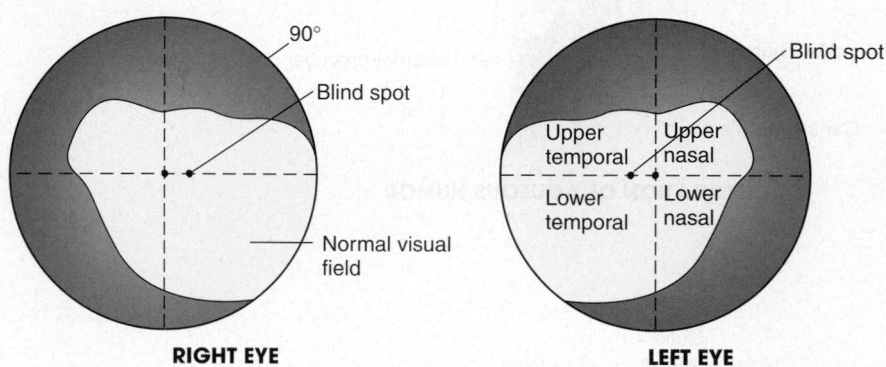

When a person is using both eyes, the two visual fields overlap in an area of binocular vision. Laterally, vision is monocular.

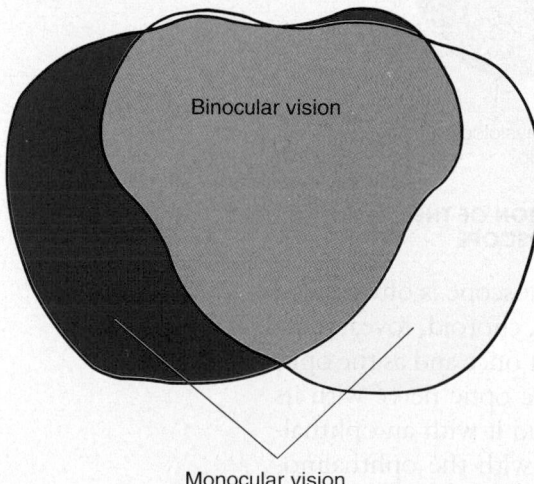

Visual Pathways. To see an image, light reflected from the image must pass through the pupil and be focused on sensory neurons in the retina. The image projected there is upside down and reversed right to left. An image from the upper nasal visual field thus strikes the lower temporal quadrant of the retina.

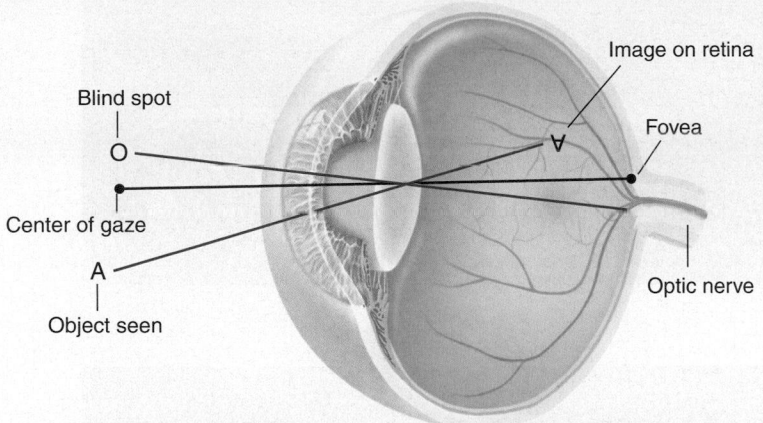

Nerve impulses, stimulated by light, are conducted through the retina, optic nerve, and optic tract on each side, then on through a curving tract called the *optic radiation*. This ends in the visual cortex, a part of the occipital lobe.

Pupillary Reactions.   Pupillary size changes in response to light and to the effort of focusing on a near object.

The Light Reaction. A light beam shining onto one retina causes pupillary constriction both in that eye, termed the *direct reaction* to light, and in the opposite eye, the *consensual reaction*. The initial sensory pathways are similar to those described for vision: retina, optic nerve, and optic tract. The pathways diverge in the midbrain, however, and impulses are transmitted through the oculomotor nerve, CN III, to the constrictor muscles of the iris of each eye.

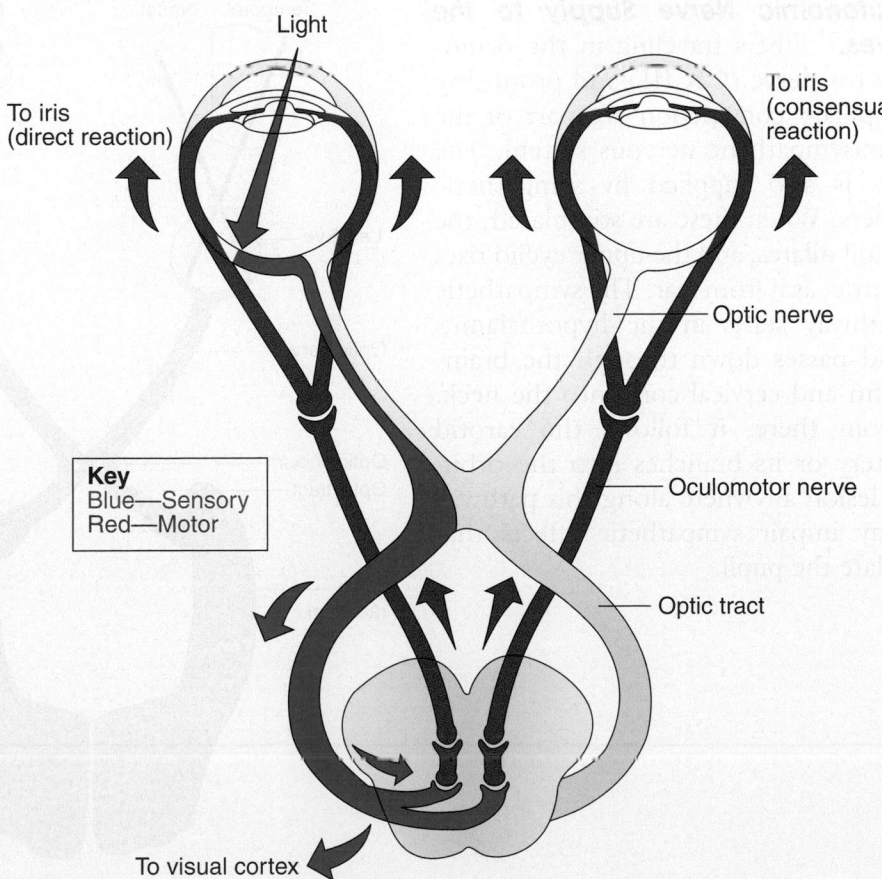

PATHWAYS OF THE LIGHT REACTION

The Near Reaction. When a person shifts gaze from a far object to a near one, the pupils constrict. This response, like the light reaction, is mediated by the oculomotor nerve (CN III). At the same time as the *pupillary constriction,* but not a part of it, are (1) *convergence* of the eyes, an extraocular movement; and (2) *accommodation,* an increased convexity of the lenses caused by contraction of the ciliary muscles. This change in shape of the lenses brings near objects into focus but is not visible to the examiner.

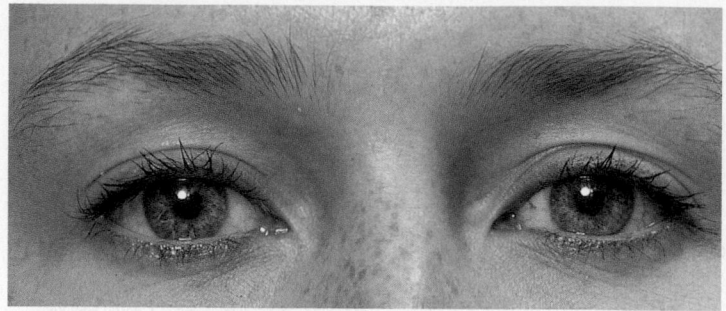

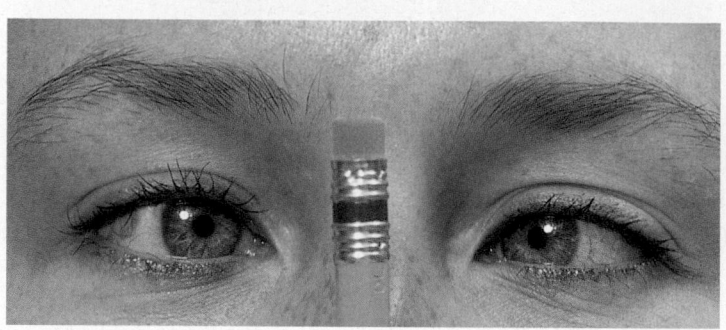

Autonomic Nerve Supply to the Eyes. Fibers traveling in the oculomotor nerve (CN III) and producing pupillary constriction are part of the parasympathetic nervous system. The iris is also supplied by sympathetic fibers. When these are stimulated, the pupil dilates, and the upper eyelid rises a little, as if from fear. The sympathetic pathway starts in the hypothalamus and passes down through the brainstem and cervical cord into the neck. From there, it follows the carotid artery or its branches into the orbit. A lesion anywhere along this pathway may impair sympathetic effects that dilate the pupil.

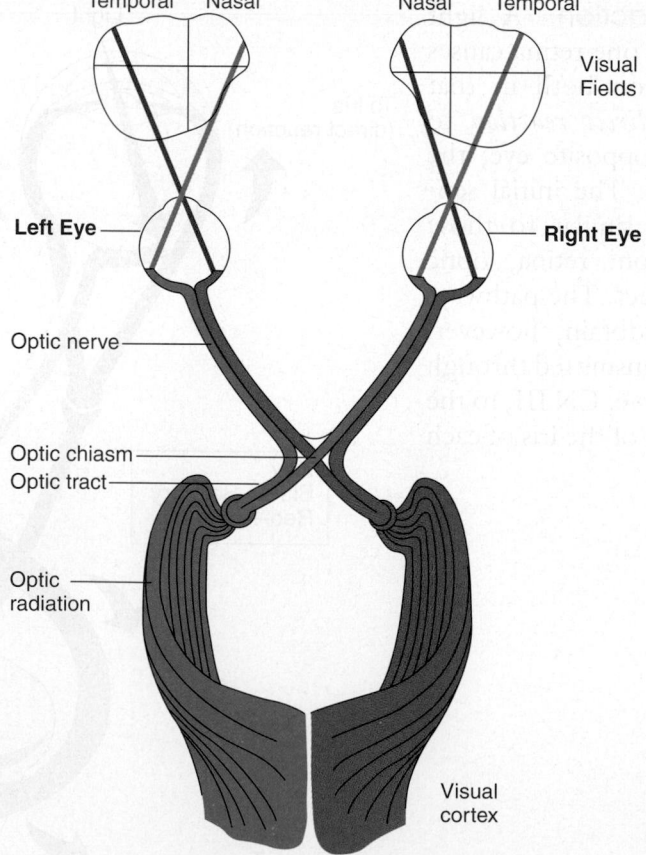

VISUAL PATHWAYS FROM THE RETINA TO THE VISUAL CORTEX

Extraocular Movements. The coordinated action of six muscles: the four rectus (superior, lateral, medial, and inferior) and two oblique (inferior and superior), control the eye. To test the function of each muscle and the nerve that supplies it, ask the patient to move the eye in the direction controlled by that muscle. There are six *cardinal directions*, indicated by the lines on the figure below. When a person looks down and to the right, for example, the right inferior rectus (CN III) is principally responsible for moving the right eye, whereas the left superior oblique (CN IV) is principally responsible for moving the left. If one of these muscles is paralyzed, the eye will deviate from its normal position in that direction of gaze and the eyes will no longer appear conjugate, or parallel.

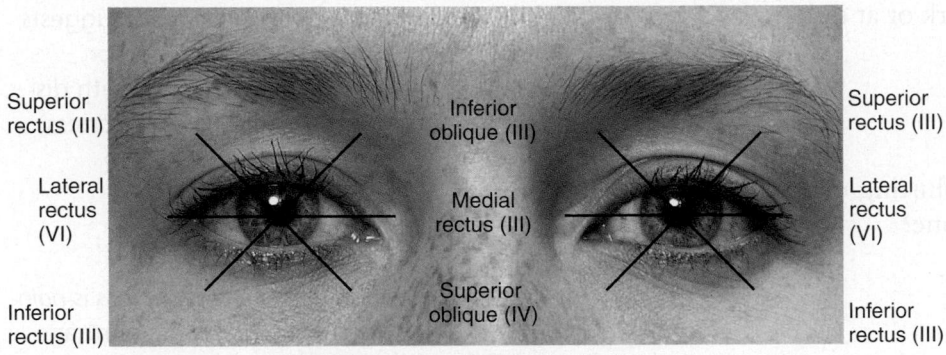

CARDINAL DIRECTIONS OF GAZE

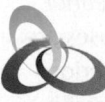 # THE HEALTH HISTORY

COMMON OR CONCERNING SYMPTOMS

- Changes in vision:
  - Hyperopia
  - Presbyopia
  - Myopia
  - Scotomas
- Double vision or diplopia
- Strabismus
- Blurring
- Redness
- Itching
- Discharge
- Pain
- Tearing
- Edema
- Lesions
- Visual disturbances
- Photophobia

A scotoma is an area of lost or depressed vision within the visual field and is surrounded by an area of normal vision.

Photophobia or light sensitivity is usually from excess light entering the eye, which may overexcite the photoreceptors in the retina.

The purpose of the health history is to identify changes in the eyes. The nurse should begin the inquiry about the eyes with a broad, open-ended question such as: "Have you noticed any changes with your eyes?" The patient may have developed symptoms gradually and learned to live with changes. Older patients may assume vision changes are a part of aging. They may not realize that they could be seeing better and may not answer the questions in the health history relative to the objective assessment revelations. Further investigation is crucial and more in-depth questioning should be pursued. For example: "Is your vision as good now as previously?"

If changes in vision are revealed then continue:

Is the **difficulty** during close work or at distances?

> Difficulty with close work suggests *hyperopia* (farsightedness) or *presbyopia* (aging vision) with distances, *myopia* (nearsightedness).

Is there **blurred** vision? Is the blurring of the entire field of vision or only parts of it? Both eyes or one?
Is the onset sudden or gradual?
Is it **painful** or painless?

> If sudden *unilateral* visual loss is *painless*, consider vitreous hemorrhage from diabetes or trauma, *macular degeneration, retinal detachment, retinal vein occlusion,* or *central retinal artery occlusion.* If *painful,* causes are usually in the cornea and anterior chamber as in *corneal ulcer, uveitis, traumatic hyphema,* and *acute glaucoma. Optic neuritis* from multiple sclerosis may also be painful.[1] Immediate referral may be warranted.[2]

> If *bilateral and painless,* medications that change refraction such as cholinergics, anticholinergics, and steroids may contribute. If bilateral and painful, consider chemical or radiation exposures. If the onset of bilateral visual loss is gradual, this usually arises from *cataracts* or *macular degeneration.*

If the visual field defect is partial, is it central, peripheral, or only on one side?

> Slow central loss in nuclear cataract (p. 239), *macular degeneration*[3]; peripheral loss in advanced *open-angle glaucoma* (p. 238); one-sided loss in *hemianopsia* and *quadrantic defects* (p. 222).

Do lights **flash** across the field of vision?

Flashing lights or new vitreous floaters suggest detachment of vitreous from retina. Prompt eye consultation is indicated.

Do **floaters** accompany this symptom?

Does it feel like a curtain is falling?

Are there **specks** in the vision or areas where you are unable to see (scotoma)? If so, do they move in the visual field with shifts of gaze or are they fixed?

Moving specks or strands suggest vitreous floaters; fixed defects (*scotomas*) suggest lesions in the retina or visual pathways.

Do you have **double vision (diplopia)**?

Are the images side by side (horizontal diplopia) or on top of each other (vertical diplopia)? Does this persist with one eye closed? Which eye is affected?

One kind of horizontal diplopia is physiologic. Hold one finger upright approximately 6 inches in front of your face, a second at arm's length. When you focus on either finger, the image of the other is double. A patient who notices this phenomenon can be reassured.

Diplopia in adults may arise from a lesion in the brainstem or cerebellum, or from weakness or paralysis of one or more extraocular muscles, as in horizontal diplopia from palsy of CN III or VI, or vertical diplopia from palsy of CN III or IV. Diplopia in one eye, with the other closed, suggests a problem in the cornea or lens.

Do you experience:
  Redness?
  Excessive tearing?
  Discharge?
  Crusting?

Infection or allergic reaction

Do you have or have you ever had lesions or growths on your eyelids or eyes?

Are your eyes painful or uncomfortable when you are in the sun or well-lit places?

Photophobia

Eye History

Do you have any past history of eye problems or eye disease?

Do you have a history of:
  Premature birth?
  Trauma or injury to the eye?
  Eye surgery? Related to injury, congenital causes, or cosmetic reasons?

Eye infections?
Strabismus?
Amblyopia?
Cataracts?
Glaucoma?
Diabetes?
Retinal detachment?
Macular degeneration?
Blindness?
When was your last eye examination? Test for color blindness?
Do you wear glasses or contact lenses? Hard or soft lenses?
When did you begin to wear them?
Are they corrective or cosmetic?
How do you care for your contacts?
Do you share contacts?
How long are the contacts in your eye? Day hours? Night hours?

Family History

Do you have a family history of congenital eye diseases, cataracts, glaucoma, macular degeneration, or diabetes?

Lifestyle Habits

Do you smoke?
Do you wear sunglasses?
Do you use goggles or protective eyewear? When?
Are you on any medications/drugs that dry out the eye?

 # PHYSICAL EXAMINATION

Preparation of the Patient

Preparation of the patient and the environment is crucial to obtain correct findings during the eye examination. If the Snellen chart is located outside the exam room, then the patient should do this portion of the examination prior to changing into a patient gown if a complete examination is being performed. The area should be well lit and free of distractions. The remainder of the examination will be in a quiet, well-lit room with all necessary equipment in the room.

The components of the eye examination include:
  Vision tests: distal, near, and peripheral
  Inspection of the eye, eyebrows, lids, conjunctiva and sclera, cornea, lens, iris, and pupils
  Inspection and palpation of the lacrimal apparatus
  Extraocular movements: assessment of cardinal fields, convergence, corneal light test, cover–uncover test

Inspection of the fundi including the optic disc and cup, retina, and retinal vessels

EQUIPMENT FOR EXAMINATION

Snellen chart or "E" card
Rosenbaum, near-vision card
Index card
Penlight
Ophthalmoscope

Vision Tests

Visual Acuity (Distal).   To test the acuity of central vision, use a Snellen
eye chart, if possible, and light it well. Position the patient 20 feet from the
chart. Patients who use glasses or contacts other than for reading should
wear them for the examination. Ask the patient to cover one eye with an
index card (to prevent peeking through the fingers) and to read the smallest line of print possible. Coaxing to attempt the next line may improve performance. A patient who cannot read the largest letter should be positioned
closer to the chart; note the intervening distance. Determine the smallest
line of print from which the patient can identify more than half the letters.
Record the visual acuity designated at the side of this line, along with use of
glasses or contacts, if any. Visual acuity is expressed as two numbers (e.g.,
20/30): the numerator indicates the distance of the patient from the chart
and this number should always be 20 unless the patient moved closer to see,
and the denominator is the distance at which a normal eye can read the line
of letters.

Vision of 20/200 means that at 20
feet the patient can read print that
a person with normal vision could
read at 200 feet. The larger the
second number, the worse the
vision. "20/40 corrected" means
the patient could read the 40 line
with glasses (a correction).

Myopia is impaired far vision.

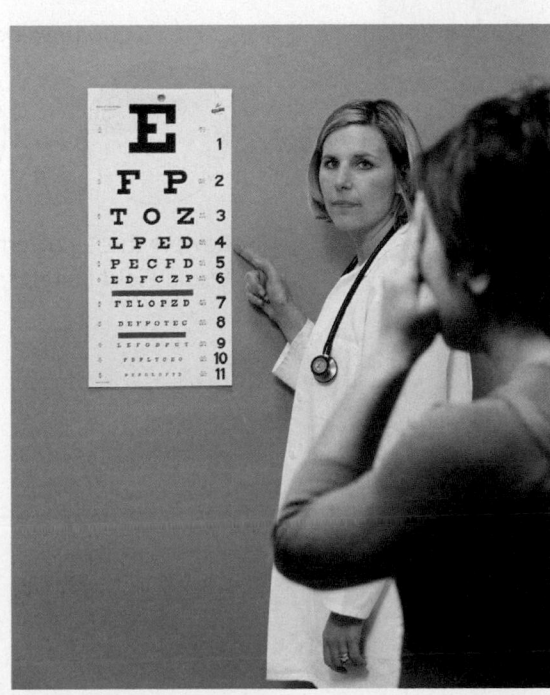

Near Vision. Testing near vision with a special hand-held card, the Rosenbaum chart, helps identify the need for reading glasses or bifocals in patients older than 45 years. This card can be utilized to test visual acuity at the bedside. Held 14 inches from the patient's eyes, the card simulates a Snellen chart. However, patients may choose their own distance.

If there are not any charts, screen visual acuity with any available print (e.g., newspaper) held at 14-16 inches away from the eyes. If patients cannot read even the largest letters, test their ability to count your upraised fingers and distinguish light (such as your flashlight) from dark.

Presbyopia is the impaired near vision found in middle-aged and older people. A presbyopic person often sees better when the card is farther away.

In the United States, a person is usually considered legally blind when vision in the better eye, corrected by glasses, is 20/200 or less. Legal blindness also results from a constricted field of vision: 20° or less in the better eye.

Peripheral Vision
Peripheral Visual Fields by Confrontation

SCREENING. Screening starts in the temporal fields because most defects involve these areas. Imagine the patient's visual fields projected onto a glass bowl that encircles the front of the patient's head. 1) Ask the patient to look with both eyes into your eyes. 2) While you return the patient's gaze, place your hands about 2 feet apart, lateral to the patient's ears. 3) Instruct the patient to point to your fingers as soon as they are seen. 4) Then slowly move the wiggling fingers of both your hands along the imaginary bowl towards the line of gaze until the patient points to them. 5) Repeat this pattern in the upper and lower temporal quadrants. Usually a person sees both sets of fingers at the same time. If so, fields are usually normal.

Field defects that are all or partly temporal include:

Homonymous Hemianopsia

Bitemporal Hemianopsia

Quadrantic Defects

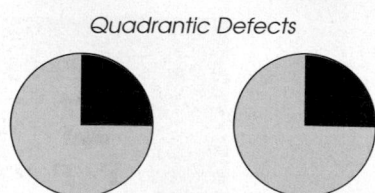

Review these patterns in Table 11-1, Visual Field Defects, p. 236.

FURTHER TESTING. If you find a defect, try to establish its boundaries. Test one eye at a time. If you suspect a temporal defect in the left visual field, for example, ask the patient to cover the right eye and, with the left one, to look into your eye directly opposite. Then slowly move your wiggling fingers from the defective area toward the better vision, noting where the patient first responds. Repeat this at several levels to define the border.

When the patient's left eye repeatedly does not see your fingers until they have crossed the line of gaze, a left *temporal hemianopsia* is present. Hemianopsia is when the patient is unable to see in half of the visual field and is generally on one side. This can occur after a cerebrovascular accident or stroke. The patient is unable to distinguish objects to the side of the visual midline. The loss is contralateral, which is on the opposite side of the brain lesion.

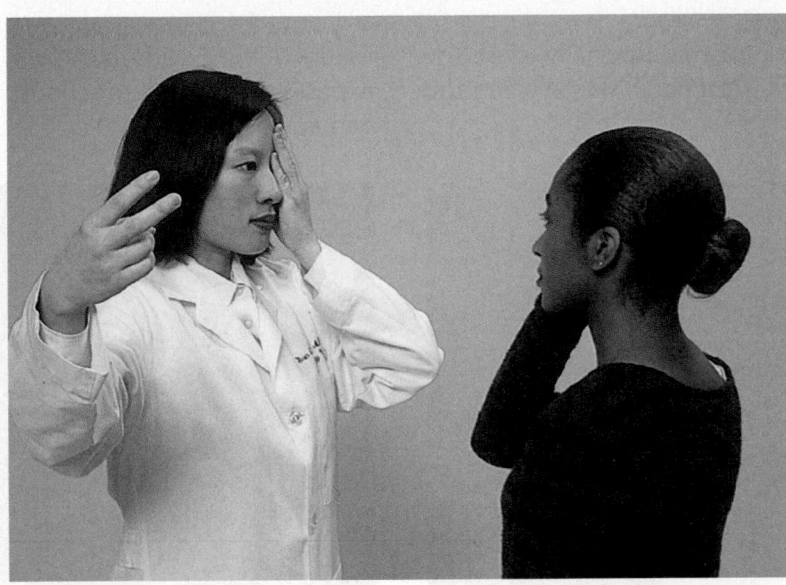

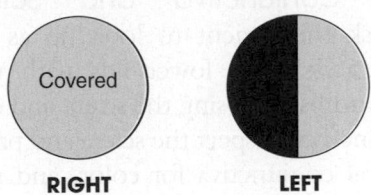

RIGHT   **LEFT**

A left *homonymous hemianopsia* may thus be established.

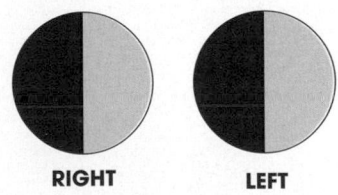

RIGHT   **LEFT**

A temporal defect in the visual field of one eye suggests a nasal defect in the other eye. To test this hypothesis, examine the other eye in a similar way, again moving from the anticipated defect toward the better vision.

Small visual field defects and enlarged blind spots require a finer stimulus. Using a small red object such as a red-headed matchstick or the red eraser on a pencil, test one eye at a time. As the patient looks into your eye directly opposite, move the object about in the visual field. The normal blind spot can be found 15° temporal to the line of gaze—the small red object disappears. (Find your own blind spots for practice.)

An enlarged blind spot occurs in conditions affecting the optic nerve such as *glaucoma, optic neuritis,* and *papilledema.*[2]

External Eye

Position and Alignment of the Eyes. Stand in front of the patient and survey the eyes for position and alignment. If one or both eyes seem to protrude, assess them from above.

Inward or outward deviation of the eyes; abnormal protrusion in *Graves disease* or ocular tumors

Eyebrows. Inspect the eyebrows, noting their quantity and distribution and any scaliness of the underlying skin.

Scaliness in *seborrheic dermatitis;* lateral sparseness in *hypothyroidism*

Eyelids. Note the position of the lids in relation to the eyeballs. Inspect for the following:

See Table 11-2, Variations and Abnormalities of the Eyelids (p. 237).

● Width of the palpebral fissures—open area between the upper and lower eyelids

Upstarting palpebral fissures in *Down syndrome*

- Edema of the lids

- Color of the lids

- Lesions

- Condition and direction of the eyelashes

- Adequacy with which the eyelids close. Look for this especially when the eyes are unusually prominent, when there is facial paralysis, or when the patient is unconscious.

Red inflamed lid margins in *blepharitis,* often with crusting

Failure of the eyelids to close exposes the corneas to serious damage.

Conjunctiva and Sclera. Ask the patient to look up as you depress both lower lids with your thumbs, exposing the sclera and conjunctiva. Inspect the sclera and palpebral conjunctiva for color, and note the vascular pattern against the white scleral background. Look for any nodules or swelling.

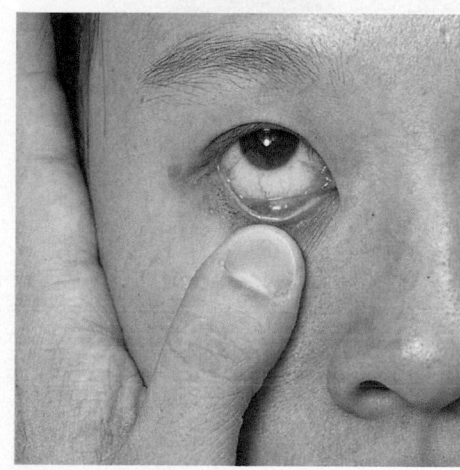

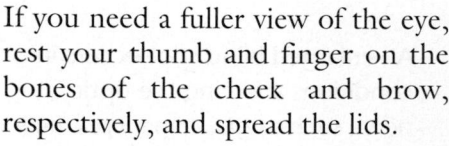

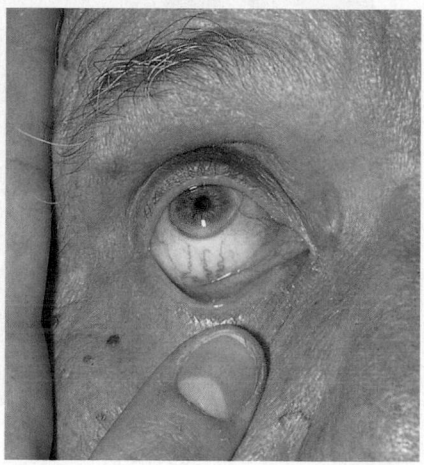

A yellow sclera indicates jaundice.

If you need a fuller view of the eye, rest your thumb and finger on the bones of the cheek and brow, respectively, and spread the lids.

Ask the patient to look to each side and down. This technique gives you a good view of the sclera and bulbar conjunctiva, but not of the palpebral conjunctiva of the upper lid. For this purpose, you need to evert the lid (see p. 233).

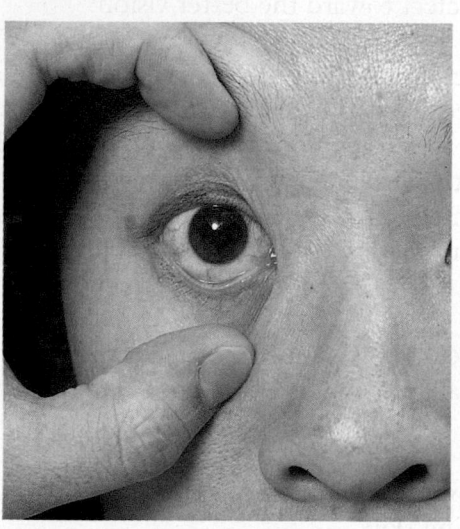

The local redness below is from *nodular episcleritis,* often self-limiting in younger adults; also seen in *rheumatoid arthritis* and *system lupus erythematosus (SLE).*

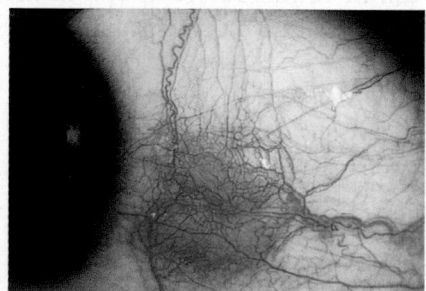

For comparisons, see Table 11-3, Red Eyes (p. 238).

Cornea and Lens. With oblique lighting, inspect the cornea of each eye for opacities and note any opacities in the lens that may be visible through the pupil.

See Table 11-4, Opacities of the Cornea and Lens (p. 239).

Iris. At the same time, inspect each iris. The markings should be clearly defined. With your light shining directly from the temporal side, look for a crescentic shadow on the medial side of the iris. Because the iris is normally fairly flat and forms a relatively open angle with the cornea, this lighting casts no shadow.

Occasionally the iris bows abnormally far forward, forming a very narrow angle with the cornea. The light then casts a crescentic shadow.

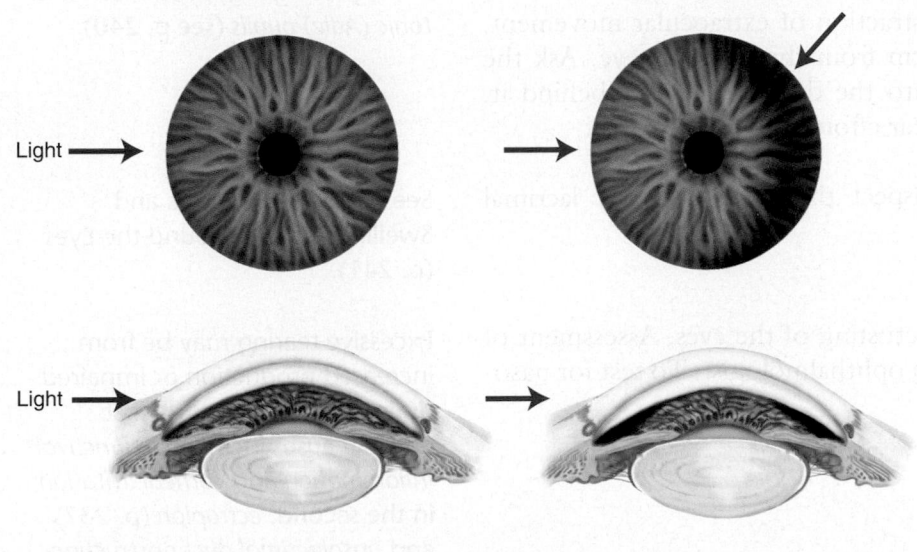

This narrow angle increases the risk for acute *narrow-angle glaucoma*—a sudden increase in intraocular pressure when drainage of the aqueous humor is blocked.

In *open-angle glaucoma*—the common form of glaucoma—the normal spatial relation between iris and cornea is preserved and the iris is fully lit.

Pupils. Inspect the *size*, *shape*, and *symmetry* of the pupils. If the pupils are large (>5 mm), small (<3 mm), or unequal, measure them. A pupil guide with black circles of varying sizes facilitates measurement.

Miosis refers to constriction of the pupils, *mydriasis* to dilation.

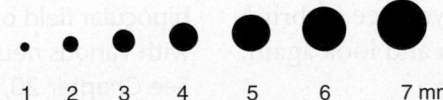

1   2   3   4   5   6   7 mm

Pupillary inequality of <0.5 mm (*anisocoria*) is visible in approximately 20% of normal people. If pupillary reactions are normal, anisocoria is considered benign.

Compare benign anisocoria with *Horner syndrome, oculomotor nerve paralysis,* and *tonic pupil.* See Table 11-5, Pupillary Abnormalities (p. 240).

Test the *pupillary reaction to light.* Ask the patient to look into the distance, and shine a bright light obliquely into each pupil in turn. (Both the distant gaze and the oblique lighting help to prevent a near reaction.) Look for:

- The *direct reaction* (pupillary constriction in the same eye)

- The *consensual reaction* (pupillary constriction in the opposite eye)

Always darken the room and use a bright light before deciding that a light reaction is absent.

If the reaction to light is impaired or questionable, test the *near reaction* in normal room light. Testing one eye at a time makes it easier to concentrate on pupillary responses, without the distraction of extraocular movement. Hold your finger or pencil about 10 cm from the patient's eye. Ask the patient to look alternately at it and into the distance directly behind it. Watch for pupillary constriction with near effort.

> Testing the near reaction is helpful in diagnosing *Argyll Robertson* and *tonic (Adie) pupils* (see p. 240).

Lacrimal Apparatus. Briefly inspect the regions of the lacrimal gland and lacrimal sac for swelling.

> See Table 11-6, Lumps and Swellings in and Around the Eyes (p. 241).

Look for excessive tearing, dryness, or crusting of the eyes. Assessment of dryness may require special testing by an ophthalmologist. To test for naso-lacrimal duct obstruction, see p. 232.

> Excessive tearing may be from increased production or impaired drainage of tears. In the first group, causes include *conjunctival inflammation* and *corneal irritation*; in the second, *ectropion* (p. 237) and *nasolacrimal duct obstruction*.

Extraocular Muscles

1. Assess. *Assess the extraocular movements,* looking for:

   - The normal *conjugate movements* of the eyes in each direction, or any *deviation* from normal

   > See Table 11-7, Dysconjugate Gaze (p. 242).

   - *Nystagmus,* a fine rhythmic oscillation of the eyes. A few beats of nystagmus on extreme lateral gaze are normal. If you see it, bring your finger in to within the field of binocular vision and look again.

   > Sustained nystagmus within the binocular field of gaze is seen with various neurologic conditions. See Chapter 20, Nystagmus (pp. 631).

   - *Lid lag* as the eyes move from up to down.

   > In lid lag of *hyperthyroidism,* a rim of sclera is visible above the iris with downward gaze.

2. Cardinal fields. *To test the six extraocular movements (EOMs), ask the patient to follow your finger or pencil* as you sweep through the six cardinal directions of gaze. Making a wide H in the air, lead the patient's gaze (1) to the patient's extreme right, (2) to the right and upward, and (3)

down on the right; then (4) without pausing in the middle, to the extreme left, (5) to the left and upward, and (6) down on the left. Pause during upward and lateral gaze to detect nystagmus. Move your finger or pencil at 12"–18" from the patient. Because middle-aged or older people may have difficulty focusing on near objects, make this distance greater for them than for young people. Some patients move their heads to follow your finger. If necessary, hold the head in the proper midline position.

Deviations in movements can signal a brain tumor or injury. The change depends on the location of the lesion or injury. In paralysis of the CN VI, illustrated below, the eyes are conjugate in right lateral gaze but not in left lateral gaze.

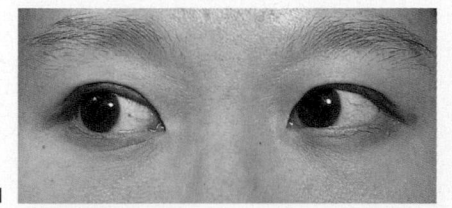
1

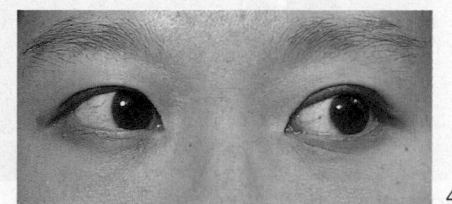
4

LOOKING RIGHT

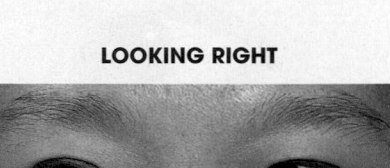

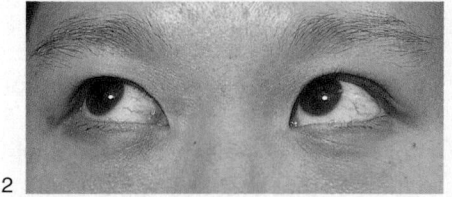
2

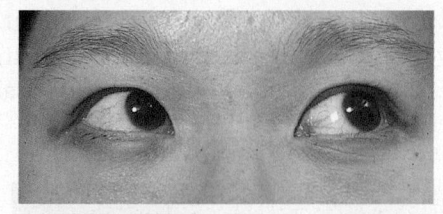
5

LOOKING LEFT

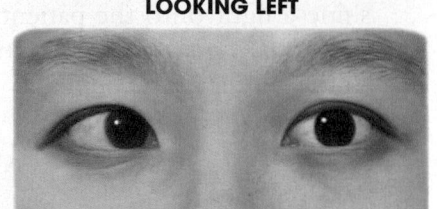

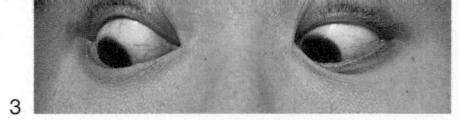
3

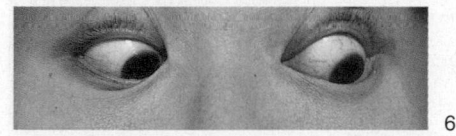
6

If you suspect lid lag or hyperthyroidism, ask the patient to follow your finger again as you move it slowly from up to down in the midline. The lid should overlap the iris slightly throughout this movement.

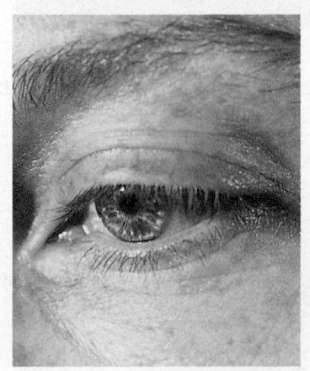

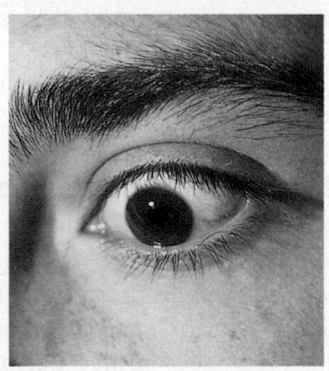

Note the rim of sclera from *proptosis,* an abnormal protrusion of the eyeball in *hyperthyroidism,* leading to a characteristic "stare" on frontal gaze.

2a. Convergence. Finally, test for *convergence*. Ask the patient to follow your finger or pencil as you move it in toward the bridge of the nose. The converging eyes normally follow the object to within 5 cm to 8 cm of the nose.

Poor convergence in *hyperthyroidism*

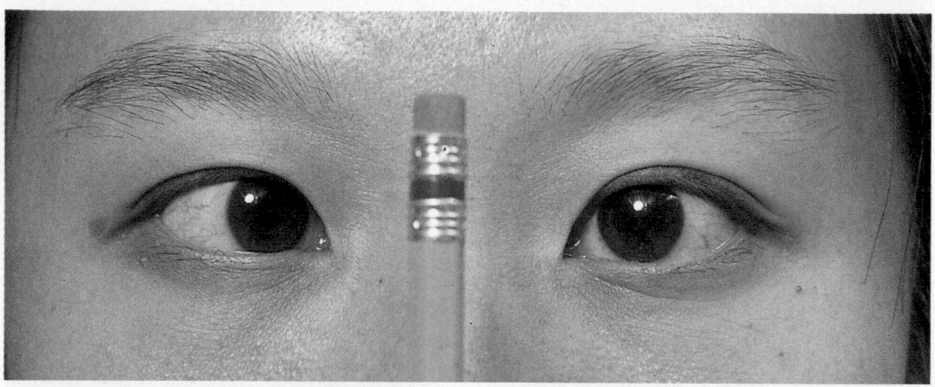

CONVERGENCE

3. *Corneal light reflex.* From about 2 feet directly in front of the patient, shine a light onto the patient's eyes and ask the patient to look at it. *Inspect the reflections in the corneas.* They should be visible slightly nasal to the center of the pupils.

Asymmetry of the corneal reflections indicates a deviation from normal ocular alignment. A temporal light reflection on one cornea, for example, indicates a nasal deviation of that eye. See Table 11-7, Dysconjugate Gaze (p. 242).

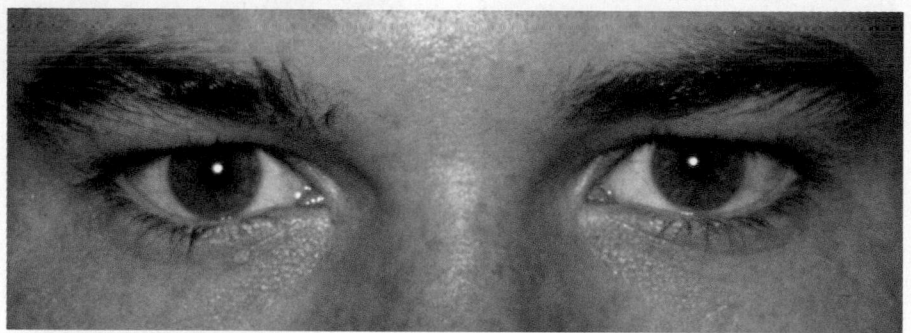

4. A *cover–uncover test* may reveal a slight or latent muscle imbalance not otherwise seen (see p. 242).

Ophthalmoscopic Examination.
The nurse would examine the patients eyes *without dilating the pupils.* The view is therefore limited to the posterior structures of the retina. To see more peripheral structures, to evaluate the macula well, or to investigate unexplained visual loss, ophthalmologists dilate the pupils with mydriatic drops unless this is contraindicated.

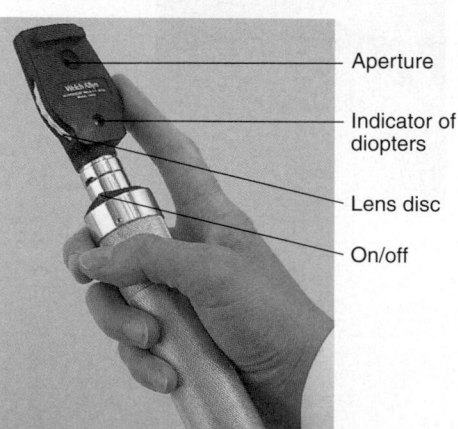

Aperture

Indicator of diopters

Lens disc

On/off

Contraindications for mydriatic drops include (1) head injury and coma, in which continuing observations of pupillary reactions are essential, and (2) any suspicion of narrow-angle glaucoma.

At first, using the ophthalmoscope may seem awkward, and it may be difficult to visualize the fundus. With patience and practice of proper technique, the fundus will come into view, and the ability to assess important structures such as the optic disc and the retinal vessels becomes easier.

The optic disc's yellowish orange to creamy pink oval or round structure may fill the field of gaze or even exceed it. Of interest, the ophthalmoscope magnifies the normal retina about 15 times and the normal iris about 4 times. The optic disc actually measures about 1.5 mm. Follow the next steps for this important segment of the physical examination.

When the lens has been removed surgically, its magnifying effect is lost. Retinal structures then look much smaller than usual, and you can see a much larger expanse of the fundus.

Steps for Examining the Optic Disc

To begin utilizing the ophthalmoscope for assessment, the nurse needs to be aware of how it functions as there are different types. Familiarize yourself with the dials and know how to turn it on. Initially, the scope needs to be set on:

- The brightest light

- The white light (ignore the other colors)

- The circle (ignore the slits and crosses)

- "0"

If the nurse wears glasses or contacts they can remain on for the examination. If the patient wears glasses they should be removed, although contacts may remain in.

Room lighting should be decreased or turned off without making the room too dark.

Explain to the patient that the ophthalmoscope light will be bright and the importance of focusing on a specific point so the eyes do not wander during the examination. Choose a point on the wall over your shoulder that the patient should stare at (you might pick a curtain or determine a spot on the wall behind you). The patient should continue to look in that direction even if you step in the line of view.

Positioning. When looking into the patient's right eye the nurse holds the scope with the right hand and uses the right eye; when looking into the patient's left eye the nurse holds the scope with the left hand and utilizes the left eye. Try to keep your other eye open during the examination. Utilizing the nondominant hand and eye will take practice. It is important to master this, as it decreases the likelihood of the nurse's nose touching the patient's nose. In addition, the hand not holding the scope can brace the thumb and forefinger on the patient's eyebrow to determine the proximity to the patient and to assist with opening the patient's eye if it tends to close.

The Examination. The nurse will shine the light into the patient's eye from 6 inches away and at a 25° angle and will be able to see the red reflex. Follow this into the eye, resting the ophthalmoscope on your eyebrow and standing about 1.5 to 2 inches away from the patient. (It is important to get close to the patient as you will have a wider field of view.) Here the optic disc, arteries, and veins are visible. If you are unable to visualize the optic disc and vessels, keep your head still and move the diopter dial (which your index finger has been resting on) either way. If the disc becomes more clear keep turning the dial; if it becomes blurry then turn the dial in the opposite direction.

STEPS FOR EXAMINING THE OPTIC DISC AND THE RETINA

The Optic Disc
- Initially the red reflex comes into view; the nurse needs to be able to look through the red reflex to visualize the arteries and veins.
- Follow the blood vessels as they get wider. Follow the vessels medially toward the nose and look for the round yellowish orange structure described earlier as the optic disc.

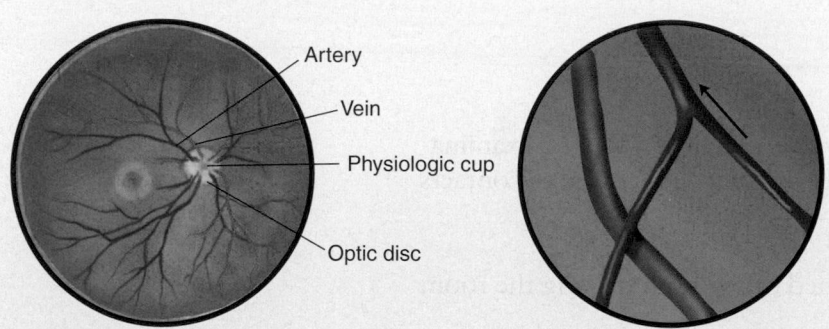

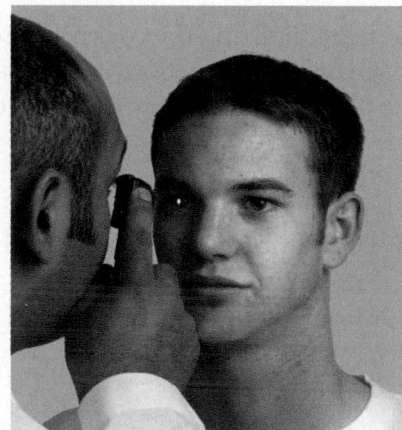

EXAMINER AT 15° ANGLE FROM PATIENT'S LINE OF VISION, ELICITING RED REFLEX

- Now, *bring the optic disc into sharp focus* by adjusting the lens of your ophthalmoscope. If both you and the patient have no refractive errors, the retina should be in focus at 0 diopters. If structures are blurred, rotate the lens disc until you find the sharpest focus.

    For example, if the patient is myopic (nearsighted), rotate the lens disc counterclockwise to the minus diopters (red); in a hyperopic (far-sighted) patient, move the disc clockwise to the plus diopters (black). You can correct your own refractive error in the same way.
- *Inspect the optic disc.* Note the following features:
  – *The sharpness or clarity of the disc outline.* The nasal portion of the disc margin may be somewhat blurred, a normal finding.
  – *The color of the disc,* normally yellowish orange to creamy pink. White or pigmented crescents may ring the disc, a normal finding.

In a *refractive error*, light rays from a distance do not focus on the retina. In *myopia*, they focus anterior to it; in *hyperopia*, posterior to it. Retinal structures in a myopic eye look larger than normal.

See Table 11-8, p. 243, Normal Variations of the Optic Disc (and Table 11-9, p. 244, Abnormalities of the Optic Disc).

(continued)

STEPS FOR EXAMINING THE OPTIC DISC AND THE RETINA (continued)

– *The size of the central physiologic cup,* if present. It is usually yellowish white. The horizontal diameter is usually less than half the horizontal diameter of the disc.

– *The comparative symmetry* of the eyes and findings in the fundi.

Detecting Papilledema.   *Papilledema* describes swelling of the optic disc and anterior bulging of the physiologic cup. Increased intracranial pressure is transmitted to the optic nerve, causing edema of the optic nerve. Papilledema often signals serious disorders of the brain, such as meningitis, subarachnoid hemorrhage, trauma, and mass lesions, so searching for this important disorder is a priority during all your funduscopic examinations.

The Retina—Arteries, Veins, Fovea, and Macula

- *Inspect the retina,* including arteries and veins as they extend to the periphery, arteriovenous crossings, the fovea, and the macula. Distinguish arteries from veins based on the features listed below.

	Arteries	Veins
Color	Light red	Dark red
Size	Smaller (⅔ to ¾ the diameter of veins)	Larger
Light reflex (*reflection*)	Bright	Inconspicuous or absent

- *Follow the vessels peripherally in each of four directions,* noting their relative sizes and the character of the arteriovenous crossings.

    Identify any lesions of the surrounding *retina* and note their size, shape, color, and distribution. As you search the retina, *move your head and instrument as a unit,* using the patient's pupil as an imaginary fulcrum. At first, you may repeatedly lose your view of the retina because your light falls out of the pupil. You will improve with practice.

    Lesions of the retina can be measured in terms of "disc diameters" from the optic disc.

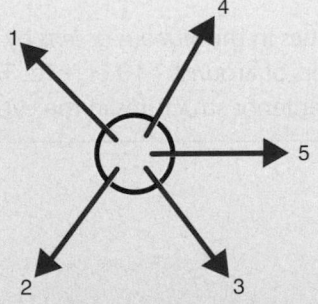

Sequence of inspection from disc to macula

LEFT EYE

(continued)

An enlarged cup suggests *chronic open-angle glaucoma.*

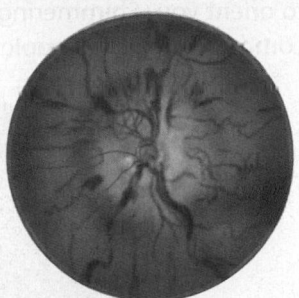

PAPILLEDEMA

See Table 11-10, p. 245, Retinal Arteries and Arteriovenous Crossings: Normal and Hypertensive Table 11-11, p. 246, Ocular Fundi: Normal and Hypertensive Retinopathy; and Table 11-12, p. 247, Ocular Fundi: Diabetic Retinopathy.

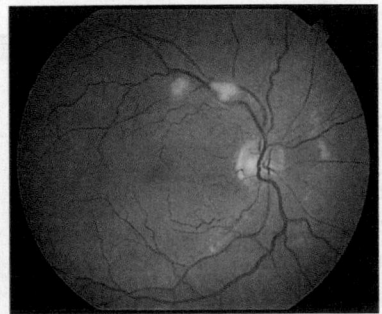

COTTON-WOOL PATCHES

Note the irregular patches between 11 and 12 o'clock, 1 to 2 disc diameters from the disc. Each measures about one-half by one-half disc diameters.

STEPS FOR EXAMINING THE OPTIC DISC AND THE RETINA (continued)

- Inspect the *fovea and surrounding macula.* Direct your light beam laterally or by asking the patient to look directly into the light. Except in older people, the tiny bright reflection at the center of the fovea helps to orient you. Shimmering light reflections in the macular area are common in young people.

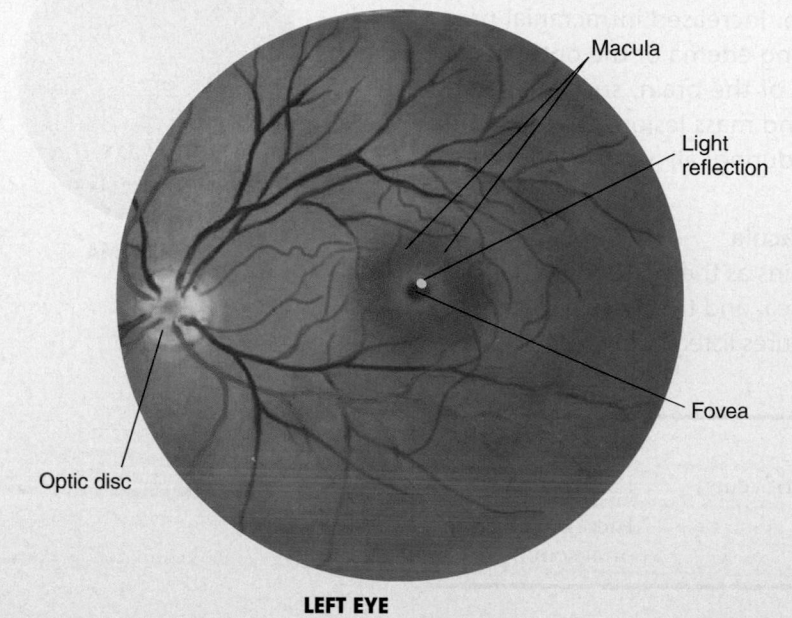

LEFT EYE

- *Inspect the anterior structures.* Look for opacities in the *vitreous* or *lens* by rotating the lens disc progressively to diopters of around +10 or +12. This technique allows you to focus on the more anterior structures in the eye.

Macular degeneration is an important cause of poor central vision in the elderly. Types include *dry atrophic* (more common but less severe) and *wet exudative,* or neovascular. Undigested cellular debris, called *drusen,* may be hard and sharply defined, as seen below, or soft and confluent with altered pigmentation.

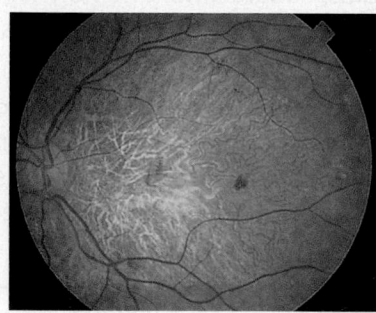

Photo from Tasman W, Jaeger E (eds). The Wills Eye Hospital Atlas of Clinical Ophthalmology, 2nd ed. Philadelphia: Lippincott Williams & Wilkins, 2001.

Vitreous floaters may be seen as dark specks or strands between the fundus and the lens. Cataracts are densities in the lens (see p. 239).

SPECIAL TECHNIQUES

For Nasolacrimal Duct Obstruction. This test helps identify the cause of excessive tearing. Ask the patient to look up. Press on the lower lid close to the medial canthus, just inside the rim of the bony orbit— this compresses the lacrimal sac. Look for fluid regurgitated out of the puncta into the eye. Avoid this test if the area is inflamed and tender.

Discharge of mucopurulent fluid from the puncta suggests an obstructed nasolacrimal duct.

For Inspection of the Upper Palpebral Conjunctiva. Adequate examination of the eye in search of a foreign body requires eversion of the upper eyelid. Follow these steps:

- Instruct the patient to look down. Get the patient to relax the eyes—by reassurance and by gentle, assured, and deliberate movements. Raise the upper eyelid slightly so that the eyelashes protrude, and then grasp the upper eyelashes and pull them gently down and forward.

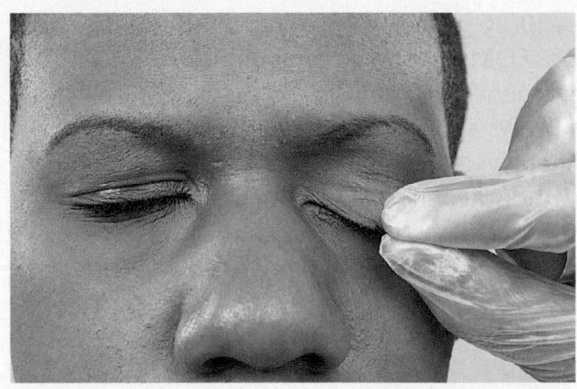

- Place a small stick such as an applicator or a tongue blade at least 1 cm above the lid margin (and therefore at the upper border of the tarsal plate). Push down on the stick as you raise the edge of the lid, thus everting the eyelid or turning it "inside out." Do not press on the eyeball itself.

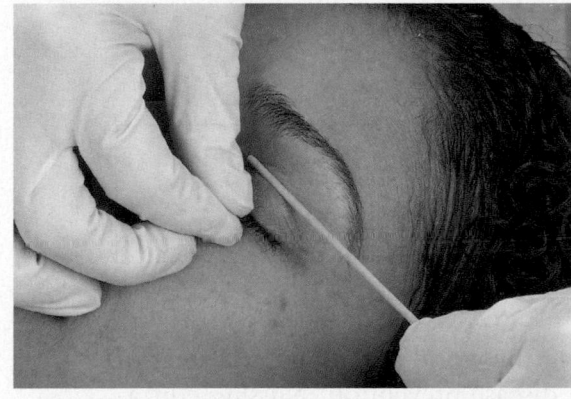

- Secure the upper lashes against the eyebrow with your thumb and inspect the palpebral conjunctiva. After your inspection, grasp the upper eyelashes and pull them gently forward. Ask the patient to look up. The eyelid will return to its normal position.

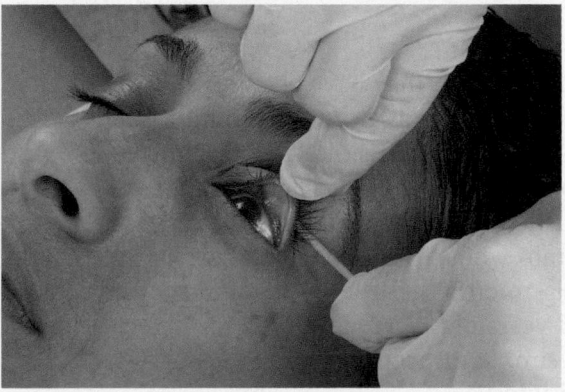

This view allows you to see the upper palpebral conjunctiva and look for a foreign body that might be lodged there.

RECORDING THE PHYSICAL EXAMINATION—THE EYE

> Eyes: near vision—14/14, distal vision—20/20 bilaterally, peripheral vision—visual fields full by confrontation. EOMs intact. No nystagmus. No deviations on cover–uncover test. Convergence to 7 cm.
>
> Thick and equal hair distribution on brows and lids. Lids tan and without lesions. Palpebral fissures equal bilaterally. No edema or ptosis. Lacrimal apparatus nontender, moist without tearing or crusting. Conjunctiva pink and sclera white bilaterally. No opacities in cornea or lens bilaterally. PERRLA. Disc yellowish orange with sharp margins. No hemorrhages or exudates. No arteriolar narrowing.

HEALTH PROMOTION, DISEASE PREVENTION, AND EDUCATION

Important Topics

- Vision screening
- Eye protection
- Care of contact lenses

Vision is a critical sense for experiencing the world around us, and areas of importance are health promotion and disease prevention. Nursing education is vital in maintaining vision and a healthy outlook for clients.

Vision Screening

Changes in vision shift with age. Young children may have changes and the U.S. Preventive Task Force (USPSTF) recommends vision screening for all children at least once between the ages of 3 and 5 years old to detect amblyopia or its risk factors. Amblyopia, also known as "lazy eye", affects approximately 2–4% or preschool children. This loss of vision is due to an alteration in neural pathways in the developing brain which in turn decreases use of the affected eye. Strabismus is eye misalignment; these are found most frequently in infants and children up to 5 years old. Screening tests for detecting strabismus and amblyopia include simple inspection, the cover uncover test, corneal light reflex and visual acuity tests.

The most common visual change in school-age children, adolescents, and young adults is refractive errors. Most school-age children are screened in school, and young adults present to their health care provider when they have changes in vision or are tested for driving exams, employment, or physicals. The Snellen vision chart is utilized for the screening examination.

Up to 25% of adults older than 65 years have refractive errors; however, cataracts, macular degeneration, and glaucoma become more prevalent.[4] These disorders reduce awareness of the social and physical environment and contribute to falls and injuries. To improve detection of visual defects, test visual acuity with a Snellen chart or Rosenbaum card. Examine the lens and fundi for clouding of the lens (*cataracts*); mottling of the *macula;* variations in the retinal pigmentation; subretinal hemorrhage or exudate (*macular degeneration*); and change in size and color of the optic cup or visual field defects (*glaucoma*).

Eye Protection

Eye injuries and trauma can occur in the home, during recreational activities, and in the place of employment. Protective eyewear should be utilized when there is a chance of injury to the eye. Eye injury can result from numerous causes, for example: chemical splashes from cleaning supplies, metal shards or rocks flying when mowing the lawn, sports (e.g., lacrosse) injuries, body fluids entering the eye—the list is endless. The activities and environment in which people work and play should be assessed and precautions taken to avoid eye injury and promote healthy habits. Emergency eye care education is important for individuals to react when something enters the eye such as chemicals or a blunt object or when there is a cut around the eye. Additional education includes: avoidance of direct sunlight and use of sunglasses to protect the eyes from ultraviolet radiation and individuals working with chemicals should be taught how to use devices to flush eyes and/or skin if they come in contact with chemicals.

Care of Contact Lenses

Infections can occur and injure the eye if contact lenses are not taken care of properly. Patients should remember to wash their hands when inserting or removing lenses, to wear and remove them as prescribed by the health care provider, and to keep them clean and not share contacts. If patients are using solutions, they should discard unused portions at the expiration date. Contact lens wearers may become too familiar with the routine and may need reminders that putting anything into the eye, including contacts, may cause damage if not done correctly. Contact lenses should be inspected by a lens specialist once a year for scratches or damage that can injure the eye.

TABLE
11-1

Visual Field Defects

Visual Field Defects

1 Horizontal Defect Occlusion of a branch of the central retinal artery may cause a horizontal (altitudinal) defect. Ischemia of the optic nerve also can produce a similar defect.

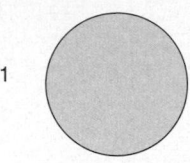 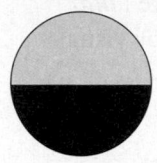

2 Blind Right Eye (right optic nerve) A lesion of the optic nerve, and of course of the eye itself, produces unilateral blindness.

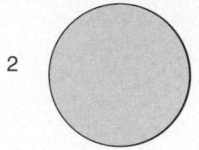 

3 Bitemporal Hemianopsia (optic chiasm) A lesion at the optic chiasm may involve only fibers crossing over to the opposite side. Since these fibers originate in the nasal half of each retina, visual loss involves the temporal half of each field.

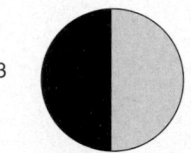 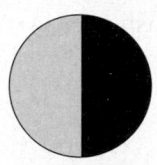

4 Left Homonymous Hemianopsia (right optic tract) A lesion of the optic tract interrupts fibers originating on the same side of both eyes. Visual loss in the eyes is therefore similar (homonymous) and involves half of each field (hemianopsia).

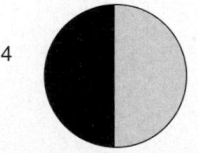 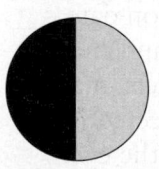

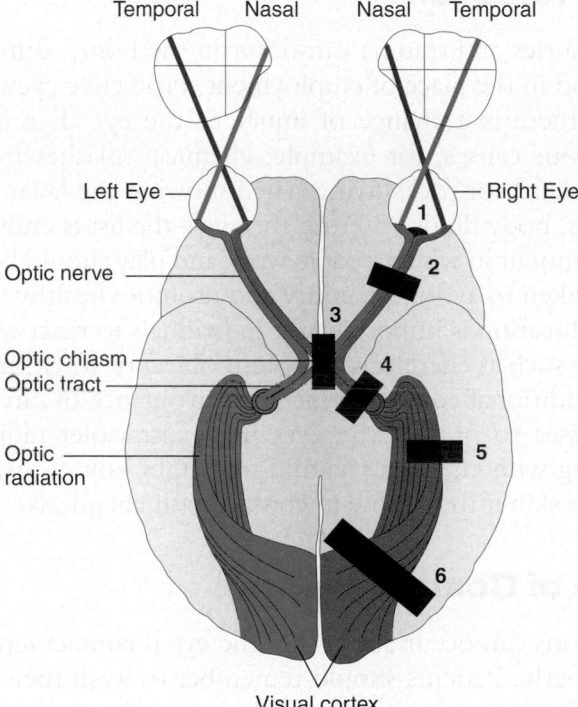

Temporal — Nasal — Nasal — Temporal

Left Eye — Right Eye

Optic nerve
Optic chiasm
Optic tract
Optic radiation
Visual cortex

5 Homonymous Left Superior Quadrantic Defect (right optic radiation, partial) A partial lesion of the optic radiation in the temporal lobe may involve only a portion of the nerve fibers, producing, for example, a homonymous quadrantic defect.

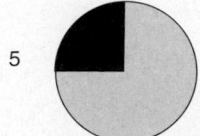 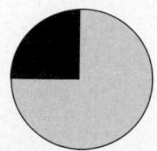

6 Left Homonymous Hemianopsia (right optic radiation) A complete interruption of fibers in the optic radiation produces a visual defect similar to that produced by a lesion of the optic tract.

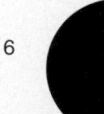 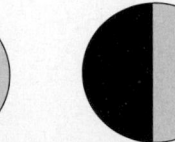

TABLE
11-2

Variations and Abnormalities of the Eyelids

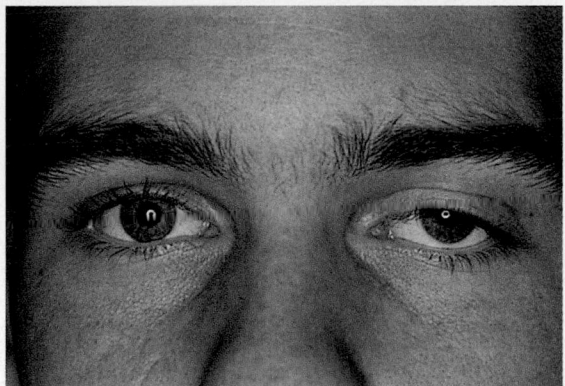

Ptosis

Ptosis is a drooping of the upper lid. Causes include myasthenia gravis, damage to the oculomotor nerve, and damage to the sympathetic nerve supply (*Horner syndrome*). A weakened muscle, relaxed tissues, and the weight of herniated fat may cause senile ptosis. Ptosis may also be congenital.

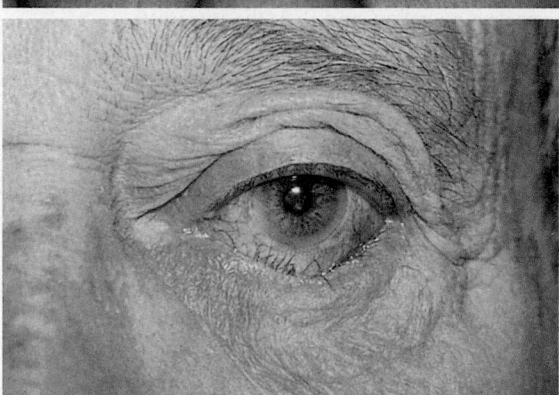

Entropion

Entropion, more common in the elderly, is an inward turning of the lid margin. The lower lashes, which are often invisible when turned inward, irritate the conjunctiva and lower cornea. Asking the patient to squeeze the lids together and then open them may reveal an entropion that is not obvious.

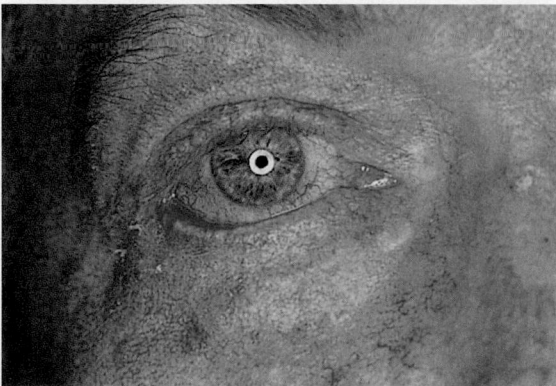

Ectropion

In ectropion the margin of the lower lid is turned outward, exposing the palpebral conjunctiva. When the punctum of the lower lid turns outward, the eye no longer drains satisfactorily, and tearing occurs. Ectropion is more common in the elderly.

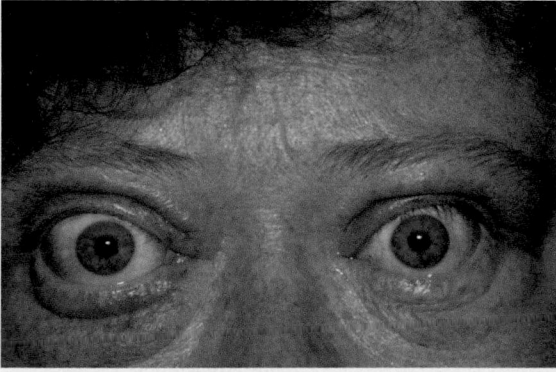

Lid Retraction and Exophthalmos

A wide-eyed stare suggests retracted eyelids. Note the rim of sclera between the upper lid and the iris. Retracted lids and a lid lag (p. 227) are often due to hyperthyroidism.

In exophthalmos the eyeball protrudes forward. When bilateral, it suggests the infiltrative ophthalmopathy of Graves hyperthyroidism. Edema of the eyelids and conjunctival injection may be associated. Unilateral exophthalmos is seen in Graves disease or a tumor or inflammation in the orbit.

(Source of photos: *Ptosis, Ectropion, Entropion*—Tasman W, Jaeger E, eds. The Wills Eye Hospital Atlas of Clinical Ophthalmology, 2nd ed. Philadelphia: Lippincott Williams & Wilkins, 2001.)

TABLE 11-3

Red Eyes[5]

Conjunctivitis

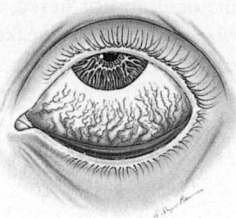

Subconjunctival Hemorrhage

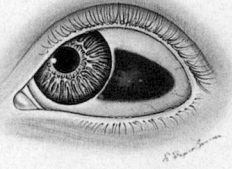

	Conjunctivitis	Subconjunctival Hemorrhage
Pattern of Redness	Conjunctival injection: diffuse dilatation of conjunctival vessels with redness that tends to be maximal peripherally	Leakage of blood outside of the vessels, producing a homogeneous, sharply demarcated, red area that fades over days to yellow and then disappears
Pain	Mild discomfort rather than pain	Absent
Vision	Not affected except for temporary mild blurring due to discharge	Not affected
Ocular Discharge	Watery, mucoid, or mucopurulent	Absent
Pupil	Not affected	Not affected
Cornea	Clear	Clear
Significance	Bacterial, viral, and other infections; allergy; irritation	Often none. May result from trauma, bleeding disorders, or a sudden increase in venous pressure, as from cough

Corneal Injury or Infection

Acute Iritis

Glaucoma

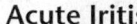
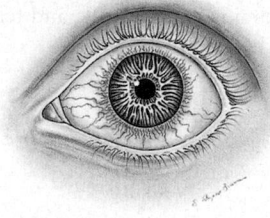
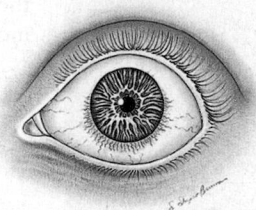
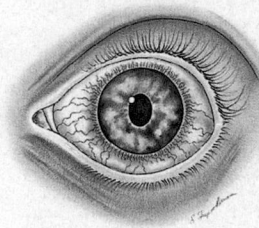

	Corneal Injury or Infection	Acute Iritis	Glaucoma
Pattern of Redness	Ciliary injection: dilation of deeper vessels that are visible as radiating vessels or a reddish violet flush around the limbus. Ciliary injection is an important sign of these three conditions but may not be apparent. The eye may be diffusely red instead. Other clues of these more serious disorders are pain, decreased vision, unequal pupils, and a less than perfectly clear cornea.		
Pain	Moderate to severe, superficial	Moderate, aching, deep	Severe, aching, deep
Vision	Usually decreased	Decreased	Decreased
Ocular Discharge	Watery or purulent	Absent	Absent
Pupil	Not affected unless iritis develops	May be small and, with time, irregular	Dilated, fixed
Cornea	Changes depending on cause	Clear or slightly clouded	Steamy, cloudy
Significance	Abrasions, and other injuries; viral and bacterial infections	Associated with many ocular and systemic disorders	Acute increase in intraocular pressure—an emergency

TABLE
11-4

Opacities of the Cornea and Lens

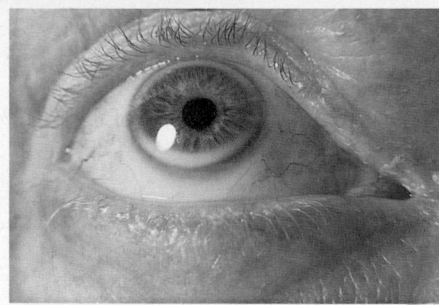

Corneal Arcus. A thin grayish white arc or circle not quite at the edge of the cornea. Accompanies normal aging but also seen in younger people, especially African-Americans. In young people, suggests possible hyperlipoproteinemia. Usually benign.

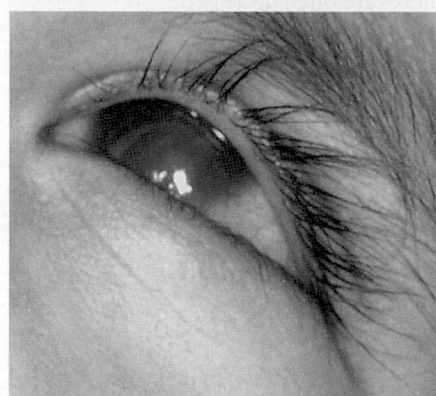

Corneal Scar. A superficial grayish white opacity in the cornea, secondary to an old injury or to inflammation. Size and shape are variable. Do not confuse with the opaque lens of a cataract, visible on a deeper plane and only through the pupil.

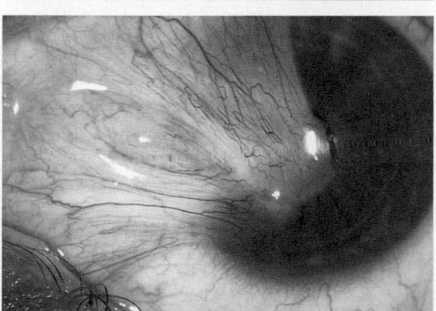

Pterygium. A triangular thickening of the bulbar conjunctiva that grows slowly across the outer surface of the cornea, usually from the nasal side. Reddening may occur. May interfere with vision as it encroaches on the pupil.

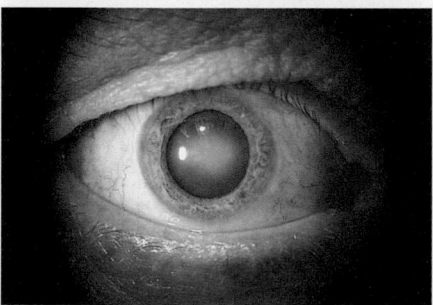

Cataracts. Opacities of the lenses visible through the pupil; most common in old age.

Nuclear cataract. A nuclear cataract looks gray when seen by a flashlight. If the pupil is widely dilated, the gray opacity is surrounded by a black rim.

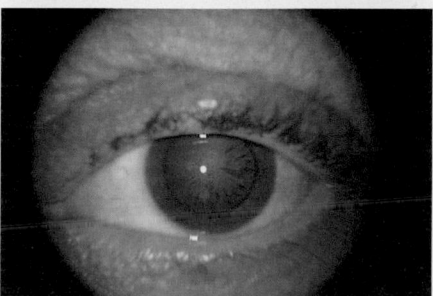

Peripheral cataract. Produces spoke-like shadows that point inward—gray against black, as seen with a flashlight, or black against red with an ophthalmoscope. A dilated pupil, as shown here, facilitates this observation.

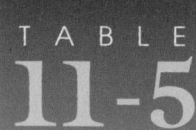
Pupillary Abnormalities

Unequal Pupils *(Anisocoria)*—When anisocoria is greater in bright light than in dim light, the larger pupil cannot constrict properly. Causes include blunt trauma to the eye, open-angle glaucoma (p. 238), and impaired parasympathetic nerve supply to the iris, as in tonic pupil, oculomotor nerve paralysis, brain injury, or brain tumors. When anisocoria is greater in dim light, the smaller pupil cannot dilate properly, as in Horner syndrome, caused by an interruption of the sympathetic nerve supply. See also Table 20-12, Pupils in Comatose Patients, p. 679.

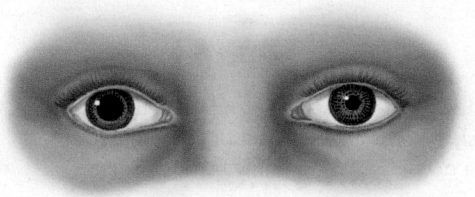

Tonic Pupil *(Adie Pupil).* Pupil is large, regular, and usually unilateral. Reaction to light is severely reduced and slowed, or even absent. Near reaction, although very slow, is present. Slow accommodation causes blurred vision. Deep tendon reflexes are often decreased.

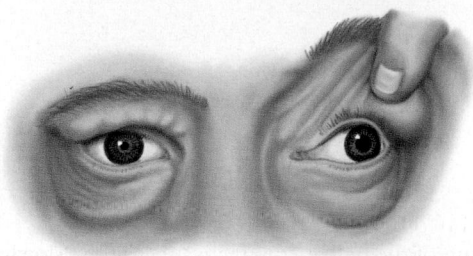

Oculomotor Nerve (CN III) Paralysis. The dilated pupil is fixed to light and near effort. Ptosis of the upper eyelid and lateral deviation of the eye are almost always present.

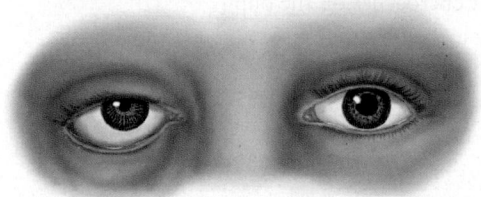

Horner Syndrome. The affected pupil, though small, reacts briskly to light and near effort. Ptosis of the eyelid is present, perhaps with loss of sweating on the forehead. In congenital Horner syndrome, the involved iris is lighter in color than its fellow (*heterochromia*).

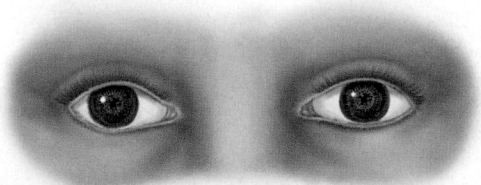

Small, Irregular Pupils. Small, irregular pupils that accommodate but do not react to light indicate *Argyll Robertson pupils*. Seen in central nervous system syphilis.

Equal Pupils and One Blind Eye. Unilateral blindness does not cause anisocoria as long as the sympathetic and parasympathetic innervation to both irises is normal. A light directed into the seeing eye produces a direct reaction in that eye and a consensual reaction in the blind eye. A light directed into the blind eye, however, causes no response in either eye.

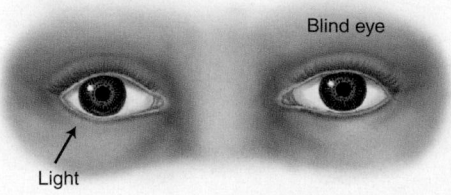

Blind eye

Light

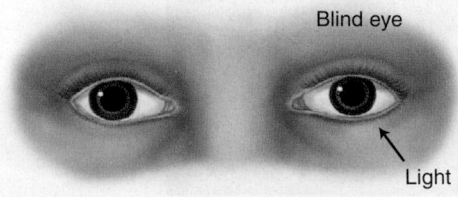

Blind eye

Light

TABLE
11-6

Lumps and Swellings in and Around the Eyes

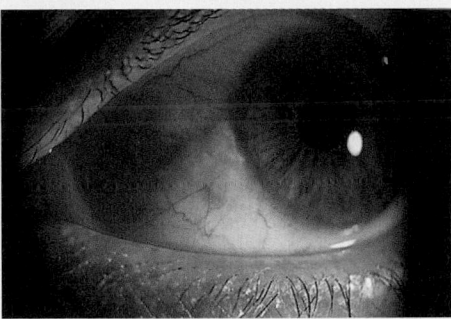

Pinguecula

A harmless yellowish triangular nodule in the bulbar conjunctiva on either side of the iris. Appears frequently with aging, first on the nasal and then on the temporal side.

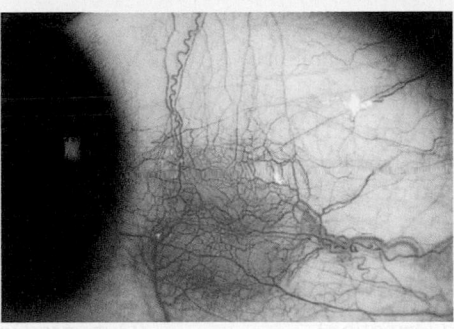

Episcleritis

A localized ocular redness from inflammation of the episcleral vessels. Vessels appear pink and are movable over the scleral surface. May be nodular, as shown, or may show only redness and dilated vessels.

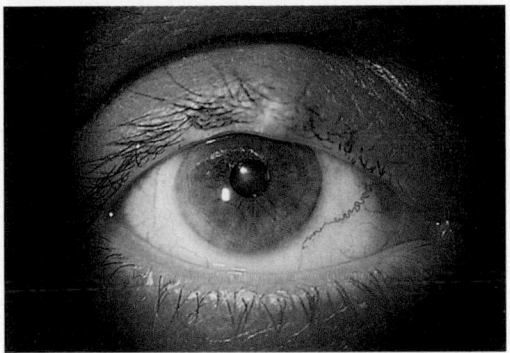

Sty (Hordeolum)

A painful, tender red infection in a gland at the margin of the eyelid.

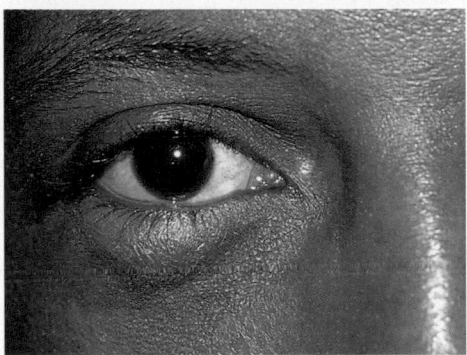

Chalazion

A subacute nontender and usually painless nodule involving a meibomian gland. May become acutely inflamed but, unlike a sty, usually points inside the lid rather than on the lid margin.

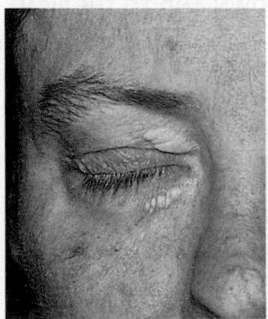

Xanthelasma

Slightly raised, yellowish, well-circumscribed plaques that appear along the nasal portions of one or both eyelids. May accompany lipid disorders.

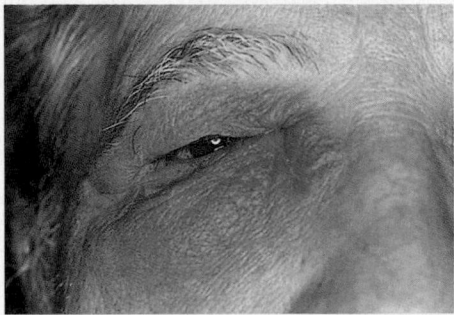

Inflammation of the Lacrimal Sac (Dacryocystitis)

A swelling between the lower eyelid and nose. An *acute* inflammation (illustrated) is painful, red, and tender. *Chronic* inflammation is associated with obstruction of the nasolacrimal duct. Tearing is prominent, and pressure on the sac produces regurgitation of material through the puncta of the eyelids.

(Source of photos: Tasman W, Jaeger E, eds. The Wills Eye Hospital Atlas of Clinical Ophthalmology, 2nd ed. Philadelphia: Lippincott Williams & Wilkins, 2001.)

TABLE
11-7

Dysconjugate Gaze

There are a variety of gaze abnormality patterns that give nurses clues about developmental disorders and cranial nerve abnormalities.

Developmental Disorders

Developmental dysconjugate gaze is caused by an imbalance in ocular muscle tone. This imbalance has many causes, may be hereditary, and usually appears in early childhood. These gaze deviations are classified according to direction:

Esotropia
(Inward Deviation)

Exotropia
(Outward Deviation)

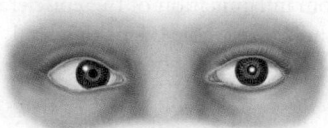 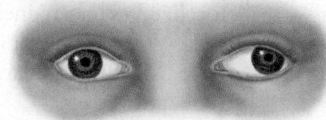

Cover–Uncover Test

A cover–uncover test may be helpful. Here is what you would see in the right monocular esotropia illustrated above.

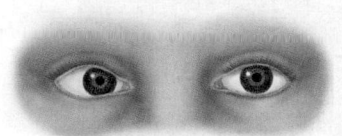

Corneal reflections are asymmetric.

COVER

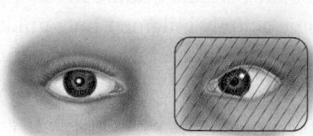

UNCOVER

The right eye moves outward to fix on the light. (The left eye is not seen but moves inward to the same degree.)

The left eye moves outward to fix on the light. The right eye deviates inward again.

Disorders of Cranial Nerves

New onset of dysconjugate gaze in adult life is usually the result of cranial nerve injuries, lesions, or abnormalities from such causes as trauma, multiple sclerosis, syphilis, and others.

A Left Cranial Nerve VI Paralysis

LOOKING TO THE RIGHT

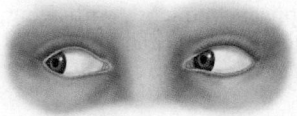

Eyes are conjugate.

LOOKING STRAIGHT AHEAD

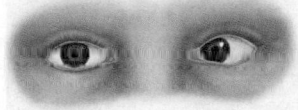

Esotropia appears.

LOOKING TO THE LEFT

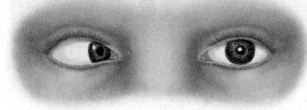

Esotropia is maximum.

A Left Cranial Nerve IV Paralysis

LOOKING DOWN AND TO THE RIGHT

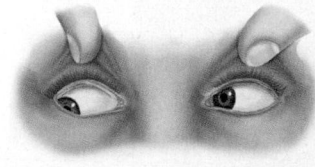

The left eye cannot look down when turned inward. Deviation is maximum in this direction.

A Left Cranial Nerve III Paralysis

LOOKING STRAIGHT AHEAD

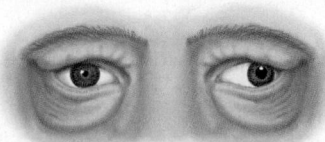

The eye is pulled outward by action of the 6th nerve. Upward, downward, and inward movements are impaired or lost. Ptosis and pupillary dilation may be associated.

TABLE
11-8

Normal Variations of the Optic Disc

Physiologic Cupping

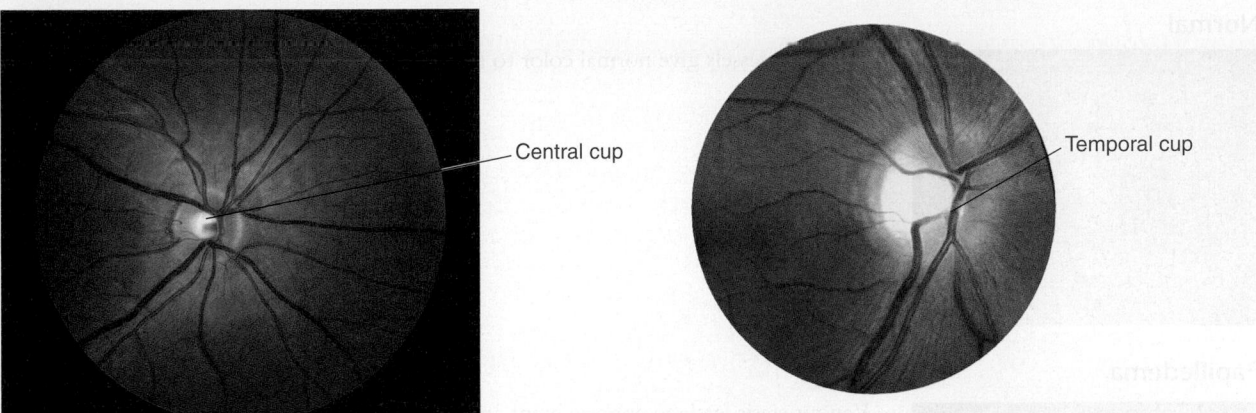

Central cup

Temporal cup

The physiologic cup is a small whitish depression in the optic disc, from which the retinal vessels appear to emerge. Although sometimes absent, the cup is usually visible either centrally or toward the temporal side of the disc. Grayish spots are often seen at its base.

Rings and Crescents

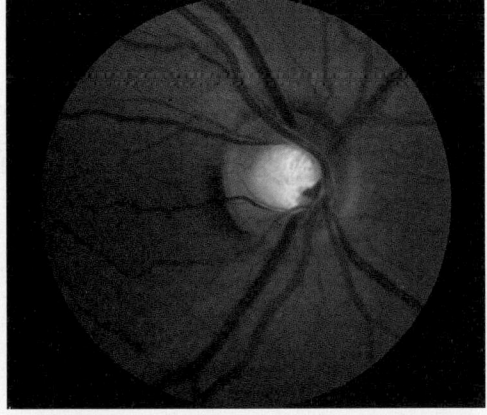

Rings and crescents are often seen around the optic disc. These are developmental variations in which you can glimpse either white sclera, black retinal pigment, or both, especially along the temporal border of the disc. Rings and crescents are not part of the disc itself and should not be included in your estimates of disc diameters.

Medullated Nerve Fibers

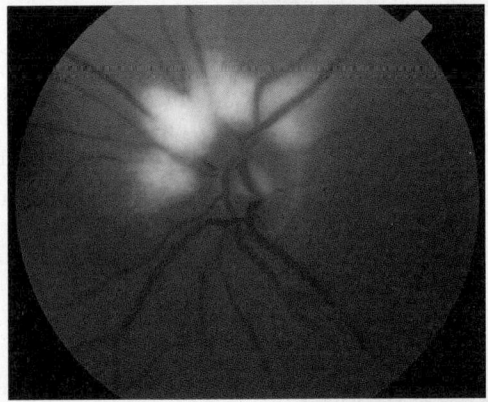

Medullated nerve fibers are a much less common but dramatic finding. Appearing as irregular white patches with feathered margins, they obscure the disc edge and retinal vessels. They have no pathologic significance.

TABLE 11-9

Abnormalities of the Optic Disc

	Process	Appearance
Normal 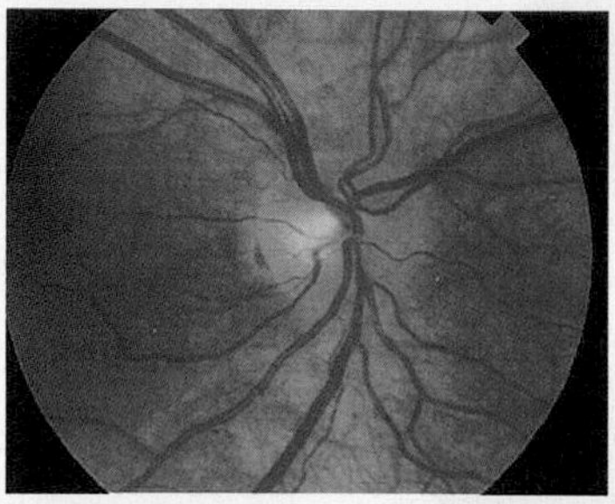	Tiny disc vessels give normal color to the disc.	Color yellowish orange to creamy pink Disc vessels tiny Disc margins sharp (except perhaps nasally) The physiologic cup is located centrally or somewhat temporally. It may be conspicuous or absent. Its diameter from side to side is usually less than half that of the disc.
Papilledema 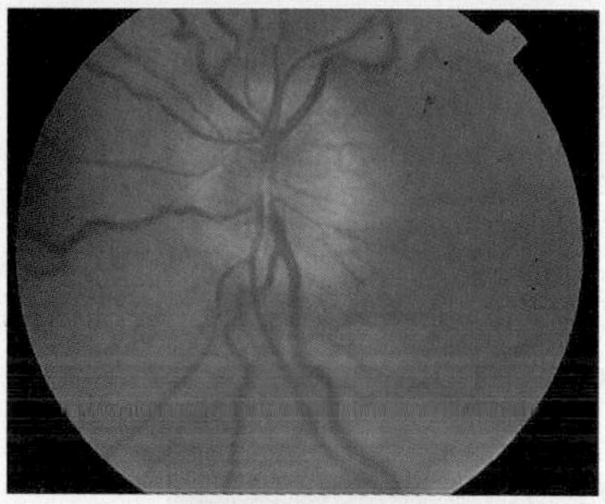	Venous stasis leads to engorgement and swelling.	Color pink, hyperemic Often with loss of venous pulsations Disc vessels more visible, more numerous, curve over the borders of the disc Disc swollen with margins blurred The physiologic cup is not visible.
Glaucomatous Cupping 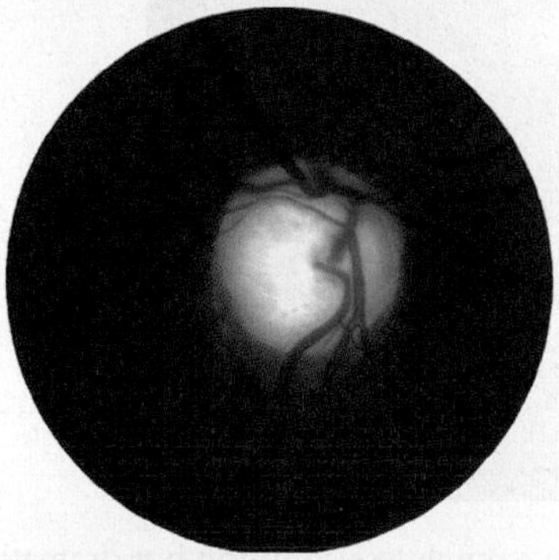	Increased pressure within the eye leads to increased cupping (backward depression of the disc) and atrophy. The base of the enlarged cup is pale.	The physiologic cup is enlarged, occupying more than half of the disc's diameter, at times extending to the edge of the disc. Retinal vessels sink in and under it, and may be displaced nasally.
Optic Atrophy 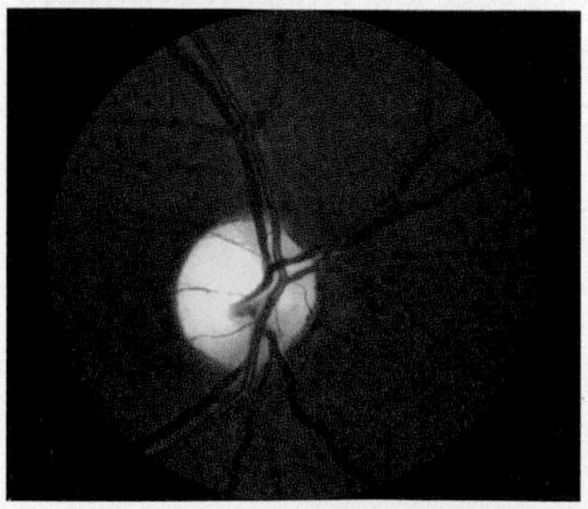	Death of optic nerve fibers leads to loss of the tiny disc vessels.	Color white Tiny disc vessels absent

(Sources of photos for *Normal*—Tasman W, Jaeger E, eds. The Wills Eye Hospital Atlas of Clinical Ophthalmology, 2nd ed. Philadelphia: Lippincott Williams & Wilkins, 2001; *Papilledema, Glaucomatous Cupping, Optic Atrophy*—Courtesy of Ken Freedman, MD.)

TABLE
11-10

Retinal Arteries and Arteriovenous Crossings: Normal and Hypertensive

Normal Retinal Artery and Arteriovenous (A-V) Crossing

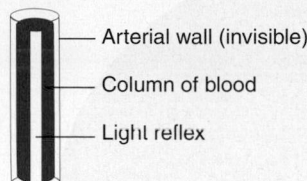

- Arterial wall (invisible)
- Column of blood
- Light reflex

The normal arterial wall is transparent. Only the column of blood within it can usually be seen. The normal light reflex is *narrow—about one-fourth the diameter of the blood column.* Because the arterial wall is transparent, a vein crossing beneath the artery can be seen right up to the column of blood on either side.

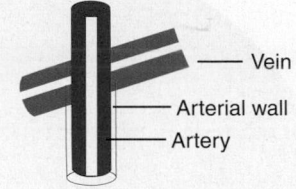

- Vein
- Arterial wall
- Artery

Retinal Arteries in Hypertension

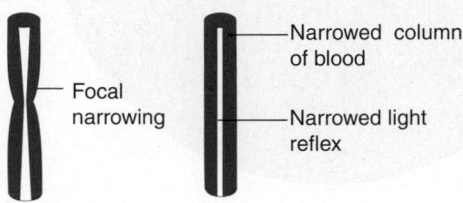

- Focal narrowing
- Narrowed column of blood
- Narrowed light reflex

Copper Wiring

Silver Wiring

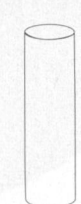

In hypertension, the arteries may show areas of focal or generalized narrowing. The light reflex is also narrowed. The arterial wall thickens and becomes less transparent.

Sometimes the arteries, especially those close to the disc, become full and somewhat tortuous and develop an increased light reflex with a bright coppery luster.

Occasionally a portion of a narrowed artery develops such an opaque wall that no blood is visible within it. It is then called a silver wire artery.

Arteriovenous Crossing

When the arterial walls lose their transparency, changes appear in the arteriovenous crossings. Decreased transparency of the retina probably also contributes to the first two changes shown below.

CONCEALMENT OR A-V NICKING

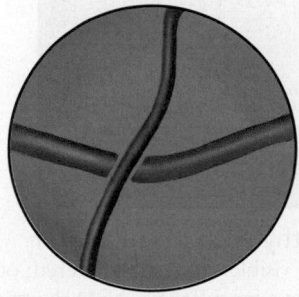

The vein appears to stop abruptly on either side of the artery.

TAPERING AND BANKING

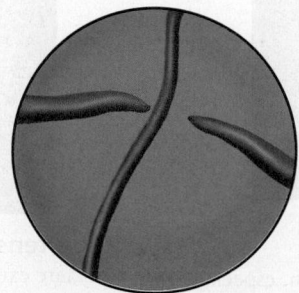

Tapering. The vein appears to taper down on either side of the artery.

BANKING

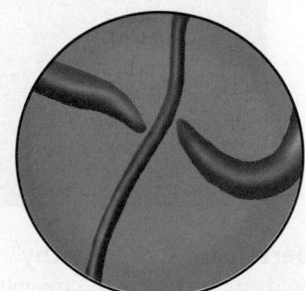

Banking. The vein is twisted on the distal side of the artery and forms a dark, wide knuckle.

TABLE
11-11

Ocular Fundi: Normal and Hypertensive Retinopathy[6]

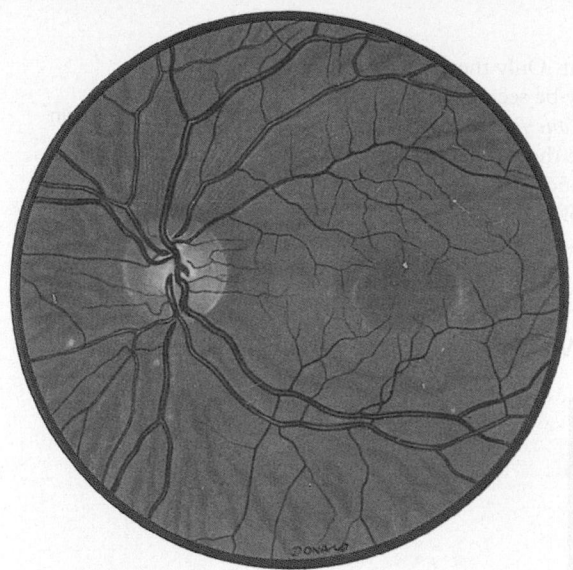

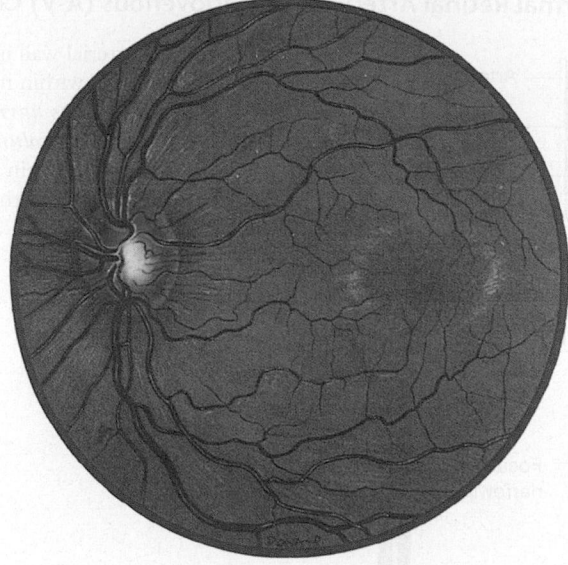

Normal Fundus of a Fair-Skinned Person

Inspect the optic disc. Follow the major vessels in four directions, noting their relative sizes and any arteriovenous crossings—both normal here. Inspect the macular area. The slightly darker fovea is just discernible; no light reflex is visible in this subject. Look for any lesions in the retina. Note the striped, or tessellated, character of the fundus, especially in the lower field, that comes from normal underlying choroidal vessels.

Normal Fundus of a Dark-Skinned Person

Again, inspect the disc, vessels, macula, and retina. The ring around the fovea is a normal light reflection. The color of the fundus has a grayish brown, almost purplish cast, which comes from pigment in the retina and the choroid that characteristically obscures the choroidal vessels; no tessellation is visible. The fundus of a light-skinned person with brunette coloring is redder.

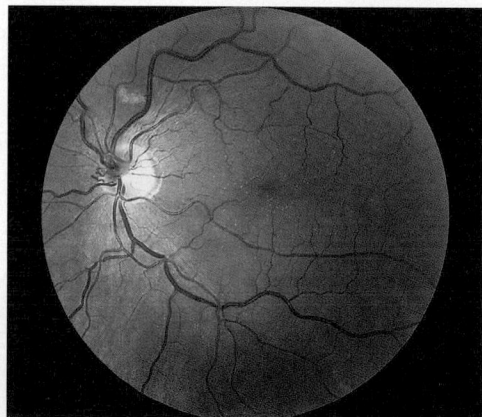

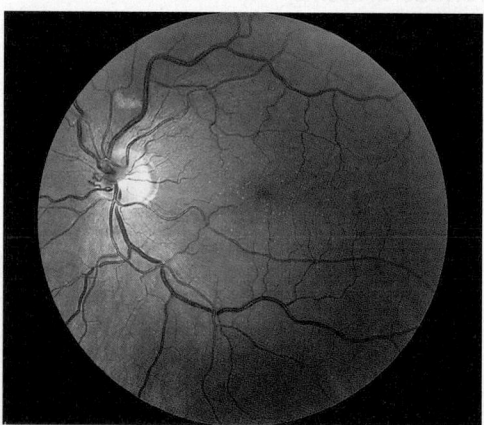

Hypertensive Retinopathy[6]

Marked arteriolar-venous crossing changes are seen, especially along the inferior vessels. Copper wiring of the arterioles is present. A cotton-wool spot is seen just superior to the disc. Incidental disc drusen are also present but are unrelated to hypertension.

Hypertensive Retinopathy with Macular Star

Punctate exudates are readily visible: some are scattered; others radiate from the fovea to form a macular star. Note the two small, soft exudates about 1 disc diameter from the disc. Find the flame-shaped hemorrhages sweeping toward 7 o'clock and 8 o'clock; a few more may be seen toward 10 o'clock. These fundi show changes typical of accelerated (malignant) hypertension and are often accompanied by a papilledema (p. 231).

(Source of photos: *Hypertensive Retinopathy, Hypertensive Retinopathy With Macular Star*—Tasman W, Jaeger E, eds. The Wills Eye Hospital Atlas of Clinical Ophthalmology, 2nd ed. Philadelphia: Lippincott Williams & Wilkins, 2001.)

TABLE
11-12

Ocular Fundi: Diabetic Retinopathy[7]

Diabetic Retinopathy

Study carefully the fundi in the series of photographs below. They represent a national standard used by ophthalmologists to assess diabetic retinopathy.

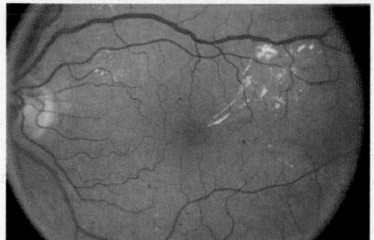

Nonproliferative Retinopathy, Moderately Severe

Note tiny red dots or microaneurysms. Note also the ring of hard exudates (white spots) located superotemporally. Retinal thickening or edema in the area of the hard exudates can impair visual acuity if it extends into the center of the macula (detection requires specialized stereoscopic examination).

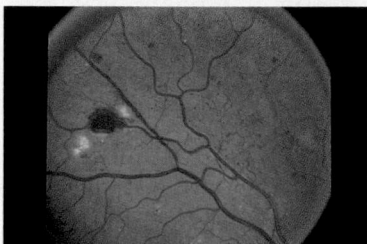

Nonproliferative Retinopathy, Severe

In the superior temporal quadrant, note the large retinal hemorrhage between two cotton-wool patches, beading of the retinal vein just above them, and tiny tortuous retinal vessels above the superior temporal artery.

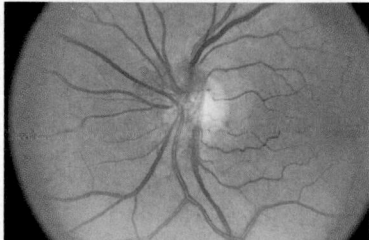

Proliferative Retinopathy, With Neovascularization

Note new preretinal vessels arising on the disc and extending across the disc margins. Visual acuity is still normal, but the risk for visual loss is high (photocoagulation reduces this risk by >50%).

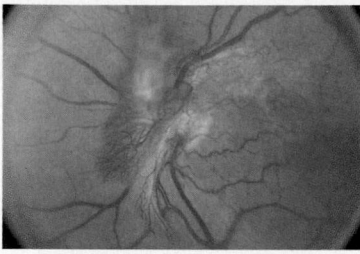

Proliferative Retinopathy, Advanced

This is the same eye, but 2 years later and without treatment. Neovascularization has increased, now with fibrous proliferations, distortion of the macula, and reduced visual acuity.

(Source of photos: *Nonproliferative Retinopathy, Moderately Severe; Proliferative Retinopathy, With Neovascularization; Nonproliferative Retinopathy, Severe; Proliferative Retinopathy, Advanced*—Early Treatment Diabetic Retinopathy Study Research Group. Courtesy of MF Davis, MD, University of Wisconsin, Madison.)

BIBLIOGRAPHY

CITATIONS

1. Coleman AC. Glaucoma. Lancet 20:1803–1810, 1999.
2. Balcer LJ. Optic neuritis. N Engl J Med 354(12):1273–1280, 2006.
3. deJong PTVM. Age-related macular degeneration. N Engl J Med 355(14):1474–1485, 2006.
4. U.S. Preventive Services Task Force. Screening for visual impairment. Available at: http://www.uspreventiveservices taskforce.org/uspstf11/vischildren/vischildrs.htm. Accessed April 9. 2011
5. Leibowitz HM. The red eye. N Engl J Med 342(5):345–351, 2000.
6. Wong TY, Mitchell P. Hypertensive retinopathy. N Engl J Med 351(22):2310–2317, 2004.
7. Frank RB. Diabetic retinopathy. N Engl J Med 350(1):48–58, 2004.

ADDITIONAL REFERENCES

Albert DM, Miller JW, Azar DT. Albert & Jakobiec's Principles and Practice of Ophthalmology, 3rd ed. Philadelphia: Saunders Elsevier, 2008

Congdon N, O'Colmain B, Klaver CC, et al. Causes and prevalence of visual impairment among adults in the United States. Arch Ophthalmol 122(4):477–485, 2004.

Ehlers JP, Shah CP, Chirag P, et al., eds. The Wills Eye Manual: Office and Emergency Room Diagnosis and Treatment of Eye Disease. Philadelphia: Lippincott Williams & Wilkins, 2008.

Fong DS, Aiello LP, Ferris FL, et al. Diabetic retinopathy. Diabetes Care 27(10):2540–2553, 2004.

Gold DH, Weingeist TA. Color Atlas of the Eye in Systemic Disease. Philadelphia: Lippincott Williams & Wilkins, 2001.

Katlinowski MA. "Eye"Dentifying Vision Impairment in the Geriatric Patient. Geriatric Nursing 29:125–132, 2008.

McCluskey PJ, Towler HM, Lightman S. Management of chronic uveitis. BMJ 320(7234):555–558, 2000.

Mohamed Q, Gillies MC, Wong TY. Management of diabetic retinopathy. JAMA 298(8):902–916, 2007.

Ostler HB, Maibach HI, Hoke AW, et al. Diseases of the Eye and Skin: A Color Atlas. Philadelphia: Lippincott Williams & Wilkins, 2004.

Spoor TC, ed. Atlas of Neuro-ophthalmology. New York: Taylor & Francis, 2004.

Tasman W, Jaeger EA. The Wills Eye Hospital Atlas of Clinical Ophthalmology, 2nd ed. Philadelphia: Lippincott Williams & Wilkins, 2001.

Yanoff M, Duker JS. Ophthalmology, 2nd ed. St. Louis: Mosby, 2004.

Ears, Nose, Mouth, and Throat

LEARNING OBJECTIVES

The student will:

1. Identify the structures and function of the ear, nose, mouth, and throat.
2. Collect an accurate health history of the ear, nose, mouth, and throat.
3. Describe the physical examination techniques performed to evaluate the ear, nose, mouth, and throat.
4. Demonstrate how to use the otoscope.
5. Identify the measures for prevention or early detection of ear, sinus, and throat infections; hearing loss; change in balance; and maintenance of oral health.
6. Perform a complete ear, nose, mouth and throat examination.
7. Document a complete ear, nose, mouth, and throat assessment utilizing information from the health history and the physical examination.

The ear is the sensory organ of hearing. Critical functions of the ear are hearing and balance. During the assessment there are various signs and symptoms that signal changes in the ears. The nurse's role is to detect changes and work with the health care team to prevent infections or loss of hearing.

The nose is the sensory organ of smell. The nurse assesses changes in the sense of smell as well as changes in breathing patterns and signs of sinus infections.

The mouth and throat are the first part of the digestive system and the nurse assesses for changes in taste, eating patterns, and oral hygiene. Voice quality is also assessed. In all components of the system, the nurse assesses the patient for deviations from normal and teaches preventative practices to maintain these sensory organs.

THE EAR

ANATOMY AND PHYSIOLOGY

The ear has three compartments: the external ear, the middle ear, and the inner ear.

The *external ear* is composed of the auricle and ear canal. The *auricle* consists chiefly of cartilage covered by skin and has a firm elastic consistency. Its prominent curved outer ridge is the *helix*. Parallel and anterior to the helix is another curved prominence, the *antihelix*. Inferiorly lies the fleshy projection of the earlobe, or *lobule*. The ear canal opens behind the *tragus*, a triangular nodular eminence that points backward over the entrance to the canal.

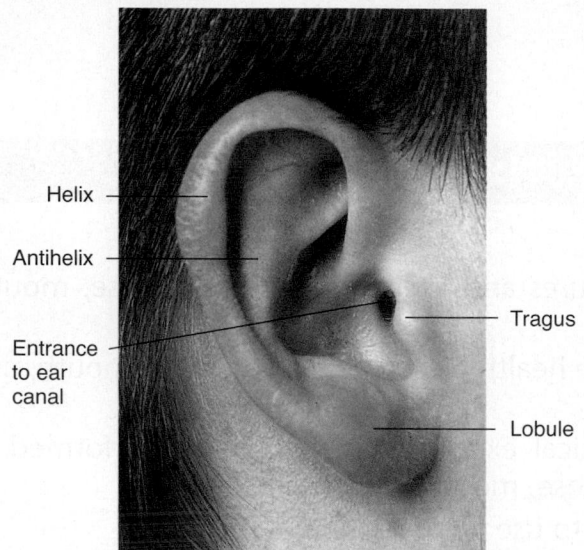

The function of the **auricle** is to gather sound waves and funnel them down the ear canal.

The *ear canal* or the auditory meatus curves inward and is approximately 24 mm long in adults. Cartilage surrounds its outer portion. The skin in this outer portion is hairy and contains glands that produce cerumen (wax). The inner portion of the canal is surrounded by bone and lined by thin, hairless skin. Pressure on this latter area causes pain—a point to remember when you examine the ear.

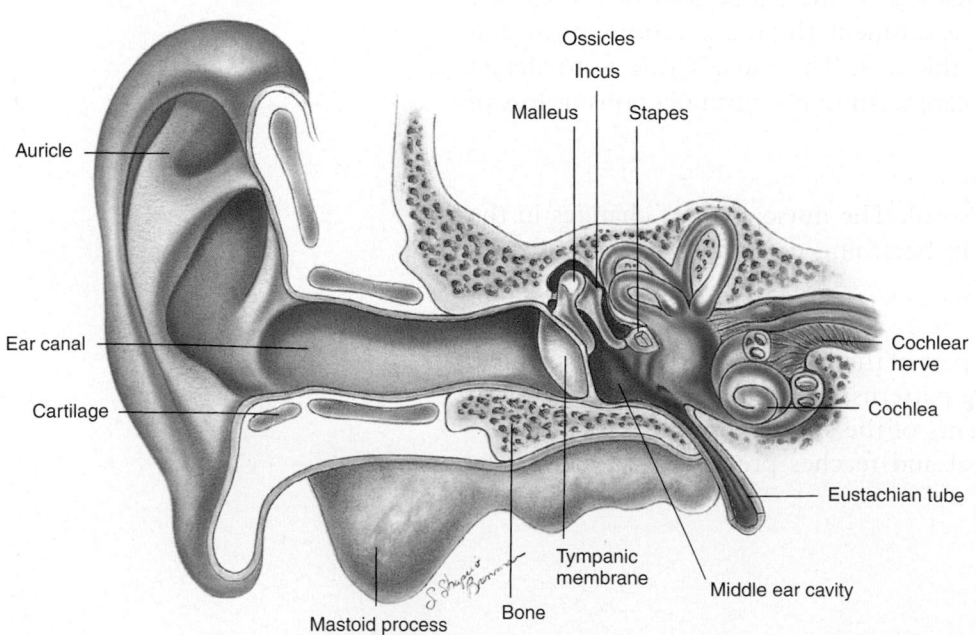

Behind and below the ear canal is the mastoid part of the temporal bone. The lowest portion of this bone, the *mastoid process,* is palpable behind the lobule.

At the end of the ear canal lies the *tympanic membrane,* or eardrum, marking the lateral limits of the middle ear. The *middle ear* is an air-filled cavity that transmits sound by way of three tiny bones, the *ossicles.* It is connected by the *eustachian tube* to the nasopharynx.

The eardrum is an oblique membrane held inward at its center by the *malleus,* one of its three ossicles. The *handle* and the *short process* of the malleus are the two chief landmarks. From the *umbo,* where the eardrum meets the tip of the malleus, a light reflection called the *cone of light* fans downward and anteriorly. Above the short process lies a small portion of the eardrum called the *pars flaccida.* The remainder of the drum is the *pars tensa.* Anterior and posterior malleolar folds, which extend obliquely upward from the short process, separate the pars flaccida from the pars tensa but are usually invisible unless the eardrum is retracted. A second ossicle, the *incus,* can sometimes be seen through the drum and the third ossicle, the *stapes* is not visible.

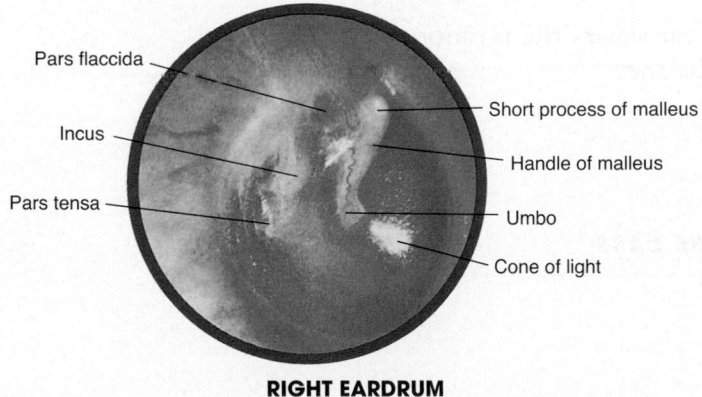

Pars flaccida
Incus
Pars tensa
Short process of malleus
Handle of malleus
Umbo
Cone of light

RIGHT EARDRUM

Much of the middle ear and all of the inner ear are inaccessible to direct examination. Some inferences concerning their condition can be made, however, by testing auditory function.

Pathways of Hearing. Vibrations of sound pass through the air of the external ear and are transmitted through the eardrum and ossicles of the middle ear to the *cochlea,* a part of the inner ear. The cochlea senses and codes the vibrations, and nerve impulses are sent to the brain through the cochlear nerve. The first part of this pathway—from the external ear through the middle ear—is known as the *conductive* phase, and a disorder here causes *conductive hearing loss.* The second part of the pathway, involving the cochlea and the cochlear nerve, is called the *sensorineural* phase; a disorder here causes *sensorineural hearing loss.*

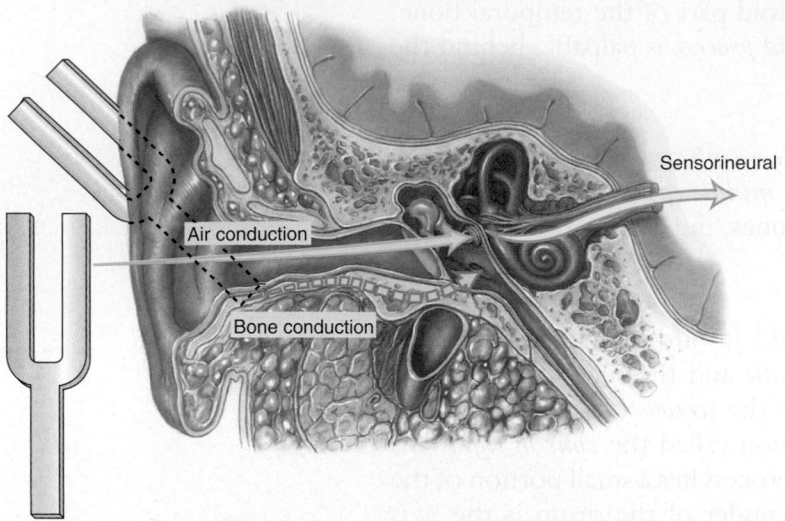

Air conduction describes the normal first phase in the hearing pathway. An alternate pathway, known as *bone conduction,* bypasses the external and middle ear and is used for testing purposes. A vibrating tuning fork, placed on the head, sets the bone of the skull into vibration and stimulates the cochlea directly. In a normal person, air conduction is more sensitive than bone conduction.

Equilibrium. The labyrinth within the inner ear senses the position and movements of the head and helps to maintain balance.

 ## THE HEALTH HISTORY

COMMON OR CONCERNING SYMPTOMS OF THE EARS

- Hearing loss
- Earache
- Discharge
- Tinnitus
- Vertigo

The purpose of the nursing health history of the ears is to detect changes in the patient's hearing, ears, and balance. The opening questions are:

"How is your hearing?"
"Have you had any trouble with your ears?"

If the patient has noticed a hearing change then further assessment utilizing the mnemonic "OLD CART" is helpful.

Hearing Loss
Onset: When did you first notice the change in your ears/hearing?
Location: Does it involve the left ear, right ear, or both ears?

Duration: How long has this been going on? Did it start suddenly or gradually? Is it temporary or constant?

Characteristic Symptoms: Do you notice any other symptoms when this occurs?

Have you put anything in your ear (e.g., food, dislodged pencil eraser)?

Has anything ever crawled/flown in your ear (i.e., bugs)?

Do you clean your ears with cotton swabs?

Do you scratch the inside of your ear? With what?

Associated Manifestations: Does anything else seem to be going on at the same time? Nausea? Dizziness?

What happened prior to the hearing loss? Did anything precipitate the loss?

Relieveing Factors: Does anything make it better?

Treatment: Have you seen anyone for this?

Ear History

Do you have a history of *hearing loss?*

Hearing loss may also be congenital, from single gene mutations.[1]

Try to distinguish between two basic types of hearing impairment: *conductive loss,* which results from problems in the external or middle ear, and *sensorineural loss,* from problems in the inner ear, the cochlear nerve, or its central connections in the brain. Two questions may be helpful: Does the patient have special difficulty understanding you as they talk? What difference does a noisy environment make?

People with sensorineural loss have particular trouble understanding speech, often complaining that others mumble; noisy environments make hearing worse. In conductive loss, noisy environments may help.

Symptoms associated with hearing loss, such as earache or vertigo, help you to assess likely causes. In addition, inquire specifically about medications that might affect hearing and ask about sustained exposure to loud noise.

Medications that affect hearing include aminoglycosides, aspirin, nonsteroidal anti-inflammatory drugs (NSAIDs), quinine, furosemide, and others.

Earache

Complaints of *earache,* or *pain in the ear,* are especially common. Ask about associated fever, sore throat, cough, and concurrent upper respiratory infection.

Pain suggests a problem in the external ear, such as *otitis externa,* or, if associated with symptoms of respiratory infection, in the inner ear, as in *otitis media.*[2] It may also be referred from other structures in the mouth, throat, or neck.

Do you have frequent earaches?

Onset. When did the last earache occur? How often do you have earaches?

Location: Which ear was affected?

Duration: How long did it last?

Characteristic Symptoms: Did you have any other symptoms?

Associated Manifestations: What additional symptoms were occurring or what might have preceded the earache?

Did you or anyone around you have a cold?

When was the last time you were swimming? Took a bath? Went in a hot tub? Did you go underwater?

Relieving Factors: What relieves the pain?

Treatment: Has this been treated previously? Currently?

Discharge

Ask about *discharge from the ear,* especially if associated with earache or trauma.

Unusually soft wax, debris from inflammation or rash in the ear canal, or discharge through a perforated eardrum may be secondary to *acute* or *chronic otitis media.*

Have you noticed any discharge?

When did you first notice the discharge?

In which ear?

Describe the discharge.

Color?

Consistency?

Amount?

Constant or intermittent drainage?

Does anything stop the discharge? Has it gotten worse or better?

Are you noting any other symptoms

Sore throat?

Cough?

Respiratory infection?

Fever?

Dizziness?

Headaches?

Does anything make it better?

Discharge from the ear may be associated with earaches or trauma.

Tinnitus

Tinnitus is a perceived sound that has no external stimulus and commonly is heard as musical ringing or a rushing or roaring noise. It can involve one or both ears. Tinnitus may accompany hearing loss and often remains unexplained. Occasionally, popping sounds originate in the temporomandibular joint, or vascular noises from the neck may be audible.

Tinnitus is a common symptom, increasing in frequency with age. When associated with hearing loss and vertigo, it suggests *Ménière's disease.*

Do you have tinnitus (ringing) in your ear?

When did this begin?

Is it in the left ear, right ear, or both ears?

Is this temporary or constant?

Do you notice any other symptoms when this occurs?

Vertigo

Vertigo refers to the perception that the patient or the environment is rotating or spinning. These sensations point primarily to a problem in the labyrinths of the inner ear, peripheral lesions of cranial nerve (CN) VIII, or lesions in its central pathways or nuclei in the brain.

See Table 12-1, Dizziness and Vertigo, p. 277.

Vertigo is a challenging symptom for you as a nurse, because patients differ widely in what they mean by the word "dizzy." "Are there times when you feel dizzy?" is an appropriate first question, but patients often find it difficult to be more specific. Ask "Do you feel unsteady, as if you are going to fall or black out? . . . Or do you feel the room is spinning (true vertigo)?" Get the story without biasing it. You may need to offer the patient several choices of wording. Ask if the patient feels pulled to the ground or off to one side, and if the dizziness is related to a change in body position. Pursue any associated feelings of clamminess or flushing, nausea, or vomiting. Check if any medications may be contributing.

Feeling unsteady, lightheaded, or "dizzy in the legs" sometimes suggests a cardiovascular etiology.

A feeling of being pulled suggests true vertigo from an inner ear problem or a central or peripheral lesion of CN VIII.

Do you have vertigo (dizziness)?
   When did this begin?
   Is this temporary or constant?
   How long does it last?
   What other symptoms do you experience at this time?
   How does it affect your daily life?
   What makes it feel better? Or go away?
   What activities of daily living are impacted due to the vertigo (e.g., avoiding steps or driving a car)?
When was the last ear exam?
   What were the results?
   Was any further testing necessary?

Past History

Congenital hearing loss
Removal of cerumen
Ear surgery
Trauma or injury to your ear(s)
Infection
Exposure to hazardous noise levels (work, home, war)
History of syphilis, rubella, meningitis

Family History

Hearing loss
Otitis media
Allergies
Smoking or exposure to cigarette smoke

Lifestyle Habits

Are you exposed to loud noises?
   What is your occupation? Hobbies (e.g. hunting)?
   Do you attend concerts? Bars? Loud places?
   Do you use headphones or earbuds to listen to music?
   Do you use an iPod? How often? On what level?
   Do you use lawn mower? Power tools? Firearms?
   Do you live near a busy road or train tracks?
   Have you ever used ear plugs/protectors? Currently?

Have you ever used hearing aid(s)? Which ear? Currently? At all times? Brand?

Have you used medications or drugs that interfere with how you hear or cause dizziness? Any medications that cause ototoxicity (e.g., large doses of antibiotics infused rapidly)?

THE NOSE AND PARANASAL SINUSES

 ## ANATOMY AND PHYSIOLOGY

The nose has four primary functions.

1. It is the site of inspiration and expiration.

2. It filters, warms, and adds moisture to the air exchanged.

3. It is the sensory organ for smell.

4. It is the site of speech resonance.

Terms used to describe the external anatomy of the nose are depicted for review.

Approximately the upper third of the nose is supported by bone, the lower two thirds by cartilage. Air enters the nasal cavity by way of the *anterior naris* on either side, then passes into a widened area known as the *vestibule* and on through the narrow nasal passage to the nasopharynx.

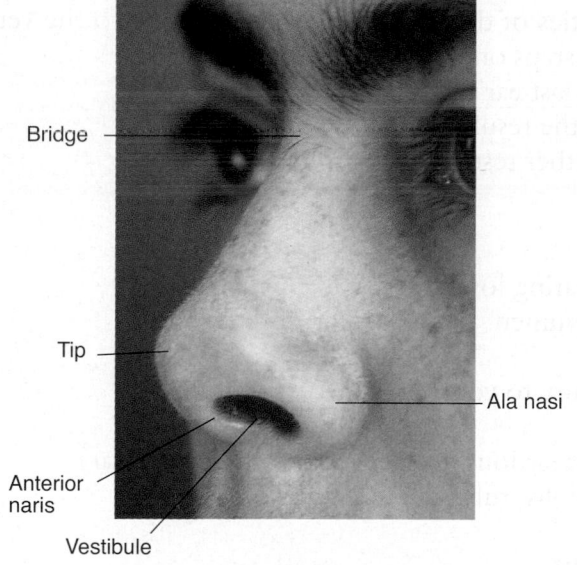

Bridge

Tip

Ala nasi

Anterior naris

Vestibule

The medial wall of each nasal cavity is formed by the *nasal septum,* which, like the external nose, is supported by both bone and cartilage. It is covered by a mucous membrane well supplied with blood. The vestibule, unlike the rest of the nasal cavity, is lined with hair-bearing skin, not mucosa.

Laterally, the anatomy is more complex. Curving bony structures, the *turbinates,* covered by a highly vascular mucous membrane protrude into the nasal cavity. Below each turbinate is a groove, or meatus, each named according to the turbinate above it. The nasolacrimal duct

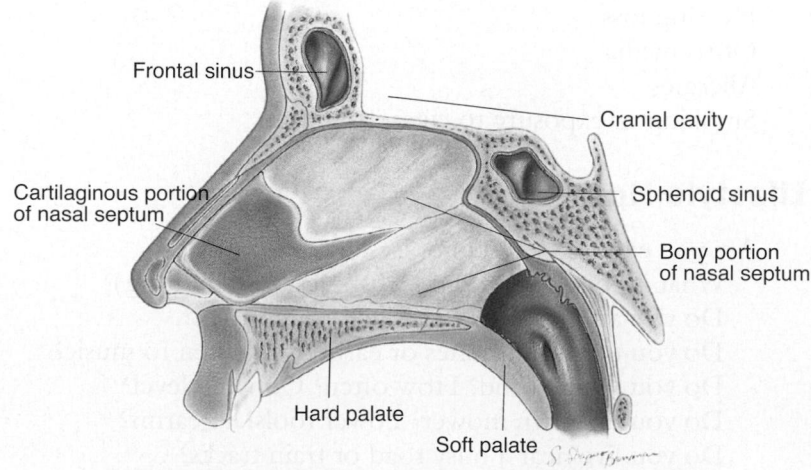

Frontal sinus

Cranial cavity

Sphenoid sinus

Cartilaginous portion of nasal septum

Bony portion of nasal septum

Hard palate

Soft palate

MEDIAL WALL—LEFT NASAL CAVITY (MUCOSA REMOVED)

drains into the inferior meatus and most of the paranasal sinus drains into the middle meatus. Their openings are not usually visible.

The additional surface area provided by the turbinates and the mucosa covering them aids the nasal cavities in their principal functions: cleansing, humidification, and temperature control of inspired air.

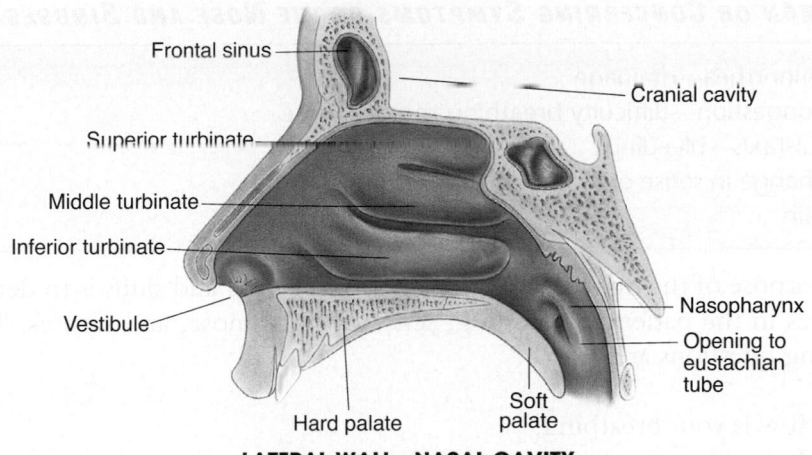

LATERAL WALL—NASAL CAVITY

The *paranasal sinuses* are air-filled cavities within the bones of the skull. Like the nasal cavities into which they drain, they are lined with mucous membranes. The paranasal sinuses are air filled and make the skull lighter and add to speech resonance. Their locations are diagrammed below. Only the frontal and maxillary sinuses are readily accessible to clinical examination.

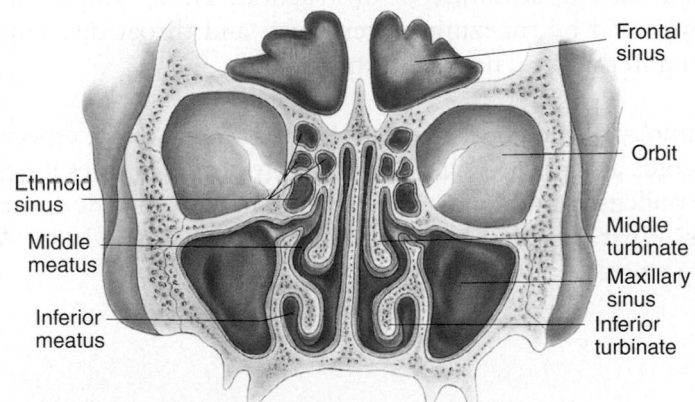

CROSS SECTION OF NASAL CAVITY—ANTERIOR VIEW

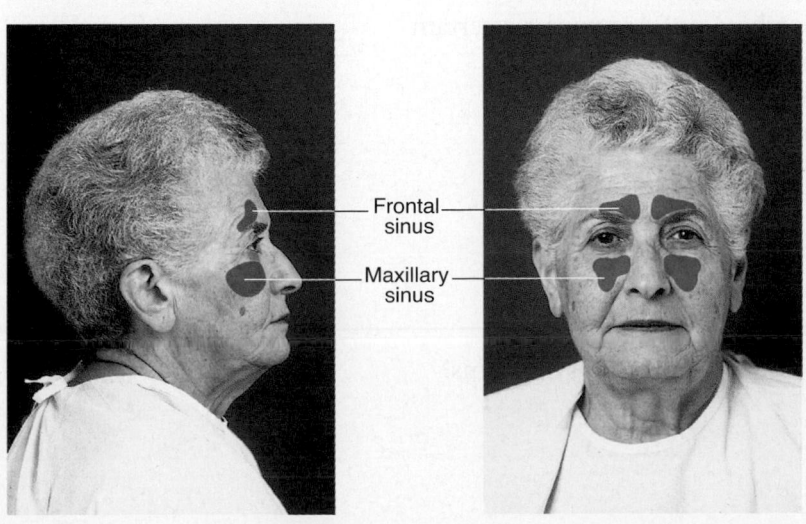

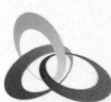

THE HEALTH HISTORY

COMMON OR CONCERNING SYMPTOMS OF THE NOSE AND SINUSES

- Rhinorrhea—drainage
- Congestion—difficulty breathing through nose
- Epistaxis—bleeding
- Change in sense of smell
- Pain

The purpose of the nursing health history of the nose and sinus is to detect changes in the patient's breathing, sense of smell, nose, and sinuses. The opening questions are:

"How is your breathing?"
"Have you noticed any changes with your nose or sinuses?"

Rhinorrhea refers to drainage from the nose and is often associated with *nasal congestion,* a sense of stuffiness or obstruction. These symptoms are frequently accompanied by sneezing, watery eyes, and throat discomfort, and also by itching in the eyes, nose, and throat.[3]

Causes include viral infections, *allergic rhinitis* ("hay fever"), and *vasomotor rhinitis.* Itching favors an allergic cause.

Assess the chronology of the illness. Does it last for a week or so, especially when common colds and related syndromes are prevalent, or does it occur seasonally when pollens are in the air? Is it associated with specific contacts or environments? What remedies has the patient used? For how long? And how well do they work?

Relation to seasons or environmental contacts suggests allergy.[3]

Excessive use of decongestants can worsen symptoms, causing *rhinitis medicamentosa.*

Rhinorrhea

Have you noticed any rhinorrhea or discharge?
  Onset: When did you first notice the runny nose (rhinorrhea)?
    Does it occur when pollen is in the air? When you are exposed to others with colds?
    What brings the runny nose (rhinorrhea) on? Are you at a certain place when it occurs? Does it occur at a certain time?
  Location: In which side does it occur? Both?
  Duration: How long does it last? A day? A week? A season?
    Does it interfere with sleep? Work? Activities of daily living?
  Characteristic Symptoms: Describe the runny nose (rhinorrhea).
    What color is the discharge?
    Consistency?
    Amount?
    Constant or intermittent drainage?
  Associated Manifestations: Have you noticed any other symptoms?
    Sore throat?
    Cough?
    Respiratory infection?
    Fever?

Headache?

Tenderness over the sinuses?

Relieving Factors/Treatment: Does anything stop the runny nose (rhinorrhea)? Has it gotten worse or better? Does anything make it better? What remedies have worked? For how long? How well do they work?

Congestion

Did symptoms appear after an upper respiratory infection (URI)? Is there pain on bending forward or a maxillary toothache? Fever or local headache? Tenderness over the sinuses?

Together these suggest *acute bacterial sinusitis*. Sensitivity and specificity are highest for symptoms appearing after a URI (~90% and ~80%).[4-6]

Inquire about drugs that might cause stuffiness.

Examples are: Oral contraceptives, reserpine, and alcohol

Is the patient's nasal congestion limited to one side? If so, you may be dealing with a different problem that requires careful physical examination.

Consider a deviated nasal septum, foreign body, or tumor.

How long have you noticed the congestion on one side?

Have you injured your nose?

Do you remember putting anything in your nose?

Have you had surgery on your nose?

Do you have a history of polyps? Family history?

What medications are you currently taking?

Oral contraceptives, reserpine, guanethidine, and alcohol may cause stuffiness.

Epistaxis means bleeding from the nose. The blood usually originates from the nose itself, but may come from a paranasal sinus or the nasopharynx. The history is usually quite graphic! However, in patients who are lying down or have bleeding that originates in posterior structures, blood may pass into the throat instead of out the nostrils. You must identify the source of the bleeding carefully—is it from the nose, or has it been coughed up or vomited? Assess the site of bleeding, its severity, and associated symptoms. Carefully differentiate epistaxis from *hemoptysis* or *hematemesis*, because each has different causes. Is it a recurrent problem? Has there been easy bruising or bleeding elsewhere in the body?

Local causes of epistaxis include trauma (especially nose picking), inflammation, drying and crusting of the nasal mucosa, tumors, and foreign bodies.

Bleeding disorders may contribute to epistaxis.

Epistaxis

O*nset:* When did you first notice the bloody nose (epistaxis)?

What caused the bloody nose? (injury, dry room, an object?)

L*ocation:* In which side does it occur? Both?

D*uration:* How long does it last? How often do the nosebleeds occur?

C*haracteristic Symptoms:* Describe the nosebleeds.

What color is the blood? Bright red? Black? Dark red-brown?

Consistency?

Amount?

Constant or intermittent drainage?

Associated Manifestations: Have you noticed any other symptoms?
  Injury to the nose?
  Recent surgery—nose or adenoids?
  Inflammation?
  Drying of the mucous membrane?
Relieving Factors/Treatment: What makes the bleeding stop? Is it difficult to stop?
  What medications are you currently taking?

Assess if the patient is on anticoagulation therapy or aspirin, which interfere with clotting. Nasal sprays, if overused, can contribute to the rebound effect, causing inflammation and congestion.

Change in Sense of Smell

Onset: When did you first notice the change in sense of smell? What triggered this?
  Was there any illness prior to the change in smell? Injury?
Location: In which side did the change of smell occur? Both?
Duration: Is it constant or intermittent?
Characteristic Symptoms: Are there any smells you can detect? Which ones?
Associated Manifestations: Have you noticed any other symptoms?
Relieving Factors/Treatment: Does anything relieve this or is it permanent?

Past History

Sinus infections
Upper respiratory infections
Allergies
Trauma or injury
Nasal or sinus surgery
Polyps
Dental history

Family History

Allergies
Asthma
Cancer of the nose or sinus

Lifestyle Habits

Air quality: at home and work, how often filters are changed, age of home and work or school site, rugs
Pets: what kind? How many? Are they in the house or outside? Do they sleep in bed with the patient?
Alcohol: what kind? How much?
Tobacco use: what kind? how often? how many?
Recreational drugs: what kind? route? How often?

Snorting cocaine can perforate the nasal mucous membrane. Frequent use can cause chronic rhinitis.

MOUTH AND PHARYNX

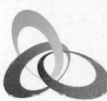

ANATOMY AND PHYSIOLOGY

The *lips* are muscular folds that surround the entrance to the mouth. When opened, the gums (gingiva) and teeth are visible. Note the scalloped shape of the *gingival margins* and the pointed *interdental papillae*.

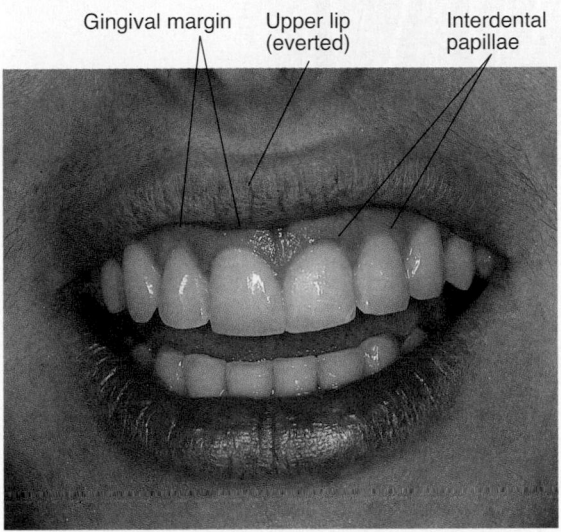

Gingival margin Upper lip (everted) Interdental papillae

The *gingiva* is firmly attached to the teeth and to the maxilla or mandible in which they are seated. In lighter-skinned people, the gingiva is pale or coral pink and lightly stippled. In darker-skinned people, it may be diffusely or partly brown, as shown. A midline mucosal fold, called a *labial frenulum*, connects each lip with the gingiva. A shallow *gingival sulcus* between the gum's thin margin and each tooth is not readily visible (but is probed and measured by dentists). Adjacent to the gingiva is the *alveolar mucosa*, which merges with the *labial mucosa* of the lip.

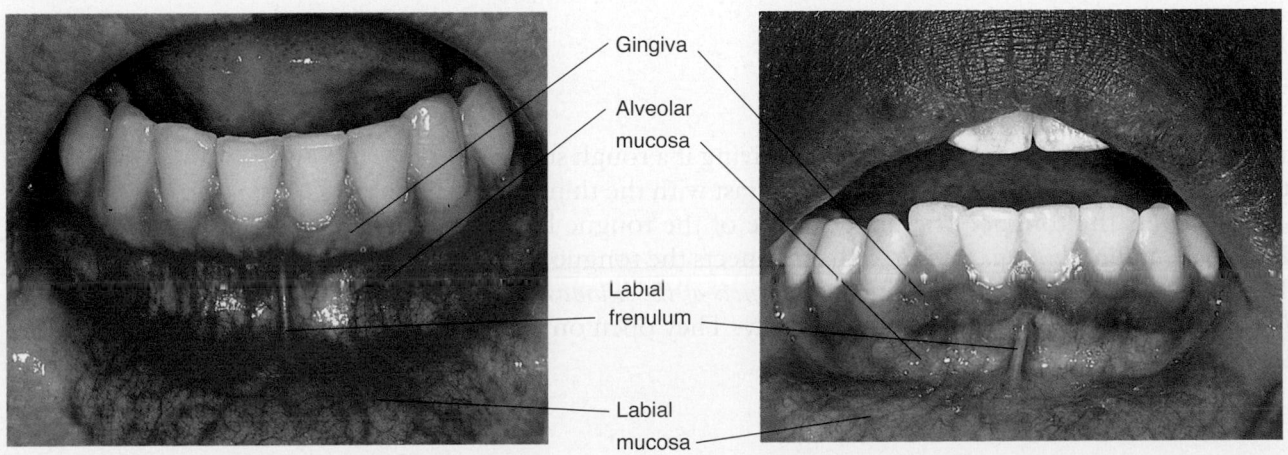

Gingiva

Alveolar mucosa

Labial frenulum

Labial mucosa

Each tooth, composed chiefly of dentin, lies rooted in a bony socket with only its enamel-covered crown exposed. Small blood vessels and nerves enter the tooth through its apex and pass into the pulp canal and pulp chamber.

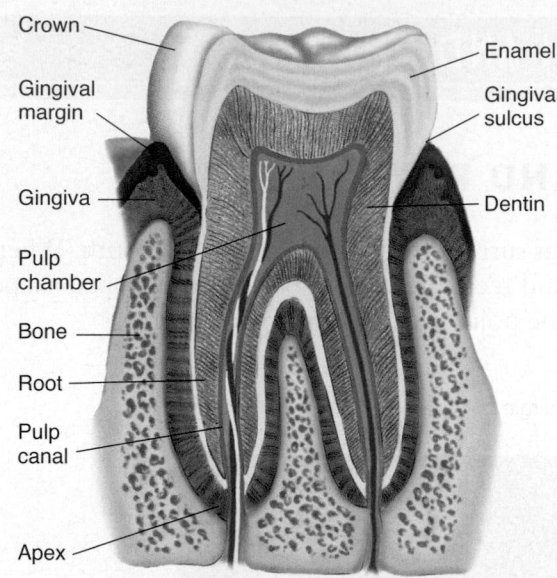

Note the terms designating the 32 adult teeth, 16 in each jaw.

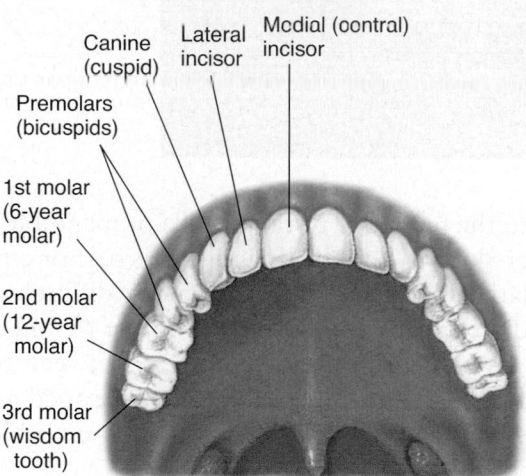

The dorsum of the *tongue* is covered with papillae, giving it a rough surface. Some of these papillae look like red dots, which contrast with the thin white coat that often covers the tongue. The undersurface of the tongue has no papillae. Note the midline *lingual frenulum* that connects the tongue to the floor of the mouth. At the base of the tongue the *ducts of the submandibular gland* (Wharton ducts) pass forward and medially. They open on papillae that lie on each side of the lingual frenulum.

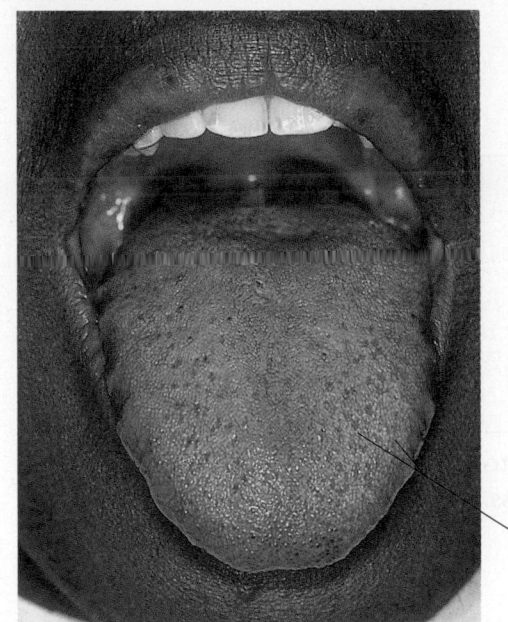

Papillae

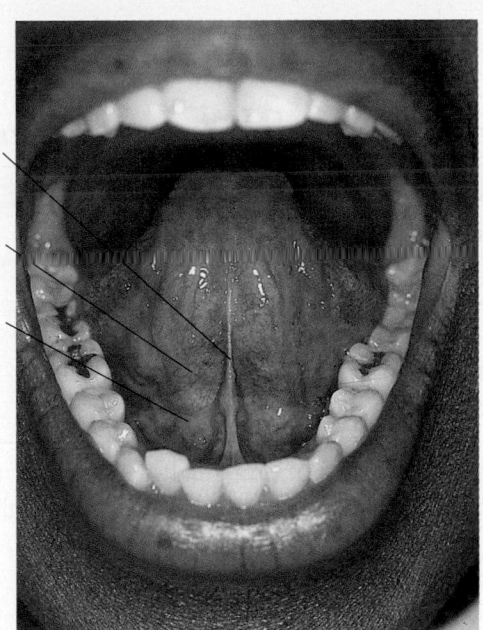

Lingual frenulum

Vein

Duct of submandibular gland

Above and behind the tongue rises an arch formed by the *anterior* and *posterior pillars*, the *soft palate*, and the *uvula*. A meshwork of small blood vessels may web the soft palate. The *pharynx* is visible in the recess behind the soft palate and tongue.

In the adjacent photograph, note the right tonsil protruding from the hollowed *tonsillar fossa*, or cavity, between the anterior and posterior pillars. In adults, tonsils are often small or absent, as in the empty left tonsillar fossa here.

The *buccal mucosa* lines the cheeks. Each *parotid duct*, sometimes termed the *Stensen duct*, opens onto the buccal mucosa near the upper second molar. Its location is frequently marked by its own small papilla.

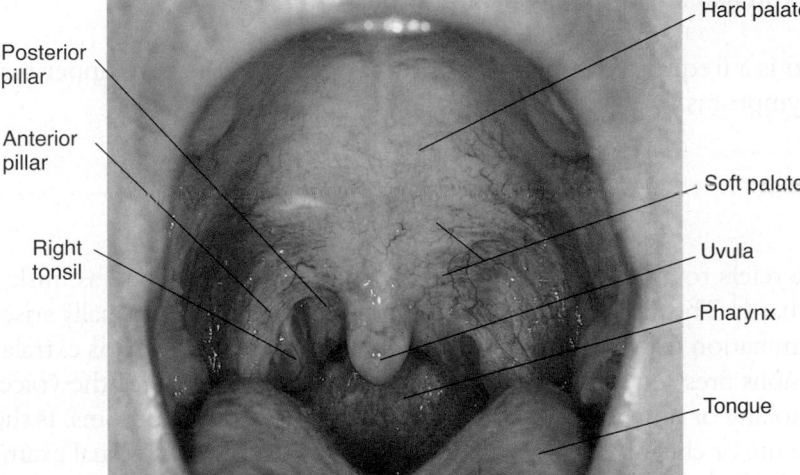

Posterior pillar

Anterior pillar

Right tonsil

Hard palate

Soft palate

Uvula

Pharynx

Tongue

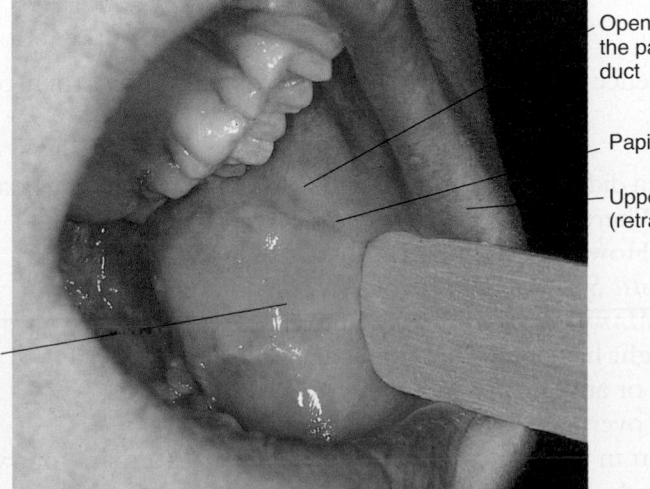

Opening of the parotid duct

Papilla

Upper lip (retracted)

Buccal mucosa

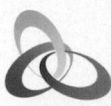

THE HEALTH HISTORY

COMMON OR CONCERNING SYMPTOMS OF THE MOUTH AND THROAT

- Sore throat
- Hoarseness
- Lesions
- Sore tongue
- Bleeding gums
- Toothache
- Dysphagia

The purpose of the nursing health history of the mouth and throat is to detect changes in skin integrity, speech, or swallowing; infection; or illness.

The opening questions are:

> Have you noticed any changes in your mouth or throat?
> Have you had any difficulty eating? Swallowing?

Sore throat is a frequent complaint, usually associated with acute upper respiratory symptoms.

Fever, pharyngeal exudates, and anterior lymphadenopathy, especially in the absence of cough, suggest *streptococcal pharyngitis,* or *strep throat* (p. 284).[7,8]

Hoarseness refers to an altered quality of the voice, often described as husky, rough, or harsh. The pitch may be lower than before. Hoarseness usually arises from inflammation or infection of the larynx but may also develop as extralaryngeal lesions press on the laryngeal nerves. Check for overuse of the voice, allergy, smoking or other inhaled irritants, and any associated symptoms. Is the problem acute or chronic? If hoarseness lasts more than 2 weeks, visual examination of the larynx by indirect or direct laryngoscopy is advisable.

Overuse of the voice (as in cheering) and acute infections are the most likely causes.

Causes of chronic hoarseness include smoking, allergy, voice abuse, *hypothyroidism,* chronic infections such as *tuberculosis,* and *tumors.*

Hoarseness

Do you experience hoarseness? If the answer is affirmative then continue the assessment.

> **O**nset: When did the hoarseness begin? How often do you have hoarseness?
> **L**ocation: Where in the throat do you feel this?
> **D**uration: How long did it last?
> **C**haracteristic Symptoms: Did you have any other symptoms?
> **A**ssociated Manifestations: What additional symptoms were occurring or what might have preceded the hoarseness?
> Did you or anyone around you have a cold? Cough?
> Did you overuse your voice?
> Were you in a situation in which you needed to raise your voice or scream (e.g., concert, crowded area, jack hammers)?

Do you smoke? If yes, what, how many per day, and since when?
   Are you around others who smoke?
Reli*eving Factors:* What relieves the hoarseness?
Treat*ment:* Has this been treated previously? Currently?

Additional questions for the mouth assessment would include:

A *sore tongue* may result from local lesions as well as systemic illness.

Aphthous ulcers (p. 272); sore smooth tongue of nutritional deficiency (p. 289)

How long have you had the sore tongue? Describe it?

Bleeding from the gums is a common symptom, especially when brushing teeth. Ask what type of toothbrush is used? Hard or soft? Ask about local lesions and any tendency to bleed or bruise elsewhere.

Bleeding gums are most often caused by *gingivitis* (p. 287).

Do you have *bleeding gums*?
   When did this begin?
   Where is the bleeding?
   Is this temporary or constant?
   Do you notice any other symptoms when this occurs?

Tell me about the *toothache.*
   When was the last dental exam?
   What were the results?
   Were any further visits necessary?

Do you have *dysphagia* (difficulty swallowing)?
   When did this begin?
   What brought it on?
   Is this temporary or constant?
   What other symptoms do you experience at this time?
   How does it affect your daily life?
   What makes it feel better or go away?
   How has this changed what you eat? How has it changed who you eat with?

Do you have a history of lesions in your mouth?
   When did you first notice the lesions?
   Where are the lesions located? Are there any others?
   Describe the lesions.
      Size?
      Shape?
      Color?
      Discharge?
      Pain?
      Relationship to other lesions?
   Have you noticed any other symptoms?
      Itching?
      Cough?
      Respiratory infection?

Fever?
Dizziness?
Headaches?
Does anything make it better?

Past History

Sore throat
Loss of voice
Dental, mouth, or throat surgery
Trauma or injury to teeth, mouth, or throat
History of infections
Oral cancer
Sexually transmitted disease (STD)

Family History

Allergies
Smoking or exposure to cigarette smoke
Stroke
Tuberculosis

Lifestyle Habits

How many times a day do you brush your teeth?
Do you floss? How often?
Do you use tobacco? Cigarettes, cigars, a pipe, or chewing tobacco?
    How many per day? Since when?
Do you smoke marijuana? Crack? Inhale any other product?
Do you drink alcohol? What? How many ounces per day?
What is your occupation?
Do you use dental dams?

PHYSICAL EXAMINATION OF THE EAR

The Auricle.   Inspect the auricle and surrounding tissue for deformities, lumps, or skin lesions.

See Table 12-2, Lumps on or Near the Ear (p. 278).

If ear pain, discharge, or inflammation is present, move the auricle up and down, press the tragus, and press firmly just behind the ear.

Movement of the auricle and tragus (the "tug test") is painful in acute *otitis externa* (inflammation of the ear canal), but not in *otitis media* (inflammation of the middle ear). Tenderness behind the ear may be present in *otitis media*.

EQUIPMENT FOR THE EXAMINATION INCLUDES:

- Tuning fork (512 Hz preferred for hearing assessment)
- Otoscope
- Speculum
- Tongue blade
- Gloves
- Penlight

Ear Canal and Drum. To see the ear canal and drum, use an otoscope with the largest ear speculum that the canal will accommodate and the brightest light. Position the patient's head so that you can see comfortably through the instrument. To straighten the ear canal, grasp the auricle firmly but gently and pull it upward, backward, and slightly away from the head. Caution the patient to remain still.

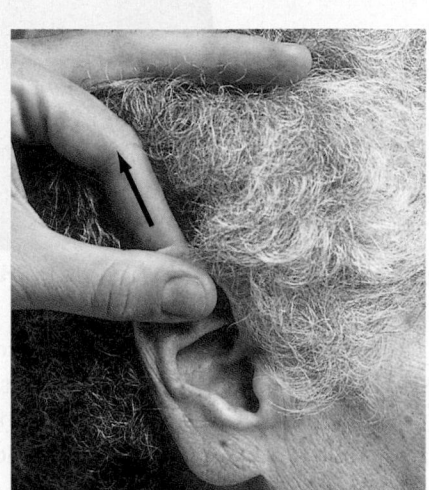

There are two common techniques utilized to hold an otoscope: the pencil grip and the hammer grip. Determine which is most comfortable.

1. Pencil grip: Hold the otoscope handle between your thumb and fingers, and brace your hand against the patient's face. Your hand and instrument thus follow unexpected movements by the patient. (If you are uncomfortable switching hands for the left ear, as shown below, you may reach over that ear to pull it up and back with your left hand and rest your otoscope-holding right hand on the head behind the ear.) This should be used in examining patients with tender ear canals or young children.

2. Hammer grip: Hold the otoscope with the battery portion facing down or up. This technique should be used cautiously in a patient who moves unexpectedly. This is often the more natural technique but there is less control; therefore, it may increase the risk of pain if the speculum comes in contact with the canal wall.

Insert the speculum gently into the ear canal about a quarter inch, directing it somewhat down and forward and through the hairs, if any, toward the eardrum.

Nontender nodular swellings covered by normal skin deep in the ear canals suggest *exostoses*. These are nonmalignant overgrowths, which may obscure the drum.

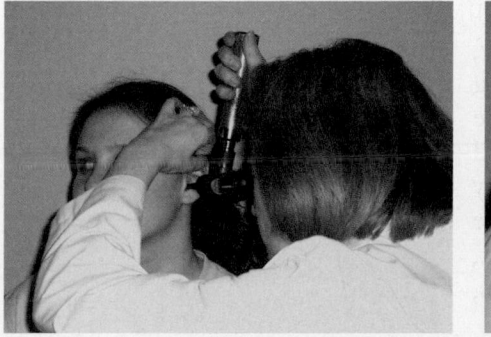

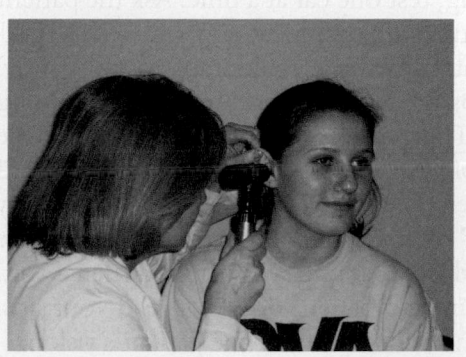

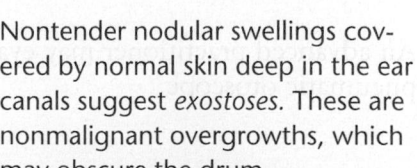

Inspect the ear canal, noting any discharge, foreign bodies, redness of the skin, or swelling. Cerumen, which varies in color and consistency from yellow and flaky to brown and sticky or even to dark and hard, may wholly or partly obscure your view.

In acute *otitis externa*, shown below, the canal is often swollen, narrowed, moist, pale, and tender. It may be reddened.

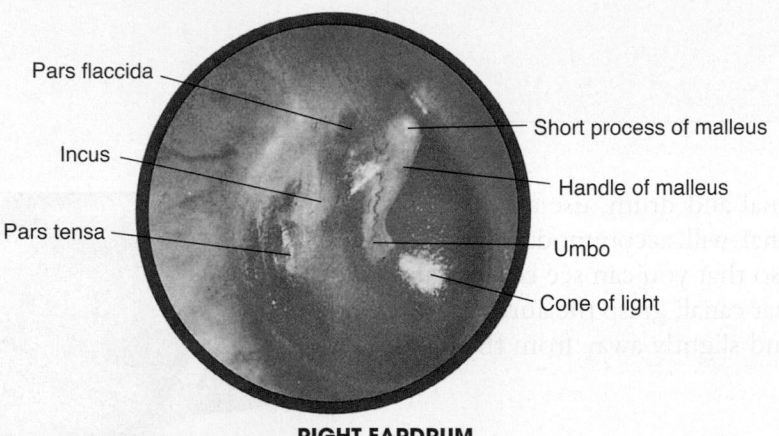

RIGHT EARDRUM

Pars flaccida

Incus

Pars tensa

Short process of malleus

Handle of malleus

Umbo

Cone of light

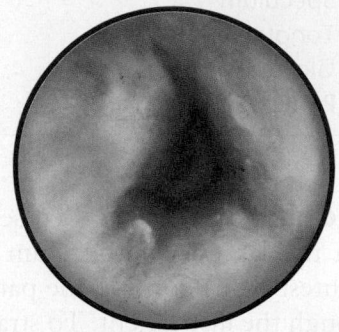

In *chronic otitis externa*, the skin of the canal is often thickened, red, and itchy.

Inspect the eardrum, noting its color and contour. The cone of light—usually easy to see—helps to orient you. The examiner is unable to visualize the entire eardrum at once but finds a landmark such as the cone of light and follows upward to see the handle of the malleus.

Red bulging drum of acute purulent *otitis media*[2]; amber drum of a serous effusion. See Table 12-3, Abnormalities of the Eardrum (pp. 279–280).

Identify the *handle of the malleus,* noting its position, and inspect the *short process of the malleus.*

An unusually prominent short process and a prominent handle that looks more horizontal suggest a retracted drum.

Gently move the speculum so that you can see as much of the drum as possible, including the *pars flaccida* superiorly and the margins of the *pars tensa.* Look for any perforations. The anterior and inferior margins of the drum may be obscured by the curving wall of the ear canal.

An advanced practitioner may evaluate the mobility of the eardrum with a pneumatic otoscope.

A serous effusion, a thickened drum, or purulent *otitis media* may decrease mobility.

Auditory Acuity.   To estimate hearing, test one ear at a time. Ask the patient to occlude one ear with a finger, or better still, occlude it yourself. When auditory acuity on the two sides is different, move your finger rapidly, but gently, in the occluded canal. This noise helps prevent the occluded ear from doing the work of the ear you wish to test. Then, standing 1 or 2 feet away, exhale fully (so as to minimize the intensity of your voice) and whisper softly toward the unoccluded ear. Choose numbers or other words with two equally accented syllables, such as "nine-four," or "baseball." If necessary, increase the intensity of your voice to a medium whisper, a loud whisper, and then a soft, medium, and loud voice. To make sure the patient does not read your lips, stand behind the patient, cover your mouth or obstruct the patient's vision.

Air and Bone Conduction. If hearing is diminished, *try to distinguish conductive from sensorineural hearing loss.* You need a quiet room and a tuning fork, preferably of 512 Hz or possibly 1024 Hz. These frequencies fall within the range of human speech (300 Hz to 3000 Hz)—functionally the most important range. Forks with lower pitches may lead to overestimating bone conduction and can also be felt as vibration.

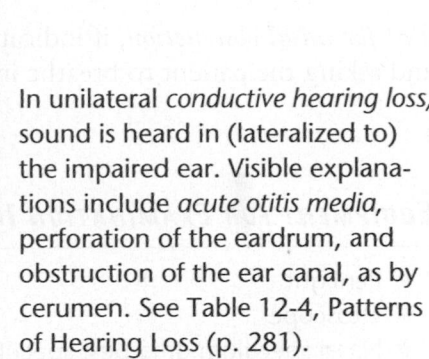

Set the fork into light vibration by briskly stroking it between the thumb and index finger (⇌) or by tapping it on your knuckles.

● *Test for lateralization* (Weber test). Place the base of the lightly vibrating tuning fork firmly on top of the patient's head or on the midforehead.

In unilateral *conductive hearing loss,* sound is heard in (lateralized to) the impaired ear. Visible explanations include *acute otitis media,* perforation of the eardrum, and obstruction of the ear canal, as by cerumen. See Table 12-4, Patterns of Hearing Loss (p. 281).

Ask where the patient hears it: on one or both sides? Normally the sound is heard in the midline or equally in both ears. If nothing is heard, try again, pressing the fork more firmly on the head. Because patients with normal hearing may lateralize, this test should be restricted to those with hearing loss.

In unilateral *sensorineural hearing loss,* sound is heard in the good ear.

● *Compare air conduction (AC) and bone conduction (BC)* (Rinne test). Place the base of a lightly vibrating tuning fork on the mastoid bone, behind the ear and level with the canal. When the patient can no longer hear the sound, quickly place the fork close to the ear canal and ascertain whether the sound can be heard again. Here the "U" of the fork should face forward, thus maximizing its sound for the patient. Normally the sound is heard longer through air than through bone (AC > BC).

In *conductive hearing loss,* sound is heard through bone as long as or longer than it is through air (BC = AC or BC > AC). In *sensorineural hearing loss,* sound is heard longer through air (AC > BC).

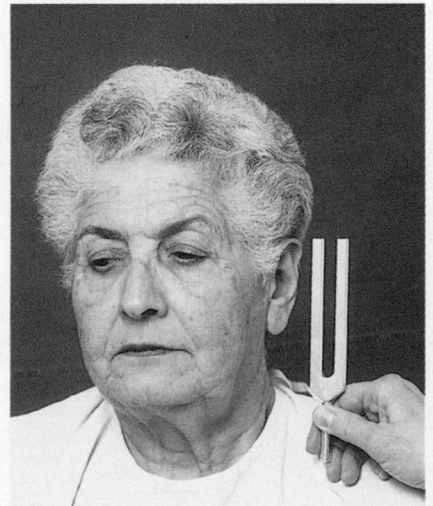

PHYSICAL EXAMINATION OF THE NOSE

Inspect the anterior and inferior surfaces of the nose. Gentle pressure on the tip of the nose with your thumb usually widens the nostrils and, with the aid of a penlight or otoscope light, you can get a partial view of each nasal *vestibule*. If the tip is tender, be particularly gentle and manipulate the nose as little as possible.

Note any asymmetry or deformity of the nose.

Test for nasal obstruction, if indicated, by pressing on each ala nasi in turn and asking the patient to breathe in.

Tenderness of the nasal tip or alae suggests local infection such as a furuncle.

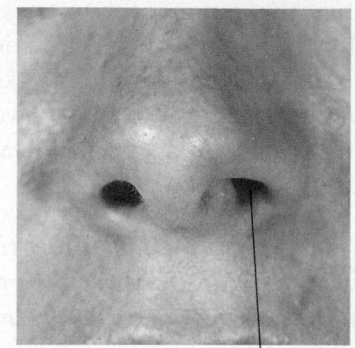

Vestibule

EQUIPMENT FOR EXAMINATION INCLUDES:

- Penlight
- Otoscope
- Nasal speculum or largest speculum available
- Gloves

Inspect the inside of the nose with an otoscope and the largest ear speculum available. Tilt the patient's head back a bit and insert the speculum gently into the vestibule of each nostril, avoiding contact with the sensitive nasal septum. Hold the otoscope handle to one side to avoid the patient's chin and improve your mobility. By directing the speculum posteriorly, then upward in small steps, try to see the inferior and middle turbinates, the nasal septum, and the narrow nasal passage between them. Some asymmetry of the two sides is normal.

Deviation of the lower septum is common and may be easily visible, as illustrated in the previous photo. Deviation seldom obstructs air flow.

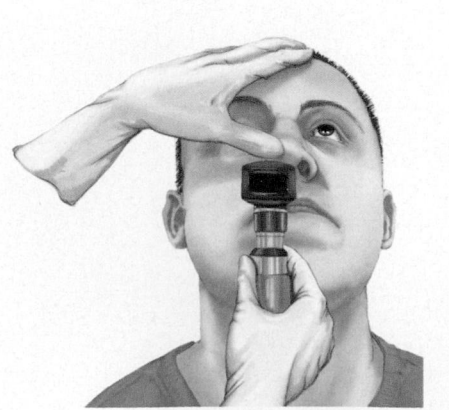

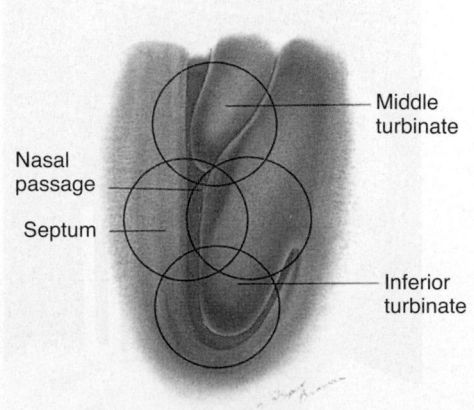

Middle turbinate

Nasal passage

Septum

Inferior turbinate

Observe the nasal mucosa, the nasal septum, and any abnormalities.

- The *nasal mucosa* that covers the septum and turbinates. Note its color and any swelling, bleeding, or exudate. If exudate is present, note its character: clear, mucopurulent, or purulent. The nasal mucosa is normally somewhat redder than the oral mucosa.

  In *viral rhinitis* the mucosa is reddened and swollen; in *allergic rhinitis* it may be pale, bluish, or red.

- The *nasal septum*. Note any deviation, inflammation, or perforation of the septum. The lower anterior portion of the septum (where the patient's finger can reach) is a common source of *epistaxis* (nosebleed).

  Fresh blood or crusting may be seen. Causes of septal perforation include trauma, surgery, and the intranasal use of cocaine or amphetamines.

- Any *abnormalities* such as ulcers or polyps.

  Polyps are pale, semitranslucent masses that usually come from the middle meatus. Ulcers may result from nasal use of cocaine.

Inspection of the nasal cavity through the anterior naris is usually limited to the vestibule, the anterior portion of the septum, and the lower and middle turbinates. Examination with a nasopharyngeal mirror is required for detection of posterior abnormalities. This technique is used by otorhinolaryngologists (ear, nose, and throat [ENT] specialists).

Make it a habit to dispose of all nasal and ear specula after use. (Check the policies of your institution.)

Palpate for sinus tenderness. Press up on the *frontal sinuses* from under the bony brows, avoiding pressure on the eyes. Then press up on the *maxillary sinuses.*

Local tenderness, together with symptoms such as pain, fever, and nasal discharge, suggest *acute sinusitis* involving the frontal or maxillary sinuses.[4-6] Transillumination may be diagnostically useful.

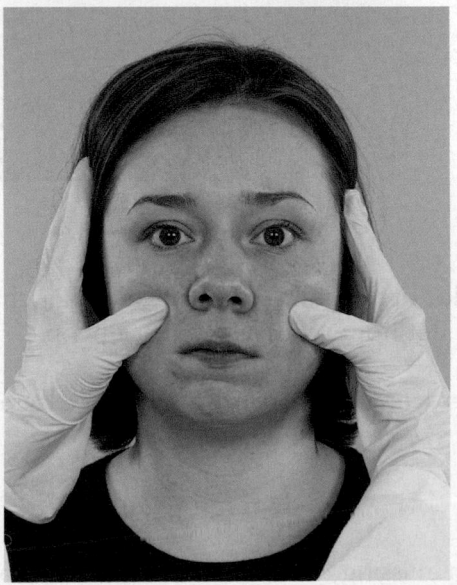

PHYSICAL EXAMINATION OF THE MOUTH AND THROAT

EQUIPMENT FOR EXAMINATION INCLUDES:

- Equipment for the examination includes:
- Penlight
- Tongue blade
- Gloves
- Gauze pad

If the patient wears dentures, offer a paper towel and ask the patient to remove them so that you can see the mucosa underneath. If you detect any suspicious ulcers or nodules, put on a glove and palpate any lesions, noting especially any thickening or infiltration of the tissues that might suggest malignancy.

Bright red edematous mucosa underneath a denture suggests denture sore mouth. There may be ulcers or papillary granulation tissue.

Inspect the following:

The Lips. Observe their color and moisture, and note any lumps, ulcers, cracking, or scaliness.

Cyanosis, pallor. See Table 12-5, Abnormalities of the Lips (pp. 282–283).

The Oral Mucosa. Look into the patient's mouth and, with a good light and the help of a tongue blade, inspect the oral mucosa for color, ulcers, white patches, and nodules. The wavy white line on this buccal mucosa developed where the upper and lower teeth meet. Irritation from sucking or chewing may cause or intensify it.

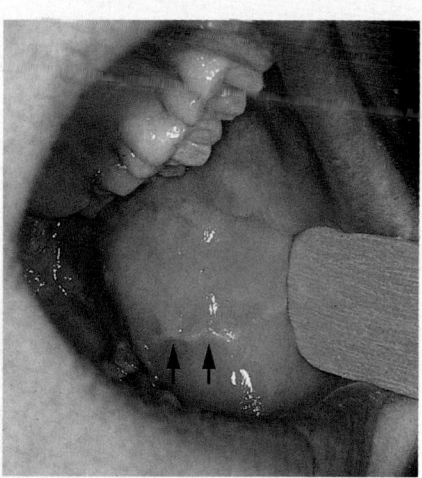

This patient has an *aphthous ulcer* (or canker sore) on the labial mucosa.

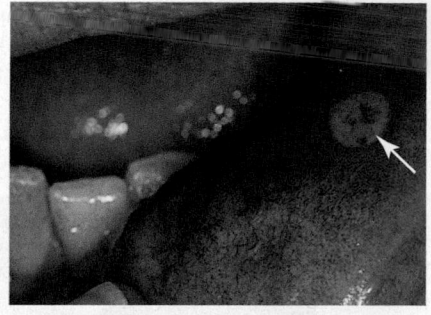

See Table 12-6, Findings in the Pharynx, Palate, and Oral Mucosa (pp. 284–286).

The Gums and Teeth. Note the color of the gums, normally pink. Patchy brownness may be present, especially but not exclusively in black people.

Redness of *gingivitis,* black line of *lead poisoning*

Inspect the gum margins and the interdental papillae for swelling or ulceration.

Swollen interdental papillae in *gingivitis.* See Table 12-7, Findings in the Gums and Teeth (pp. 287–288).

Inspect the teeth. Are any of them missing, discolored, misshapen, or abnormally positioned? You can check for looseness with your gloved thumb and index finger. Look for malocclusion of the teeth.

The Roof of the Mouth. Inspect the color and architecture of the hard palate.

Torus palatinus, a benign midline lump (see p. 285)

The Tongue and the Floor of the Mouth. Ask the patient to put out his or her tongue. Inspect it for symmetry—a test of the hypoglossal nerve (cranial nerve XII).

Note the color and texture of the dorsum of the tongue.

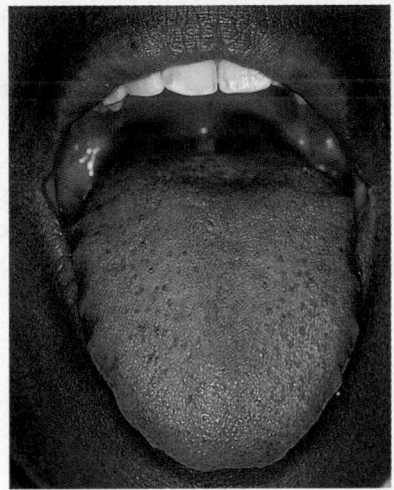
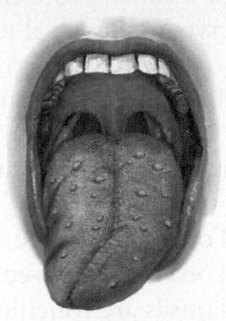

Asymmetric protrusion suggests a lesion of CN XII, as shown below.

Inspect the sides and undersurface of the tongue and the floor of the mouth. These are the areas where cancer most often develops. Note any white or reddened areas, nodules, or ulcerations. Because cancer of the tongue is more common in men older than 50 years, especially in smokers and drinkers of alcohol, palpation is indicated.[9] Explain what you plan to do and put on gloves. Ask the patient to protrude his or her tongue. With your right hand, grasp the tip of the tongue with a square of gauze and gently pull it to the patient's left. Inspect the side of the tongue, and then palpate it with your gloved left hand, feeling for any induration (hardness).[9] Reverse the procedure for the other side.

Cancer of the tongue is the second most common cancer of the mouth, second only to cancer of the lip. Any persistent nodule or ulcer, red or white, must be suspect. Induration of the lesion further increases the possibility of malignancy. Cancer occurs most often on the side of the tongue, next most often at its base.

See Table 12-8, Findings in or Under the Tongue (pp. 289–290).

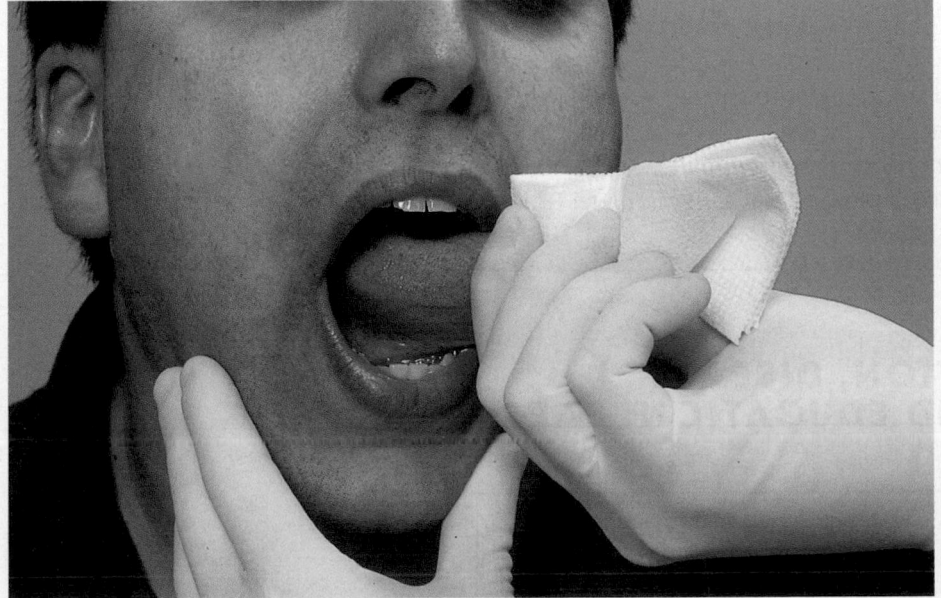

The Pharynx. Now, with the patient's mouth open but the tongue not protruded, ask the patient to say "ah" or yawn. This action may let you see the pharynx well. If not, press a tongue blade firmly down upon the midpoint of the arched tongue—far enough back to get good visualization of the pharynx but not so far that you cause gagging. Simultaneously, ask for an "ah" or a yawn. Note the rise of the soft palate and the uvula—a test of cranial nerve X (the vagal nerve).

Inspect the soft palate, anterior and posterior pillars, uvula, tonsils, and pharynx. Note their color and symmetry and look for exudate, swelling, ulceration, or tonsillar enlargement. Tonsils are graded based on size:

+1: Tonsils are visible.
+2: Tonsils are between the tonsillar pillars and the uvula.
+3: Tonsils are touching the uvula.
+4: Tonsils are touching each other.

If possible, palpate any suspicious area for induration or tenderness. Tonsils have crypts, or deep infoldings of squamous epithelium. Whitish spots of normal exfoliating epithelium may sometimes be seen in these crypts.

Discard your tongue blade and gloves after use and wash hands.

In CN X paralysis, the soft palate fails to rise and the uvula deviates to the opposite side.

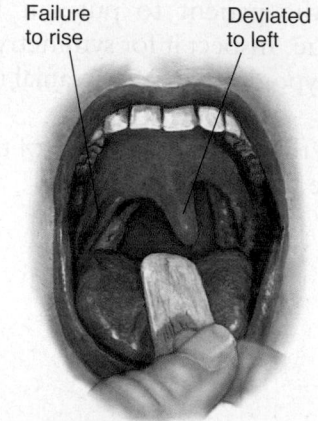

Failure to rise   Deviated to left

See Table 12-6, Findings in the Pharynx, Palate, and Oral Mucosa (pp. 284–286)

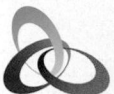

RECORDING YOUR FINDINGS

RECORDING THE PHYSICAL EXAMINATION—EARS, NOSE, AND THROAT

Ears—Acuity to whispered voice: L, "baseball"; R, "99." Tympanic membranes (TMs) intact, pearly grey, with cone of light at 7:00, L ear; 5:00, R ear. Weber midline. AC > BC. *Nose*—Nasal mucosa pink, septum midline; no sinus tenderness. *Throat (or Mouth)*—Oral mucosa pink, dentition 32 teeth, white, visible decay, pharynx without exudates.

OR

Ears—Acuity diminished to whispered voice; intact to spoken voice, L decreased to "baseball." TMs intact, pearly grey. *Nose*—Mucosa swollen with erythema and clear drainage. Septum midline. Tender over maxillary sinuses. *Throat*—Oral mucosa pink, dental caries in lower molars, pharynx erythematous, no exudates.

HEALTH PROMOTION, DISEASE PREVENTION, AND EDUCATION: EARS

IMPORTANT TOPICS

- Hearing screening
- Ear protection

Hearing is a critical sense for experiencing the world around us, and areas of importance are health promotion and disease prevention. Nursing education is vital in maintaining hearing and a healthy outlook for clients.

Hearing Screening.   Hearing screening tests provide a quick and cost-effective way to separate people into two groups: a pass group and a fail group. Hearing screening should be completed before an infant leaves the hospital. Without such programs, the average age of detection of significant hearing loss is approximately 14 months.[10] Language development is delayed when there is a hearing deficit. A child may not be ready for school if he or she has an undetected hearing deficit, but this is not the case for the child who has early intervention and is able to function at grade level.

Periodic screenings are recommended because of the increased potential for hearing loss due to overexposure to high levels of noise. As nurses, prevention is key, and patients should be reminded to utilize ear plugs when exposed to loud noises in their daily lives (e.g., lawnmowers, leaf blowers, chainsaws, concerts, train stations, battlefields, and sirens) and to limit exposure (iPod buds and cell phones).

Hearing Loss.   Hearing loss can also trouble the later years.[11,12] More than a third of adults older than 65 years have detectable hearing deficits, contributing to emotional isolation and social withdrawal. These losses may go undetected—unlike vision prerequisites for driving, there is no mandate for widespread testing of hearing, and many seniors avoid use of hearing aids. Questionnaires and hand-held audioscopes work well for periodic screening. Less sensitive are the clinical "whisper test," rubbing fingers, or use of the tuning fork. Groups at risk are those who have a history of congenital or familial hearing loss, receive intravenous antibiotics, or are exposed to syphilis, rubella, or meningitis.

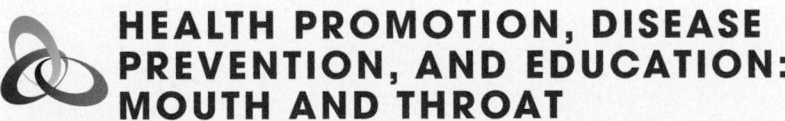

HEALTH PROMOTION, DISEASE PREVENTION, AND EDUCATION: MOUTH AND THROAT

IMPORTANT TOPICS

- Oral and dental screening
- Cancer prevention

More than one third (36.8%) of poor children ages 2 to 9 have one or more untreated decayed primary teeth, compared to 17.3% of nonpoor children.[13] This issue persists, as the 50 to 69 year old age group has at least one tooth with periodontal disease. The rate is highest for non-Hispanic blacks (31.2%), Mexican Americans (28.2%), and non-Hispanic whites (16.9%). As these groups age, the percentages rise to 47.1%, 32.0%, and 24.1%, respectively.[13]

Oral Health.   Nurses should play an active role in promoting oral health. Effective screening begins with careful examination of the mouth. Inspect the oral cavity for decayed or loose teeth, inflammation of the gingiva, and signs of periodontal disease (bleeding, pus, recession of the gums, and bad breath). Inspect the mucous membranes, the palate, the oral floor, and the surfaces of the tongue for ulcers and leukoplakia, warning signs for oral cancer and HIV disease. Use of dental dams during oral sex will act as a barrier to bodily fluids and help reduce transmission of STDs such as herpes, genital warts, and HIV.

To improve oral health, counsel patients to adopt daily hygiene measures. Use of fluoride-containing toothpaste reduces tooth decay, and brushing and flossing daily retard periodontal disease by removing bacterial plaques. Urge patients to seek dental care at least annually to receive the benefits of more specialized preventive care such as scaling, planing of roots, and topical fluorides.

Diet, tobacco and alcohol use, changes in salivary flow from medication, and proper use of dentures should also be addressed. As with children, adults should avoid excessive intake of foods high in refined sugars such as sucrose, which enhance attachment and colonization of cariogenic bacteria. Use of all tobacco products and excessive alcohol, the principal risk factors for oral cancers, should be avoided.

Saliva cleanses and lubricates the mouth. Many medications reduce salivary flow, increasing risk for tooth decay, mucositis, and gum disease from *xerostomia,* especially for the elderly. For those wearing dentures, dental examinations should be scheduled annually, and patients should be counseled about the importance of removing and cleaning the dentures each night to reduce bacterial plaque and risk of malodor. Regular massage of the gums relieves soreness and pressure from dentures on the underlying soft tissue.

TABLE
12-1

Dizziness and Vertigo[14-18]

"Dizziness" is a nonspecific term used by patients encompassing several disorders that clinicians must carefully sort out. A detailed history usually identifies the primary etiology. It is important to learn the specific meanings of the following terms or conditions:

Vertigo—a spinning sensation accompanied by nystagmus and ataxia; usually from *peripheral vestibular dysfunction* (~40% of "dizzy" patients) but may be from a *central brainstem lesion* (~10%; causes include atherosclerosis, multiple sclerosis, vertebrobasilar migraine, or transient ischemic attack [TIA])

Presyncope—a near faint from "feeling faint or lightheaded"; causes include orthostatic hypotension, especially from medication, arrhythmias, and vasovagal attacks (~5%)

Dysequilibrium—unsteadiness or imbalance when walking, especially in older patients (see p. 848); causes include fear of walking, visual loss, weakness from musculoskeletal problems, and peripheral neuropathy (up to 15%)

Psychiatric—causes include anxiety, panic disorder, hyperventilation, depression, somatization disorder, and alcohol and substance abuse (~10%)

Multifactorial or unknown—(up to 20%)

Peripheral and Central Vertigo

	Onset	Duration and Course	Hearing	Tinnitus	Additional Features
Peripheral Vertigo					
Benign Positional Vertigo	Sudden, on rolling onto affected side or tilting head up	Onset a few seconds to <1 minute Lasts a few weeks, may recur	Not affected	Absent	Sometimes nausea, vomiting nystagmus
Vestibular Neuronitis (acute labyrinthitis)	Sudden	Onset hours to up to 2 weeks May recur over 12–18 months	Not affected	Absent	Nausea, vomiting, nystagmus
Ménière's Disease	Sudden	Onset several hours to ≥1 day Recurrent	Sensorineural hearing loss–recurs, eventually progresses	Present, fluctuating	Pressure or fullness in affected ear; nausea, vomiting, nystagmus
Drug Toxicity	Insidious or acute–linked to loop diuretics, aminoglycosides, salicylates, alcohol	May or may not be reversible Partial adaptation occurs	May be impaired	May be present	Nausea, vomiting
Acoustic Neuroma	Insidious from CN VIII compression, vestibular branch	Variable	Impaired, one side	Present	May involve CN V and VII
Central Vertigo	Often sudden (see causes above)	Variable but rarely continuous	Not affected	Absent	Usually with other brainstem deficits— dysarthria, ataxia, crossed motor and sensory deficits

TABLE
12-2

Lumps on or Near the Ear

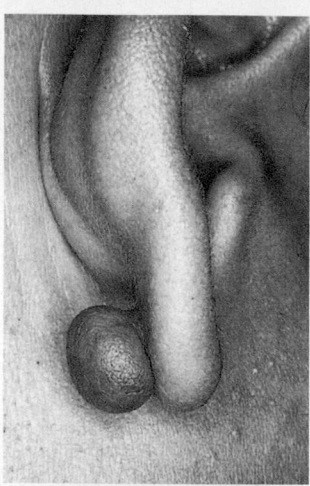

Keloid. A firm, nodular, hypertrophic mass of scar tissue extending beyond the area of injury. It may develop in any scarred area but is most common on the shoulders and upper chest. A keloid on a pierced earlobe may have troublesome cosmetic effects. Keloids are more common in darker-skinned people. Recurrence may follow treatment.

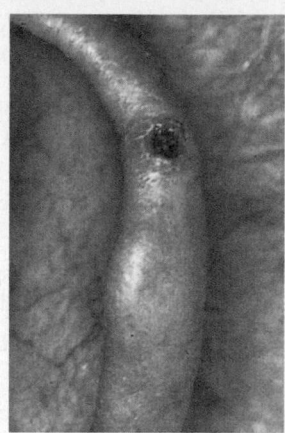

Chondrodermatitis Helicis. This chronic inflammatory lesion starts as a painful, tender papule on the helix or antihelix. Here the upper lesion is at a later stage of ulceration and crusting. Reddening may occur. Biopsy is needed to rule out carcinoma.

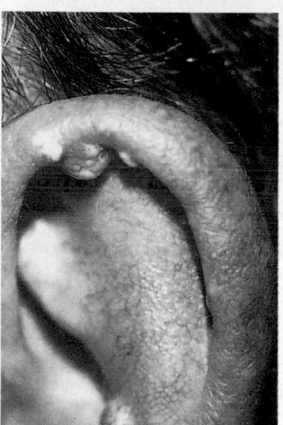

Tophi. A deposit of uric acid crystals characteristic of chronic tophaceous gout. It appears as hard nodules in the helix or antihelix and may discharge chalky white crystals through the skin. It also may appear near the joints, hands (p. 589), feet, and other areas. It usually develops after chronic sustained high blood levels of uric acid.

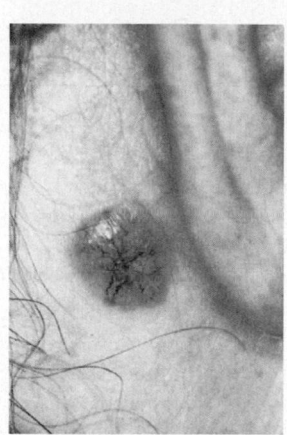

Basal Cell Carcinoma. This raised nodule shows the lustrous surface and telangiectatic vessels of basal cell carcinoma, a common slow-growing malignancy that rarely metastasizes. Growth and ulceration may occur. These are more frequent in fair-skinned people overexposed to sunlight.

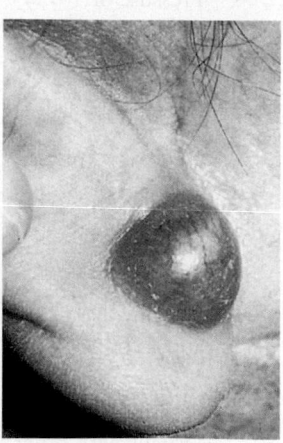

Cutaneous Cyst. Formerly called a *sebaceous cyst,* a dome-shaped lump in the dermis forms a benign closed firm sac attached to the epidermis. A dark dot (blackhead) may be visible on its surface. Histologically, it is usually either (1) an *epidermoid* cyst, common on the face and neck, or (2) a *pilar (trichilemmal)* cyst, common in the scalp. Both may become inflamed.

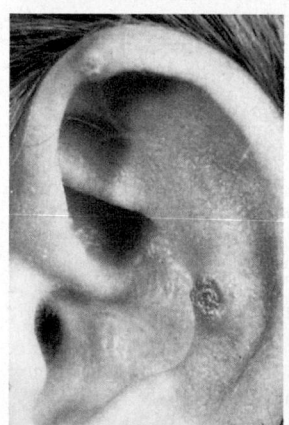

Rheumatoid Nodules. In chronic rheumatoid arthritis, look for small lumps on the helix or antihelix and additional nodules elsewhere on the hands, along the surface of the ulna distal to the elbow, and on the knees and heels. Ulceration may result from repeated injuries. Such nodules may antedate the arthritis.

(Sources of photos: *Keloid*—Sams WM Jr, Lynch PJ, eds. Principles and Practice of Dermatology. Edinburgh: Churchill Livingstone, 1990; *Tophi*—du Vivier A. Atlas of Clinical Dermatology, 2nd ed. London: Gower Medical Publishing, 1993; *Cutaneous Cyst, Chondrodermatitis Helicis*—Young EM, Newcomer VD, Kligman AM. Geriatric Dermatology: Color Atlas and Practitioner's Guide. Philadelphia: Lea & Febiger, 1993; *Basal Cell Carcinoma*—N Engl J Med, 326:169–170, 1992; *Rheumatoid Nodules*—Champion RH, Burton JL, Ebling FJG, eds. Rook/Wilkinson/Ebling Textbook of Dermatology, 5th ed. Oxford, UK: Blackwell Scientific, 1992.)

TABLE 12-3	**Abnormalities of the Eardrum**

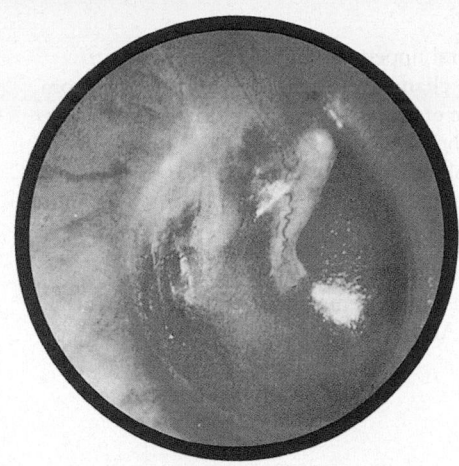

Normal Eardrum (Right)

This normal right eardrum (tympanic membrane) is pinkish gray. Note the malleus lying behind the upper part of the drum. Above the short process lies the *pars flaccida*. The remainder of the drum is the *pars tensa*. From the umbo, the bright cone of light fans anteriorly and downward. Posterior to the malleus, part of the incus is visible behind the drum. The small blood vessels along the handle of the malleus are normal.

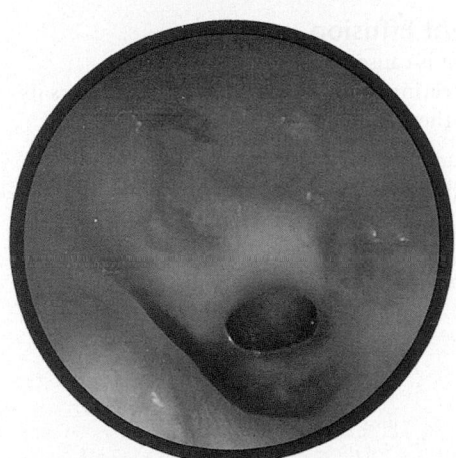

Perforation of the Drum

Perforations are holes in the eardrum that usually result from purulent infections of the middle ear. They are classified as *central* perforations, which do not extend to the margin of the drum, and *marginal* perforations, which do involve the margin.

The more common central perforation is illustrated here. A reddened ring of granulation tissue surrounds the perforation, indicating chronic infection. The eardrum itself is scarred, and no landmarks are visible. Discharge from the infected middle ear may drain out through such a perforation. A perforation often closes in the healing process, as in the next photo. The membrane covering the hole may be exceedingly thin and transparent.

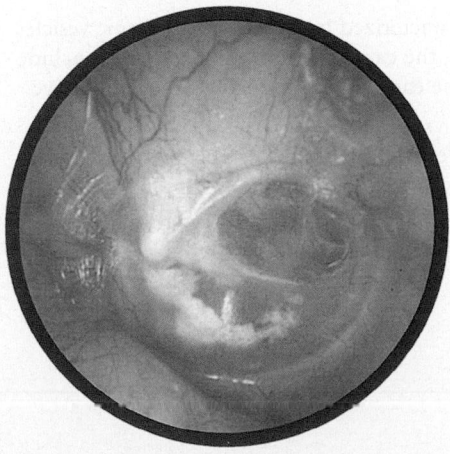

Tympanosclerosis

In the inferior portion of this left eardrum, there is a large, chalky white patch with irregular margins. It is typical of tympanosclerosis: a deposition of hyaline material within the layers of the tympanic membrane that sometimes follows a severe episode of otitis media. It does not usually impair hearing and is seldom clinically significant.

Other abnormalities in this eardrum include a *healed perforation* (the large oval area in the upper posterior drum) and signs of a *retracted drum*. A retracted drum is pulled medially, away from the examiner's eye, and the malleolar folds are tightened into sharp outlines. The short process often protrudes sharply, and the handle of the malleus, pulled inward at the umbo, looks foreshortened and more horizontal.

(Sources of photos: *Normal Eardrum*—Hawke M, Keene M, Alberti PW. Clinical Otoscopy: A Text and Colour Atlas. Edinburgh: Churchill Livingstone, 1984; *Perforation of the Drum, Tympanosclerosis*—Courtesy of Michael Hawke, MD, Toronto, Canada.)

(table continues on page 280)

| TABLE |
| 12-3 |

Abnormalities of the Eardrum (continued)

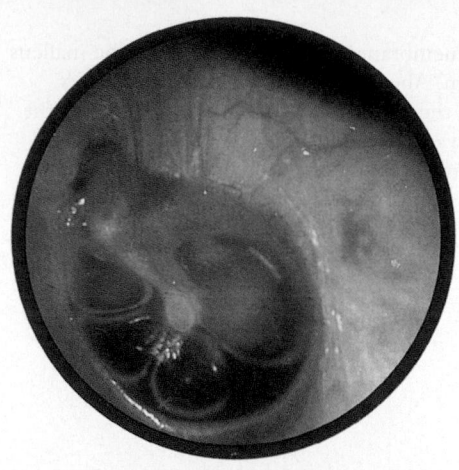

Serous Effusion

Serous effusions are usually caused by viral upper respiratory infections (*otitis media with serous effusion*) or by sudden changes in atmospheric pressure as from flying or diving (*otitic barotrauma*). The eustachian tube cannot equalize the air pressure in the middle ear with that of the outside air. Air is partly or completely absorbed from the middle ear into the bloodstream, and serous fluid accumulates there instead. Symptoms include fullness and popping sensations in the ear, mild conduction hearing loss, and perhaps some pain.

Amber fluid behind the eardrum is characteristic, as in this patient with otitic barotrauma. A fluid level, a line between air above and amber fluid below, can be seen on either side of the short process. Air bubbles (not always present) can be seen here within the amber fluid.

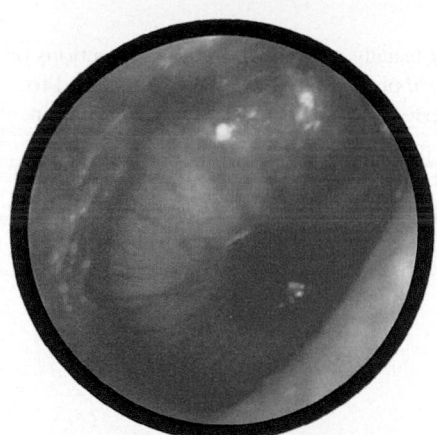

Acute Otitis Media With Purulent Effusion

Acute otitis media with purulent effusion is caused by bacterial infection. Symptoms include earache, fever, and hearing loss. The eardrum reddens, loses its landmarks, and bulges laterally, toward the examiner's eye.

Here the eardrum is bulging, and most landmarks are obscured. Redness is most obvious near the umbo, but dilated vessels can be seen in all segments of the drum. A diffuse redness of the entire drum often develops. Spontaneous rupture (perforation) of the drum may follow, with discharge of purulent material into the ear canal.

Hearing loss is of the conductive type. Acute purulent otitis media is much more common in children than in adults.

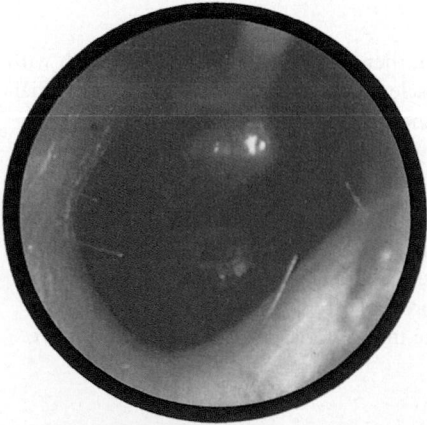

Bullous Myringitis

Bullous myringitis is a viral infection characterized by painful hemorrhagic vesicles that appear on the tympanic membrane, the ear canal, or both. Symptoms include earache, blood-tinged discharge from the ear, and hearing loss of the conductive type.

In this right ear, at least two large vesicles (bullae) are discernible on the drum. The drum is reddened, and its landmarks are obscured.

Several different viruses may cause this condition, including mycoplasma.

(Sources of photos: *Serous Effusion*—Hawke M, Keene M, Alberti PW. Clinical Otoscopy: A Text and Colour Atlas. Edinburgh: Churchill Livingstone, 1984; *Acute Otitis Media, Bullous Myringitis*—The Wellcome Trust, National Medical Slide Bank, London, UK.)

TABLE
12-4

Patterns of Hearing Loss

	Conductive Loss	Sensorineural Loss
	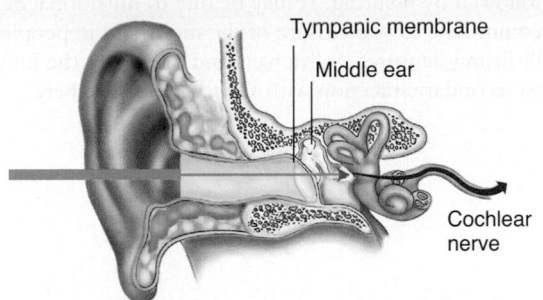	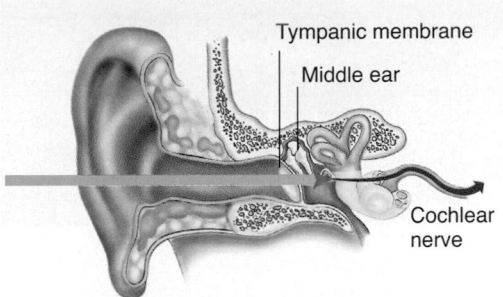
Pathophysiology	External or middle ear disorder impairs sound conduction to inner ear. Causes include foreign body, *otitis media,* perforated eardrum, and otosclerosis of ossicles.	Inner ear disorder involves cochlear nerve and neuronal impulse transmission to the brain. Causes include loud noise exposure, inner ear infections, trauma, tremors, congenital and familial disorders, and aging.
Usual Age of Onset	Childhood and young adulthood, up to age 40	Middle or later years
Ear Canal and Drum	Abnormality usually visible, except in otosclerosis	Problem not visible
Effects	• Little effect on sound • Hearing seems to improve in noisy environment • Voice becomes soft because inner ear and cochlear nerve are intact	• Higher registers are lost, so sound may be distorted. • Hearing worsens in noisy environment. • Voice may be loud because hearing is difficult.
Weber Test *(in unilateral hearing loss)*	• Tuning fork at vertex • Sound lateralizes to *impaired ear*—room noise not well heard, so detection of vibrations *improves.*	• Tuning fork at vertex • Sound lateralizes to *good ear*—inner ear or cochlear nerve damage impairs transmission to affected ear.
Rinne Test	• Tuning fork at external auditory meatus then on mastoid bone • Bone conduction longer than or equal to air conduction (BC ≥ AC). While air conduction through the external or middle ear is impaired, vibrations through bone bypass the problem to reach the cochlea.	• Tuning fork at external auditory meatus then on mastoid bone • Air conduction longer than bone conduction (AC > BC). The inner ear or cochlear nerve is less able to transmit impulses regardless of how the vibrations reach the cochlea. The normal pattern prevails.

TABLE 12-5

Abnormalities of the Lips

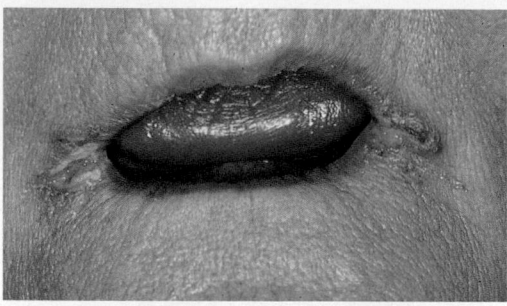

Angular Cheilitis

Angular cheilitis starts with softening of the skin at the angles of the mouth, followed by fissuring. It may be due to nutritional deficiency or, more commonly, to overclosure of the mouth, as in people with no teeth or with ill-fitting dentures. Saliva wets and macerates the infolded skin, often leading to secondary infection with *Candida*, as seen here.

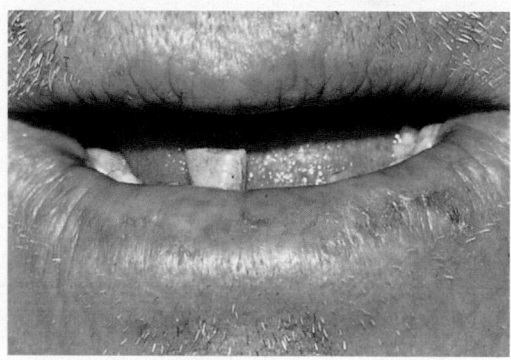

Actinic Cheilitis

Actinic cheilitis results from excessive exposure to sunlight and affects primarily the lower lip. Fair-skinned men who work outdoors are most often affected. The lip loses its normal redness and may become scaly, somewhat thickened, and slightly everted. Because solar damage also predisposes to carcinoma of the lip, be alert to this possibility.

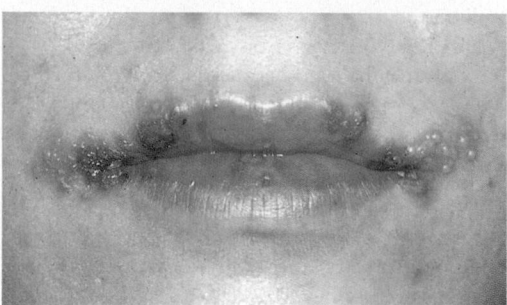

Herpes Simplex *(Cold Sore, Fever Blister)*

The herpes simplex virus (HSV) produces recurrent and painful vesicular eruptions of the lips and surrounding skin. A small cluster of vesicles first develops. As these break, yellow-brown crusts form, and healing ensues within 10 to 14 days. Both of these stages are visible here.

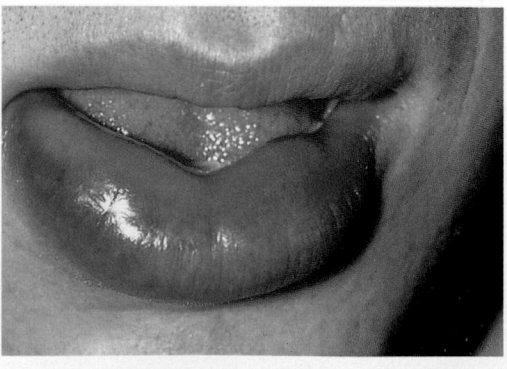

Angioedema

Angioedema is a diffuse, nonpitting, tense swelling of the dermis and subcutaneous tissue. It develops rapidly, and typically disappears over subsequent hours or days. Although usually allergic in nature and sometimes associated with hives, angioedema does not itch.

(Sources of photos: *Angular Cheilitis, Herpes Simplex, Angioedema*—Neville B, et al. Color Atlas of Clinical Oral Pathology. Philadelphia: Lea & Febiger, 1991; Used with permission; *Actinic Cheilitis*—Langlais RP, Miller CS. Color Atlas of Common Oral Diseases. Philadelphia: Lea & Febiger, 1992; Used with permission.)

(table continues on page 283)

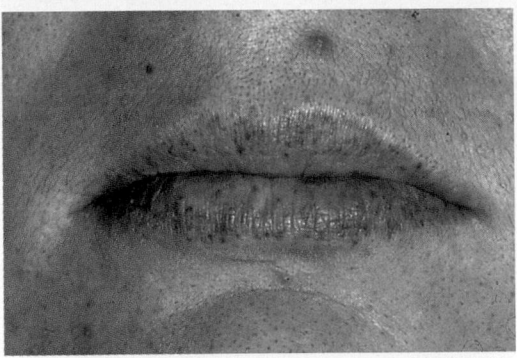

Hereditary Hemorrhagic Telangiectasia

Multiple small red spots on the lips strongly suggest hereditary hemorrhagic telangiectasia. Spots may also be visible on the face and hands and in the mouth. The spots are dilated capillaries and may bleed when traumatized. Affected people often have nosebleeds and gastrointestinal bleeding.

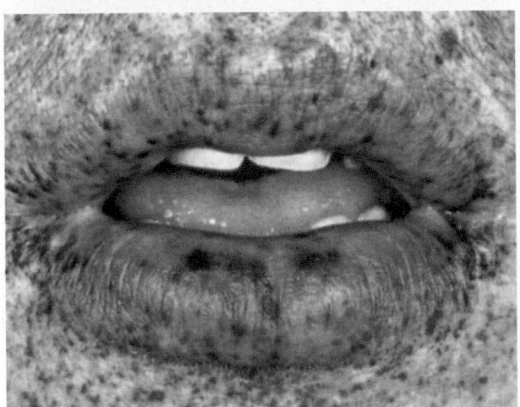

Peutz-Jeghers Syndrome

When pigmented spots on the lips are more prominent than freckling of the surrounding skin, suspect this syndrome. Pigment in the buccal mucosa helps to confirm the diagnosis. Pigmented spots may also be found on the face and hands. Multiple intestinal polyps are often associated.

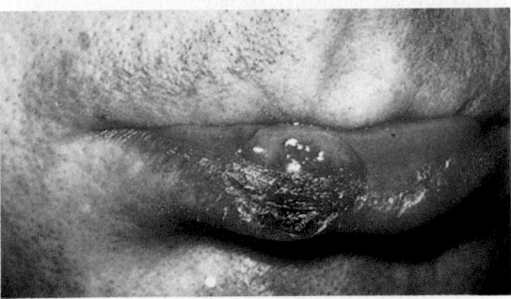

Chancre of Syphilis

This lesion of primary syphilis may appear on the lip rather than on the genitalia. It is a firm, button-like lesion that ulcerates and may become crusted. A chancre may resemble a carcinoma or a crusted cold sore. Because it is infectious, use gloves to feel any suspicious lesion.

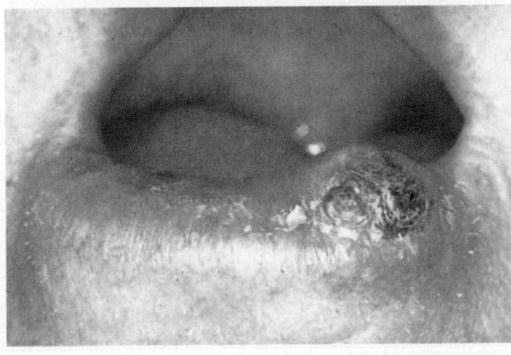

Carcinoma of the Lip

Like actinic cheilitis, carcinoma usually affects the lower lip. It may appear as a scaly plaque, as an ulcer with or without a crust, or as a nodular lesion, illustrated here. Fair skin and prolonged exposure to the sun are common risk factors.

(Sources of photos: *Hereditary Hemorrhagic Telangiectasia*—Langlais RP, Miller CS. Color Atlas of Common Oral Diseases. Philadelphia: Lea & Febiger, 1992; Used with permission; *Peutz-Jeghers Syndrome*—Robinson HBG, Miller AS. Colby, Kerr, and Robinson's Color Atlas of Oral Pathology. Philadelphia: JB Lippincott, 1990; *Chancre of Syphilis*—Wisdom A. A Colour Atlas of Sexually Transmitted Diseases, 2nd ed. London: Wolfe Medical Publications, 1989; *Carcinoma of the Lip*—Tyldesley WR. A Colour Atlas of Orofacial Diseases, 2nd ed. London: Wolfe Medical Publications, 1991.)

TABLE
12-6

Findings in the Pharynx, Palate, and Oral Mucosa

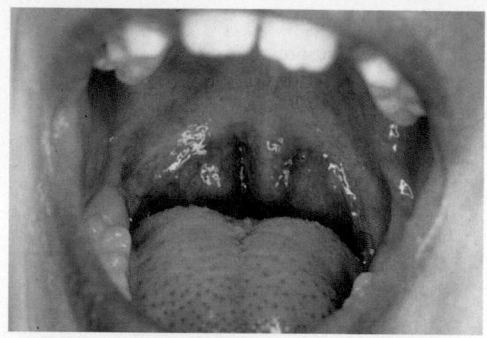

Large Normal Tonsils

Normal tonsils may be large without being infected, especially in children. They may protrude medially beyond the pillars and even to the midline. Here they touch the sides of the uvula and obscure the pharynx. Their color is pink. The white marks are light reflections, not exudate.

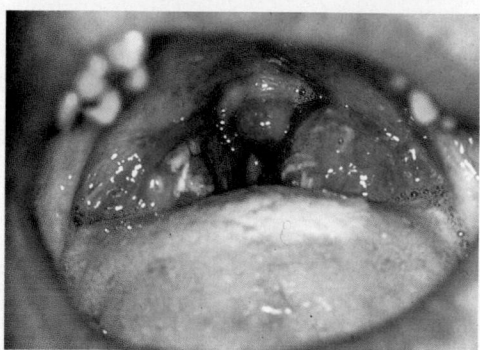

Exudative Tonsillitis

This red throat has a white exudate on the tonsils. This, together with fever and enlarged cervical nodes, increases the probability of *group A streptococcal infection* or *infectious mononucleosis*. Anterior cervical lymph nodes are usually enlarged in the former, posterior nodes in the latter.

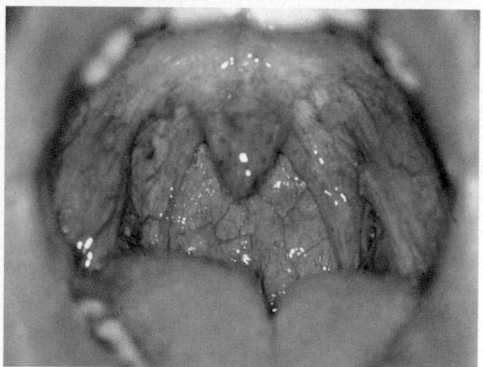

Pharyngitis

These two photos show reddened throats without exudate.

In **A**, redness and vascularity of the pillars and uvula are mild to moderate.

A

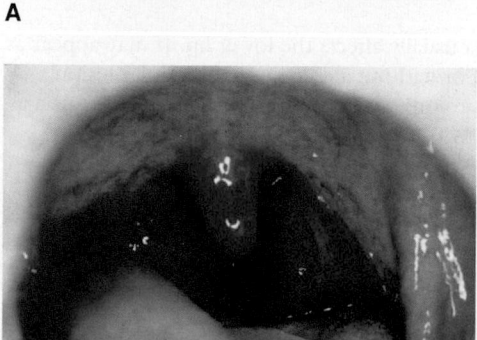

In **B**, redness is diffuse and intense. Each patient would probably complain of a sore throat, or at least a scratchy one. Possible causes include several kinds of viruses and bacteria. If the patient has no fever, exudate, or enlargement of cervical lymph nodes, the chances of infection by either of two common causes—*group A streptococci* and *Epstein-Barr virus* (infectious mononucleosis)—are very small.

B

(Sources of photos: *Large Normal Tonsils, Exudative Tonsillitis, Pharyngitis [A and B]*—The Wellcome Trust, National Medical Slide Bank, London, UK.)

(*table continues on page 285*)

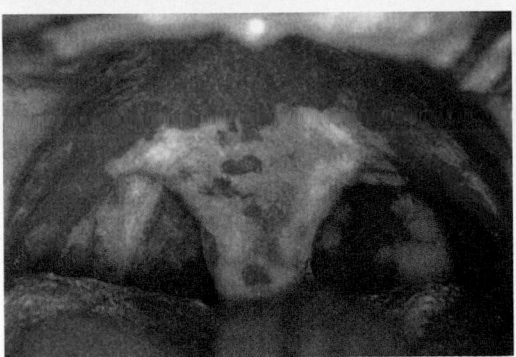

Diphtheria

Diphtheria (an acute infection caused by *Corynebacterium diphtheriae*) is now rare but still important. Prompt diagnosis may lead to life-saving treatment. The throat is dull red, and a gray exudate (pseudomembrane) is present on the uvula, pharynx, and tongue. The airway may become obstructed.

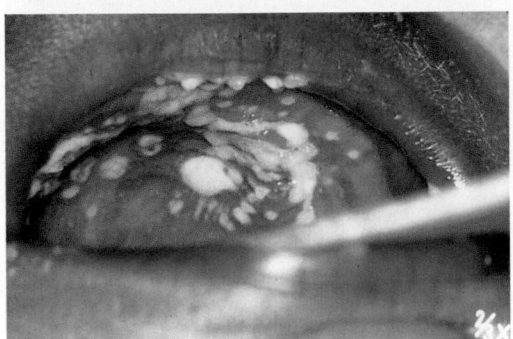

Thrush on the Palate (Candidiasis)

Thrush is a yeast infection due to *Candida*. Shown here on the palate, it may appear elsewhere in the mouth (see p. 289). Thick, white plaques are somewhat adherent to the underlying mucosa. Predisposing factors include (1) prolonged treatment with antibiotics or corticosteroids and (2) AIDS.

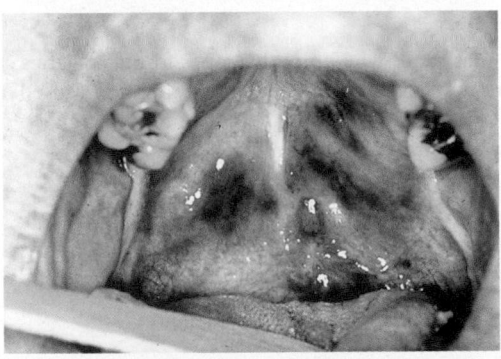

Kaposi Sarcoma in AIDS

The deep purple color of these lesions, although not necessarily present, strongly suggests Kaposi sarcoma. The lesions may be raised or flat. Among people with AIDS, the palate, as illustrated here, is a common site for this tumor.

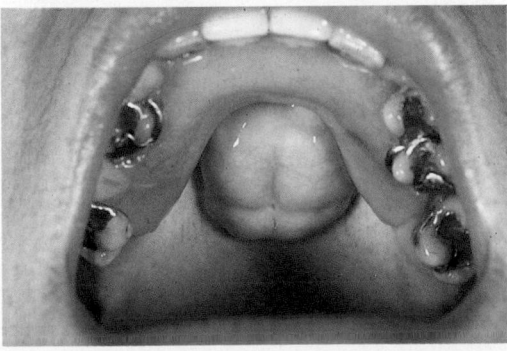

Torus Palatinus

A torus palatinus is a midline bony growth in the hard palate that is fairly common in adults. Its size and lobulation vary. Although alarming at first glance, it is harmless. In this example, an upper denture has been fitted around the torus.

(Sources of photos: *Diphtheria*—Harnisch JP, et al. Diphtheria among alcoholic urban adults. Ann Intern Med 111:77, 1989; *Thrush on the Palate*—The Wellcome Trust, National Medical Slide Bank, London, UK; *Kaposi's Sarcoma in AIDS*—Ioachim HL. Textbook and Atlas of Disease Associated With Acquired Immune Deficiency Syndrome. London: Gower Medical Publishing, 1989.)

(table continues on page 286)

TABLE
12-6

Findings in the Pharynx, Palate, and Oral Mucosa (continued)

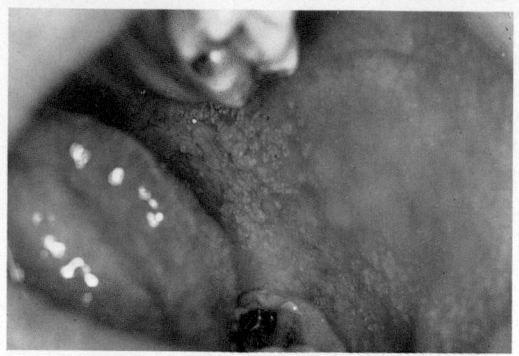

Fordyce Spots (Fordyce Granules)

Fordyce spots are normal sebaceous glands that appear as small yellowish spots in the buccal mucosa or on the lips. A worried person who has suddenly noticed them may be reassured. Here they are seen best anterior to the tongue and lower jaw. These spots are usually not so numerous.

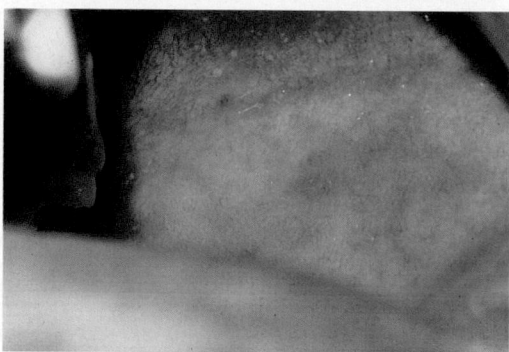

Koplik Spots

Koplik spots are an early sign of measles (rubeola). Search for small white specks that resemble grains of salt on a red background. They usually appear on the buccal mucosa near the first and second molars. In this photo, look also in the upper third of the mucosa. The rash of measles appears within a day.

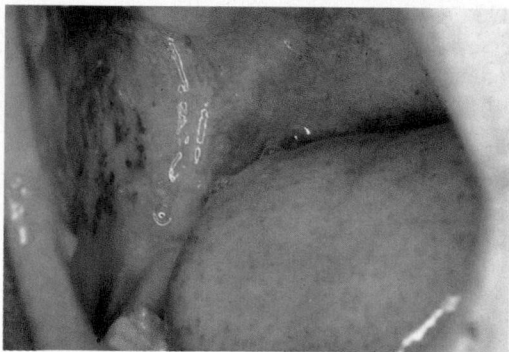

Petechiae

Petechiae are small red spots that result when blood escapes from capillaries into the tissues. Petechiae in the buccal mucosa, as shown, are often caused by accidentally biting the cheek. Oral petechiae may be due to infection or decreased platelets, as well as to trauma.

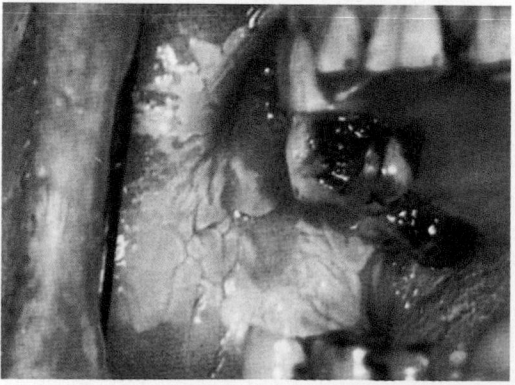

Leukoplakia

A thickened white patch (*leukoplakia*) may occur anywhere in the oral mucosa. The extensive example shown on this buccal mucosa resulted from frequent chewing of tobacco, a local irritant. This kind of irritation may lead to cancer.

(Sources of photos: *Fordyce Spots*—Neville B, et al. Color Atlas of Clinical Oral Pathology. Philadelphia: Lea & Febiger, 1991; Used with permission; *Koplik's Spots, Petechiae*—The Wellcome Trust, National Medical Slide Bank, London, UK; *Leukoplakia*—Robinson HBG, Miller AS. Colby, Kerr, and Robinson's Color Atlas of Oral Pathology. Philadelphia: JB Lippincott, 1990.)

TABLE
12-7

Findings in the Gums and Teeth

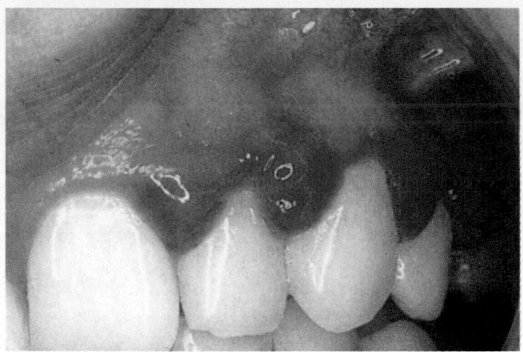

Marginal Gingivitis

Marginal gingivitis is common among teenagers and young adults. The gingival margins are reddened and swollen, and the interdental papillae are blunted, swollen, and red. Brushing the teeth often makes the gums bleed. *Plaque*—the soft white film of salivary salts, protein, and bacteria that covers the teeth and leads to gingivitis—is not readily visible.

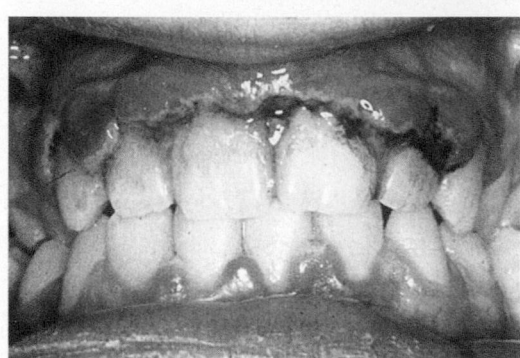

Acute Necrotizing Ulcerative Gingivitis

This uncommon form of gingivitis occurs suddenly in adolescents and young adults and is accompanied by fever, malaise, and enlarged lymph nodes. Ulcers develop in the interdental papillae. Then the destructive (necrotizing) process spreads along the gum margins, where a grayish pseudomembrane develops. The red, painful gums bleed easily; the breath is foul.

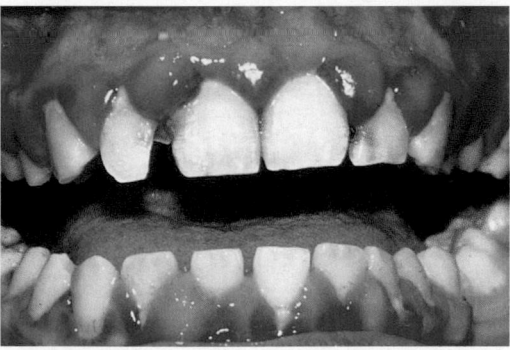

Gingival Hyperplasia

Gums enlarged by hyperplasia are swollen into heaped-up masses that may even cover the teeth. The redness of inflammation may coexist, as in this example. Causes include Dilantin therapy (as in this case), puberty, pregnancy, and leukemia.

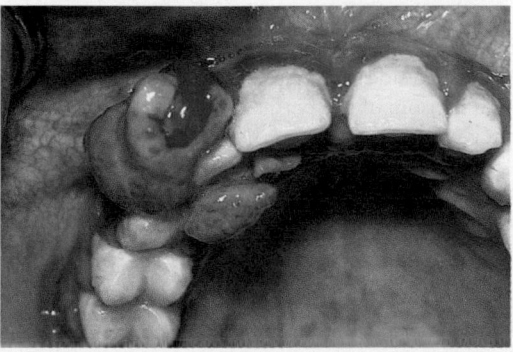

Pregnancy Tumor (Epulis, Pyogenic Granuloma)

Gingival enlargement may be localized, forming a tumor-like mass that usually originates in an interdental papilla. It is red and soft and usually bleeds easily. The estimated incidence of this lesion in pregnancy is about 1%. Note the accompanying gingivitis in this example.

(Sources of photos: *Marginal Gingivitis, Acute Necrotizing Ulcerative Gingivitis*—Tyldesley WR. A Colour Atlas of Orofacial Diseases, 2nd ed. London: Wolfe Medical Publications, 1991; *Gingival Hyperplasia*—Courtesy of Dr. James Cottone; *Pregnancy Tumor*—Langlais RP, Miller CS. Color Atlas of Common Oral Diseases. Philadelphia: Lea & Febiger, 1992; Used with permission.)

(table continues on page 288)

TABLE 12-7

Findings in the Gums and Teeth (continued)

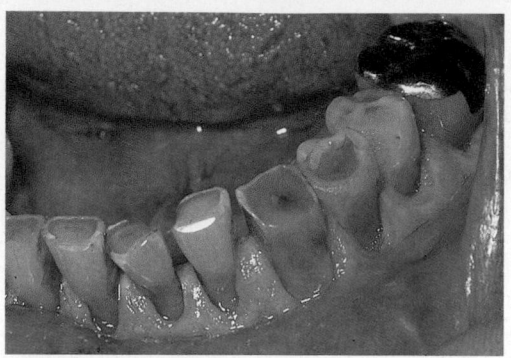

Attrition of Teeth; Recession of Gums

In many elderly people, the chewing surfaces of the teeth have been worn down by repetitive use so that the yellow-brown dentin becomes exposed—a process called *attrition*. Note also the *recession of the gums,* which has exposed the roots of the teeth, giving a "long in the tooth" appearance.

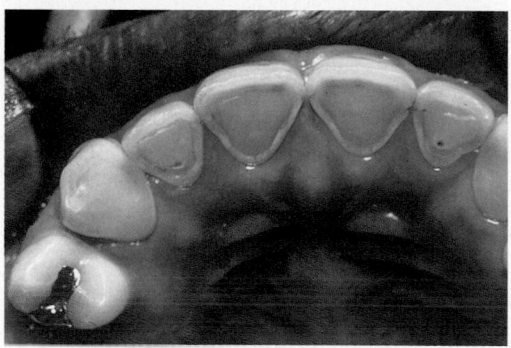

Erosion of Teeth

Teeth may be eroded by chemical action. Note here the erosion of the enamel from the lingual surfaces of the upper incisors, exposing the yellow-brown dentin. This results from recurrent regurgitation of stomach contents, as in bulimia.

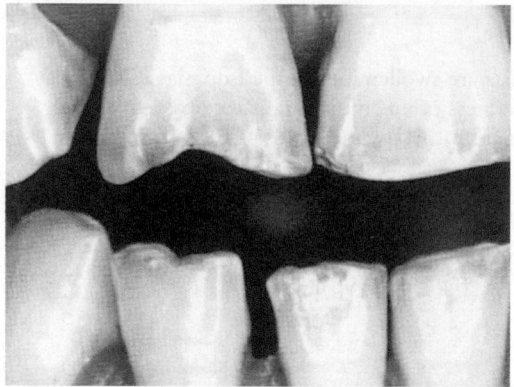

Abrasion of Teeth With Notching

The biting surface of the teeth may become abraded or notched by recurrent trauma, such as holding nails or opening bobby pins between the teeth. Unlike Hutchinson teeth, the sides of these teeth show normal contours; size and spacing of the teeth are unaffected.

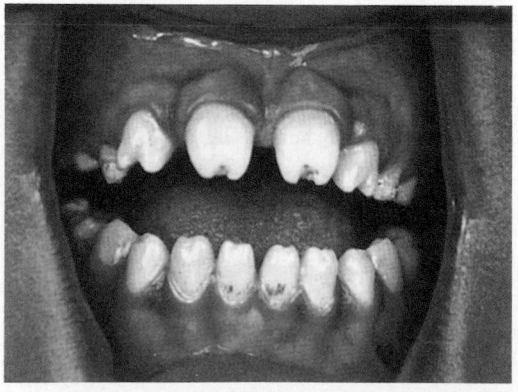

Hutchinson Teeth

Hutchinson teeth are smaller and more widely spaced than normal and are notched on their biting surfaces. The sides of the teeth taper toward the biting edges. The upper central incisors of the permanent (not the deciduous) teeth are most often affected. These teeth are a sign of congenital syphilis.

(Sources of photos: *Attrition of Teeth, Erosion of Teeth*—Langlais RP, Miller CS. Color Atlas of Common Oral Diseases. Philadelphia: Lea & Febiger, 1992; Used with permission; *Abrasion of Teeth, Hutchinson Teeth*—Robinson HBG, Miller AS. Colby, Kerr, and Robinson's Color Atlas of Oral Pathology. Philadelphia: JB Lippincott, 1990.)

TABLE
12-8

Findings in or Under the Tongue

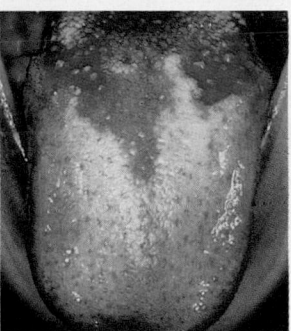

Geographic Tongue. In this benign condition, the dorsum shows scattered smooth red areas denuded of papillae. Together with the normal rough and coated areas, they give a maplike pattern that changes over time.

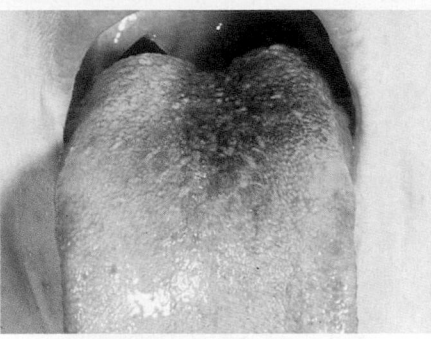

Hairy Tongue. Note the "hairy" yellowish to brown or black elongated papillae on the tongue's dorsum. This benign condition may follow antibiotic therapy; it also may occur spontaneously.

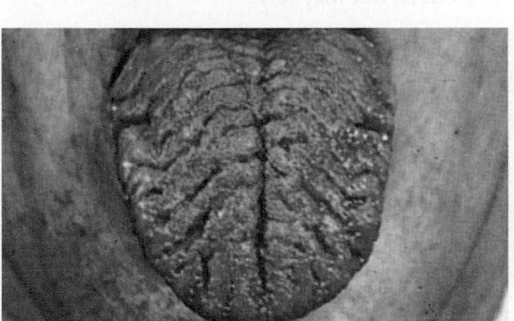

Fissured Tongue. Fissures appear with increasing age, sometimes termed *scrotal tongue*. Food debris may accumulate in the crevices and become irritating, but a fissured tongue is benign.

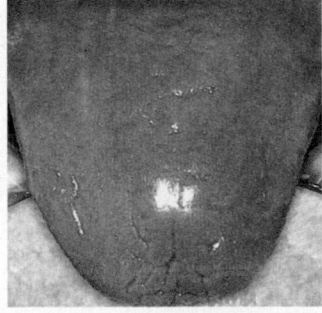

Smooth Tongue (Atrophic Glossitis). A smooth and often sore tongue that has lost its papillae suggests a deficiency in riboflavin, niacin, folic acid, vitamin B_{12}, pyridoxine, or iron, or treatment with chemotherapy.

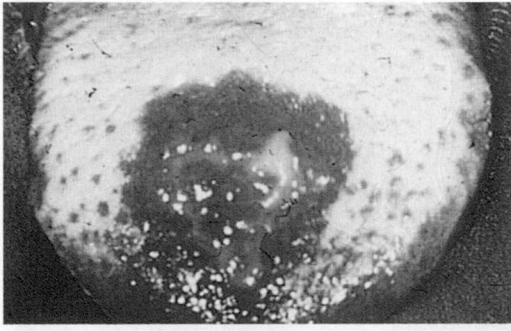

Candidiasis. Note the thick white coating from *Candida* infection. The raw red surface is where the coat was scraped off. Infection may also occur without the white coating. It is seen in immunosuppressed conditions.

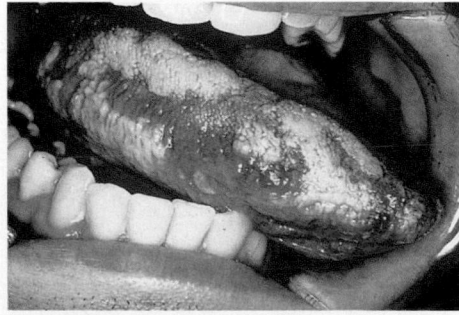

Hairy Leukoplakia. These whitish raised areas with a feathery or corrugated pattern most often affect the sides of the tongue. Unlike candidiasis, these areas cannot be scraped off. They are seen with HIV and AIDS.

(*table continues on page 290*)

TABLE 12-8

Findings in or Under the Tongue (continued)

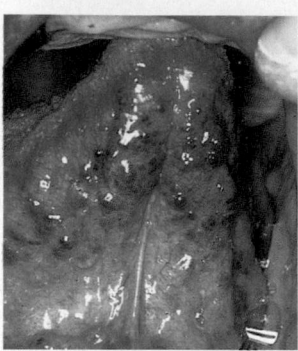

Varicose Veins. Small purplish or blue-black round swellings appear under the tongue with age. These dilatations of the lingual veins have no clinical significance.

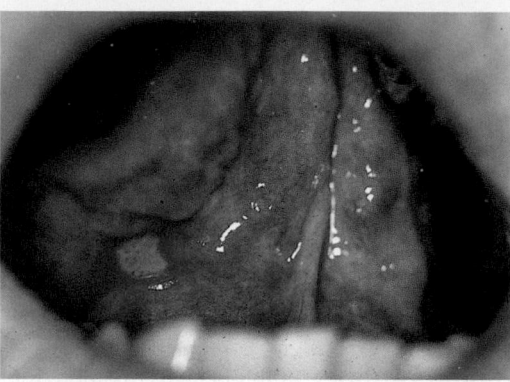

Aphthous Ulcer (Canker Sore). A painful, round or oval ulcer that is white or yellowish gray and surrounded by a halo of reddened mucosa. It may be single or multiple. It heals in 7–10 days, but may recur.

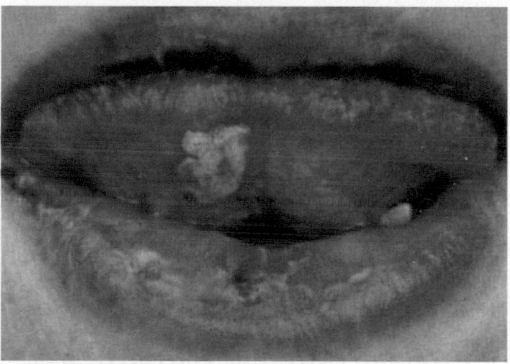

Mucous Patch of Syphilis. This painless lesion in the secondary stage of syphilis is highly infectious. It is slightly raised, oval, and covered by a grayish membrane. It may be multiple and occur elsewhere in the mouth.

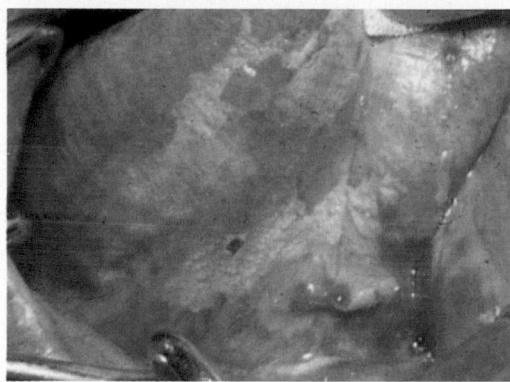

Leukoplakia. With this persisting painless white patch in the oral mucosa, the undersurface of the tongue appears painted white. Patches of any size raise the possibility of malignancy and require a biopsy.

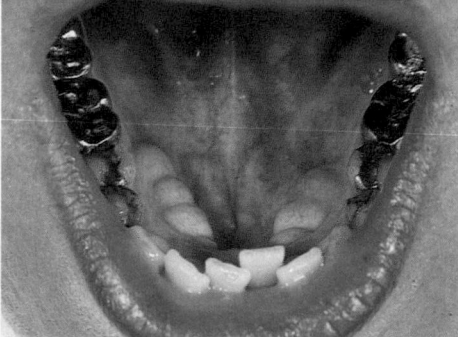

Tori Mandibulares. Rounded bony growths on the inner surfaces of the mandible are typically bilateral, asymptomatic, and harmless.

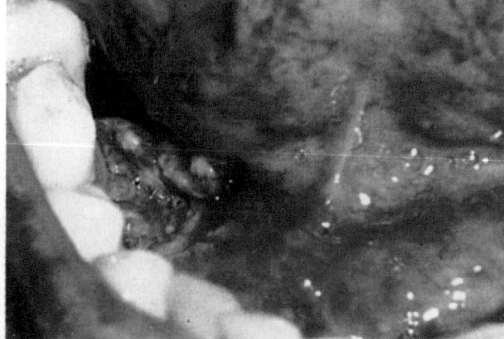

Carcinoma, Floor of the Mouth. This ulcerated lesion is in a common location for carcinoma. Medially, note the reddened area of mucosa, called *erythroplakia*, suggesting possible malignancy.

(Sources of photos: *Fissured Tongue, Candidiasis, Mucous Patch, Leukoplakia, Carcinoma*—Robinson HBG, Miller AS. Colby, Kerr, and Robinson's Color Atlas of Oral Pathology. Philadelphia, JB Lippincott, 1990; *Smooth Tongue*—Courtesy of Dr. R. A. Cawson, from Cawson RA. Oral Pathology, 1st ed. London, UK: Gower Medical Publishing, 1987; *Geographic Tongue*—The Wellcome Trust, National Medical Slide Bank, London, UK; *Hairy Leukoplakia*—Ioachim HL. Textbook and Atlas of Disease Associated With Acquired Immune Deficiency Syndrome. London, UK: Gower Medical Publishing, 1989; *Varicose Veins*—Neville B, et al. Color Atlas of Clinical Oral Pathology. Philadelphia, Lea & Febiger, 1991. Used with permission.)

BIBLIOGRAPHY

CITATIONS

1. Willems PJ. Genetic causes of hearing loss. N Engl J Med 342(15):1101–1109, 2000.
2. Hendley JO. Otitis media. N Engl J Med 347(15):1169–1174, 2002.
3. Plaut M, Valentine MD. Allergic rhinitis. N Engl J Med 353(18):1934–1944, 2005.
4. Piccirillo JF. Acute bacterial sinusitis. N Engl J Med 351(9): 902–910, 2004.
5. Spector SL, Bernstein IL, Li JT, et al. Parameters for the diagnosis and management of sinusitis. J Allergy Clin Immunol 102(6, Part 2):S107–S144, 1998.
6. Williams JW, Simel DL, Roberts L, et al. Clinical evaluation for sinusitis: making the diagnosis by history and physical examination. Ann Intern Med 117(9):705–710, 1992.
7. Cooper RJ, Hoffman JR, Bartlett JG, et al. Principles of appropriate antibiotic use for acute pharyngitis in adults: background. Ann Intern Med 134(6):509–517, 2001.
8. McGinn TG, Deluca J, Ahlawat SK, et al. Validation and modification of streptococcal pharyngitis clinical prediction rules. Mayo Clin Proc 78(3):289–293, 2003.
9. Gupta R, Pery M. Digital examination for oral cancer. BMJ 319:1113–1114, 1999.
10. Task Force on Newborn and Infant Hearing. Newborn and infant hearing loss: detection and intervention. Pediatrics 103(2):527–530, 1999.
11. Jackler JK. A 73-year-old man with hearing loss. JAMA 289(12): 1557–1565, 2003.
12. U.S. Preventive Services Task Force. Screening for hearing impairment. Available at: http://www.uspreventiveservices taskforce.org/uspstf/uspshear.htm. Accessed April 11, 2011.
13. Stanton MW, Rutherford MK. Dental care: improving access and quality. Research in Action Issue #13. AHRQ Pub No. 03-0040. Rockville, MD: Agency for Healthcare Research and Quality, 2003.
14. Kroenke K, Lucas CA, Rosengerg ML, et al. Causes of persistent dizziness: a prospective study of 100 patients in ambulatory care. Ann Intern Med 117(11):898–904, 1992.
15. Kroenke K, Hoffman RM, Einstadter D. How common are various causes of dizziness? A critical review. South Med J 93(2):160–167, 2000.
16. Tusa RJ. Vertigo. Neurol Clin 19(1):23–55, 2001.
17. Lockwood AH, Salvi RJ, Burkard RF. Tinnitus. N Engl J Med 347(12):904–910, 2002.
18. Matthies C, Samii M. Management of 1000 vestibular schwannomas (acoustic neuromas): clinical presentation. Neurosurgery 1:1–10, 1997.

ADDITIONAL REFERENCES

The Ears, Nose, and Throat

Bagai A, Thavendiranathan P, Detsky AS. Does this patient have hearing impairment? JAMA 295(4):416–428, 2006.

Bevan Y, Shapiro N, MacLean CH, et al. Screening and management of adult hearing loss in primary care: scientific review. JAMA 289(15):1976–1985, 2003.

Bull TR. Color Atlas of ENT Diagnosis, 4th ed. New York: Thieme, 2003.

Cady RK, Dodick DW, Levine HL, et al. Sinus headache: a neurology, otolaryngology, allergy, and primary care consensus on diagnosis and treatment. Mayo Clin Proc 80(7):908–916, 2005.

Ebell MH, Smith MA, Barry HC, et al. Does this patient have strep throat? JAMA 284(22):2912–2918, 2000.

Hendley JO. Otitis media. N Engl J Med 347(15):1169–1174, 2002.

Institute of Medicine Report. Advancing Oral Health in America. Released April 4, 2011. Available at: http://www.iom.edu/reports/2011/advancing-oral-health-in-america/report-brief.aspx. Accessed April 9, 2011.

Kennedy DW. A 48-year-old man with recurrent sinusitis. JAMA 283(16):2143–2150, 2000.

O'Donoghue GM, Narula AA, Bates GJ. Clinical ENT: An Illustrated Textbook, 2nd ed. San Diego: Singular Publishing Group, 2000.

Patil SP, Schneider H, Schwartz AR, et al. Adult obstructive sleep apnea: pathophysiology and diagnosis. Chest 132(1):325–337, 2007.

Young T, Skatrud J, Peppard PE. Risk factors for obstructive sleep apnea in adults. JAMA 291(16):2013–2016, 2004.

The Mouth

Field EA, Longman L, Tyldesley WR, et al. Tyldesley's Oral Medicine, 5th ed. New York: Oxford University Press, 2003.

Langlais RP, Miller CS. Color Atlas of Common Oral Diseases, 3rd ed. Philadelphia: Lippincott Williams & Wilkins, 2003.

Newman MF, Carranza FA, Takei H, et al. Carranza's Clinical Periodontology, 10th ed. Philadelphia: Saunders–Elsevier, 2006.

Regezi JA, Sciubba JJ, Jordan RCK. Oral Pathology: Clinical Pathologic Correlations, 5th ed. St. Louis: Saunders–Elsevier, 2008.

CHAPTER 13

The Respiratory System

LEARNING OBJECTIVES

The student will:

1. Describe the structure and functions of the airways, alveoli, lungs, and pleura.
2. Identify the locations of each lung lobe using landmarks on the thorax.
3. Describe the mechanics of breathing.
4. Identify the percussion and auscultation sites for assessment of the lungs.
5. Describe the normal lung sounds and their location.
6. Describe adventitious sounds and voice sounds and their origin.
7. Obtain an accurate history of the respiratory system.
8. Appropriately prepare and position the patient for the respiratory examination.
9. Describe the equipment necessary to perform a respiratory examination.
10. Correctly inspect, palpate, percuss, and auscultate the anterior and posterior thorax.
11. Discuss risk factors for respiratory disease.
12. Discuss risk reduction and health promotion strategies to reduce respiratory disease.

ANATOMY AND PHYSIOLOGY

Study the *anatomy of the chest wall*, identifying the structures illustrated. Note that an intercostal space between two ribs is numbered by the rib above it.

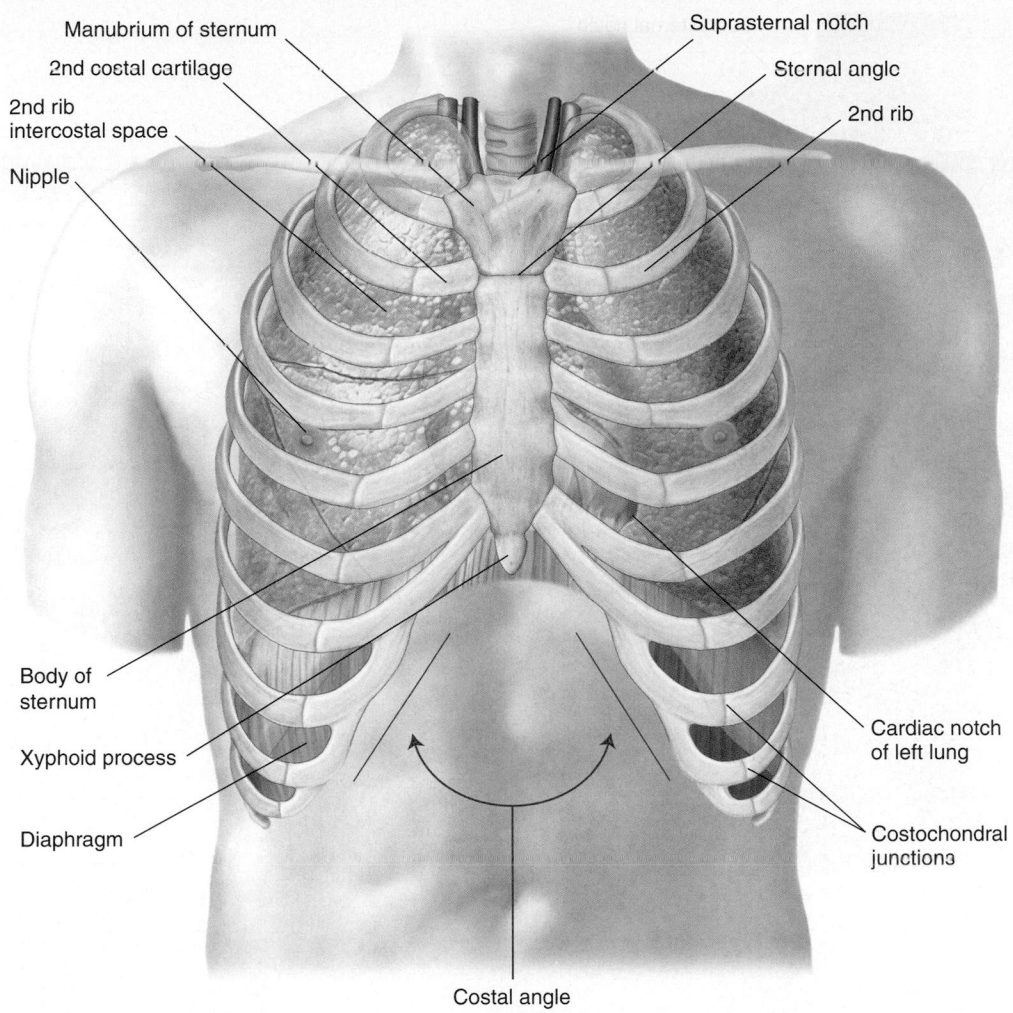

Manubrium of sternum

2nd costal cartilage

2nd rib
intercostal space

Nipple

Suprasternal notch

Sternal angle

2nd rib

Body of
sternum

Xyphoid process

Diaphragm

Cardiac notch
of left lung

Costochondral
junctions

Costal angle

Locating Findings on the Chest. Abnormalities of the chest are described in two dimensions: *along the vertical axis* and *around the circumference of the chest.*

To make *vertical* locations, count the ribs and intercostal spaces. The *sternal angle,* also termed the angle of Louis, is the best guide: place your finger in the hollow curve of the suprasternal notch, and then move your finger down approximately 5 cm to the horizontal bony ridge joining the manubrium to the body of the sternum. Then move your finger laterally and find the adjacent 2nd rib and costal cartilage. From here, using two fingers, "walk down" the intercostal spaces, one space at a time, on an oblique line, illustrated by the red numbers on page 294. Do not try to count intercostal spaces along the lower edge of the sternum; the ribs there are too close together. In a woman, to find the intercostal spaces, either displace the breast laterally or palpate closer to the sternum. Avoid pressing too hard on tender breast tissue.

Note special landmarks: 2nd intercostal space for needle insertion for tension pneumothorax; 4th intercostal space for chest tube insertion.

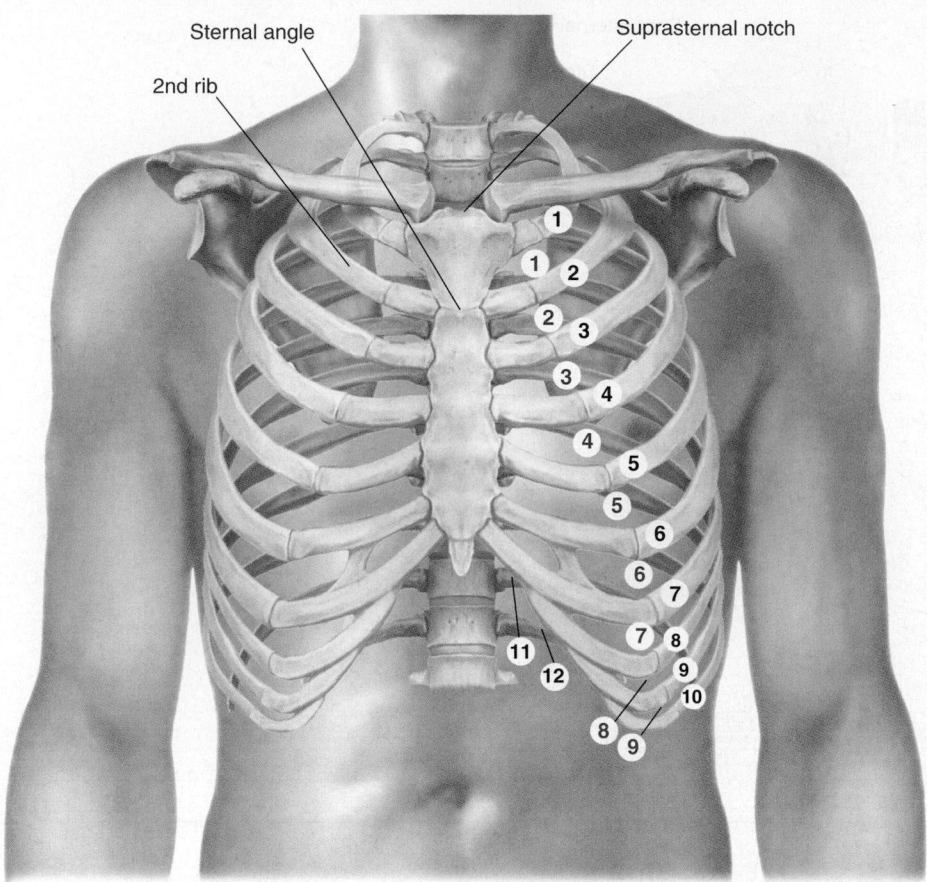

Note that the costal cartilages of the first seven ribs articulate with the sternum; the cartilages of the 8th, 9th, and 10th ribs articulate with the costal cartilages just above them. The 11th and 12th ribs, the "floating ribs," have no anterior attachments. The cartilaginous tip of the 11th rib usually can be felt laterally, and the 12th rib may be felt posteriorly. On palpation, costal cartilages and ribs feel identical.

Posteriorly, the 12th rib is another possible starting point for counting ribs and intercostal spaces: it helps locate findings on the lower posterior chest and provides an option when the anterior approach is unsatisfactory. With the fingers of one hand, press in and up against the lower border of the 12th rib, then "walk up" the intercostal spaces numbered in red on page 295, or follow a more oblique line up and around to the front of the chest.

The inferior tip of the scapula is another useful bony landmark—it usually lies at the level of the 7th rib or intercostal space.

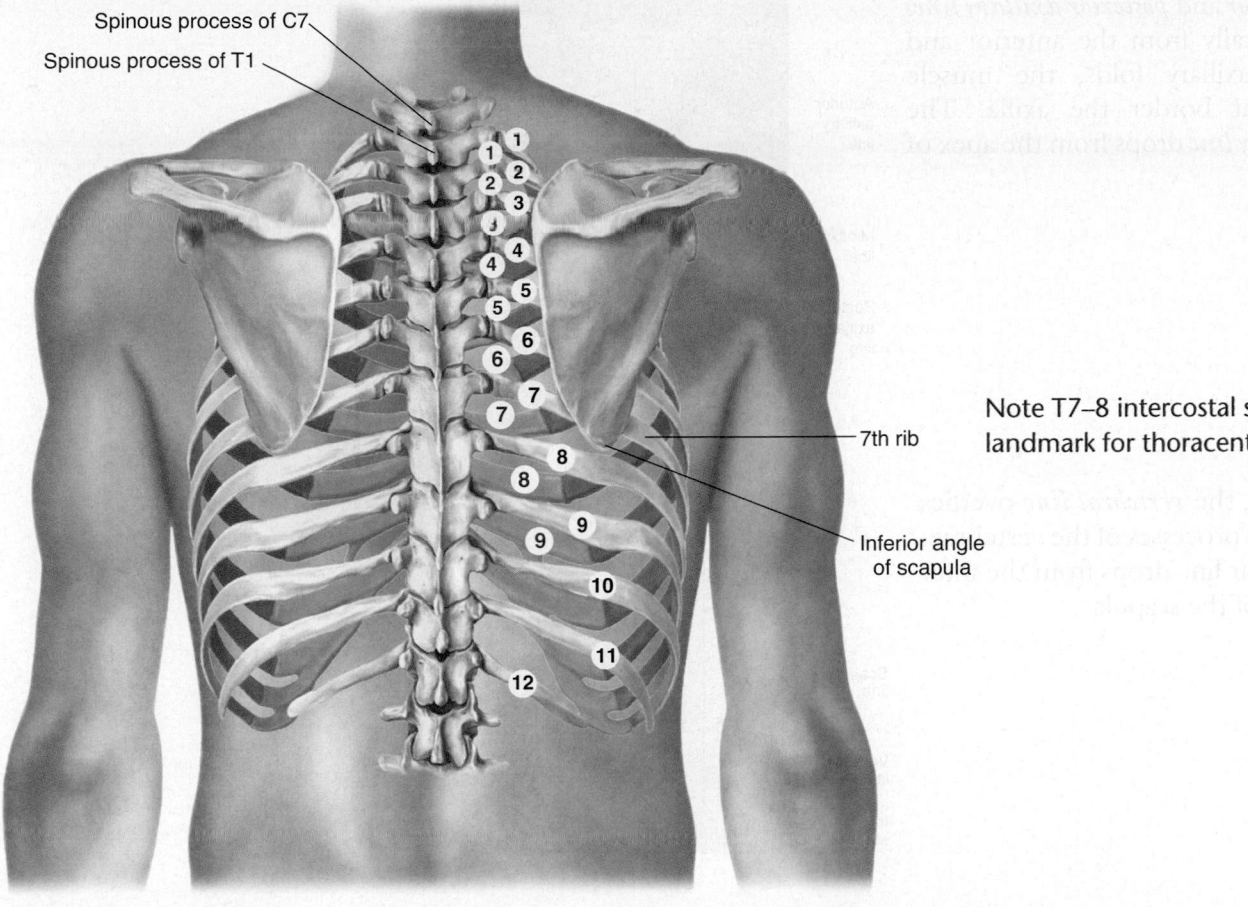

Spinous process of C7

Spinous process of T1

7th rib

Inferior angle
of scapula

Note T7–8 intercostal space as
landmark for thoracentesis.

The spinous processes of the vertebrae are also useful anatomic landmarks.
When the neck is flexed forward, the most protruding process is usually the
vertebra of C7, known as the vertebral prominens. If two processes are
equally prominent, they are C7 and T1. You can often palpate and count
the processes below them, especially when the spine is flexed.

To locate findings around the *circumference of the chest,* use a series
of vertical lines, shown in the adjacent illustrations. The *midsternal*
and *vertebral lines* are precise; the
others are estimated. The *midclavicular line* drops vertically from the
midpoint of the clavicle. To find it,
you must identify both ends of the
clavicle accurately (see p. 530).

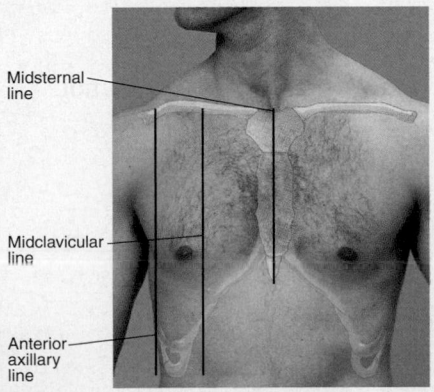

Midsternal
line

Midclavicular
line

Anterior
axillary
line

The *anterior* and *posterior axillary lines* drop vertically from the anterior and posterior axillary folds, the muscle masses that border the axilla. The *midaxillary line* drops from the apex of the axilla.

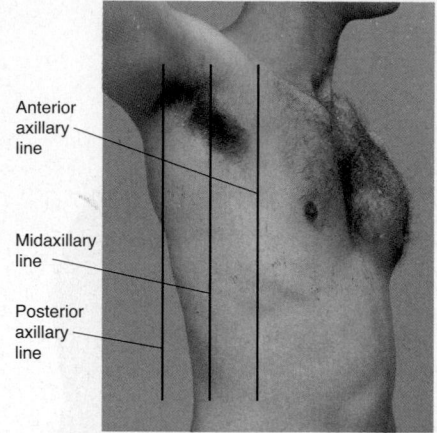

Anterior axillary line

Midaxillary line

Posterior axillary line

Posteriorly, the *vertebral line* overlies the spinous processes of the vertebrae. The scapular line drops from the inferior angle of the scapula.

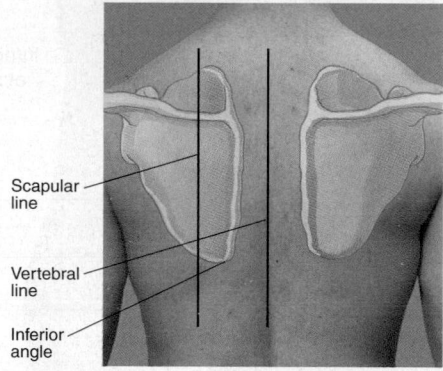

Scapular line

Vertebral line

Inferior angle

Lungs, Fissures, and Lobes.   Picture the lungs and their fissures and lobes on the chest wall. Anteriorly, the apex of each lung rises approximately 2 cm to 4 cm above the inner third of the clavicle. The lower border of the lung crosses the 6th rib at the midclavicular line and the 8th rib at the midaxillary line. Posteriorly, the lower border of the lung lies at about the level of the T10 spinous process. On inspiration, it descends farther.

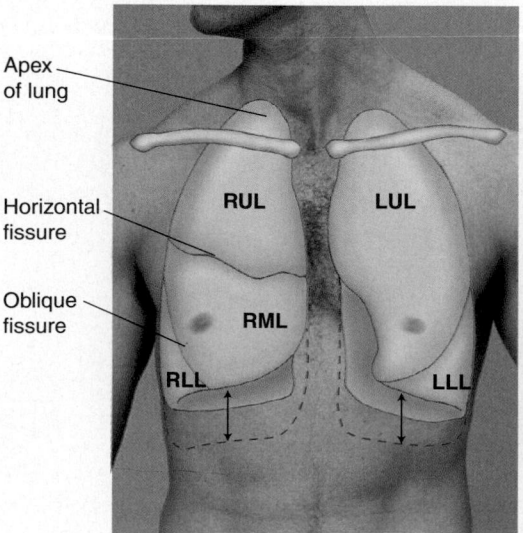

Apex of lung

Horizontal fissure

Oblique fissure

RUL   LUL

RML

RLL   LLL

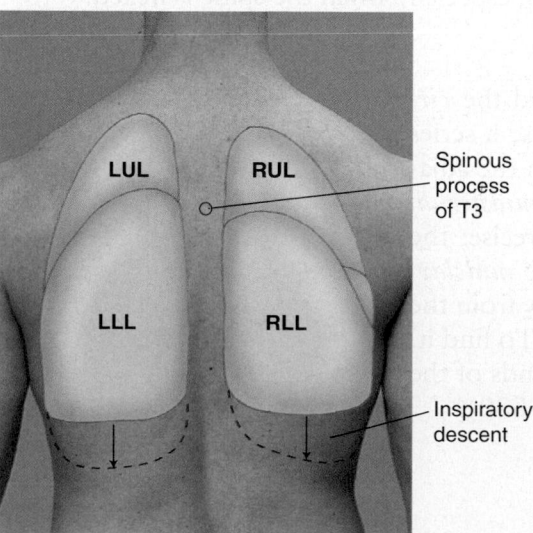

LUL   RUL

Spinous process of T3

LLL   RLL

Inspiratory descent

Each lung is divided roughly in half by an *oblique (major) fissure*. This fissure may be approximated by a string that runs from the T3 spinous process obliquely down and around the chest to the 6th rib at the midclavicular line. The right lung is further divided by the *horizontal (minor) fissure*. Anteriorly, this fissure runs close to the 4th rib and meets the oblique fissure in the midaxillary line near the 5th rib. The *right lung* is thus divided into *upper, middle,* and *lower lobes*. The *left lung* has only *two lobes*, upper and lower.

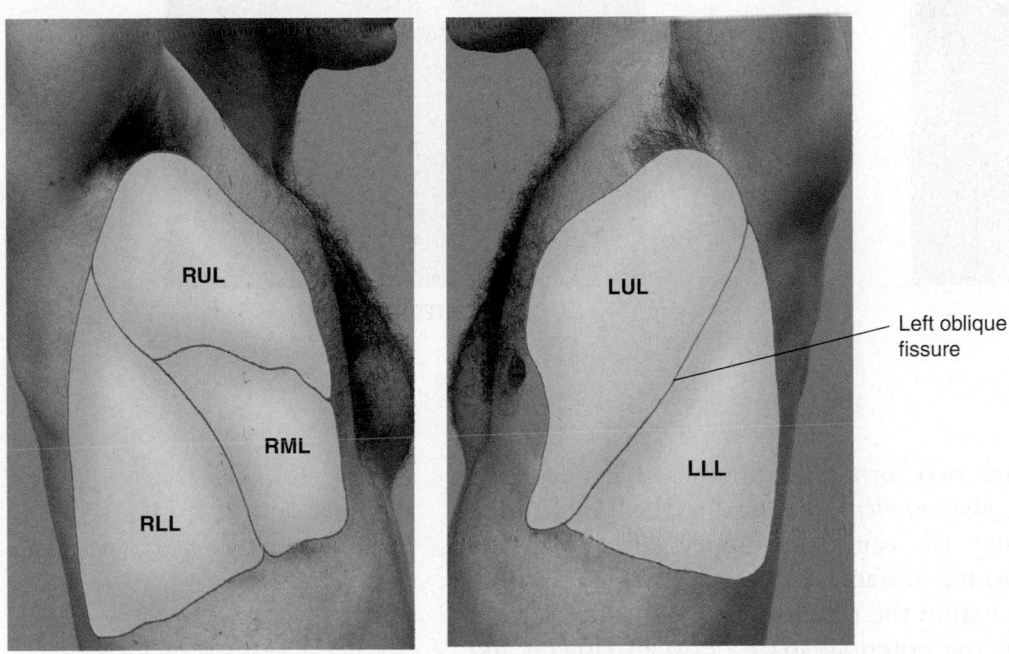

Left oblique fissure

Locations on the Chest.
Learn the general anatomic terms used to locate chest findings, such as:

Supraclavicular—above the clavicles
Infraclavicular—below the clavicles
Interscapular—between the scapulae
Infrascapular—below the scapulae
Bases of the lungs—the lowermost portions
Upper, middle, and lower lung fields

You may then infer which parts of the lungs are affected by an abnormal process. Signs in the right upper lung field, for example, almost certainly originate in the right upper lobe. Signs in the right middle lung field laterally, however, could come from any of three different lobes.

The Trachea and Major Bronchi.
Breath sounds over the trachea and bronchi have a different quality than breath sounds over the lung parenchyma. Be sure you know the location of these structures. The trachea bifurcates into its mainstem bronchi at the levels of the sternal angle anteriorly and the T4 spinous process posteriorly.

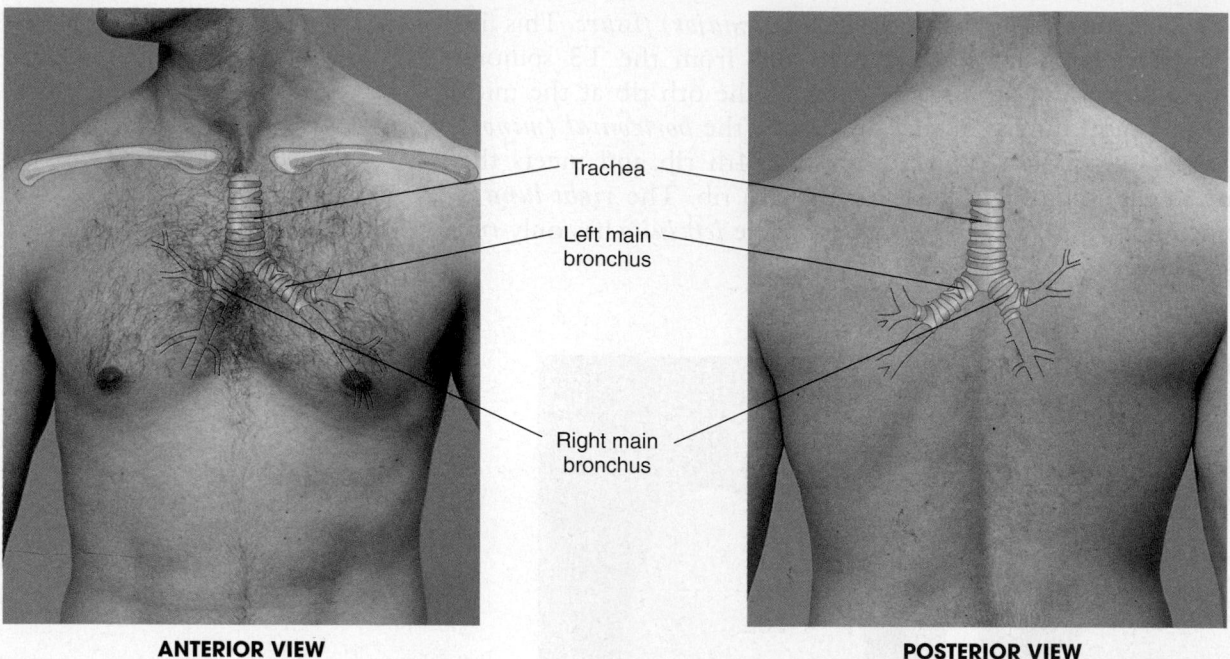

Trachea

Left main
bronchus

Right main
bronchus

ANTERIOR VIEW

POSTERIOR VIEW

The Pleurae. The pleurae are two serous membranes that cover the outer surface of each lung. The *visceral pleura* lies next to the lung and the *parietal pleura* lines the inner rib cage and upper surface of the diaphragm. Their smooth opposing surfaces, lubricated by pleural fluid, allow the lungs to move easily within the rib cage during inspiration and expiration. The *pleural space* is the potential space between visceral and parietal pleurae.

Breathing. Breathing is largely an automatic act, controlled in the brainstem and mediated by the muscles of respiration in response to cellular demands for oxygen. The dome-shaped *diaphragm* is the primary muscle of inspiration. When it contracts, it descends in the chest and enlarges the thoracic cavity. At the same time, it compresses the abdominal contents, pushing the abdominal wall outward. Muscles in the rib cage and neck expand the thorax during inspiration, especially the *parasternals,* which run obliquely from sternum to ribs, and the *scalenes,* which run from the cervical vertebrae to the first two ribs.

During inspiration, as these muscles contract, the thorax expands. Intrathoracic pressure decreases, drawing air through the tracheobronchial tree into the *alveoli,* or distal air sacs, and expanding the lungs. Oxygen diffuses into the blood of adjacent pulmonary capillaries, and carbon dioxide diffuses from the blood into the alveoli.

After inspiratory effort stops, the expiratory phase begins. The chest wall and lungs recoil, the diaphragm relaxes and rises passively, air flows outward, and the chest and abdomen return to their resting positions.

Normal breathing is quiet and easy—barely audible near the open mouth as a faint whish. When a healthy person lies supine, the breathing movements of the thorax are relatively slight. In contrast, the abdominal movements are usually easy to see. In the sitting position, movements of the thorax become more prominent.

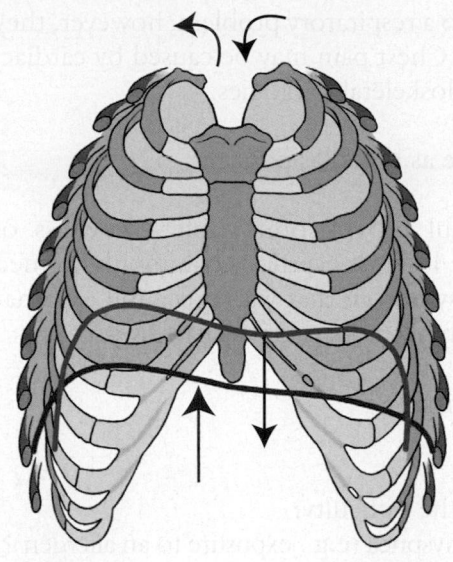

During exercise and in certain diseases, extra work is required to breathe, and accessory muscles join the inspiratory effort. The *sternomastoids* are the most important of these, and the *scalenes* may become visible. Abdominal muscles assist in expiration.

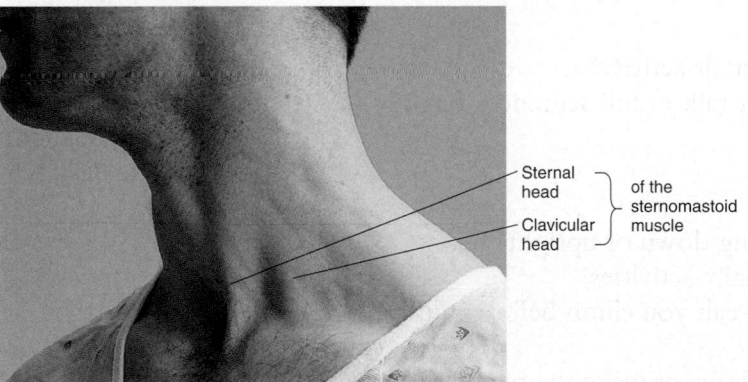

Sternal head
Clavicular head

of the sternomastoid muscle

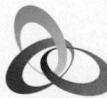 ## THE HEALTH HISTORY

COMMON OR CONCERNING SYMPTOMS

- Shortness of breath (dyspnea)
- Wheezing
- Cough
- Blood-streaked sputum (hemoptysis) or purulent sputum
- Chest pain

Overview

The thorax houses several organs and structures, and the nurse must use astute questioning to ascertain the patient's problem. Dyspnea, wheezing, cough, and hemoptysis usually point to a respiratory problem; however, they may also indicate a cardiac condition. Chest pain may be caused by cardiac, respiratory, gastrointestinal, or musculoskeletal etiologies.

The initial history questions should be as broad as possible.

Dyspnea is air hunger, a nonpainful but uncomfortable awareness of breathing that is inappropriate to the level of exertion, commonly termed shortness of breath. This is a serious symptom that warrants a full explanation and assessment. It can result from pulmonary or cardiac disease. Ask:

Have you had any difficulty breathing?

See Table 13-1, Dyspnea, pp. 324–325.

    O*nset:* When did you first notice the difficulty?
- Did anything precipitate the dyspnea (e.g., exposure to an allergen)?

    L*ocation:* Is the difficulty in your throat or neck area or chest?
    D*uration:* Does this occur at a particular time of day?
- Did it come on suddenly or gradually?

Sudden onset may indicate anaphylaxis or pulmonary embolism (both emergencies), spontaneous pneumothorax, or anxiety.

- Is it continuous or intermittent?
- Does it occur at rest or with exercise or activity?

    C*haracteristic Symptoms:* Can the patient talk in full sentences or only short phrases?

Determine the severity of the dyspnea based on the patient's ability to talk and complete daily activities.

    Is the dyspnea worse when you are lying down or upright?
    Has dyspnea altered your lifestyle or daily activities?
- How many steps or flights of stairs can you climb before pausing for breath?
- Can you carry groceries, mop the floor, or make the bed without dyspnea?

    A*ssociated Manifestations:* Are there any associated symptoms, such as wheezing or cough? Chest pain? Nausea?
    R*elieveing Factors:* Does anything make it better?
    T*reatment:* Have you seen anyone or tried any medications or treatments?

Anxious patients present a different picture. They may describe difficulty taking a deep-enough breath, or a smothering sensation with the inability to get enough air. If they are hyperventilating they may report *paraesthesias,* or sensations of tingling or "pins and needles" around the lips or in the hands and feet.

Anxious patients may have episodic dyspnea during both rest and exercise, and hyperventilation, or rapid shallow breathing. At other times, they may sigh frequently.

Wheezes are musical respiratory sounds that may be audible to the patient and others.

Wheezing suggests partial airway obstruction from secretions, tissue inflammation, or a foreign body.

Are you experiencing wheezing?

O*nset:* When did you first notice the wheeze?
- Did anything precipitate the wheezing (e.g., exposure to an allergen, cold, etc.)?

L*ocation:* Is it from your throat area or chest?

D*uration:* Does this occur at a particular time of day?
- Did it come on suddenly or gradually?
- Is it continuous or intermittent?
- Does it occur at rest or with exercise or activity?

C*haracteristic Symptoms:* Does the wheeze occur during inspiration or expiration or both?

A*ssociated Manifestations:* Are there any associated symptoms, such as dyspnea or cough?

R*elieveing Factors:* Does anything make it better?

T*reatment:* Have you seen anyone or tried any medications or treatments?

Cough is typically a reflex response to stimuli that irritate receptors in the larynx, trachea, or large bronchi. These stimuli include mucus, pus, blood, dust, foreign bodies, and even extremely hot or cold air. Coughing may also be caused by inflammation of the respiratory mucosa or tension in the air passages from a tumor or enlarged peribronchial lymph nodes. Patients with asthma may experience a cough without wheezing. The narrowed airways trigger a cough on expiration as the patient tries to fully exhale the trapped air.

Do you have a cough?

O*nset:* When did you first notice the cough?
- Did anything precipitate the cough (e.g., a cold or respiratory infection)?
- Have you begun any medications recently?

L*ocation:* Does it seem to originate from your throat or chest?

D*uration:* Does this occur at a particular time of day?

- Did it come on suddenly or gradually?

See Table 13-2, p. 326, Cough and Hemoptysis

Cough can be a symptom of *left-sided heart failure.*

Viral upper respiratory infections are the most common cause of *acute cough;* other causes include acute bronchitis, pneumonia, asthma, or foreign body. Postinfectious cough, bacterial sinusitis, or asthma in *subacute cough;* postnasal drip, asthma, gastroesophageal reflux, chronic bronchitis, bronchiectasis in *chronic cough.*[26,30,31]

Mucoid sputum is translucent, white or grey; *purulent* sputum is yellowish or greenish.

Foul-smelling sputum in anaerobic lung abscess; tenacious sputum in cystic fibrosis.

Large volumes of purulent sputum in bronchiectasis or lung abscess.

An acute cough lasts <3 weeks, subacute 3 to 8 weeks, and chronic >8 weeks.

- Is it continuous or intermittent?
- Does it occur at rest or with exercise or activity?
- Does it wake you at night?

Characteristic Symptoms: Do you feel the urge to cough with inspiration or expiration?

Do you cough up mucus or phlegm?

- If yes, ask the patient to describe the color, odor, consistency, and amount.
- To quantify mucus volume, ask: How much mucus do you think you cough up in 24 hours: a teaspoon, tablespoon, quarter cup, half cup, cupful?
- Have you noticed blood in the mucus?

Hemoptysis is coughing up of blood from the lungs; it may vary from blood-streaked phlegm to frank blood. Blood or blood-streaked material may originate in the mouth, pharynx, or gastrointestinal tract and is easily mislabeled.

- Describe the color and amount of blood.
- Have you had any mouth injuries or nosebleeds recently? Any ulcers?
- If the patient is actively coughing ask him or her to cough into a tissue in order to examine its characteristics.

Associated Manifestations: Are there any associated symptoms, such as dyspnea or wheezing?

Some medications such as angiotensin-converting enzyme (ACE) inhibitors produce a cough as a side effect.

Relieving Factors: Does anything make it better?

Treatment: Have you seen anyone or tried any medications or treatments?

Chest pain may be caused by cardiac, respiratory, gastrointestinal, or musculoskeletal etiologies. See Table 13-3, pp. 327–328, Chest Pain. The nurse should carefully ask follow-up questions using the "OLD CART" mnemonic to identify the source of the pain. Lung tissue itself has no pain fibers. Pain in lung conditions, such as pneumonia or pulmonary infarction, usually arises from inflammation of the adjacent parietal pleura. Sources of chest pain are listed below.

- Trachea and large bronchi

  Bronchitis

- Parietal pleura

  Pericarditis, pneumonia

- Chest wall, including the musculoskeletal system and skin

  Costochondritis, herpes zoster

- Myocardium

  Angina pectoris, myocardial infarction

- Pericardium

  Pericarditis

● Aorta

Dissecting aortic aneurysm

● Esophagus

Reflux esophagitis, esophageal spasm

● Extrathoracic structures: neck, gallbladder, and stomach

Cervical arthritis, biliary colic, gastritis

● Anxiety (the mechanism of pain remains obscure)

This chapter will focus on pulmonary complaints. See Chapter 14, The Cardiovascular System, and Chapter 16, The Gastrointestinal and Renal Systems, for history questions related to nonpulmonary chest pain.

Do you have chest pain?

> *Onset:* When did the pain begin?
> > ● Have you experienced chest pain previously? When?
> > ● Is this the same pain?
> > ● Did you fall or have any chest injuries prior to the pain?
>
> *Location:* Where in your chest do you feel the pain?
> *Duration:* Does it occur with breathing? Is the pain continuous or intermittent?
> *Characteristic Symptoms:* Describe your pain. Is your chest tender to touch? Rate the pain on a scale of 1 to 10.
> *Associated Manifestations:* When you have the chest pain, does anything else happen, e.g., loss of consciousness, nausea, numbness or tingling?
> *Relieving Factors:* Does anything make it better?
> *Treatment:* Have you seen anyone or tried any medications or treatments?

Past History

● Have you had any prior respiratory problems, such as respiratory infections, asthma, bronchitis, emphysema, pneumonia, tuberculosis, collapsed lung (pneumothorax), or cystic fibrosis?

  ● If yes, ask about onset, duration, treatment, and sequelae.

● Have you had thoracic surgery, biopsy, or trauma to your chest?

  ● If yes, ask the purpose, date, and outcome of the event.

● Do you have any allergies that affect your breathing or respiratory system?

  ● If yes, ask the patient to describe his or her symptoms and treatment.

● Have you had tuberculosis skin testing (purified protein derivative [PPD]) or a chest x-ray? When? What were the results?

Ask clients born outside the United States if they received the bacillus Calmette-Guerin (BCG) vaccine. This vaccine is given in some countries to reduce the risk of contracting tuberculosis.

- Have you had any other pulmonary testing? When? What were the results?

- Have you had an influenza immunization? When?

- Have you had the Tdap version of the tetanus immunization?

Immunity to pertussis from the childhood (DPT) vaccine has been shown to be weakening. Vaccination with the Tdap vaccine is recommended.

- If the patient is over 65 years, inquire: did you have pneumococcal or varicella zoster immunizations.

- Have you traveled outside the United States within the last 6 months? If yes, where?

- Have you been in contact with anyone with severe acute respiratory syndrome (SARS) or suspected of having SARS?

Family History

- Does anyone in your family currently have a respiratory infection or disease?

- Has anyone had lung cancer, asthma, or cystic fibrosis?

- Did anyone smoke in your home when you were growing up? Who?

Lifestyle and Personal Habits

- Do you smoke or have you ever smoked tobacco or marijuana?

  - How many cigarettes or packs per day do you smoke?

  - When did you start? How long have you smoked/did you ever smoke?

- Do you use or have you ever used snuff?

- Do you chew or have you ever chewed tobacco?

- Are you exposed to second-hand smoke? Where?

  - How many hours per day? For how many years?

- Are you exposed to any environmental conditions at home or work that affect your breathing (e.g., mold, sawdust, asbestos, coal dust, insecticides, radon, paint, or pollution)?

- Are you taking any prescription, herbal, or over-the-counter (OTC) medications for breathing or respiratory problems?

- Do you use oxygen or other treatments for breathing problems (e.g., nebulizer treatments)?

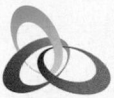

PHYSICAL EXAMINATION
Overview

It is helpful to examine the posterior thorax and lungs while the patient is sitting, and the anterior thorax and lungs with the patient supine. Proceed in an orderly fashion: inspect, palpate, percuss, and auscultate. Try to visualize the underlying lobes, and compare one side with the other, so that the patient serves as his or her own control. For men, arrange the patient's gown so that you can see the chest fully. For women, cover the anterior chest when you examine the back. For the anterior examination, drape the gown over each half of the chest as you examine the other half.

- *With the patient sitting,* examine the posterior thorax and lungs. The patient's arms should be folded across the chest with hands resting, if possible, on the opposite shoulders. This position moves the scapulae partly out of the way and increases your access to the lung fields. Following the posterior thorax examination, ask the patient to lie down.

- *With the patient supine,* examine the anterior thorax and lungs. The supine position makes it easier to examine women because the breasts can be gently displaced. Furthermore, wheezes, if present, are more likely to be heard. (Some clinicians prefer to examine both the back and the front of the chest with the patient sitting. This technique is also satisfactory.)

- *For patients who cannot sit up without aid,* try to get help so that you can examine the posterior chest in the sitting position. If this is impossible, roll the patient to one side and then to the other. Percuss the upper lung, and auscultate both lungs in each position. Because ventilation is relatively greater in the dependent (i.e., lower) lung, your chances of hearing abnormal wheezes or crackles are greater on the dependent side (see Characteristics of Breath Sounds p. 313).

Hospitalized or long-term care patients who cannot sit up for routine lung assessment every shift may be examined using this technique.

INITIAL SURVEY OF RESPIRATION AND THE THORAX

Observation and documentation of the rate, rhythm, depth, and effort of breathing is the first step of the respiratory assessment. This may have been done already with the vital signs. A healthy adult breathes quietly and regularly about 12 to 20 times a minute. An occasional sigh is to be expected. Note whether expiration lasts longer than usual. See Chapter 7, p. 116 for information on assessing respiratory rate and rhythm.

See Table 7-1, p. 124, Abnormalities in Rate and Rhythm of Breathing.

Always inspect the patient for any signs of respiratory difficulty.

- *Observe the patient's facial expression*—it should be relaxed and calm.

Low oxygenation produces anxiety and restlessness.

- *Observe level of consciousness.*

Decreased level of consciousness indicates poor oxygenation to the brain.

- *Assess the patient's color* for cyanosis, especially the face, mucous membranes, and nail beds. Recall any relevant findings from earlier parts of your examination, such as the shape of the fingernails.

Cyanosis signals hypoxia. Clubbing of the nails (see Table 9-14, pp. 183–184.) in, *cystic fibrosis,* or *congenital heart disease.*

- *Listen to the patient's breathing.* Are there any audible sounds (e.g., *wheezing* or *stridor*)? If so, where do they fall in the respiratory cycle?

Audible stridor, a high-pitched inspiratory sound, is an ominous sign of airway obstruction in the larynx or trachea. Audible wheezing indicates severe asthma.

- *Inspect the neck.* During inspiration, is there contraction of the accessory muscles, namely, the sternomastoid and scalene muscles, or supraclavicular retraction? Is the trachea midline?

Inspiratory contraction of the sternomastoids and scalenes at rest signals severe difficulty in breathing. Lateral displacement of the trachea in *pneumothorax, pleural effusion,* or *atelectasis.*

Also *observe the shape of the chest.* The anteroposterior (AP) diameter may increase with aging, compared with the lateral chest diameter. Usually there is a 2:1 ratio of transverse to anteroposterior diameters.

The AP diameter also may increase in *chronic obstructive pulmonary disease* (COPD), although evidence is not definitive.[1]

EXAMINATION OF THE POSTERIOR CHEST

Inspection

From a midline position behind the patient, note the *shape of the chest* and *how the chest moves,* including:

- Deformities or asymmetry

See Table 13-4, p. 329, Deformities of the Thorax.

- Abnormal retraction of the intercostal spaces during inspiration. Retraction is most apparent in the lower intercostal spaces.

Retraction is seen in severe *asthma, COPD,* or upper airway obstruction.

● Impaired respiratory movement on one or both sides or a unilateral lag (or delay) in movement.

Unilateral impairment or lagging of respiratory movement suggests disease of the underlying lung or pleura.

Palpation

As you palpate the chest, focus on areas of tenderness and abnormalities in the overlying skin, muscles and ribs, respiratory expansion, and fremitus.

Intercostal tenderness over inflamed pleura.

● *Identify tender areas.* Carefully palpate any area where pain has been reported or where lesions or bruises are evident.

Bruises or tenderness over a fractured rib.

● *Assess any observed abnormalities* such as masses

● *Test chest expansion.* Place your thumbs at about the level of the 10th ribs, with your fingers loosely grasping and parallel to the lateral rib cage. As you position your hands, slide them medially just enough to raise a loose fold of skin on each side between your thumb and the spine.

Ask the patient to inhale deeply. Watch the distance between your thumbs as they move apart during inspiration, and feel for the range and symmetry of the rib cage as it expands and contracts. Your thumbs should move equally apart.

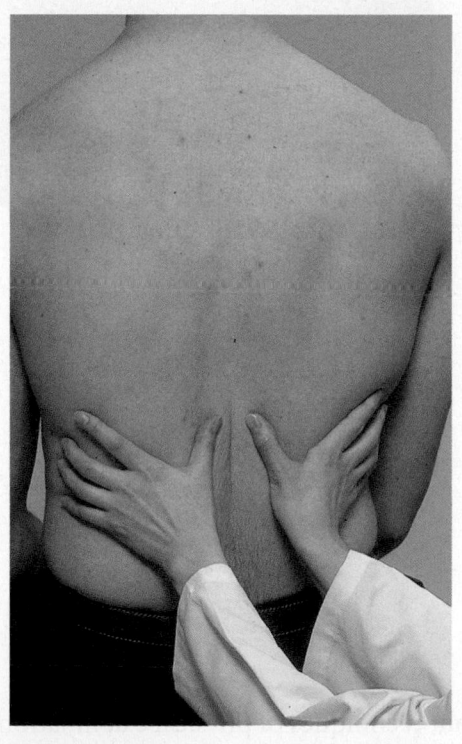

Causes of unilateral decrease or delay in chest expansion include *chronic fibrosis* of the underlying lung or pleura, *pleural effusion, lobar pneumonia,* pleural pain with associated splinting, and unilateral bronchial obstruction.

● *Feel for tactile fremitus.* Fremitus refers to the palpable vibrations transmitted through the bronchopulmonary tree to the chest wall as the patient is speaking. To detect fremitus, use either the ball (the bony part of the palm at the base of the fingers) or the ulnar surface of your hand to optimize the vibratory sensitivity of the bones in your hand. Ask the patient to repeat the words "ninety-nine" or "one-one-one." If fremitus is faint, ask the patient to speak more loudly or in a deeper voice.

Fremitus is decreased or absent when the voice is soft or when the transmission of vibrations from the larynx to the surface of the chest is impeded. Causes include a very thick chest wall; an obstructed bronchus; *COPD*; and separation of the pleural surfaces by fluid (*pleural effusion*), fibrosis (*pleural thickening*), air (*pneumothorax*), or an infiltrating tumor.

Use one hand until you have learned the feel of fremitus. Some clinicians find using one hand more accurate. The simultaneous use of both hands to compare sides, however, increases your speed and may facilitate detection of differences.

● *Palpate and compare symmetric areas* of the lungs in the pattern shown in the photograph. Identify and locate any areas of increased, decreased, or absent fremitus. Fremitus is typically more prominent in the interscapular area than in the lower lung fields and is often more prominent on the right side than on the left. It disappears below the diaphragm.

Look for *asymmetric* fremitus: asymmetric *decreased* fremitus in unilateral pleural effusion, pneumothorax, neoplasm from decreased transmission of low-frequency sounds; asymmetric *increased* fremitus in unilateral pneumonia from increased transmission.[1]

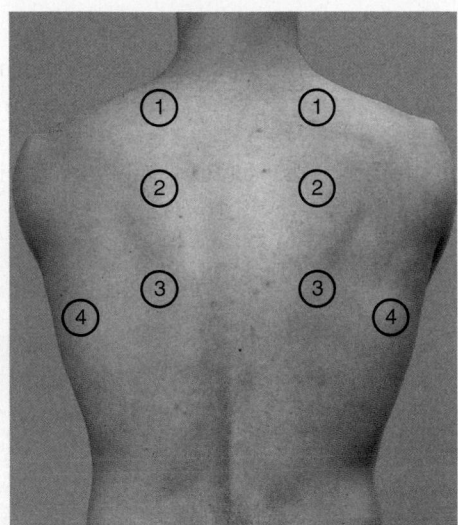

LOCATIONS FOR FEELING FREMITUS

Tactile fremitus is a somewhat imprecise assessment tool, but as a scouting technique, It directs your attention to possible abnormalities. Later in the examination you will check any suggested findings by listening for breath sounds, voice sounds, and whispered voice sounds. All these attributes tend to increase or decrease together.

Percussion

Percussion is one of the most important techniques of physical examination. Percussion sets the chest wall and underlying tissues in motion, producing audible sound and palpable vibrations. Percussion helps to establish whether the underlying tissues are air filled, fluid filled, or solid. It penetrates only 5 cm to 7 cm into the chest, however, and will not help detect deep-seated lesions.

The technique of percussion can be practiced on any surface. As you practice, listen for changes in percussion notes over different types of materials or different parts of the body. The key points for good technique, described for a right-handed person, are as follows:

- Hyperextend the middle finger of your left hand, known as the *pleximeter finger*. Press its distal interphalangeal joint firmly on the surface to be percussed. *Avoid surface contact by any other part of the hand, because this dampens out vibrations.* Note that the thumb and 2nd, 4th, and 5th fingers are not touching the chest.

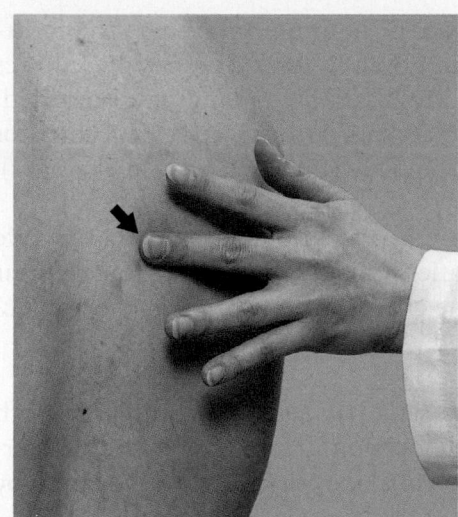

- Position your right forearm quite close to the surface, with the hand cocked upward. The middle finger should be partially flexed, relaxed, and poised to strike.

- With a *quick, sharp but relaxed wrist motion,* strike the pleximeter finger with the right middle finger, or plexor finger. Aim at your distal interphalangeal joint. You are trying to transmit vibrations through the bones of this joint to the underlying chest wall.

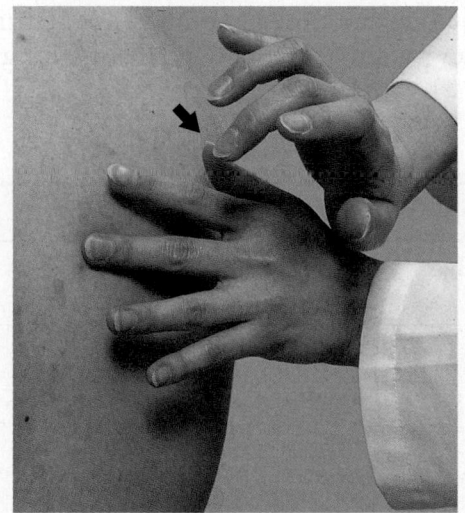

- Strike using the *tip of the plexor finger,* not the finger pad. Your finger should be almost at right angles to the pleximeter. A short fingernail is recommended to avoid self-injury.

- Withdraw your striking finger quickly to avoid damping the vibrations you have created.

In summary, the movement is at the wrist. It is directed, brisk yet relaxed, and a bit bouncy.

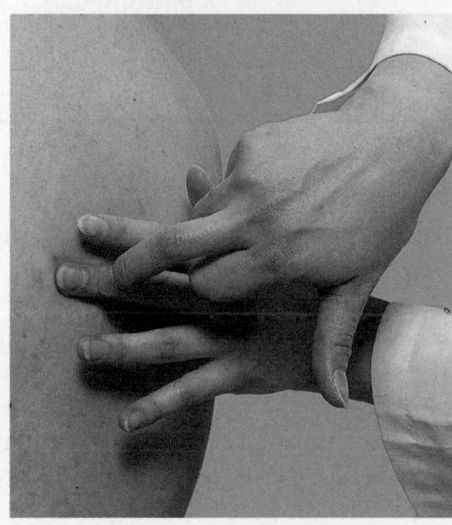

Percussion Notes. With your plexor or tapping finger, use the lightest percussion that produces a clear note. A thick chest wall requires stronger percussion than a thin one. However, if a *louder* note is needed, apply more pressure with the *pleximeter* finger (this is more effective for increasing percussion note volume than tapping harder with the plexor finger).

● *When percussing the lower posterior chest,* stand somewhat to the side rather than directly behind the patient. This allows you to place your pleximeter finger more firmly on the chest and your plexor is more effective, making a better percussion note.

● *When comparing two areas,* use the same percussion technique in both areas. Percuss or strike twice in each location. It is easier to detect differences in percussion notes by comparing one area with another than by striking repetitively in one place.

● *Learn to identify five percussion notes.* You can practice four of them on yourself. These notes differ in their basic qualities of sound: intensity, pitch, and duration. Train your ear to distinguish these differences by concentrating on one quality at a time as you percuss first in one location, then in another. Review the table below. Healthy lungs are *resonant.*

● **Percussion Notes and Their Characteristics**					**Pathologic Examples**
	Relative Intensity	Relative Pitch	Relative Duration	Example of Location	
Flatness	Soft	High	Short	Thigh	Large pleural effusion
Dullness	Medium	Medium	Medium	Liver	Lobar pneumonia
Resonance	Loud	Low	Long	Healthy lung	Simple chronic bronchitis
Hyperresonance	Very loud	Lower	Longer	Usually none	COPD, pneumothorax
Tympany	Loud	High*	*	Gastric air bubble or puffed-out cheek	Large pneumothorax

*Distinguished mainly by its musical timbre.

While the patient keeps both arms crossed in front of the chest, percuss the thorax in symmetric locations from the apex to the base.

● *Alternate percussing one side of the chest and then the other at each level* in a ladder-like pattern, as shown by the numbers below. Begin above the scapula. Omit the areas over the scapulae—the thickness of muscle and bone alters the percussion notes of the lungs. The lateral numbers 6 and 7 should be percussed on the midaxillary line. Identify and locate the area and quality of any abnormal percussion note.

Dullness replaces resonance when fluid or solid tissue replaces air-containing lung or occupies the pleural space beneath your percussing fingers. Examples include *lobar pneumonia,* in which the

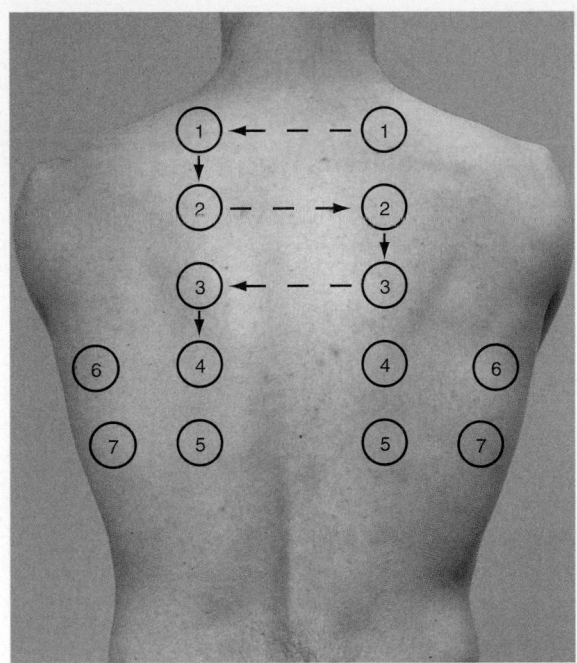

"LADDER" PATTERN FOR PERCUSSION AND AUSCULTATION

alveoli are filled with fluid and blood cells; and pleural accumulations of serous fluid (*pleural effusion*), blood (*hemothorax*), pus (*empyema*), fibrous tissue, or tumor.

Generalized hyperresonance may be heard over the hyperinflated lungs of COPD or *asthma,* but is not a reliable sign. *Unilateral hyperresonance* suggests a large pneumothorax or possibly a large air-filled bulla in the lung.

● *Identify the descent of the diaphragm, or **diaphragmatic excursion.** First, determine the level of diaphragmatic dullness* during quiet respiration. Holding the pleximeter finger *above and parallel* to the expected level of dullness, percuss downward in progressive steps until dullness clearly replaces resonance. Confirm this level of change by percussion near the middle of the hemithorax and also more laterally.

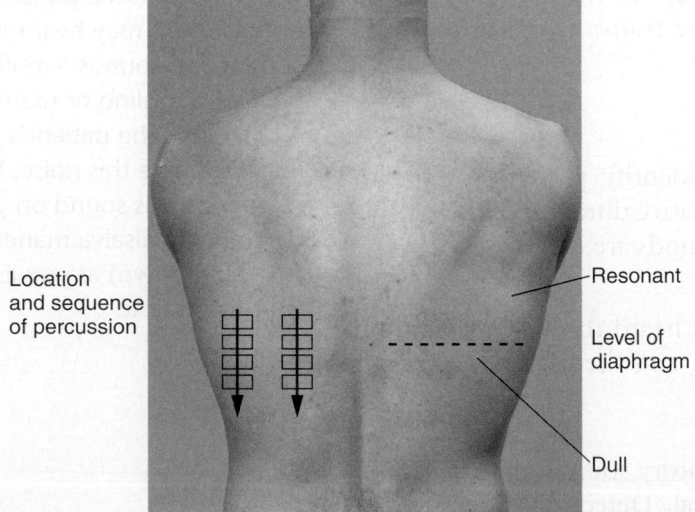

Location and sequence of percussion

Resonant

Level of diaphragm

Dull

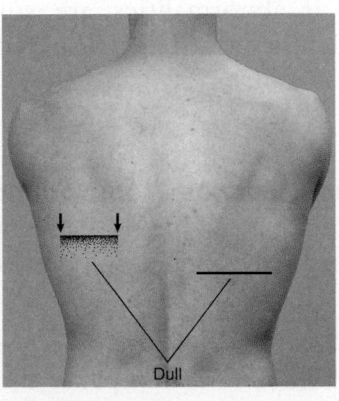

An abnormally high level suggests *pleural effusion,* or a high diaphragm as in *atelectasis* or *diaphragmatic paralysis.*

Note that with this technique, you are identifying the boundary between the resonant lung tissue and the duller structures below the diaphragm. You are not percussing the diaphragm itself. You can infer the probable location of the diaphragm from the level of dullness.

Now, *estimate the extent of diaphragmatic excursion* by determining the distance between the level of dullness on full expiration and the level of dullness on full inspiration, normally about 3 to 5 cm.

- Ask the patient to breathe in, then out fully and hold his or her breath.

- Percuss down to dullness and mark this point on the patient's back with a pen.

- Next ask the patient to breathe in fully and hold his or her breath, and continue percussing down until dullness is heard; mark this point.

- Repeat on the opposite side.

- Measure the distances; they should be equal through the right side, maybe 1 cm higher due to the liver.

The diaphragmatic excursion should be 3 cm to 5 cm in adults, although in athletes it may be up to 7 cm to 8 cm.

Auscultation

Auscultation is the most important examination technique for assessing air flow through the tracheobronchial tree. Together with percussion, it also helps the nurse assess the condition of the surrounding lungs and pleural space. Auscultation involves (1) listening to the sounds generated by breathing, (2) listening for any adventitious (extra) sounds, and (3) if abnormalities are suspected, listening to the sounds of the patient's spoken or whispered voice as they are transmitted through the chest wall.

Sounds from bedclothes, paper gowns, and the chest itself can generate confusion in auscultation. Hair on the chest may cause crackling sounds. Either press harder or wet the hair. If the patient is cold or tense, you may hear muscle contraction sounds—muffled, low-pitched rumbling or roaring noises. A change in the patient's position may eliminate this noise. You can reproduce this sound on yourself by doing a Valsalva maneuver (straining down) as you listen to your own chest.

Breath Sounds (Lung Sounds). Learn to identify patterns of breath sounds by their intensity, their pitch, and the relative duration of their inspiratory and expiratory phases. Normal breath sounds are:

- *Vesicular,* or soft and low pitched. They are heard through inspiration, continue without pause through expiration, and then fade away about one third of the way through expiration.

- *Bronchovesicular,* with inspiratory and expiratory sounds about equal in length, at times separated by a silent interval. Detecting differences in pitch and intensity is often easier during expiration.

- *Bronchial,* or louder and higher in pitch, with a short silence between inspiratory and expiratory sounds. Expiratory sounds last longer than inspiratory sounds.

The characteristics of these three kinds of breath sounds are summarized in the next table. Also shown are the *tracheal* breath sounds—very loud, harsh sounds that are heard by listening over the trachea in the neck.

● Characteristics of Breath Sounds[2]

	Duration of Sounds	Intensity of Expiratory Sound	Pitch of Expiratory Sound	Locations Where Heard Normally
Vesicular*	Inspiratory sounds last longer than expiratory ones.	Soft	Relatively low	Over most of both lungs
Broncho-vesicular	Inspiratory and expiratory sounds are about equal.	Intermediate	Intermediate	Often in the 1st and 2nd intercostal spaces anteriorly and between the scapulae
Bronchial	Expiratory sounds last longer than inspiratory ones.	Loud	Relatively high	Over the manubrium, if heard at all
Tracheal	Inspiratory and expiratory sounds are about equal.	Very loud	Relatively high	Over the trachea in the neck

*The thickness of the bars indicates intensity; the steeper their incline, the higher the pitch.

If bronchovesicular or bronchial breath sounds are heard in locations distant from those listed, suspect that air-filled lung has been replaced by fluid-filled or solid lung tissue. See Table 13-5, p. 330 Normal and Altered Breath and Voice Sounds.

Listen to the breath sounds with the diaphragm of a stethoscope after instructing the patient to breathe deeply through an open mouth. Use the pattern suggested for percussion, moving from one side to the other and comparing symmetric areas of the lungs. If you hear or suspect abnormal sounds, auscultate adjacent areas so that you can fully describe the extent of any abnormality. Listen to at least one full breath in each location. Be alert for patient discomfort resulting from hyperventilation (e.g., lightheadedness, faintness), and allow the patient to rest as needed.

Note the *intensity* of the breath sounds. Breath sounds are usually louder in the lower posterior lung fields and may also vary from area to area. If the breath sounds seem faint, ask the patient to breathe more deeply. You may then hear them easily. When patients do not breathe deeply enough or have a thick chest wall, as in obesity, breath sounds may remain diminished.

Breath sounds may be decreased when air flow is decreased (as in obstructive lung disease or muscular weakness) or when the transmission of sound is poor (as in *pleural effusion, pneumothorax, or COPD*).

Is there a *silent gap* between the inspiratory and expiratory sounds?

A gap suggests bronchial breath sounds.

Listen for the *pitch, intensity, and duration of the expiratory and inspiratory sounds.* Are vesicular breath sounds distributed throughout the chest wall? Or are there bronchovesicular or bronchial breath sounds in unexpected places? If so, where are they?

Adventitious (Extra) Sounds. Listen for any extra, or adventitious, sounds that are superimposed on the usual breath sounds. Detection of adventitious sounds—*crackles* (sometimes called *rales*), *wheezes,* and *rhonchi*—is an important part of your examination, often leading to diagnosis of cardiac and pulmonary conditions. The most common kinds of these sounds are described below.

For further discussion and other added sounds, see Table 13-6, p. 331, Adventitious (Added) Lung Sounds: Causes and Qualities.

● **Adventitious or Added Breath Sounds[2]**

Crackles (or Rales)	Wheezes and Rhonchi
● **Discontinuous**	● **Continuous**
● Intermittent, nonmusical, and brief	● ≥250 msec, musical, prolonged (but not necessarily persisting throughout the respiratory cycle)
● Like dots in time	● Like dashes in time
● *Fine crackles:* soft, high-pitched, very brief (5–10 msec)	● *Wheezes:* relatively high pitched (≥400 Hz) with hissing or shrill quality
· · · · ·	wwwww
● *Coarse crackles:* somewhat louder, lower in pitch, brief (20–30 msec)	● *Rhonchi:* relatively low pitched (≤200 Hz) with snoring quality
● ● ● ● ●	⋀⋀⋀

Crackles may be from abnormalities of the lungs (*pneumonia, fibrosis, early congestive heart failure*) or of the airways (bronchitis, bronchiectasis).

Wheezes suggest narrowed airways, as in *asthma, COPD,* or *bronchitis.*

Rhonchi suggest secretions in large airways.

If you hear *crackles,* especially those that do not clear after coughing, listen carefully for the following characteristics.[2-5] These are clues to the underlying condition:

● Loudness, pitch, and duration (summarized as fine or coarse crackles)

Fine late inspiratory crackles that persist from breath to breath suggest abnormal lung tissue.

● Number (few to many)

● Timing in the respiratory cycle

● Location on the chest wall

● Persistence of their pattern from breath to breath

● Any change after a cough or a change in the patient's position

Clearing of crackles, wheezes, or rhonchi after coughing or position change suggests thickened secretions, as in *bronchitis* or *atelectasis*.

In some normal people, crackles may be heard at the lung bases anteriorly after maximal expiration. Crackles in dependent portions of the lungs may also occur after prolonged recumbency.

If you hear *wheezes* or *rhonchi*, note their timing (inspiratory, expiratory, or both) and location. Do they change with deep breathing or coughing?

Findings predictive of *COPD* include combinations of symptoms and signs, especially wheezing by self-report or examination, plus history of smoking, age, and decreased breath sounds. Diagnosis requires pulmonary function tests such as spirometry.[6–11]

Transmitted Voice Sounds. If you hear abnormally located bronchovesicular or bronchial breath sounds or adventitious sounds, assess transmitted voice sounds. With a stethoscope, listen in symmetric areas over the chest wall as you:

Increased transmission of voice sounds suggests that air-filled lung has become airless. See Table 13-5, p. 330, Normal and Altered Breath and Voice Sounds.

● Ask the patient to say "ninety-nine." Normally the sounds transmitted through the chest wall are muffled and indistinct.

Louder, clearer voice sounds are called **bronchophony.**

● Ask the patient to say "ee." You will normally hear a muffled long E sound.

When "ee" is heard as "ay," an *E-to-A change* **(egophony)** is present, as in lobar consolidation from *pneumonia*. The quality sounds nasal.

● Ask the patient to whisper "ninety-nine" or "one-two-three." The whispered voice is normally heard faintly and indistinctly, if at all.

Louder, clearer whispered sounds are called **whispered pectoriloquy.**

EXAMINATION OF THE ANTERIOR CHEST

When examined in the supine position, the patient should lie comfortably with arms somewhat abducted. A patient who is having difficulty breathing should be examined in the sitting position or with the head of the bed elevated to a comfortable level.

Persons with severe *COPD* may prefer to sit leaning forward, with lips pursed during exhalation and arms supported on their knees or a table. This is called *tripod* position.

Inspection

Observe *the shape of the patient's chest* and *the movement of the chest wall.* Note:

1. Deformities or asymmetry

See Table 13-4, p. 329, Deformities of the Thorax.

2. Work of breathing: abnormal retraction of the lower intercostal spaces during inspiration. Supraclavicular or substernal retraction is often present.

Severe *asthma, COPD,* or upper airway obstruction.

3. Local lag or impairment in respiratory movement

Underlying disease of lung or pleura.

Palpation

Palpation has four potential uses:

1. *Identification of tender areas*

Tender pectoral muscles or costal cartilages corroborate, but do not prove, that chest pain has a musculoskeletal origin.

2. *Assessment of observed abnormalities*

3. *Further assessment of chest expansion.* Place your thumbs along each costal margin, your hands along the lateral rib cage. As you position your hands, slide them medially a bit to raise loose skin folds between your thumbs. Ask the patient to inhale deeply (as the thorax expands; see picture on page 317). Observe how far your thumbs diverge and feel for the extent and symmetry of respiratory movement.

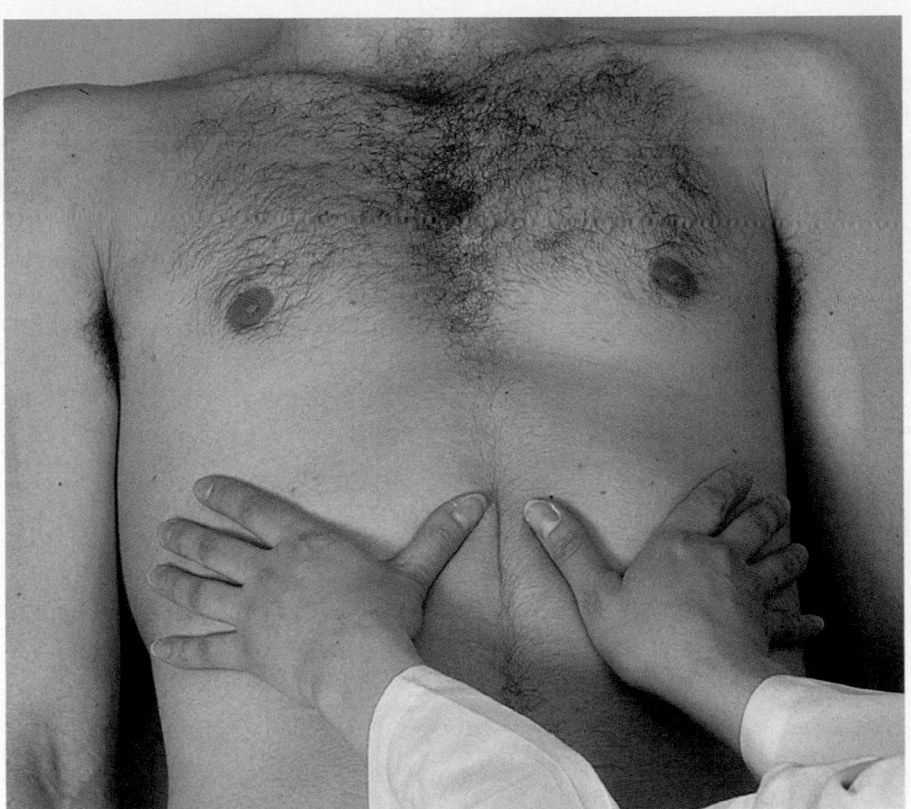

CHEST EXPANSION HAND POSITION

4. *Assessment of tactile fremitus.* Compare both sides of the chest, using the ball or ulnar surface of your hand. Fremitus is usually decreased or absent over the precordium. When examining a woman, gently displace the breasts as necessary.

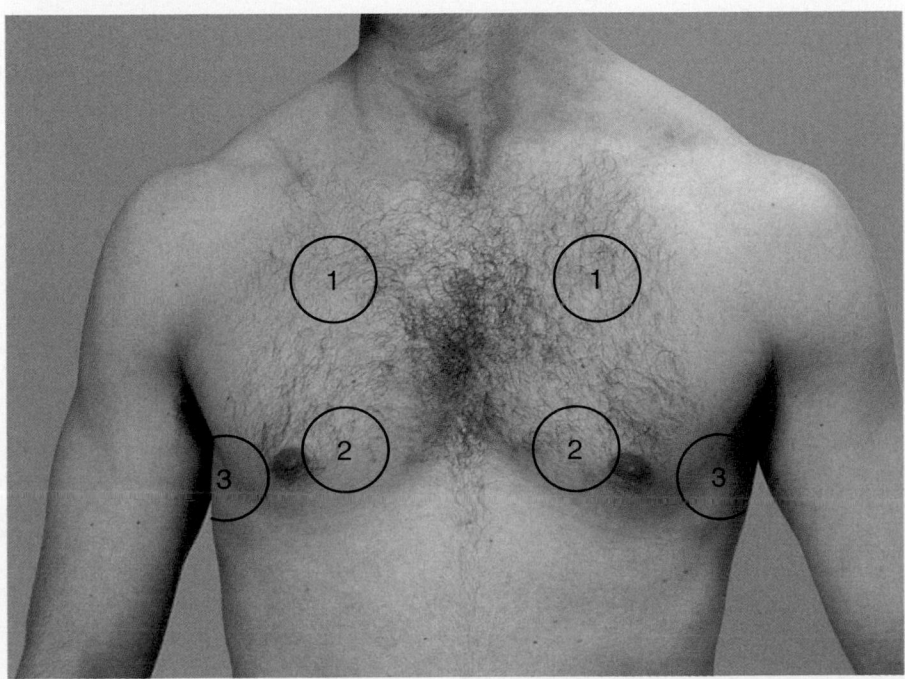

LOCATIONS FOR FEELING FREMITUS

Percussion

1. Percuss the anterior and lateral chest, again comparing both sides. The heart normally produces an area of dullness to the left of the sternum from the 3rd to the 5th intercostal spaces. Percuss the left lung lateral to it.

Dullness replaces resonance when fluid or solid tissue replaces air-containing lung or occupies the pleural space. Because pleural fluid usually sinks to the lowest part of the pleural space (posteriorly in a supine patient), only a very large effusion can be detected anteriorly.

The hyperresonance of *COPD* may totally replace cardiac dullness.

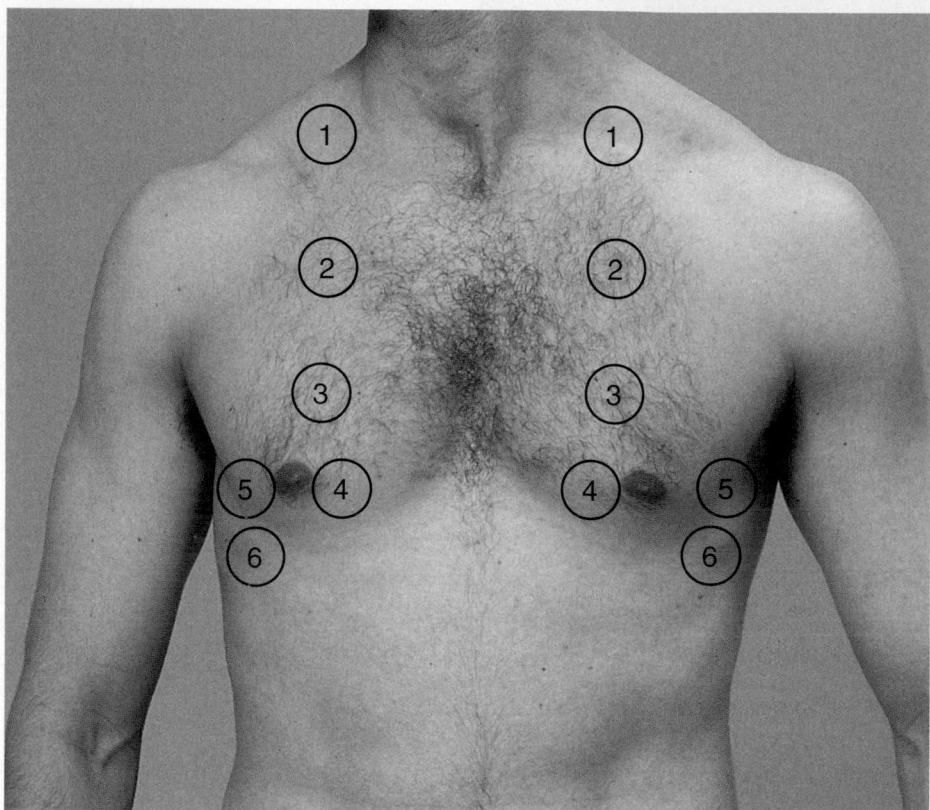

LOCATIONS FOR PERCUSSION AND AUSCULTATION

In a woman, to enhance percussion, gently displace the breast with your left hand while percussing with the right.

The dullness of right middle lobe pneumonia typically occurs behind the right breast. Unless you displace the breast, you may miss the abnormal percussion note.

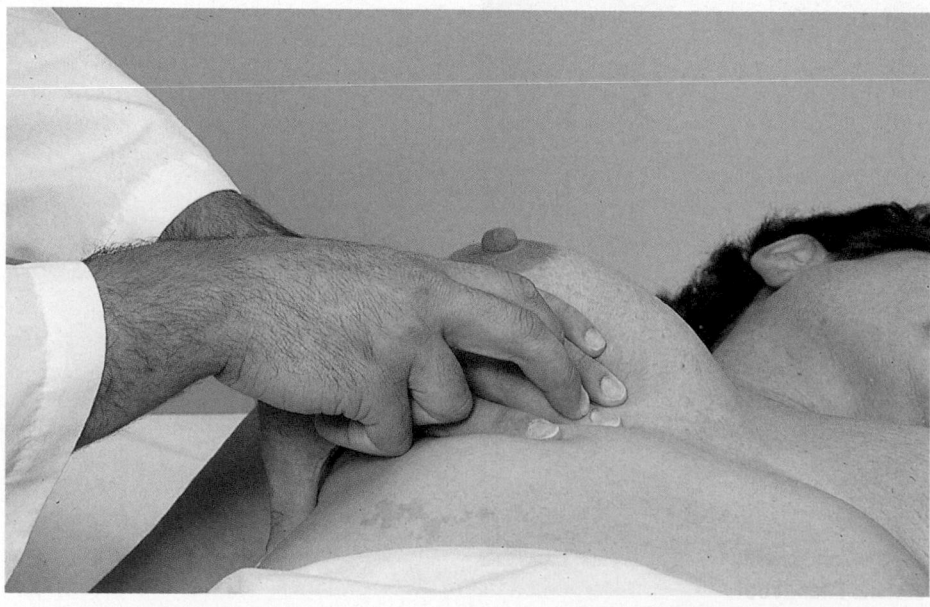

Alternatively, you may ask the patient to move her breast for you.

Identify and locate any area with an abnormal percussion note.

2. With your pleximeter finger above and parallel to the expected upper border of liver dullness, percuss in progressive steps downward in the right midclavicular line. Identify the upper border of liver dullness. Later, during the abdominal examination, you will use this method to estimate the size of the liver. As you percuss down the chest on the left, the resonance of normal lung usually changes to the tympany of the gastric air bubble.

A lung affected by *COPD* often displaces the upper border of the liver downward. It also lowers the level of diaphragmatic dullness posteriorly.

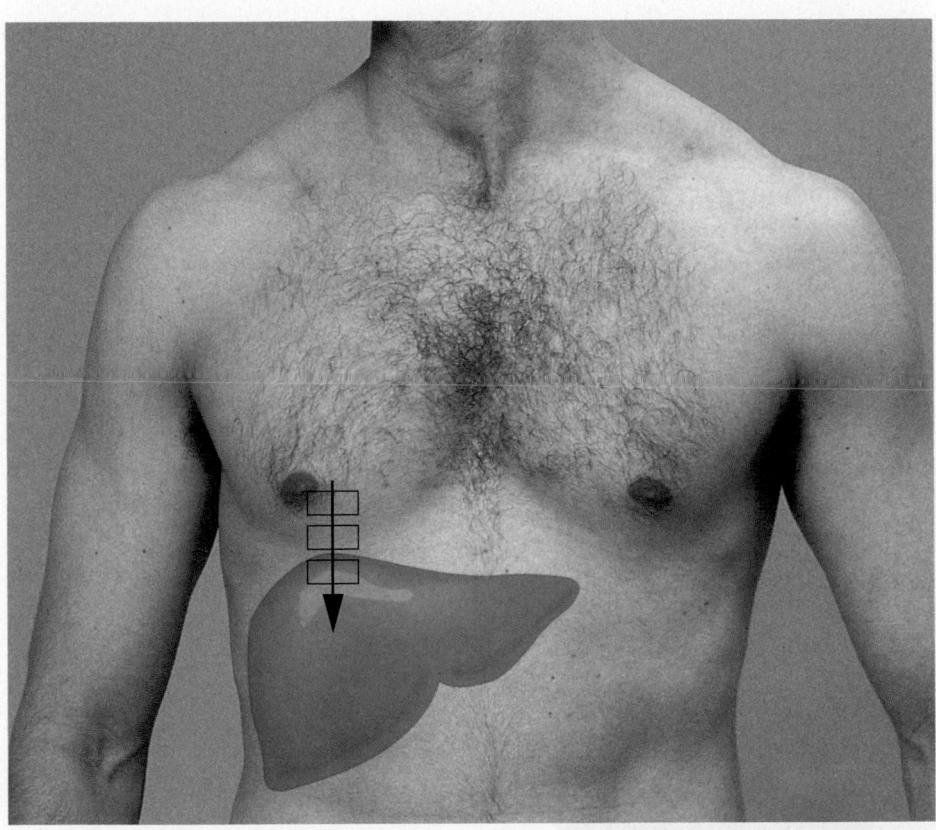

Auscultation

Listen to the chest anteriorly and laterally as the patient breathes with mouth open, somewhat more deeply than normal. Compare symmetric areas of the lungs, using the pattern suggested for percussion and extending it to adjacent areas as indicated.

1. *Listen to the breath sounds,* noting their intensity and identifying any variations from normal vesicular breathing. Breath sounds are usually louder in the upper anterior lung fields. Bronchovesicular breath sounds may be heard over the large airways, especially on the right.

2. *Identify any adventitious sounds,* time them in the respiratory cycle, and locate them on the chest wall. Do they clear with deep breathing?

See Table 13-6, p. 331, Adventitious (Added) Lung Sounds: Causes and Qualities, and Table 13-7, pp. 332–333, Physical Findings in Selected Chest Disorders.

3. If indicated, *listen for transmitted voice sounds.*

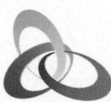 ## SPECIAL TECHNIQUES

Pulse Oximetry.   Pulse oximetry measures the arterial oxygenation saturation, or SpO_2. A probe is placed on the patient's finger or earlobe. The toe is used for infants and young children. A diode emits light and a detector on the opposite side of the probe measures the amount of light absorbed by oxyhemoglobin. The oximeter compares the amount of light emitted to the amount absorbed and calculates the percentage of oxygen saturation. A healthy person has an SpO_2 of 97% to 100%. Poor perfusion, hypotension, dyshemoglobinemias, dyes in some nail polishes, and excessive ambient light may cause inaccurate readings.

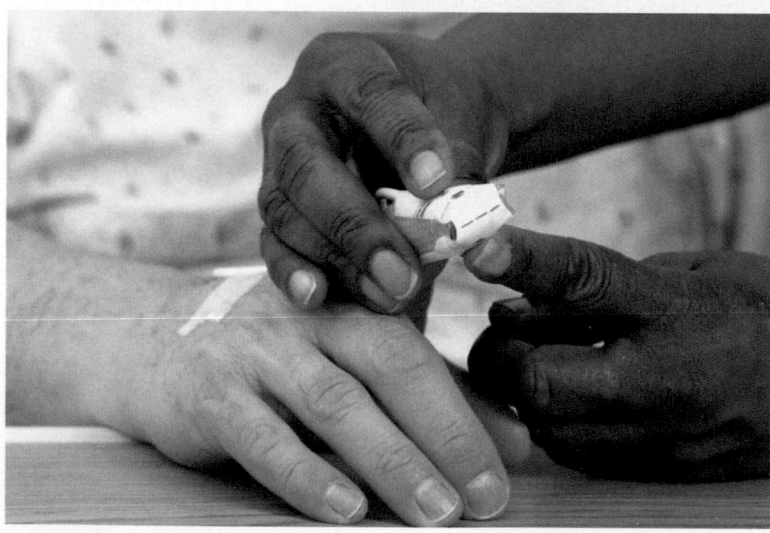

Clinical Assessment of Pulmonary Function.   A simple but informative way to assess the pulmonary function is "the walk test." Time an 8-foot walk at the patient's normal pace. Repeat the walk and note the faster time. Also observe the rate, effort, and sound of the patient's breathing.

Nondisabled older adults taking 5.6 seconds or longer are more likely to be disabled over time than those taking 3.1 seconds or fewer. Early intervention may prevent onset of subsequent disability.[12]

Forced Expiratory Time. This test assesses the expiratory phase of breathing, which is typically slowed in obstructive pulmonary disease. Ask the patient to take a deep breath in and then breathe out as quickly and completely as possible with mouth open. Listen over the trachea with the diaphragm of a stethoscope and time the audible expiration. Try to get three consistent readings, allowing a short rest between efforts if necessary.

Patients older than 60 years with a forced expiratory time of 6 to 8 seconds are twice as likely to have COPD.[13]

Identification of a Fractured Rib. Local pain and tenderness of one or more ribs raise the question of fracture. By anteroposterior compression of the chest, you can help to distinguish a fracture from soft-tissue injury. With one hand on the sternum and the other on the thoracic spine, squeeze the chest. Is this painful, and where?

An increase in the local pain (distant from your hands) suggests rib fracture rather than just soft-tissue injury.

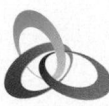

RECORDING YOUR FINDINGS

RECORDING THE PHYSICAL EXAMINATION—THE THORAX AND LUNGS

> "Thorax is symmetric with equal expansion. Lungs resonant. Anterior and posterior breath sounds clear bilaterally. Diaphragm descends 4 cm bilaterally."
>
> **OR**
>
> "Thorax symmetric with moderate kyphosis and increased AP diameter, decreased expansion. Lungs are hyperresonant. Breath sounds distant with delayed expiratory phase and scattered expiratory wheezes. Fremitus decreased; no bronchophony, egophony, or whispered pectoriloquy. Diaphragm descends 2 cm bilaterally."

Suggests *COPD*.[6–11]

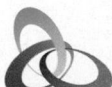

HEALTH PROMOTION AND COUNSELING

IMPORTANT TOPICS FOR HEALTH PROMOTION AND COUNSELING

- Tobacco cessation
- Immunizations

Tobacco Cessation. Despite declines in smoking over the past several decades, in 2008 20.6% of U.S. adults continue to smoke.[14] Smoking rates are highest among young adults 18 to 24 years. Approximately 80% of smokers start by 18 years, with one in five U.S. high school students reported smoking cigarettes in the last 30 days.[15] Smoking causes extensive risks of disease and accounts for one in five deaths each year in the United States.

● Adverse Effects of Smoking on Health and Disease

Condition	Increased Risk Compared with Nonsmokers
● Coronary artery disease	2–4 times higher
● Stroke	2–4 times higher
● COPD mortality	12–13 times higher
● Lung cancer mortality	23 times higher in men
	13 times higher in women

(Source: Centers for Disease Control and Prevention, DHHS. Smoking and tobacco use. Fact sheet. Health effects of cigarette smoking. Available at: http://www.cdc.gov/tobacco/data_statistics/Factsheets/health_effects.htm. Accessed March 27, 2011.

In addition, smoking contributes to many types of cancer and increases risk of infertility, preterm birth, low birth weight, and sudden infant death syndrome. Nonsmokers exposed to smoke also have increased risk of lung cancer, ear and respiratory infections, asthma, and residential fires.

Smoking is the leading preventable cause of death. Although a number of tests, such as helical computerized tomography, have been studied, screening for lung cancer is currently not recommended.[16] Instead, nurses should focus on prevention and cessation, especially in teenagers and pregnant women.[17] Health care providers should advise smokers to quit during every visit. This advice has been shown to raise quit rates by 30%.[18–19] Use the "5 A's" framework or the Stages of Change model (precontemplation, contemplation, preparation, action, maintenance)[20] to assess readiness to quit.

Nicotine is highly addicting, comparable to heroin and cocaine, and quitting tobacco use is difficult. Cognitive therapy techniques will help patients recognize signs of withdrawal such as irritability, difficulty concentrating, anxiety, and depressed mood.[18] Guide patients to better understand craving, triggers for smoking, and strategies for managing withdrawal, coping with stress, and preventing relapse. Combining counseling with pharmacotherapy is recommended. Three drugs have been shown to improve and sustain quit rates: nicotine replacement therapies; bupropion, a norepinephrine and dopamine reuptake inhibitor and nicotinic receptor antagonist; and more recently, varenicline, a nicotinic receptor partial agonist that stimulates dopamine release, thought to relieve craving.[21–22]

ASSESSING READINESS TO QUIT SMOKING: THE "5 A'S"

1. *Ask* about tobacco use.
2. *Advise* to quit through clear, personalized messages.
3. *Assess* willingness to quit.
4. *Assist* to quit.
5. *Arrange* follow-up and support.

(Source: U.S. Preventive Services Task Force. Counseling and Interventions to prevent tobacco use and tobacco caused Diseases in Adults and Pregnant Women: recommendation statement. Rockville, MD: Agency for Healthcare Research and Quality, 2009. Available at: http://www.uspreventiveservicestaskforce.org/uspstf09/tobacco/tobaccosum2.htm. (Accessed March 27, 2011.)

Immunizations (Adults). *Influenza* causes more than 36,000 deaths and 200,000 hospitalizations annually, especially during the late fall and winter, peaking in February.[23] The CDC Advisory Committee on Immunization Practices updates its recommendations for vaccination annually. Two types of vaccine are available: the "flu shot," an inactivated vaccine containing killed virus, and a nasal-spray vaccine containing attenuated live viruses, approved only for healthy people between 5 and 49 years. Because influenza viruses change from year to year, each vaccine contains three vaccine strains and is modified yearly. All people wishing to reduce risk of infection should be vaccinated, especially these groups:

- Adults with chronic pulmonary conditions and chronic medical illnesses, and adults who are immunosuppressed

- Residents of nursing homes and chronic care facilities

- Health care personnel

- Healthy household contacts and caregivers of children younger than 5 years and adults 50 years or older, particularly those with medical conditions placing them at higher risk for complications from influenza

Streptococcus pneumoniae causes approximately 175,000 cases of U.S. pneumococcal pneumonia each year; 25% to 30% of these cases are accompanied by sepsis.[24] Incubation is as short as 1 to 3 days, and fatalities are 5%. There are an additional 3,000 to 6,000 cases of pneumococcal meningitis annually, many in children. The two types of *pneumococcal vaccine*, polysaccharide and conjugated, are both inactivated. The CDC recommends the pneumococcal vaccine for these groups:

- All adults 65 years and older

- People between the ages of 2 and 64 with chronic illnesses specifically associated with increased risk from pneumococcal infection, such as sickle cell anemia, cardiovascular and pulmonary disease, diabetes, cirrhosis, or leaks of cerebrospinal fluid

- Anyone with or about to receive a cochlear implant

- Persons 2 years or older who are immunocompromised, including those with HIV infection or AIDS and those receiving steroids, radiation, or chemotherapy

- Alaska natives of certain Native American groups

- Healthy children older than 6 months

TABLE
13-1

Dyspnea[25]

Problem	Process	Timing
Left-Sided Heart Failure *(left ventricular failure or mitral stenosis)*	Elevated pressure in pulmonary capillary bed with movement of fluid into interstitial spaces and alveoli, decreased compliance (increased stiffness) of the lungs, increased work of breathing	Dyspnea may progress slowly, or suddenly as in acute pulmonary edema.
Chronic Bronchitis*[26]	Excessive mucus production in bronchi, followed by chronic obstruction of airways	Chronic productive cough followed by slowly progressive dyspnea
Chronic Obstructive Pulmonary Disease (COPD)*[6–11]	Overdistention of air spaces distal to terminal bronchioles, with destruction of alveolar septa and chronic obstruction of the airways	Slowly progressive dyspnea; relatively mild cough later
Asthma[27]	Bronchial hyperresponsiveness involving release of inflammatory mediators, increased airway secretions, and bronchoconstriction	Acute episodes, separated by symptom-free periods. Nocturnal episodes common
Diffuse Interstitial Lung Diseases *(such as sarcoidosis, widespread neoplasms, asbestosis, and idiopathic pulmonary fibrosis)*	Abnormal and widespread infiltration of cells, fluid, and collagen into interstitial spaces between alveoli. Many causes	Progressive dyspnea, which varies in its rate of development with the cause
Pneumonia[28]	Inflammation of lung parenchyma from the respiratory bronchioles to the alveoli	An acute illness, timing varies with the causative agent
Spontaneous Pneumothorax	Leakage of air into pleural space through blebs on visceral pleura, with resulting partial or complete collapse of the lung	Sudden onset of dyspnea
Acute Pulmonary Embolism[29]	Sudden occlusion of all or part of pulmonary arterial tree by a blood clot that usually originates in deep veins of legs or pelvis	Sudden onset of dyspnea
Anxiety With Hyperventilation	Overbreathing, with resultant respiratory alkalosis and fall in the partial pressure of carbon dioxide in the blood	Episodic, often recurrent

*Chronic bronchitis and chronic obstructive pulmonary disease (COPD) may coexist.

Factors That Aggravate	Factors That Relieve	Associated Symptoms	Setting
Exertion, lying down	Rest, sitting up, though dyspnea may become persistent	Often cough, orthopnea, paroxysmal nocturnal dyspnea; sometimes wheezing	History of heart disease or its predisposing factors
Exertion, inhaled irritants, respiratory infections	Expectoration; rest, though dyspnea may become persistent	Chronic productive cough, recurrent respiratory infections; wheezing may develop	History of smoking, air pollutants, recurrent respiratory infections
Exertion	Rest, though dyspnea may become persistent	Cough, with scant mucoid sputum	History of smoking, air pollutants, sometimes a familial deficiency in α_1-antitrypsin
Variable, including allergens, irritants, respiratory infections, exercise, and emotion	Separation from aggravating factors	Wheezing, cough, tightness in chest	Environmental and emotional conditions
Exertion	Rest, though dyspnea may become persistent	Often weakness, fatigue. Cough less common than in other lung diseases	Varied. Exposure to one of many substances may be causative.
		Pleuritic pain, cough, sputum, fever, though not necessarily present	Varied
		Pleuritic pain, cough	Often a previously healthy young adult
		Often none. Retrosternal oppressive pain if the occlusion is massive. Pleuritic pain, cough, and hemoptysis may follow an embolism if pulmonary infarction ensues. Symptoms of anxiety (see below)	Postpartum or postoperative periods; prolonged bed rest; congestive heart failure, chronic lung disease, and fractures of hip or leg; deep venous thrombosis (often not clinically apparent)
More often occurs at rest than after exercise. An upsetting event may not be evident.	Breathing in and out of a paper or plastic bag sometimes helps the associated symptoms.	Sighing, lightheadedness, numbness or tingling of the hands and feet, palpitations, chest pain	Other manifestations of anxiety may be present.

TABLE
13-2

Cough[30] and Hemoptysis*

Problem	Cough and Sputum	Associated Symptoms and Setting
Acute Inflammation		
Laryngitis	Dry cough (without sputum), may become productive of variable amounts of sputum	An acute, fairly minor illness with hoarseness. Often associated with viral nasopharyngitis
Tracheobronchitis	Dry cough, may become productive	An acute, often viral illness, with burning retrosternal discomfort
Mycoplasma and Viral Pneumonias[28]	Dry hacking cough, often becoming productive of mucoid sputum	An acute febrile illness, often with malaise, headache, and possibly dyspnea
Bacterial Pneumonias[28]	Pneumococcal: sputum mucoid or purulent; may be blood streaked, diffusely pinkish, or rusty	An acute illness with chills, high fever, dyspnea, and chest pain. Often preceded by acute upper respiratory infection
	Klebsiella: similar; or sticky, red, and jelly-like	Typically occurs in older alcoholic men
Chronic Inflammation		
Postnasal Drip	Chronic cough; sputum mucoid or mucopurulent	Repeated attempts to clear the throat. Postnasal discharge may be sensed by patient or seen in posterior pharynx. Associated with chronic rhinitis, with or without sinusitis
Chronic Bronchitis[26]	Chronic cough; sputum mucoid to purulent, may be blood streaked or even bloody	Often long-standing cigarette smoking. Recurrent superimposed infections. Wheezing and dyspnea may develop.
Bronchiectasis[31]	Chronic cough; sputum purulent, often copious and foul smelling; may be blood streaked or bloody	Recurrent bronchopulmonary infections common; sinusitis may coexist.
Pulmonary Tuberculosis[32]	Cough dry or sputum that is mucoid or purulent; may be blood streaked or bloody	Early, no symptoms. Later, anorexia, weight loss, fatigue, fever, and night sweats
Lung Abscess	Sputum purulent and foul smelling; may be bloody	A febrile illness. Often poor dental hygiene and a prior episode of impaired consciousness
Asthma[27]	Cough, with thick mucoid sputum, especially near end of an attack	Episodic wheezing and dyspnea, but cough may occur alone. Often a history of allergy
Gastroesophageal Reflux	Chronic cough, especially at night or early in the morning	Wheezing, especially at night (often mistaken for asthma), early morning hoarseness, and repeated attempts to clear the throat. Often a history of heartburn and regurgitation
Neoplasm		
Cancer of the Lung	Cough dry to productive; sputum may be blood streaked or bloody	Usually a long history of cigarette smoking. Associated manifestations are numerous.
Cardiovascular Disorders		
Left Ventricular Failure or Mitral Stenosis	Often dry, especially on exertion or at night; may progress to the pink frothy sputum of pulmonary edema or to frank hemoptysis	Dyspnea, orthopnea, paroxysmal nocturnal dyspnea
Pulmonary Emboli[29]	Dry to productive; may be dark, bright red, or mixed with blood	Dyspnea, anxiety, chest pain, fever; factors that predispose to deep venous thrombosis
Irritating Particles, Chemicals, or Gases	Variable. There may be a latent period between exposure and symptoms.	Exposure to irritants. Eyes, nose, and throat may be affected.

*Characteristics of hemoptysis are printed in red.

TABLE
13-3

Chest Pain

Problem	Process	Location	Quality	Severity	Timing	Factors That Aggravate	Factors That Relieve	Associated Symptoms
Pulmonary								
Tracheobronch- itis	Inflammation of trachea and large bronchi	Upper sternal or on either side of the sternum	Burning	Mild to moderate	Variable	Coughing	Lying on the involved side may relieve it.	Cough
Pleuritic Pain	Inflammation of the parietal pleura, as in pleurisy, pneumonia, pulmonary infarction, or neoplasm	Chest wall overlying the process	Sharp, knife-like	Often severe	Persistent	Inspiration, coughing, movements of the trunk		Of the underlying illness
Cardiovascular								
Angina Pectoris	Temporary myocardial ischemia, usually secondary to coronary atherosclerosis	Retrosternal or across the anterior chest, sometimes radiating to the shoulders, arms, neck, lower jaw, or upper abdomen	Pressing, squeezing, tight, heavy, occasionally burning	Mild to moderate, sometimes perceived as discomfort rather than pain	Usually 1–3 min but up to 10 min. Prolonged episodes up to 20 min	Exertion, especially in the cold; meals; emotional stress. May occur at rest	Rest, nitroglycerin	Sometimes dyspnea, nausea, sweating
Myocardial Infarction	Prolonged myocardial ischemia, resulting in irreversible muscle damage or necrosis	Same as in angina	Same as in angina	Often but not always a severe pain	20 min to several hours			Nausea, vomiting, sweating, weakness
Pericarditis	• Irritation of parietal pleura adjacent to the pericardium	Precordial, may radiate to the tip of the shoulder and to the neck	Sharp, knife-like	Often severe	Persistent	Breathing, changing position, coughing, lying down, sometimes swallowing	Sitting forward may relieve it.	Of the underlying illness
	• Mechanism unclear	Retrosternal	Crushing	Severe	Persistent			

(table continues on page 328)

TABLE
13-3
Chest Pain (continued)

Problem	Process	Location	Quality	Severity	Timing	Factors That Aggravate	Factors That Relieve	Associated Symptoms
Dissecting Aortic Aneurysm	A splitting within the layers of the aortic wall, allowing passage of blood to dissect a channel	Anterior chest, radiating to the neck, back, or abdomen	Ripping, tearing	Very severe	Abrupt onset, early peak, persistent for hours or more	Hypertension		Of the underlying illness Syncope, hemiplegia, paraplegia

Gastrointestinal and Other

Problem	Process	Location	Quality	Severity	Timing	Factors That Aggravate	Factors That Relieve	Associated Symptoms
Reflex Esophagitis	Inflammation of the esophageal mucosa by reflux of gastric acid	Retrosternal, may radiate to the back	Burning, may be squeezing	Mild to severe	Variable	Large meal; bending over, lying down	Antacids, sometimes belching	Sometimes regurgitation, dysphagia
Diffuse Esophageal Spasm	Motor dysfunction of the esophageal muscle	Retrosternal, may radiate to the back, arms, and jaw	Usually squeezing	Mild to severe	Variable	Swallowing of food or cold liquid; emotional stress	Sometimes nitroglycerin	Dysphagia
Chest Wall Pain, Costochondritis	Variable, often unclear	Often below the left breast or along the costal cartilages; also elsewhere	Stabbing, sticking, or dull, aching	Variable	Fleeting to hours or days	Movement of chest, trunk, arms		Often local tenderness
Anxiety	Unclear	Precordial, below the left breast, or across the anterior chest	Stabbing, sticking, or dull, aching	Variable	Fleeting to hours or days	May follow effort, emotional stress		Breathlessness, palpitations, weakness, anxiety

Note: Remember that chest pain may be referred from extrathoracic structures such as the neck (*arthritis*) and abdomen (*biliary colic, acute cholecystitis*). Pleural pain may be from abdominal conditions such as *subdiaphragmatic abscess*.

TABLE 13-4

Deformities of the Thorax

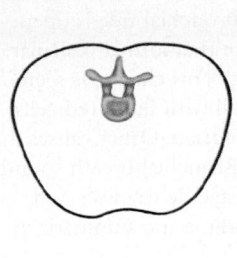
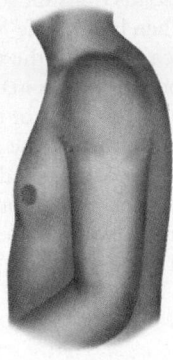

Normal Adult

The thorax in the normal adult is wider than it is deep. Its lateral diameter is larger than its anteroposterior diameter.

Funnel Chest (*Pectus Excavatum*)

Note depression in the lower portion of the sternum. Compression of the heart and great vessels may cause murmurs.

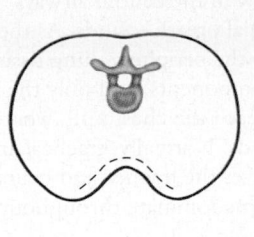
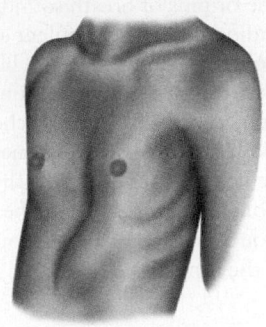

Depressed costal cartilages

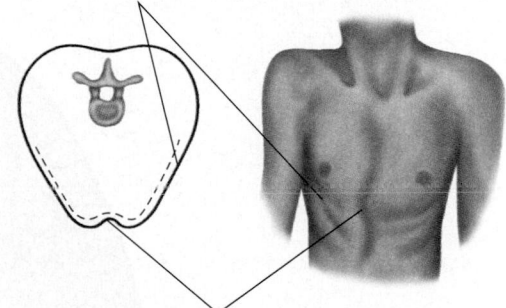

Anteriorly displaced sternum

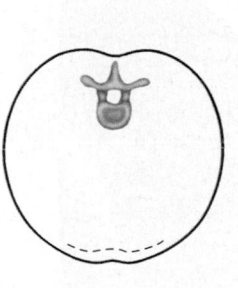
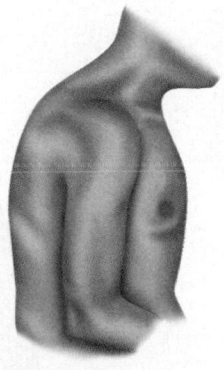

Barrel Chest

There is an increased anteroposterior diameter. This shape is normal during infancy, and often accompanies aging and chronic obstructive pulmonary disease.

Pigeon Chest (*Pectus Carinatum*)

The sternum is displaced anteriorly, increasing the anteroposterior diameter. The costal cartilages adjacent to the protruding sternum are depressed.

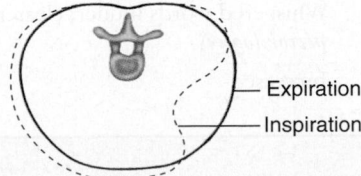

Expiration
Inspiration

Traumatic Flail Chest

Multiple rib fractures may result in paradoxical movements of the thorax. As descent of the diaphragm decreases intrathoracic pressure, on inspiration the injured area caves inward; on expiration, it moves outward.

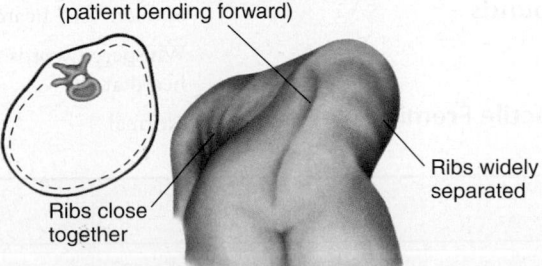

Spinal convexity to the right (patient bending forward)

Ribs widely separated

Ribs close together

Thoracic Kyphoscoliosis

Abnormal spinal curvatures and vertebral rotation deform the chest. Distortion of the underlying lungs may make interpretation of lung findings very difficult.

TABLE
13-5

Normal and Altered Breath and Voice Sounds

The origins of breath sounds are still unclear. According to leading theories, turbulent air flow in the central airways produces the tracheal and bronchial breath sounds. As these sounds pass through the lungs to the periphery, lung tissue filters out their higher-pitched components, and only the soft and lower-pitched components reach the chest wall, where they are heard as vesicular breath sounds. Normally, tracheal and bronchial sounds may be heard over the trachea and mainstem bronchi; vesicular breath sounds predominate throughout most of the lungs.

Fluids and solids transmit sound and vibration waves better than air. When lung tissue loses its air, it transmits high-pitched sounds much better. If the tracheobronchial tree is open, bronchial breath sounds may replace the normal vesicular sounds over airless areas of the lung. This change is seen in lobar pneumonia when the alveoli fill with fluid, red cells, and white cells—a process called *consolidation*. Other causes include pulmonary edema or hemorrhage. Bronchial breath sounds usually correlate with an increase in tactile fremitus and transmitted voice sounds. These findings are summarized below.

	Normal Air-Filled Lung	**Airless Lung, as in Lobar Pneumonia**
	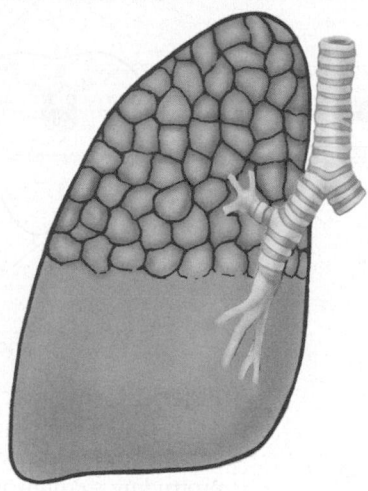	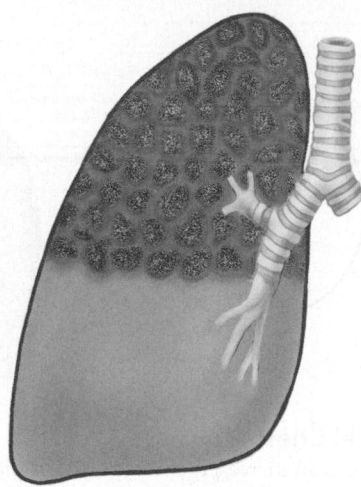
Breath Sounds	Predominantly vesicular	Bronchial or bronchovesicular over the involved area
Transmitted Voice Sounds	Spoken words muffled and indistinct Spoken "ee" heard as "ee" Whispered words faint and indistinct, if heard at all	Spoken words louder, clearer (*bronchophony*) Spoken "ee" heard as "ay" (*egophony*) Whispered words louder, clearer (*whispered pectoriloquy*)
Tactile Fremitus	Normal	Increased

TABLE
13-6

Adventitious (Added) Lung Sounds: Causes and Qualities[2–5]

Crackles

Crackles have two leading explanations. (1) They result from a series of tiny explosions when small airways, deflated during expiration, pop open during inspiration. This mechanism probably explains the late inspiratory crackles of interstitial lung disease and early congestive heart failure. (2) Crackles result from air bubbles flowing through secretions or lightly closed airways during respiration. This mechanism probably explains at least some coarse crackles.

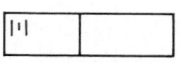

Inspiration   Expiration

Late inspiratory crackles may begin in the first half of inspiration but must continue into late inspiration. They are usually fine and fairly profuse, and persist from breath to breath. They appear first at the bases of the lungs, spread upward as the condition worsens, and shift to dependent regions with changes in posture. Causes include *interstitial lung disease* (such as fibrosis) and early *congestive heart failure*.

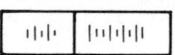

Early inspiratory crackles appear and end soon after the start of inspiration. They are often coarse and relatively few in number. Expiratory crackles are sometimes associated. Causes include *chronic bronchitis* and *asthma*.

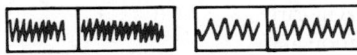

Midinspiratory and expiratory crackles are heard in *bronchiectasis* but are not specific for this diagnosis. Wheezes and rhonchi may be associated.

Wheezes and Rhonchi

Wheezes occur when air flows rapidly through bronchi that are narrowed nearly to the point of closure. They are often audible at the mouth as well as through the chest wall. Causes of wheezes throughout the chest include *asthma, chronic bronchitis, COPD,* and *congestive heart failure* (cardiac asthma). In *asthma*, wheezes may be heard only in expiration or in both phases of the respiratory cycle. Rhonchi suggest secretions in the larger airways. In chronic bronchitis, wheezes and rhonchi often clear with coughing.

Occasionally in severe obstructive pulmonary disease, the patient is unable to force enough air through the narrowed bronchi to produce wheezing. The resulting *silent chest* is ominous and warrants immediate attention.

Persistent localized wheezing suggests partial obstruction of a bronchus, as by a tumor or foreign body. It may be inspiratory, expiratory, or both.

Stridor

A high-pitched harsh sound that is entirely or predominantly inspiratory is called *stridor*. It is often heard without a stethoscope louder in the neck than over the chest wall. It indicates a partial obstruction of the larynx or trachea, and demands immediate attention. It is sometimes described as a seal's bark.

Pleural Rub

Inflamed and roughened pleural surfaces grate against each other as they are momentarily and repeatedly delayed by increased friction. These movements produce creaking sounds known as a *pleural rub* (or pleural friction rub).

Pleural rubs resemble crackles acoustically, although they are produced by different pathologic processes. The sounds may be discrete, but sometimes are so numerous that they merge into a seemingly continuous sound. A rub is usually confined to a relatively small area of the chest wall, and typically is heard in both phases of respiration. When inflamed pleural surfaces are separated by fluid, the rub often disappears.

TABLE
13-7

Physical Findings in Selected Chest Disorders

The red boxes in this table suggest a framework for clinical assessment. Start with the three boxes under Percussion Note: resonant, dull, and hyperresonant. Then move from each of these to other boxes that emphasize some of the key differences among various conditions. The changes described vary with the extent and severity of the disorder. Abnormalities deep in the chest usually produce fewer signs than superficial ones, and may cause no signs at all. Use the table for the direction of typical changes, not for absolute distinctions.

Condition	Percussion Note	Trachea	Breath Sounds	Adventitious Sounds	Tactile Fremitus and Transmitted Voice Sounds
Normal The tracheobronchial tree and alveoli are clear; pleurae are thin and close together; mobility of the chest wall is unimpaired.	**Resonant**	Midline	Vesicular, except perhaps bronchovesicular and bronchial sounds over the large bronchi and trachea, respectively	None, except perhaps a few transient inspiratory crackles at the bases of the lungs	Normal
Chronic Bronchitis The bronchi are chronically inflamed and a productive cough is present. Airway obstruction may develop.	**Resonant**	Midline	Vesicular (normal)	None; or scattered coarse *crackles* in early inspiration and perhaps expiration; or *wheezes* or *rhonchi*	Normal
Left-Sided Heart Failure *(Early)* Increased pressure in the pulmonary veins causes congestion and interstitial edema (around the alveoli); bronchial mucosa may become edematous.	**Resonant**	Midline	Vesicular	*Late inspiratory crackles* in the dependent portions of the lungs; possibly *wheezes*	Normal
Consolidation Alveoli fill with fluid or blood cells, as in pneumonia, pulmonary edema, or pulmonary hemorrhage.	**Dull** over the airless area	Midline	*Bronchial* over the involved area	*Late inspiratory crackles* over the involved area	*Increased* over the involved area, with *bronchophony, egophony,* and *whispered pectoriloquy*
Atelectasis *(Lobar Obstruction)* When a plug in a mainstem bronchus (as from mucus or a foreign object) obstructs air flow, affected lung tissue collapses into an airless state.	**Dull** over the airless area	May be *shifted toward involved side*	*Usually absent* when bronchial plug persists. Exceptions include right upper lobe atelectasis, where adjacent tracheal sounds may be transmitted.	None	Usually absent when the bronchial plug persists. In exceptions (e.g., right upper lobe atelectasis) may be increased

Condition	Percussion Note	Trachea	Breath Sounds	Adventitious Sounds	Tactile Fremitus and Transmitted Voice Sounds
Pleural Effusion Fluid accumulates in the pleural space and separates air-filled lung from the chest wall, blocking the transmission of sound.	**Dull** to flat over the fluid	*Shifted toward opposite side* in a large effusion	*Decreased to absent,* but bronchial breath sounds may be heard near top of large effusion.	None, except a *possible pleural* rub	*Decreased to absent, but may be increased* toward the top of a large effusion
Pneumothorax When air leaks into the pleural space, usually unilaterally, the lung recoils from the chest wall. Pleural air blocks transmission of sound.	**Hyperresonant** or tympanitic over the pleural air	*Shifted toward opposite side* if much air	*Decreased to absent* over the pleural air	None, except a *possible pleural rub*	*Decreased to absent* over the pleural air
Chronic Obstructive Pulmonary Disease (COPD) Slowly progressive disorder in which the distal air spaces enlarge and lungs become hyperinflated. Chronic bronchitis is often associated.	Diffusely **hyperresonant**	Midline	*Decreased to absent*	None, or the crackles, wheezes, and rhonchi of associated chronic bronchitis	*Decreased*
Asthma Widespread narrowing of the tracheobronchial tree diminishes air flow to a fluctuating degree. During attacks, air flow decreases further, and lungs hyperinflate.	**Resonant** to diffusely **hyperresonant**	Midline	*Often obscured by wheezes*	*Wheezes, possibly crackles*	*Decreased*

BIBLIOGRAPHY

CITATIONS

1. McGee S. Evidence-Based Physical Diagnosis, 2nd ed. Philadelphia: Saunders: 314, 2007.

2. Loudon R, Murphy LH. Lungs sounds. Am Rev Respir Dis 130(4):663–673, 1994.

3. Epler GR, Carrrington CB, Gaensler EA. Crackles (rales) in the interstitial pulmonary diseases. Chest 73(3):333–339, 1978.

4. Nath AR, Capel LH. Inspiratory crackles and mechanical events of breathing. Thorax 29(6):695–698, 1974.

5. Nath AR, Capel LH. Lung crackles in bronchiectasis. Thorax 35(9):694–699, 1980.

6. Badgett RG, Tanaka DJ, Hunt DK, et al. Can moderate chronic obstructive pulmonary disease be diagnosed by historical and physical findings alone? Am J Med 94(2):188–196, 1993.

7. Holleman DR, Simel DL. Does the clinical examination predict airflow limitation? JAMA 273(4):63–68, 1995.

8. Straus SE, McAlister FA, Sackett DL, et al. The accuracy of patient history, wheezing, and laryngeal measurements in diagnosing obstructive airway disease. JAMA 283(14):1853–1857, 2000.

9. Pauwels RA, Buist AS, Calverley PM, et al. GOLD Scientific Committee. Global strategy for the diagnosis, management, and prevention of chronic obstructive pulmonary disease: NHLBI/WHO Global Initiative for Chronic Obstructive Lung Disease (GOLD) workshop summary. Am J Respir Crit Care Med 163(5):1256–1276, 2001.

10. Sin DD, McAlister FA, Man WEP, et al. Contemporary management of chronic obstructive pulmonary disease: scientific review. JAMA 290(17):2310–2312, 2003.

11. Sutherland ER, Cherniack RM. Management of chronic obstructive pulmonary disease. N Engl J Med 350(26):2689–2697, 2004.

12. Gurlanik JM, Ferrucci L, Simonsick EM, et al. Lower extremity function in persons over the age of 70 years as a predictor of subsequent disability. N Engl J Med 332(9):556–561, 1995.

13. Schapira RM, Schapira MM, Funahashi A, et al. The value of the forced expiratory time in the physical diagnosis of obstructive airway disease. JAMA 270(6):731–736, 1993.

14. CDC, MMWR: Cigarette Smoking Among Adults and Trends in Smoking Cessation—United States, 2008. Available at: http://www.cdc.gov/mmwr/preview/mmwrhtml/mm5844a2.htm. Accessed April 10, 2011.

15. CDC, MMWR: Vital Signs: Current Cigarette Smoking Among Adults Aged ≥18 Years—United States, 2009, September 10, 2010 / 59(35);1135–1140. Available at: http://www.cdc.gov/mmwr/preview/mmwrhtml/mm5935a3.htm?s_cid=mm5935a3_w. Accessed April 10, 2011.

16. U.S. Preventive Services Task Force. *Lung Cancer Screening*, Topic Page. May 2004. http://www.uspreventiveservicestaskforce.org/uspstf/uspslung.htm. Accessed March 27, 2011.

17. U.S. Public Health Service. Clinical Practice Guideline: Treating tobacco use and dependence: 2008 Update. May 2008. Available at: http://www.surgeongeneral.gov/tobacco/treating_tobacco_use08.pdf. Accessed April 10, 2011.

18. Centers for Disease Control and Prevention, DHHS. Fact sheet: smoking and tobacco use. Cessation. Available at: http://www.cdc.gov/tobacco/data_statistics/Factsheets/cessation2.htm. Accessed April 10, 2011.

19. Ranney L, Melvin C, Lux L, et al. Systematic review: smoking cessation intervention strategies for adults and adults in special populations. Ann Intern Med 145(11):845–856, 2006.

20. Norcross JC, Prochaska JO. Using the stages of change. Harvard Mental Health Letter May 5–7, 2002.

21. Varenicline (Chantix) for tobacco dependence. Med Lett Drugs Ther 48(1241–1242):66–68, 2006.

22. Cahill K, Stead LF, Lancaster T. Nicotine receptor partial agonists for smoking cessation. Cochrane Database of Systematic Reviews, 2011 (2).

23. Advisory Committee on Immunization Practices (ACIP), Centers for Disease Control and Prevention. Prevention and control of influenza: recommendations of the ACIP. MMWR Morb Mortal Wkly Rep 56(RR-6):1–54, 2007.

24. Centers for Disease Control and Prevention. Vaccines and preventable diseases: pneumococcal vaccination. Available at: http://www.cdc.gov/vaccines/vpdvac/pneumo/default.htm# recs. Accessed April 10, 2011.

25. American Thoracic Society. Dyspnea—mechanisms, assessment, and management: a consensus statement. Am J Respir Crit Care Med 159(1):321–340, 1999.

26. Wenzel RP, Fowler AA. Acute bronchitis. N Engl J Med 355(20):2125–2130, 2006.

27. Panettieri RA. In the clinic. Asthma. Ann Intern Med 146(11):ITC6-1–ITC6-14, 2007.

28. Metlay JP, Kapoor WN, Fine MJ. Does this patient have community-acquired pneumonia? Diagnosing pneumonia by history and physical examination. JAMA 378(17):1440–1445, 1997.

29. Chunilal SD, Eikelboom JW, Attia J, et al. Does this patient have pulmonary embolism? JAMA 290(21):2849–2858, 2003.

30. Irwin RS, Madison JM. The diagnosis and treatment of cough. N Engl J Med 3432(3):1715–1721, 2000.

31. Barker A. Bronchiectasis. N Engl J Med 346(18):1383–1393, 2002.

32. American Thoracic Society. Diagnostic standards/classification of TB in adults and children. Am J Respir Crit Care Med 161:1376–1395, 2000.

33. Ware LB, Matthay MA. Acute pulmonary edema. N Engl J Med 353(26):2788–2796, 2005.

ADDITIONAL REFERENCES

Examination of the Lungs

Bettancourt PE, DelBono EA, Speigelman D, et al. Clinical utility of chest auscultation in common pulmonary disease. Am J Resp Crit Care Med 150:1921, 1994.

BIBLIOGRAPHY

Committee on Infectious Diseases. Recommendations for Prevention and Control of Influenza in Children, 2010–2011. Pediatrics 126(4):816–826, October 2010. Available at: http://pediatrics.aappublications.org/content/126/4/816.1.full.html. Accessed June 12. 2011.

Cugell DW. Lung sound nomenclature. Am Rev Respir Dis 136:1016, 1987.

Koster MEY, Baughmann RP, Loudon RG. Continuous adventitious lung sounds. J Asthma 27:237, 1990.

Kraman SS. Lung sounds for the clinician. Arch Intern Med 146:1411, 1986.

Lehrer S. Understanding Lung Sounds, 3rd ed. Philadelphia: WB Saunders, 2002.

Pulmonary Conditions

Chung KF, Pavord ID. Prevalence, pathogenesis, and causes of chronic cough. Lancet 371(9621):1364–1374, 2008.

Eder W, Ege MJ, Mutius E. The asthma epidemic. N Engl J Med 355(21):2226–2235, 2006.

Fiore MC, Jaén CR, Baker TB, et al. Treating Tobacco Use and Dependence: 2008 Update. Rockville, MD: U.S. Department of Health and Human Services, May 2008. Available at: http://www.ahrq.gov/path/tobacco.htm#Clinic. Accessed April 10, 2011.

Ware LB, Matthay MA. Acute pulmonary edema. N Engl J Med 353(26):2788–2796, 2005.

The Cardiovascular System

The student will:

1. Describe the structure and functions of the heart and great vessels.
2. Identify the landmarks and key auscultation sites of the precordium.
3. Describe the electrical conduction system of the heart.
4. Explain the normal electrocardiogram waveform pattern.
5. Describe the two phases of the mechanical heart cycle.
6. Describe the normal heart sounds and their origin.
7. Describe extra heart sounds and their origin.
8. Obtain an accurate history of the cardiovascular system.
9. Appropriately prepare and position the patient for the cardiovascular examination.
10. Describe the equipment necessary to perform a cardiovascular examination.
11. Inspect, palpate, and auscultate the jugular veins and carotid arteries of the neck.
12. Inspect, palpate, and auscultate the precordium to evaluate cardiovascular status.
13. Discuss risk factors for coronary heart disease.
14. Discuss risk reduction and health promotion strategies to reduce coronary heart disease.

The cardiovascular system is made up of the heart and blood vessels. The main functions of this system are delivering oxygen and nutrients to the cells of the body, removing waste products, and maintaining perfusion to the organs and tissues. The heart is the pump that drives circulation of the blood and the blood vessels are the pathways to and from the tissues. To assess a patient's cardiovascular health the nurse gathers a thorough focused health history and uses this information to perform an appropriate physical examination of the patient's heart and blood vessels. This chapter will discuss the assessment of the heart and great vessels, aorta, pulmonary artery, vena cavae, and pulmonary veins. Chapter 15 will cover the assessment of the peripheral blood vessels and lymph system.

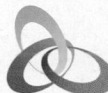

ANATOMY AND PHYSIOLOGY

In order to perform an accurate assessment of the cardiovascular system the nurse must have a thorough understanding of the anatomy and physiology of the system including the heart muscle, chambers, valves, great vessels, conduction system of the heart, peripheral arteries and veins, capillaries, and lymph system.

Location of the Heart and Great Vessels

The heart is a hollow muscular organ a little larger than the patient's fist. It lies in the pericardial cavity in the mediastinum under the sternum and between the 2nd and 5th intercostal spaces. About two thirds of the heart lies to the left of the midline of the sternum.

The area of the exterior chest that overlays the heart and great vessels is called the *precordium*. It is helpful to visualize the underlying structures of the heart as you examine the precordium. Note that the heart is rotated so that the *right ventricle* occupies most of the anterior cardiac surface. This chamber and the pulmonary artery form a wedge-shaped structure behind and to the left of the sternum, outlined in black.

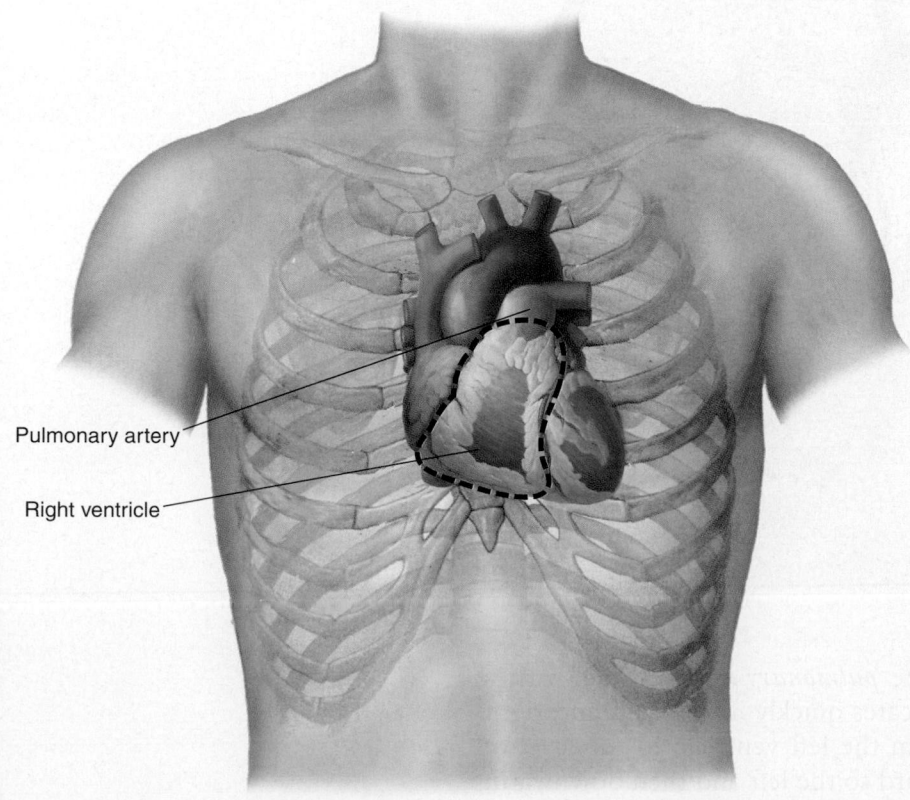

Pulmonary artery

Right ventricle

The inferior border of the right ventricle lies at the junction of the sternum and the xiphoid process. The right ventricle narrows as it rises to meet the pulmonary artery just below the sternal angle. This is called the *"base of the heart"* and is located at the right and left 2nd intercostal spaces next to the sternum.

The *left ventricle,* behind the right ventricle and to the left, outlined below in black, forms the left margin of the heart. Its tapered inferior tip is often termed the *cardiac "apex."* It is clinically important because it produces the apical impulse, identified during palpation of the precordium as the *point of maximal impulse,* or *PMI.* This impulse locates the left border of the heart and is normally found in the 5th intercostal space 7 cm to 9 cm lateral to the midsternal line, at or just medial to the left midclavicular line. The PMI may not be readily felt in a healthy patient with a normal heart, however.

The apical impulse is easily palpated in children and slender adults, but as the anteroposterior chest diameter increases it becomes more difficult to feel. Obesity or a thick chest wall also makes palpation of the apical impulse difficult.[1]

- In supine patients the *diameter of the PMI* may be as large as a quarter, approximately 1 cm to 2.5 cm. A PMI >2.5 cm is evidence of left ventricular hypertrophy (LVH), or enlargement.

- Similarly, *displacement of the PMI* lateral to the midclavicular line or >10 cm lateral to the midsternal line also suggests LVH, or enlargement.

Note that in some patients the most prominent precordial impulse may not be at the apex of the left ventricle. For example, in patients with chronic obstructive pulmonary disease, the most prominent palpable impulse or PMI may be in the xiphoid or epigastric area as a result of *right ventricular hypertrophy.*

Aorta
Pulmonary artery
Right pulmonary artery
Left pulmonary artery
Left ventricle
Superior vena cava
Right atrium
Apical impulse
Right ventricle

Above the heart lie the *great vessels.* The *pulmonary artery,* which carries unoxygenated blood to the lungs, bifurcates quickly into its left and right branches. The *aorta* curves upward from the left ventricle to the level of the sternal angle, where it arches backward to the left and then downward.

On the medial border, the *superior* and *inferior venae cavae* channel venous blood from the upper and lower portions of the body, respectively, into the right atrium.

The Heart Wall

The wall of the heart is composed of several layers. The *pericardium,* the outermost layer, is composed of two tough fibrous membranes that enclose and protect the heart. A few milliliters of serous fluid between the membranes provide lubrication for smooth movement of the heart. The *myocardium* is the heart muscle that does the pumping. The *endocardium* is a thin, smooth layer of endothelial tissue that lines the inner surface of the chambers and valves of the heart.

Cardiac Chambers, Valves, and Circulation

Circulation through the heart is shown in the diagram which identifies the cardiac chambers, valves, and direction of blood flow. Blood from the body's organs and tissues returns to the heart via the superior and inferior vena cavae; empties into the right atrium; and travels through the tricuspid valve into the right ventricle, which pumps it through the pulmonary valve into the pulmonary artery. After passage through the lungs the blood returns to the left atrium through the pulmonary veins and passes through the mitral valve into the left ventricle, where it is pumped into the aorta for distribution of oxygenated blood throughout the body. Because of their positions, the *tricuspid* and *mitral valves* are often called *atrioventricular valves.* The *aortic* and *pulmonic valves* are called *semilunar valves* because each of their leaflets is shaped like a half moon. Although this diagram shows all valves in an open position, they do not open simultaneously in the living heart.

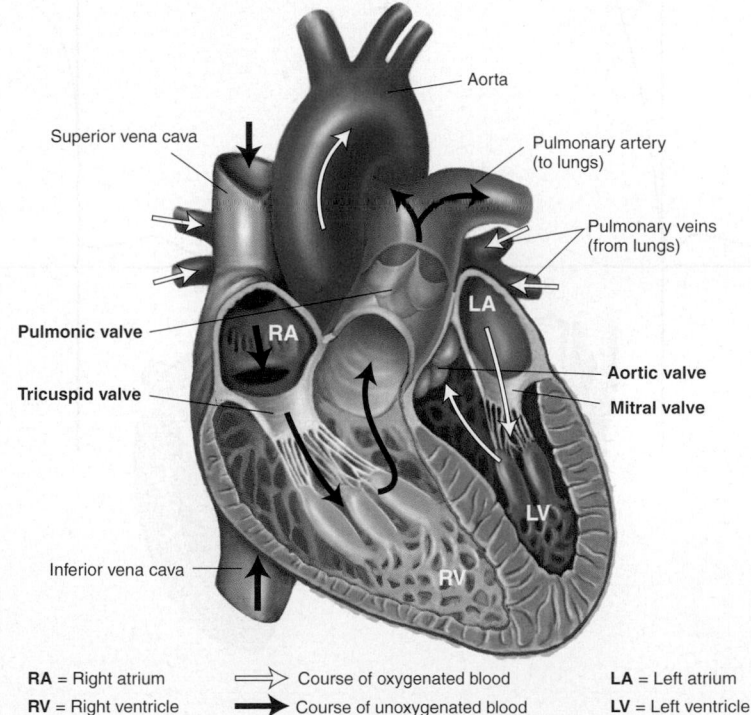

Aorta
Superior vena cava
Pulmonary artery (to lungs)
Pulmonary veins (from lungs)
LA
Pulmonic valve
RA
Tricuspid valve
Aortic valve
Mitral valve
LV
Inferior vena cava
RV

RA = Right atrium	⟹ Course of oxygenated blood	**LA** = Left atrium
RV = Right ventricle	⟶ Course of unoxygenated blood	**LV** = Left ventricle

As the heart valves close, the heart sounds arise from vibrations emanating from the leaflets, the adjacent cardiac structures, and the flow of blood. Study carefully the positions and movements of the valves in relation to events in the cardiac cycle in order to understand the heart sounds.

The Cardiac Cycle

Ventricular Pressures.   The heart serves as a pump that generates varying pressures as its chambers contract and relax. *Systole is the period of ventricular contraction*. In the diagram below, pressure in the left ventricle rises from less than 5 mm Hg in its resting state to a normal peak of 120 mm Hg. After the ventricle ejects much of its blood into the aorta, the pressure levels off and starts to fall. *Diastole is the period of ventricular relaxation*. Ventricular pressure falls to below 5 mm Hg, and blood flows from atrium to ventricle. Late in diastole, ventricular pressure rises slightly during inflow of blood from atrial contraction.

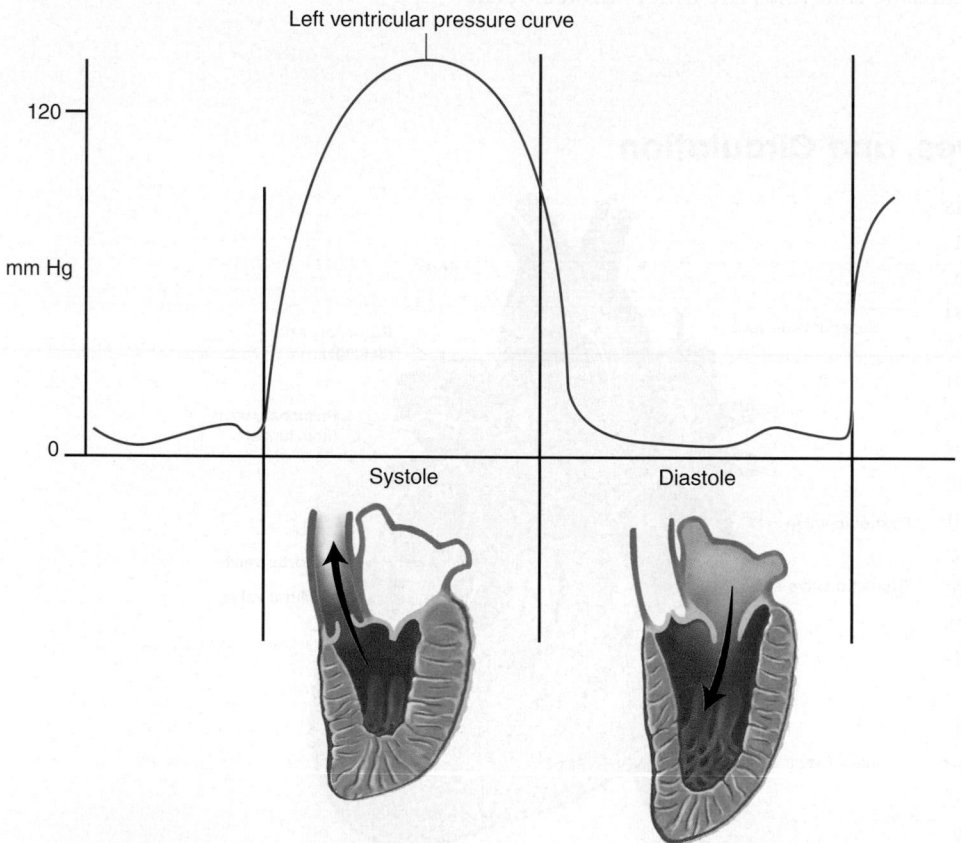

Left ventricular pressure curve

120 —

mm Hg

0 —

Systole   Diastole

Valve Openings and Closings.   Note that during *systole* the aortic valve is open, allowing ejection of blood from the left ventricle into the aorta. The mitral valve is closed, preventing blood from regurgitating (leaking) back into the left atrium. In contrast, during *diastole* the aortic valve is closed, preventing regurgitation of blood from the aorta back into the left ventricle. The mitral valve is open, allowing blood to flow from the left atrium into the relaxed left ventricle.

Understanding the interrelationships of the *pressures* in the left atrium, left ventricle, and aorta together with the position and movement of the valves is fundamental to understanding heart sounds. Trace these changing pressures and sounds through one cardiac cycle. Note that during auscultation the first and second heart sounds define the duration of *systole* and *diastole*.

During *diastole,* pressure in the blood-filled left atrium slightly exceeds that in the relaxed left ventricle, and blood flows from left atrium to left ventricle across the open mitral valve. Just before the onset of ventricular systole, atrial contraction empties the atrium and produces a slight pressure rise in both chambers.

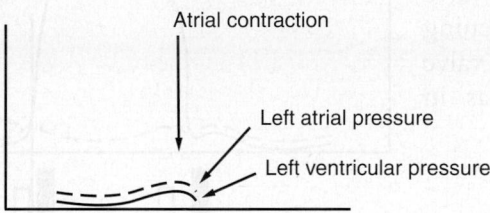

During *systole,* the left ventricle starts to contract and ventricular pressure rapidly exceeds left atrial pressure, shutting the mitral valve. *Closure of the mitral valve produces the first heart sound, S_1.*

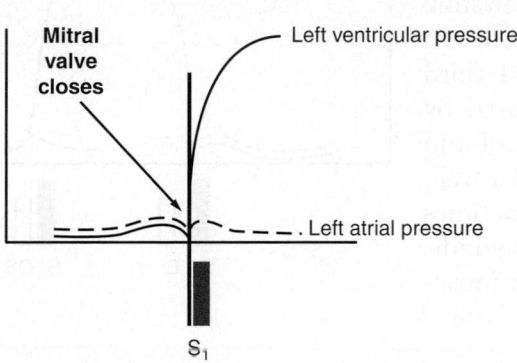

As left ventricular pressure continues to rise, it quickly exceeds the pressure in the aorta and forces the aortic valve open. *Normally, maximal left ventricular pressure corresponds to systolic blood pressure.*

In some pathologic conditions, an early systolic ejection sound (E_j) accompanies the opening of the aortic valve.

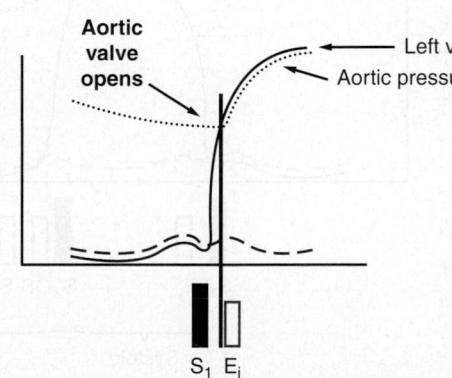

After the left ventricle ejects most of its blood, ventricular pressure begins to fall. When left ventricular pressure drops below aortic pressure, the aortic valve shuts. *Aortic valve closure produces the second heart sound, S_2, and another diastole begins.*

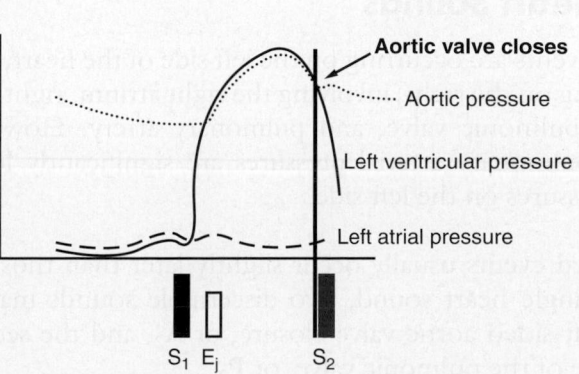

In *diastole,* left ventricular pressure continues to drop and falls below left atrial pressure. The mitral valve silently opens. However, an opening snap (OS) may be heard if valve leaflet motion is restricted, as in mitral stenosis.

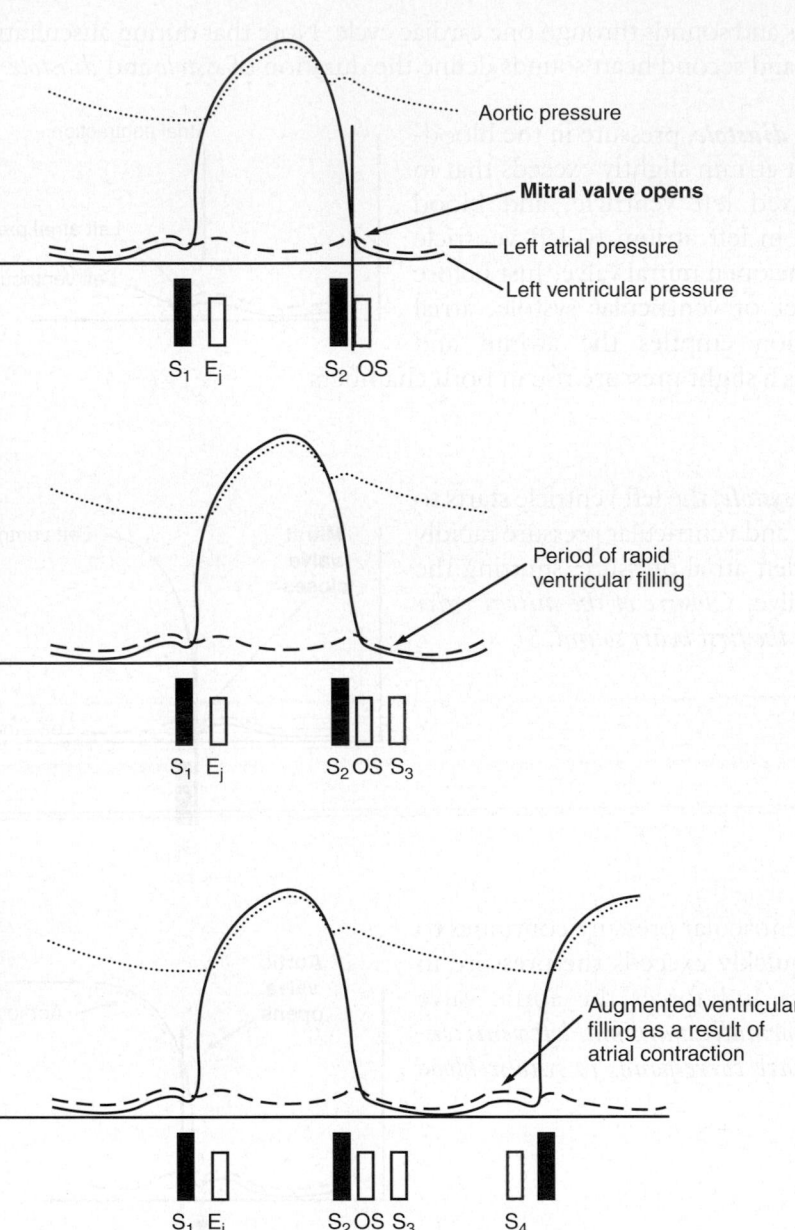

Aortic pressure

Mitral valve opens

Left atrial pressure

Left ventricular pressure

S_1 E_j S_2 OS

Period of rapid ventricular filling

S_1 E_j S_2 OS S_3

After the mitral valve opens, there is a period of early rapid ventricular filling as blood flows early in diastole from left atrium to left ventricle. In children and young adults, a third heart sound, S_3, may be caused by the rapid deceleration of the column of blood against the ventricular wall. In older adults, an S_3, sometimes termed "an S_3 gallop," usually indicates a pathologic change in ventricular compliance.

Finally, although not often heard in healthy adults, a fourth heart sound, S_4, marks atrial contraction. It immediately precedes S_1 of the next beat and also reflects a pathologic change in ventricular compliance.

Compliance is the ease with which the heart muscle relaxes as it fills with blood. Poor compliance produces a stiff ventricle with reduced ability to expand as it receives blood.

Augmented ventricular filling as a result of atrial contraction

S_1 E_j S_2 OS S_3 S_4

Systole   Diastole

The Splitting of Heart Sounds

Split S_2. While these events are occurring on the left side of the heart, similar changes are occurring on the right, involving the right atrium, right ventricle, tricuspid valve, pulmonic valve, and pulmonary artery. However, right ventricular and pulmonary arterial pressures are significantly lower than corresponding pressures on the left side.

Furthermore, right-sided events usually occur slightly later than those on the left. Instead of a single heart sound, two discernible sounds may be heard, the first from left-sided aortic valve closure, or A_2, and the second from right-sided closure of the pulmonic valve, or P_2.

S_2, and its two components, A_2 and P_2, are caused by the closure of the aortic and pulmonary valves, respectively. During inspiration the filling time of the right heart increases, thereby increasing the *stroke volume* and lengthening the duration of right ventricle emptying compared to the left ventricle. This delays closure of the pulmonic valve, P_2, **splitting** S_2 into its two audible components.[2]

During expiration, these two components fuse into a single sound, S_2.

The split S may be difficult to hear in obese individuals or people with increased anteroposterior diameter chest walls.

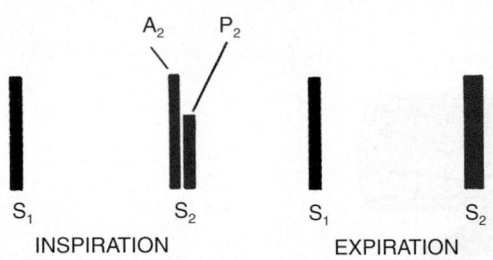

Stroke volume is the amount of blood ejected by the ventricle with each heartbeat.

Vein walls contain less muscle so they are more distensible than arteries and can store more blood. During inspiration the pulmonary vascular bed has more capacity, which contributes to the increased filling time and delays closure of P_2.

Of the two components of the S_2, A_2 is normally louder, reflecting the high pressure in the aorta. It is heard throughout the precordium. P_2, in contrast, is relatively soft, reflecting the lower pressure in the pulmonary artery. It is heard best in its own area—the 2nd and 3rd left intercostal spaces close to the sternum. It is here that you should search for splitting of the S_2. See the diagram on p. 345.

Split S_1. S_1 also has two components, an earlier mitral and a later tricuspid sound. The mitral sound, its principal component, is much louder, again reflecting the high pressures on the left side of the heart. It can be heard throughout the precordium and is loudest at the cardiac apex. The softer tricuspid component is heard best at the lower left sternal border, and it is here that you may hear a split S_1. The earlier, louder mitral component may mask the tricuspid sound, however, and splitting is not always detectable. Splitting of S_1 does not vary with respiration.

Heart Murmurs

Heart murmurs are distinguishable from heart sounds by their longer duration. They are attributed to turbulent blood flow and may be "innocent," as with flow murmurs of young adults, or diagnostic of valvular or congenital heart disease. A *stenotic valve* has an abnormally narrowed valvular orifice that obstructs blood flow, as in *aortic stenosis,* and causes a characteristic murmur. A valve that fails to fully close, as in *aortic regurgitation* or *insufficiency,* allows blood to leak backward in a retrograde direction and produces a *regurgitant* murmur.

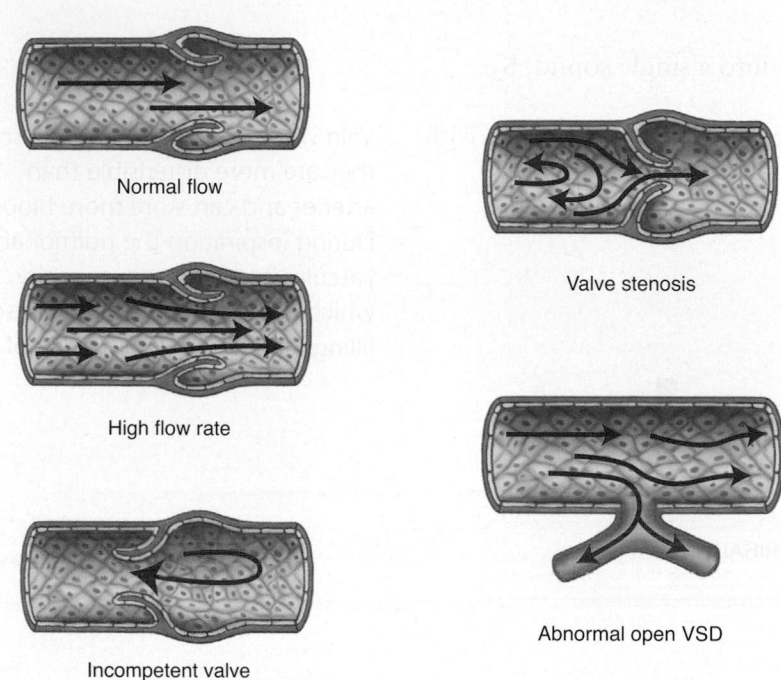

Normal flow

High flow rate

Incompetent valve

Valve stenosis

Abnormal open VSD

In the section on Physical Examination, the characteristics of murmurs, including intensity, pitch, duration, and direction of radiation, will be discussed (see pp. 372–375).

Relation of Auscultatory Findings to the Chest Wall

The locations on the chest wall where heart sounds and murmurs are heard help to identify the valve or chamber where they originate. The sounds produced by the heart valves travel with the flow of blood. As you review the locations on the diagram (p. 345), picture the direction of blood flow between the upper and lower chambers and through the pulmonary artery and aorta. Sounds and murmurs arising from the mitral valve are usually heard best at and around the cardiac apex. Those originating in the tricuspid valve are heard best at or near the lower left sternal border. Murmurs arising from the pulmonic valve are usually heard best in the 2nd and 3rd left intercostal spaces close to the sternum but at times may also be heard at higher or lower levels. Murmurs originating in the aortic valve may be heard anywhere from the right 2nd intercostal space to the apex. *These areas overlap,* as illustrated, and you will need to correlate auscultatory findings with other cardiac examination findings to identify sounds and murmurs accurately.

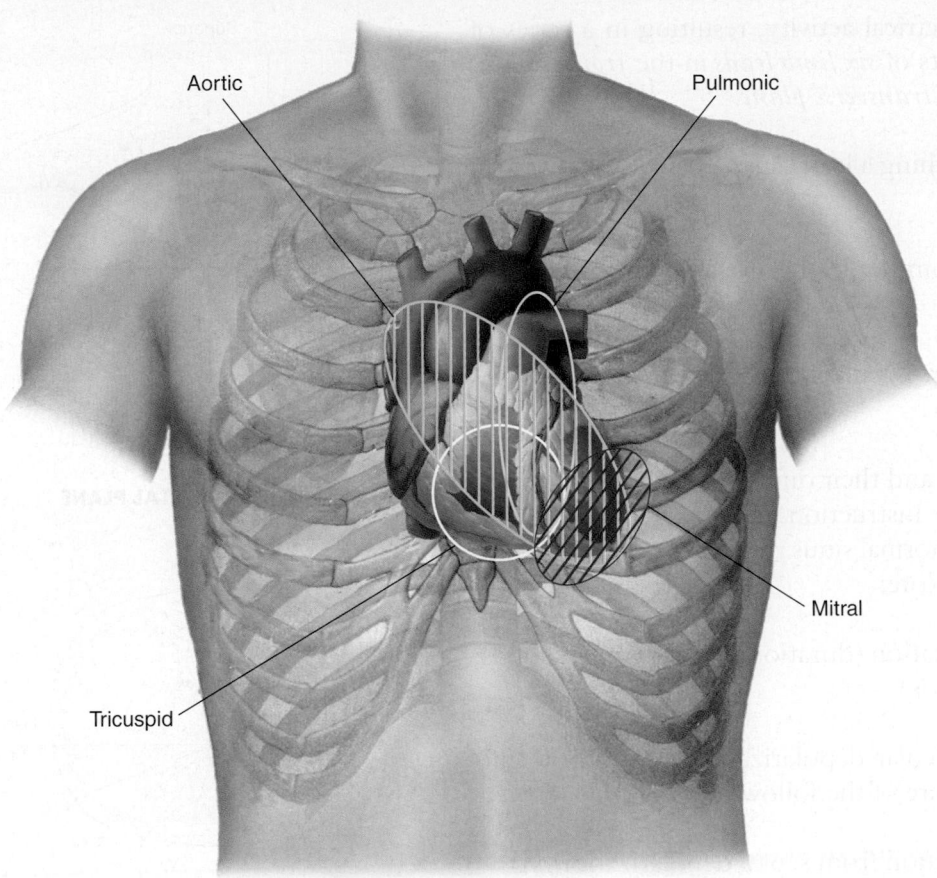

Aortic

Pulmonic

Mitral

Tricuspid

The Conduction System

An electrical conduction system stimulates and coordinates the contraction of cardiac muscle.

Each electrical impulse is initiated in the *sinus node*, a group of specialized cardiac cells located in the right atrium near the junction of the vena cava. The sinus node acts as the cardiac pacemaker and automatically discharges an impulse about 60 to 100 times a minute. This impulse travels through both atria to the *atrioventricular node*, a specialized

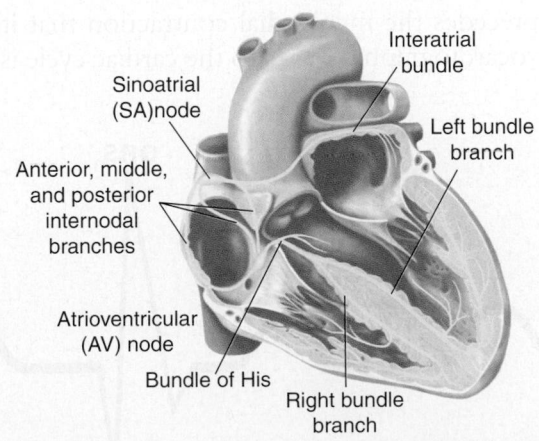

Sinoatrial
(SA)node

Interatrial
bundle

Left bundle
branch

Anterior, middle,
and posterior
internodal
branches

Atrioventricular
(AV) node

Bundle of His

Right bundle
branch

group of cells located low in the atrial septum. Here the impulse is delayed before passing down the bundle of His and its branches to the ventricular myocardium. Muscular contraction follows: first the atria, then the ventricles. The normal conduction pathway is diagrammed above in simplified form. The electrocardiogram, or ECG, records these events. Contraction of cardiac smooth muscle produces electrical activity, resulting in a series of waves on the ECG. The ECG consists of *six limb leads* in the *frontal plane* and *six chest or precordial leads* in the *transverse plane*.

- Electrical vectors (signals) approaching a lead cause a *positive, or upward, deflection*.

- Electrical vectors moving away from the lead cause a *negative, or downward, deflection*.

- When positive and negative vectors balance, they are *isoelectric*, appearing as a straight line.

The components of the *normal ECG* and their duration are briefly summarized here, but you will need further instruction and practice to interpret recordings from patients. The term "normal sinus rhythm" (NSR) is used to describe normal ECG transmission. Note:

- The small *P wave* of atrial depolarization (duration up to 80 milliseconds; *PR interval* 120 to 200 milliseconds)

- The larger *QRS complex* of ventricular depolarization (up to 100 milliseconds), consisting of one or more of the following:

  - The *Q wave*, a downward deflection from septal depolarization
  - The *R wave*, an upward deflection from ventricular depolarization
  - The S wave, a downward deflection following an R wave

- A *T wave* of ventricular repolarization, or recovery (duration relates to QRS)

The electrical impulse slightly precedes the myocardial contraction that it stimulates. The relation of electrocardiographic waves to the cardiac cycle is shown below.

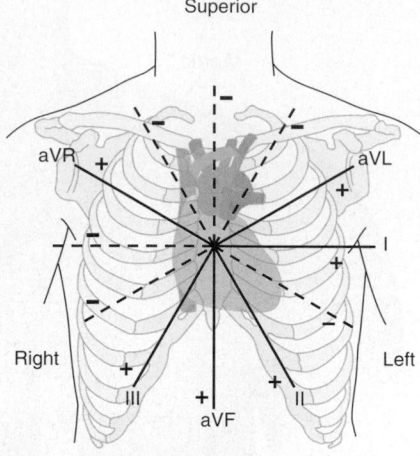

LIMB LEADS: FRONTAL PLANE

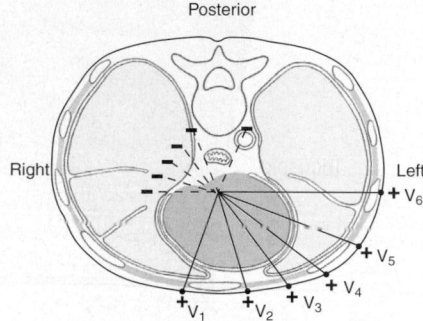

CHEST LEADS: TRANSVERSE PLANE

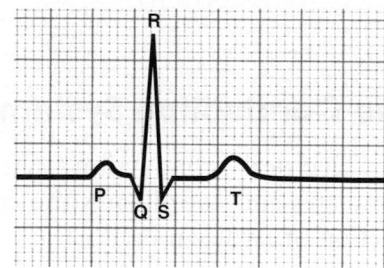

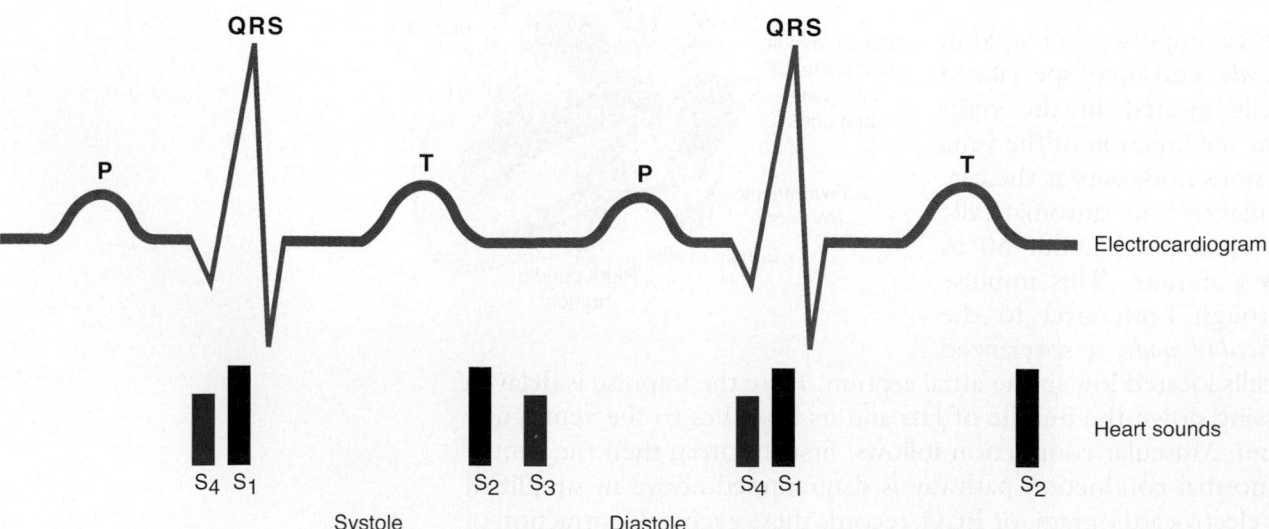

The Heart as a Pump

The left and right ventricles pump blood into the systemic and pulmonary arterial trees, respectively. *Cardiac output,* the volume of blood ejected from each ventricle during 1 minute, is the product of *heart rate* and *stroke volume.* Stroke volume (the volume of blood ejected with each heartbeat) depends in turn on preload, myocardial contractility, and afterload.

- *Preload* refers to the load that stretches the cardiac muscle before contraction. The volume of blood in the right ventricle at the end of diastole, then, constitutes its preload for the next beat. Right ventricular preload is increased by increasing venous return to the right heart. Physiologic causes include inspiration and the increased volume of blood flow from exercising muscles. The increased blood volume in a dilated right ventricle of congestive heart failure also increases preload. Causes of decreased right ventricular preload include exhalation, decreased left ventricular output, and pooling of blood in the capillary bed or the venous system.

- *Myocardial contractility* refers to the ability of the cardiac muscle, when given a load, to contract or shorten. Contractility increases when stimulated by the sympathetic nervous system and decreases when blood flow or oxygen delivery to the myocardium is impaired.

- *Afterload* refers to the degree of vascular resistance to ventricular contraction. Sources of resistance to left ventricular contraction include the tone in the walls of the aorta, the large arteries, and the peripheral vascular tree (primarily the small arteries and arterioles), as well as the volume of blood already in the aorta. Increased arterial blood pressure causes increased afterload.

Pathologic increases in preload and afterload, called *volume overload* and *pressure overload,* respectively, produce changes in ventricular function that may be clinically detectable. These changes include alterations in ventricular impulses, detectable by palpation, and in normal heart sounds. Pathologic heart sounds and murmurs may also develop.

The term *heart failure* is now preferred over "congestive heart failure" because not all patients have volume overload on initial presentation.[3]

Arterial Pulses and Blood Pressure

With each contraction, the left ventricle ejects a volume of blood into the aorta and on into the arterial tree. The ensuing pressure wave moves rapidly through the arterial system, where it is felt as the *arterial pulse.* Although the pressure wave travels quickly—many times faster than the blood itself—a palpable delay between ventricular contraction and peripheral pulses makes the pulses in the arms and legs unsuitable for timing events in the cardiac cycle.

Blood pressure in the arterial system varies during the cardiac cycle, peaking in systole and falling to its lowest trough in diastole. These are the levels that are measured with the blood pressure cuff, or sphygmomanometer. The difference between systolic and diastolic pressures is known as the *pulse pressure.*

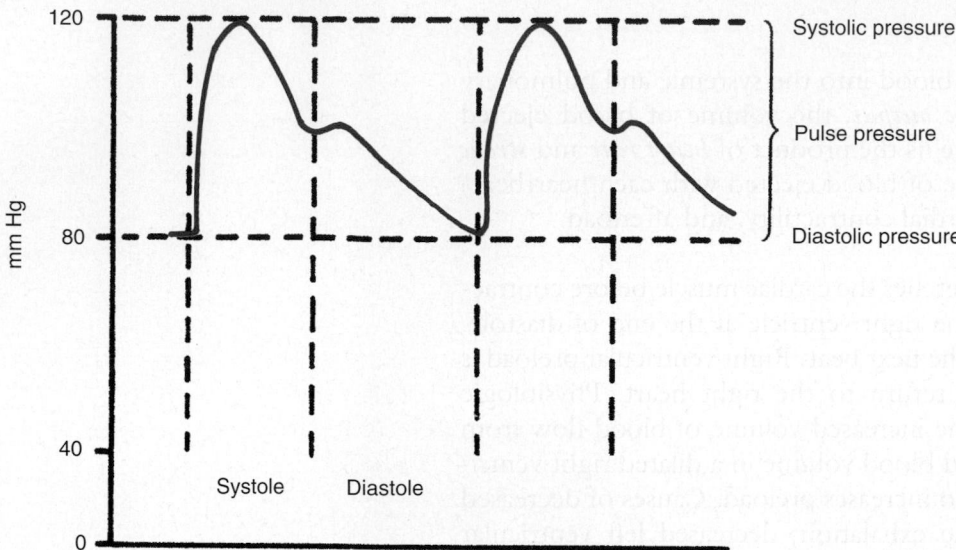

FACTORS INFLUENCING ARTERIAL PRESSURE

- Left ventricular stroke volume
- Distensibility of the aorta and the large arteries
- Peripheral vascular resistance, particularly at the arteriolar level
- Volume of blood in the arterial system.

Changes in any of these four factors alter systolic pressure, diastolic pressure, or both. Blood pressure levels fluctuate strikingly throughout any 24-hour period, varying with physical activity; emotional state; pain; noise; environmental temperature; use of coffee, tobacco, and other drugs; and even time of day.

Jugular Venous Undulations

The oscillations visible in the internal jugular veins, and often in the externals, reflect changing pressures within the right atrium. Careful observation reveals that the undulating pulsations of the internal jugular veins, and sometimes the externals, are composed of two quick peaks (a and v) and two troughs (x and y).

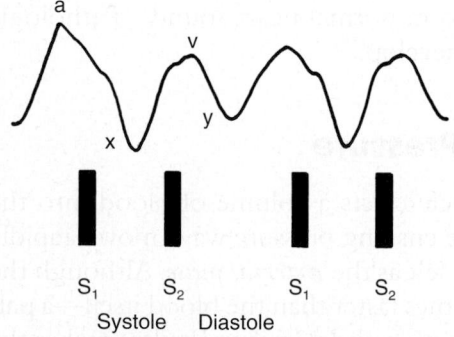

Jugular Venous Pressure

The jugular veins provide an important clinical index of right heart pressures and cardiac function. *Jugular venous pressure (JVP)* reflects right atrial pressure, which in turn equals *central venous pressure (CVP)* and right ventricular end-diastolic pressure. The JVP is best estimated from the *right internal jugular vein,* which has a more direct anatomic channel into the right atrium. Contrary to widely held views, a recent study has reaffirmed inspection of the *right external jugular vein* as a useful and accurate method for estimating CVP.[4-6]

Pressure changes from right atrial filling, contraction, and emptying cause fluctuations in the JVP and its waveforms that are visible to the examiner. Careful observation of changes in these fluctuations yields clues about volume status, right and left ventricular function, patency of the tricuspid and pulmonary valves, pressures in the pericardium, and arrhythmias. For example, JVP falls with loss of blood and increases with right or left heart failure, pulmonary hypertension, tricuspid stenosis, and pericardial compression or tamponade.

The internal jugular veins lie under the sternomastoid muscles in the neck and are not directly visible, so the nurse must learn to identify the *undulations* of the *internal jugular vein* or *external jugular vein* that are transmitted to the surface of the neck, making sure to carefully distinguish these venous undulations from the crisp pulsations of the carotid artery.

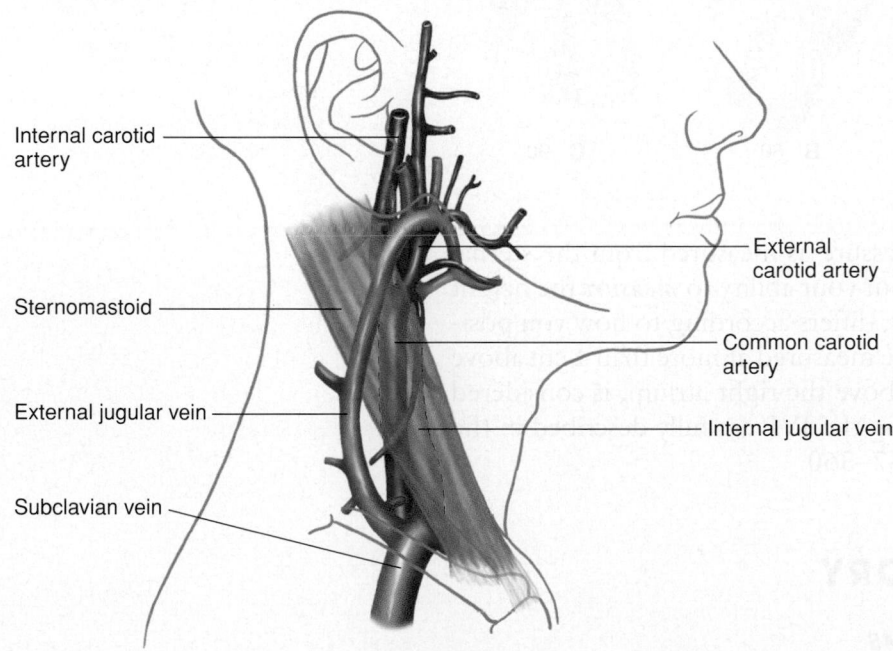

Internal carotid artery

Sternomastoid

External jugular vein

Subclavian vein

External carotid artery

Common carotid artery

Internal jugular vein

To estimate the level of the JVP, find the *highest point of undulation in the internal jugular vein* or, if necessary, the point above which the external jugular vein appears collapsed. The JVP is usually measured in vertical distance above the *sternal angle,* the bony ridge adjacent to the second rib where the manubrium joins the body of the sternum.

Study the illustrations below. Note that regardless of the patient's position, the sternal angle remains roughly 5 cm above the right atrium. In this patient, however, the pressure in the internal jugular vein is somewhat elevated.

● In *Position A,* the head of the bed is raised to the usual level, approximately 30°, but the JVP cannot be measured because undulation is above the jaw and therefore not visible.

- In *Position B,* the head of the bed is raised to 60°. The "top" of the internal jugular vein is now easily visible, so the vertical distance from the sternal angle or right atrium can now be measured.

- In *Position C,* the patient is upright and the veins are barely discernible above the clavicle, making measurement impossible.

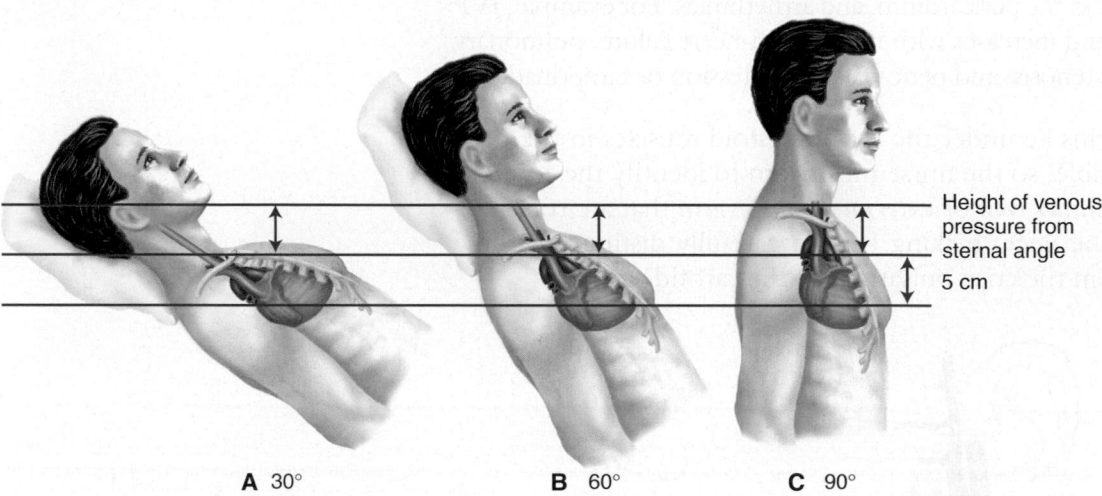

Height of venous pressure from sternal angle

5 cm

A 30°   B 60°   C 90°

Note that the height of the venous pressure as measured from the sternal angle is the *same* in all three positions, but your ability to *measure* the height of the column of venous blood, or JVP, differs according to how you position the patient. Jugular venous pressure measured at more than 4 cm above the sternal angle, or more than 9 cm above the right atrium, is considered abnormal. The techniques for measuring the JVP are fully described in the Physical Examination section on pp. 357–360.

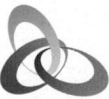 **THE HEALTH HISTORY**

COMMON OR CONCERNING SYMPTOMS

- Chest pain
- Pain or discomfort radiating to the neck, left shoulder or arm, and back
- Nausea
- Diaphoresis
- Arrhythmias: skipped beats, palpitations
- Dyspnea
- Orthopnea or paroxysmal nocturnal dyspnea
- Cough
- Edema
- Nocturia
- Fatigue
- Cyanosis or pallor

Assessing Cardiac Symptoms—Overview and Comparison With Baseline Activity Levels.

Chest symptoms may be caused by cardiac, respiratory, gastrointestinal, or musculoskeletal etiologies. The nurse differentiates the cause of the symptoms through astute history questioning. This section focuses on chest symptoms from a cardiac standpoint. Cardiac symptoms reflect the heart's ability to function (i.e., to pump blood through the body and remove waste products).

Start the inquiry about the heart with broad open-ended questions. For each symptom it is important to habitually ask the patient to quantify how it affects lifestyle or baseline level of activity. For example, in patients with chest pain, does the pain occur with walking? If yes, how far can you walk before the pain begins—50 feet, one block, more?

Chest Pain

Chest pain is one of the most serious and important symptoms and often signals *coronary heart disease*, which currently affects 16.5 million people in the United States.[7] Approximately 9 million of these people have *angina pectoris*, and 8 million have had a *myocardial infarction*. Coronary heart disease is the leading cause of death for both men and women, and accounted for one in every six U.S. deaths in 2007. Death rates are highest in African-American men and women, compared with other ethnic groups.

Classic exertional pain, pressure, or discomfort in the chest, shoulder, back, neck, or arm in *angina pectoris*, seen in 50% of patients with acute myocardial infarction; atypical descriptors also are common, such as cramping, grinding, pricking; rarely, tooth or jaw pain.[8,9] Annual incidence of *exertional angina* is 1 per 1000 in the population 30 years or older.

Your initial questions should be broad: **Do you have any pain or discomfort in your chest?**

Acute coronary syndrome is increasingly used to refer to any of the clinical syndromes caused by acute myocardial ischemia, including *unstable angina, non-ST elevation myocardial infarction,* and *ST elevation infarction.*[10]

- Ask the patient to point to the pain and to describe its attributes.

- Move on to more specific questions, such as:

  - Is the pain related to exertion?

  - What kinds of activities bring on the pain?

  - How intense is the pain, on a scale of 1 to 10?

  - Does it radiate into the neck, shoulder, or back or down your arm?

  - Are there any associated symptoms such as shortness of breath, sweating, palpitations, or nausea?

  - Does it ever wake you up at night?

  - What do you do to make it better?

Anterior chest pain, often tearing or ripping, often radiating into the back or neck, in *acute aortic dissection.*[11]

Palpitations

Palpitations involve an unpleasant awareness of the heartbeat. When describing palpitations, patients use terms such as skipping, racing, fluttering, pounding, or stopping of the heart.

Palpitations may result from an irregular heartbeat, from rapid acceleration or slowing of the heart, or from increased forcefulness of cardiac contraction. Such perceptions also depend on how patients respond to their own body sensations. Palpitations do not necessarily mean heart disease. In contrast, the most serious dysrhythmias, such as ventricular tachycardia, often do not produce palpitations.

Do you ever have palpitations?

If the patient does not understand your question, reword it. Are you ever aware of your heartbeat? What is it like? How long did the palpitations last? Did they start and stop suddenly or come on gradually?

Shortness of Breath

Shortness of breath is a common patient concern and may represent *dyspnea, orthopnea,* or *paroxysmal nocturnal dyspnea.*

Dyspnea is an uncomfortable awareness of breathing that is inappropriate to a given level of exertion.

Do you ever have difficulty breathing or shortness of breath?

● When does it occur?

● What were you doing when you became short of breath?

● How many pillows do you use to sleep?

Orthopnea is dyspnea that occurs when the patient is lying down and improves when the patient sits up. Make sure, however, that the reason the patient uses extra pillows or sleeps upright is shortness of breath and not other causes.

● Have you ever awoken suddenly due to shortness of breath?

Paroxysmal nocturnal dyspnea, or *PND,* describes episodes of sudden dyspnea and orthopnea that awaken the patient from sleep, usually 1 or 2 hours after going to bed, prompting the patient to sit up, stand up, or go to a window for air. There may be associated wheezing and coughing. The episode usually subsides but may recur at about the same time on subsequent nights.

Cough

Cough can result from fluid leaking into the lungs.

- Do you ever have a cough?

- Describe your cough.

- Do you cough up mucus? If yes, describe the mucus.

- When does it occur? Any particular time of day?

Left-sided heart failure can cause fluid to leak into the lungs. Fine crackles or rales may be heard on auscultation.

Edema

Edema refers to the accumulation of excessive fluid in the extravascular interstitial space. Focus your questions on the location, timing, and setting of the swelling, and on associated symptoms.

- Have you had any swelling anywhere?

- Where? Anywhere else?

- When does it occur?

- Is it worse in the morning or at night?

- Do your shoes get tight?

- Are the rings tight on your fingers?

- Are your eyelids puffy or swollen in the morning?

- Have you had to let out your belt?

Dependent edema appears in the lowest body parts: the feet and lower legs when sitting, or the sacrum when bedridden. Causes may be cardiac (*congestive heart failure*), nutritional (*hypoalbuminemia*), or positional.

Nocturia

Nocturia is dependent edema that is mobilized at night and returned to the kidneys for excretion during the night when the patient is reclining.

- Do you get up more than once during the night to urinate?

- How many times?

Fatigue

Fatigue is an overwhelming sustained sense of exhaustion.

- Do you feel more tired than previously?

- Are you able to perform your usual activities without resting?

Fatigue signals that the heart is not adequately supplying the body with oxygen and nutrients.

Cyanosis or pallor

Cyanosis or pallor indicates poor oxygentation of the body.

- Have you ever noticed your facial skin, lips, or fingers become blue or pale?

- How long did it last?

Cyanosis and pallor also indicate that the heart is not adequately circulating blood.

Past History

Do you have a history of heart problems or heart disease?
Do you have a history of:
    Heart murmur?
    Congenital heart disease?
    Rheumatic fever?
    Hypertension?
    Elevated cholesterol or triglycerides?
    Peripheral arterial disease?
    Cerebral arterial disease?
    Diabetes?

When were your last ECG, cholesterol measurement? Results?

Have you had any other heart tests? When? Results?

Family History

Is there any family history of coronary artery disease, hypertension, sudden death at younger than 60 years of age? Stroke? Diabetes? Obesity?
(Family refers primarily to first-degree blood relatives [i.e., parent, sibling, or child]. However, information on grandparents, aunts, uncles, and first cousins can be useful as well.)

Lifestyle Habits

    Nutrition
    Smoking
    Alcohol
    Exercise: Describe your daily or weekly exercise: type and amount
    Medications/drugs

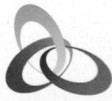 # PHYSICAL EXAMINATION

Preparation of the Patient

Appropriate preparation of the patient is essential to obtain accurate findings during the cardiovascular examination. The patient should be comfortable and calm as anxiety may elevate the blood pressure or change the heart rate or rhythm. Review the examination procedure with the patient before putting on the examination gown. Explain why visualization of the anterior chest is important for data gathering. The examination gown has the opening in the front, which enables the nurse to open the gown only as necessary during the examination. Assist the patient onto the examination table, if necessary, and immediately drape with a sheet. Perform the examination from the patient's right side.

EQUIPMENT NEEDED FOR EXAMINATION

- Stethoscope with a bell and diaphragm
- Sphygmomanometer
- Two 15-cm rulers
- Watch with second hand
- Examination light for tangential lighting

Blood Pressure and Heart Rate.   As you begin the cardiovascular examination, review the blood pressure and heart rate recorded during the General Survey and Vital Signs at the start of the physical examination. If you need to repeat these measurements, or if they have not already been done, take the time to measure the blood pressure and heart rate using optimal technique (see Chapter 7, Beginning the Physical Examination: General Survey, Vital Signs, and Pain, especially pp. 109–118).[12–16]

The components of the cardiovascular examination include:

- Examination of the face

- Examination of the great vessels of the neck

- Inspection and palpation of the precordium

- Auscultation of heart sounds

- Inspection for peripheral edema

Face

As you are taking the patient's history inspect the face, noting its color and the presence of any orbital edema. Look for signs of anxiety. Pallor or cyanosis may indicate poor perfusion of oxygen and orbital edema may indicate heart failure. Anxiety occurs during heart attacks.

Infants may exhibit circumoral cyanosis with feeding.

Great Vessels of the Neck

The Carotid Artery Pulse.   The carotid pulse provides valuable information about cardiac function and is especially useful for detecting stenosis or insufficiency of the aortic valve.

For irregular rhythms, see Table 14-1, p. 384, Selected Heart Rates and Rhythms, and Table 14-2, p. 385, Selected Irregular Rhythms

Amplitude and Contour.   To assess *amplitude and contour* of the carotid pulse, the patient should be lying down with the head of the bed elevated to about 30°. First inspect the neck for carotid pulsations. These may be visible just medial to the sternomastoid muscles. Then place your index

A tortuous and kinked carotid artery may produce a unilateral pulsatile bulge.

and middle fingers on the right carotid artery in the lower third of the neck, press posteriorly, and feel for pulsations.

Press just inside the medial border of a well-relaxed sternomastoid muscle, roughly at the level of the cricoid cartilage. Avoid pressing on the *carotid sinus,* which lies at the level of the top of the thyroid cartilage. For the left carotid artery, use your right fingers. Never press both carotids at the same time. This may decrease blood flow to the brain and induce syncope.

Causes of decreased pulsations include decreased stroke volume and local factors in the artery such as atherosclerotic narrowing or occlusion.

Pressure on the carotid sinus may cause a reflex drop in pulse rate or blood pressure.

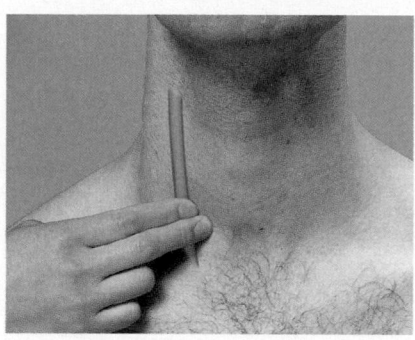 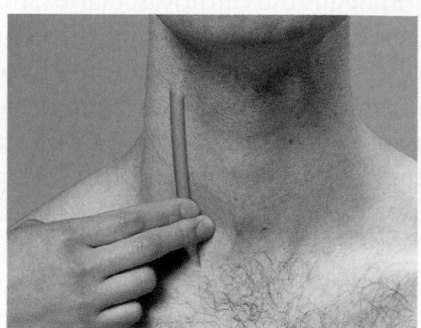

Slowly increase pressure until the maximal pulsation is felt, and then slowly decrease pressure until you best sense the arterial pressure and contour. Try to assess:

See Table 15-5, Abnormalities of the Arterial Pulse and Pressure Waves (p. 429).

● The *amplitude of the pulse.* This correlates reasonably well with the pulse pressure.

Small, thready, or weak pulse in *cardiogenic shock; bounding* pulse in *aortic insufficiency* (see p. 429)

● The *contour of the pulse wave,* namely, the speed of the upstroke, the duration of its summit, and the speed of the downstroke. The normal upstroke is *brisk*. It is smooth and rapid and follows S_1 almost immediately. The summit is smooth, rounded, and roughly midsystolic. The downstroke is less abrupt than the upstroke.

Delayed carotid upstroke in *aortic stenosis*

● Any *variations in amplitude,* either from beat to beat or with respiration.

Pulsus alternans (see Table 15-5 , p. 429, bigeminal pulse (beat-to-beat variation); paradoxical pulse (respiratory variation)

● *The timing of the carotid upstroke in relation to S_1 and S_2.* Note that the normal carotid upstroke follows S_1 and precedes S_2. This relationship is very helpful in correctly identifying S_1 and S_2, especially when the heart rate is increased and the duration of diastole, normally shorter than systole, is shortened and approaches the duration of systole.

Thrills and Bruits. During palpation of the carotid artery, humming vibrations, or *thrills,* that feel like the throat of a purring cat may be detected. Routinely, but especially in the presence of a thrill, listen over both carotid arteries with the bell of the stethoscope for a *bruit,* a murmur-like sound of vascular rather than cardiac origin.

Note that an aortic valve murmur may radiate to the neck and sound like a carotid bruit.

Listen for carotid bruits if the patient is middle-aged or elderly or if cerebrovascular disease is suspected. Ask the patient to hold breathing for a moment so that breath sounds do not obscure the vascular sound, and then listen with the bell. Heart sounds alone do not constitute a bruit.

The prevalence of asymptomatic carotid bruits increases with age, reaching 8% in people 75 years or older, with a threefold increased risk of ischemic heart disease and stroke. Presence of a carotid bruit does not predict the degree of underlying stenosis, so pursue further investigation.[17]

Further examination of arterial pulses is described in Chapter 15, The Peripheral Vascular System.

The Brachial Artery. The carotid arteries reflect aortic pulsations more accurately, but in patients with carotid obstruction, kinking, or thrills, they are unsuitable. If so, assess the pulse in the *brachial artery,* applying the techniques described above for determining amplitude and contour.

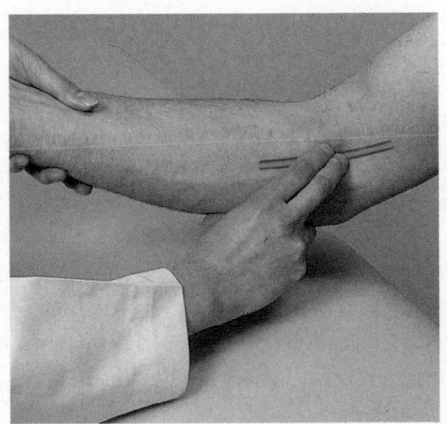

Use the index and middle fingers to feel for the pulse just medial to the biceps tendon. The patient's arm should rest with the elbow extended, palm up. With your free hand, you may need to flex the elbow to a varying degree to get optimal muscular relaxation.

Jugular Venous Pressure. The JVP provides valuable information about the patient's volume status and cardiac function. As you have learned, the JVP reflects pressure in the right atrium, or central venous pressure, and is best assessed from undulations in the right internal jugular vein.

Note, however, that the jugular veins are difficult to see in children younger than 12 years, so they are not useful for evaluating the cardiovascular system in this age group.

At the beginning of the assessment, consider the patient's volume status and how high the head of the bed or examining table needs to be elevated.

- The usual starting point for assessing the JVP is to elevate the head of the bed to 30°. Identify the external jugular vein on each side, and then find the internal jugular venous undulations transmitted from deep in the neck to the overlying soft tissues. The JVP is the highest point of the jugular venous undulation that is usually evident in euvolemic patients.

- In patients who are *hypovolemic, the JVP may be low*, necessitating lowering *the head of the bed*, sometimes even to 0°, to see the point of undulation best.

- Likewise, in volume-overloaded or *hypervolemic* patients, *the JVP may be high*, requiring raising *the head of the bed*.

- When documenting the JVP, record the height of the head of the bed.

A hypovolemic patient may have to lie flat before you see the neck veins. In contrast, when jugular venous pressure is increased, an elevation up to 60° or even 90° may be required. In all these positions, the sternal angle usually remains about 5 cm above the right atrium, as diagrammed on p. 350.

STEPS FOR ASSESSING THE JVP

- Make the patient comfortable. *Raise the head slightly on a pillow* to relax the sternomastoid muscles.
- *Raise the head of the bed or examining table to about 30°. Turn the patient's head slightly away from the side you are inspecting.*
- Use *tangential lighting* and examine both sides of the neck. Identify the external jugular vein on each side, and then find the internal jugular venous pulsations.
- *If necessary, raise or lower the head of the bed* until you can see the undulations of the internal jugular vein in the lower half of the neck.
- Focus on the *right internal jugular vein*. Look for undulations in the suprasternal notch, between the attachments of the sternomastoid muscle on the sternum and clavicle, or just posterior to the sternomastoid. The table below helps you distinguish internal jugular undulations from those of the carotid artery.
- *Identify the highest point of undulation in the right internal jugular vein.* Extend a long rectangular object or card horizontally from this point and a centimeter ruler vertically from the sternal angle, making an exact right angle. Measure the vertical distance in centimeters above the sternal angle where the horizontal object crosses the ruler. *This distance, measured in centimeters above the sternal angle or the right atrium, is the JVP* (See picture p. 360).

The following features help to distinguish jugular undulations from carotid artery pulsations[4]:

● Distinguishing Internal Jugular Undulations and Carotid Pulsations

Internal Jugular Undulations	Carotid Pulsations

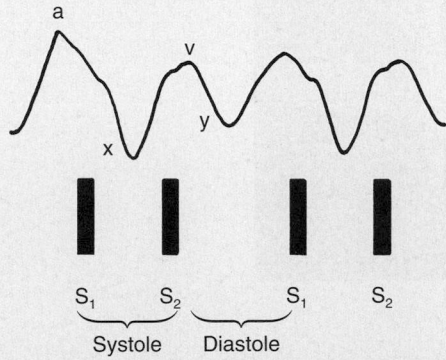

Jugular venous pulsations

a
v
x
y

S₁ S₂ S₁ S₂

Systole Diastole

Jugular venous pressure curves

a = atrial contraction
x = descent in right atrium following *a*
v = passive venous filling of atria from the vena cavae
y = descent during atrial resting phase before contraction

Internal Jugular Undulations	Carotid Pulsations
Rarely palpable	Palpable
Soft, biphasic, undulating quality, usually with two elevations and two troughs per heartbeat	A more vigorous thrust with a *single outward component*
Pulsations eliminated by light pressure on the vein(s) just above the sternal end of the clavicle	Pulsations not eliminated by this pressure
Height of undulations changes with position, dropping as the patient becomes more upright	Height of pulsations unchanged by position
Height of undulations usually falls with inspiration	Height of pulsations not affected by inspiration

Establishing the true vertical and horizontal lines to measure the JVP is difficult, much like the problem of hanging a picture straight when you are close to it. Place your ruler on the sternal angle and line it up with something in the room that you know to be vertical. Then place a card or rectangular object at an exact right angle to the ruler. This constitutes your horizontal line. Move it up or down—still horizontal—so that the lower edge rests at the top of the jugular pulsations, and read the vertical distance on the ruler. Round your measurement off to the nearest centimeter.

Increased pressure suggests *right-sided heart failure* or, less commonly, *constrictive pericarditis, tricuspid stenosis,* or *superior vena cava obstruction.*[18,19]

In patients with obstructive lung disease, venous pressure may appear elevated on expiration only; the veins collapse on inspiration. This finding does not indicate congestive heart failure.

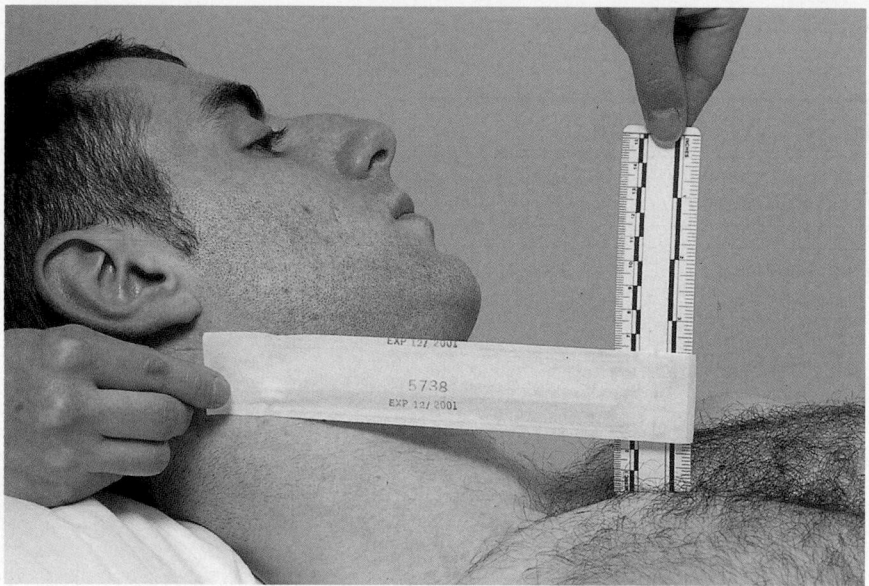

Venous pressure measured at >3 cm or possibly 4 cm above the sternal angle, or more than 8 cm or 9 cm in total distance above the right atrium, is considered *abnormal*.

An elevated JVP is 98% specific for an increased left ventricular end-diastolic pressure and low left ventricular ejection fraction, and it increases risk of death from heart failure.[20,21]

If undulations in the internal jugular vein cannot be seen, look for them in the external jugular vein. If there is no undulation, use *the point above which the external jugular veins appear to collapse*. Make this observation on each side of the neck. Measure the vertical distance of this point from the sternal angle.

Local kinking or obstruction is the usual cause of unilateral distention of the external jugular vein.

The highest point of venous undulations may lie below the level of the sternal angle. Under these circumstances, venous pressure is not elevated and seldom needs to be measured.

Hepatojugular Reflux.   If heart failure is suspected from the patient history or physical examination or if the jugular venous pressure is elevated, perform the hepatojugular reflux maneuver. Position the patient supine with the head of the bed at the same angle used for the jugular venous pressure examination. Place your right hand with fingers pointing toward the patient's head over the right upper quadrant of the patient's abdomen just below the costal margin as seen on the next page. Press deeply in and upward and hold the pressure for 30 seconds. This maneuver forces the hepatic venous blood into the vena cavae, elevating the venous blood volume and pressure. While you are applying pressure, watch the patient's jugular vein level. The healthy person is able to pump the extra blood through the heart within a few seconds. The jugular vein pressure will rise for a few seconds and then rapidly diminish to previous levels.

If heart failure is present the jugular venous pressure will remain elevated as long as the pressure is maintained.

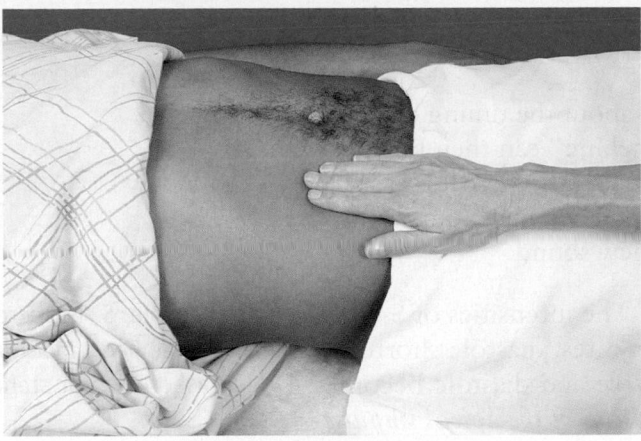

The Heart

For much of the cardiac examination, the patient should be *supine*, with the upper body raised by elevating the head of the bed or table to about 30°. Two other positions are also needed: (1) *turning to the left side* and (2) *sitting and leaning forward*. These positions bring the ventricular apex and left ventricular outflow tract closer to the chest wall, enhancing detection of the PMI and aortic insufficiency. *The examiner should stand at the patient's right side.*

During the cardiac examination, remember to correlate the findings with the patient's jugular venous pressure and carotid pulse. It is also important to document both the anatomic location of findings with their timing in the cardiac cycle.

- Note the *anatomic location* of sounds in terms of intercostal spaces and their distance from the midsternal or midclavicular lines. The midsternal line offers the most reliable zero point for measurement, but some feel that the midclavicular line accommodates the different sizes and shapes of patients.

- Identify the *timing of impulses or sounds* in relation to the cardiac cycle. Timing of sounds is often possible through auscultation alone. In most people with normal or slow heart rates, it is easy to identify the paired heart sounds by listening through a stethoscope. S_1 is the first of these sounds, S_2 is the second, and the relatively long diastolic interval separates one pair from the next.

S_1 is sometimes called "lub" and S_2 "dub." Listen for the lub-dub sequence to distinguish the two sounds.

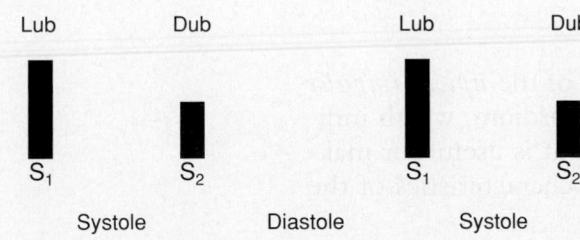

The relative intensity of these sounds is also helpful. *S_1 is usually louder than S_2 at the apex; S_2 is usually louder than S_1 at the base.*

Even experienced nurses are sometimes uncertain about the timing of heart sounds, especially extra sounds and murmurs. "Inching" can then be helpful. Return to a place on the chest—most often the base—where it is easy to identify S_1 and S_2. Get their rhythm clearly in mind. Then inch your stethoscope down the chest in steps until you hear the new sound.

Auscultation alone, however, can be misleading. The intensities of S_1 and S_2, for example, may be abnormal. At rapid heart rates, diastole shortens, and at about a rate of 120, the durations of systole and diastole become indistinguishable. *Use palpation of the carotid pulse or of the apical impulse to help determine whether the sound or murmur is systolic or diastolic.* Because both the carotid upstroke and the apical impulse occur in systole, right after S_1, sounds or murmurs coinciding with them are systolic; sounds or murmurs occurring after the carotid upstroke or apical impulse are diastolic.

For example, S_1 is decreased in *first-degree heart block*, and S_2 is decreased in *aortic stenosis*.

Sequence of Cardiac Examination. The table below summarizes patient positions and a suggested sequence for the examination.

● Sequence of the Cardiac Examination

Patient Position	Examination	Accentuated Findings
Supine, with the head elevated 30°	Inspect and palpate the precordium: the 2nd right and left intercostal spaces; the right ventricle; and the left ventricle, including the apical impulse (diameter, location, amplitude, duration).	
	Listen at the 2nd right and left intercostal spaces, along the left sternal border, across to the apex with the *diaphragm*.	
Left lateral decubitus	Palpate the apical impulse if not previously detected. Listen at the apex with the *bell* of the stethoscope.	Low-pitched extra sounds such as an S_3, opening snap, diastolic rumble of *mitral stenosis*
Sitting, leaning forward, after full exhalation	Listen at the right sternal border for tricuspid murmurs and sounds with the *bell*.	Soft decrescendo diastolic murmur of *aortic insufficiency*

Inspection

Carefully *inspect* the anterior chest for the location of the *apical impulse* or *point of maximal impulse* or heaves over the precordium, which indicate increased ventricular movement. Tangential light is useful for making this observation. Use *palpation* to confirm the characteristics of the apical impulse.

Palpation

● Begin with general palpation of the chest wall. First palpate for *heaves*, *(lifts)*, using your *fingerpads*. Hold them flat or obliquely on the body surface. Ventricular impulses may heave or lift your fingers.

● Check for *thrills*, formed by the turbulence of underlying murmurs, by pressing the *ball of your hand* firmly on the chest. If subsequent auscultation reveals a loud murmur, go back to that area and check for thrills again.

Thrills may accompany loud, harsh, or rumbling murmurs as in *aortic stenosis, patent ductus arteriosus, ventricular septal defect*, and, less commonly, *mitral stenosis*. They are palpated more easily in patient positions that accentuate the murmur.

On rare occasions, a patient has *dextrocardia*—a heart situated on the right side. The apical impulse will then be found on the right. If you cannot find an apical impulse, percuss for the dullness of the heart and liver and for the tympany of the stomach. In *situs inversus*, all three of these structures are on opposite sides from normal. A right-sided heart with a normally placed liver and stomach is usually associated with congenital heart disease.

Right 2nd intercostal space: Aortic area

Left 2nd intercostal space: Pulmonic area

Left 3rd intercostal space 2nd pulmonic area (Erb's point)

Left 4th and 5th intercostal space: Left sternal border

5th intercostal space LMCL: Apex

Epigastric (subxiphoid)

● Be sure to assess the *right ventricle* by palpating the right ventricular area at the lower left sternal border and in the subxiphoid area, the pulmonary artery in the left 2nd intercostal space, and the aortic area in the right 2nd intercostal space (see the diagram with palpation areas indicated.

Palpable pulsations of the right ventricle may indicate an enlarged right ventricle.

The Apical Impulse or Point of Maximal Impulse. The apical impulse represents the brief early pulsation of the left ventricle as it moves anteriorly during contraction and touches the chest wall.

Note that in most examinations the apical impulse is the point of maximal impulse, or PMI; however, some pathologic conditions may produce a pulsation that is more prominent than the apex beat, such as an enlarged right ventricle, a dilated pulmonary artery, or an aneurysm of the aorta.

If you cannot identify the apical impulse with the patient supine, ask the patient to roll partly onto the left side—this is the *left lateral decubitus* position. Palpate again, using the palmar surfaces of several fingers. If you cannot find the apical impulse, ask the patient to exhale fully and stop breathing for a few seconds. When examining a woman, it may be helpful to displace the left breast upward or laterally as necessary; alternatively, ask her to do this for you.

The apex beat is palpable in only 25% to 40% of healthy adults in the supine position and in 50% of healthy adults in the left lateral decubitus position, especially those who are thin.[1]

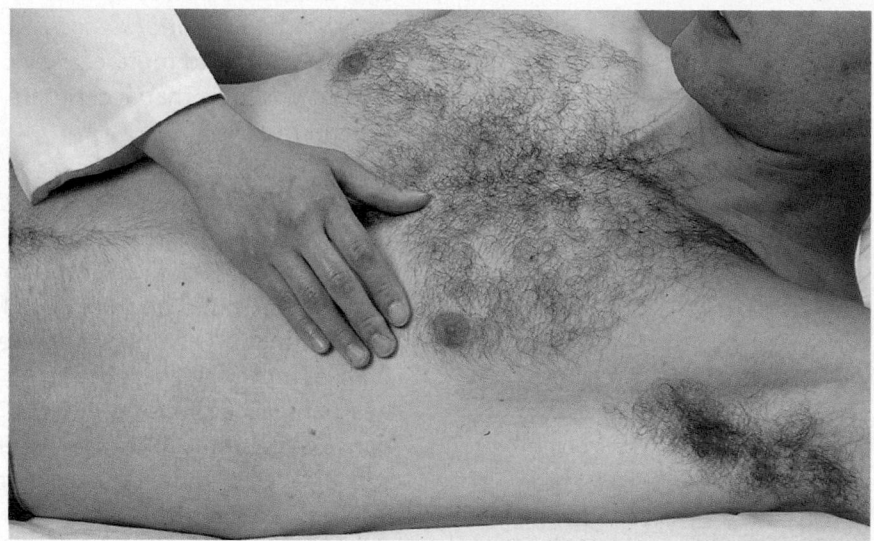

Once the apical impulse is found, make finer assessments with the fingertips, and then with one finger.

Obesity, a very muscular chest wall, or an increased anteroposterior diameter of the chest, however, may make it undetectable. Some apical impulses hide behind the rib cage, despite positioning.

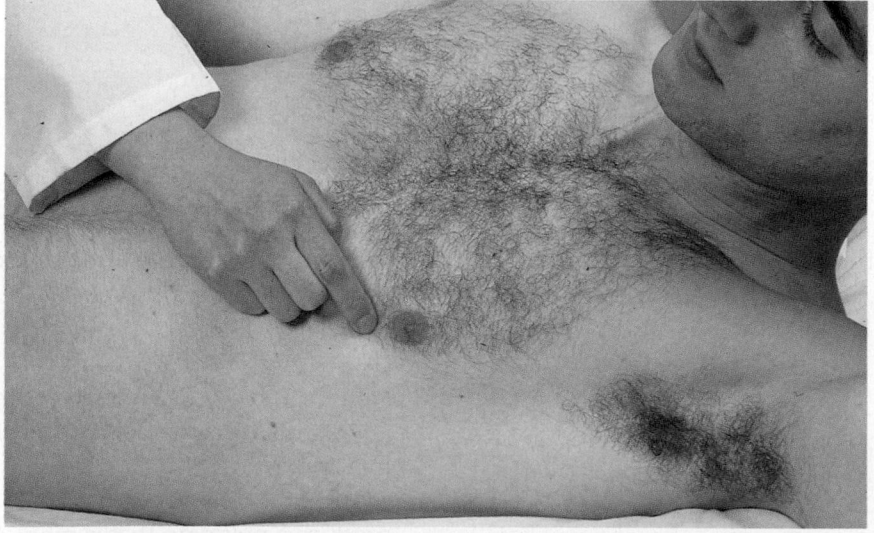

Now assess the location, diameter, amplitude, and duration of the apical impulse. You may wish to have the patient breathe out and briefly stop breathing to check your findings.

See Table 14-3, p 386, Variations and Abnormalities of the Apical Impulse

● **Location.** Try to assess location with the patient *supine,* because the left lateral decubitus position displaces the apical impulse to the left. Locate two points: the intercostal spaces, usually the 5th or possibly the 4th, which give the vertical location; and the distance in centimeters from the *midsternal line,* which gives the horizontal location.

Some authors recommend measurement from the *midclavicular line,* because the apical impulse falls roughly at this line. Clinicians using this line should use a ruler to mark the midpoint between the sternoclavicular and acromioclavicular joints; otherwise, use of this line is less reproducible because of variations in estimating the midpoint of the clavicle.

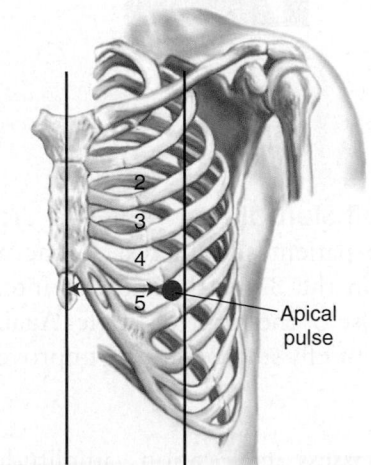

Midsternal   Midclavicular
line   line

Apical pulse

Pregnancy or a high left diaphragm may displace the apical impulse upward and to the left.

Lateral displacement from cardiac enlargement in *congestive heart failure, cardiomyopathy, ischemic heart disease.* Displacement in deformities of the thorax and mediastinal shift.

Lateral displacement outside the midclavicular line increases the likelihood of cardiac enlargement and a low-left ventricular ejection fraction by 3–4 and 10, respectively.[1]

● **Diameter.** Palpate the diameter of the apical impulse. In the supine patient, it usually measures less than 2.5 cm and occupies only one intercostal space. It may feel larger in the left lateral decubitus position.

In the left lateral decubitus position, a *diffuse* PMI with a diameter >3 cm indicates left ventricular enlargement.[22]

● **Amplitude.** Estimate the amplitude of the impulse. It is usually small and feels *brisk* and *tapping.* Some young people have an increased amplitude, or hyperkinetic impulse, especially when excited or after exercise; its duration, however, is normal.

Increased amplitude may also reflect *hyperthyroidism, severe anemia,* pressure overload of the left ventricle (as in *aortic stenosis*), or volume overload of the left ventricle (as in *mitral regurgitation*).

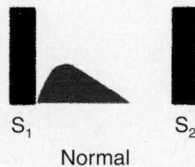

S₁   S₂

Normal

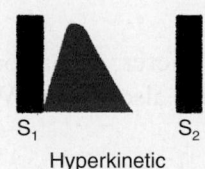

S₁   S₂

Hyperkinetic

● **Duration.** Duration is the most useful characteristic of the apical impulse for identifying hypertrophy of the left ventricle. To assess duration, listen to the heart sounds as you feel the apical impulse, or watch the movement of your stethoscope as you listen at the apex. Estimate the proportion of systole occupied by the apical impulse. Normally it lasts through the first two thirds of systole, and often less, but does not continue to the second heart sound.

A *sustained*, high-amplitude impulse that is normally located suggests left ventricular hypertrophy from pressure overload (as in *hypertension*). If such an impulse is displaced laterally, consider volume overload.

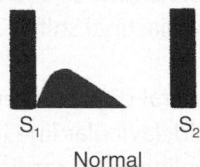

S_1 S_2

Normal

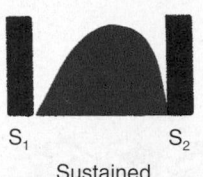

S_1 S_2

Sustained

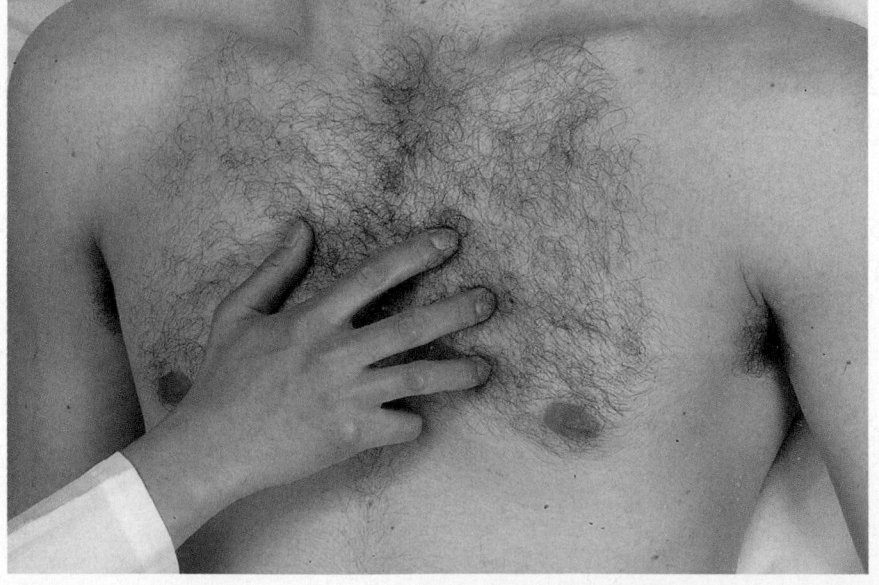

S_1 S_2

A sustained low-amplitude (hypokinetic) impulse may result from *dilated cardiomyopathy.*

Right Ventricular Area—The Left Sternal Border in the 3rd, 4th, and 5th Intercostal Spaces. The patient should rest supine at 30°. Place the tips of your curved fingers in the 3rd, 4th, and 5th intercostal spaces and try to feel the systolic impulse of the right ventricle. Again, asking the patient to breathe out and then briefly stop breathing improves your observation.

If an impulse or heave is palpable, assess its location, amplitude, and duration.

A marked increase in amplitude with little or no change in duration occurs in chronic volume overload of the right ventricle, as from an *atrial septal defect*. An impulse with increased amplitude and duration occurs with pressure overload of the right ventricle, as in *pulmonic stenosis* or *pulmonary hypertension*.

In patients with an increased anteroposterior (AP) diameter, palpation of the *right ventricle* in the *epigastric* or *subxiphoid area* is also useful. With your hand flattened, press your index finger just under the rib cage and up toward the left shoulder and try to feel right ventricular pulsations.

In obstructive pulmonary disease, hyperinflated lung may prevent palpation of an enlarged right ventricle in the left parasternal area. The impulse is felt easily, however, high in the epigastrium where heart sounds are also often heard best.

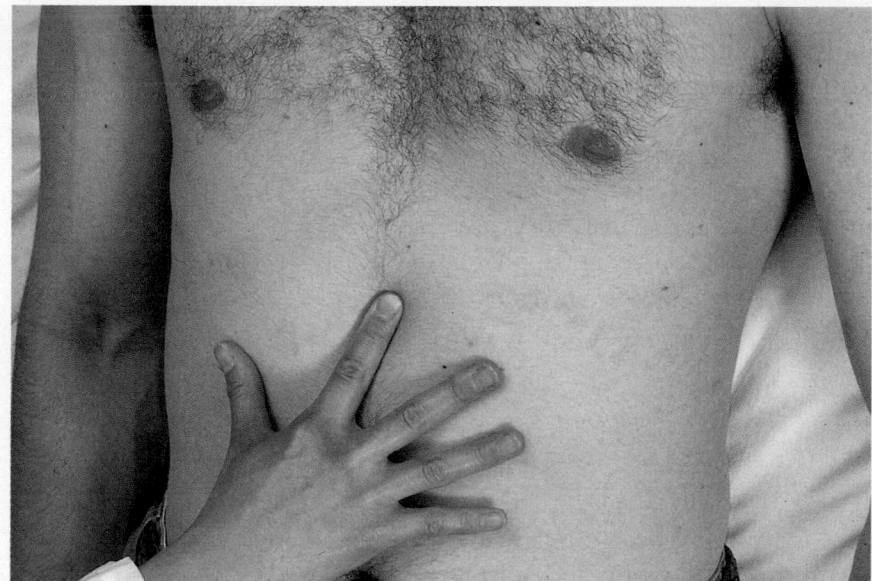

Asking the patient to inhale and briefly stop breathing is helpful. The inspiratory position moves your hand well away from the pulsations of the abdominal aorta, which might otherwise be confusing.

Pulmonic Area—The Left 2nd Intercostal Space.

This intercostal space overlies the *pulmonary artery*. As the patient holds expiration, look and feel for an impulse and feel for possible heart sounds. In thin or shallow-chested patients, the pulsation of a pulmonary artery may sometimes be felt here, especially after exercise or with excitement.

A prominent pulsation here often accompanies dilatation or increased flow in the pulmonary artery. A palpable S_2 suggests increased pressure in the pulmonary artery (*pulmonary hypertension*).

Aortic Area—The Right 2nd Intercostal space.

This intercostal space overlies the aortic outflow tract. Search for pulsations and palpable heart sounds.

A palpable S_2 suggests systemic *hypertension*. A pulsation here suggests a dilated or aneurysmal aorta.

Percussion

Percussion is rarely used today to estimate cardiac size. X-rays, ECG, and echocardiography provide accurate measurement. Palpation of the apical impulse can provide a rough size estimate. When you cannot feel the apical impulse, however, percussion may be your only tool, but may not be reliable. Under these circumstances, cardiac dullness often occupies a large area. Starting well to the left on the chest, percuss from resonance toward cardiac dullness in the 3rd, 4th, 5th, and possibly 6th

A markedly dilated failing heart may have a hypokinetic apical impulse that is displaced far to the left. A large pericardial effusion may make the impulse undetectable.

intercostal spaces. It is especially difficult to obtain accurate findings in women. Ask the woman to lift her breast up and back before attempting percussion.

Auscultation

Overview.   Auscultation of heart sounds and murmurs is an important skill of physical examination that leads directly to several clinical diagnoses. In this section, you will learn the techniques for identifying S_1 and S_2, extra heart sounds in systole and diastole, and systolic and diastolic murmurs. Review the auscultatory areas on the next page with the following caveats: (1) many authorities discourage use of names such as "aortic area," because murmurs may be loudest in other areas; and (2) these areas may not apply to patients with cardiac enlargement, anomalies of the great vessels, or dextrocardia. It is best to use locations such as "base of the heart," apex, or parasternal border to describe your findings.

Know Your Stethoscope!   It is important to understand the uses of both the diaphragm and the bell.

- *The diaphragm.* The diaphragm is better for picking up the relatively high-pitched sounds of S_1 and S_2, the murmurs of aortic and mitral regurgitation, and pericardial friction rubs. *Listen throughout the precordium* with the diaphragm, pressing it firmly against the chest.

- *The bell.* The bell is more sensitive to the low-pitched sounds of S_3 and S_4 and the murmur of mitral stenosis. Apply the bell lightly, with just enough pressure to produce an air seal with its full rim. *Use the bell at the apex, and then move medially along the lower sternal border.* Resting the heel of your hand on the chest like a fulcrum may help you to maintain light pressure.

Pressing the bell firmly on the chest makes it function more like the diaphragm by stretching the underlying skin. Low-pitched sounds such as S_3 and S_4 may disappear with this technique—an observation that may help to identify them. In contrast, high-pitched sounds such as a midsystolic click, an ejection sound, or an opening snap will persist or get louder.

There are three types of stethoscope heads. The simplest has only a diaphragm. This type is unsuitable for a full cardiac examination. The second type has a diaphragm on one side and a bell on the opposite side. The head of the stethoscope is rotated to open either the bell or the diaphragm. Lightly tapping on each side with the stethoscope in one's ears will reveal which side is open. The third type of head combines the diaphragm and bell on one side. The bell is activated by very light pressure (no ring should be seen on the skin when the stethoscope is removed) and with increased pressure it becomes a diaphragm. (A ring of blanched skin will remain for a few seconds.) This version comes as either a single-sided stethoscope or a double-sided stethoscope with a pediatric and adult side.

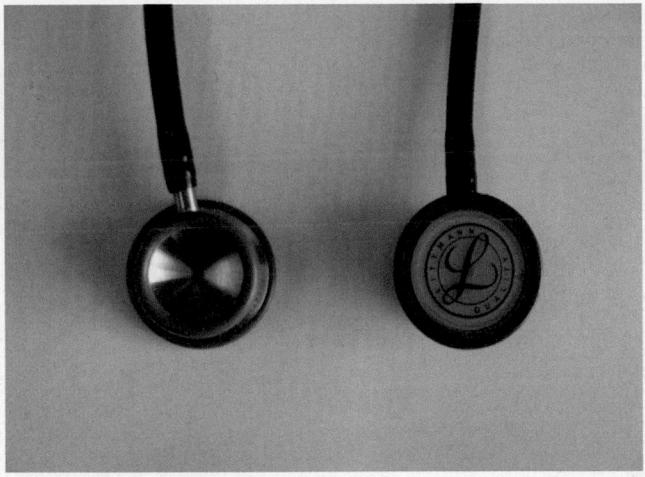

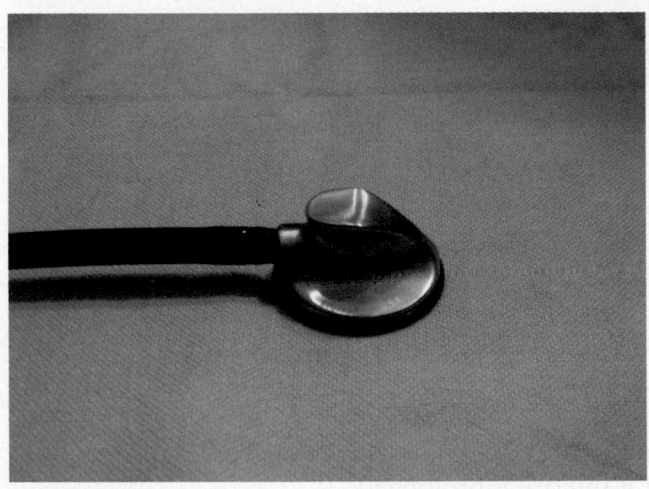

"Inching" Your Stethoscope. In a quiet room, listen to the heart with your stethoscope, starting at either the base or apex. Either pattern is satisfactory.

- Some experts recommend *starting at the apex and inching to the base:* move the stethoscope from the PMI medially to the left sternal border, superiorly to the 2nd intercostal space, then across the sternum to the 2nd intercostal space at the right sternal border.

- Alternatively, you can *start at the base and inch your stethoscope to the apex:* with your stethoscope in the right 2nd intercostal space close to the sternum, move along the left sternal border in each intercostal space from the 2nd through the 5th, and then to the apex.

Heart sounds and murmurs that originate in the four valves range widely, as illustrated. Use anatomic location rather than valve area to describe where murmurs and sounds are best heard.

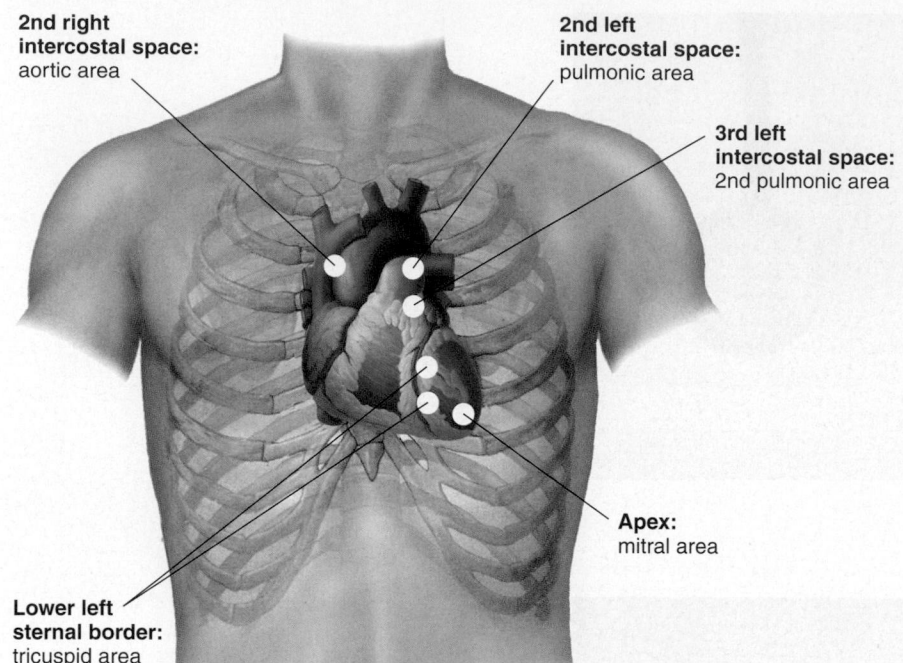

2nd right intercostal space: aortic area

2nd left intercostal space: pulmonic area

3rd left intercostal space: 2nd pulmonic area

Apex: mitral area

Lower left sternal border: tricuspid area

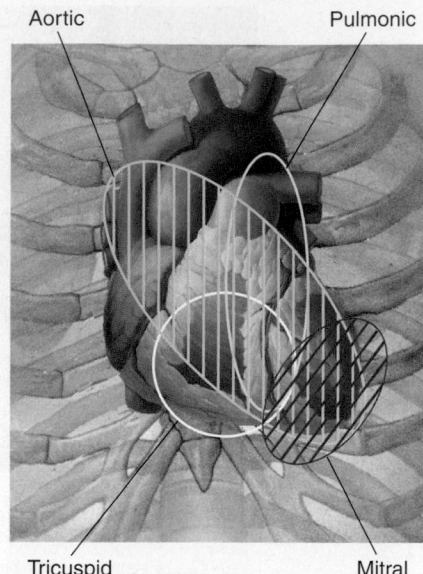

Aortic

Pulmonic

Tricuspid

Mitral

(Redrawn from Leatham A: Introduction to the Examination of the Cardiovascular System, 2nd ed. Oxford, Oxford University Press, 1979.)

The Importance of Timing S_1 and S_2. Regardless of the direction you move your stethoscope, keep your left index and middle fingers on the right carotid artery in the lower third of the neck to facilitate correct identification of S_1, just before the carotid upstroke, and S_2, which follows the carotid upstroke. Be sure to compare the intensities of S_1 and S_2 as you move your stethoscope through the listening areas above.

● At the base S_2 is louder than S_1 and may split with respiration. At the apex, S_1 is usually louder than S_2 unless the PR interval is prolonged.

● By carefully noting the intensities of S_1 and S_2, you will confirm each of these sounds and thereby correctly identify *systole*, the interval between S_1 and S_2, and *diastole*, the interval between S_2 and S_1.

When listening to the extra sounds of S_3 and S_4 and to murmurs, timing systole and diastole is an absolute prerequisite to the correct identification of these events in the cardiac cycle.

Listen to the entire precordium with the patient supine. For new patients and patients needing a complete cardiac examination, use two other important positions to listen for S_3, S_4, and the murmurs of mitral stenosis and aortic regurgitation.

USE IMPORTANT MANEUVERS. Ask the patient to *roll partly onto the left side into the left lateral decubitus position*, bringing the left ventricle close to the chest wall. Place the bell of your stethoscope lightly on the apical impulse.

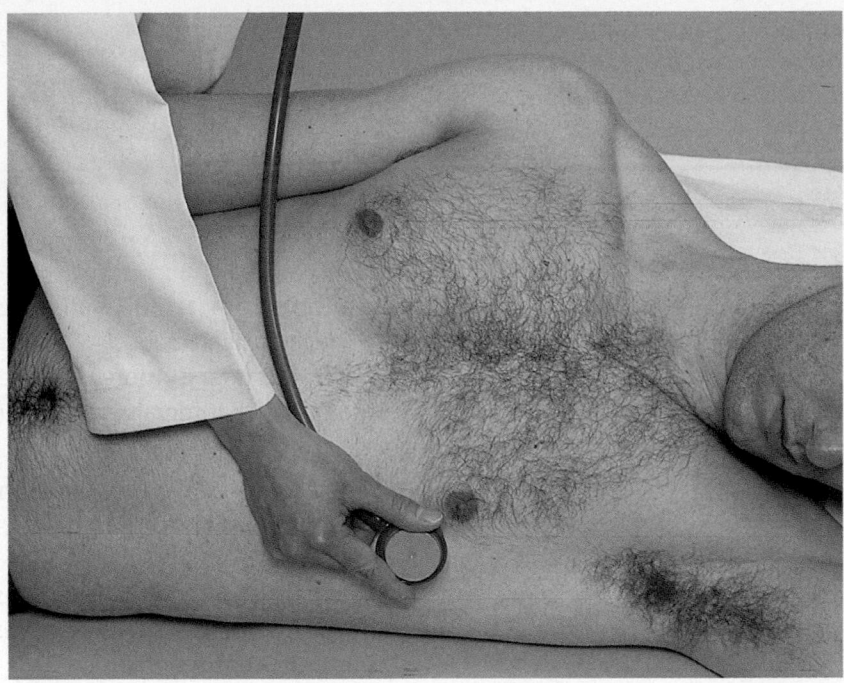

This position accentuates or brings out a left-sided S_3 and S_4 and mitral murmurs, especially *mitral stenosis*. Otherwise, you may miss these important findings.

Ask the patient to *sit up, lean forward, exhale completely, and stop breathing in expiration*. Pressing the diaphragm of your stethoscope on the chest, listen along the left sternal border and at the apex, pausing periodically so the patient may breathe.

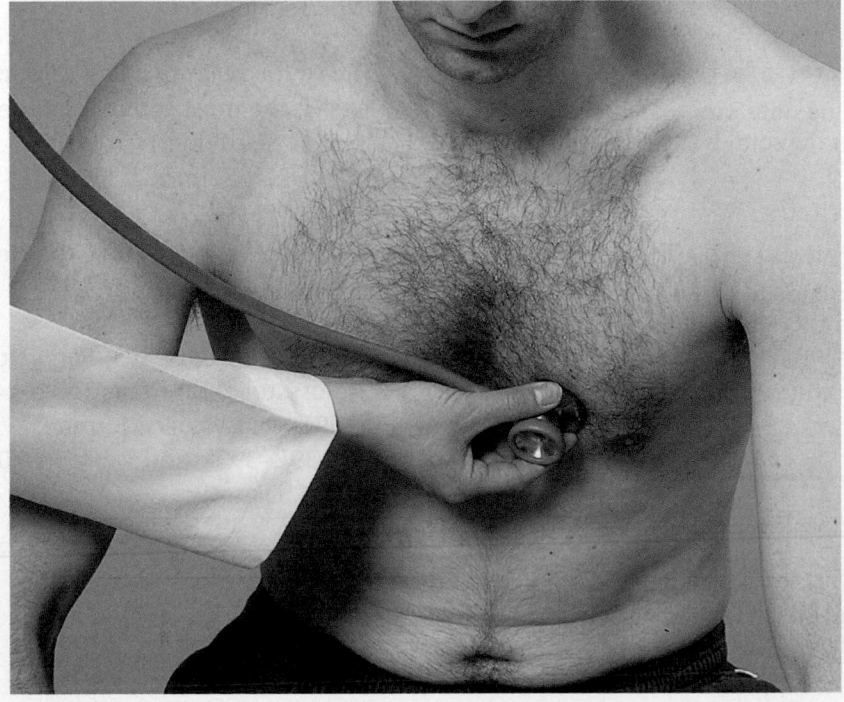

This position accentuates or brings out aortic murmurs. You may easily miss the soft diastolic murmur of *aortic regurgitation* unless you listen at this position.

Listening for Heart Sounds. Throughout your examination, take your time at each auscultatory area. Concentrate on each of the events in the cardiac cycle listed below and sounds heard in systole and diastole.

Heart Sounds	Guides to Auscultation	
● Auscultatory Sounds		
S_1	Note its intensity and any apparent splitting. Normal splitting is detectable along the lower left sternal border.	See Table 14-4, p. 387, Variations in the First Heart Sound—S_1 Note that S_1 is louder at more rapid heart rates (and PR intervals are shorter).
S_2	Note its intensity.	
Split S_2	Listen for splitting of this sound in the 2nd and 3rd left intercostal spaces. Ask the patient to breathe quietly, and then slightly more deeply than normal. Does S_2 split into its two components, as it normally does? If not, ask the patient to (1) breathe a little more deeply or (2) sit up. Listen again. A thick chest wall may make the pulmonic component of S_1 inaudible.	See Table 14-5, p. 388, Variations in the Second Heart Sound—S_2
	Width of split. How wide is the split? It is normally quite narrow.	When either A_2 or P_2 is absent, as in disease of the respective valves, S_2 is persistently single.
	Timing of split. When in the respiratory cycle do you hear the split? It is normally heard late in inspiration.	Expiratory splitting suggests an abnormality
	Does the split disappear as it should, during exhalation? If not, listen again with the patient sitting up.	Persistent splitting results from delayed closure of the pulmonic valve or early closure of the aortic valve.
	Intensity of A_2 and P_2. Compare the intensity of the two components, A_2 and P_2. A_2 is usually louder.	A loud P_2 suggests pulmonary hypertension.
Extra Sounds in Systole	Such as ejection sounds or systolic clicks	The systolic click of mitral valve prolapse is the most common of these sounds. See Table 14-6, p. 389, Extra Heart Sounds in Systole
	Note their location, timing, intensity, and pitch, and the effects of respiration on the sounds.	
Extra Sounds in Diastole	Such as S_3, S_4, or an opening snap	See Table 14-7, p. 390, Extra Heart Sounds in Diastole
	Note the location, timing, intensity, and pitch, and the effects of respiration on the sounds. (An S_3 or S_4 in athletes is a normal finding.)	
Systolic and Diastolic Murmurs	Murmurs are differentiated from heart sounds by their longer duration.	See Table 14-8, p. 391, Pansystolic (Holosystolic) Murmurs Table 14-9, p. 391, Midsystolic Murmurs (pp. 392–393), and Table 14-10, p. 394, Diastolic

Correctly Identifying Heart Murmurs. Correctly identifying heart murmurs requires a logical and systematic approach, a thorough understanding of cardiac anatomy and physiology, and *dedication to the study, practice, and mastery of techniques of examination.* Whenever possible, compare your findings with those of an experienced clinician to improve your clinical acumen.

● *Timing.* First decide if you are hearing a *systolic murmur*, falling between S_1 and S_2, or a *diastolic murmur*, falling between S_2 and S_1. Palpating the carotid pulse as you listen can help you with timing. *Murmurs that coincide with the carotid upstroke are systolic.*

Diastolic murmurs usually indicate valvular heart disease. Systolic murmurs may indicate valvular disease but often occur when the heart valves are normal.

Systolic murmurs are usually *midsystolic* or *pansystolic.* Late systolic murmurs may also be heard.

TIPS FOR IDENTIFYING HEART MURMURS

- Time the murmur—is it in systole or diastole?
- Locate where the murmur is loudest on the precordium—at the base, along the sternal border, at the apex?
- Conduct any necessary maneuvers, such as having the patient lean forward and exhale or turn to the left lateral decubitus position.
- Determine the shape of the murmur—for example, is it crescendo or decrescendo, is it holosystolic?
- Grade the intensity of the murmur from 1 to 6.
- Identify associated features such as the quality of S_1 and S_2; the presence of extra sounds such as S_3, S_4, or an opening snap; or the presence of additional murmurs.
- Be sure to listen in a quiet room!

A *midsystolic murmur* begins after S_1 and stops before S_2. Brief gaps are audible between the murmur and the heart sounds. Listen carefully for the gap just before S_2. It is heard more easily and, if present, usually confirms the murmur as midsystolic, not pansystolic.

S_1 S_2 S_1

Midsystolic murmurs typically arise from blood flow across the semilunar (aortic and pulmonic) valves. See Table 14-9, pp. 392–393, Midsystolic Murmurs

A *pansystolic (holosystolic) murmur* starts with S_1 and stops at S_2, without a gap between murmur and heart sounds.

S_1 S_2 S_1

Pansystolic murmurs often occur with regurgitant (backward) flow across the atrioventricular valves. See Table 14-8, p. 391, Pansystolic (Holosystolic) Murmurs

A *late systolic murmur* usually starts in mid- or late systole and persists up to S_2.

S_1 S_2 S_1

This is the murmur of mitral valve prolapse and is often, but not always, preceded by a systolic click

Diastolic murmurs may be early *diastolic, middiastolic,* or *late diastolic.*

An *early diastolic murmur* starts immediately after S_2, without a discernible gap, and then usually fades into silence before the next S_1.

 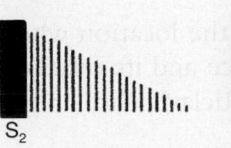

S_1 S_2 S_1

Early diastolic murmurs typically accompany regurgitant flow across incompetent semilunar valves.

A *middiastolic murmur* starts a short time after S_2. It may fade away, as illustrated, or merge into a late diastolic murmur.

 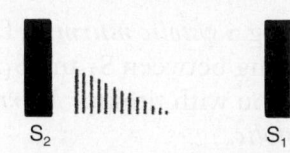

Middiastolic and presystolic murmurs reflect turbulent flow across the atrioventricular valves. See Table 14-10, p. 394, Diastolic Murmurs

A *late diastolic (presystolic) murmur* starts late in diastole and typically continues up to S_1.

  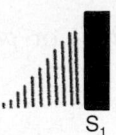

The murmur of a patent ductus arteriosus starts in systole and continues without pause through S_2, into but not necessarily throughout diastole. It is called a *continuous murmur*. Other cardiovascular sounds, such as pericardial friction rubs or venous hums, have *both systolic and diastolic components*. Observe and describe these sounds according to the characteristics used for systolic and diastolic murmurs.

See Table 14-11, p. 395, Cardiovascular Sounds With Both Systolic and Diastolic Components

● *Shape.* The shape or configuration of a murmur's shape is the most difficult for a novice to determine. Concentrate on learning the other characteristics of murmurs first. As your ears become attuned to listening, shape will become identifiable.

A *crescendo murmur* grows louder.

 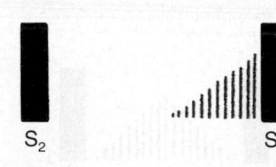

The late diastolic murmur of *mitral stenosis* in normal sinus rhythm

A *decrescendo murmur* grows softer.

 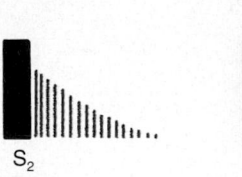

The early diastolic murmur of *aortic regurgitation*

A *crescendo–decrescendo murmur* first rises in intensity, then falls.

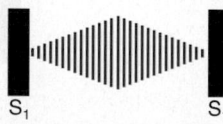

The midsystolic murmur of *aortic stenosis* and *innocent flow murmurs*

A *plateau murmur* has the same intensity throughout.

The pansystolic murmur of *mitral regurgitation*

● *Location of Maximal Intensity.* Find the location where the murmur is heard in terms of the intercostal space and its relation to the sternum, the apex, or the midsternal, the midclavicular, or one of the axillary lines.

For example, a murmur best heard in the 2nd right intercostal space often originates at or near the aortic valve.

● *Radiation or Transmission From the Point of Maximal Intensity.* This reflects not only the site of origin but also the intensity of the murmur and the direction of blood flow. Explore the area around a murmur and determine where else you can hear it.

● *Intensity.* This is usually graded on a 6-point scale and expressed as a fraction. The numerator describes the intensity of the murmur wherever it is loudest; the denominator indicates the scale you are using. Intensity is influenced by the thickness of the chest wall and the presence of intervening tissue.

A loud murmur of *aortic stenosis* often radiates into the neck (in the direction of arterial flow), especially on the right side.

An identical degree of turbulence would cause a louder murmur in a thin person than in a very muscular or obese person. Emphysematous lungs may diminish the intensity of murmurs.

Learn to grade murmurs using the 6-point scale below. Note that grades 4 through 6 require the added presence of a palpable thrill.

● Grades of Murmurs	
Grade	**Description**
Grade 1	Very faint, heard only after listener has "tuned in"; may not be heard in all positions
Grade 2	Quiet, but heard immediately after placing the stethoscope on the chest
Grade 3	Moderately loud
Grade 4	Loud, with palpable thrill
Grade 5	Very loud, with thrill. May be heard when the stethoscope is partly off the chest
Grade 6	Very loud, with thrill. May be heard with stethoscope entirely off the chest

● *Pitch.* This is categorized as high, medium, or low.

● *Quality.* This is described in terms such as blowing, harsh, rumbling, and musical.

A fully described murmur might be: a "medium-pitched, grade 2/6, blowing decrescendo diastolic murmur, heard best in the 4th left intercostal space, with radiation to the apex" (*aortic regurgitation*).

Other characteristics of murmurs include variation with respiration or with the position of the patient. Document the position(s) of the patient or respiratory variation with the other characteristics.

Murmurs originating in the right side of the heart tend to vary with respiration more than left-sided murmurs.

Functional murmurs are short, early, midsystolic murmurs that decrease in intensity with maneuvers that reduce left ventricular volume, such as standing, sitting up, and straining during the Valsalva maneuver.

Peripheral Edema

Inspect the patient's feet, ankles and legs for edema. See Chapter 15 for the examination techniques.

Peripheral edema may indicate heart failure.

Integrating Cardiovascular Assessment

A good cardiovascular examination requires more than observation. The nurse utilizes diagnostic reasoning to integrate individual observations, fit them together in a logical pattern, and correlate cardiac findings with the patient's blood pressure, arterial pulses, venous pulsations, jugular venous pressure, the remainder of the physical examination findings, and the patient's history.

Evaluating the common systolic murmur illustrates this point. In examining an asymptomatic teenager, for example, the nurse might hear a grade 2/6 midsystolic murmur in the 2nd and 3rd left intercostal spaces. Because this suggests a murmur of pulmonic origin, assess the size of the right ventricle by carefully palpating the left parasternal area. Because pulmonic stenosis and atrial septal defects can occasionally cause such murmurs, listen carefully to the splitting of the second heart sound and try to hear any ejection sounds. Listen to the murmur after the patient sits up. Look for evidence of anemia, hyperthyroidism, or pregnancy that could produce such a murmur by increasing the flow across the aortic or the pulmonic valve. If all your findings are normal, your patient probably has an *innocent* or *functional murmur*—one with no pathologic significance.

In a 60-year-old person with angina, you might hear a harsh 3/6 midsystolic crescendo–decrescendo murmur in the right 2nd intercostal space radiating to the neck. These findings suggest *aortic stenosis* but could arise from *aortic sclerosis* (leaflets sclerotic but not stenotic), a dilated aorta, or increased flow across a normal valve. Assess any delay in the carotid upstroke and the intensity of A_2 for evidence of *aortic stenosis*. Check the apical impulse for left ventricular hypertrophy. Listen for *aortic regurgitation* as the patient leans forward and exhales.

Put all this information together to make a hypothesis about the origin of the murmur.

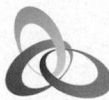

RECORDING YOUR FINDINGS

Recording the Physical Examination—The Cardiovascular Examination

"Carotid upstrokes are brisk, without bruits. JVP is 3 cm above the sternal angle with the head of bed elevated to 30°. Jugular venous distension diminishes rapidly with hepatojugular reflex. The apical impulse is 2 cm in diameter and tapping, 7 cm lateral to the midsternal line in the 5th intercostal space. Crisp S_1 and S_2. At the base S_2 is $>S_1$ and split with respiration, with $A_2 >P_2$. At the apex S_1 is $>S_2$ and constant. No murmurs or extra sounds."

OR

"Carotid upstrokes are brisk; a bruit is heard over the left carotid artery. The JVP is 5 cm above the sternal angle with the head of bed elevated to 50°. Venous distension diminishes over 10 seconds with hepatojugular reflux. The apical impulse is diffuse, 3 cm in diameter, palpated at the anterior axillary line in the 5th and 6th intercostal spaces. S_1 and S_2 are soft. S_3 present at the apex. High-pitched harsh 2/6 holosystolic murmur best heard at the apex, radiating to the axilla."

Suggests *congestive heart failure with volume overload* with possible *left carotid occlusion* and *mitral regurgitation*.[23–25]

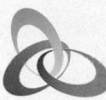 **HEALTH PROMOTION**

Health Promotion Topics

- Coronary heart disease and stroke prevention
- Hypertension prevention and management
- Hyperlipidemia prevention and management

Key roles for the nurse in health promotion are:

- Screening patients for disease and risk factors

- Teaching patients the relationship of risk factors to diseases

- Educating patients on lifestyle changes to reduce risk factors

- Encouraging patients to adhere to healthy lifestyles and medical regimens to reduce the incidence of disease morbidity

Incidence

Cardiovascular disease (CVD) affects 82.6 million U.S. adults and includes hypertension, coronary heart disease (CHD), heart failure, stroke, peripheral vascular disease, and congenital cardiovascular defects. CVD remains the leading cause of death for both men and women, accounting for approximately one third of all U.S. deaths.[7]

According to the U.S. Preventative Services Task Force, hypertension accounts for "35% of all myocardial infarctions and strokes, 49% of all episodes of heart failure, and 24% of all premature deaths."[26] Primary hypertension has no known cause and few symptoms, but is responsible for approximately 95% of adult hypertension. The classifications for blood pressure were modified by the Joint National Committee (JNC) and the old "high-normal" category changed to prehypertension to reflect the tougher standards for hypertension control.

● Blood Pressure (BP) Classification		
Normal	BP <120/80 mm Hg	No treatment required
Prehypertension	Systolic BP between 120 and 139 or diastolic BP between 80 and 88 mm Hg	Lifestyle modifications advised
Stage 1 hypertension	Systolic BP of 140–159 or diastolic BP of 90–99 mm Hg	Lifestyle modifications plus drug therapy
Stage 2 hypertension	Systolic BP ≥160 or diastolic BP ≥100 mm Hg	Lifestyle modifications plus drug therapy, frequently two-drug combination required

(Source: 7th Report of the Joint National Committee on Prevention, Detection, Evaluation, and Treatment of High Blood Pressure [JNC-7].)

HYPERTENSION FACTS

- "Individuals who are normotensive at 55 years have a 90% lifetime risk for developing hypertension."[27]
- "More than 1 of every 2 adults older than 60 years of age has hypertension,"[28] and only 34% of those with hypertension have achieved blood pressure goals.[27]
- "For individuals aged 40 to 70 years, each increment of 20 mm Hg in systolic BP or 10 mm Hg in diastolic BP doubles the risk of CVD."[27,29]
- Recent large population studies of cardiovascular risk factors reveal two striking findings[30]:
  1. Only 4.8% to 9.9% of the young and middle-aged population is at low risk for CVD.
  2. The benefits of low-risk status are enormous: a 72% to 85% reduction in mortality from all causes, leading to a gain of 5.8 to 9.5 years in life expectancy. This gain "holds for both African-Americans and whites, and for those of lower and higher socioeconomic status."[30]
- Identifying and treating people with risk factors are not enough. *A population-wide strategy is critical to prevent and reduce the magnitude of all the major risk factors* so that people develop favorable behaviors in childhood *and remain at low risk for life.*[30]

High serum cholesterol and related lipid disorders are continuously correlated with an elevated risk for CHD in many of the world's populations.[31]

Diabetes and metabolic syndrome increase a person's risk for CVD. Metabolic syndrome is a group of lipid and nonlipid risk factors of metabolic origin that increases the risk of heart disease, stroke, and diabetes.[32,33] It is closely linked to the metabolic insulin resistance disorder.

A client with three or more of these findings may have metabolic syndrome:

- Large waist circumference (abdominal obesity)

  Men: waist circumference of 40 inches or more
  Women: waist circumference of 35 inches or more

- High blood pressure—130/85 mm Hg or higher

- High fasting blood sugar—fasting glucose of 100 mg/dL or higher

- High triglycerides—150 mg/dL or higher

- Low high-density lipoprotein (HDL; good) cholesterol

  Men: <40 mg/dL
  Women: <50 mg/dL

Smoking is also a risk factor for metabolic syndrome.

Risk Reduction

Identification of the patient's risk factors for CVD is a primary nursing function and a part of the history. The risks for cardiac disorders and hypertension overlap, as can be seen below. The more risk factors an individual has, the greater is the chance of developing heart disease. Also, the greater the level of each risk factor, the greater is the risk (e.g., a low-density lipoprotein [LDL] cholesterol of 160 is a greater risk than one of 135). Decreasing the number and severity of risk factors reduces the risk of developing heart disease.

CORONARY HEART DISEASE RISK FACTORS

Modifiable Risk Factors
  Diabetes
  Systolic and/or diastolic hypertension
  Elevated cholesterol and/or triglycerides
  Smoking
  Obesity
  Physical inactivity

Nonmodifiable Factors
  Increasing age
  History of cardiovascular disease
  Family history of early heart disease (younger than 55 years for men and
    65 years for women)

HYPERTENSION RISK FACTORS[27]

Modifiable Risk Factors
  Obesity
  Physical inactivity
  Smoking
  Microalbuminuria or a glomerular filtration rate of <60 mL/min
  Excess dietary sodium
  Insufficient intake of potassium
  Excess alcohol consumption

Nonmodifiable Factors
  Age
  Family history of hypertension or early CVD

The National Cholesterol Education Program (NCEP) wrote a report titled *Detection, Evaluation, and Treatment of High Cholesterol in Adults (Adult Treatment Panel III) or* ATP III that provides guidelines on how to prevent, detect, evaluate, and treat high blood cholesterol.

The 7th Report of the Joint National Committee on Prevention, Detection, Evaluation, and Treatment of High Blood Pressure (JNC-7) describes how to prevent, detect, evaluate, and treat high blood pressure.

Risk assessment is a key element of the report. Screening for adults should begin at 20 years, and the American Pediatric Association is recommending screening children for cholesterol levels and hypertension, especially in families with heart disease histories.[34] Adults 40 years and older should have their *10-year global risk* for heart disease estimated to help them keep their risk as low as possible.

RISK FACTORS USED TO ASSESS THE 10-YEAR CORONARY HEART DISEASE RISK SCORE

Age
Gender
Height, weight, waist circumference (or body mass index [BMI])
Smoking
History of cardiovascular disease or diabetes
Systolic and diastolic blood pressure
Total cholesterol, LDL and HDL cholesterol
Triglycerides
Family history of early heart disease*

*Family is a blood-related parent, sibling, or child.

Risk assessment tools for CHD and metabolic syndrome were developed from the ATP III national guidelines based on research from the Framingham Heart Study.

The CHD tool predicts a patient's risk of suffering a heart attack or dying of heart disease over the next 10 years. For example, if the patient scores a 10% risk, it means in a group of 100 people with similar risk factors about 10 will have a heart attack or die from heart disease (CHD) in the next 10 years.

The metabolic syndrome tool gives 1 point for each of the five risk factors for the syndrome. The goal is to have <3 points.

These tools can be found on the following Web sites.

http://www.heart.org/HEARTORG/Conditions/HeartAttack/Heart AttackToolsResources/Heart-Attack-Risk-Assessment_UCM_303944_ Article.jsp

http://hp2010.nhlbihin.net/atpiii/calculator.asp?usertype=prof

A more sensitive assessment tool called the Reynolds Risk Score was developed for women. This tool is based on data from both the Framingham Heart Study and the Women's Health Study from Harvard. The researchers added C-reactive protein to the risk analysis.[35,36]

This tool can be found at www.reynoldsriskscore.org.

Screening for hypertension, cardiovascular disease, hyperlipidemia, metabolic syndrome, and other risk factors should be carried out routinely. A suggested schedule is below; however, if a condition is present, more frequent screening is recommended. The nurse should encourage patients to obtain regular screening.[37]

● Risk Factors and Screening Frequency for Adults Beginning at 20 Years	
Risk Factor	**Frequency**
Family history of coronary heart disease (CHD)	Update regularly
Smoking status	
Diet	At each routine visit
Alcohol intake	
Physical activity	
Blood pressure	
Body mass index	At each routine visit (at least every 2 years)
Waist circumference	
Pulse (to detect atrial fibrillation)	
Fasting lipoprotein profile	At least every 5 years
Fasting glucose	If risk factors for hyperlipidemia or diabetes present, every 2 years

(Source: Pearson TA, Blair SN, Daniels SR, et al. AHA guidelines for primary prevention of cardiovascular disease and stroke: 2000 update. Circulation 106(3):388–391, 2002.)

Healthy Lifestyles

Educating patients about healthy lifestyle choices and encouraging them to make changes is an important nursing role. It is helpful to obtain a picture of the client's lifestyle before "preaching" changes. Many patients will already include healthy choices in their lives. A nutrition history (see pp. 132–133) and a "typical day" record can help the nurse identify good diet choices and where improvements can be made. Healthy choices should be affirmed. The nurse can then work with the patient to identify where further change is needed and create a mutually agreed upon change plan. The nurse can also supply resources that may help the patient achieve goals. For example, if the patient's goal is to stop smoking, the nurse can explain aids available to decrease the desire for nicotine. Prochaska and DiClemente's Stages of Change Model can be used during a patient assessment to help the nurse determine interventions appropriate to the patient's level.[38]

LIFESTYLE MODIFICATIONS TO PREVENT OR MANAGE HYPERTENSION

- Maintenance of an optimal weight or BMI of 18.5 to 24.9 kg/m^2
- Salt intake of <6 grams of sodium chloride or 2.4 grams of sodium per day. However individuals with hypertension, ≥40 years or are African-American should consume no more than 1500 mg of sodium per day.[39]
- Regular aerobic exercise, such as brisk walking for at least 30 minutes per day, most days of the week
- Moderate alcohol consumption per day of two drinks or fewer for men and one drink or fewer for women (two drinks = 1 oz. ethanol, 24 oz. beer, 10 oz. wine, or 2–3 oz. whiskey)
- Dietary intake of more than 3,500 mg of potassium
- Diet rich in fruits, vegetables, and low-fat dairy products with reduced content of saturated and total fat

(Source: Whelton PK, He J, Appel LJ, et al. Primary prevention of hypertension. Clinical and Public Health Advisory from the National High Blood Pressure Education Program. JAMA 288[15]:1882–1888, 2002.)

LIFESTYLE MODIFICATIONS TO PREVENT CARDIOVASCULAR DISEASE AND STROKE

- Complete cessation of smoking
- Optimal blood pressure control
- Healthy eating—see diet recommendations
- Lipid management
- Regular aerobic exercise—see previous page
- Optimal weight—see previous page
- Diabetes management so that fasting glucose level is below 110 mg/dL and HgA1C is <7%
- Conversion of atrial fibrillation to normal sinus rhythm or, if chronic, anticoagulation

(Source: Pearson TA, Blair SN, Daniels SR, et al. AHA guidelines for primary prevention of cardiovascular disease and stroke: 2002 update. Circulation 106[3]:388–391, 2002.)

Healthy Eating. Begin with a nutrition history (see pp. 129–130), and then target low intake of cholesterol and total fat, especially less saturated and *trans* fat. Foods with monounsaturated fats, polyunsaturated fats, and omega-3 fatty acids in fish oils help to lower blood cholesterol. Review the food sources of these healthy and unhealthy fats on the next page.

FOOD SOURCES OF HEALTHY AND UNHEALTHY FATS

Healthy Fats

- *Foods high in monounsaturated fat:* nuts, such as almonds, pecans, and peanuts; sesame seeds; avocados; canola oil; olive and peanut oil; peanut butter
- *Foods high in polyunsaturated fat:* corn, safflower, cottonseed, and soybean oil; walnuts; pumpkin or sunflower seeds; soft (tub) margarine; mayonnaise; salad dressings
- *Foods high in omega-3 fatty acids:* albacore tuna, herring, mackerel, rainbow trout, salmon, sardines

Unhealthy Fats

- *Foods high in trans fat:* snacks and baked goods with hydrogenated or partially hydrogenated oil, stick margarines, shortening, french fries
- *Foods high in cholesterol:* dairy products, egg yolks, liver and organ meats, high-fat meat and poultry
- *Foods high in saturated fat:* high-fat dairy products—cream, cheese, ice cream, whole and 2% milk, butter, and sour cream; bacon; chocolate; coconut oil; lard and gravy from meat drippings; high-fat meats like ground beef, bologna, hot dogs, and sausage

Counseling About Weight and Exercise. *The Healthy People 2020 Nutrition and Weight Status* reports that dietary factors are associated with 4 of the 10 leading causes of death—coronary heart disease, some types of cancer, stroke, and type 2 diabetes—as well as with high blood pressure and osteoporosis.[40] More than 60% of all Americans are now obese or overweight, with a BMI ≥25.

Counseling about weight has become a nursing imperative. Assess BMI as described in Chapter 8, pp. 134–135. Discuss the principles of healthy eating—patients with high fat intake are more likely to accumulate body fat than patients with high intake of protein and carbohydrate. Review the patient's eating habits and weight patterns in the family. Set realistic goals that will help the patient maintain healthy eating habits *for life*.

Exercise is a critical adjunct to weight control for maintaining health. *Healthy People 2020's* overview on Physical Activity notes that "Regular physical activity can improve the health and quality of life of Americans of all ages, regardless of the presence of a chronic disease or disability. Among adults and older adults, physical activity can lower the risk of early death, coronary heart disease, stroke, high blood pressure, type 2 diabetes, breast and colon cancer, falls, and depression."[42] To reduce the risk for CHD, counsel patients to pursue aerobic exercise, or exercise that increases muscle oxygen uptake, for at least 30 minutes on most days of the week. Spur motivation by emphasizing the immediate benefits to health and well-being. Deep breathing, sweating in cool temperatures, and pulse rates exceeding 60% of the maximum normal age-adjusted heart rate, or 220 minus the person's age, are markers that help patients recognize onset of aerobic metabolism. Be sure to evaluate any cardiovascular, pulmonary, or musculoskeletal conditions that present risks before selecting an exercise regimen.

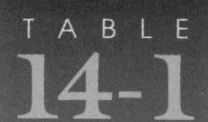
Selected Heart Rates and Rhythms

Cardiac rhythms may be classified as *regular or irregular*. When rhythms are irregular or rates are fast or slow, an ECG should be obtained to identify the origin of the beats (sinus node, AV node, atrium, or ventricle) and the pattern of conduction. Note that with AV (atrioventricular) block, arrhythmias may have a fast, normal, or slow ventricular rate. Some authors consider 90 beats/minute the upper limit of normal.

	ECG Pattern	Usual Resting Rate
WHAT IS THE RATE?		
FAST (>100)	Sinus tachycardia	100–180
	Supraventricular (atrial or nodal) tachycardia	150–250
	Atrial flutter with a regular ventricular response	100–175
	Ventricular tachycardia	110–250
OR		
NORMAL (60–100)	Normal sinus rhythm	60–90
	Second-degree AV block	60–100
	Atrial flutter with a regular ventricular response	75–100
OR		
SLOW (<60)	Sinus bradycardia	<60
	Second-degree AV block	30–60
	Complete heart block	<40

REGULAR

IS THE RHYTHM REGULAR OR IRREGULAR?

IRREGULAR

RHYTHMIC OR SPORADIC	With early beats, atrial or nodal (supraventricular) premature contraction OR ventricular premature contractions	
	Sinus arrhythmia	See Table 14-2
OR		
TOTAL	Atrial fibrillation	
	Atrial flutter with varying block	

WHAT IS THE PATTERN OF IRREGULARITY?

Selected Irregular Rhythms

Type of Rhythm	ECG Waves and Heart Sounds	
Atrial or Nodal Premature Contractions (*Supraventricular*)	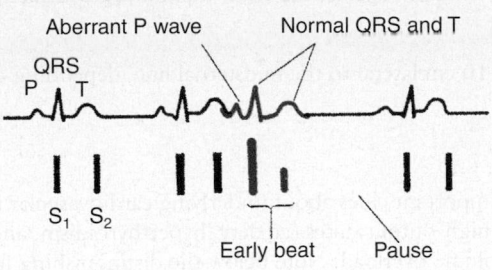	**Rhythm.** A beat of atrial or nodal origin comes earlier than the next expected normal beat. A pause follows, and then the rhythm resumes. **Heart Sounds.** S_1 may differ in intensity from the S_1 of normal beats, and S_2 may be decreased.
Ventricular Premature Contractions	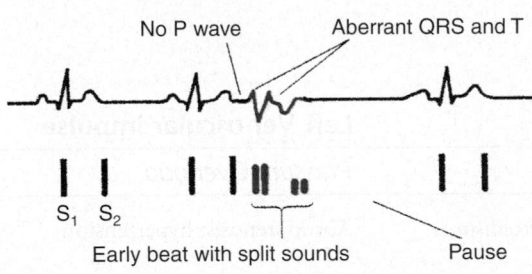	**Rhythm.** A beat of ventricular origin comes earlier than the next expected normal beat. A pause follows, and the rhythm resumes. **Heart Sounds.** S_1 may differ in intensity from the S_1 of the normal beats, and S_2 may be decreased. Both sounds are likely to be split.
Sinus Arrhythmia	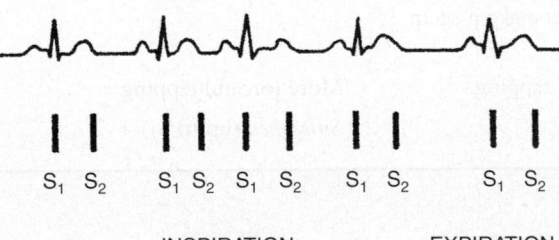	**Rhythm.** The heart varies cyclically, usually speeding up with inspiration and slowing down with expiration. **Heart Sounds.** Normal, although S_1 may vary with the heart rate.
Atrial Fibrillation and Atrial Flutter With Varying AV Block	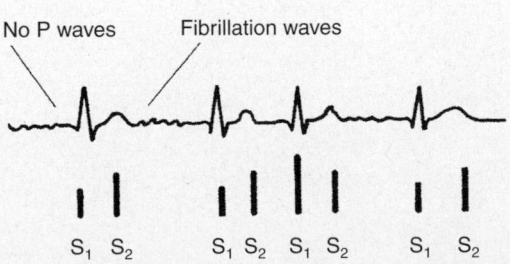	**Rhythm.** The ventricular rhythm is totally irregular, although short runs of the irregular ventricular rhythm may seem regular. **Heart Sounds.** S_1 varies in intensity.

For the Atrial or Nodal Premature Contractions diagram: Aberrant P wave, Normal QRS and T, QRS, P, T, S_1, S_2, Early beat, Pause

For the Ventricular Premature Contractions diagram: No P wave, Aberrant QRS and T, S_1, S_2, Early beat with split sounds, Pause

For the Sinus Arrhythmia diagram: S_1 S_2 S_1 S_2 S_1 S_2 S_1 S_2 S_1 S_2, INSPIRATION, EXPIRATION

For the Atrial Fibrillation diagram: No P waves, Fibrillation waves, S_1 S_2 S_1 S_2 S_1 S_2 S_1 S_2

TABLE
14-3

Variations and Abnormalities of the Apical Impulse

In the healthy heart, the apical impulse or *left ventricular impulse* is usually the *point of maximal impulse,* or *PMI.* This brief impulse is generated by the movement of the ventricular apex against the chest wall during contraction. The classical descriptors of the apical impulse are:

- *Location:* in the 4th or 5th intercostal space, ~7–10 cm lateral to the midsternal line, depending on the diameter of the chest
- *Diameter: discrete,* or ≤2 cm
- *Amplitude: brisk* and *tapping*
- *Duration:* ≤2/3 of systole

Careful examination of the apical impulse gives you important clues about underlying cardiovascular hemodynamics. The quality of the impulse changes as the left ventricle adapts to high-output states (anxiety, hyperthyroidism, and severe anemia) and to the more pathologic conditions of chronic pressure or volume overload. Note below the distinguishing features of three types of apical impulses: the *hyperkinetic impulse* from transiently increased stroke volume—this change does not necessarily indicate heart disease; the *sustained* impulse of ventricular hypertrophy from chronic pressure load, known as *increased afterload* (see p. 347); and the *diffuse* impulse of ventricular dilation from chronic volume overload, or *increased preload.*

	Left Ventricular Impulse		
	Hyperkinetic	*Pressure Overload*	*Volume Overload*
Examples of Causes	Anxiety, hyperthyroidism, severe anemia	Aortic stenosis, hypertension	Aortic or mitral regurgitation
Location	Normal	Normal	Displaced to the left and possibly downward
Diameter	~2 cm, though increased amplitude may make it seem larger	>2 cm	>2 cm
Amplitude	More forceful tapping	More forceful tapping	*Diffuse*
Duration	<2/3 systole	*Sustained* (up to S_2)	Often slightly sustained

Variations in the First Heart Sound—S_1

Normal

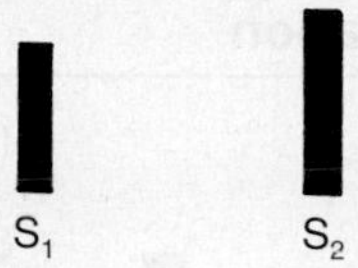

S_1 is softer than S_2 at the *base* (right and left 2nd intercostal spaces).

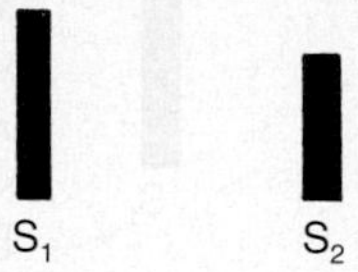

S_1 is often but not always louder than S_2 at the *apex*.

Accentuated S_1

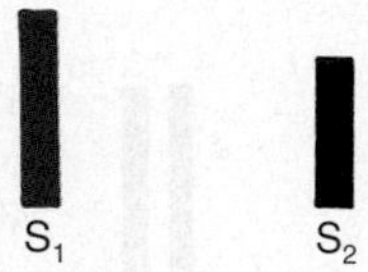

S_1 is accentuated in (1) tachycardia, rhythms with a short PR interval, and high cardiac output states (e.g., exercise, anemia, hyperthyroidism) and (2) mitral stenosis. In these conditions, the mitral valve is still open wide at the onset of ventricular systole and then closes quickly.

Diminished S_1

S_1 is diminished in first-degree heart block (delayed conduction from atria to ventricles). Here the mitral valve has had time after atrial contraction to float back into an almost closed position before ventricular contraction shuts it. It closes more quietly. S_1 is also diminished (1) when the mitral valve is calcified and relatively immobile, as in mitral regurgitation, and (2) when left ventricular contractility is markedly reduced, as in congestive heart failure or coronary heart disease.

Varying S_1

S_1 varies in intensity (1) in complete heart block, when atria and ventricles are beating independently of each other, and (2) in any totally irregular rhythm (e.g., atrial fibrillation). In these situations, the mitral valve is in varying positions before being shut by ventricular contraction. Its closure sound, therefore, varies in loudness.

Split S_1

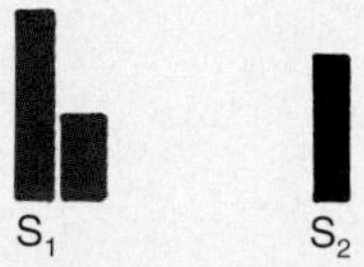

S_1 may be split normally along the lower left sternal border where the tricuspid component, often too faint to be heard, becomes audible. This split may sometimes be heard at the apex, but if heard it should be differentiated from an S_4, an aortic ejection sound, or an early systolic click. Abnormal splitting of both heart sounds may be heard in right bundle branch block and in premature ventricular contractions.

TABLE
14-5

Variations in the Second Heart Sound—S_2

	Inspiration	Expiration	

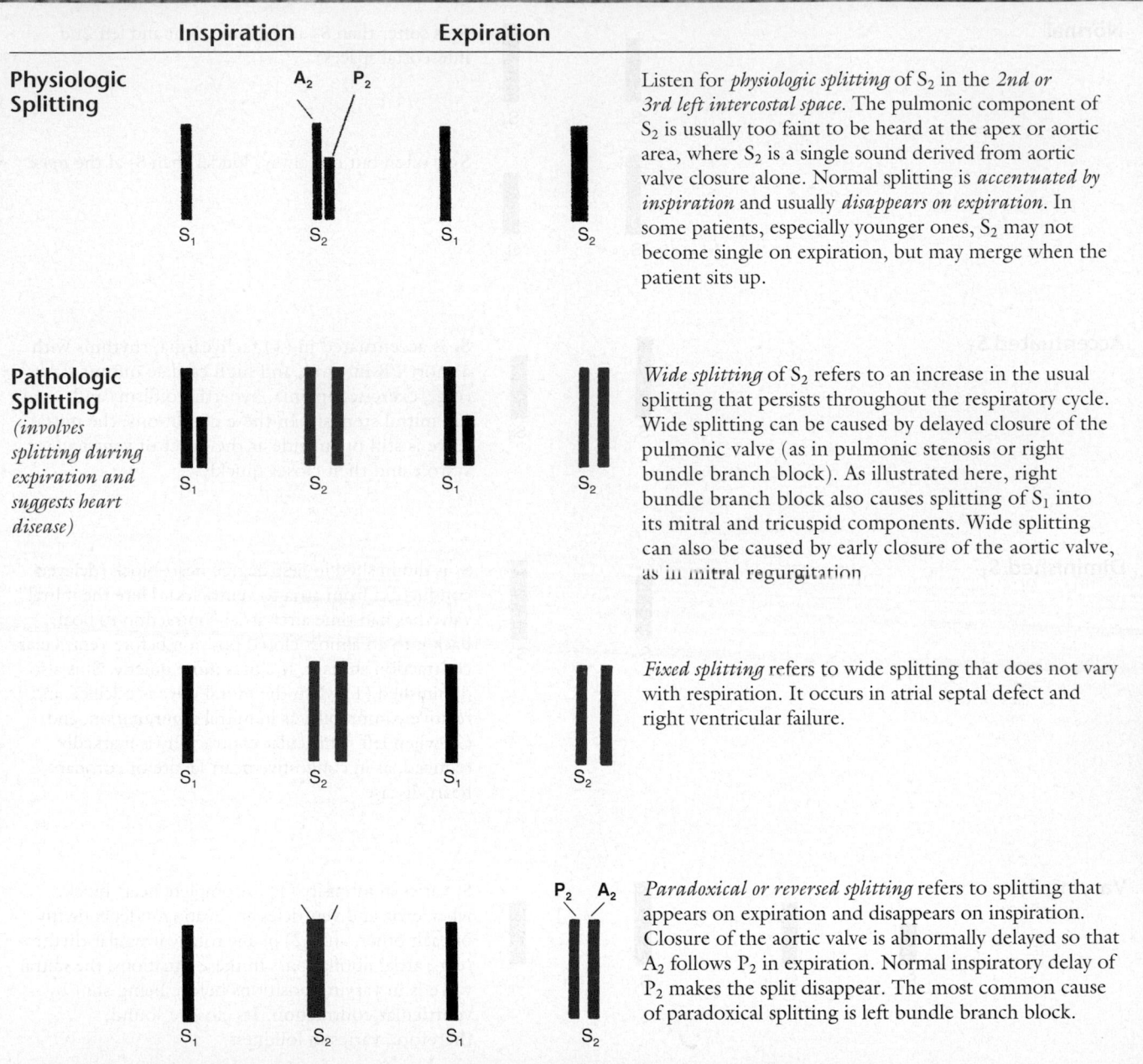

Physiologic Splitting

Listen for *physiologic splitting* of S_2 in the *2nd or 3rd left intercostal space*. The pulmonic component of S_2 is usually too faint to be heard at the apex or aortic area, where S_2 is a single sound derived from aortic valve closure alone. Normal splitting is *accentuated by inspiration* and usually *disappears on expiration*. In some patients, especially younger ones, S_2 may not become single on expiration, but may merge when the patient sits up.

Pathologic Splitting
(involves splitting during expiration and suggests heart disease)

Wide splitting of S_2 refers to an increase in the usual splitting that persists throughout the respiratory cycle. Wide splitting can be caused by delayed closure of the pulmonic valve (as in pulmonic stenosis or right bundle branch block). As illustrated here, right bundle branch block also causes splitting of S_1 into its mitral and tricuspid components. Wide splitting can also be caused by early closure of the aortic valve, as in mitral regurgitation

Fixed splitting refers to wide splitting that does not vary with respiration. It occurs in atrial septal defect and right ventricular failure.

Paradoxical or reversed splitting refers to splitting that appears on expiration and disappears on inspiration. Closure of the aortic valve is abnormally delayed so that A_2 follows P_2 in expiration. Normal inspiratory delay of P_2 makes the split disappear. The most common cause of paradoxical splitting is left bundle branch block.

TABLE
14-6

Extra Heart Sounds in Systole

There are two kinds of extra heart sounds in systole: (1) early ejection sounds and (2) clicks, commonly heard in mid- and late systole.

Early Systolic Ejection Sounds

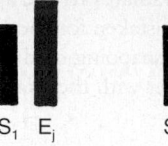

S_1 E_j S_2

Early systolic ejection sounds occur shortly after S_1, coincident with opening of the aortic and pulmonic valves. They are relatively high in pitch; have a sharp, clicking quality, and are heard better with the diaphragm of the stethoscope. An ejection sound indicates cardiovascular disease.

Listen for an *aortic ejection sound* at both the base and apex. It may be louder at the apex and usually does not vary with respiration. An aortic ejection sound may accompany a dilated aorta, or aortic valve disease from congenital stenosis or a bicuspid valve.

A *pulmonic ejection sound* is heard best in the 2nd and 3rd left intercostal spaces. When S_1, usually relatively soft in this area, appears to be loud, you may be hearing a pulmonic ejection sound. Its intensity often *decreases with inspiration*. Causes include dilatation of the pulmonary artery, pulmonary hypertension, and pulmonic stenosis.

Systolic Clicks

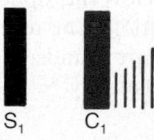

S_1 C_1 S_2

Systolic clicks are usually caused by *mitral valve prolapse*—an abnormal systolic ballooning of part of the mitral valve into the left atrium. The clicks are usually mid- or late systolic. Prolapse of the mitral valve is a common cardiac condition, affecting about 5% of the general population. There is equal prevalence in men and women.

The click is usually single, but you may hear more than one, usually *at or medial to the apex,* but also *at the lower left sternal border.* It is high-pitched, so listen with the diaphragm. The click is often followed by a late systolic murmur from mitral regurgitation—a flow of blood from left ventricle to left atrium. The murmur usually crescendos up to S_2. Auscultatory findings are notably variable. Most patients have only a click, some have only a murmur, and some have both. Systolic clicks may also be of extracardial or mediastinal origin.

TABLE
14-7

Extra Heart Sounds in Diastole

Opening Snap

S_1	S_2 OS	S_1

The *opening snap* is a very early diastolic sound usually produced by the opening of a *stenotic mitral valve*. It is heard best just medial to the apex and along the lower left sternal border. When it is loud, an opening snap radiates to the apex and to the pulmonic area, where it may be mistaken for the pulmonic component of a split S_2. Its high pitch and snapping quality help to distinguish it from an S_2. It is heard better with the *diaphragm*.

S_3

S_1	S_2 S_3	S_1

You will detect *physiologic* S_3 frequently in children and in young adults to the age of 35 or 40. It is common during the last trimester of pregnancy. Occurring early in diastole during rapid ventricular filling, it is later than an opening snap, dull and low in pitch, and heard best at the apex in the left lateral decubitus position. The *bell* of the stethoscope should be used with very light pressure.

A *pathologic S_3* or *ventricular gallop* sounds just like a physiologic S_3. An S_3 in a person over age 40 (possibly a little older in women) is almost certainly pathologic, arising from altered left ventricular compliance at the end of the rapid filling phase of diastole.[42] Causes include decreased myocardial contractility, congestive heart failure, and volume overloading of a ventricle, as in mitral or tricuspid regurgitation. A *left-sided* S_3 is heard typically at the apex in the left lateral decubitus position. A *right-sided* S_3 is usually heard along the lower left sternal border or below the xiphoid with the patient supine, and is louder on inspiration. The term *gallop* comes from the cadence of three heart sounds, especially at rapid heart rates, and sounds like "Kentucky."

S_4

S_1	S_2	S_4 S_1

An S_4 (*atrial sound* or *atrial gallop*) occurs just before S_1. It is dull, low in pitch, and heard better with the bell. An S_4 is heard occasionally in an apparently normal person, especially in trained athletes and older age groups. More commonly, it is due to increased resistance to ventricular filling following atrial contraction. This increased resistance is related to decreased compliance (increased stiffness) of the ventricular myocardium.[43]

Causes of a left-sided S_4 include hypertensive heart disease, coronary artery disease, aortic stenosis, and cardiomyopathy. A *left-sided* S_4 is heard best at the apex in the left lateral position; it may sound like "Tennessee." The less common *right-sided* S_4 is heard along the lower left sternal border or below the xiphoid. It often gets louder with inspiration. Causes of a right-sided S_4 include pulmonary hypertension and pulmonic stenosis.

An S_4 may also be associated with delayed conduction between the atria and ventricles. This delay separates the normally faint atrial sound from the louder S_1 and makes it audible. An S_4 is never heard in the absence of atrial contraction, which occurs with atrial fibrillation.

Occasionally, a patient has both an S_3 and an S_4, producing a *quadruple rhythm* of four heart sounds. At rapid heart rates, the S_3 and S_4 may merge into one loud extra heart sound, called a *summation gallop*.

TABLE
14-8

Pansystolic (Holosystolic) Murmurs

Pansystolic (holosystolic) murmurs are pathologic, arising from blood flow from a chamber with high pressure to one of lower pressure, through a valve or other structure that should be closed. The murmur begins immediately with S_1 and continues up to S_2.

	Mitral Regurgitation[44,45]	Tricuspid Regurgitation	Ventricular Septal Defect
Murmur	*Location.* Apex	*Location.* Lower left sternal border	*Location.* 3rd, 4th, and 5th left intercostal spaces
	Radiation. To the left axilla, less often to the left sternal border	*Radiation.* To the right of the sternum, to the xiphoid area, and perhaps to the left midclavicular line, but not into the axilla	*Radiation.* Often wide
	Intensity. Soft to loud; if loud, associated with an apical thrill	*Intensity.* Variable	*Intensity.* Often very loud, with a thrill
	Pitch. Medium to high	*Pitch.* Medium	*Pitch.* High, holosystolic
	Quality. Harsh, holosystolic	*Quality.* Blowing, holosystolic	*Quality.* Often harsh
	Aids. Unlike tricuspid regurgitation, it does not become louder in inspiration.	*Aids.* Unlike mitral regurgitation, the intensity may increase slightly with inspiration.	
Associated Findings	S_1 normal (75%), loud (12%), soft (12%)	The right ventricular impulse is increased in amplitude and may be sustained.	S_2 may be obscured by the loud murmur.
	An apical S_3 reflects volume overload of the left ventricle.	An S_3 may be audible along the lower left sternal border. The jugular venous pressure is often elevated, with large *v* waves in the jugular veins.	Findings vary with the severity of the defect and with associated lesions.
	The apical impulse is increased in amplitude (diffuse), is laterally displaced, and may be sustained.		
Mechanism	When the *mitral valve fails to close fully in systole,* blood regurgitates from left ventricle to left atrium, causing a murmur. This leakage creates volume overload on the left ventricle, with subsequent dilatation.	When the *tricuspid valve fails to close fully in systole,* blood regurgitates from right ventricle to right atrium, producing a murmur. The most common cause is right ventricular failure and dilatation, with resulting enlargement of the tricuspid orifice. Either pulmonary hypertension or left ventricular failure is the usual initiating cause.	A ventricular septal defect is a congenital abnormality in which *blood flows from the relatively high-pressure left ventricle into the low-pressure right ventricle through a hole.*

TABLE
14-9

Midsystolic Murmurs

Midsystolic ejection murmurs are the most common kind of heart murmur. They may be (1) *innocent*—without any detectable physiologic or structural abnormality; (2) *physiologic*—from physiologic changes in body metabolism; or (3) *pathologic*—arising from a structural abnormality in the heart or great vessels.[44,45] Midsystolic murmurs tend to peak near midsystole and usually stop before S_2. The crescendo–decrescendo or "diamond" shape is not always audible, but the gap between the murmur and S_2 helps to distinguish midsystolic from pansystolic murmurs.

	Innocent Murmurs	**Physiologic Murmurs**
	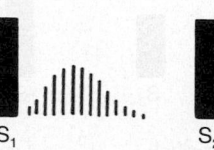	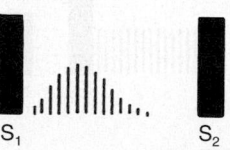
Murmur	*Location.* 2nd to 4th left intercostal spaces between the left sternal border and the apex	Similar to innocent murmurs
	Radiation. Little	
	Intensity. Grade 1 to 2, possibly 3	
	Pitch. Soft to medium	
	Quality. Variable	
	Aids. Usually decreases or disappears on sitting	
Associated Findings	None: normal splitting, no ejection sounds, no diastolic murmurs, and no palpable evidence of ventricular enlargement. Occasionally, both an innocent murmur and another kind of murmur are present.	Possible signs of a likely cause
Mechanism	Innocent murmurs result from turbulent blood flow, probably generated by ventricular ejection of blood into the aorta from the left and occasionally the right ventricle. Very common in children and young adults—may also be heard in older people. There is no underlying cardiovascular disease.	Turbulence due to a temporary increase in blood flow in predisposing conditions such as anemia, pregnancy, fever, and hyperthyroidism.

Pathologic Murmurs

Aortic Stenosis[46,47]

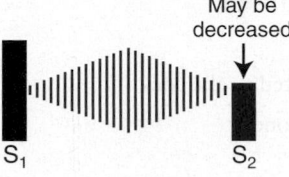

Location. Right 2nd intercostal space

Radiation. Often to the carotids, down the left sternal border, even to the apex

Intensity. Sometimes soft but often loud, with a thrill

Pitch. Medium, harsh; crescendo–decrescendo may be higher at the apex

Quality. Often harsh; may be more musical at the apex

Aids. Heard best with the patient sitting and leaning forward

A_2 decreases as aortic stenosis worsens. A_2 may be delayed and merge with $P_2 \rightarrow$ single S_2 on expiration or paradoxical S_2 split. Carotid upstroke may be *delayed*, with slow rise and small amplitude. Hypertrophied left ventricle may $\rightarrow$ *sustained* apical impulse and an S_4 from decreased compliance.

Significant aortic valve stenosis impairs blood flow across the valve, causing turbulence, and increases left ventricular afterload. Causes are congenital, rheumatic, and degenerative; findings may differ with each cause. Other conditions mimic aortic stenosis without obstructing flow: *aortic sclerosis*, a stiffening of aortic valve leaflets associated with aging; a *bicuspid aortic valve*, a congenital condition that may not be recognized until adulthood; *a dilated aorta*, as in arteriosclerosis, syphilis, or Marfan syndrome; *pathologically increased flow across the aortic valve* during systole can accompany aortic regurgitation.

Hypertrophic Cardiomyopathy

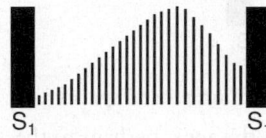

Location. 3rd and 4th left intercostal spaces

Radiation. Down the left sternal border to the apex, possibly to the base, but not to the neck

Intensity. Variable

Pitch. Medium

Quality. Harsh

Aids. Decreases with squatting, increases with straining down from Valsalva and standing

S_3 may be present. An S_4 is often present at the apex (unlike mitral regurgitation). The apical impulse may be *sustained* and have two palpable components. The carotid pulse rises *quickly*, unlike the pulse in aortic stenosis.

Massive ventricular hypertrophy is associated with unusually rapid ejection of blood from the left ventricle during systole. Outflow tract obstruction of flow may coexist. Accompanying distortion of the mitral valve may cause mitral regurgitation.

Pulmonic Stenosis

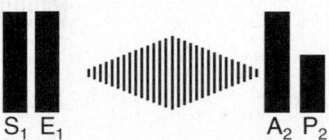

Location. 2nd and 3rd left intercostal spaces

Radiation. If loud, toward the left shoulder and neck

Intensity. Soft to loud; if loud, associated with a thrill

Pitch. Medium; crescendo–decrescendo

Quality. Often harsh

In severe stenosis, S_2 is widely split, and P_2 is diminished or inaudible. An early pulmonic ejection sound is common. May hear a right-sided S_4. Right ventricular impulse often increased in amplitude and *sustained*.

Pulmonic valve stenosis impairs flow across the valve, increasing right ventricular afterload. Congenital and usually found in children. In an *atrial septal defect*, the systolic murmur from pathologically increased flow across the pulmonic valve may mimic pulmonic stenosis.

TABLE
14-10

Diastolic Murmurs

Diastolic murmurs almost always indicate heart disease. There are two basic types. *Early decrescendo diastolic murmurs* signify regurgitant flow through an incompetent semilunar valve, more commonly the aortic. *Rumbling diastolic murmurs in mid- or late diastole* suggest stenosis of an atrioventricular valve, usually the mitral.

	Aortic Regurgitation[69]	**Mitral Stenosis**
	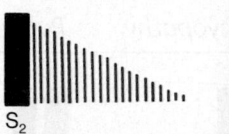 S$_2$ S$_1$	Accentuated S$_2$ OS S$_1$
Murmur	*Location.* 2nd to 4th left intercostal spaces	*Location.* Usually limited to the apex
	Radiation. If loud, to the apex, perhaps to the right sternal border	*Radiation.* Little or none
	Intensity. Grade 1 to 3	*Intensity.* Grade 1 to 4
	Pitch. High. *Use the diaphragm.*	*Pitch.* Decrescendo low-pitched rumble. *Use the bell.*
	Quality. Blowing decrescendo; may be mistaken for breath sounds	
	Aids. The murmur is heard best with the *patient sitting, leaning forward,* with breath held after exhalation.	*Aids.* Placing the bell exactly on the apical impulse, turning the patient into a *left lateral position,* and mild exercise all help to make the murmur audible. It is heard better in exhalation.
Associated Findings	An ejection sound may be present.	S$_1$ is accentuated and may be palpable at the apex.
	An S$_3$ or S$_4$, if present, suggests severe regurgitation.	An opening snap (OS) often follows S$_2$ and initiates the murmur.
	Progressive changes in the apical impulse include increased amplitude, displacement laterally and downward, widened diameter, and increased duration.	If pulmonary hypertension develops, P$_2$ is accentuated, and the right ventricular impulse becomes palpable.
	The pulse pressure increases, and *arterial pulses are often large and bounding.* A midsystolic flow murmur or an Austin Flint murmur suggests large regurgitant flow.	Mitral regurgitation and aortic valve disease may be associated with mitral stenosis.
Mechanism	The leaflets of the aortic valve fail to close completely during diastole, and blood regurgitates from the aorta back into the left ventricle. Volume overload on the left ventricle results. Two other murmurs may be associated: (1) a midsystolic murmur from the resulting increased forward flow across the aortic valve and (2) a mitral diastolic (*Austin Flint*) murmur, attributed to diastolic impingement of the regurgitant flow on the anterior leaflet of the mitral valve.	When the leaflets of the mitral valve thicken, stiffen, and become distorted from the effects of rheumatic fever, the *mitral valve fails to open sufficiently in diastole.* The resulting murmur has two components: (1) middiastolic (during rapid ventricular filling) and (2) presystolic (during atrial contraction). The latter disappears if atrial fibrillation develops, leaving only a middiastolic rumble.

TABLE
14-11

Cardiovascular Sounds With Both Systolic and Diastolic Components

Some cardiovascular sounds extend beyond one phase of the cardiac cycle. Three examples, further described below, are: (1) a *venous hum*, a benign sound produced by turbulence of blood in the jugular veins—common in children; (2) a *pericardial friction rub*, produced by inflammation of the pericardial sac; and (3) *patent ductus arteriosus*, a congenital abnormality in which an open channel persists between the aorta and pulmonary artery. *Continuous murmurs* begin in systole and extend through S_2 into all or part of diastole, as in *patent ductus arteriosus*.

	Venous Hum	Pericardial Friction Rub	Patent Ductus Arteriosus
	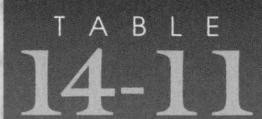		
Timing	Continuous murmur without a silent interval. Loudest in diastole	May have three short components, each associated with friction from cardiac movement in the pericardial sac: (1) atrial systole, (2) ventricular systole, and (3) ventricular diastole. Usually the first two components are present; all three make diagnosis easy; only one (usually the systolic) invites confusion with a murmur.	Continuous murmur in both systole and diastole, often with a silent interval late in diastole. Loudest in late systole, obscures S_2, and fades in diastole
Location	Above the medial third of the clavicles, especially on the right	Variable, but usually heard best in the 3rd interspace to the left of the sternum	Left 2nd intercostal space
Radiation	1st and 2nd intercostal spaces	Little	Toward the left clavicle
Intensity	Soft to moderate. Can be obliterated by pressure on the jugular veins	Variable. May increase when the patient leans forward, exhales, and holds breath (in contrast to pleural rub)	Usually loud, sometimes associated with a thrill
Quality	Humming, roaring	Scratchy, scraping	Harsh, machinery-like
Pitch	Low (heard better with the *bell*)	High (heard better with the *diaphragm*)	Medium

BIBLIOGRAPHY

CITATIONS

1. McGee S. Palpation of the heart. In: Evidence-Based Physical Diagnosis, 2nd ed. St. Louis: Saunders, 2007:400–404.

2. O'Rourke RA, Braunwald E. Physical examination of the cardiovascular system. In: Kasper DL, Braunwald E, Hauser S, et al., eds. Harrison's Principles of Internal Medicine, 16th ed. New York: McGraw-Hill, 2005:1307.

3. Hunt SA, Abraham WT, Chin MH, et al. ACC/AHA 2005 guideline update for the diagnosis and management of chronic heart failure in the adult—summary article. Circulation 112(12): 154–235, 2005.

4. Cook DJ, Simel DL. Does this patient have abnormal central venous pressure? JAMA 275(8):630–654, 1996.

5. Vinayak AG, Levitt J, Gehlbach B, et al. Usefulness of the external jugular vein examination in detecting abnormal central venous pressure in critically ill patients. Arch Intern Med 166(19):2132–2137, 2006.

6. Davison R, Cannon R. Estimation of central venous pressure by examination of jugular veins. Am Heart J 87(3):279–282, 1974.

7. Roger V et al. American Heart Association Heart Disease and Stroke Statistics 2011 Update: A Report from the American Heart Association. Circulation 2011;123;e18-e209; originally published online Dec 15, 2010; Available at http://circ.aha journals.org/cgi/reprint/CIR.0b013e3182009701. Accessed April 12, 2011.

8. Hofgren C, Karlson BW, Gaston-Johansson F, et al. Word descriptors in suspected acute myocardial infarction: a comparison between patients with and without confirmed myocardial infarction. Heart Lung 23(5):397–403, 1994.

9. Abrams J. Chronic stable angina. N Engl J Med 352(24): 2524–2533, 2005.

10. Gibbons RJ, Abrams J, Chatterjee K, et al. ACC/AHA 2002 ACC/AHA 2002 guideline update for the management of patients with chronic stable angina—summary article. Circulation 107(1):149–158, 2003.

11. Klompas M. Does this patient have an acute thoracic aortic dissection? JAMA 287(17): 2262–2272, 2002.

12. Beevers G, Lip GY, O'Brien E. ABC of hypertension: blood pressure measurement. Part I. Sphygmomanometry: factors common in all techniques. BMJ 322(7292):981–985, 2001.

13. Beevers G, Lip GY, O'Brien E. ABC of hypertension: blood pressure measurement. Part II Conventional sphygmomanometry: technique of auscultatory blood pressure measurement. BMJ 322(7293):1043–1047, 2001.

14. McAlister FA, Straus SE. Evidence-based treatment of hypertension. Measurement of blood pressure: an evidence based review. BMJ 322(7292):908–911, 2001.

15. Tholl U, Forstner K, Anlauf M. Measuring blood pressure: pitfalls and recommendations. Nephrol Dial Transplant 19(4):766–770, 2004.

16. Edmonds ZV, Mower WR, Lovato LM, et al. The reliability of vital sign measurements. Ann Emerg Med 39(3):233–237, 2002.

17. Sauve JS, Laupacis A, Feagan B, et al. Does this patient have a clinically important carotid bruit? JAMA 270(23):2843–2845, 1993.

18. Lange RA, Hillis LD. Acute pericarditis. N Engl J Med 351(21):2195–2202, 2004.

19. Aurigemma GP, Gasach WH. Diastolic heart failure. N Engl J Med 351(11): 1097–1104, 2004.

20. McGee S. Inspection of the neck veins. In: Evidence-Based Physical Diagnosis, 2nd ed. St. Louis: Saunders, 2007:378.

21. Drazner MH, Rame E, Stevenson LW, et al. Prognostic importance of elevated jugular venous pressure and a third heart sound in patients with heart failure. N Engl J Med 345(8):574–581, 2001.

22. Dans AL, Bossone EF, Guyatt GH, et al. Evaluation of the reproducibility and accuracy of apex beat measurement in the detection of echocardiographic left ventricular dilation. Can J Cardiol 11(6):493–407, 1995.

23. Halder AW, Larson MG, Franklin SS, et al. Systolic blood pressure, diastolic blood pressure, and pulse pressure as predictors of risk for congestive heart failure in the Framingham Heart Study. Ann Intern Med 138(1):10–16, 2003.

24. Thomas JT, Kelly RF, Thomas SJ, et al. Utility of history, physical examination, electrocardiogram, and chest radiograph for differentiating normal from decreased systolic function in patients with heart failure. Am J Med 112(6):437–445, 2002.

25. Fonarow GC, Adams KF, Abraham WT, et al. Risk stratification for in-hospital mortality in acutely decompensated heart failure: classification and regression tree analysis. JAMA 293(5):572–580, 2005.

26. U.S. Preventive Services Task Force. Evidence for the Reaffirmation of the U.S. Preventive Services Task Force Recommendation on Screening for High Blood Pressure. December 2007. First published in Ann Intern Med 2007;147(11):787– 91. http://www.uspreventiveservicestaskforce.org/uspstf07/hbp/ hbparticle.htm. Accessed April 13, 2011

27. Chobanion AV, Bakris GL, Black HR, et al. The Seventh Report of the Joint National Committee on Prevention, Detection, Evaluation, and Treatment of High Blood Pressure—The JNC 7 Report. JAMA 289(19):2560–2572, 2003. Available at: http://www.nhlbi.nih.gov/guidelines/ hypertension/jnc7full.htm Accessed April 13, 2011.

28. Whelton PK, He J, Appel LJ, et al. Primary prevention of hypertension. Clinical and Public Health Advisory from the National High Blood Pressure Education Program. JAMA 288(15):1882–1888, 2002.

29. Vasan RS, Larson MG, Leip EP, et al. Impact of high-normal blood pressure on the risk of cardiovascular disease. N Engl J Med 345(18):1291–1297, 2001.

30. Stamler J, Stamler R, Neaton JD, et al. Low risk-factor profile and long-term cardiovascular and noncardiovascular mortality and life expectancy—findings for 5 large cohorts of young adult and middle-aged men and women. JAMA 282(21): 2012–2018, 1999.

31. Grundy SM, Cleeman JI, Merz NB, et al, for the Coordinating Committee of the National Cholesterol Education Program. Implications of recent clinical trials for the National Cholesterol Education Program Adult Treatment Panel III guidelines. Circulation 110(2):227–239, 2004.

32. Third Report of the National Cholesterol Education Program (NCEP) Expert Panel. Detection, evaluation, and treatment of high blood cholesterol in adults: executive summary. National Cholesterol Education Program, National Heart, Lung, and Blood Institute, National Institutes of Health. NIH Publication No. 01-3670. May 2001. Available at: www.nhlbi.nih.gov/ guidelines/cholesterol/index.htm. Accessed April 13, 2011

33. National Cholesterol Education Panel. Third report of the National Cholesterol Education Program (NCEP) Expert Panel on detection, evaluation, and treatment of high blood cholesterol in adults (Adult Treatment Panel III) final report. Circulation 106(25):3143–3421, 2002.

34. Daniels SR, Greer FR, Committee on Nutrition. Lipid screening and cardiovascular health in childhood. Pediatrics 122:198–208, 2008.

35. Bassuk SB. The Reynolds risk score – improving cardiovascular risk prediction in women. AAOHN J 56(4):180, 2008.

36. Ridker PM, Buring JE, Rifai N, et al. Development and validation of improved algorithms for the assessment of global cardiovascular risk in women. JAMA 297(6):611–619, 2007.

37. Pearson TA, Blair SN, Daniels SR, et al. AHA guidelines for primary prevention of cardiovascular disease and stroke: 2002 update. Circulation 106(3):388–391, 2002.

38. Prochaska JO, DiClemente CC. Stages and processes of self-change in smoking: towards an integrative model of change. J Consult Clin Psychol 51:390–395, 1983.

39. Center for Disease Control and Prevention. CDC Features: Most Americans Should Consume Less Sodium (1,500 mg./Day or Less. Available at: http://www.cdc.gov/Features/Sodium/. Accessed March 21, 2011.

40. Healthy People 2020. 2020 Topics and Objectives: Nutrition and Weight Status U.S. Department of Health and Human Services. Available at: http://www.healthypeople.gov/ 2020/topicsobjectives2020/ebr.aspx?topicid=29. Accessed April 13, 2011.

41. Healthy People 2020. 2020 Topics and Objectives: Physical Activity.. U.S. Department of Health and Human Services. Available at: http://www.healthypeople.gov/2020/topicsobjectives2020/overview.aspx?topicid=33/. Accessed April 13, 2011.

42. Pierard LA, Lancellotti P. The role of ischemic mitral regurgitation in the pathogenesis of acute pulmonary edema. N Engl J Med 351(16):1627–1634, 2004.

43. Otto CM. Evaluation and management of chronic mitral regurgitation. N Engl J Med 345(10):740–746, 2001.

44. Lembo NJ, Dell'Italia LJ, Crawford MH, et al. Bedside diagnosis of systolic murmurs. N Engl J Med 318(24):1572–1578, 1988.

45. Etchells E, Bell C, Robb K. Does this patient have an abnormal systolic murmur? JAMA 277(7):564–571, 1997.

46. Etchells E, Glenns V, Shadowitz S, et al. A bedside clinical prediction rule for detecting moderate or severe aortic stenosis. J Gen Intern Med 13(10):699–704, 1998.

47. Carabello BA. Aortic stenosis. N Engl J Med 356(9):677–682, 2001.

48. Enriquez-Serano M, Tajik AJ. Aortic regurgitation. N Engl J Med 351(15):1539–1546, 2004.

ADDITIONAL REFERENCES

Bassuk SB. The Reynolds risk score:Improving cardiovascular risk prediction in women. AAOHN Journal 56(4): 180, 2008.

Beckman JA, Creager MA, Libby P. Diabetes and atherosclerosis: epidemiology, pathophysiology, and management. JAMA 287(19):2570–2581, 2002.

Capuzzi DM, Freeman JS. C-reactive protein and cardiovascular risk in the metabolic syndrome and type 2 diabetes: controversy and challenge. Clin Diabetes 25(1):16–22, 2007.

Carnici PG, Crea F. Coronary microvascular dysfunction. N Engl J Med 356(8):830–840, 2007.

Cohn JN, Hoke L, Whitwam W, et al. Screening for early detection of cardiovascular disease in asymptomatic individuals. Am Heart J 146(4):679–685, 2003.

Crane PB, Wallace DC. Cardiovascular risks and physical activity in middle-aged and elderly African American women. J Cardiovasc Nurs 22(4):297–303, 2007.

Criley JM. The Physiological Origins of Heart Sounds and Murmurs: The Unique Interactive Guide to Cardiac Diagnosis. English/Spanish (CD-ROM). Palo Alto, CA: Blaufuss Multimedia, 1997.

de Ferranti S, Ludwig D. Storm over statins—the controversy surrounding pharmacologic treatment of children. N Engl J Med 359(13):1309–1312, 2008.

Fischer Aggarwal BA, Liao M, Mosca L. Physical activity as a potential mechanism through which social support may reduce cardiovascular disease risk. J Cardiovasc Nurs 23(2): 90–96, 2008.

Fuster V, Alexander RW, O'Rourke RA, et al. Hurst's The Heart, 11th ed. New York: McGraw-Hill, Medical Publishing Division, 2004.

Hansson GK. Inflammation, atherosclerosis, and coronary artery disease. N Engl J Med 352(16):1685–1695, 2005.

Kuperstein R, Feinberg MS, Eldar M, et al. Physical determinants of systolic murmur intensity in aortic stenosis. Am J Cardiol 95(6):774–776, 2005.

Libby P, ed. Braunwald's Heart Disease: A Textbook of Cardiovascular Medicine, 8th ed. Philadelphia: Elsevier–Saunders, 2008.

Maron BJ, Thompson PD, Ackerman MJ, et al. Recommendations and considerations related to preparticipation screening for cardiovascular abnormalities in competitive athletes: 2007 update. A scientific statement from the American Heart Association Council on Nutrition, Physical Activity, and Metabolism, endorsed by the American College of Cardiology Foundation. Circulation 115(12):1643–1655, 2007.

McCauley KM. Modifying women's risk for cardiovascular disease. J Obstet Gynecol Neonatal Nurs 36(2):116–124, 2007.

National Cholesterol Education Program. Risk Assessment Tool for Estimating 10-year Risk of Developing Hard CHD (Myocardial Infarction and Coronary Death). Available at: http:// hp2010. nhlbihin.net /atpiii/calculator.asp?usertype= prof. Accessed May 30, 2008.

Neubauer S. The failing heart: an engine out of fuel. N Engl J Med 356(11):1140–1151, 2007.

Schroetter SA, Peck SD. Women's risk of heart disease: promoting awareness and prevention—a primary care approach. Medsurg Nurs 17(2):107–113, 2008.

Sebastian TP, Kostis JB, Cassazza L, et al. Heart rate and blood pressure response in adult men and women during exercise and sexual activity. Am J Cardiol 100(12):1795–1801, 2007.

Selvanayagam J, De Pasquale C, Arnolda L. Usefulness of clinical assessment of the carotid pulse in the diagnosis of aortic stenosis. Am J Cardiol 93(4):493–495, 2004.

Sherman C. Reducing the risk of heart disease in women. The Clinical Advisor: For Nurse Practitioners 11(1):49–50,53, 2008.

Sinisalo J, Rapola J, Rossinen J, et al. Simplifying the estimation of jugular venous pressure. Am J Cardiol 100(12):1779–1781, 2007.

Sipahi I, Tuzcu EM, Schoenhagen P, et al. Effects of normal, prehypertensive, and hypertensive blood pressure levels on progression of coronary atherosclerosis. J Am Coll Cardiol 48(4):833–838, 2006.

The Peripheral Vascular System and Lymphatic System

LEARNING OBJECTIVES

The student will:

1. Identify the locations of the peripheral pulses.
2. Obtain an accurate history of the peripheral vascular system.
3. Describe the structure and functions of arteries, veins, and lymph vessels and nodes.
4. Appropriately prepare and position the patient for the peripheral vascular examination.
5. Describe the equipment necessary to perform a peripheral vascular examination.
6. Evaluate and interpret variations in pulse rhythm, rate, and amplitude.
7. Discuss risk factors for peripheral artery disease, chronic venous stasis, and thromboembolic disease.
8. Discuss risk reduction and health promotion strategies to reduce peripheral vascular disease.

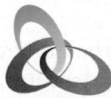

ANATOMY AND PHYSIOLOGY

Careful assessment of the peripheral vascular system is essential for detection of **peripheral arterial disease** (PAD), found in approximately 30% of the adult population, but "silent" in roughly half of those affected.[1] PAD is defined by the American Heart Association as stenotic, occlusive, and aneurysmal disease of the aorta, its visceral arterial branches, and the arteries of the lower extremities, but not the coronary arteries.

Venous thrombosis or thrombophlebitis is the presence of a thrombus or clot in a vein that is accompanied by an inflammatory response in the vein wall. Thrombi in the superficial veins are usually a response to vessel injury and rarely cause complications. Deep vein thrombosis (DVT) poses a grave

Dislodgement of the thrombus produces an embolus that can travel to the lungs, causing pulmonary embolism and possible death.

danger to patients. Each year, 2 million cases of DVT are diagnosed in the United States.[2]

Chronic venous insufficiency is caused by incompetent vein valves secondary to deep vein thrombosis or prolonged increased venous pressure as seen in prolonged standing or pregnancy. This can lead to varicose veins and skin changes.

Arteries

Arteries contain three concentric layers of tissue: the *intima*, the *media*, and the *adventitia* (or the externa).

Injury to vascular endothelial cells can provoke thrombus formation, atheromas, and the vascular lesions of hypertension.[3]

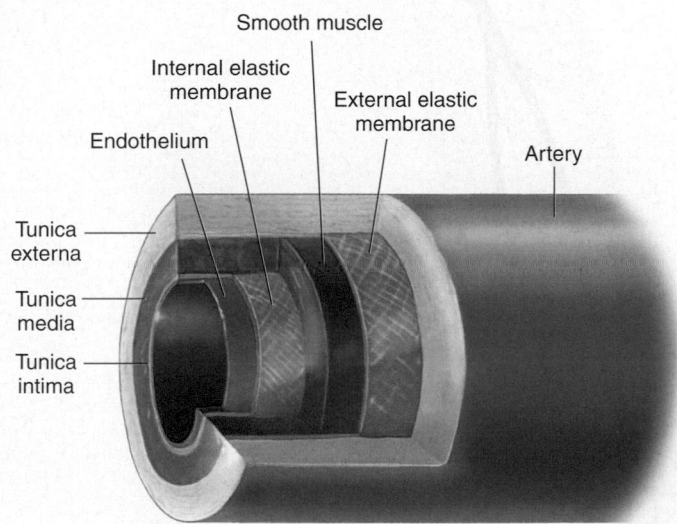

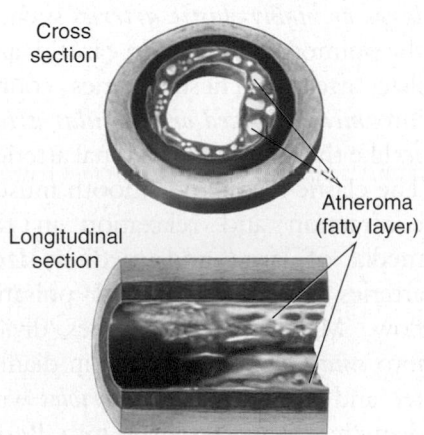

The innermost layer of all blood vessels is the ***intima,*** a single continuous lining of the endothelial cells, which synthesize regulators of clotting, modulate blood flow through synthesis of vasoconstrictors and vasodilators, and regulate immune and inflammatory reactions.

An *atheroma* is a fatty thickening in the walls of arteries. It begins in the intima as lipid-filled foam cells, then fatty streaks. *Complex atheromas* are thickened asymmetric plaques that narrow the lumen, reducing blood flow, and weaken the underlying media. They have a soft lipid core and a fibrous cap of smooth muscle cells and a collagen-rich matrix. Plaque rupture may precede thrombosis formation and lead to arterial occlusions in peripheral coronary or cerebral arteries.[3,4]

The *media* is composed of smooth muscle cells that dilate and constrict to accommodate blood pressure and flow. Its inner and outer boundaries are membranes of elastic fibers, or *elastin*, called *internal and external elastic laminae*. Small arterioles called the *vasa vasorum* perfuse the media. The outer layer of the artery is the *adventitia*, connective tissue containing nerve fibers and the vasa vasorum.

Arteries must respond to the variations that cardiac systole and diastole generate in cardiac output. Their anatomy and size vary according to their distance from the heart. The aorta and its immediate branches are *large or highly elastic arteries* such as the pulmonary, common carotid, and iliac arteries. These arteries course into *medium-sized or muscular arteries* like the coronary and renal arteries. The elastic recoil and smooth muscle contraction and relaxation in the media of large and medium-sized arteries propagate arterial pulsatile flow. Medium-sized arteries divide into *small arteries* <2 mm in diameter and even smaller *arterioles* with diameters from 20 to 100 mm. Resistance to blood flow occurs primarily in the arterioles. From the arterioles blood flows into the vast network of *capillaries,* each the diameter of a single red blood cell, only 7 to 8 microns across. Capillaries have an endothelial cell lining but no media, facilitating rapid diffusion of oxygen and carbon dioxide.

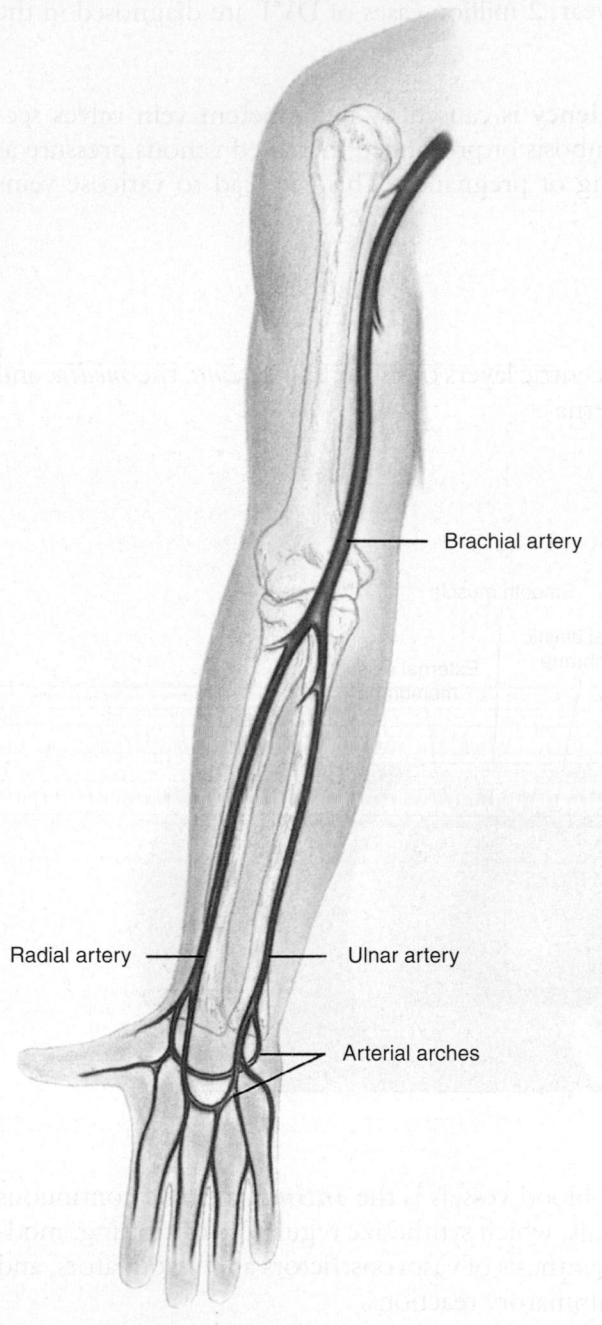

Brachial artery

Radial artery — Ulnar artery

Arterial arches

Arterial pulses are palpable in arteries lying close to the body surface. In the arms, note pulsations in:

- The *brachial artery* at the bend of the elbow just medial to the biceps tendon

- The *radial artery* on the lateral flexor surface

- The *ulnar artery* on the medial flexor surface, although overlying tissues may obscure the ulnar artery

Two vascular arches within the hand interconnect the radial and ulnar arteries, doubly protecting circulation to the hand and fingers against possible arterial occlusion.

In the legs, the pulsations are found in:

- The *femoral artery* just below the inguinal ligament, midway between the anterior superior iliac spine and the symphysis pubis

- The *popliteal artery,* an extension of the femoral artery that passes medially behind the femur, palpable just behind the knee. The popliteal artery divides into the two arteries perfusing the lower leg and foot, namely:

  - The *dorsalis pedis artery* on the dorsum of the foot just lateral to the extensor tendon of the big toe

  - The *posterior tibial artery* behind the medial malleolus of the ankle. An interconnecting arch between its two chief arterial branches protects circulation to the foot.

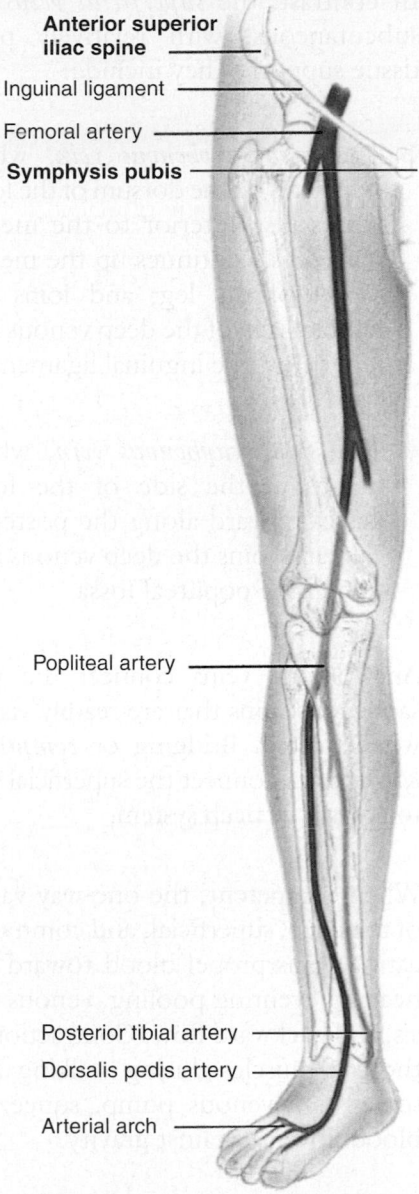

Anterior superior iliac spine

Inguinal ligament

Femoral artery

Symphysis pubis

Popliteal artery

Posterior tibial artery

Dorsalis pedis artery

Arterial arch

Veins

Unlike arteries, veins are thin-walled and highly distensible, with a capacity for up to two thirds of circulating blood flow. The *venous intima* consists of nonthrombogenic endothelium. Protruding into the lumen are valves that promote unidirectional venous return to the heart. The *media* contains circumferential rings of elastic tissue and smooth muscle that change vein diameter in response to even minor changes in venous pressure.[3,5]

Veins from the arms, upper trunk, and head and neck drain into the *superior vena cava,* which empties into the right atrium. Veins from the legs and lower trunk drain upward into the *inferior vena cava.* Because of their weaker wall structure, the leg veins are susceptible to irregular dilatation (varicosities), compression, ulceration, and invasion by tumors and warrant special attention.

Deep and Superficial Venous System (Legs).   The *deep veins* of the legs carry approximately 90% of venous return from the lower extremities. They are well supported by surrounding tissues.

In contrast, the *superficial veins* are subcutaneous, with relatively poor tissue support. They include:

● The *great saphenous vein*, which originates on the dorsum of the foot, passes just anterior to the medial malleolus, continues up the medial aspect of the leg, and joins the femoral vein of the deep venous system below the inguinal ligament

● The *small saphenous vein*, which begins at the side of the foot, passes upward along the posterior calf, and joins the deep venous system in the popliteal fossa

Anastomotic veins connect the two saphenous veins that are readily visible when dilated. Bridging or *communicating veins* connect the superficial system with the deep system.

When competent, the one-way valves of the deep, superficial, and communicating veins propel blood toward the heart, preventing pooling, venous stasis, and backward flow. Contraction of the calf muscles during walking also serves as a venous pump, squeezing blood upward against gravity.

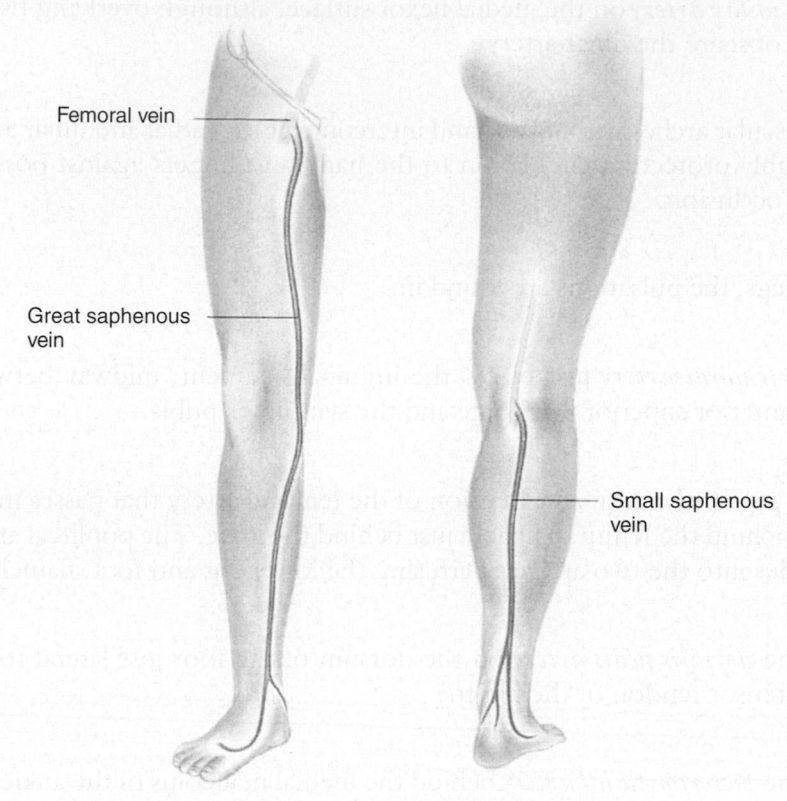

Femoral vein

Great saphenous vein

Small saphenous vein

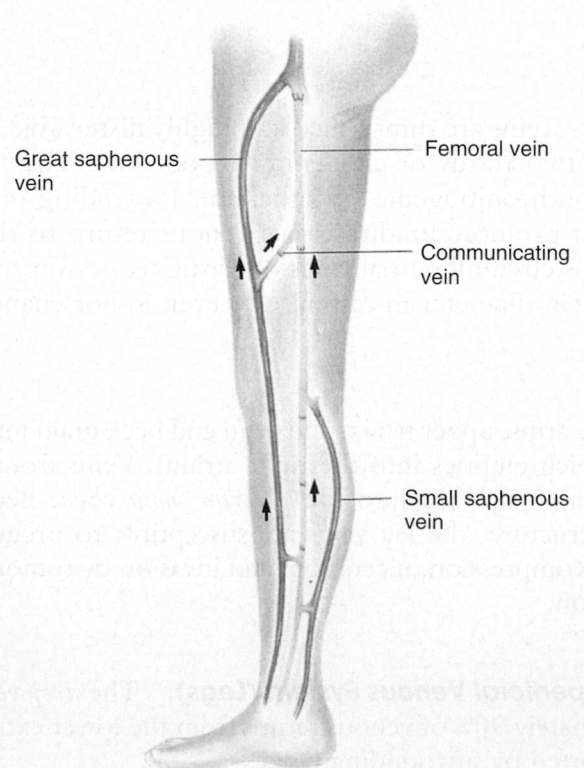

Great saphenous vein

Femoral vein

Communicating vein

Small saphenous vein

The Lymphatic System and Lymph Nodes

The lymphatic system is an extensive vascular network that drains lymph fluid from body tissues and returns it to the venous circulation. The system starts peripherally as blind lymphatic capillaries; continues centrally as thin vascular channels, then collecting ducts; and empties into the major veins at the neck. Lymph fluid transported through these channels is filtered through lymph nodes interposed along the way.

Lymph nodes are round, oval, or bean-shaped structures that vary in size according to their location. Some lymph nodes, such as the preauriculars, if palpable at all, are typically very small. The inguinal nodes, in contrast, are relatively larger—often 1 cm in diameter and occasionally even 2 cm in an adult.

In addition to its vascular functions, the lymphatic system plays an important role in the body's immune system. Cells within the lymph nodes engulf cellular debris and bacteria and produce antibodies.

Only the superficial lymph nodes are accessible to physical examination. These include the head and cervical nodes (pp. 195, 198), the clavicular nodes, the axillary nodes (p. 493), and the epitrochlear and inguinal nodes.

Recall that the axillary lymph nodes drain most of the arm. Lymphatics from the ulnar surface of the forearm and hand, the little and ring fingers, and the adjacent surface of the middle finger, however, drain first into the *epitrochlear nodes*. These are located on the medial surface of the arm approximately 3 cm above the elbow. Lymphatics from the rest of the arm drain mostly into the axillary nodes. A few may go directly to the infraclaviculars.

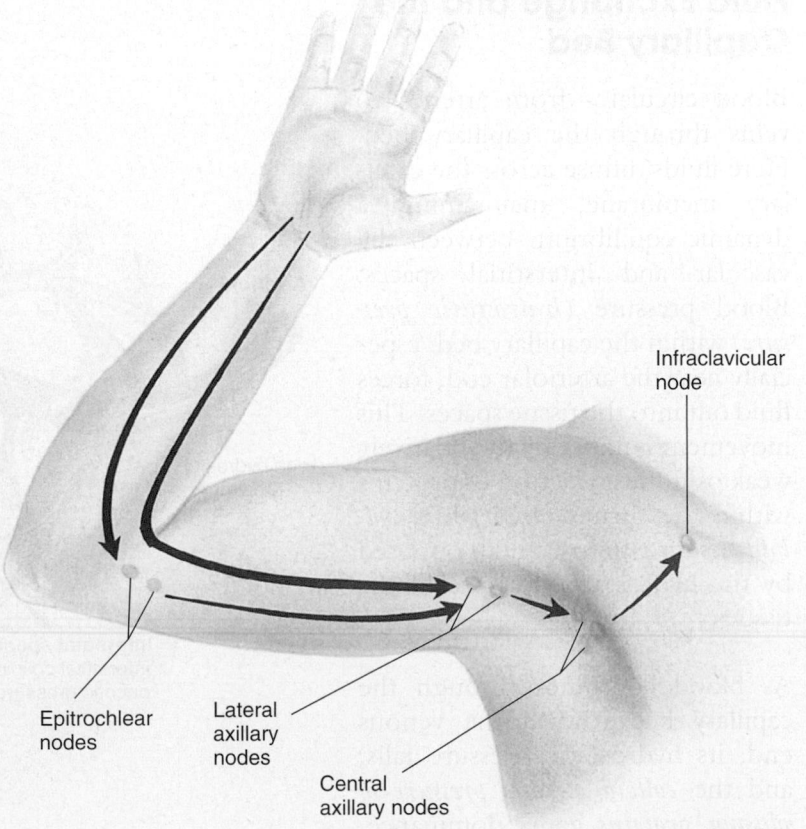

Infraclavicular node

Epitrochlear nodes

Lateral axillary nodes

Central axillary nodes

The lymphatics of the lower limb follow the veins and consist of both deep and superficial systems. Only the superficial nodes are palpable. The *superficial inguinal nodes* include two groups. The *horizontal group* lies in a chain high in the anterior thigh below the inguinal ligament. It drains the superficial portions of the lower abdomen and buttock, the external genitalia (but not the testes), the anal canal and perianal area, and the lower vagina.

The *vertical group* clusters near the upper part of the saphenous vein and drains a corresponding region of the leg.

In contrast, lymphatics from the heel and outer aspect of the foot join the deep system at the level of the popliteal space. Lesions in this area, therefore, are not usually associated with palpable inguinal lymph nodes.

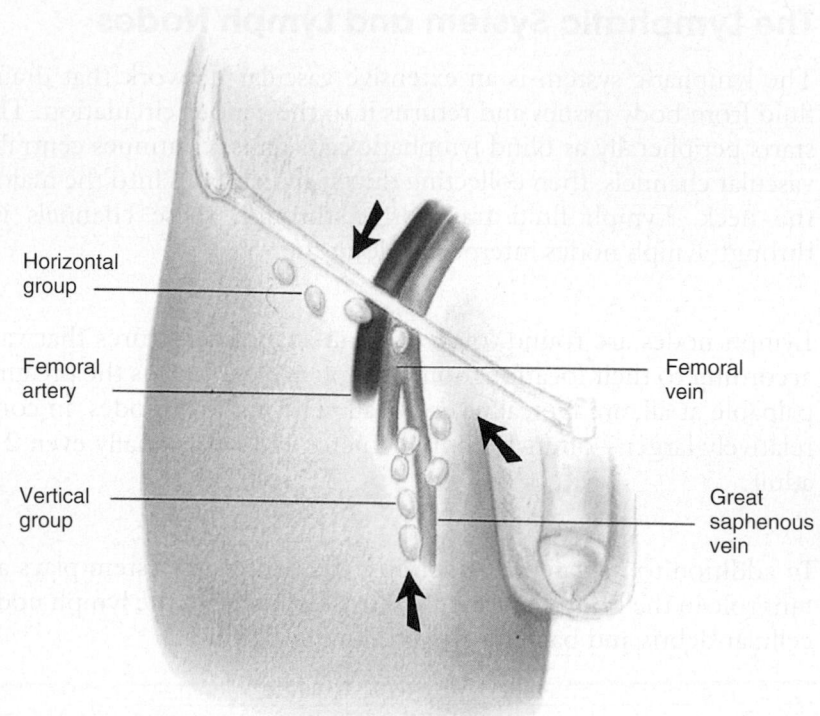

Horizontal group

Femoral artery

Vertical group

Femoral vein

Great saphenous vein

Fluid Exchange and the Capillary Bed

Blood circulates from arteries to veins through the capillary bed. Here fluids diffuse across the capillary membrane, maintaining a dynamic equilibrium between the vascular and interstitial spaces. Blood pressure (*hydrostatic pressure*) within the capillary bed, especially near the arteriolar end, forces fluid out into the tissue spaces. This movement is aided by the relatively weak osmotic attraction of proteins within the tissues (*interstitial colloid oncotic pressure*) and is opposed by the hydrostatic pressure of the tissues.

As blood continues through the capillary bed toward the venous end, its hydrostatic pressure falls, and the *colloid oncotic pressure of plasma proteins* gains dominance,

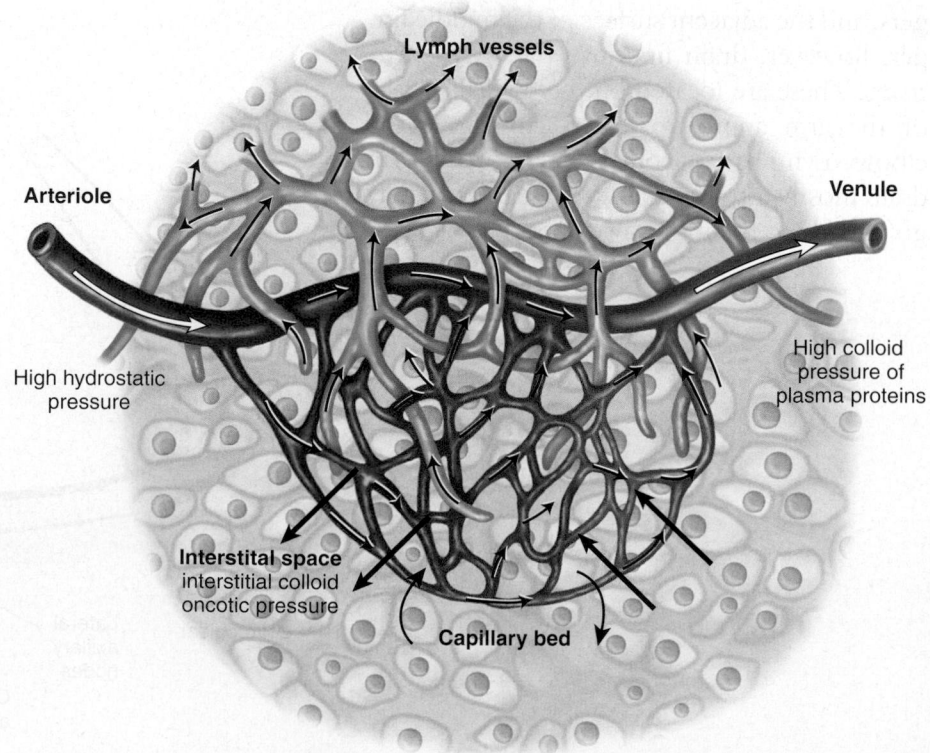

Lymph vessels

Arteriole

Venule

High hydrostatic pressure

High colloid pressure of plasma proteins

Interstitial space interstitial colloid oncotic pressure

Capillary bed

pulling fluid back into the vascular tree. Net flow of fluid, which was directed outward on the arteriolar side of the capillary bed, reverses and turns inward on the venous side. Lymphatic capillaries, which also play an important role in this equilibrium, remove excessive fluid, including protein, from the interstitial space.

Lymphatic dysfunction or disturbances in capillary bed fluid exchange commonly result in **edema,** the presence of excess fluid in the interstitial spaces. Four mechanisms produce edema: (1) increased capillary blood pressure (increased hydrostatic pressure), which may be caused by venous insufficiency or congestive heart failure; (2) increased capillary membrane permeability (capillary leak syndrome), caused by burns, snake bites, angioedema, or allergic reactions; (3) low plasma protein levels (creating low colloid osmotic pressure), caused by renal disorders; and (4) blockage or removal of lymphatic drainage, as seen in lymph node removal. This is termed lymphedema and is usually nonpitting.

Edema may be pitting or nonpitting. In pitting edema the interstitial water is mobile and can be translocated with the pressure exerted by a finger. A "pit" or depression is left for 5 to 30 seconds. The degree of pitting is measured on a 1 to 4 scale.

Scale	Depression
1+	2 mm
2+	4 mm
3+	6 mm
4+	8 mm

Nonpitting edema reflects a condition in which serum proteins have accumulated in the interstitial space with the water and coagulated. This is frequently seen with local infection or trauma and is called brawny edema.

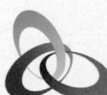 **THE HEALTH HISTORY**

COMMON OR CONCERNING SYMPTOMS

- Pain in the arms or legs
- Intermittent claudication
- Cold, numbness, or pallor in the legs; hair loss
- Swelling in the calves, legs, or feet
- Swelling with redness or tenderness

The purpose of the history questions is to identify symptoms of peripheral arterial and venous disease.

Because most patients with peripheral vascular diseases report minimal symptoms, asking specifically about the symptoms below is recommended, especially in patients older than 50 years and those with risk factors, especially smoking, diabetes, hypertension, elevated cholesterol, or coronary artery disease:

- Do you have pain or cramping in your legs during walking or exertion? (This is termed intermittent claudication.)

  These symptoms are caused by insufficient arterial supply to the legs, which may be caused by atherosclerosis.

  - Is it relieved by rest within 10 minutes?

  - If present, identify the location and the distance the patient walks before symptoms occur.

- Do you have coldness, numbness, or pallor in the legs or feet?

- Do you have hair on your shins?

- Do you have aching or pain at rest in the lower leg or foot?

  - Is pain alleviated by elevating the legs?

- Do you have fatigue or aching in the lower legs with prolonged standing?

- Do you have swelling of the feet or legs? If present, identify:

  Edema, varicose veins, and aching in the legs are symptoms of venous stasis.

  - Location

  - Time of day it is present

  - Whether it is bilateral or unilateral

- Do you have any varicose veins?

  - Where are they located?

  - How long have you had them?

  - Do you have any discomfort from them?

- Do you have any wounds of the legs or feet that will not heal or heal very slowly?

  Ulcers may be of venous or arterial origin.

  - Where is the wound located?

  - How long have you had the wound?

  - What precipitated the wound (e.g., an injury)?

- Do your fingertips or toes change color in cold weather?

May be caused by Raynaud disease: the small arteries spasm in response to cold.

- Have you experienced erectile dysfunction?

Poor blood supply to the penile arteries can cause erectile dysfunction.

- Do you have abdominal pain after meals?
  - Does it prevent you from eating?

Atherosclerosis of the mesenteric or celiac arteries can cause intestinal ischemia, producing abdominal pain and "food fear," where the patient is fearful of eating.

- Do you have tender or swollen lymph nodes (glands)?

Swollen nodes may indicate an infection or tumor.

Past History

- Medications, especially oral contraceptives or hormone replacement therapy

Estrogen use and pregnancy increase one's risk for blood clots.

- Pregnancy or recent childbirth

- Inflammatory diseases such as lupus, rheumatoid arthritis, or irritable bowel disease

Inflammation contributes to clot formation.

- Active cancer

- Coronary artery disease (CAD)

Coronary artery disease and cerebral artery disease are also caused by atherosclerosis; an individual with either is at risk for PAD.

- Heart attack

- Congestive heart failure

- Stroke (cerebral arterial disease)

- Clotting disorders

- Hypertension

- Diabetes

- Problems in circulation, such as blood clots, leg ulcers, swelling, or poor healing of wounds

- Major surgery or fracture of a long bone in the last 4 weeks

- **Risk factors**

  - Obesity

  - Smoking

  - Hyperlipidemia

  - Constrictive clothing

  - Central venous lines

Family History

- Peripheral vascular disease

- Varicose veins

- Abdominal aortic aneurysm

- CAD

- Sudden death younger than 60 years of age

- Diabetes

Lifestyle or Health Patterns

- Job requiring prolonged standing or sitting

- Sedentary lifestyle

- Decreased mobility such as paralysis or cast

PHYSICAL EXAMINATION

EQUIPMENT LIST

- Tape measure
- Doppler ultrasound device
- Tourniquet or blood pressure cuff

Important Areas of Examination

The Arms	The Legs
• Size, symmetry, skin color	• Size, symmetry, skin color, tenderness
• Radial pulse, brachial pulse	• Femoral pulse and inguinal lymph nodes
• Epitrochlear lymph nodes	• Popliteal, dorsalis pedis, and posterior tibial pulses
	• Peripheral edema

The American College of Cardiology and the American Heart Association have urged clinicians to intensify their focus when examining the peripheral vascular system.[6] Recall that peripheral arterial disease is often asymptomatic and underdiagnosed, leading to significant morbidity and mortality.

Arms

Inspection. *Inspect both arms* from the fingertips to the shoulders. Note:

1. Their size, symmetry, swelling, and any lesions

2. The venous pattern

3. The color of the skin and nail beds and the texture of the skin

Palpation
1. Palpate the temperature of the arms and hands simultaneously with the backs of your fingers. Compare the temperature of the arms simultaneously.

2. *Palpate the radial pulse* with the pads of your fingers on the flexor surface of the wrist laterally. Partially flexing the patient's wrist may help you feel this pulse. Compare the pulses in both arms. Pulses may be palpated simultaneously to facilitate comparison.

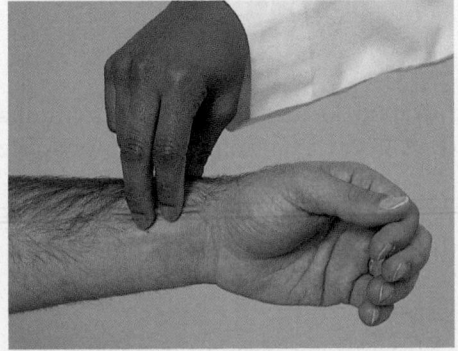

(Source: Marks R: Skin Disease in Old Age. Philadelphia: JB Lippincott, 1987)

Lymphedema of the arm and hand may follow axillary node dissection and radiation therapy.

Prominent veins in an edematous arm suggest venous obstruction.

In *Raynaud disease,* wrist pulses are typically normal, but spasm of more distal arteries causes episodes of sharply demarcated pallor of the fingers (see Table 15-1, pp. 424–425, Painful Peripheral Vascular Disorders and Their Mimics).

There are two common systems for grading the amplitude of the arterial pulses. One system uses a scale of 0 to 3, as below.[6] The other system uses a scale of 0 to 4. You should check to see what scale your institution uses.

Note that if an artery is widely dilated, it is *aneurysmal.*

● **Recommended Grading of Pulses**[6]	
3+	Bounding
2+	Brisk, expected (normal)
1+	Diminished, weaker than expected
0	Absent, unable to palpate

Bounding carotid, radial, and femoral pulses in *aortic insufficiency*; asymmetric diminished pulses in *arterial occlusion* from atherosclerosis or embolism

If you suspect arterial insufficiency, feel for the *brachial pulse.* Flex the patient's elbow slightly, and palpate the artery just medial to the biceps tendon at the antecubital crease. The brachial artery can also be felt higher in the arm in the groove between the biceps and triceps muscles.

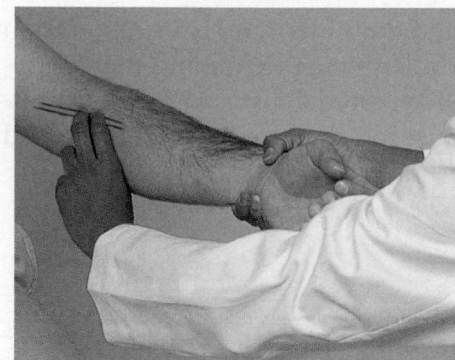

Feel for the *epitrochlear nodes.* With the patient's elbow flexed to about 90° and the forearm supported by your hand, reach around behind the arm and feel in the groove between the biceps and triceps muscles, about 3 cm above the medial epicondyle. If a node is present, note its size, consistency, and tenderness.

An enlarged epitrochlear node may arise from local or distal infection or may be associated with generalized lymphadenopathy.

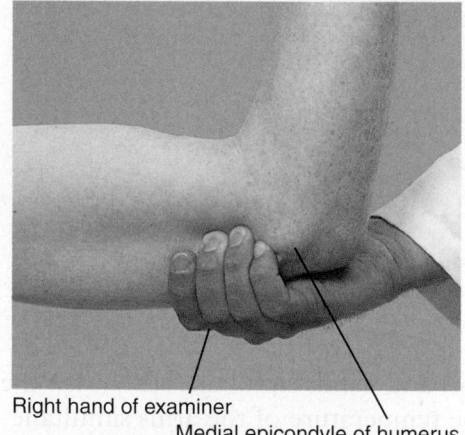

Right hand of examiner
Medial epicondyle of humerus
MEDIAL ASPECT, LEFT ARM

Epitrochlear nodes are difficult or impossible to identify in most normal people.

Legs

The patient should be lying down and draped so that the external genitalia are covered and the legs fully exposed. A good examination is impossible through stockings or socks!

Inspection. Inspect both legs from the groin and buttocks to the feet. Note:

1. Their size, symmetry, and edema. Measure leg circumferences in centimeters if discrepancy is suspected.

See Table 15-2, p. 426, Chronic Insufficiency of Arteries and Veins.

2. The venous pattern and any venous enlargement or varicosities

3. Pigmentation, rashes, scars, or ulcers

See Table 15-3, p. 427, Common Ulcers of the Ankles and Feet.

4. The color and texture of the skin and the color of the nail beds

5. The distribution of hair on the lower legs, feet, and toes.

6. Look for brownish areas (or increased pigmentation on dark-skinned clients) near the ankles. The brown discoloration is caused by hemosiderin released from the red blood cells that seep into the skin with edema and break down.

Brownish discoloration or ulcers just above the malleolus suggest *chronic venous insufficiency.*

7. Note the location, size, and depth of any ulcers in the skin. Are the edges of the wound well demarcated? Is there bleeding?

Palpation

1. Palpate the temperature of both legs and feet simultaneously with the backs of your hands. Compare the temperature of the legs. Bilateral coolness is most often caused by a cold environment or anxiety.

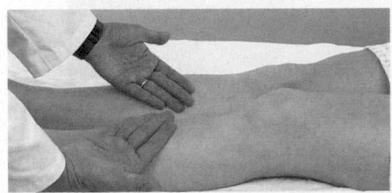

Coldness, especially when unilateral or associated with other signs, suggests arterial insufficiency from inadequate arterial circulation.

2. Palpate for edema. Compare one foot and leg with the other, noting their relative size and the prominence of veins, tendons, and bones.

Edema causes swelling that may obscure the veins, tendons, and bony prominences.

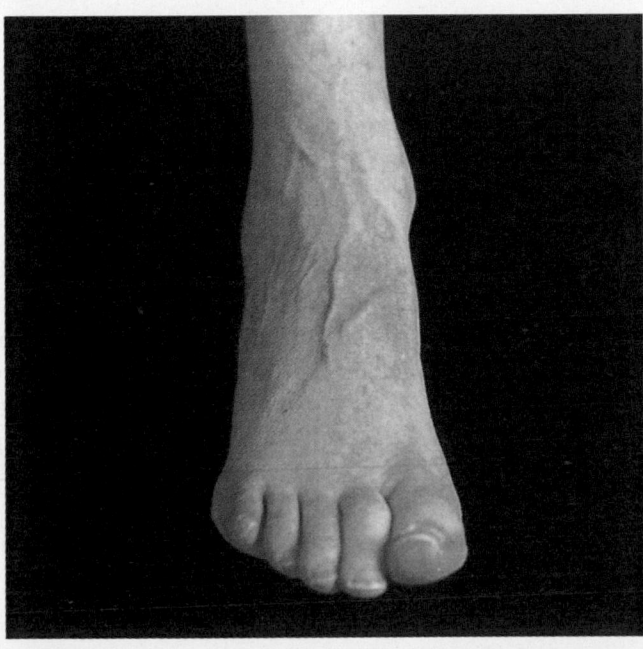

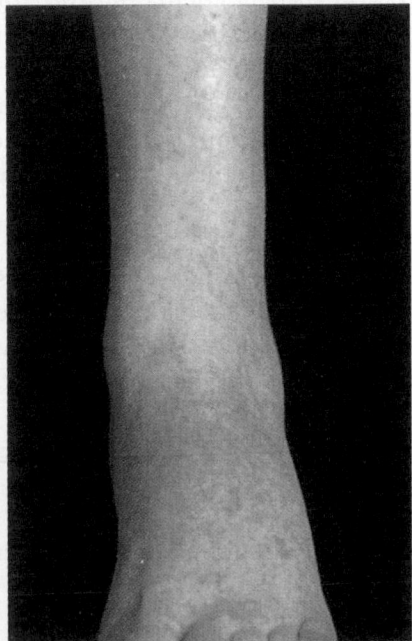

Palpate for pitting edema. Press firmly but gently with your thumb for at least 5 seconds (1) over the dorsum of each foot, (2) behind each medial malleolus, and (3) over the shins. Look for *pitting*—a depression caused by pressure from your thumb. Normally there is none. The severity of edema is graded on a four-point scale (see p. 405).

See Table 15-4, p. 428 Some Peripheral Causes of Edema

Shown below is 3+ pitting edema.

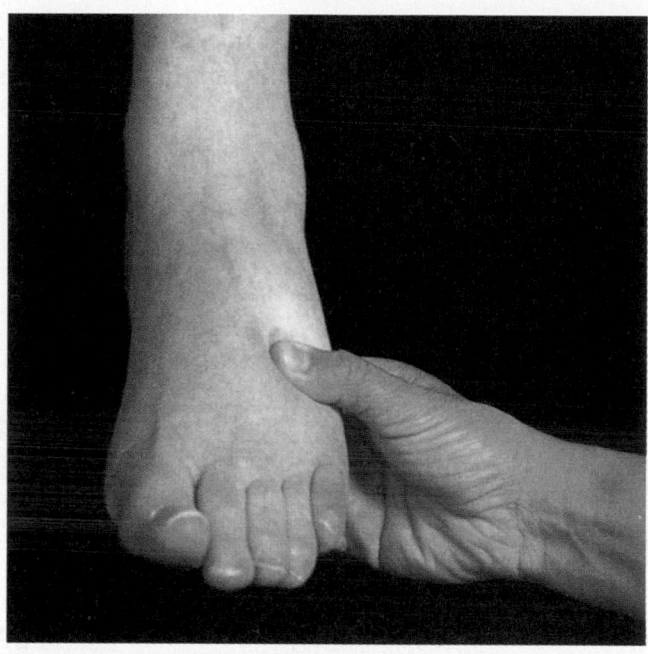
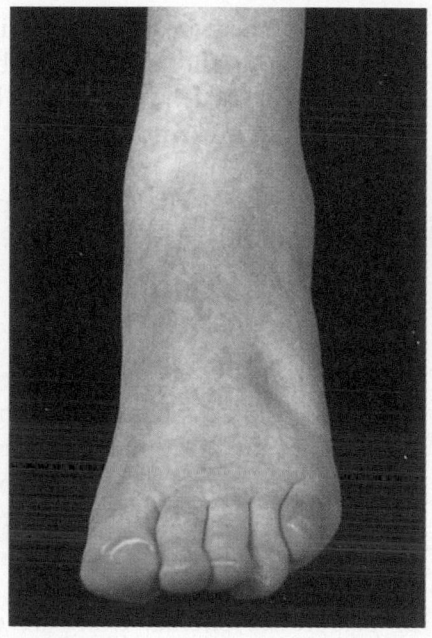

If you suspect edema, *measure the legs* to identify the edema and to follow its course. With a flexible tape, measure (1) the forefoot, (2) the smallest possible circumference above the ankle, (3) the largest circumference at the calf, and (4) the midthigh, a measured distance above the patella with the knee extended. Compare one side with the other. A difference of more than 1 cm just above the ankle or 2 cm at the calf is unusual and suggests edema.

Conditions such as muscular atrophy can also cause different circumferences in the legs.

If edema is present, look for possible causes in the peripheral vascular system. These include (1) recent deep venous thrombosis, (2) chronic venous insufficiency from previous deep venous thrombosis or incompetence of the venous valves, and (3) lymphedema. Note the extent of the swelling and how far up the leg it goes.

In *deep venous thrombosis,* the extent of edema suggests the location of the occlusion: the popliteal vein when the lower leg or the ankle is swollen; the iliofemoral veins when the entire leg is swollen.

Is the swelling unilateral or bilateral? Are the veins unusually prominent?

Venous distention suggests a venous cause of edema.

If risk factors for DVT are present, try to identify any venous tenderness that may accompany deep venous thrombosis. Very faintly palpate the groin just medial to the femoral pulse for tenderness of the femoral vein. Next, with the patient's leg flexed at the knee and relaxed, palpate the calf. With your fingerpads, very gently compress the calf muscles against the tibia, and search for any tenderness or cords. Deep venous thrombosis, however, may have no demonstrable signs, and diagnosis often depends on high clinical suspicion and other testing. *Firm palpation or massage over a DVT may dislodge the clot, causing a pulmonary embolus or death.*

A painful, pale swollen leg, together with tenderness in the groin over the femoral vein, suggests deep *iliofemoral thrombosis.* Only half of patients with *deep venous thrombosis* in the calf have tenderness and cords deep in the calf. Calf tenderness is nonspecific and may be present without thrombosis.

3. Feel the thickness of the skin.

Thickened brawny skin suggests lymphedema and advanced venous insufficiency.

4. Palpate areas of local redness, noting the skin temperature, and then gently palpate for the firm cord of a thrombosed vein in the area. The calf is most often involved.

Local swelling, redness, warmth, and a subcutaneous cord suggest *superficial thrombophlebitis.*

5. *Palpate the pulses* to assess the arterial circulation.

A diminished or absent pulse indicates partial or complete occlusion proximally; for example, at the popliteal level, the dorsalis pedis and posterior tibial pulses are typically affected. Chronic arterial occlusion, usually from atherosclerosis, causes *intermittent claudication.*

- *The femoral pulse.* Press deeply, below the inguinal ligament and about midway between the anterior superior iliac spine and the symphysis pubis. As in deep abdominal palpation, the use of two hands, one on top of the other, may facilitate this examination, especially in obese patients.

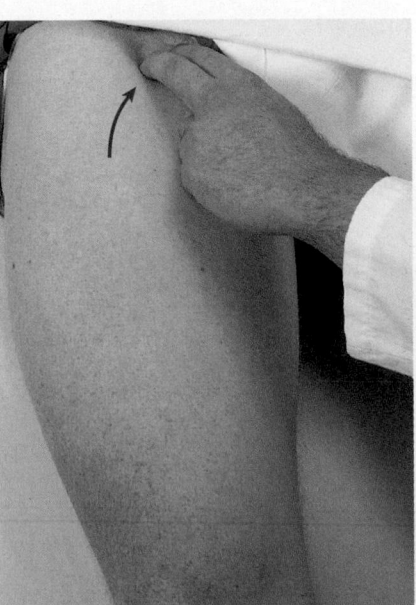

An exaggerated, widened femoral pulse suggests a *femoral aneurysm,* a pathologic dilatation of the artery.

● *The popliteal pulse.* The patient's knee should be somewhat flexed, with the leg relaxed. Place the fingertips of both hands so that they meet in the midline behind the knee and press deeply into the popliteal fossa. The popliteal pulse is often more difficult to find than other pulses. It is deeper and feels more diffuse.

An exaggerated, widened popliteal pulse suggests an aneurysm of the popliteal artery. Popliteal and femoral aneurysms are not common. They are usually caused by atherosclerosis and occur primarily in men older than 50 years.

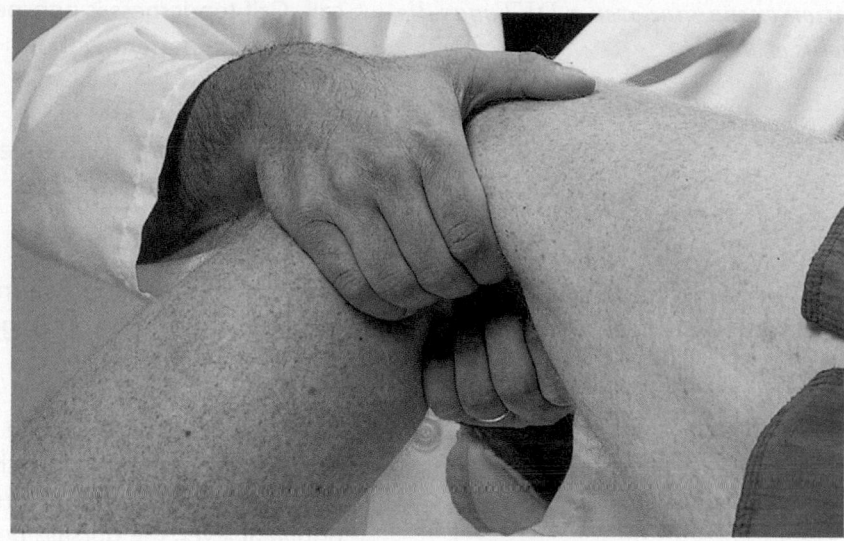

If you cannot feel the popliteal pulse with this approach, try with the patient prone. Flex the patient's knee to about 90°, let the lower leg relax against your shoulder or upper arm, and press your two thumbs deeply into the popliteal fossa.

Atherosclerosis (arteriosclerosis obliterans) most commonly obstructs arterial circulation in the thigh. The femoral pulse is then normal, the popliteal decreased or absent.

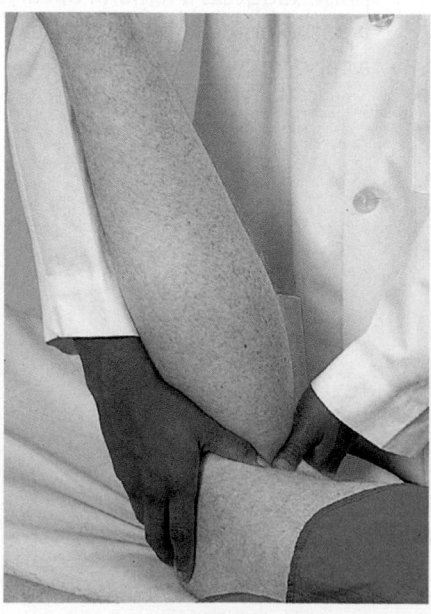
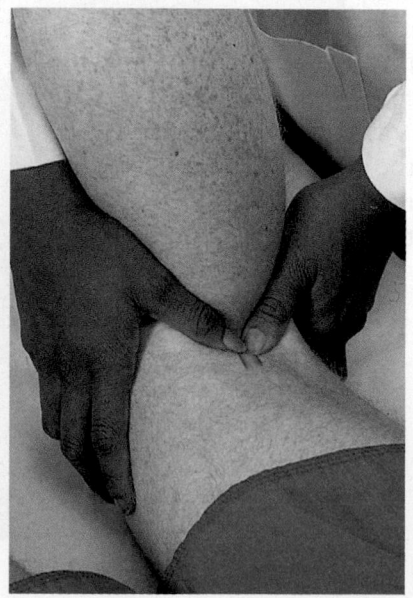

● *The dorsalis pedis pulse.* Feel the dorsum of the foot (not the ankle) just lateral to the extensor tendon of the great toe. If you cannot feel a pulse, explore the dorsum of the foot more laterally.

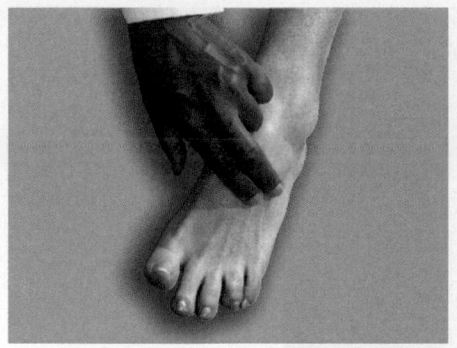

The dorsalis pedis artery may be congenitally absent or may branch higher in the ankle. Search for a pulse more laterally.

Decreased or absent pedal pulses (assuming a warm environment) with normal femoral and popliteal pulses suggest occlusive disease in the lower popliteal artery or its branches—often seen in *diabetes mellitus.*

● *The posterior tibial pulse.* Curve your fingers behind and slightly below the medial malleolus of the ankle. (This pulse may be hard to feel in a fat or edematous ankle.)

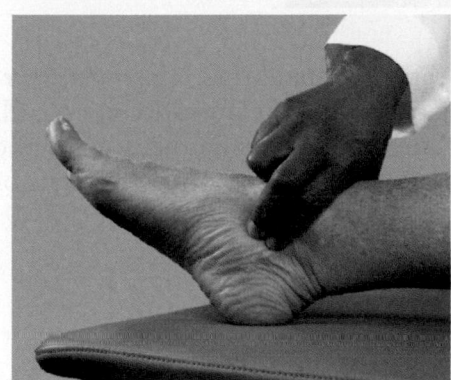

Sudden arterial occlusion from embolism or thrombosis causes pain and numbness or tingling. The limb distal to the occlusion becomes cold, pale, and pulseless. Emergency treatment is required. If collateral circulation is good, only numbness and coolness may result.

TIPS FOR FEELING DIFFICULT PULSES

1. Position your body and examining hand comfortably; awkward positions decrease your tactile sensitivity.
2. Place your hand properly and linger there, varying the pressure of your fingers to pick up a weak pulsation. If unsuccessful, then explore the area deliberately.
3. Do not confuse the patient's pulse with your own pulsating fingertips. If you are unsure, count your own heart rate and compare it with the patient's. The rates are usually different. Your carotid pulse is convenient for this comparison.

6. Palpate the *superficial inguinal nodes,* including both the horizontal and the vertical groups. Note their size, consistency, and discreteness, and note any tenderness. Nontender, discrete inguinal nodes up to 1 cm or even 2 cm in diameter are frequently palpable in normal people. See page 404.

Lymphadenopathy refers to enlargement of the nodes, with or without tenderness.

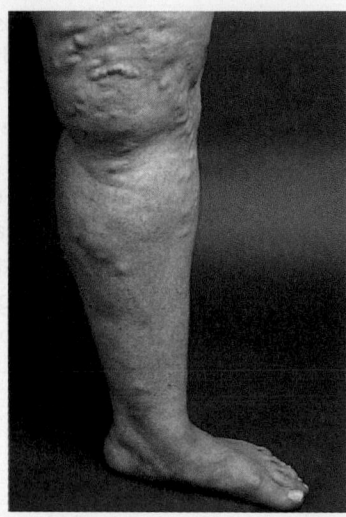

Varicose veins are dilated and tortuous. Their walls may feel somewhat thickened. Many varicose veins can be seen in the leg in the picture on the left.

At the end of the examination, ask the patient to stand, and *inspect the saphenous system for varicosities*. The standing posture allows any varicosities to fill with blood and makes them visible. You can easily miss them when the patient is in a supine position. Feel for any varicosities, noting any signs of thrombophlebitis.

 ## RECORDING YOUR FINDINGS

Recall that the written description of lymph nodes appears in Chapter 10, The Head and Neck (see p. 202). Likewise, assessment of the carotid pulse is recorded in Chapter 14, The Cardiovascular System (see p. 374).

RECORDING THE PHYSICAL EXAMINATION—THE PERIPHERAL VASCULAR SYSTEM

"Extremities are warm and without edema. No varicosities or stasis changes. Calves are supple and nontender. No femoral or abdominal bruits. Brachial, radial, femoral, popliteal, dorsalis pedis (DP), and posterior tibial (PT) pulses are 2+ and symmetric."

OR

"Extremities are pale below the midcalf, with notable hair loss. Rubor noted when legs dependent but no edema or ulceration. Bilateral femoral bruits; no abdominal bruits heard. Brachial and radial pulses 2+; femoral, popliteal, DP, and PT pulses 1+ bilaterally." (Alternatively, pulses can be recorded as below.)

Suggests atherosclerotic *peripheral arterial disease*

	Radial	Brachial	Femoral	Popliteal	Dorsalis Pedis	Posterior Tibial
RT	2+	2+	1+	1+	1+	1+
LT	2+	2+	1+	1+	1+	1+

(continued)

RECORDING THE PHYSICAL EXAMINATION—THE PERIPHERAL VASCULAR SYSTEM (continued)

OR

A stick figure with the pulse amplitude values may be used.

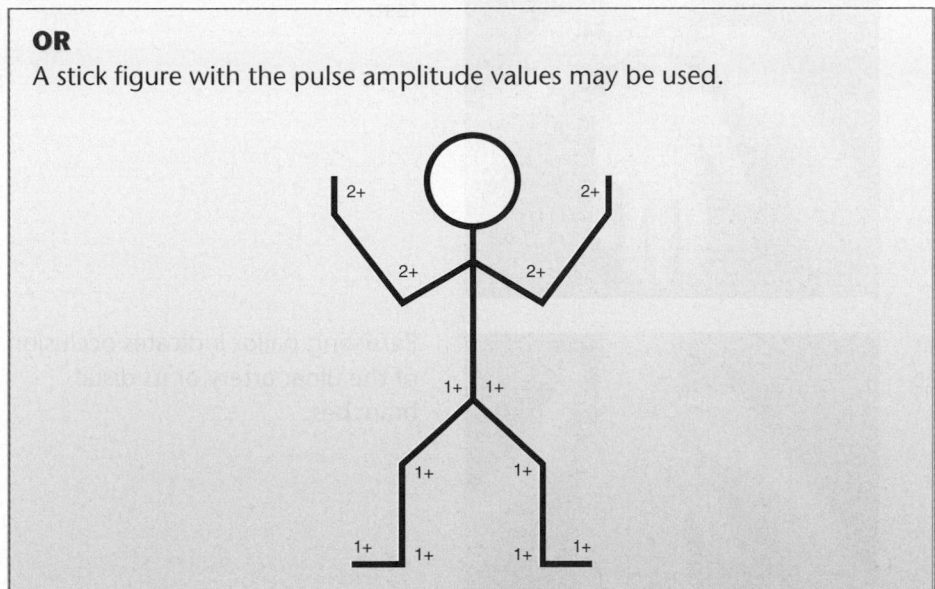

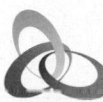 **SPECIAL TECHNIQUES**

Evaluating the Arterial Supply to the Hand. To assess for arterial insufficiency in the arm or hand, try to feel the *ulnar pulse* as well as the radial and brachial pulses. Feel for it deeply on the flexor surface of the wrist medially. Partially flexing the patient's wrist may help you. The pulse of a normal ulnar artery, however, may not be palpable.

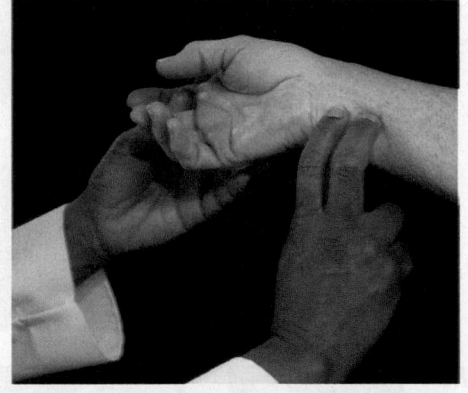

Arterial occlusive disease is much less common in the arms than in the legs. Absent or diminished pulses at the wrist are found in acute embolic occlusion and in *Buerger disease,* or *thromboangiitis obliterans.*

Allen Test. The *Allen test* gives further information. This test is also useful to ensure the patency of the ulnar artery before puncturing the radial artery for blood samples or arterial lines. The patient should rest with hands in lap, palms up.

Ask the patient to make a tight fist with one hand; then compress both radial and ulnar arteries firmly between your thumbs and fingers.

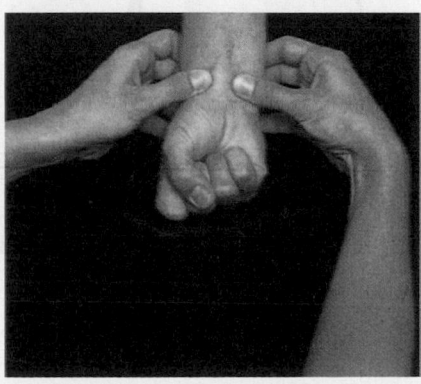

Next, ask the patient to open the hand into a relaxed, slightly flexed position. The palm is pale.

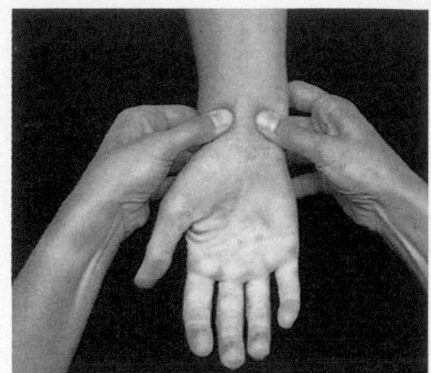

Extending the hand fully may cause pallor and a falsely positive test.

Release your pressure over the ulnar artery. If the ulnar artery is patent, the palm flushes within 3 to 5 seconds.

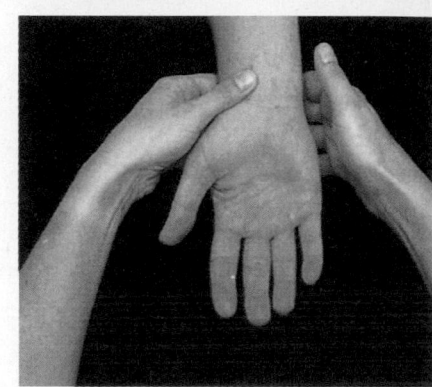

Persisting pallor indicates occlusion of the ulnar artery or its distal branches.

Patency of the radial artery may be tested by repeating the test and releasing the radial artery while still compressing the ulnar artery.

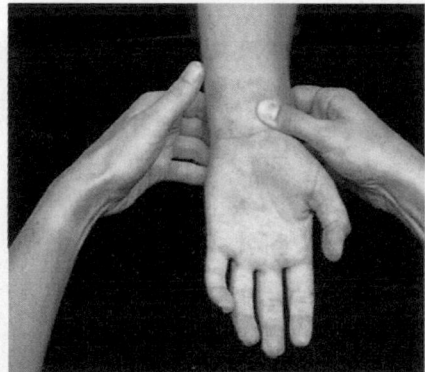

Evaluating Arterial Supply to the Legs. If pain or diminished pulses suggest arterial insufficiency, look for postural color changes. With the patient lying down, raise both legs, as shown to about 60° until maximal pallor of the feet develops—usually within a minute. Have the patient flex the ankles up and down to drain venous blood. In light-skinned persons, either maintenance of normal color, as seen in this right foot, or slight pallor is normal. In dark-skinned persons, evaluate the soles of the feet or nail beds for pallor.

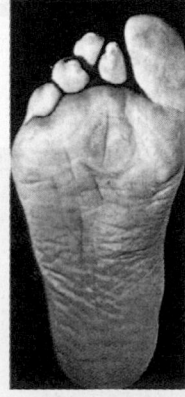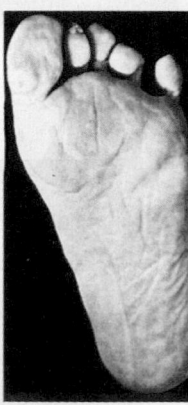

Marked pallor on elevation suggests *arterial insufficiency.*

Then ask the patient to sit up and dangle the legs over the side of the examination table. Compare both feet, noting the time required for:

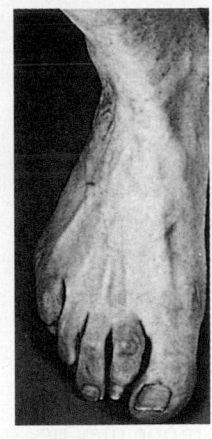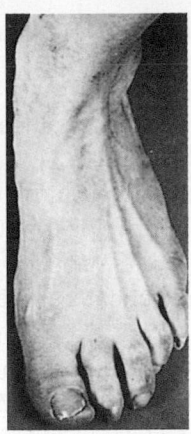

The foot above is still pale, and the veins are just starting to fill—signs of arterial insufficiency.

- Return of pinkness to the skin, normally about 10 seconds or less

- Filling of the veins of the feet and ankles, normally about 15 seconds

This right foot has normal color and the veins on the foot have filled. These normal responses suggest an adequate circulation.

Look for any unusual *rubor* (dusky redness) to replace the pallor of the dependent foot. Rubor may take a minute or more to appear.

Normal responses accompanied by diminished arterial pulses suggest that a good collateral circulation has developed around an arterial occlusion.

Persisting rubor on dependency suggests arterial insufficiency. When veins are incompetent, dependent rubor and the timing of color return and venous filling are not reliable tests of arterial insufficiency.

ANKLE–BRACHIAL INDEX

If the patient has risk factors for peripheral artery disease, an ankle–brachial index (ABI) screening should be performed. ABI is a noninvasive method to assess lower extremity arterial blood flow by comparing systolic blood pressure in the ankle to arm systolic pressure.

Equipment
Doppler device with 8-MHz probe (For obese individuals, a 4-MHz probe may be necessary.)
Doppler gel
Blood pressure cuffs for arm and leg; cuffs should be 40% of limb circumference (or 20% of the limb diameter).

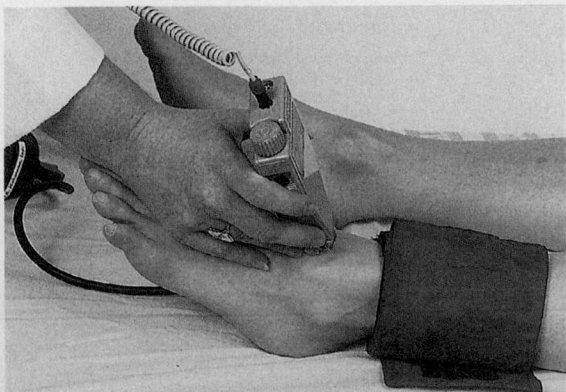

(Source of foot photos: Kappert A, Winsor T: Diagnosis of Peripheral Vascular Disease. Philadelphia, FA Davis, 1972.)

(continued)

ANKLE–BRACHIAL INDEX (continued)

Procedure

1. Patient should avoid caffeine and tobacco for at least 1 hour prior to the procedure.
2. Explain the procedure to the patient and position him or her in the supine position. The client should rest supine for 10 to 20 minutes before the procedure.
3. Apply the blood pressure cuff to the patient's arm and feel for the brachial pulse.
4. Apply a small mound of gel over the pulse; turn on the Doppler.
5. Place the tip of the Doppler probe in the gel at a 45° angle and listen for the "whooshing" sound, indicating the pulse. (The probe may be adjusted between 30° and 60° to maximize the sound.)
6. Inflate the blood pressure cuff until the sound is no longer heard, and then inflate it 20 to 30 mm Hg above that point.
7. Deflate the cuff at a rate of 2 to 4 mm Hg/second until the sound returns. This is the systolic blood pressure. Repeat the procedure in the other arm.
8. Place the ankle blood pressure cuff just above the malleoli. Locate the posterior tibial pulse with the Doppler and inflate the cuff 20–30 mm Hg above the number the pulse is last heard. Slowly release the pressure until the pulse is heard. This is the systolic pressure. Repeat the procedure using the dorsalis pedis pulse.
9. Obtain the systolic pressure for both pulses on the opposite ankle.

NOTE: The ankle blood pressure cuff must be the appropriate size in order to obtain accurate readings. Artery pressure is measured at the site of the cuff; if the cuff is placed higher on the leg a false high systolic reading will be obtained.

Calculation

Divide the higher systolic pressure from each leg by the higher brachial systolic pressure.

Interpretation

ABI	Interpretation
1.0	Normal
≤0.9	Mild ischemia
0.6–0.8	Borderline perfusion
0.50–0.75	Severe ischemia
≤0.49	Critical ischemia, rest pain, or gangrene
>1.0	Unreliable. Calcium in arterial walls prevents compression of the artery during the test. Frequently seen in diabetic patients. Refer for a toe–brachial index test. Toe arteries rarely have calcified walls. Bonham

Bonham PA. Get the LEAD out: noninvasive assessment for lower extremity arterial disease using ankle brachial index and tow brachial index measurements. J Wound Ostomy Continence Nurs 33(1):30–41, 2006.

Evaluating the Competency of Venous Valves. By the *retrograde filling (Trendelenburg) test,* you can assess the valvular competency in both the communicating veins and the saphenous system. Start with the patient supine. Elevate one leg to about 90° to empty it of venous blood.

Next, occlude the great saphenous vein in the upper thigh by manual compression or tourniquet, using enough pressure to occlude this vein but not the deeper vessels. Ask the patient to stand. While you keep the vein occluded, watch for venous filling in the leg. Normally the saphenous vein fills from below, taking about 35 seconds as blood flows through the capillary bed into the venous system.

> Rapid filling of the superficial veins while the saphenous vein is occluded indicates incompetent valves in the communicating veins. Blood flows quickly in a retrograde direction from the deep to the saphenous system.

After the patient stands for 20 seconds, release the compression and look for sudden additional venous filling. Normally there is none; competent valves in the saphenous vein block retrograde flow. Slow venous filling continues.

> Sudden additional filling of superficial veins after release of compression indicates incompetent valves in the saphenous vein.

When both steps of this test are normal, the response is termed negative–negative. Negative–positive and positive–negative responses may also occur.

> When both steps are abnormal, the test is positive–positive.

Pulsus Alternans. In *pulsus alternans,* the rhythm of the pulse remains regular, but the *force* of the arterial pulse alternates because of alternating strong and weak ventricular contractions. *Pulsus alternans* almost always indicates severe left-sided heart failure and is usually best felt by applying light pressure on the radial or femoral arteries.[7] Use a blood pressure cuff to confirm your finding. After raising the cuff pressure, lower it slowly to the systolic level—the initial Korotkoff sounds are the strong beats. As you lower the cuff, you will hear the softer sounds of the alternating weak beats.

> Alternately loud and soft Korotkoff sounds or a sudden doubling of the apparent heart rate as the cuff pressure declines indicates a *pulsus alternans* (see p. 429).

> The upright position may accentuate the alternation.

Paradoxical Pulse. If you have noted that the pulse varies in amplitude with respiration or if you suspect pericardial tamponade (because of increased jugular venous pressure, a rapid and diminished pulse, and dyspnea, for example), use a blood pressure cuff to check for a *paradoxical pulse.* This is a greater than normal drop in systolic pressure during inspiration. As the patient breathes, quietly if possible, lower the cuff pressure slowly to the systolic level. Note the pressure level at which the first sounds can be heard. Then drop the pressure very slowly until sounds can be heard throughout the respiratory cycle. Again note the pressure level. The difference between these two levels is normally no greater than 3 or 4 mm Hg.

> The level identified by first hearing Korotkoff sounds is the highest systolic pressure during the respiratory cycle. The level identified by hearing sounds throughout the cycle is the lowest systolic pressure. A difference between these levels of more than 10 mm Hg indicates a paradoxical pulse and suggests *pericardial tamponade,* possible *constrictive pericarditis,* but most commonly *obstructive airway disease* (see p. 429).

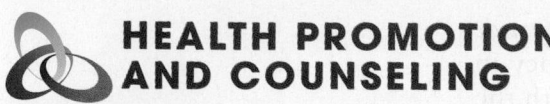

HEALTH PROMOTION AND COUNSELING

Important Topics for Health Promotion and Counseling

Arterial Disease
- Smoking cessation
- Weight control
- Exercise program
- Hypertension control
- Hyperlipidemia control
- Diabetes management
- Limiting alcohol intake
- Foot care

Venous Disease
- Avoidance of prolonged sitting and standing
- Avoidance of constrictive clothing, including girdles and tight hose
- Exercise program
- Weight control
- Foot care
- Dehydration prevention

Diseases of the peripheral vascular system, peripheral arterial disease, venous stasis, and thromboembolic disorders can severely affect the lifestyle and quality of life of patients. Identifying modifiable risk factors and providing health promotion counseling can prevent or delay long-term complications, such as decreased mobility and amputation. Helping the patient understand the effects of smoking, obesity, hypertension, hyperlipidemia, and diabetes and the need for exercise encourages the patient to institute lifestyle changes that promote peripheral and cardiovascular health.

PAD has the same underlying pathology as coronary artery disease. PAD is a common manifestation of atherosclerosis, affecting from 12% to 29% of community populations.[1,8] The presence of PAD increases with age and the presence of cardiovascular risk factors. PAD and cardiovascular disease overlap in 16% of patients. Nineteen percent of patients 70 years or older have PAD.[9] Controlling risk factors will help prevent or decrease the complications of both diseases.

Early identification of peripheral vascular diseases and modification of risk factors are important nursing functions. Careful and thorough history taking is essential to identify early peripheral vascular disease, especially in patients older than 50 years. Identification of risk factors should be performed with every patient. The nurse can use the ABI to assess peripheral arterial disease. Serial ABI testing will document any progression of the disease.

Since atherosclerotic renal arterial disease and abdominal aortic aneurysm often accompany peripheral vascular disease, patients with risk factors should be referred to their physicians for screening of these diseases. Atherosclerotic renal arterial disease affects 7% of adults older than 65 years, and rises to 22% to 55% of those with PAD and 30% of those with documented coronary artery disease.[6,10] Patients with worsening hypertension despite medication or new worsening of renal function should be evaluated. Abdominal aortic aneurysms (AAAs) are rarely symptomatic and the mortality rate for ruptured aneurysms is high. Risk factors for AAA include a history of ever smoking, family history, PAD, coronary artery disease, hypertension, elevated cholesterol, and age older than 65 years.

Prevention and early identification of DVT are critical nursing tasks, especially in the care of hospitalized patients and patients with reduced mobility. The Virchow triad—venous stasis, hypercoagulability, and vessel wall damage—set the stage for the development of a DVT. Most commonly immobility, compression of the vein, and increased blood viscosity (as seen in dehydration) lead to blood stasis, usually within the pockets of the vein valves. A thrombus forms and the patient is at risk for an embolism.[2] The Homan sign, with the patient's knee flexed and the ankle forcibly dorsiflexed, was the classic assessment maneuver; however, research has found this test very unreliable, yielding many false positives and negatives.[11] It should not be used. Almost every hospitalized patient is at risk for DVT. DVT risk assessment tools for hospitalized patients have been developed. The tools identify and rank risk factors and become part of the patient chart. Prevention strategies can then be initiated.[12]

Patients should be educated about the risk of DVT outside the hospital as well. Conditions that produce dehydration, cramped positioning, or immobility, such as long plane travel, can cause a DVT to form. Patients with sedentary jobs should be advised to walk or flex their legs at their desks at least every hour. Ergonomic furniture may reduce the effects of prolonged flexion of the legs.

TABLE
15-1

Painful Peripheral Vascular Disorders and Their Mimics[6,13]

Problem	Process	Location of Pain
Arterial Disorders *Atherosclerosis (arteriosclerosis obliterans)*		
• Intermittent claudication	Episodic muscular ischemia induced by exercise, due to atherosclerosis of large or medium-sized arteries	Usually calf muscles, but also may be in the buttock, hip, thigh, or foot, depending on the level of obstruction
• Rest pain	Ischemia even at rest	Distal pain, in the toes or forefoot
Acute Arterial Occlusion	Embolism or thrombosis, possibly superimposed on arteriosclerosis obliterans	Distal pain, usually involving the foot and leg
Raynaud Disease and Phenomenon	*Raynaud disease:* Episodic spasm of the small arteries and arterioles; no vascular occlusion *Raynaud phenomenon:* Syndrome secondary to other conditions such as collagen vascular disease, arterial occlusion, trauma, drugs	Distal portions of one or more fingers. Pain is usually not prominent unless fingertip ulcers develop. Numbness and tingling are common.
Venous Disorders *Superficial Thrombophlebitis*	Clot formation and acute inflammation in a superficial vein	Pain in a local area along the course of a superficial vein, most often in the saphenous system
Deep Venous Thrombosis (DVT)	Clot formation in a deep vein	Tight, bursting pain, if present, usually in the calf; may be painless
Chronic Venous Insufficiency (deep)	Chronic venous engorgement secondary to venous occlusion or incompetency of venous valves	Diffuse aching of the leg(s)
Thromboangiitis Obliterans (Buerger disease)	Inflammatory and thrombotic occlusions of small arteries and also of veins, occurring in smokers	• Intermittent claudication, particularly in the arch of the foot • Rest pain in the fingers or toes
Compartment Syndrome	Pressure builds from trauma or bleeding into one of the four major muscle compartments between the knee and ankle. Each compartment is enclosed by fascia and thus cannot expand to accommodate increasing pressure.	Tight, bursting pain in calf muscles, usually in the anterior tibial compartment, sometimes with overlying dusky red skin
Acute Lymphangitis	Acute bacterial infection (usually streptococcal) spreading up the lymphatic channels from a portal of entry such as an injured area or an ulcer	An arm or a leg
Mimics* *Acute Cellulitis*	Acute bacterial infection of the skin and subcutaneous tissues	Arms, legs, or elsewhere

*Mistaken primarily for acute superficial thrombophlebitis.

Timing	Factors That Aggravate	Factors That Relieve	Associated Manifestations
Fairly brief; pain usually forces the patient to rest.	Exercise such as walking	Rest usually stops the pain in 1–3 min.	Local fatigue, numbness, diminished pulses, often signs of arterial insufficiency (see p. 426)
Persistent, often worse at night	Elevation of the feet, as in bed	Sitting with legs dependent	Numbness, tingling, trophic signs and color changes of arterial insufficiency (see p. 426)
Sudden onset; associated symptoms may occur without pain.			Coldness, numbness, weakness, absent distal pulses
Relatively brief (minutes) but recurrent	Exposure to cold, emotional upset	Warm environment	Color changes in the distal fingers: severe pallor (essential for the diagnosis) followed by cyanosis and then redness
An acute episode lasting days or longer			Local redness, swelling, tenderness, a palpable cord, possibly fever
Often hard to determine because of lack of symptoms	Walking	Elevation speeds relief.	Possible swelling of the foot and calf, local calf tenderness. Prior history of DVT
Chronic, increasing as the day wears on	Prolonged standing	Elevation of the leg(s)	Chronic edema, pigmentation, possibly ulceration (see p. 426)
• Fairly brief but recurrent • Chronic, persistent, may be worse at night	• Exercise	• Rest • Permanent cessation of smoking helps both kinds of pain (but patients seldom stop).	Distal coldness, sweating, numbness, and cyanosis; ulceration and gangrene at the tips of fingers or toes; migratory thrombophlebitis
Several hours if *acute* (pressure must be relieved to overt necrosis). During exercise if *chronic*	*Acute:* anabolic steroids; surgical complication; crush injury. *Chronic:* occurs with exercise	*Acute:* surgical incision to relieve pressure *Chronic:* avoiding exercise; ice elevation	Tingling, burning sensations in calf; muscles may feel tight, full, numbness, paralysis if unrelieved
An acute episode lasting days or longer			Red streak(s) on the skin, with tenderness, enlarged, tender lymph nodes, and fever
An acute episode lasting days or longer			A local area of diffuse swelling, redness, and tenderness with enlarged, tender lymph nodes and fever; no palpable cord

TABLE 15-2	Chronic Insufficiency of Arteries and Veins

Chronic Arterial Insufficiency (Advanced)	Chronic Venous Insufficiency (Advanced)

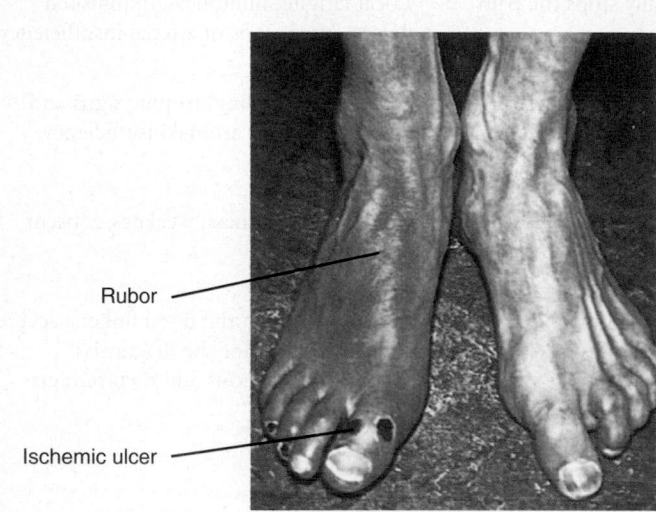

Rubor

Ischemic ulcer

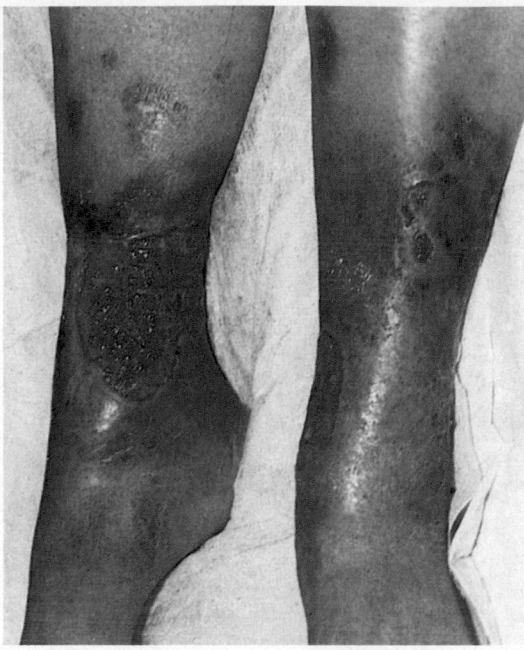

	Chronic Arterial Insufficiency (Advanced)	Chronic Venous Insufficiency (Advanced)
Pain	Intermittent claudication, progressing to pain at rest	Ulcer often painful[17], generalized leg aching, especially at end of day
Mechanism	Tissue ischemia	Venous hypertension
Pulses	Decreased or absent	Normal, though may be difficult to feel through edema
Color	Pale, especially on elevation; dusky red on dependency	Normal, or cyanotic on dependency Petechiae and then brown pigmentation appear with chronicity.
Temperature	Cool	Normal
Edema	Absent or mild; may develop as the patient tries to relieve rest pain by lowering the leg	Present, often marked
Skin Changes	Trophic changes: thin, shiny, atrophic skin; loss of hair over the foot and toes; nails thickened and ridged	Often brown pigmentation around the ankle, stasis dermatitis, and possible thickening of the skin and narrowing of the leg as scarring develops
Ulceration	If present, involves toes or points of trauma on feet	If present, develops at sides of ankle, especially medially
Gangrene	May develop	Does not develop

(Sources of photos: *Arterial Insufficiency*—Kappert A, Winsor T. Diagnosis of Peripheral Vascular Disease. Philadelphia: FA Davis, 1972; *Venous Insufficiency*—Marks R. Skin Disease in Old Age. Philadelphia: JB Lippincott, 1987.)

TABLE
15-3

Common Ulcers of the Ankles and Feet

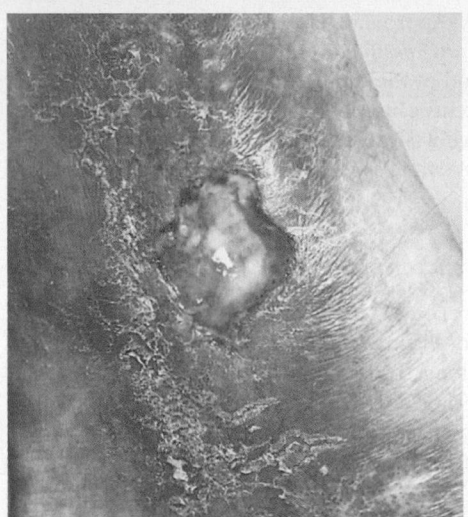

Chronic Venous Insufficiency Ulcer

This condition usually appears over the medial and sometimes the lateral malleolus. The ulcer contains small, painful granulation tissue and fibrin; necrosis or exposed tendons are rare. Borders are irregular, flat, or slightly steep. Pain affects quality of life in 75% of patients. Associated findings include edema, reddish pigmentation and purpura, venous varicosities, the eczematous changes of stasis dermatitis (redness, scaling, and pruritus), and at times cyanosis of the foot when dependent. Gangrene is rare.[13]

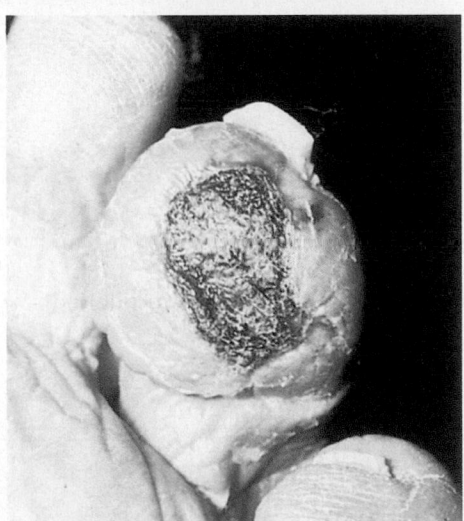

Arterial Insufficiency Ulcer

This condition occurs in the toes, feet, or possibly areas of trauma (e.g., the shins). Surrounding skin shows no callus or excess pigment, although it may be atrophic. Pain often is severe unless neuropathy masks it. Gangrene may be associated, along with decreased pulses, trophic changes, foot pallor on elevation, and dusky rubor on dependency.

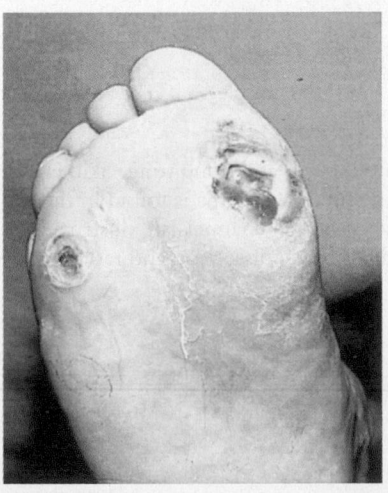

Neuropathic Ulcer

This condition develops in pressure points of areas with diminished sensation; seen in diabetic neuropathy, neurologic disorders, and Hansen disease. Surrounding skin is calloused. There is no pain, so the ulcer may go unnoticed. In uncomplicated cases, there is no gangrene. Associated signs include decreased sensation and absent ankle jerks.

(Source of photos: Marks R. Skin Disease in Old Age. Philadelphia: JB Lippincott, 1987.)

TABLE
15-4

Some Peripheral Causes of Edema

Approximately one third of total body water is extracellular, or outside the body's cells. Approximately 25% of extracellular fluid is plasma; the remainder is interstitial fluid. At the arteriolar end of the capillaries, *hydrostatic pressure* in the blood vessels and *colloid oncotic pressure* in the interstitium cause fluid to move into the tissues; at the venous end of the capillaries and in the lymphatics, hydrostatic pressure in the interstitium and the colloid oncotic pressure of plasma proteins cause fluid to return to the vascular compartment. Several clinical conditions disrupt this balance, resulting in *edema,* or a clinically evident accumulation of interstitial fluid. Not depicted below is *capillary leak syndrome,* in which protein leaks into the interstitial space, seen in burns, angioedema, snake bites, and allergic reactions.

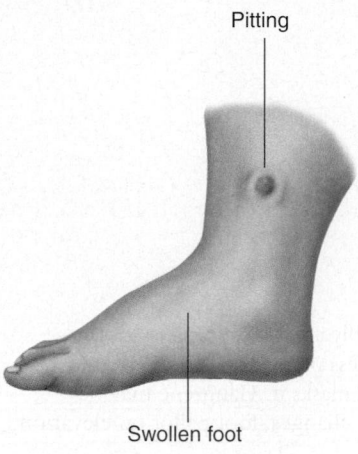

Pitting

Swollen foot

Pitting Edema

Edema is soft, bilateral, with pitting on pressure, on the anterior tibiae and feet. There is no skin thickening, ulceration, or pigmentation. Pitting edema results from several conditions: when legs are dependent from prolonged standing or sitting, which leads to increased hydrostatic pressure in the veins and capillaries; congestive heart failure leading to decreased cardiac output; nephrotic syndrome, cirrhosis, or malnutrition leading to low albumin and decreased intravascular colloid oncotic pressure; and drug use.

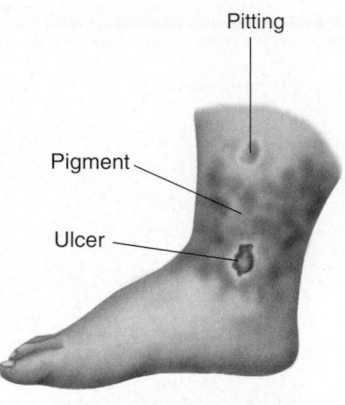

Pitting

Pigment

Ulcer

Chronic Venous Insufficiency

Edema is soft, with pitting on pressure, and occasionally bilateral. Look for brawny changes and skin thickening, especially near the ankle. Ulceration, brownish pigmentation, and edema in the feet are common. Arises from chronic obstruction and from incompetent valves in the deep venous system.

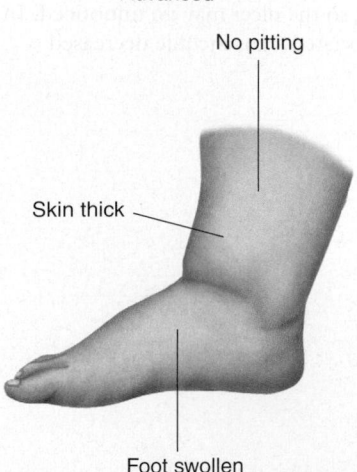

Advanced
No pitting

Skin thick

Foot swollen

Lymphedema

Edema is soft in the early stages, then becomes indurated, hard, and nonpitting. Skin is markedly thickened; ulceration is rare. There is no pigmentation. Edema is found in the extremities, often bilaterally. Lymphedema develops when lymph channels are obstructed by tumor, fibrosis, or inflammation, and in cases of axillary node dissection and radiation.

TABLE 15-5

Abnormalities of the Arterial Pulse and Pressure Waves

Normal

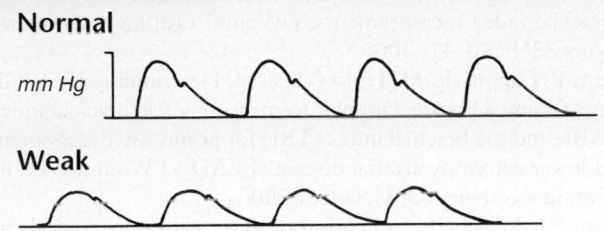

mm Hg

The pulse pressure is approximately 30–40 mm Hg. The pulse contour is smooth and rounded. (The notch on the descending slope of the pulse wave is not palpable.)

Weak

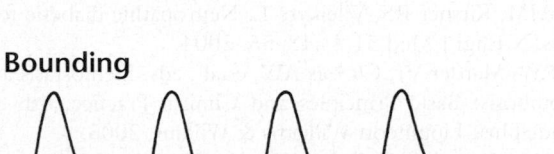

The pulse pressure is diminished, and the pulse feels weak and small. The upstroke may feel slowed, the peak prolonged. Causes include (1) decreased stroke volume, as in heart failure, hypovolemia, and severe aortic stenosis, and (2) increased peripheral resistance, as in exposure to cold and severe congestive heart failure.

Bounding

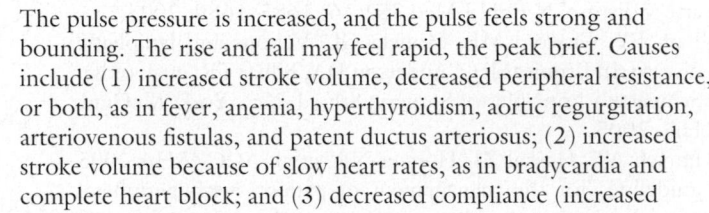

The pulse pressure is increased, and the pulse feels strong and bounding. The rise and fall may feel rapid, the peak brief. Causes include (1) increased stroke volume, decreased peripheral resistance, or both, as in fever, anemia, hyperthyroidism, aortic regurgitation, arteriovenous fistulas, and patent ductus arteriosus; (2) increased stroke volume because of slow heart rates, as in bradycardia and complete heart block; and (3) decreased compliance (increased stiffness) of the aortic walls, as in aging or atherosclerosis.

Bisferiens

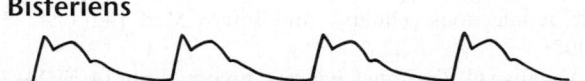

A bisferiens pulse is an increased arterial pulse with a double systolic peak. Causes include pure aortic regurgitation and aortic stenosis with regurgitation.

Pulsus Alternans

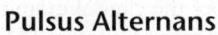

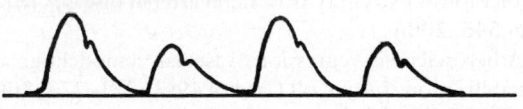

The pulse alternates in amplitude from beat to beat even though the rhythm is regular. When the difference between stronger and weaker beats is slight, it can be detected only by sphygmomanometry. Pulsus alternans indicates left ventricular failure and is usually accompanied by a left-sided S3.

Bigeminal Pulse

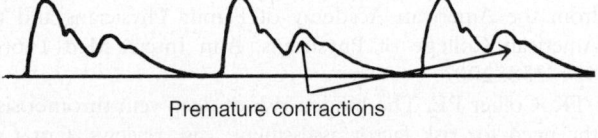

Premature contractions

This disorder of rhythm may mimic pulsus alternans. A bigeminal pulse is caused by a normal beat alternating with a premature contraction. The stroke volume of the premature beat is diminished in relation to that of the normal beats, and the pulse varies in amplitude accordingly.

Paradoxical Pulse

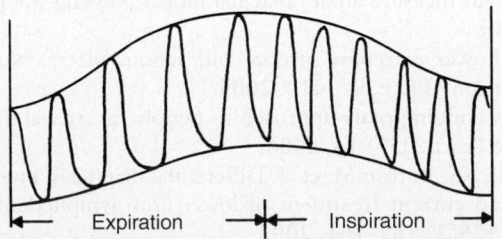

Expiration   Inspiration

A palpable decrease in the pulse's amplitude with quiet inspiration. A blood pressure cuff may be needed to detect the difference in amplitude. Systolic pressure decreases by more than 10 mm Hg during inspiration. A paradoxical pulse is found in pericardial tamponade, constrictive pericarditis (though less commonly), and obstructive lung disease.

BIBLIOGRAPHY

CITATIONS

1. Hirsch AT, Criqui MH, Treat-Jacobsen D, et al. Peripheral arterial disease detection, awareness, and treatment in primary care. JAMA 286(11):1317–1324, 2001.
2. Fox JC. Diagnostic and therapeutic keys to deep vein thrombosis. Emerg Med 38(2):14–20, 2006.
3. Schoen FJ. Blood vessels. In Kumar VK, Fausto N, Abbas AK (eds). Robbins and Cotran Pathologic Basis of Disease, 7th ed. Philadelphia: Elsevier, 2005.
4. Hansson GK. Inflammation, atherosclerosis, and coronary artery disease. N Engl J Med 352(16):1685–1689, 2005.
5. Lam EY, Giswold ME, Moneta GL. Venous and lymphatic disease. In Brunicardi C, Anderson DA, Billiar TR, et al. (eds). Schwartz's Principles of Surgery, 8th ed. New York: McGraw Hill, 2005.
6. Hirsch AT, Haskal ZJ, Hertzer NR, et al. ACC/AHA 2005 guidelines for the management of patients with peripheral arterial disease (lower extremity, renal, mesenteric, and abdominal aortic): a collaborative report from the American Association for Vascular Surgery/Society for Vascular Surgery, Society for Cardiovascular Angiography and Interventions, Society for Vascular Medicine and Biology, Society of Interventional Radiology, and the ACC/AHA Task Force on Practice Guidelines (Writing Committee to Develop Guidelines for the Management of Patients With Peripheral Arterial Disease). Available at: http://circ.ahajournals.org/cgi/reprint/113/11/e463. Accessed June 21, 2011.
7. Cha K, Falk RH. Images in clinical medicine: pulsus alternans. N Engl J Med 334(13):834, 1996.
8. Newman AB. Peripheral arterial disease: insights from population studies of older adults. J Am Ger Soc 48(9):1157–1162, 2000.
9. Kanel WB. The demographics of claudication and the aging of the American population. Vasc Med 1:60–64, 1986.
10. Balk E, Raman G, Chung M, et al, Effectiveness of management strategies for renal artery senosis: a systematic review. Ann Intern Med 146(10): 699–706, 2007.
11. Urbano FL. Homan's sign in the diagnosis of deep vein thrombosis. Hospital Physician March:22–24, 2001.
12. McCaffrey R, Bishop M, Adonis-Rizzo M, et al. Development and testing of a DVT risk assessment tool: providing evidence of validity and reliability. Worldviews Evid Based Nurs 4(1): 14–20, 2007.
13. De Araujo T, Valencia I, Federman D, et al. Managing the patient with venous ulcers. Ann Intern Med 138(4):326–334, 2003.

ADDITIONAL REFERENCES

Bates SM, Ginsberg JS. Treatment of deep-vein thrombosis. N Engl J Med 351(3):268–277, 2004.

Bonham PA. Get the LEAD out: noninvasive assessment for lower extremity arterial disease using ankle brachial index and tow brachial index measurements. J Wound Ostomy Continence Nurs 33(1):30–41, 2006.

Bonham P, Cappuccio M, Hulsey T, et al. Determining the validity of using a pocket Doppler to measure ankle brachial index (ABI) and toe brachial index (TBI) for noninvasive assessment of lower extremity arterial disease (LEAD). J Wound Ostomy Continence Nurs 33(3):S5–S5, 2006.

Bonham PA, Kelechi T. Evaluation of lower extremity arterial circulation and implications for nursing practice. J Cardiovasc Nurs 23(2):144–152, 2008.

Boulton AJM, Kirsner RS, Vileikyte L. Neuropathic diabetic foot ulcers. N Engl J Med 51(1):48–55, 2004.

Colman RW, Marder VJ, Clowes AW, et al., eds. Hemostasis and Thrombosis: Basic Principles and Clinical Practice, 4th ed. Philadelphia: Lippincott Williams & Wilkins, 2005.

Creager MA, Loscalzo J, Dzau VJ, eds. Vascular Medicine: A Companion to Braunwald's Heart Disease. Philadelphia: WB Saunders, 2006.

Douketis JD. Use of a clinical prediction score in patients with suspected deep venous thrombosis: two steps forward, one step back? Ann Intern Med 143(2):140–141, 2005.

Falagas ME, Vergidis PI. Narrative review: diseases that masquerade as infectious cellulitis. Ann Intern Med 142(1):47–55, 2005.

Hoyle-Vaughan G. Treating leg ulcers. Emerg Nurse 14(5):24–27, 2006.

Khan NA, Rahim SA, Anand SS, et al. Does the clinical examination predict lower extremity peripheral arterial disease? JAMA 295:536–545, 2006.

Klein LW. Atherosclerosis regression, vascular remodeling, and plaque stabilization. J Am Coll Cardiol 49(2):271–273, 2007.

Olson K, Treat-Jacobson D. Symptoms of peripheral arterial disease: a critical review. J Vasc Nurs 22(3):72–77, 2004.

Qaseem A, Snow V, Barry P, et al. Current diagnosis of venous thromboembolism in primary care: a clinical practice guideline from the American Academy of Family Physicians and the American College of Physicians. Ann Intern Med 146(6): 454–458, 2007.

Race TK, Collier PE. The hidden risk of deep vein thrombosis—the need for risk factor assessment: case reviews. Crit Care Nurs Q 30(3):245–254, 2007.

Rice K L. How to measure ankle/brachial index. Nursing 35(1): 56–57, 2005.

Sieggreen M. Lower extremity arterial and venous ulcers. Nurs Clin North Am 40(2):391–410, 2005.

Sieggreen M. A contemporary approach to peripheral arterial disease. Nurse Pract 31(7):14, 2006.

Tiwari A, Cheng KS, Button M, et al. Differential diagnosis, investigation, and current treatment of lower limb lymphedema. Arch Surg 138(2):152–161, 2003.

Wigley FM. Raynaud's phenomenon. N Engl J Med 347(13): 1001–1008, 2002.

The Gastrointestinal and Renal Systems

LEARNING OBJECTIVES

The student will:

1. Identify the structures and function of the gastrointestinal and renal systems.
2. Identify the four quadrants and the organs in each quadrant.
3. Collect an accurate health history of the gastrointestinal and renal systems.
4. Describe the physical examination techniques and the order performed to evaluate the gastrointestinal and renal systems.
5. Determine the health promotion and counseling measures related to alcohol abuse, hepatitis, colorectal cancer, and urinary incontinence.
6. Perform a complete gastrointestinal and renal system examination.
7. Document a complete gastrointestinal and renal system assessment utilizing information from the health history and the physical examination.

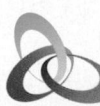 **ANATOMY AND PHYSIOLOGY**

The gastrointestinal and renal systems encompass many organs of the body. It is important to be familiar with the site and function of each organ and in which quadrant each is located for the assessment. The landmarks of the abdominal wall and pelvis are illustrated. The rectus abdominis muscles become more prominent when the patient raises the head and shoulders from the supine position.

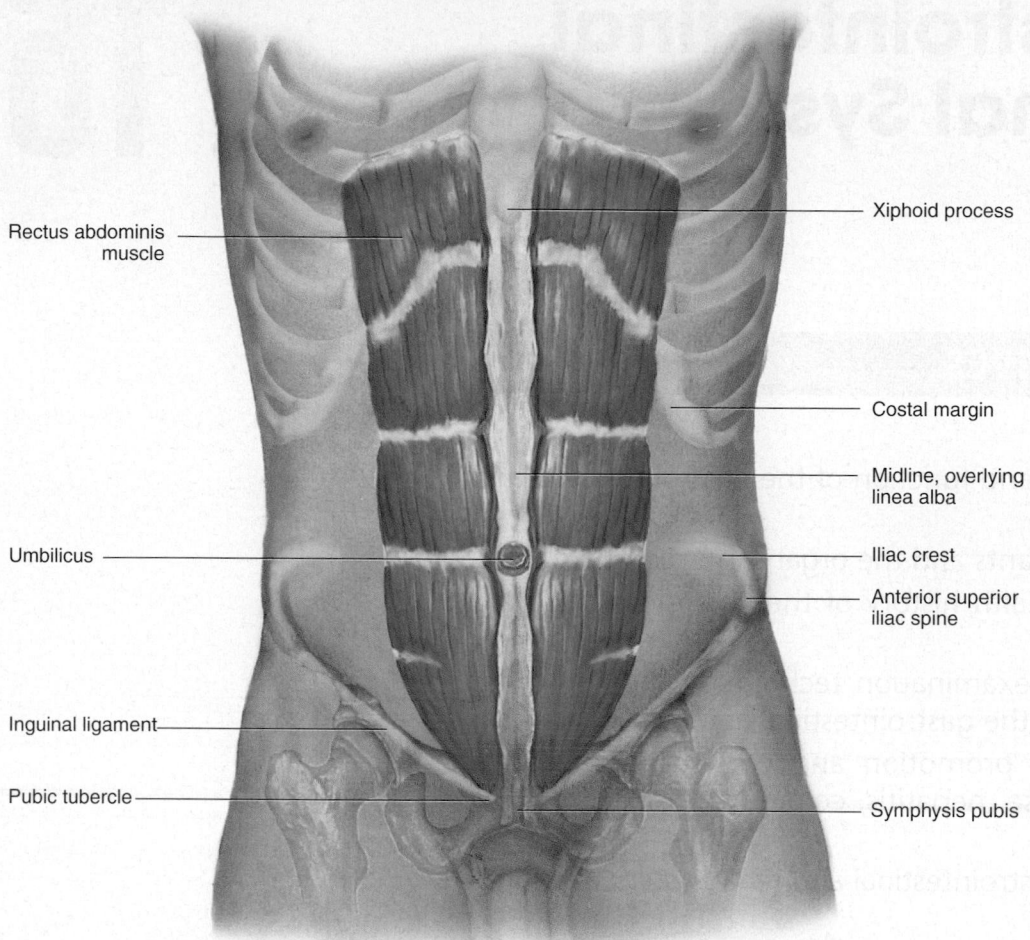

Rectus abdominis muscle

Umbilicus

Inguinal ligament

Pubic tubercle

Xiphoid process

Costal margin

Midline, overlying linea alba

Iliac crest

Anterior superior iliac spine

Symphysis pubis

For descriptive purposes, the abdomen is often divided by imaginary lines crossing at the umbilicus, forming the right upper quadrant (RUQ), right lower quadrant (RLQ), left upper quadrant (LUQ), and left lower quadrant (LLQ).

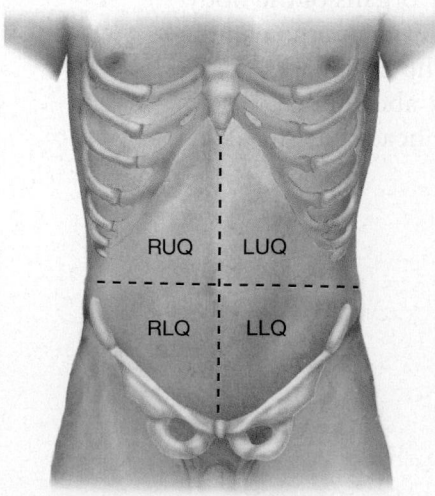

RUQ | LUQ

RLQ | LLQ

When examining the abdomen and moving in a clockwise rotation, several organs are often palpable. Exceptions are the stomach and much of the liver and spleen. The abdominal cavity extends up under the rib cage to the dome of the diaphragm, placing these organs in a protected location, beyond the reach of the palpating hand.

In the *right upper quadrant,* the soft consistency of the *liver* makes it difficult to feel through the abdominal wall. The lower margin of the liver, the liver edge, is often palpable at the right costal margin. The *gallbladder,* which rests against the inferior surface of the liver, and the more deeply lying *duodenum* are generally not palpable. At a deeper level, the *lower pole of the right kidney* may be felt, especially in thin people with relaxed abdominal muscles. Moving medially, the examiner encounters the rib cage, which protects the stomach; the *xiphoid process* lies in the midline. The *abdominal aorta* often has visible pulsations and is usually palpable in the upper abdomen.

In the *left upper quadrant,* the *spleen* is lateral to and behind the stomach, just above the left kidney in the left midaxillary line. Its upper margin rests against the dome of the diaphragm. The 9th, 10th, and 11th ribs protect most of the spleen. The tip of the spleen may be palpable below the left costal margin in a small percentage of adults. The *pancreas* in healthy people escapes detection.

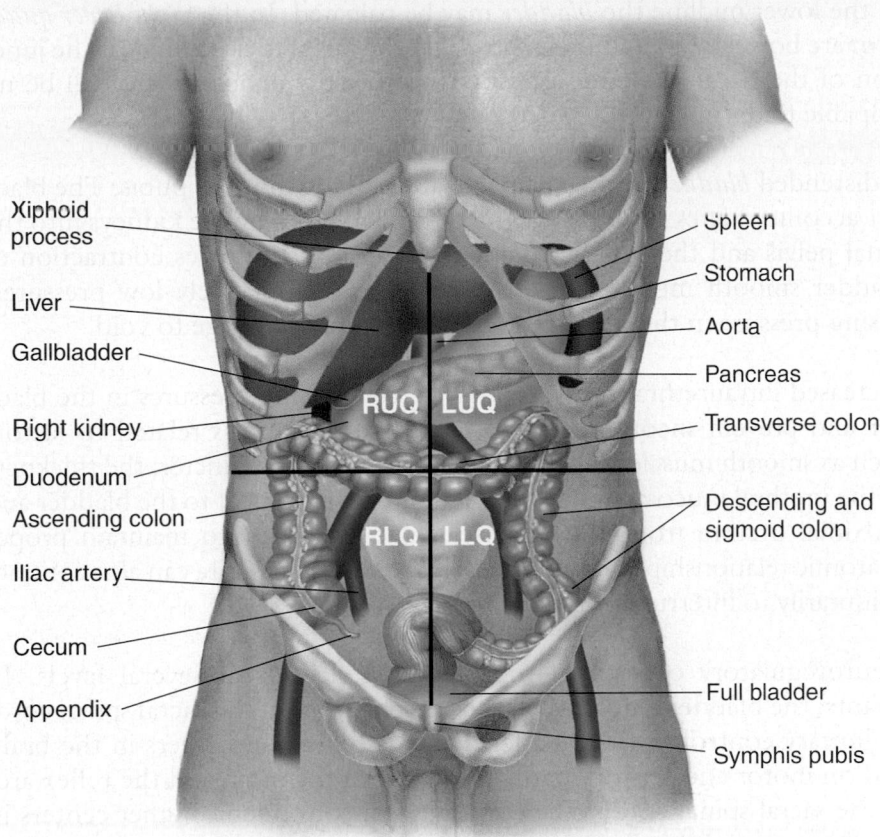

Labels (left): Xiphoid process, Liver, Gallbladder, Right kidney, Duodenum, Ascending colon, Iliac artery, Cecum, Appendix

Quadrant labels: RUQ, LUQ, RLQ, LLQ

Labels (right): Spleen, Stomach, Aorta, Pancreas, Transverse colon, Descending and sigmoid colon, Full bladder, Symphis pubis

Right Upper Quadrant (RUQ)	Left Upper Quadrant (LUQ)
Ascending colon	Descending colon
Duodenum	Left kidney
Gallbladder	Pancreas (body and tail)
Right kidney	Spleen
Liver	Stomach
Pancreas (head)	Transverse colon
Transverse colon	Ureter (left)
Ureter (right)	
Right Lower Quadrant (RLQ)	**Left Lower Quadrant (LLQ)**
Appendix	Bladder
Ascending colon	Descending colon
Bladder	Ovary, uterus, fallopian tube (female)
Cecum	Prostate and spermatic cord (male)
Rectum	Small intestine
Ovary, uterus and fallopian tube (female)	Sigmoid colon
Prostate and spermatic cord (male)	Ureter (left)
Small intestine	
Ureter (right)	

In the *left lower quadrant* the firm, narrow, tubular sigmoid *colon* is often felt and portions of the transverse and descending colon may also be palpable.

In the lower midline the *bladder* may be palpated. In the *right lower quadrant* are bowel loops and the *appendix* at the tail of the cecum near the junction of the small and large intestines. In healthy people, there will be no palpable findings.

A distended *bladder* may be palpable above the symphysis pubis. The bladder accommodates roughly 300 ml of urine filtered by the kidneys into the renal pelvis and the ureters. Bladder expansion stimulates contraction of bladder smooth muscle, the *detrusor muscle,* at relatively low pressures. Rising pressure in the bladder triggers the conscious urge to void.

Increased intraurethral pressure can overcome rising pressures in the bladder and prevent incontinence. Intraurethral pressure is related to factors such as smooth muscle tone in the internal urethral sphincter, the thickness of the urethral mucosa, and in women, sufficient support to the bladder and proximal urethra from pelvic muscles and ligaments to maintain proper anatomic relationships. Striated muscle around the urethra can also contract voluntarily to interrupt voiding.

Neuroregulatory control of the bladder functions at several levels. In infants, the bladder empties by reflex mechanisms in the sacral spinal cord. Voluntary control of the bladder depends on higher centers in the brain and on motor and sensory pathways between the brain and the reflex arcs of the sacral spinal cord. When voiding is inconvenient, higher centers in the brain can inhibit detrusor contractions until the capacity of the bladder, approximately 400 to 500 ml, is exceeded. The integrity of the sacral nerves that innervate the bladder can be tested by assessing perirectal and perineal sensation in the S2, S3, and S4 dermatomes (see pp. 643–644).

The *kidneys* are posterior organs. The ribs protect their upper portions. The *costovertebral angle*—the angle formed by the lower border of the 12th rib and the transverse processes of the upper lumbar vertebrae—defines the region to assess for kidney tenderness.

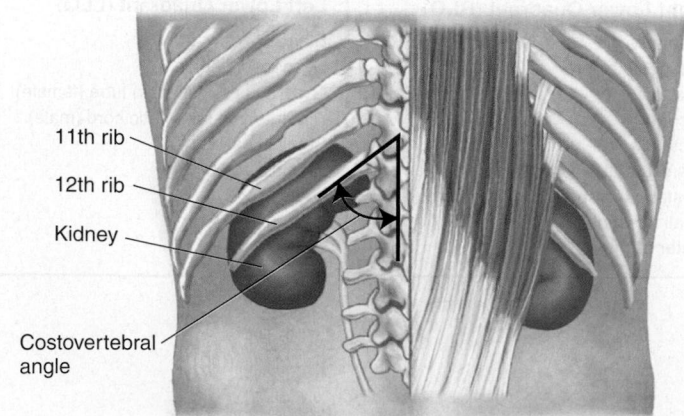

11th rib

12th rib

Kidney

Costovertebral angle

POSTERIOR VIEW

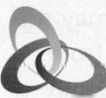

THE HEALTH HISTORY

COMMON OR CONCERNING SYMPTOMS

Gastrointestinal	Urinary and Renal
• Abdominal pain, acute and chronic	• Suprapubic pain
• Indigestion, nausea, vomiting including blood, loss of appetite, early satiety	• Dysuria, urgency, or frequency
	• Hesitancy, decreased stream in males
• Dysphagia and/or odynophagia	• Polyuria or nocturia
• Change in bowel function	• Urinary incontinence
• Diarrhea, constipation	• Hematuria
• Jaundice	• Kidney or flank pain
	• Ureteral colic

Gastrointestinal complaints rank high among reasons for office and emergency room visits. Patients complain of a wide variety of upper gastrointestinal symptoms, including abdominal pain, heartburn, nausea and vomiting, difficulty or pain with swallowing, vomiting of stomach contents or blood, loss of appetite, and jaundice. Lower gastrointestinal complaints are also common: diarrhea, constipation, change in bowel habits, and blood in the stool, often described as either bright red or dark and tarry.

Numerous symptoms also originate in the *genitourinary tract:* difficulty urinating, urgency and frequency, hesitancy and decreased stream in men, high urine volume, urinating at night, incontinence, blood in the urine, and flank pain and colic from renal stones or infection.

Often you will need to cluster several findings from both the patient's story and your examination as you sort through various explanations for the patient's symptoms. Your skills in history taking and examination will be needed for sound clinical reasoning.

Patterns and Mechanisms of Abdominal Pain.
Before exploring gastrointestinal and genitourinary symptoms, review the mechanisms and clinical patterns of abdominal pain. Be familiar with three broad categories of abdominal pain:

See Table 16-1, Abdominal Pain (pp. 472–473).

• *Visceral pain* occurs when hollow abdominal organs such as the intestine or biliary tree contract unusually forcefully or are distended or stretched. Solid organs such as the liver can also become painful when their capsules are stretched. Visceral pain may be difficult to localize. It is typically palpable near the midline at levels that vary according to the structure involved, as illustrated on the next page.

Visceral pain in the right upper quadrant may result from liver distention against its capsule in *alcoholic hepatitis.*

Visceral pain varies in quality and may be gnawing, burning, cramping, or aching. When it becomes severe, it may be associated with sweating, pallor, nausea, vomiting, and restlessness.

Visceral periumbilical pain may signify early *acute appendicitis* from distention of an inflamed appendix. It gradually changes to parietal pain in the right lower quadrant from inflammation of the adjacent parietal peritoneum.

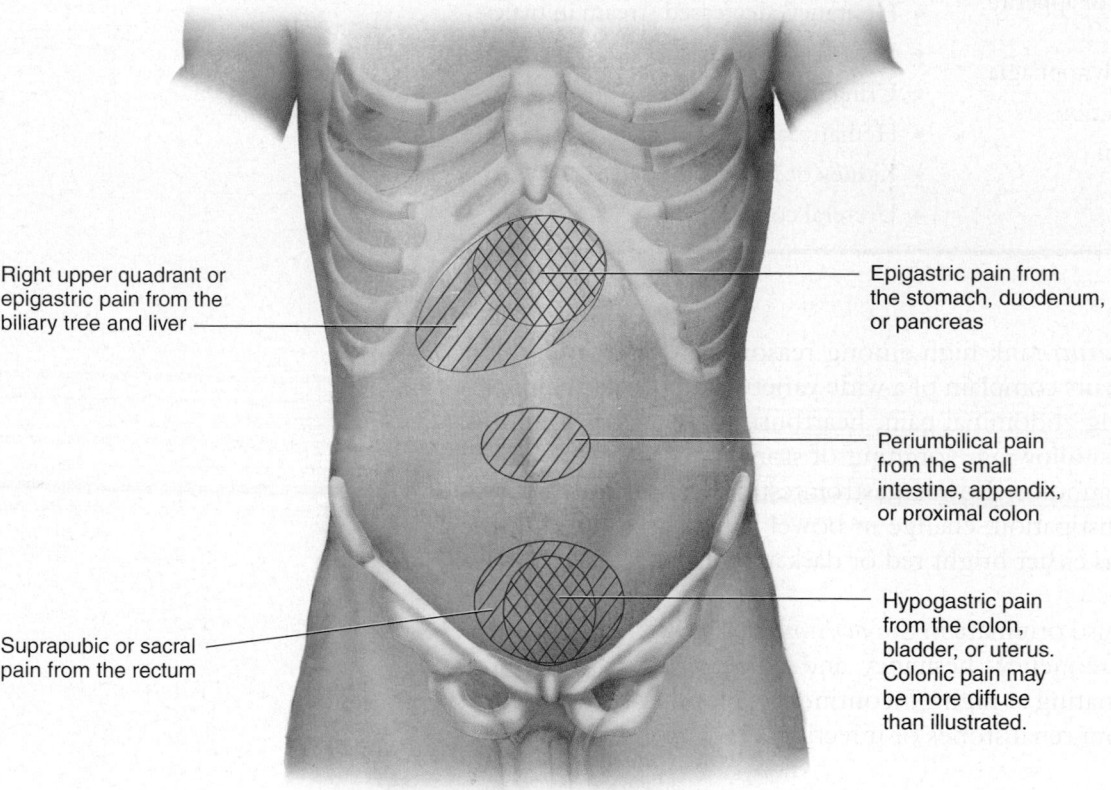

Right upper quadrant or epigastric pain from the biliary tree and liver

Epigastric pain from the stomach, duodenum, or pancreas

Periumbilical pain from the small intestine, appendix, or proximal colon

Suprapubic or sacral pain from the rectum

Hypogastric pain from the colon, bladder, or uterus. Colonic pain may be more diffuse than illustrated.

TYPES OF VISCERAL PAIN

- *Parietal pain* originates from inflammation in the parietal peritoneum. It is a steady, aching pain that is usually more severe than visceral pain and more precisely localized over the involved structure. It is typically aggravated by movement or coughing. Patients with this type of pain usually prefer to lie still.

- *Referred pain* is felt in more distant sites, which are innervated at approximately the same spinal levels as the disordered structures. Referred pain often develops as the initial pain becomes more intense and thus seems to radiate or travel from the initial site. It may be felt superficially or deeply but is usually well localized.

Pain may also be referred to the abdomen from the chest, spine, or pelvis, thus complicating the assessment of abdominal pain.

Pain of duodenal or pancreatic origin may be referred to the back; pain from the biliary tree, to the right shoulder or the right posterior chest.

Pain from *pleurisy* or *acute myocardial infarction* may be referred to the epigastric area.

The Gastrointestinal Tract

Upper Abdominal Pain, Discomfort, and Heartburn. The prevalence of recurrent upper abdominal discomfort or pain in the United States and other Western countries is approximately 25%.[1]

Acute Upper Abdominal Pain or Discomfort.

For patients complaining of abdominal pain, causes range from benign to life-threatening, so take the time to conduct a careful history.

Onset: First determine the *timing of the pain*. Is it *acute or chronic?* Acute abdominal pain has many patterns. Did the pain start suddenly or gradually? When did it begin?

> In emergency rooms 40% to 45% of patients have nonspecific pain, but 15% to 30% need surgery, usually for appendicitis, intestinal obstruction, or cholecystitis.[2]

Location: Then ask the patient to *point to the pain*. Patients are not always clear when they try to describe in words where pain is most intense. The quadrant where the pain is located can be helpful. Often underlying organs are involved. If clothes interfere, repeat the question during the physical examination.

> Epigastric pain occurs with *gastritis* or *gastroesophageal reflux disease (GERD)*. Right upper quadrant and upper abdominal pain signify *cholecystitis*.[3]

Duration: How long does it last?
What is its pattern over a 24-hour period?
Over weeks or months? Are you dealing with an acute illness or a chronic and recurring one?

Characteristic Symptoms:
- Ask patients to *describe the pain in their own words*. Pursue important details: "Where does the pain start?"

  "Does it radiate or travel anywhere?"

  "What is the pain like?"

  If the patient has trouble describing the pain, try offering several choices:

  "Is it aching, burning, gnawing . . . ?"

> Doubling over with cramping colicky pain indicates *renal stone*. Sudden knife-like epigastric pain occurs in *gallstone pancreatitis*.[4]

- Ask the patient to rank the *severity of the pain* on a scale of 1 to 10. Note that severity does not always help you to identify the cause. Sensitivity to abdominal pain varies widely and tends to diminish in older patients, masking acute abdominal conditions. Pain threshold and how patients accommodate to pain during daily activities also affect ratings of severity.

Associated Manifestations: Ask the patient if he or she is experiencing any other symptoms (e.g., nausea, vomiting, or indigestion).

Relieving Factors: As you probe *factors that aggravate or relieve the pain,* pay special attention to any association with meals, alcohol, medications (including aspirin and aspirin-like drugs and any over-the-counter medications), stress, body position, and use of antacids. Ask if indigestion or discomfort is related to exertion and relieved by rest.

Note that angina from inferior wall coronary artery disease may present as "indigestion," but is precipitated by exertion and relieved by rest. See Table 13-3, pp. 327–328, Chest Pain.

Treatment: Determine what remedies the patient has tried and the results of each.

Chronic Upper Abdominal Discomfort or Pain. For more chronic symptoms, *dyspepsia* is defined as chronic or recurrent discomfort or pain centered in the upper abdomen.[7] *Discomfort* is defined as a subjective negative feeling that is nonpainful. It can include various symptoms such as bloating, nausea, upper abdominal fullness, and heartburn.

- Note that bloating, nausea, or belching can occur alone or be associated with other disorders. When they occur alone they do not meet the criteria for dyspepsia.

Bloating may occur with *inflammatory bowel disease,* belching from *aerophagia,* or swallowing air.

- Many patients with upper abdominal discomfort or pain will have *functional, or nonulcer, dyspepsia,* defined as a 3-month history of nonspecific upper abdominal discomfort or nausea not attributable to structural abnormalities or peptic ulcer disease. Symptoms are usually recurring and typically present for more than 6 months.[3]

Multifactorial causes include delayed gastric emptying (20%–40%), gastritis from *Helicobacter pylori* (20%–60%), peptic ulcer disease (up to 15% if *H. pylori* is present), and psychosocial factors.[1]

- Many patients with chronic upper abdominal discomfort or pain complain primarily of *heartburn, acid reflux,* or *regurgitation.* If patients report these symptoms more than once a week, they are likely to have *GERD* until proven otherwise.[5,6]

These symptoms or mucosal damage on endoscopy are the diagnostic criteria for GERD. Risk factors include reduced salivary flow, which prolongs acid clearance by damping action of the bicarbonate buffer; delayed gastric emptying; selected medications; and hiatal hernia.

- *Heartburn* is a rising retrosternal burning pain or discomfort occurring weekly or more often.[1] It is typically aggravated by food such as alcohol, chocolate, citrus fruits, coffee, onions, and peppermint; or positions like bending over, exercising, lifting, or lying supine.

Note that angina from inferior wall coronary ischemia along the diaphragm may present as heartburn. See Table 13-3, pp. 327–328, Chest Pain.

- Some patients with GERD have *atypical respiratory symptoms* such as cough, wheezing, and aspiration pneumonia. Others complain of *pharyngeal symptoms,* such as hoarseness and chronic sore throat.[7]

● Some patients may have "*alarm symptoms,*" such as difficulty swallowing (dysphagia), pain with swallowing (odynophagia), recurrent vomiting, evidence of gastrointestinal bleeding, weight loss, anemia, or risk factors for gastric cancer.

Patients with uncomplicated GERD who do not respond to empiric therapy, patients older than 55 years, and those with "alarm symptoms" warrant endoscopy to detect esophagitis, peptic strictures, or Barrett esophagus (in this condition the squamocolumnar junction is displaced proximally and replaced by intestinal metaplasia, increasing the risk of esophageal cancer 30-fold).[6,8,9] Approximately 50% of patients with GERD will have no disease on endoscopy.[10]

Lower Abdominal Pain and Discomfort—Acute and Chronic. Lower abdominal pain and discomfort may be acute or chronic. Asking the patient to point to the pain and characterize all its features, combined with findings on physical examination, will help you identify possible causes. Some acute pain, especially in the suprapubic area or radiating from the flank, originates in the genitourinary tract (see p. 447).

Acute Lower Abdominal Pain. Patients may complain of *acute pain* localized to the *right lower quadrant*. Find out if it is sharp and continuous or intermittent and cramping, causing them to double over.

Right lower quadrant pain or pain that migrates from the periumbilical region, combined with abdominal wall rigidity on palpation, is most likely to predict *appendicitis*. In women other causes include *pelvic inflammatory disease, ruptured ovarian follicle,* and *ectopic pregnancy.*[11]

Cramping pain radiating to the right or left lower quadrant may be a renal stone.

When patients report acute pain in the *left lower quadrant* or *diffuse abdominal pain,* investigate associated symptoms such as fever and loss of appetite.

Left lower quadrant pain with a palpable mass may be *diverticulitis.* Diffuse abdominal pain with absent bowel sounds and firmness, guarding, or rebound on palpation indicates *small or large bowel obstruction* (see p. 454).

Chronic Lower Abdominal Pain. If there is *chronic pain* in the quadrants of the lower abdomen, ask about change in bowel habits and alternating diarrhea and constipation.

Change in bowel habits with mass lesion indicates *colon cancer.* Intermittent pain for 12 weeks of the preceding 12 months with relief from defecation, change in frequency of bowel movements, or change in form of stool (loose, watery, pellet-like), without structural or biochemical abnormalities are symptoms of *irritable bowel syndrome.*[12]

Gastrointestinal Symptoms Associated With Abdominal Pain. Patients often experience abdominal pain in conjunction with other symptoms. "How is your appetite?" is a good starting question that may lead to other concerns like *indigestion, nausea, vomiting,* and *anorexia. Indigestion* is a general term for distress associated with eating that can have many meanings. Urge your patient to be more specific.

Anorexia, nausea, and vomiting accompany many gastrointestinal disorders; these are all seen in pregnancy, *diabetic ketoacidosis, adrenal insufficiency, hypercalcemia, uremia,* liver disease, emotional states, adverse drug reactions, and other conditions. Induced vomiting without nausea is more indicative of *anorexia/bulimia.*

- *Nausea,* often described as "feeling sick to my stomach," may progress to retching and vomiting. *Retching* describes involuntary spasm of the stomach, diaphragm, and esophagus that precedes and culminates in *vomiting,* the forceful expulsion of gastric contents out of the mouth. Sudden vomiting without nausea may occur.

Sudden vomiting without nausea may be indicative of increased intracranial pressure.

Some patients may not actually vomit but raise esophageal or gastric contents without nausea or retching, called *regurgitation.*

Regurgitation occurs in *GERD, esophageal stricture,* and *esophageal cancer.*

Ask about any vomitus or regurgitated material and inspect it if possible. What color is it? What does the vomitus smell like? How much has there been? You may have to help the patient with the amount: a teaspoon? Two teaspoons? A cupful?

Vomiting and pain indicate *small bowel obstruction.* Fecal odor occurs with *small bowel obstruction.*

Ask specifically if the vomitus contains any blood, and quantify the amount. Gastric juice is clear and mucoid. Small amounts of yellowish or greenish bile are common and have no special significance. Brownish or blackish vomitus with a "coffee grounds" appearance suggests blood altered by gastric acid. Coffee-grounds emesis or red blood is termed *hematemesis.*

Hematemesis may accompany *esophageal* or *gastric varices, gastritis,* or *peptic ulcer disease.*

Is there any dehydration or electrolyte imbalance from prolonged vomiting, or significant blood loss? Do the patient's symptoms suggest any complications of vomiting, such as aspiration into the lungs, seen in debilitated, obtunded, or elderly patients?

Symptoms of blood loss such as lightheadedness or syncope depend on the rate and volume of bleeding and are rare until blood loss exceeds 500 ml.

• *Anorexia* is loss or lack of appetite. Find out if it arises from intolerance to certain foods or reluctance to eat because of anticipated discomfort. Check for associated symptoms of nausea and vomiting.

Patients may complain of unpleasant *abdominal fullness* after light or moderate meals, or *early satiety*, the inability to eat a full meal. A dietary assessment or recall may be warranted (see Chapter 8, Nutrition).

Consider *diabetic gastroparesis*, anticholinergic medications, *gastric outlet obstruction, gastric cancer;* early satiety in *hepatitis*.

Other Gastrointestinal Symptoms.   Do you have any difficulty/pain swallowing?

Dysphagia and/or Odynophagia.   Less commonly, patients may report difficulty swallowing from impaired passage of solid foods or liquids from the mouth to the stomach, or *dysphagia*. Food seems to stick, hesitate, or "not go down right," suggesting motility disorders or structural anomalies. The sensation of a lump in the throat or the retrosternal area unassociated with swallowing is not true dysphagia.

For types of dysphagia, see Table 16-2, p. 474, Dysphagia.

Indicators of *oropharyngeal dysphagia* include drooling, nasopharyngeal regurgitation, and cough from aspiration in muscular or neurologic disorders affecting motility.

Ask the patient to point to where the dysphagia occurs.

Pointing to below the sternoclavicular notch indicates *esophageal dysphagia*.

Pursue which types of foods provoke symptoms: solid foods, or solids and liquids? Establish the timing. When does the dysphagia start? Is it intermittent or persistent? Is it progressing? If so, over what time period? Are there associated symptoms and medical conditions?

If solid foods, consider structural esophageal conditions like esophageal stricture, web or Schatzki's ring, neoplasm; if solids and liquids, a motility disorder is more likely.

Is there *odynophagia*, or pain on swallowing?

Consider esophageal ulceration from radiation, caustic ingestion, or infection from *Candida, cytomegalovirus, herpes simplex,* or *HIV.* Can be pill-induced (aspirin, nonsteroidal anti-inflammatory agents).

Change in Bowel Function.   *Bowel function* is frequently assessed. Start with open-ended questions: "Have you noticed any change in your bowel movements?" "How frequent are they?" "Do you have any difficulties?" The range of normal is broad. Current parameters suggest a minimum may be as low as two bowel movements per week.

Some patients may complain of passing excessive gas, or *flatus*, normally about 600 ml per day.

Consider aerophagia, legumes or other gas-producing foods, *intestinal lactase deficiency, irritable bowel syndrome*.

Diarrhea and Constipation.   Patients vary widely in their views of diarrhea and constipation. Increased water content of the stool results in *diarrhea,* or stool volume >200 grams in 24 hours. Patients, however, usually focus on the change to loose watery stools or increased frequency.

Ask about the duration. *Acute diarrhea* lasts 2 weeks or fewer. *Chronic diarrhea* is defined as lasting 4 weeks or more.

See Table 16-3, p. 475, Constipation and Table 16-4, pp. 476–477, Diarrhea.

Acute diarrhea is usually caused by infection[13]; chronic diarrhea is typically noninfectious in origin, as in *Crohn disease* and *ulcerative colitis.*

Query the characteristics of the diarrhea, including volume, frequency, and consistency.

Is there mucus, pus, or blood? Is there associated *tenesmus*, a constant urge to defecate, accompanied by pain, cramping, and involuntary straining?

High-volume, frequent watery stools usually are from the small intestine; small-volume stools with tenesmus, or diarrhea with mucus, pus, or blood occurs in rectal inflammatory conditions.

Does diarrhea occur at night?

Nocturnal diarrhea usually has pathologic significance.

Are the stools greasy or oily? Frothy? Foul-smelling? Floating on the surface because of excessive gas?

Oily residue, sometimes frothy or floating, occurs with *steatorrhea,* or fatty diarrheal stools, from malabsorption in *celiac sprue, pancreatic insufficiency, cystic fibrosis,* or *small bowel bacterial overgrowth.*

Associated features are important in identifying possible causes. Pursue current medications, including alternative medicines and especially antibiotics, recent travel, diet patterns, baseline bowel habits, and risk factors for immunocompromise.

Diarrhea is common with use of penicillins and macrolides, magnesium-based antacids, metformin, and herbal and alternative medicines.

Another common symptom is *constipation*. Recent definitions stipulate that constipation should be present for at least 12 weeks of the prior 6 months with at least two of the following conditions: fewer than three bowel movements per week; 25% or more defecations with either straining or sensation of incomplete evacuation; lumpy or hard stools; or manual facilitation.[14]

Ask about frequency of bowel movements, passage of hard or painful stools, straining, and a sense of incomplete rectal emptying or pressure.

Check if the patient actually looks at the stool and can describe its color and bulk.

Thin, pencil-like stool occurs in an obstructing "apple core" lesion of the sigmoid colon.

What remedies has the patient tried? Do medications or stress play a role? Are there associated systemic disorders?

Consider medications such as anti-cholinergic agents, calcium channel blockers, iron supplements, and opiates. Constipation also occurs with *diabetes, hypothyroidism, hypercalcemia, multiple sclerosis, Parkinson disease,* and *systemic sclerosis.*

Occasionally there is no passage of either feces or gas, or *obstipation.*

Obstipation signifies *intestinal obstruction.*

Inquire about the color of stools. Is there *melena,* or black tarry stools, or *hematochezia,* stools that are red or maroon-colored? Pursue such important details as quantity and frequency of any blood.

See Table 16-5, Black and Bloody Stools, p. 478.

Melena may appear with as little as 100 ml of *upper gastrointestinal bleeding,* and hematochezia, is usually from *lower gastrointestinal bleeding.*

Is it mixed in with stool or on the surface? Is it streaks on the toilet paper or more copious?

Blood on the surface or toilet paper may occur with *hemorrhoids.*

Jaundice. In some patients, you will find jaundice or icterus, the yellowish discoloration of the skin and sclerae from increased levels of bilirubin, a bile pigment derived chiefly from the breakdown of hemoglobin. Normally the hepatocytes conjugate, or combine, unconjugated bilirubin with other substances, making the bile water soluble, and then excrete it into the bile. The bile passes through the cystic duct into the common bile duct, which also drains the extrahepatic ducts from the liver. More distally the common bile duct and the pancreatic ducts empty into the duodenum at the ampulla of Vater. Mechanisms of jaundice include the following:

- Increased production of bilirubin

- Decreased uptake of bilirubin by the hepatocytes

- Decreased ability of the liver to conjugate bilirubin

Predominantly unconjugated bilirubin occurs from the first three mechanisms, as in *hemolytic anemia* (increased destruction) and *Gilbert syndrome.*

- Decreased excretion of bilirubin into the bile, resulting in absorption of *conjugated* bilirubin back into the blood

Impaired excretion of conjugated bilirubin occurs with *viral hepatitis, cirrhosis, primary biliary cirrhosis,* and *drug-induced cholestasis,* as from oral contraceptives, methyl testosterone, and chlorpromazine.

Intrahepatic jaundice can be *hepatocellular,* from damage to the hepato-cytes, or *cholestatic,* from impaired excretion as a result of damaged hepato-cytes or intrahepatic bile ducts. *Extrahepatic* jaundice arises from obstruction of the extrahepatic bile ducts, most commonly the cystic and common bile ducts.

Gallstones or *pancreatic carcinoma* may obstruct the common bile duct.

As the patient with jaundice is assessed, pay special attention to the associated symptoms and the setting in which the illness occurred. What was the *color of the urine* as the patient became ill? When the level of conjugated bilirubin increases in the blood, it may be excreted into the urine, turning the urine a dark yellowish brown or tea color. Unconjugated bilirubin is not water soluble, so it is not excreted into urine.

Dark urine from bilirubin indicates impaired excretion of bilirubin into the gastrointestinal tract.

Ask also about the *color of the stools.* When excretion of bile into the intestine is completely obstructed, the stools become gray or light colored, or *acholic,* without bile.

Acholic stools may occur briefly in *viral hepatitis;* they are common in obstructive jaundice.

Does the skin itch without other obvious explanation? Is there associated pain? What is its pattern? Has it been recurrent in the past?

Itching indicates cholestatic or obstructive jaundice; pain may signify a distended liver capsule, *biliary cholic,* or *pancreatic cancer.*

Ask about risk factors for liver diseases, such as:

- *Hepatitis:* Travel or meals in areas of poor sanitation, ingestion of contaminated water or food (hepatitis A); parenteral or mucous membrane exposure to infectious body fluids such as blood, serum, semen, and vaginal fluid, especially through sexual contact with an infected partner or use of shared needles for injection drug use (hepatitis B); sharing needles of infected persons (hepatitis C)

- *Alcoholic hepatitis* or *alcoholic cirrhosis* (interview the patient carefully about alcohol use, e.g., CAGE questionnaire)

- *Toxic liver damage* from medications, industrial solvents, or environmental toxins

- *Gallbladder disease* or *surgery* that may result in extrahepatic biliary obstruction

- *Hereditary disorders* in the Family History

The Urinary Tract

General questions for a urinary history include:

> Do you have any difficulty passing your urine?
> How often do you go?
> Do you have to get up at night? How often?
> How much urine do you pass at a time?

See Table 16-6, p. 479, Frequency, Nocturia, and Polyuria

Is there any pain or burning?
Do you ever have trouble getting to the toilet in time?
Do you ever leak any urine? Or wet yourself involuntarily?
Can you sense when your bladder is full and when voiding occurs?

Involuntary voiding or lack of awareness suggests cognitive or neurosensory deficits.

Ask women:

Does sudden coughing, sneezing, or laughing make you lose urine? Roughly half of young women report this experience even before bearing children. Occasional leakage is not necessarily significant.

Stress incontinence arises from decreased intraurethral pressure (see pp. 480–481).

Ask older men:

Do you have trouble starting your stream?
Do you have to stand close to the toilet to void?
Is there a change in the force or size of your stream, or straining to void?
Do you hesitate or stop in the middle of voiding?
Is there dribbling when you're through?

These problems are common in men with partial bladder outlet obstruction from *benign prostatic hyperplasia*; also seen with *urethral stricture.*

Suprapubic Pain.   Disorders in the urinary tract may cause pain in either the abdomen or the back. Bladder disorders may cause *suprapubic pain.* In *bladder infection,* pain in the lower abdomen is typically dull and pressure-like. In sudden overdistention of the bladder, pain is often agonizing; in contrast, chronic bladder distention is usually painless.

Pain of sudden overdistention accompanies acute urinary retention.

Dysuria, Urgency, or Frequency.   Infection or irritation of either the bladder or urethra often provokes several symptoms. Frequently there is *pain on urination,* usually felt as a burning sensation. Some clinicians refer to this as *dysuria,* whereas others reserve the term *dysuria* for difficulty voiding. Women may report internal urethral discomfort, sometimes described as a pressure or an external burning from the flow of urine across irritated or inflamed labia. Men typically feel a burning sensation proximal to the glans penis. In contrast, *prostatic pain* is felt in the perineum and occasionally in the rectum.

Painful urination accompanies *cystitis* or *urethritis.*

If dysuria, consider bladder stones, foreign bodies, tumors; also *acute prostatitis.* In women, internal burning occurs in *urethritis,* and external burning in *vulvovaginitis.*

Other associated symptoms are common. Urinary *urgency* is an unusually intense and immediate desire to void, sometimes leading to involuntary voiding or *urge incontinence.* Urinary *frequency,* or abnormally frequent voiding, may occur. Ask about any related fever or chills, blood in the urine, or any pain in the abdomen, flank, or back (see illustration on p. 447). Men with partial obstruction to urinary outflow often report *hesitancy* in starting the urine stream, straining to void, reduced caliber and force of the urinary stream, or dribbling as voiding is completed.

Urgency suggests bladder infection or irritation. In men, painful urination without frequency or urgency suggests *urethritis.*

Polyuria or Nocturia.   Three additional terms describe important alterations in the pattern of urination. *Polyuria* refers to a significant increase in 24-hour urine volume, roughly defined as exceeding 3 liters. It should be distinguished from urinary frequency, which can involve voiding in high amounts, seen in polyuria, or in small amounts, as in infection. *Nocturia*

Abnormally high renal production of urine suggests polyuria. Frequency without polyuria during the day or night suggests bladder disorder or impairment to

refers to urinary frequency at night, sometimes defined as awakening the patient more than once; urine volumes may be large or small. Clarify the patient's daily fluid intake. Note any change in nocturnal voiding patterns and the number of trips to the bathroom.

flow at or below the bladder neck.

Urinary Incontinence.

Up to 30% of older patients are concerned about *urinary incontinence*, an involuntary loss of urine that may become socially embarrassing or cause problems with hygiene. If the patient reports incontinence, ask:

See Table 16-7, pp. 480–481, Urinary Incontinence.

When does it happen? How often?

Do you leak small amounts of urine with increased intra-abdominal pressure from coughing, sneezing, laughing, or lifting?

Is it difficult to hold the urine once there is an urge to void?

Is a large amount of urine lost?

Is there a sensation of bladder fullness? Frequent leakage?

Do you void small amounts of urine but have difficulty emptying the bladder?

Stress incontinence with increased intra-abdominal pressure suggests decreased contractility of urethral sphincter or poor support of bladder neck; *urge incontinence,* if unable to hold the urine, suggests detrusor overactivity; *overflow incontinence,* when the bladder cannot be emptied until bladder pressure exceeds urethral pressure, indicates anatomic obstruction by prostatic hypertrophy or stricture, or neurogenic abnormalities.

As described earlier, bladder control involves complex neuroregulatory and motor mechanisms (see p. 434). Several central or peripheral nerve lesions may affect normal voiding.

Can you sense when your bladder is full? When voiding occurs?

Although there are four broad categories of incontinence, a patient may have a combination of causes.

In addition, the patient's functional status may significantly affect voiding behaviors even when the urinary tract is intact. Is the patient mobile? Alert? Able to respond to voiding cues and reach the bathroom? Is alertness or voiding affected by medications?

Functional incontinence may arise from impaired cognition, musculoskeletal problems, or immobility.

Hematuria.

Blood in the urine, or *hematuria*, is an important cause for concern. When visible to the naked eye, it is called *gross hematuria*. The urine may appear frankly bloody. Blood may be detected only during microscopic urinalysis, known as *microscopic hematuria*. Smaller amounts of blood may tinge the urine with a pinkish or brownish cast. In women, be sure to distinguish menstrual blood from hematuria. If the urine is reddish, ask about ingestion of beets or medications that might discolor the urine. Test the urine with a dipstick and microscopic examination before you settle on the term *hematuria*.

Kidney or Flank Pain; Ureteral Colic. Disorders of the urinary tract may also cause *kidney pain*, often reported as *flank pain*, which is on the side of the body between the upper abdomen and the back. It may radiate anteriorly toward the umbilicus. Kidney pain is a visceral pain usually produced by distention of the renal capsule and typically dull, aching, and steady. *Ureteral pain* is dramatically different. It is usually severe and colicky, originating at the costovertebral angle and radiating around the trunk into the lower quadrant of the abdomen, or possibly into the upper thigh and testicle or labium. Ureteral pain results from sudden distention of the ureter and associated distention of the renal pelvis. Ask about any associated fever, chills, or hematuria.

Kidney pain, fever, and chills occur in *acute pyelonephritis*.

Renal or ureteral colic is caused by sudden obstruction of a ureter, for example, from urinary stones or blood clots.

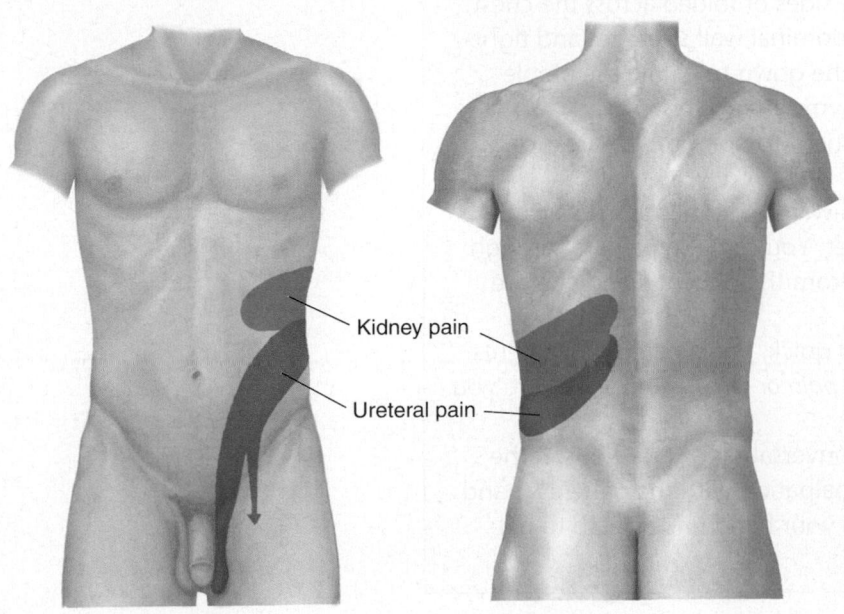

Kidney pain

Ureteral pain

PHYSICAL EXAMINATION

EQUIPMENT

- Good lighting
- Stethoscope
- Tape measure with centimeter markings

For a skilled abdominal examination, you need good light and a relaxed and well-draped patient, with exposure of the abdomen from just above the xiphoid process to the symphysis pubis. The groin should be visible. The genitalia should remain draped. The abdominal muscles should be relaxed to enhance all aspects of the examination, but especially palpation.

TIPS FOR ENHANCING EXAMINATION OF THE ABDOMEN

- Ensure tangential lighting.
- Check that the patient has an empty bladder.
- Make the patient comfortable in the supine position, with a pillow under the head and perhaps another under the knees. Slide your hand under the low back to see if the patient is relaxed and lying flat on the table.
- Ask the patient to keep the arms at the sides or folded across the chest. If the arms are above the head, the abdominal wall stretches and tightens, making palpation difficult. Move the gown to below the nipple line, and the drape to the level of the symphysis pubis.
- Before you begin palpation, ask the patient to point to any areas of pain so you can examine these areas last.
- Warm your hands and stethoscope. To warm your hands, rub them together or place them under hot water. You can also palpate through the patient's gown to absorb warmth from the patient's body before exposing the abdomen.
- Approach the patient calmly and avoid quick, unexpected movements. *Watch the patient's face for any signs of pain or discomfort.* Make sure you avoid long fingernails.
- Distract the patient if necessary with conversation or questions. If the patient is frightened or ticklish, begin palpation with the patient's hand under yours. After a few moments, slip your hand underneath to palpate directly.

An arched back thrusts the abdomen forward and tightens the abdominal muscles.

Visualize each organ in the region you are examining. Stand at the patient's right side and proceed in an orderly fashion with inspection, auscultation, percussion, and palpation. Assess the liver, spleen, kidneys, and aorta.

THE ABDOMEN

Inspection

Starting from the usual standing position at the right side of the bed, inspect the abdomen. Look at the contour of the abdomen and watch for peristalsis. It is helpful to sit or bend down to view the abdomen tangentially.

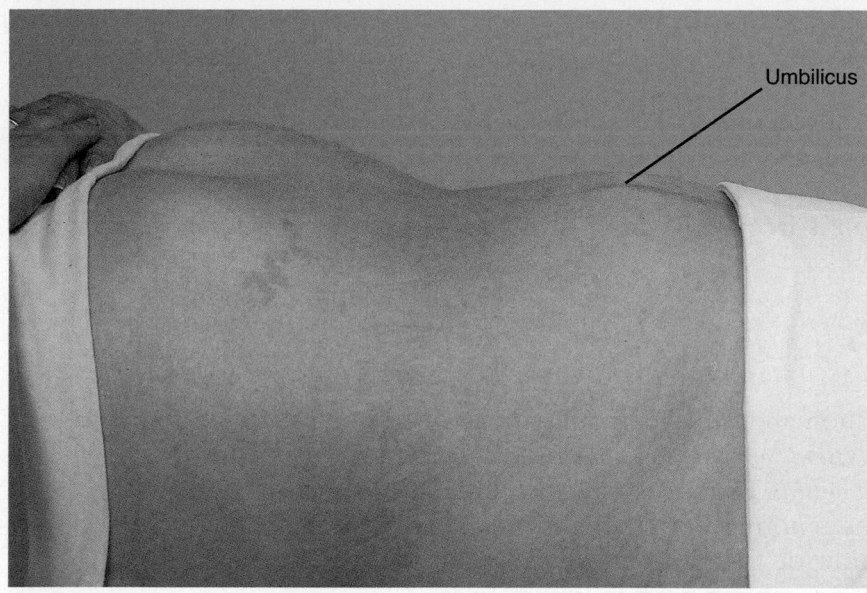

Umbilicus

Inspect the surface, contours, and movements of the abdomen, including the following:

- *The skin.* Note:

  Scars. Describe or diagram their location.

  Striae. Old silver striae or stretch marks are normal.

  Pink–purple striae of *Cushing syndrome*

  Dilated veins. A few small veins may be visible normally.

  Dilated veins of *hepatic cirrhosis* or of *inferior vena cava obstruction*

  Rashes and lesions. Describe and/or diagram.

- *The umbilicus.* Observe its contour and location and any inflammation or bulges suggesting a hernia.

  See Table 16-8, p. 482, Localized Bulges in the Abdominal Wall.

- *The contour of the abdomen*

  Is it flat, rounded, protuberant, or scaphoid (markedly concave or hollowed)?

  See Table 16-9, p. 483, Protuberant Abdomens.

  Do the flanks bulge, or are there any local bulges? Also survey the inguinal and femoral areas.

  Bulging flanks of *ascites*; suprapubic bulge of a distended bladder or pregnant uterus; hernias

  Is the abdomen symmetric?

  Asymmetry from an enlarged organ or mass

Are there visible organs or masses? Look for an enlarged liver or spleen that has descended below the rib cage.

Lower abdominal mass of an ovarian or a uterine tumor

● *Peristalsis.* Observe for several minutes if you suspect intestinal obstruction. Peristalsis may be visible normally in very thin people.

Increased peristaltic waves of *intestinal obstruction*

● *Pulsations.* The normal aortic pulsation is frequently visible in the epigastrium.

Increased pulsation of an *aortic aneurysm* or of *increased pulse pressure*

Auscultation

Auscultation provides important information about bowel motility. *Listen to the abdomen before performing percussion or palpation because these maneuvers may alter the frequency of bowel sounds.* Practice auscultation until you are thoroughly familiar with variations in normal bowel sounds and can detect changes suggestive of inflammation or obstruction. Auscultation may also reveal *bruits,* or vascular sounds resembling heart murmurs, over the aorta or other arteries in the abdomen.

See Table 16-10, Sounds in the Abdomen (p. 484).

Bruits suggest vascular occlusive disease.

Place the diaphragm of your stethoscope gently on the abdomen. Listen for bowel sounds and note their frequency and character. Normal sounds consist of clicks and gurgles, occurring at an estimated frequency of 5 to 34 per minute. Occasionally you may hear *borborygmi*—prolonged gurgles of hyperperistalsis—the familiar "stomach growling." Bowel sounds should be assessed in all four quadrants. Note if you are unable to hear bowel sounds within 2 to 3 minutes and question why this alteration exists.

Bowel sounds may be altered in diarrhea, intestinal obstruction, *paralytic ileus,* and *peritonitis.*

Abdominal Bruits and Friction Rubs.   If the patient has high blood pressure, listen in the epigastrium and in each upper quadrant for *bruits.* Later in the examination, when the patient sits up, listen also in the costovertebral angles. Epigastric bruits confined to systole may be heard normally.

A bruit in the midclavicular line that has both systolic and diastolic components strongly suggests *renal artery stenosis* as the cause of hypertension.

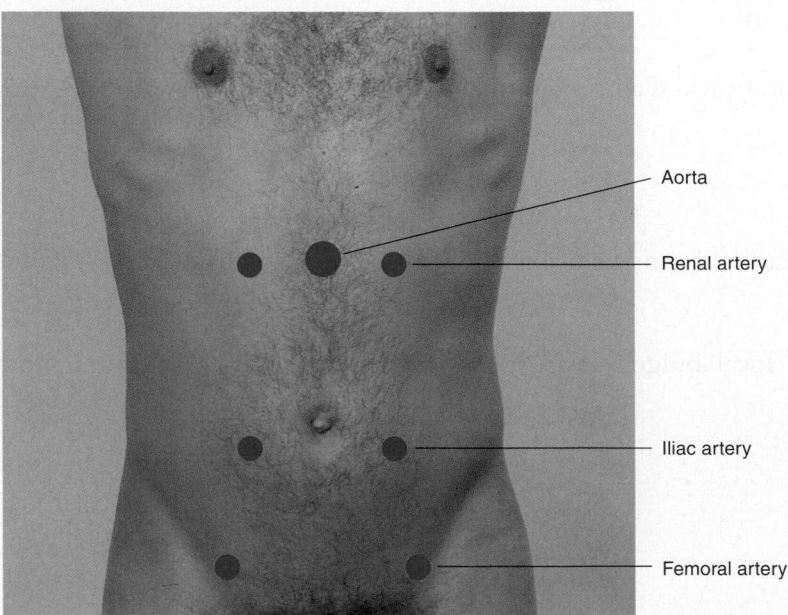

Aorta

Renal artery

Iliac artery

Femoral artery

Listen for bruits over the aorta, the iliac arteries, and the femoral arteries. Bruits confined to systole are relatively common, however, and do not necessarily signify occlusive disease.

Listening points for bruits in these vessels are illustrated.

Listen over the liver and spleen for *friction rubs*.

Bruits with both systolic and diastolic components suggest the turbulent blood flow of *partial arterial occlusion* or *arterial insufficiency*.

Friction rubs in liver tumor, gonococcal infection around the liver, splenic infarction

Percussion

Percussion helps you to assess the amount and distribution of gas in the abdomen and to identify possible masses that are solid or fluid-filled. Its use in estimating the size of the liver and spleen will be described in later sections.

Percuss the abdomen lightly in all four quadrants to assess the distribution of *tympany* and *dullness*. Tympany usually predominates because of gas in the gastrointestinal tract, but scattered areas of dullness from fluid and feces are also typical.

A protuberant abdomen that is tympanitic throughout suggests *intestinal obstruction*. See Table 16-9, p. 483, Protuberant Abdomens.

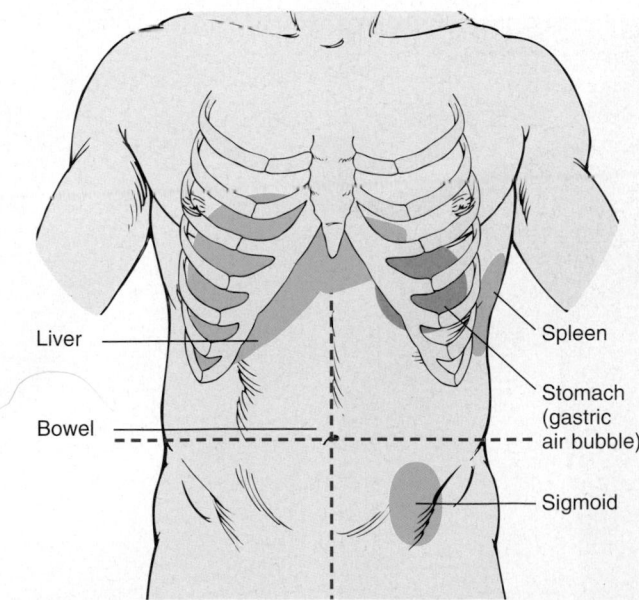

Liver

Bowel

Spleen

Stomach (gastric air bubble)

Sigmoid

- Note any large dull areas that might indicate an underlying mass or enlarged organ. This observation will guide your palpation.

Pregnant uterus, ovarian tumor, distended bladder, large liver or spleen

- On each side of a protuberant abdomen, note where abdominal tympany changes to the dullness of solid posterior structures.

Dullness in both flanks prompts further assessment for ascites (see pp. 463–464).

Briefly percuss the lower anterior chest, between the lungs above and costal margins below. On the right, you will usually find the dullness of the liver; on the left, the tympany that overlies the gastric air bubble and the splenic flexure of the colon.

In *situs inversus* (rare), organs are reversed: air bubble on the right, liver dullness on the left.

Palpation

Light Palpation. Feeling the abdomen gently is especially helpful for identifying abdominal tenderness, muscular resistance, and some superficial organs and masses. It also serves to reassure and relax the patient.

Keeping your hand and forearm on a horizontal plane, with fingers together and flat on the abdominal surface, palpate the abdomen with a light, gentle, dipping motion approximately 1 cm. When moving the hand from place to place, raise it just off the skin. Moving smoothly, feel in all quadrants.

Identify any superficial organs or masses and any area of tenderness or increased resistance to your hand. If resistance is present, try to distinguish voluntary guarding from involuntary muscular spasm. To do this:

Involuntary rigidity (muscular spasm) typically persists despite these maneuvers. It indicates *peritoneal inflammation.*

● Try utilizing relaxing methods (see p. 448).

(see p. 448)

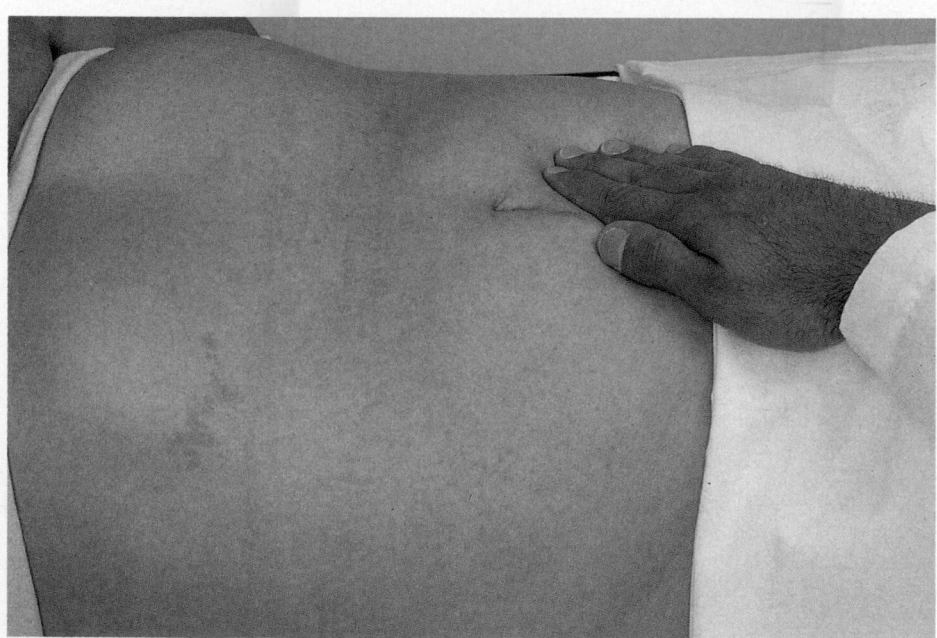

● Feel for the relaxation of abdominal muscles that normally accompanies exhalation.

● Ask the patient to mouth-breathe with the jaw dropped open.

Voluntary guarding usually decreases with these maneuvers.

Deep Palpation.　This is usually required to delineate abdominal masses. Again using the palmar surfaces of your fingers, push down about 5 to 8 cm (2 to 3 inches) and feel in all four quadrants. Identify any masses and note their location, size, shape, consistency, tenderness, pulsations, and any mobility with respiration or with the examining hand. Correlate your palpable findings with their percussion notes.

Abdominal masses may be categorized in several ways: physiologic (pregnant uterus), inflammatory (*diverticulitis* of the colon), vascular (an abdominal aortic aneurysm), neoplastic (carcinoma of the colon), or obstructive (a distended bladder or dilated loop of bowel).

Assessment for Peritoneal Inflammation.　Abdominal pain and tenderness, especially when associated with muscular spasm, suggest inflammation of the parietal peritoneum. Localize the pain as accurately as possible. First, even before palpation, *ask the patient to cough* and determine where the cough produces pain. Then, *palpate gently with one finger* to map the tender area. Pain produced by light percussion has similar localizing value. These gentle maneuvers may establish an area of peritoneal inflammation.

Abdominal pain with coughing or light percussion suggests peritoneal inflammation. See Table 16-11, pp. 485–486, Tender Abdomens

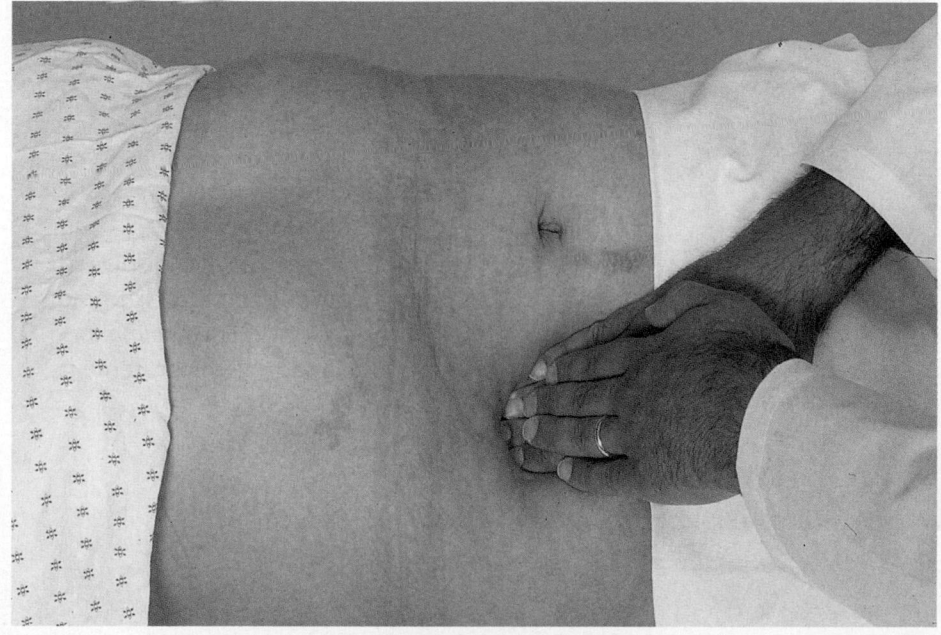

TWO-HANDED DEEP PALPATION

If not, look for *rebound tenderness*. Press down with your fingers firmly and slowly, and then withdraw them quickly. Watch and listen to the patient for signs of pain. Ask the patient, "Which hurts more, when I press or let go?" Have the patient locate the pain exactly. Pain induced or increased by quick withdrawal constitutes *rebound tenderness* caused by rapid movement of an inflamed peritoneum.

Rebound tenderness suggests peritoneal inflammation. If tenderness is felt elsewhere than where you were trying to elicit rebound, that area may be the real source of the problem.

The Liver

Because the rib cage shelters most of the liver, assessment is difficult. Liver size and shape can be estimated by percussion and perhaps palpation, however, and the palpating hand helps evaluate its surface, consistency, and tenderness.

Percussion. Measure the vertical span of liver dullness in the right midclavicular line. Locate the midclavicular line carefully to avoid inaccurate measurement from use of a "wandering landmark." Use a light to moderate percussion stroke, because examiners with a heavier stroke underestimate liver size.[17] Starting at a level below the umbilicus (in an area of tympany, not dullness), percuss upward toward the liver. Identify the *lower border of dullness* in the midclavicular line.

Next, identify the *upper border of liver dullness* in the midclavicular line. Starting at the nipple line, lightly percuss from lung resonance down toward liver dullness. Gently displace a woman's breast as necessary to be sure to start in a resonant area. The course of percussion is shown next.

The span of liver dullness is *increased* when the liver is enlarged.

The span of liver dullness is *decreased* when the liver is small, or when free air is present below the diaphragm, as from a *perforated hollow viscus.* Serial observations may show a decreasing span of dullness with resolution of *hepatitis* or *congestive heart failure* or, less commonly, with progression of *fulminant hepatitis.*

Liver dullness may be displaced downward by the low diaphragm of *chronic obstructive pulmonary disease.* Span, however, remains normal.

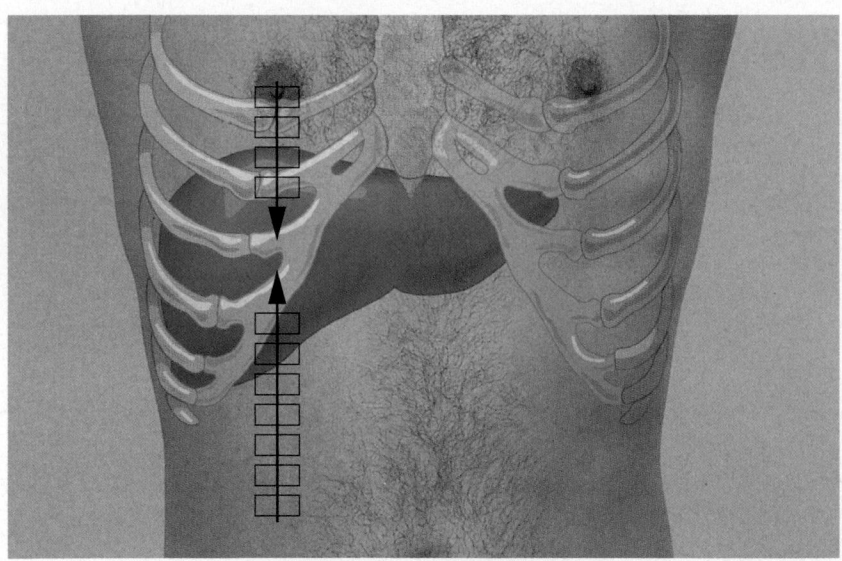

PERCUSSING LIVER SPAN

Now measure in centimeters the distance between the two points—the vertical span of liver dullness. Normal liver spans, shown below, are generally greater in men than in women and greater in tall people than in short people. If the liver seems to be enlarged, outline the lower edge by percussing in other areas.

Dullness of a right pleural effusion or consolidated lung, if adjacent to liver dullness, may falsely *increase* the estimate of liver size.

Gas in the colon may produce tympany in the right upper quadrant, obscure liver dullness, and falsely *decrease* the estimate of liver size.

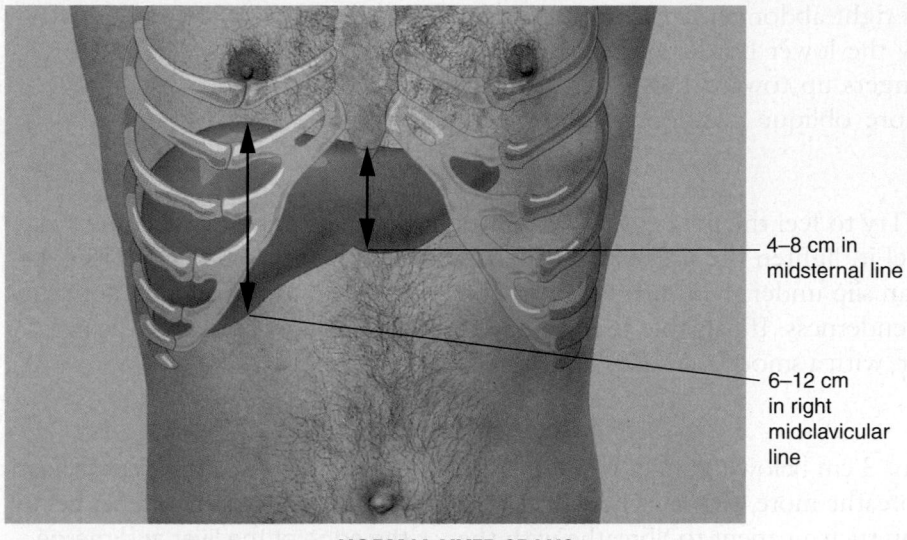

4–8 cm in midsternal line

6–12 cm in right midclavicular line

NORMAL LIVER SPANS

Measurements of liver span by percussion are more accurate when the liver is enlarged with a palpable edge.[16]

Only about half of livers with an edge below the right costal margin are palpable, but when the edge is palpable, the likelihood of hepatomegaly roughly doubles.[15]

Palpation. Place your left hand behind the patient, parallel to and supporting the right 11th and 12th ribs and adjacent soft tissues below. Remind the patient to relax on your hand if necessary. By pressing the left hand forward, the patient's liver may be felt more easily by the other hand.

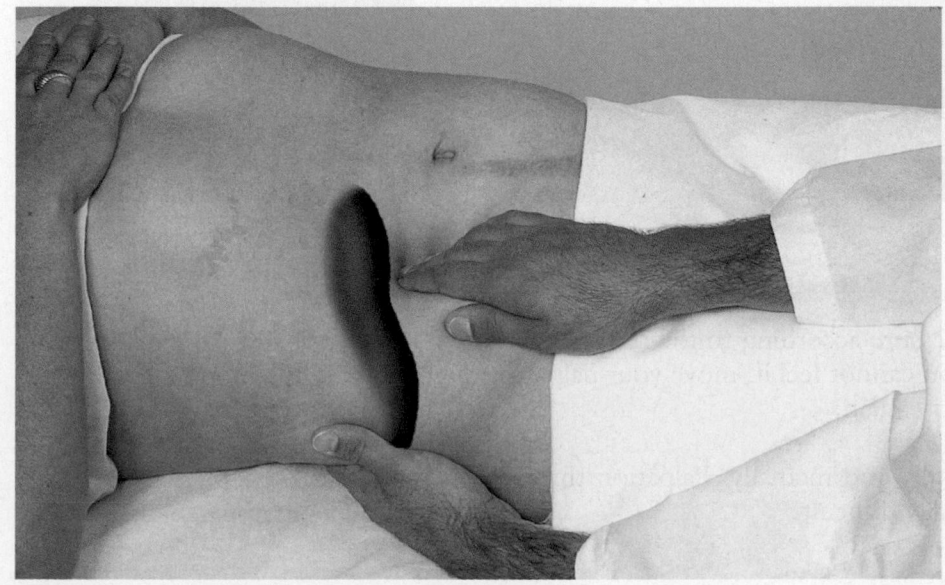

Place your right hand on the patient's right abdomen lateral to the rectus muscle, with the fingertips well below the lower border of liver dullness. Some examiners like to point their fingers up toward the patient's head, whereas others prefer a somewhat more oblique position, as shown. In either case, press gently in and up.

Ask the patient to take a deep breath. Try to feel the liver edge as it comes down to meet the fingertips. If you feel it, lighten the pressure of the palpating hand slightly so that the liver can slip under the fingerpads and you can feel its anterior surface. Note any tenderness. If palpable at all, the normal liver edge is soft, sharp, and regular, with a smooth surface. The normal liver may be slightly tender.

Firmness or hardness of the liver, bluntness or rounding of its edge, and irregularity of its contour suggest an abnormality of the liver.

On inspiration, the liver is palpable about 3 cm below the right costal margin in the midclavicular line. Some people breathe more with the chest than with the diaphragm. It may be helpful to train such a patient to "breathe with the abdomen," thus bringing the liver, as well as the spleen and kidneys, into a palpable position during inspiration.

An obstructed, distended gallbladder may form an oval mass below the edge of the liver and merge with it. It is dull to percussion.

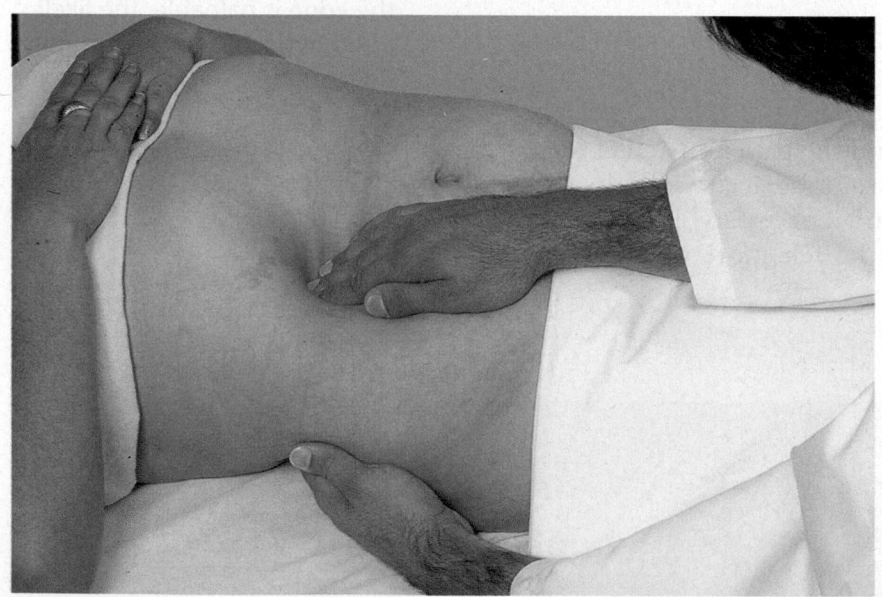

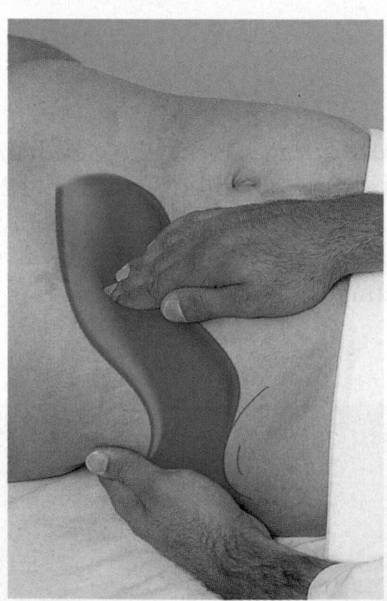

In order to feel the liver, alter the pressure according to the thickness and resistance of the abdominal wall. If you cannot feel it, move your palpating hand closer to the costal margin and try again.

The edge of an enlarged liver may be missed by starting palpation too high in the abdomen, as shown.

Try to trace the liver edge both laterally and medially. Palpation through the rectus muscles, however, is especially difficult.

See Table 16-12, p. 487, Liver Enlargement: Apparent and Real.

The "hooking technique" may be helpful. Stand to the right of the patient's chest. Place both hands, side by side, on the right abdomen below the border of liver dullness. Press in with your fingers and up toward the costal margin. Ask the patient to take a deep breath. The liver edge shown below is palpable with the fingerpads of both hands.

Tenderness over the liver suggests inflammation, as in *hepatitis*, or congestion, as in *heart failure*.

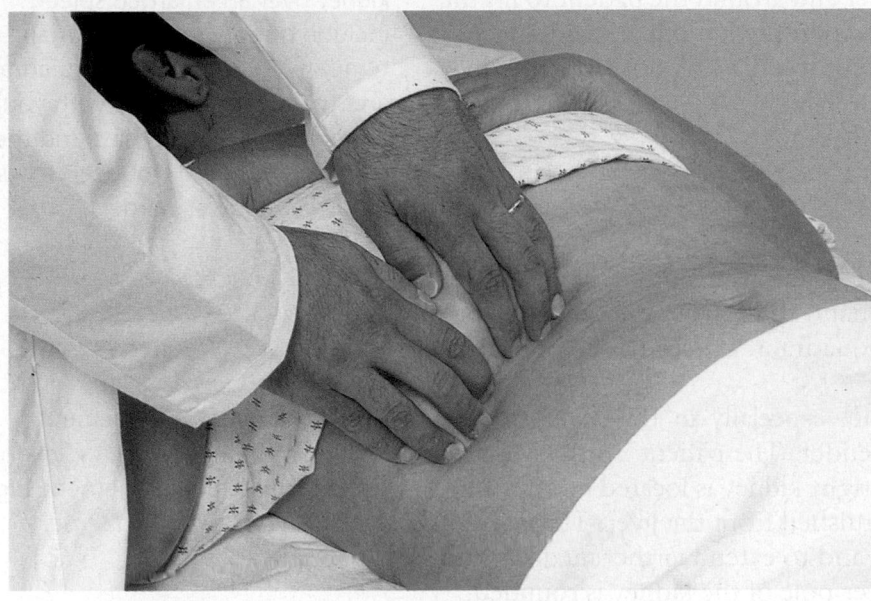
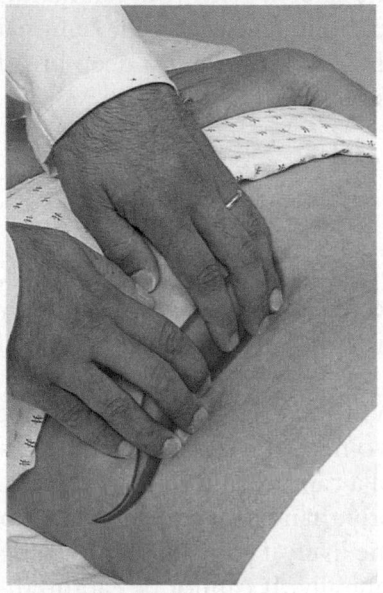

The Kidneys

Palpation. Although kidneys are not usually palpable, you should learn and practice the techniques for examination. Detecting an enlarged kidney may prove to be very important.

A left flank mass may represent marked *splenomegaly* or an enlarged left kidney. Suspect *splenomegaly* if a notch is palpated on the medial border, the edge extends beyond the midline, percussion is dull, and the fingers can probe deep to the medial and lateral borders but *not* between the mass and the costal margin. Confirm findings with further evaluation.

Palpation of the Left Kidney. Move to the patient's left side. Place your right hand behind the patient, just below and parallel to the 12th rib, with your fingertips just reaching the costovertebral angle. Lift, trying to displace the kidney anteriorly. Place the left hand gently in the left upper quadrant, lateral and parallel to the rectus muscle. Ask the patient to take a deep breath. At the peak of inspiration, press your left hand firmly and deeply into the left upper quadrant, just below the costal margin, and try to "capture" the kidney between your two hands. Ask the patient to breathe out and then to stop breathing briefly. Slowly release the pressure of your left hand, feeling at the same time for the kidney to slide back into its expiratory position. If the kidney is palpable, describe its size, contour, and any tenderness.

Alternatively, try to feel for the left kidney by a method similar to feeling for the spleen. With your left hand, reach over and around the patient to lift the left loin, and with your right hand feel deep in the left upper quadrant. Ask the patient to take a deep breath, and feel for a mass. A normal left kidney is rarely palpable.

Attributes favoring an *enlarged kidney* over an enlarged spleen include preservation of normal tympany in the left upper quadrant and the ability to probe with your fingers between the mass and the costal margin, but not deep to its medial and lower borders.

Palpation of the Right Kidney. To capture the right kidney, return to the patient's right side. Use your left hand to lift from in back, and your right hand to feel deep in the left upper quadrant. Proceed as before.

A normal right kidney may be palpable, especially in thin, well-relaxed women. It may or may not be slightly tender. The patient is usually aware of a capture and release. Occasionally, a right kidney is located more anteriorly than usual and then must be distinguished from the liver. The edge of the liver, if palpable, tends to be sharper and to extend farther medially and laterally. It cannot be captured. The lower pole of the kidney is rounded.

Causes of kidney enlargement include hydronephrosis, cysts, and tumors. Bilateral enlargement suggests *polycystic kidney disease.*

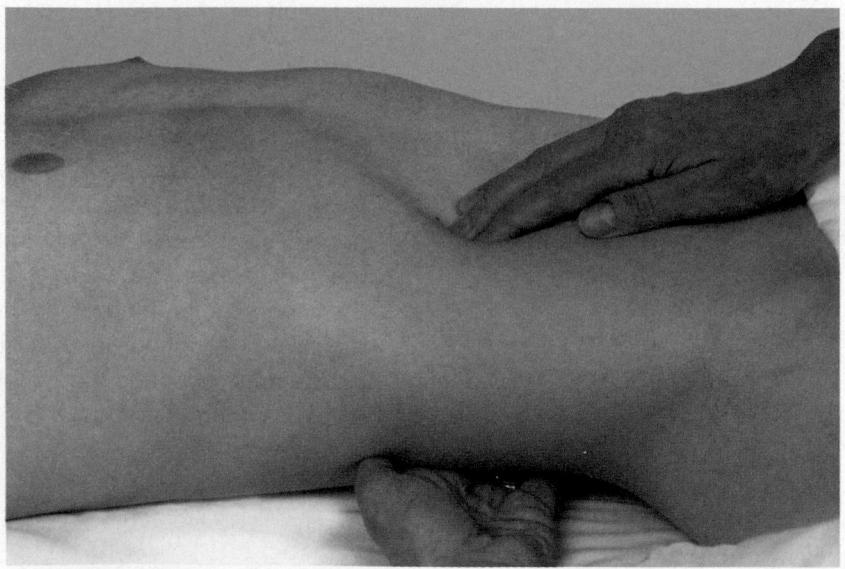

Assessing Percussion Tenderness of the Kidneys. You may note tenderness when examining the abdomen, but also search for it at each costovertebral angle. Pressure from your fingertips may be enough to elicit tenderness, but if not, use fist percussion. Place the ball of one hand in the costovertebral angle and strike it with the ulnar surface of your fist. Use enough force to cause a perceptible but painless jar or thud in a normal person.

Pain with pressure or fist percussion suggests *pyelonephritis* but may also have a musculoskeletal cause.

To save the patient needless exertion, integrate this assessment with your examination of the back.

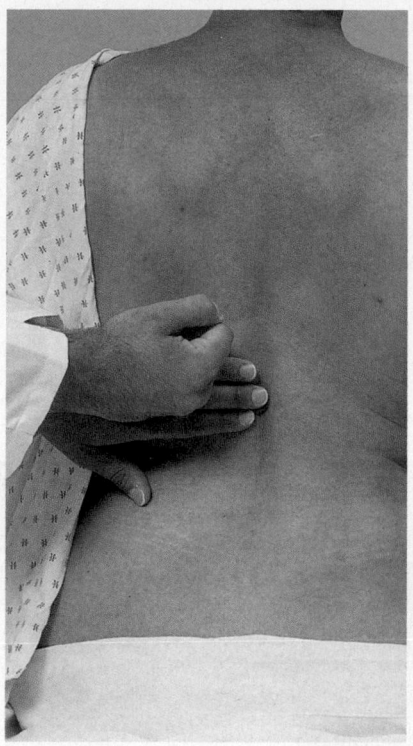

ASSESSING COSTOVERTEBRAL ANGLE TENDERNESS

The Bladder

The bladder normally cannot be examined unless it is distended above the symphysis pubis. On palpation, the dome of the distended bladder feels smooth and round. Check for tenderness. Use percussion to check for dullness and to determine how high the bladder rises above the symphysis pubis.

Bladder distention from outlet obstruction due to *urethral stricture, prostatic hyperplasia;* also from medications and neurologic disorders such as *stroke, multiple sclerosis*

Suprapubic tenderness in *bladder infection*

The Aorta

Press firmly deep in the upper abdomen, slightly to the left of the midline, and identify the aortic pulsations. In people older than age 50, assess the width of the aorta by pressing deeply in the upper abdomen with one hand on each side of the aorta, as illustrated. In this age group, a normal aorta is not more than 3.0 cm wide (average, 2.5 cm). This measurement does not include the thickness of the abdominal wall. The ease of feeling aortic pulsations varies greatly with the thickness of the abdominal wall and with the anteroposterior diameter of the abdomen.

Risk factors for abdominal aortic aneurysm (AAA) are age 65 years or older, history of smoking, male gender, and a first-degree relative with a history of AAA repair.[17,18]

A periumbilical or upper abdominal mass with expansile pulsations that is 3 cm or more wide suggests an AAA. Sensitivity of palpation increases as AAAs enlarge: for widths of 3.0–3.9 cm, 29%; 4.0–4.9 cm, 50%; ≥5.0 cm, 76%.[20]

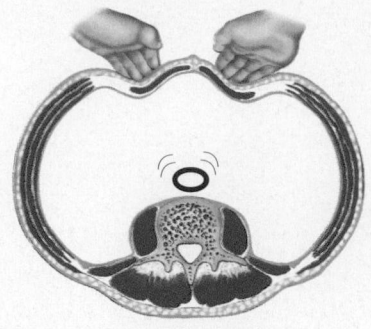
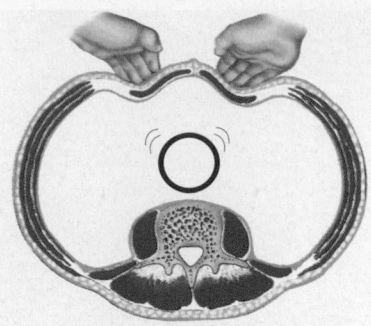

Screening by palpation followed by ultrasound decreases mortality, especially in male smokers 65 years or older. Pain may signal rupture. Rupture is 15 times more likely in AAAs >4 cm than in smaller aneurysms.[19]

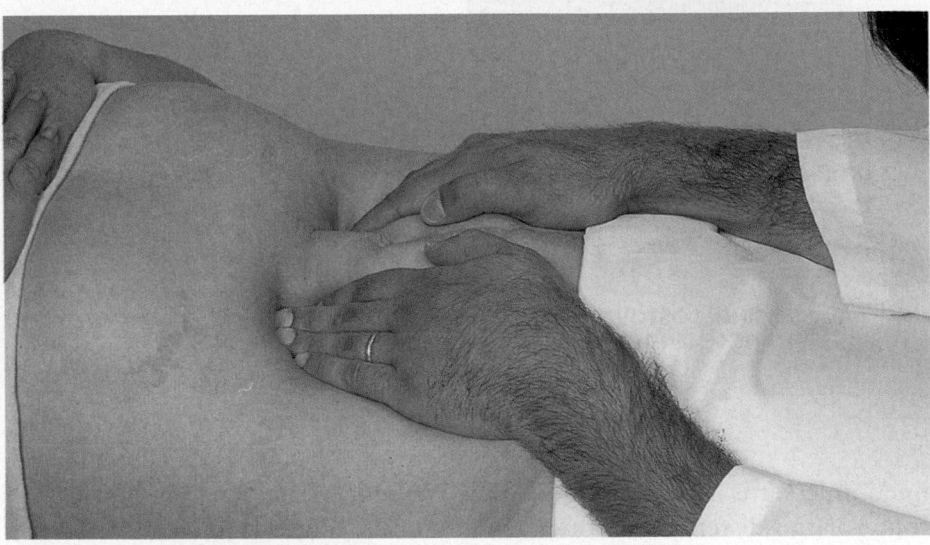

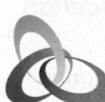

SPECIAL TECHNIQUES

ASSESSMENT TECHNIQUES FOR

- Enlarged spleen
- Ascites
- Appendicitis
- Acute cholecystitis
- Ventral hernia
- Mass in abdominal wall

The Spleen

When a spleen enlarges, it expands anteriorly, downward, and medially, often replacing the tympany of the stomach and colon with the dullness of a solid organ. It then becomes palpable below the costal margin. Percussion suggests but does not confirm splenic enlargement. Palpation can confirm the enlargement but often misses a large spleen that does not descend below the costal margin.

Percussion. Two techniques may help you to detect *splenomegaly*, an enlarged spleen:

- *Percuss the left lower anterior chest wall* between lung resonance above and the costal margin, an area termed the *Traube space*. As you percuss along the routes suggested by the arrows in the following figures, note the lateral extent of tympany. Percussion is moderately accurate in detecting splenomegaly (sensitivity, 60%–80%; specificity, 72%–94%).[20]

If percussion dullness is present, palpation correctly detects presence or absence of splenomegaly more than 80% of the time.[21]

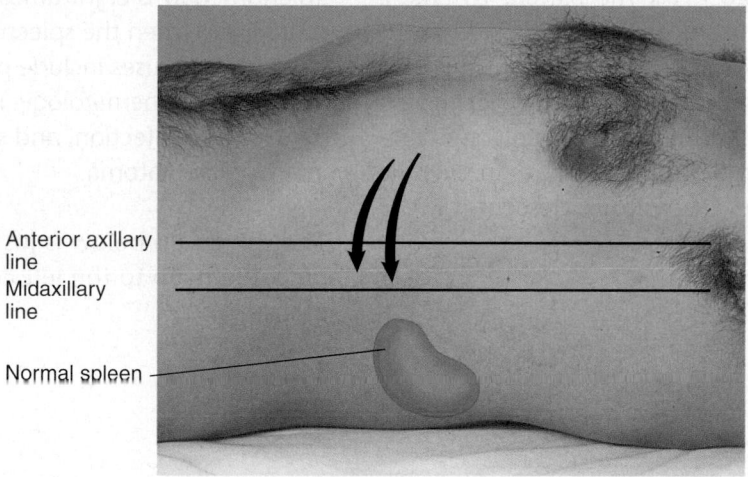

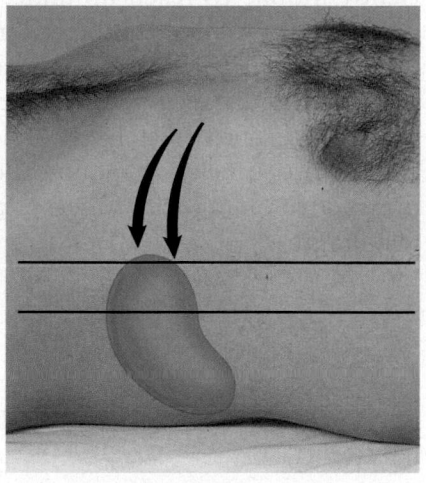

If tympany is prominent, especially laterally, splenomegaly is not likely. The dullness of a normal spleen is usually hidden within the dullness of other posterior tissues.

Fluid or solids in the stomach or colon may also cause dullness in the Traube space.

- *Check for a splenic percussion sign.* Percuss the lowest interspace in the left anterior axillary line, as shown next. This area is usually tympanitic. Then ask the patient to take a deep breath, and percuss again. When spleen size is normal, the percussion note usually remains tympanitic.

A change in percussion note from tympany to dullness on inspiration suggests splenic enlargement. This is a *positive splenic percussion sign*.

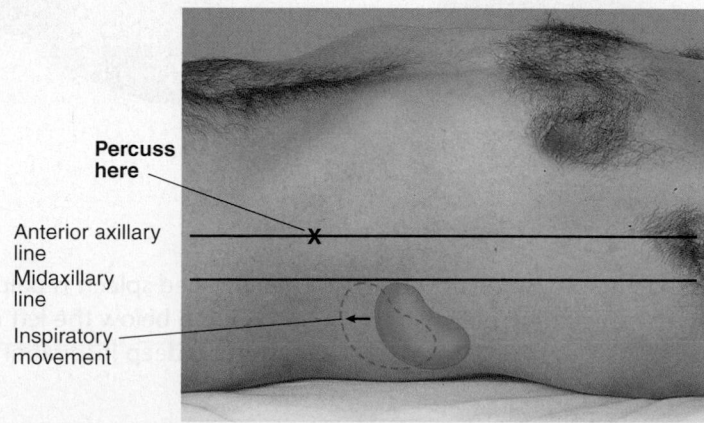

NEGATIVE SPLENIC PERCUSSION SIGN

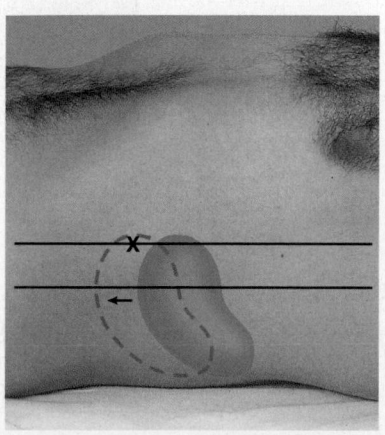

POSITIVE SPLENIC PERCUSSION SIGN

If either or both of these tests are positive, pay extra attention to palpation of the spleen.

The splenic percussion sign may also be positive when spleen size is normal.

Palpation. With your left hand, reach over and around the patient to support and press forward the lower left rib cage and adjacent soft tissue. With your right hand below the left costal margin, press in toward the spleen. Begin palpation low enough so that you are below a possibly enlarged spleen. (If your hand is close to the costal margin, moreover, it is not sufficiently mobile to reach up under the rib cage.) Ask the patient to take a deep breath. Try to feel the tip or edge of the spleen as it comes down to meet your fingertips. Note any tenderness, assess the splenic contour, and measure the distance between the spleen's lowest point and the left costal margin. In approximately 5% of normal adults, the tip of the spleen is palpable. Causes include: mononucleosis, a low, flat diaphragm, as in chronic obstructive pulmonary disease, and a deep inspiratory descent of the diaphragm.

An enlarged spleen may be missed if the examiner starts too high in the abdomen to feel the lower edge.

Splenomegaly is eight times more likely when the spleen is palpable.[17] Causes include portal hypertension, hematologic malignancies, HIV infection, and splenic infarct or hematoma.

The spleen tip below is just palpable deep to the left costal margin.

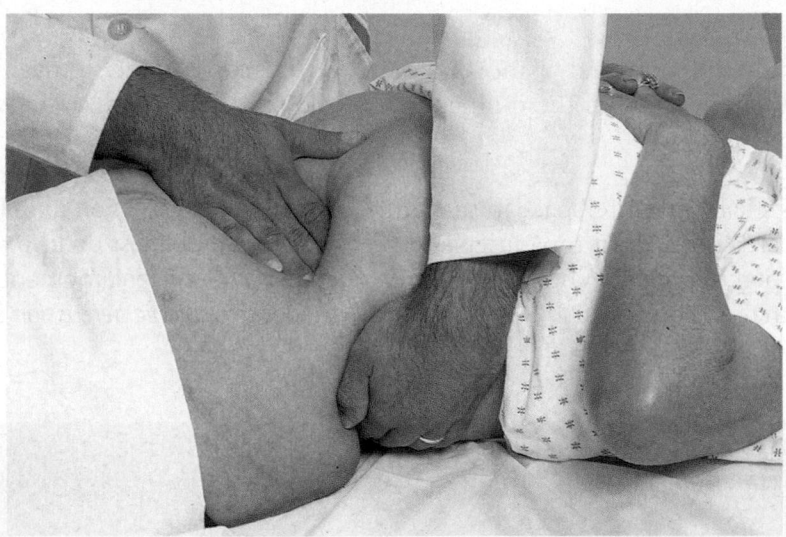
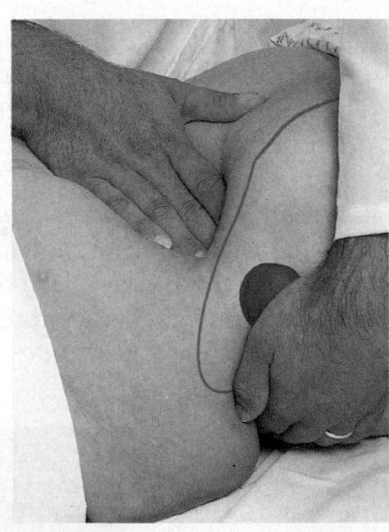

Repeat with the patient lying on the right side with legs somewhat flexed at hips and knees. In this position, gravity may bring the spleen forward and to the right into a palpable location.

The enlarged spleen is palpable about 2 cm below the left costal margin on deep inspiration.

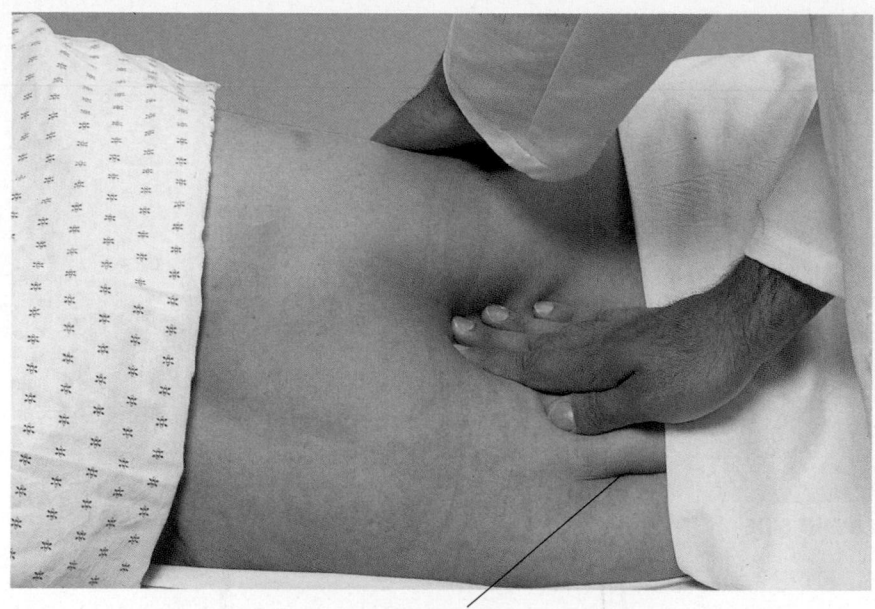

Umbilicus

PALPATING THE SPLEEN—PATIENT LYING ON RIGHT SIDE

Assessing Possible Ascites.

A protuberant abdomen with bulging flanks suggests the possibility of ascitic fluid. Because ascitic fluid characteristically sinks with gravity, whereas gas-filled loops of bowel float to the top, percussion gives a dull note in dependent areas of the abdomen. Look for such a pattern by percussing outward in several directions from the central area of tympany. Map the border between tympany and dullness.

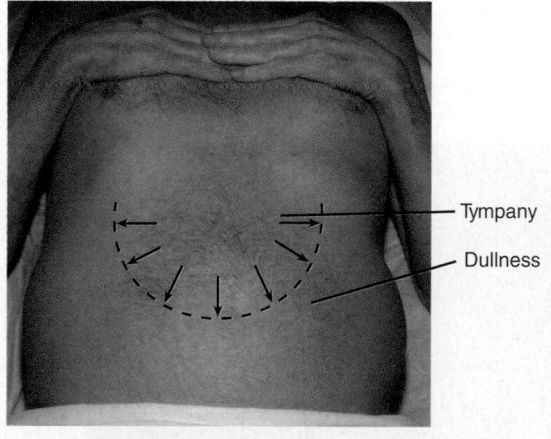

Tympany

Dullness

Ascites from increased hydrostatic pressure in cirrhosis, congestive heart failure, constrictive pericarditis, or inferior vena cava or hepatic vein obstruction; from decreased osmotic pressure in nephrotic syndrome, malnutrition. Also in ovarian cancer.

Two additional techniques help to confirm ascites, although both signs may be misleading.

● *Test for shifting dullness*. After mapping the borders of tympany and dullness, ask the patient to turn onto one side. Percuss and mark the borders again. In a person without ascites, the borders between tympany and dullness usually stay relatively constant.

In ascites, dullness shifts to the more dependent side, whereas tympany shifts to the top.

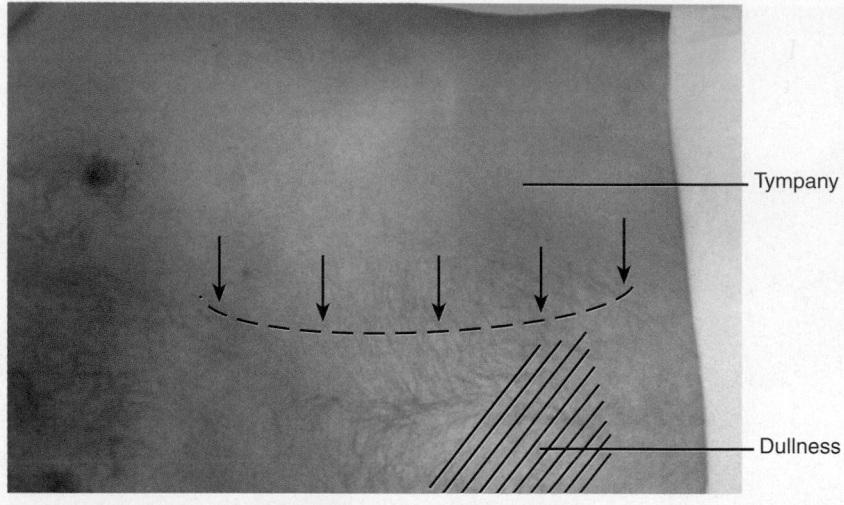

PATIENT LYING ON RIGHT SIDE

● *Test for a fluid wave.* Ask the patient or an assistant to press the edges of both hands firmly down the midline of the abdomen. This pressure helps to stop the transmission of a wave through fat. While you tap one flank sharply with your fingertips, feel on the opposite flank for an impulse transmitted through the fluid. Unfortunately, this sign is often negative until ascites is obvious, and it is sometimes positive in people without ascites.

An easily palpable impulse suggests ascites. A positive fluid wave, shifting dullness, and peripheral edema make the diagnosis of ascites highly likely (likelihood ratios of 3.0–6.0).[20]

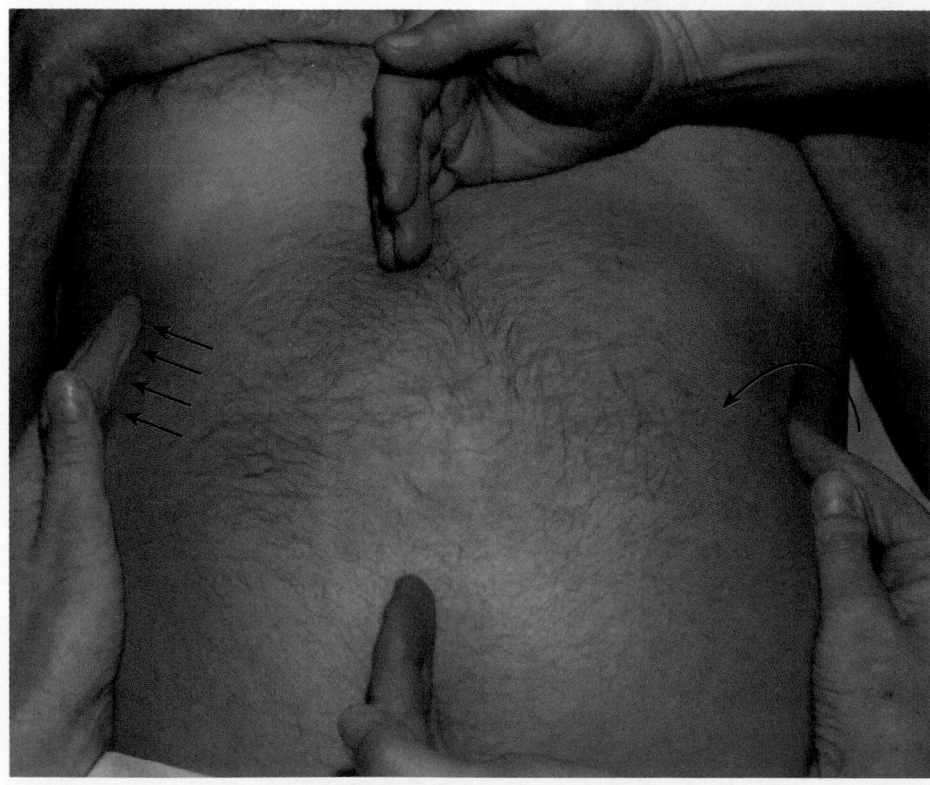

Assessing Possible Appendicitis

- Ask the patient to point to where the pain began and where it is now. Ask the patient to cough. Determine whether and where pain results.

  The pain of *appendicitis* classically begins near the umbilicus, then shifts to the right lower quadrant, where coughing increases it. Older patients report this pattern less frequently than younger ones.[11]

- Search carefully for an area of local tenderness.

  Localized tenderness anywhere in the right lower quadrant, even in the right flank, may indicate *appendicitis*.

- Feel for muscular rigidity.

  Early voluntary guarding may be replaced by involuntary muscular rigidity.

- *Perform a rectal examination and, in women, a pelvic examination.* These maneuvers may not help to discriminate between a normal and an inflamed appendix, but they may help identify an inflamed appendix atypically located within the pelvic cavity. They may also suggest other causes of the abdominal pain.

  Right-sided rectal tenderness may also be caused by an inflamed adnexa or an inflamed seminal vesicle.

Additional techniques are sometimes helpful:

- Check the tender area for rebound tenderness. (If other signs are typically positive, you can save the patient unnecessary pain by omitting this test.)

  Rebound tenderness suggests peritoneal inflammation, if *appendicitis.*

- Check for the *Rovsing sign* and for referred rebound tenderness. Press deeply and evenly in the *left* lower quadrant. Then quickly withdraw your fingers.

  Pain in the *right* lower quadrant during *left*-sided pressure suggests *appendicitis* (a positive Rovsing sign). So does right lower quadrant pain on quick withdrawal (*referred rebound tenderness*).

- Look for a *psoas sign*. Place your hand just above the patient's right knee and ask the patient to raise that thigh against your hand. Alternatively, ask the patient to turn onto the left side. Then extend the patient's right leg at the hip. Flexion of the leg at the hip makes the psoas muscle contract; extension stretches it.

  Increased abdominal pain on either maneuver constitutes a *positive psoas sign,* suggesting irritation of the psoas muscle by an inflamed appendix.

- Look for an *obturator sign*. Flex the patient's right thigh at the hip, with the knee bent, and rotate the leg internally at the hip. This maneuver stretches the internal obturator muscle. (Internal rotation of the hip is described on p. 566.)

  Right hypogastric pain constitutes a *positive obturator sign,* suggesting irritation of the obturator muscle by an inflamed appendix.

- Test for *cutaneous hyperesthesia*. At a series of points down the abdominal wall, gently pick up a fold of skin between your thumb and index

  Localized pain with this maneuver, in all or part of the right lower

finger, without pinching it. This maneuver should not normally be painful.

Assessing Possible Acute Cholecystitis.   When right upper quadrant pain and tenderness suggest acute cholecystitis, look for the *Murphy sign*. Hook your left thumb or the fingers of your right hand under the costal margin at the point where the lateral border of the rectus muscle intersects with the costal margin. Alternatively, if the liver is enlarged, hook your thumb or fingers under the liver edge at a comparable point below. Ask the patient to take a deep breath. Watch the patient's breathing and note the degree of tenderness.

Assessing Ventral Hernias.   Ventral hernias are hernias in the abdominal wall exclusive of groin hernias. If you suspect but do not see an umbilical or incisional hernia, ask the patient to raise both head and shoulders off the table.

Inguinal and femoral hernias are discussed in Chapter 21, pp 706–707, Reproductive Systems. They can give rise to important abdominal problems and must not be overlooked.

Mass in the Abdominal Wall

Distinguishing an Abdominal Mass From a Mass in the Abdominal Wall.   An occasional mass is in the abdominal wall rather than inside the abdominal cavity. Ask the patient either to raise the head and shoulders or to strain down, thus tightening the abdominal muscles. Feel for the mass again.

Right column notes:

quadrant, may accompany *appendicitis.*

A sharp increase in tenderness with a sudden stop in inspiratory effort constitutes a *positive Murphy sign* of *acute cholecystitis.* Hepatic tenderness may also increase with this maneuver but is usually less well localized.

The bulge of a hernia will usually appear with this action (see p. 707).

The cause of intestinal obstruction or peritonitis may be missed by overlooking a strangulated femoral hernia.

A mass in the abdominal wall remains palpable; an intra-abdominal mass is obscured by muscular contraction.

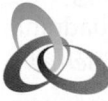

RECORDING YOUR FINDINGS

Recording the Physical Examination—The Abdomen

> "Abdomen is protuberant with active bowel sounds. Soft, nontender; no palpable masses or hepatosplenomegaly. Liver span 7 cm in ® (right) MCL (midclavicular line); edge smooth and palpable 1 cm below the right costal margin. Spleen and kidneys not felt. No costovertebral angle (CVA) tenderness."
>
> **OR**
>
> "Abdomen is flat. No bowel sounds heard. Firm, board-like, with increased tenderness, guarding, and rebound tenderness in the right midquadrant. Liver percusses 7 cm in the MCL; edge not felt. Spleen and kidneys not felt. No palpable masses. No CVA tenderness.

Suggests peritonitis from possible *appendicitis.*

HEALTH PROMOTION

Health Promotion Topics

- Screening for alcohol abuse
- Risk factors for Hepatitis A, B, and C
- Screening for colon cancer
- Prevention of urinary incontinence

Screening for Alcohol Abuse. Alert clinicians often notice clues of unhealthy alcohol use from social patterns and behavioral problems that emerge during the history. The patient may report past episodes of pancreatitis, family history of alcoholism, or arrest for driving under the influence of alcohol. Examination of the abdomen may reveal such classic findings as hepatosplenomegaly, ascites, or even *caput medusa,* a collateral pathway of recanalized umbilical veins radiating up the abdomen that decompresses portal vein hypertension.

Alcohol abuse or dependence is on the rise, affecting 8.5% of the U.S. population, or 17.6 million people.[22] Lifetime prevalence is approximately 13.5%, and in emergency rooms and trauma admissions, prevalence reaches 30% to 40% and 50%, respectively.[23,24] The addictions are increasingly viewed as chronic relapsing behavioral disorders with substance-induced rearrangements of brain neurotransmitters resulting in tolerance, physical dependence, sensitization, craving, and relapse. Alcohol addiction has numerous sequelae and is highly correlated with fatal car accidents, suicide and other mental health disorders, family disruption, violence, hypertension, cirrhosis, and malignancies of the upper gastrointestinal tract and liver.

Because early at-risk behaviors may be hard to identify, knowledge of basic alcohol screening criteria is critical. The U.S. Preventive Services Task Force recommends screening and behavioral counseling interventions for adolescents and adults in primary care settings, including pregnant women.[25] If your patient drinks alcoholic beverages, choose one of three well-validated screening tools: the CAGE questionnaire, the Alcohol Use Disorders Identification Test (AUDIT), or the screening question about heavy drinking days, "How many times in the past year have you had 4 or more drinks a day (women) or 5 or more drinks a day (men)?" Cutoffs for risky or hazardous drinking are:

- Women: ≥3 drinks per occasion and ≥7 drinks per week

- Men: ≥4 drinks per occasion and ≥14 drinks per week

Other classic findings include spider angiomas, palmar erythema, and peripheral edema.

See Chapter 19, Mental Status.

See the four CAGE questions, Chapter 4, p. 68, The Health History.

Tailor your recommendations for treatment to the severity of the problem, ranging from brief interventions to inpatient detoxification to long-term rehabilitation (see Chapter 19, Mental Status).

Risk Factors for Hepatitis A, B, and C. The mainstay for protecting adults against viral hepatitis is adherence to vaccination guidelines for hepatitis A and hepatitis B, the most effective method for preventing infection and transmission. Educating patients about how the hepatitis viruses spread and the benefits of vaccination for groups at risk is also important.

Hepatitis A. Transmission of hepatitis A is fecal–oral: fecal shedding by those handling food causes contamination of water and foods, leading to infection for those in close contact in households and extended family settings. Infected children are often asymptomatic and play a key role in spreading infection. In 2006 the Centers for Disease Control and Prevention (CDC) recommended hepatitis A vaccination for children starting at 1 year old and for persons at increased risk for infection, such as travelers to endemic areas, male–male partners, injection and illicit drug users, and persons with chronic liver disease. For immediate protection and prophylaxis for household contacts and travelers, immune serum globulin can be administered before and within 2 weeks of contact with hepatitis A. Advise handwashing with soap and water before bathroom use, changing diapers, and preparing and eating food.[26,27]

Hepatitis B. Hepatitis B poses more serious threats to patient health. Approximately 95% of infections in healthy adults are self-limited, with elimination of the virus from blood and development of immunity.[28] Chronic infection occurs in 5% of those older than 5 years, and approximately 15% of those infected after childhood die prematurely from cirrhosis or liver cancer. Most (approximately 70%) are asymptomatic until they develop advanced liver disease. The CDC has identified three risk categories:

- *Sexual contacts,* including sex partners for those already infected, people with more than one sex partner in the prior 6 months, people seeking evaluation and treatment for sexually transmitted diseases, and men having sex with men

- *People with percutaneous (through the skin) or mucosal exposure to blood,* including injection drug users, household contacts of antigen-positive persons, residents and staff of facilities for the developmentally disabled, health care workers, and people on dialysis

- *Other,* including travelers to endemic areas, people with chronic liver disease or HIV infection, and people seeking protection from hepatitis B infection

The CDC issued new recommendations for expanded hepatitis B immunization in 2006.[28] The following groups should receive vaccination:

- All adults in high-risk settings, such as STD clinics, HIV testing and treatment programs, drug-abuse treatment programs and programs for injection drug users, correctional facilities, programs for men having sex with men, chronic hemodialysis facilities and end-stage renal disease programs, and facilities for people with developmental disabilities

- In primary care and specialty settings, adults in at-risk groups or requesting the hepatitis B vaccine even without acknowledging a specific risk factor

- Adults in occupations involving exposure to blood or other potentially infectious body fluids

The U.S. Preventive Services Task Force recommends screening for all pregnant women at their first prenatal visit.[28]

Hepatitis C. Hepatitis C is transmitted by repeated percutaneous exposure to blood and is present in approximately 2% of U.S. adults. However, prevalence reaches 50% to 90% in groups at high risk.[26] The strongest risk factors are injection drug use and transfusion with clotting factors before 1987. Additional risk factors include hemodialysis, sex partners using injection drugs, blood transfusion or organ transplant before 1992, undiagnosed liver disease, infants born to infected mothers, occupational exposure, and multiple sex partners or an infected sex partner. Sexual transmission is rare. Chronic infection occurs in 55% to 85% of those infected; chronic liver disease occurs in 70% of those with chronic infections.[29] There is no vaccine for prevention, so screening for risk factors and referral of those infected, plus counseling to avoid risk factors, including tattoos, are critical.

Screening for Colorectal Cancer. Colorectal cancer is the third most common cancer in both men and women and accounts for almost 9% of all cancer deaths.[30] More than 90% of cases occur after age 50, primarily from neoplastic changes in adenomatous polyps. Mortality rates are declining, reflecting improvements in early detection and treatment. Evidence supports screening guidelines by multisociety task forces, including the American Cancer Society and places emphasis on risk stratification, use of colonoscopy, and postpolypectomy management.[31,32]

- *Assessing risk status.* Clinicians should assess risk status beginning at age 20 by asking the questions below. If 50 years or older, patients answering no to these three questions are at *average risk;* if younger than 50 years, no screening is indicated. A positive response warrants screening for increased or high colorectal cancer risk and referral for more complex patient management.[31,32]

  - Has the patient had colorectal cancer or an adenomatous polyp?

  - Does the patient have an illness such as inflammatory bowel disease that increases risk for colorectal cancer?

● Has a family member had colorectal cancer or an adenomatous polyp? If so, how many, at what age, and was it a first-degree relative (parent, sibling, or child)?

● *Screening for people at average risk.* Because no one screening option is clearly superior, beginning at age 50 average-risk patients should be offered one of the following five options:

   ● Fecal occult blood test (FOBT) annually, using six samples and tested without rehydration. Single samples have a sensitivity for detecting advanced neoplasia of approximately 5%, compared with approximately 24% using six samples, so a single-sample office test is not sufficient.[33,34] Aggressive follow-up with colonoscopy is recommended for a positive test on any specimen.

   ● Flexible sigmoidoscopy every 5 years

   ● Combined FOBT and flexible sigmoidoscopy

   ● Colonoscopy every 10 years

   ● Double-contrast barium enema every 5 years

● *Screening for people at increased risk.* Colonoscopy at the intervals noted below is indicated for the following increased risk factors:

   ● Single small adenoma (<1 cm): 3 to 6 years after initial polypectomy

   ● Single large adenoma (>1 cm), multiple adenomas, adenoma with high-grade dysplasia or villous change: within 3 years of initial polypectomy

   ● History of resection of colorectal cancer: within 1 year after resection

   ● Any first-degree relative younger than 60 years, two or more first-degree relatives with either colorectal cancer or adenomatous polyps: at age 40 or 10 years before youngest case in immediate family, whichever is earlier. Approximately 15% of those with colorectal cancer have familial disease.[37]

● *Screening for people at high risk.* High-risk factors include family history of familial adenomatous polyposis (found in ~1% of colorectal cancers); family history of hereditary nonpolyposis colon cancer (in approximately 3% to 4%); and history of inflammatory bowel disease, chronic ulcerative colitis, or Crohn disease. Referral, genetic testing, and early surveillance are recommended in these groups.[32,35,36]

Other Risk Factors for Colorectal Cancer. Some studies show possible increased risk from diabetes (approximately 30% increase), alcohol use, obesity, smoking, and high-fat diet. Some evidence suggests that several factors may be protective: diet high in fruits and vegetables; diet high in fiber; regular physical activity; and use of aspirin or nonsteroidal anti-inflammatory agents (NSAIDs). Study findings remain conflicting about the benefits of high-fiber and low-fat high-fruit and -vegetable diets.[37,40] The U.S. Preventive Services Task Force recommends *against* routine use of aspirin and NSAIDs to prevent colorectal cancer in average-risk people because of poor-quality evidence that these agents lead to a reduction in colorectal cancer mortality and good evidence of increased incidence of gastrointestinal bleeding and renal impairment.[39]

Prevention of Urinary Incontinence.   Patients at higher risk for urinary incontinence, such as postpartum women, older women, and men after prostate surgery, should be aware of prevention and how to reverse incontinence. Many patients believe incontinence is "normal." Nurses play an integral part during the health history in identifying patients in need of assistance. Teaching pelvic muscle training, pelvic muscle exercises, and biofeedback, which are all effective in reducing and eliminating urinary incontinence, will promote healthy lifestyles and quality of life for these individuals.

TABLE

16-1

Abdominal Pain

Problem	Process	Location	Quality
Peptic Ulcer and Dyspepsia[1,40]	Peptic ulcer refers to a demonstrable ulcer, usually in the duodenum or stomach. Dyspepsia causes similar symptoms but no ulceration. Infection by *Helicobacter pylori* is often present.	Epigastric, may radiate to the back	Variable: gnawing burning, boring, aching, pressing, or hunger-like
Cancer of the Stomach	Predominantly adenocarcinoma (90%–95%)	Increasingly in "cardia" and GE junction; also in distal stomach	Variable
Acute Pancreatitis[4]	An acute inflammation of the pancreas	Epigastric, may radiate to the back or other parts of the abdomen; may be poorly localized	Usually steady
Chronic Pancreatitis	Fibrosis of the pancreas secondary to recurrent inflammation	Epigastric, radiating through to the back	Steady, deep
Cancer of the Pancreas	Predominantly adenocarcinoma (95%)	Epigastric and in either upper quadrant; often radiates to the back	Steady, deep
Biliary Colic	Sudden obstruction of the cystic duct or common bile duct by a gallstone	Epigastric or right upper quadrant; may radiate to the right scapula and shoulder	Steady, aching; *not* colicky
Acute Cholecystitis[3]	Inflammation of the gallbladder, usually from obstruction of the cystic duct by a gallstone	Right upper quadrant or upper abdominal; may radiate to the right scapular area	Steady, aching
Acute Diverticulitis	Acute inflammation of a colonic diverticulum, a sac-like mucosal outpouching through the colonic muscle	Left lower quadrant	May be cramping at first, but becomes steady
Acute Appendicitis[11]	Acute inflammation of the appendix with distention or obstruction	• Poorly localized *periumbilical pain*, followed usually by • *Right lower quadrant pain*	• Mild but increasing, possibly cramping • Steady and more severe
Acute Mechanical Intestinal Obstruction	Obstruction of the bowel lumen, most commonly caused by (1) adhesions or hernias (small bowel) or (2) cancer or diverticulitis (colon)	• *Small bowel:* periumbilical or upper abdominal • *Colon:* lower abdominal or generalized	• Cramping • Cramping
Mesenteric Ischemia	Blood supply to the bowel and mesentery blocked from thrombosis or embolus (acute arterial occlusion), or reduced from hypoperfusion	May be periumbilical at first, then diffuse	Cramping at first, then steady

Timing	Factors That May Aggravate	Factors That May Relieve	Associated Symptoms and Setting
Intermittent. Duodenal ulcer is more likely than gastric ulcer or dyspepsia to cause pain that (1) wakes the patient at night and (2) occurs intermittently over a few weeks, then disappears for months, and then recurs.	Variable	Food and antacids may bring relief, but not necessarily in any of these disorders and least commonly in gastric ulcer.	Nausea, vomiting, belching, bloating; heartburn (more common in duodenal ulcer); weight loss (more common in gastric ulcer). Dyspepsia is more common in the young (20–29 yrs), gastric ulcer in those over 50 yrs, and duodenal ulcer in those 30–60 yrs.
The history of pain is typically shorter than in peptic ulcer. The pain is persistent and slowly progressive.	Often food	*Not* relieved by food or antacids	Anorexia, nausea, early satiety, weight loss, and sometimes bleeding. Most common in ages 50–70
Acute onset, persistent pain	Lying supine	Leaning forward with trunk flexed	Nausea, vomiting, abdominal distention, fever. Often a history of previous attacks and alcohol abuse or gallstones
Chronic or recurrent course	Alcohol, heavy or fatty meals	Possibly leaning forward with trunk flexed; often intractable	Symptoms of decreased pancreatic function may appear: diarrhea with fatty stools (steatorrhea) and diabetes mellitus.
Persistent pain; relentlessly progressive illness		Possibly leaning forward with trunk flexed; often intractable	Anorexia, nausea, vomiting, weight loss, and jaundice; depression
Rapid onset over a few minutes, lasts 1 to several hours and subsides gradually. Often recurrent			Anorexia, nausea, vomiting, restlessness
Gradual onset; course longer than in biliary colic	Jarring, deep breathing		Anorexia, nausea, vomiting, fever
Often a gradual onset			Fever, constipation. There may be initial brief diarrhea.

• Lasts roughly 4–6 hours			
• Depends on intervention	• Movement or cough	• If it subsides temporarily, suspect perforation of the appendix.	Anorexia, nausea, possibly vomiting, which typically follow the onset of pain; low fever
• Paroxysmal; may decrease as bowel mobility is impaired			• Vomiting of bile and mucus (high obstruction) or fecal material (low obstruction). Obstipation develops.
• Paroxysmal, though typically milder			• Obstipation early. Vomiting late if at all. Prior symptoms of underlying cause
Usually abrupt in onset, then persistent			Vomiting, diarrhea (sometimes bloody), constipation, shock

TABLE
16-2

Dysphagia

Process and Problem	Timing	Factors That Aggravate	Factors That Relieve	Associated Symptoms and Conditions
Oropharyngeal Dysphagia, *due to motor disorders affecting the pharyngeal muscles*	Acute or gradual onset and a variable course, depending on the underlying disorder	Attempts to start the swallowing process		Aspiration into the lungs or regurgitation into the nose with attempts to swallow. Neurologic evidence of stroke, bulbar palsy, or other neuromuscular conditions
Esophageal Dysphagia				
Mechanical Narrowing				
• Mucosal rings and webs	Intermittent	Solid foods	Regurgitation of the bolus of food	Usually none
• Esophageal stricture	Intermittent; may become slowly progressive	Solid foods	Regurgitation of the bolus of food	A long history of heartburn and regurgitation
• Esophageal cancer	May be intermittent at first; progressive over months	Solid foods, with progression to liquids	Regurgitation of the bolus of food	Pain in the chest and back and weight loss, especially late in the course of illness
Motor Disorders				
• Diffuse esophageal spasm	Intermittent	Solids or liquids	Maneuvers described below; sometimes nitroglycerin	Chest pain that mimics angina pectoris or myocardial infarction and lasts minutes to hours; possibly heartburn
• Scleroderma	Intermittent; may progress slowly	Solids or liquids	Repeated swallowing; movements such as straightening the back, raising the arms, or a Valsalva maneuver (straining down against a closed glottis)	Heartburn; other manifestations of scleroderma
• Achalasia	Intermittent; may progress	Solids or liquids		Regurgitation, often at night when lying down, with nocturnal cough; possibly chest pain precipitated by eating

TABLE 16-3

Constipation

Problem	Process	Associated Symptoms and Setting
Life Activities and Habits		
Inadequate Time or Setting for the Defecation Reflex	Ignoring the sensation of a full rectum inhibits the defecation reflex.	Hectic schedules, unfamiliar surroundings, bed rest
False Expectations of Bowel Habits	Expectations of "regularity" or more frequent stools than a person's norm	Beliefs, treatments, and advertisements that promote the use of laxatives
Diet Deficient in Fiber	Decreased fecal bulk	Other factors such as debilitation and constipating drugs may contribute.
Irritable Bowel Syndrome[12]	Change in frequency or form of bowel movement without structural or chemical abnormality	Small, hard stools, often with mucus; periods of diarrhea; intermittent pain for 12 weeks of preceding 12 months, relieved by defecation; stress may aggravate.
Mechanical Obstruction		
Cancer of the Rectum or Sigmoid Colon	Progressive narrowing of the bowel lumen	Change in bowel habits; often diarrhea, abdominal pain, and bleeding. In rectal cancer, tenesmus and pencil-shaped stools
Fecal Impaction	A large, firm, immovable fecal mass, most often in the rectum	Rectal fullness, abdominal pain, and diarrhea around the impaction; common in debilitated, bedridden, and often elderly patients
Other Obstructing Lesions (such as diverticulitis, volvulus, intussusception, or hernia)	Narrowing or complete obstruction of the bowel	Colicky abdominal pain, abdominal distention, and in intussusception, often "currant jelly" stools (red blood and mucus)
Painful Anal Lesions	Pain may cause spasm of the external sphincter and voluntary inhibition of the defecation reflex.	Anal fissures, painful hemorrhoids, perirectal abscesses
Drugs	A variety of mechanisms	Opiates, anticholinergics, antacids containing calcium or aluminum, and many others
Depression	A disorder of mood.	Fatigue, anhedonia, sleep disturbance, weight loss
Neurologic Disorders	Interference with the autonomic innervation of the bowel	Spinal cord injuries, multiple sclerosis, Hirschsprung disease, and other conditions
Metabolic Conditions	Interference with bowel motility	Pregnancy, hypothyroidism, hypercalcemia

TABLE
16-4

Diarrhea

Problem	Process	Characteristics of Stool
Acute Diarrhea[13]		
Secretory Infection	Infection by viruses, preformed bacterial toxins (such as *Staphylococcus aureus, Clostridium perfringens*, toxigenic *Escherichia coli, Vibrio cholerae*), cryptosporidium, *Giardia lamblia*	Watery, without blood, pus, or mucus
Inflammatory Infection	Colonization or invasion of intestinal mucosa (nontyphoid *Salmonella, Shigella, Yersinia, Campylobacter*, enteropathic *E. coli, Entamoeba histolytica*)	Loose to watery, often with blood, pus, or mucus
Drug-Induced Diarrhea	Action of many drugs, such as magnesium-containing antacids, antibiotics, antineoplastic agents, and laxatives	Loose to watery
Chronic Diarrhea		
Diarrheal Syndrome		
• Irritable bowel syndrome[12]	Change in frequency and form of bowel movements without chemical or structural abnormality	Loose; may show mucus but no blood. Small, hard stools with constipation
• Cancer of the sigmoid colon	Partial obstruction by a malignant neoplasm	May be blood-streaked
Inflammatory Bowel Disease		
• Ulcerative colitis	Inflammation of the mucosa and submucosa of the rectum and colon with ulceration; typically extends proximally from the rectum	Soft to watery, often containing blood
• Crohn disease of the small bowel (regional enteritis) or colon (granulomatous colitis)	Chronic transmural inflammation of the bowel wall, in a skip pattern typically involving the terminal ileum and/or proximal colon	Small, soft to loose or watery, usually free of gross blood (enteritis) or with less bleeding than ulcerative colitis (colitis)
Voluminous Diarrhea		
• Malabsorption syndrome	Defective absorption of fat, including fat-soluble vitamins, with steatorrhea (excessive excretion of fat) as in pancreatic insufficiency, bile salt deficiency, bacterial overgrowth	Typically bulky, soft, light yellow to gray, mushy, greasy or oily, and sometimes frothy; particularly foul-smelling; usually floats in the toilet
• Osmotic diarrhea Lactose intolerance	Deficiency in intestinal lactase	Watery diarrhea of large volume
Abuse of osmotic purgatives	Laxative habit, often surreptitious	Watery diarrhea of large volume
• Secretory diarrhea from bacterial infection, secreting villous adenoma, fat or bile salt malabsorption, hormone-mediated conditions (gastrin in Zollinger-Ellison syndrome, vasoactive intestinal peptide)	Variable	Watery diarrhea of large volume

Timing	Associated Symptoms	Setting, Persons at Risk
Duration of a few days, possibly longer. Lactase deficiency may lead to a longer course.	Nausea, vomiting, periumbilical cramping pain. Temperature normal or slightly elevated	Often travel, a common food source, or an epidemic
An acute illness of varying duration	Lower abdominal cramping pain and often rectal urgency, tenesmus; fever	Travel, contaminated food or water. Men and women who have had frequent anal intercourse.
Acute, recurrent, or chronic	Possibly nausea; usually little if any pain	Prescribed or over-the-counter medications
Often worse in the morning. Diarrhea rarely wakes the patient at night.	Crampy lower abdominal pain, abdominal distention, flatulence, nausea, constipation	Young and middle-aged adults, especially women
Variable	Change in usual bowel habits, crampy lower abdominal pain, constipation	Middle-aged and older adults, especially older than 55 yrs
Onset ranges from insidious to acute. Typically recurrent; may be persistent. Diarrhea may wake the patient at night.	Crampy lower or generalized abdominal pain, anorexia, weakness; fever if severe. May include episcleritis, uveitis, arthritis, erythema nodosum.	Often young people. Increases risk of colon cancer.
Insidious onset; chronic or recurrent. Diarrhea may wake the patient at night.	Crampy periumbilical or right lower quadrant (enteritis) or diffuse (colitis) pain, with anorexia, low fever, and/or weight loss. Perianal or perirectal abscesses and fistulas. May cause small or large bowel obstruction	Often young people, especially in late teens, but also in middle age. More common in people of Jewish descent. Increases risk of colon cancer
Onset of illness typically insidious	Anorexia, weight loss, fatigue, abdominal distention, often crampy lower abdominal pain. Symptoms of nutritional deficiencies such as bleeding (vitamin K), bone pain and fractures (vitamin D), glossitis (vitamin B), and edema (protein)	Variable, depending on cause
Follows the ingestion of milk and milk products; relieved by fasting	Crampy abdominal pain, abdominal distention, flatulence	In >50% of African-Americans, Asians, Native Americans, Hispanics; in 5%–20% of Caucasians
Variable	Often none	Persons with anorexia nervosa or bulimia nervosa
Variable	Weight loss, dehydration, nausea, vomiting, and cramping abdominal pain	Variable depending on cause

TABLE
16-5

Black and Bloody Stools

Problem	Selected Causes	Associated Symptoms and Setting
Melena Refers to passage of black, tarry (sticky and shiny) stools. Tests for occult blood are positive. Involves loss of at least 60 ml of blood into the gastrointestinal tract (less in infants and children), usually from the esophagus, stomach, or duodenum. Less commonly, when intestinal transit is slow, blood may originate in the jejunum, ileum, or ascending colon. In infants, melena may result from swallowing blood during the birth process.	Peptic ulcer	Often, but not necessarily, a history of epigastric pain
	Gastritis or stress ulcers	Recent ingestion of alcohol, aspirin, or other anti-inflammatory drugs; recent bodily trauma, severe burns, surgery, or increased intracranial pressure
	Esophageal or gastric varices	Cirrhosis of the liver or other cause of portal hypertension
		History of heartburn
	Reflux esophagitis Mallory-Weiss tear, a mucosal tear in the esophagus due to retching and vomiting	Retching, vomiting, often recent ingestion of alcohol
Black, Nonsticky Stools May result from other causes, then give negative results when tested for occult blood. (Ingestion of iron or other substances, however, may cause a positive test result in the absence of blood.) These stools have no pathologic significance.	Ingestion of iron, bismuth salts as in Pepto-Bismol, licorice, or even commercial chocolate cookies	
Red Blood in the Stools Usually originates in the colon, rectum, or anus, and much less frequently in the jejunum or ileum. Upper gastrointestinal hemorrhage may also cause red stools. The amount of blood lost is then usually large (more than a liter). Rapid transit time through the intestinal tract leaves insufficient time for the blood to turn black.	Cancer of the colon	Often a change in bowel habits
	Benign polyps of the colon	Often no other symptoms
	Diverticula of the colon	Often no other symptoms
	Inflammatory conditions of the colon and rectum	
	• Ulcerative colitis, Crohn's disease	See Table 16-4, Diarrhea.
	• Infectious diarrhea	See Table 16-4, Diarrhea.
	• Proctitis (various causes) from frequent anal intercourse	Rectal urgency, tenesmus
	Ischemic colitis	Lower abdominal pain, sometimes fever or shock in older adults. Abdomen typically soft to palpation
	Hemorrhoids	Blood on the toilet paper, on the surface of the stool, or dripping into the toilet
	Anal fissure	Blood on the toilet paper or on the surface of the stool; anal pain
Reddish but Nonbloody Stools	Ingestion of beets	Pink urine, which usually precedes the reddish stool

TABLE 16-6

Frequency, Nocturia, and Polyuria

Problem	Mechanisms	Selected Causes	Associated Symptoms
Frequency	Decreased capacity of the bladder		
	• Increased bladder sensitivity to stretch because of inflammation	*Infection*, stones, tumor, or foreign body in the bladder	Burning on urination, urinary urgency, sometimes gross hematuria
	• Decreased elasticity of the bladder wall	Infiltration by scar tissue or tumor	Symptoms of associated inflammation (see above) are common.
	• Decreased cortical inhibition of bladder contractions	Motor disorders of the central nervous system, such as a stroke	Urinary urgency; neurologic symptoms such as weakness and paralysis
	Impaired emptying of the bladder, with residual urine in the bladder		
	• Partial mechanical obstruction of the bladder neck or proximal urethra	Most commonly, benign prostatic hyperplasia; also urethral stricture and other obstructive lesions of the bladder or prostate	Prior obstructive symptoms: hesitancy in starting the urinary stream, straining to void, reduced size and force of the stream, and dribbling during or at the end of urination
	• Loss of peripheral nerve supply to the bladder	Neurologic disease affecting the sacral nerves or nerve roots (e.g., diabetic neuropathy)	Weakness or sensory defects
Nocturia			
With High Volumes	Most types of polyuria (see pp. 445–446)		
	Decreased concentrating ability of the kidney with loss of the normal decrease in nocturnal urinary output	Chronic renal insufficiency due to a number of diseases	Possibly other symptoms of renal insufficiency
	Excessive fluid intake before bedtime	Habit, especially involving alcohol and coffee	
	Fluid-retaining, edematous states. Dependent edema accumulates during the day and is excreted when the patient lies down at night.	Congestive heart failure, nephrotic syndrome, hepatic cirrhosis with ascites, chronic venous insufficiency	Edema and other symptoms of the underlying disorder. Urinary output during the day may be reduced as fluid reaccumulates in the body. See Table 15-4, p. 428 Peripheral Causes of Edema.
With Low Volumes	Frequency		
	Voiding while up at night without a real urge, a "pseudo-frequency"	Insomnia	Variable
Polyuria	Deficiency of antidiuretic hormone (diabetes insipidus)	A disorder of the posterior pituitary and hypothalamus	Thirst and polydipsia, often severe and persistent; nocturia
	Renal unresponsiveness to antidiuretic hormone (nephrogenic diabetes insipidus)	A number of kidney diseases, including hypercalcemic and hypokalemic nephropathy; drug toxicity (e.g., from lithium)	Thirst and polydipsia, often severe and persistent; nocturia
	Solute diuresis		
	• Electrolytes, such as sodium salts	Large saline infusions, potent diuretics, certain kidney diseases	Variable
	• Nonelectrolytes, such as glucose	Uncontrolled diabetes mellitus	Thirst, polydipsia, and nocturia
	Excessive water intake	Primary polydipsia	Polydipsia tends to be episodic. Thirst may not be present. Nocturia is usually absent.

TABLE 16-7

Urinary Incontinence*

Problem	Mechanisms
Stress Incontinence The urethral sphincter is weakened so that transient increases in intra-abdominal pressure raise the bladder pressure to levels that exceed urethral resistance.	In women, often a weakness of the pelvic floor with inadequate muscular support of the bladder and proximal urethra and a change in the angle between the bladder and the urethra. Causes include childbirth and surgery. Local conditions affecting the internal urethral sphincter, such as postmenopausal atrophy of the mucosa and urethral infection, may also contribute. In men, stress incontinence may follow prostatic surgery.
Urge Incontinence Detrusor contractions are stronger than normal and overcome the normal urethral resistance. The bladder is typically *small*.	• Decreased cortical inhibition of detrusor contractions from strokes, brain tumors, dementia, and lesions of the spinal cord above the sacral level • Hyperexcitability of sensory pathways, as in bladder infections, tumors, and fecal impaction • Deconditioning of voiding reflexes, as in frequent voluntary voiding at low bladder volumes
Overflow Incontinence Detrusor contractions are insufficient to overcome urethral resistance. The bladder is typically *large*, even after an effort to void.	• Obstruction of the bladder outlet, as in benign prostatic hyperplasia or tumor • Weakness of the detrusor muscle associated with peripheral nerve disease at the sacral level • Impaired bladder sensation that interrupts the reflex arc, as from diabetic neuropathy
Functional Incontinence This is a functional inability to get to the toilet in time because of impaired health or environmental conditions.	Problems in mobility resulting from weakness, arthritis, poor vision, or other conditions. Environmental factors such as an unfamiliar setting, distant bathroom facilities, bed rails, or physical restraints
Incontinence Secondary to Medications Drugs may contribute to any type of incontinence listed.	Sedatives, tranquilizers, anticholinergics, sympathetic blockers, and potent diuretics

* Patients may have more than one kind of incontinence.

Symptoms	Physical Signs
Momentary leakage of small amounts of urine with coughing, laughing, and sneezing while the person is in an upright position. A desire to urinate is not associated with pure stress incontinence.	The bladder is not detected on abdominal examination.
	Stress incontinence may be demonstrable, especially if the patient is examined before voiding and in a standing position.
	Atrophic vaginitis may be evident.
Incontinence preceded by an urge to void. The volume tends to be moderate.	The bladder is not detectable on abdominal examination.
Urgency	When cortical inhibition is decreased, mental deficits or motor signs of central nervous system disease are often, though not necessarily, present.
Frequency and nocturia with small to moderate volumes	
If acute inflammation is present, pain on urination	
Possibly "pseudo-stress incontinence"—voiding 10–20 sec after stresses such as a change of position, going up or down stairs, and possibly coughing, laughing, or sneezing	When sensory pathways are hyperexcitable, signs of local pelvic problems or a fecal impaction may be present.
A continuous dripping or dribbling incontinence	An enlarged bladder is often found on abdominal examination and may be tender. Other signs include prostatic enlargement, motor signs of peripheral nerve disease, a decrease in sensation (including perineal sensation), and diminished to absent reflexes.
Decreased force of the urinary stream	
Prior symptoms of partial urinary obstruction or other symptoms of peripheral nerve disease may be present.	
Incontinence on the way to the toilet or only in the early morning	The bladder is not detectable on physical examination. Look for physical or environmental clues to the likely cause.
Variable. A careful history and chart review are important.	Variable

TABLE
16-8

Localized Bulges in the Abdominal Wall

Localized bulges in the abdominal wall include *ventral hernias* (defects in the wall through which tissue protrudes) and subcutaneous tumors such as *lipomas*. The more common ventral hernias are umbilical, incisional, and epigastric. Hernias and a rectus diastasis usually become more evident when the patient raises head and shoulders from a supine position.

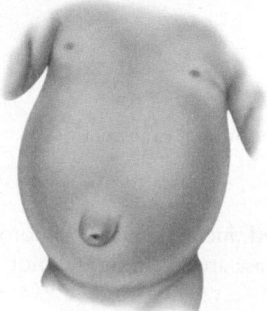

INFANT

Umbilical Hernia

A protrusion through a defective umbilical ring is most common in infants but also occurs in adults. In infants, but not in adults, it usually closes spontaneously within 1 to 2 years.

Diastasis Recti

Separation of the two rectus abdominis muscles, through which abdominal contents form a midline ridge when the patient raises head and shoulders. Often seen in repeated pregnancies, obesity, and chronic lung disease. It has no clinical consequences.

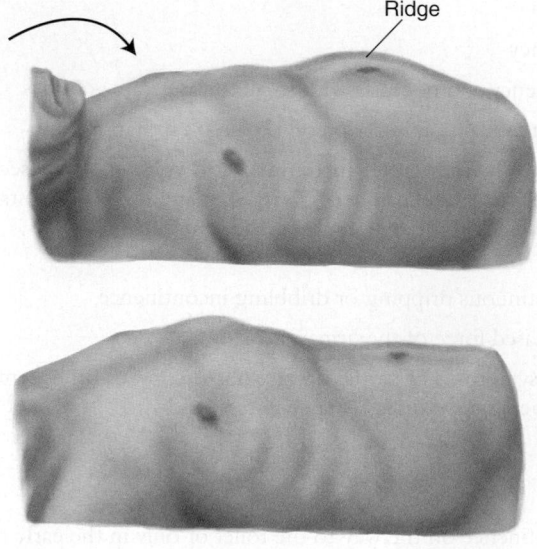

Ridge

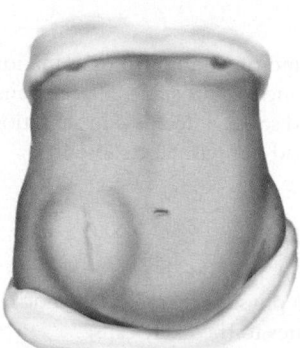

Incisional Hernia

This is a protrusion through an operative scar. Palpate to detect the length and width of the defect in the abdominal wall. A small defect, through which a large hernia has passed, has a greater risk for complications than a large defect.

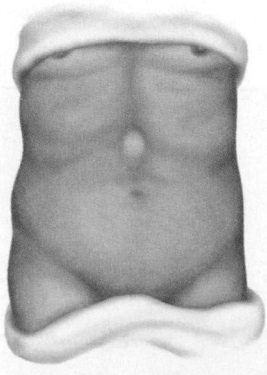

Epigastric Hernia

A small midline protrusion through a defect in the linea alba occurs between the xiphoid process and the umbilicus. With the patient's head and shoulders raised (or with the patient standing), run your fingerpad down the linea alba to feel it.

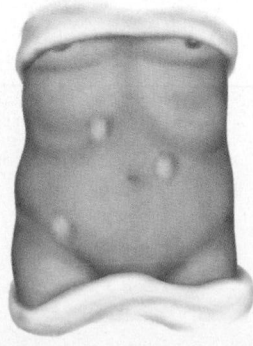

Lipoma

Common, benign, fatty tumors usually in the subcutaneous tissues almost anywhere in the body, including the abdominal wall. Small or large, they are usually soft and often lobulated. Press your finger down on the edge of a lipoma. The tumor typically slips out from under it.

TABLE	
16-9	**Protuberant Abdomens**

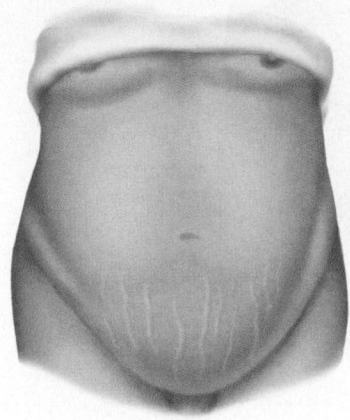

Fat

Fat is the most common cause of a protuberant abdomen. Fat thickens the abdominal wall, the mesentery, and omentum. The umbilicus may appear sunken. A *pannus,* or apron of fatty tissue, may extend below the inguinal ligaments. Lift it to look for inflammation in the skin folds or even for a hidden hernia.

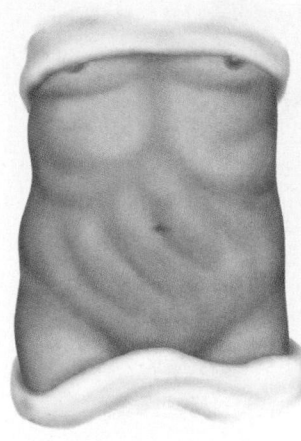

Gas

Gaseous distention may be localized or generalized. It causes a tympanitic percussion note. Increased intestinal gas production from certain foods may cause mild distention. More serious are intestinal obstruction and adynamic (paralytic) ileus. Note the location of the distention. Distention becomes more marked in colonic than in small bowel obstruction.

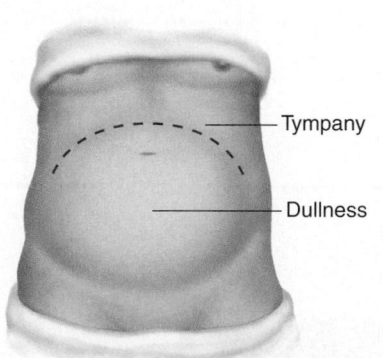

Tympany

Dullness

Tumor

A large, solid tumor, usually rising out of the pelvis, is dull to percussion. Air-filled bowel is displaced to the periphery. Causes include ovarian tumors and uterine myomata. Occasionally a markedly distended bladder may be mistaken for such a tumor.

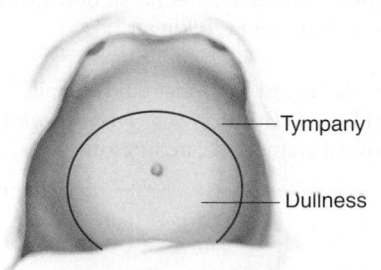

Tympany

Dullness

Pregnancy

Pregnancy is a common cause of a pelvic "mass." Listen for the fetal heart.

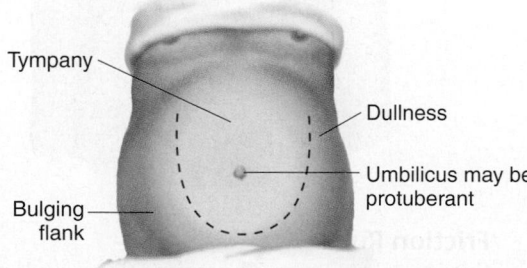

Tympany

Dullness

Umbilicus may be protuberant

Bulging flank

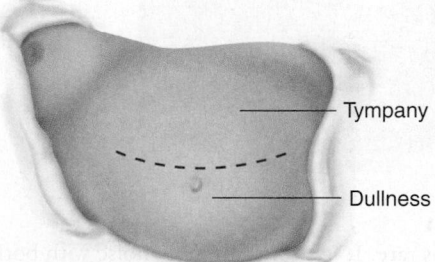

Tympany

Dullness

Ascitic Fluid[23]

Ascitic fluid seeks the lowest point in the abdomen, producing bulging flanks that are dull to percussion. The umbilicus may protrude. Turn the patient onto one side to detect the shift in position of the fluid level (shifting dullness). (See pp. 463–464 for the assessment of ascites.)

TABLE
16-10

Sounds in the Abdomen

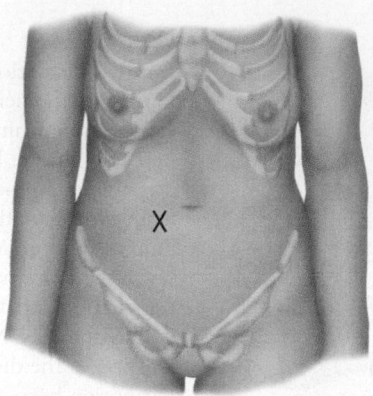

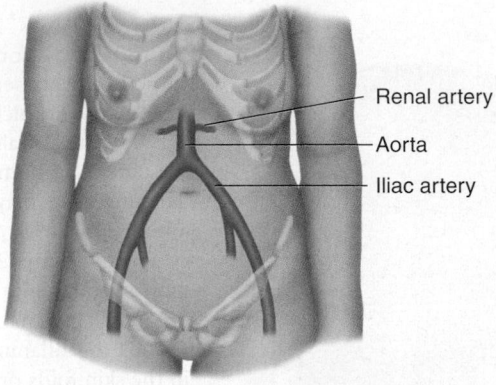

Bowel Sounds

Bowel sounds may be:

- *Increased,* as in diarrhea or *early intestinal obstruction*

- *Decreased,* then absent, as in *adynamic ileus* and *peritonitis.* Before deciding that bowel sounds are absent, sit down and listen where shown for 2–3 min or even longer.

High-pitched tinkling sounds suggest intestinal fluid and air under tension in a dilated bowel. *Rushes of high-pitched sounds* coinciding with an abdominal cramp indicate intestinal obstruction.

Bruits

A *hepatic bruit* suggests carcinoma of the liver or alcoholic hepatitis. *Arterial bruits* with both systolic and diastolic components suggest partial occlusion of the aorta or large arteries. Partial occlusion of a renal artery may explain hypertension.

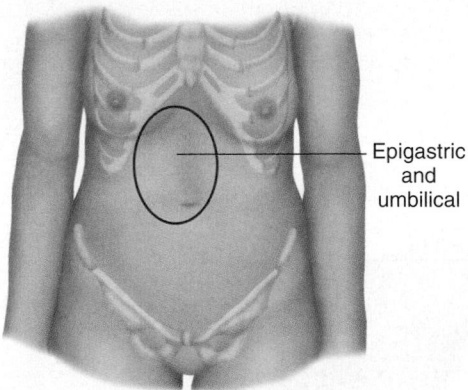

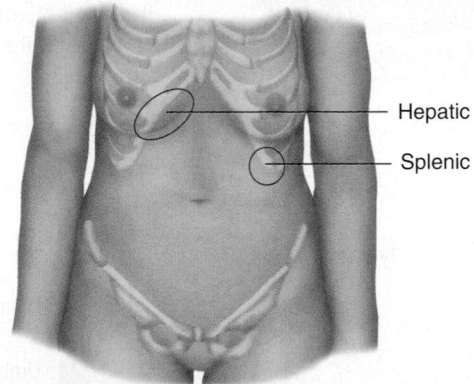

Venous Hum

A venous hum is rare. It is a soft humming noise with both systolic and diastolic components. It indicates increased collateral circulation between portal and systemic venous systems, as in hepatic cirrhosis.

Friction Rubs

Friction rubs are rare. They are grating sounds with respiratory variation. They indicate inflammation of the peritoneal surface of an organ, as in liver cancer, chlamydial or gonococcal perihepatitis, recent liver biopsy, or splenic infarct. When a systolic bruit accompanies a hepatic friction rub, suspect carcinoma of the liver.

TABLE
16-11

Tender Abdomens

Abdominal Wall Tenderness

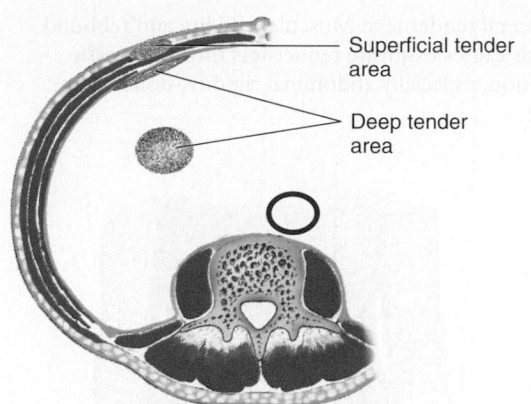

Superficial tender area

Deep tender area

Tenderness may originate in the abdominal wall. When the patient raises the head and shoulders, this tenderness persists, whereas tenderness from a deeper lesion (protected by the tightened muscles) decreases.

Visceral Tenderness

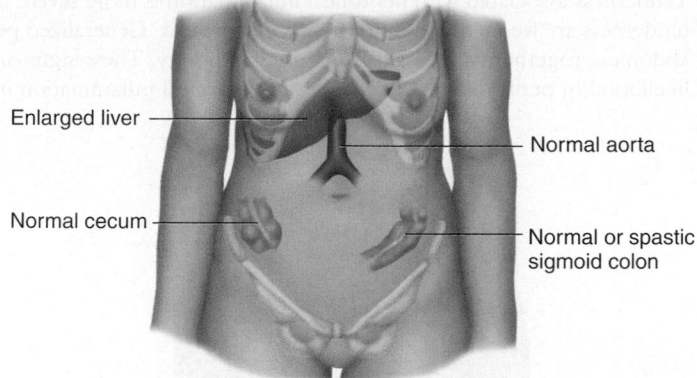

Enlarged liver

Normal cecum

Normal aorta

Normal or spastic sigmoid colon

The structures shown may be tender to deep palpation. Usually the discomfort is dull with no muscular rigidity or rebound tenderness. A reassuring explanation to the patient may prove quite helpful.

Tenderness From Disease in the Chest and Pelvis

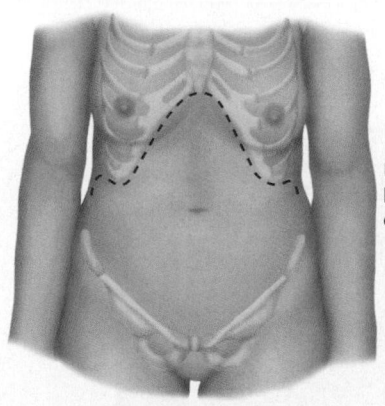

Unilateral or bilateral, upper or lower abdomen

Acute Pleurisy

Abdominal pain and tenderness may result from acute pleural inflammation. When unilateral, it may mimic acute cholecystitis or appendicitis. Rebound tenderness and rigidity are less common; chest signs are usually present.

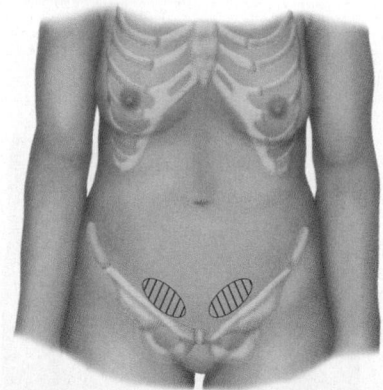

Acute Salpingitis

Frequently bilateral, the tenderness of acute salpingitis (inflammation of the fallopian tubes) is usually maximal just above the inguinal ligaments. Rebound tenderness and rigidity may be present. On pelvic examination, motion of the uterus causes pain.

(table continues on page 486)

TABLE
16-11

Tender Abdomens (continued)

Tenderness of Peritoneal Inflammation

Tenderness associated with peritoneal inflammation is more severe than visceral tenderness. Muscular rigidity and rebound tenderness are frequently but not necessarily present. Generalized peritonitis causes exquisite tenderness throughout the abdomen, together with board-like muscular rigidity. These signs on palpation, especially abdominal rigidity, double the likelihood of peritonitis.[17] Local causes of peritoneal inflammation include:

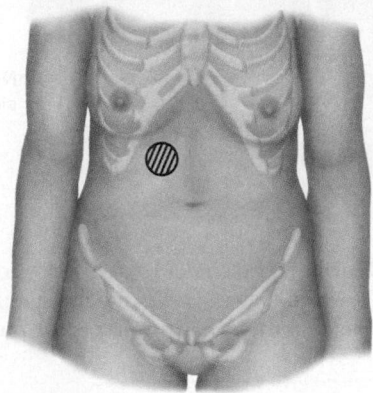

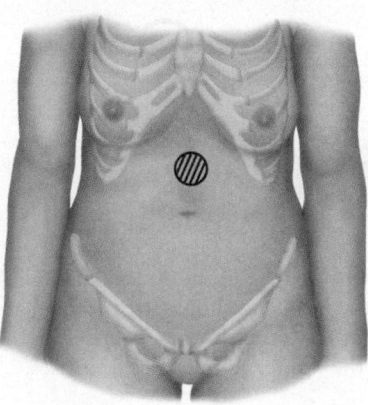

Acute Cholecystitis[3]

Signs are maximal in the right upper quadrant. Check for the Murphy sign (see p. 466).

Acute Pancreatitis[4]

In acute pancreatitis, epigastric tenderness and rebound tenderness are usually present, but the abdominal wall may be soft.

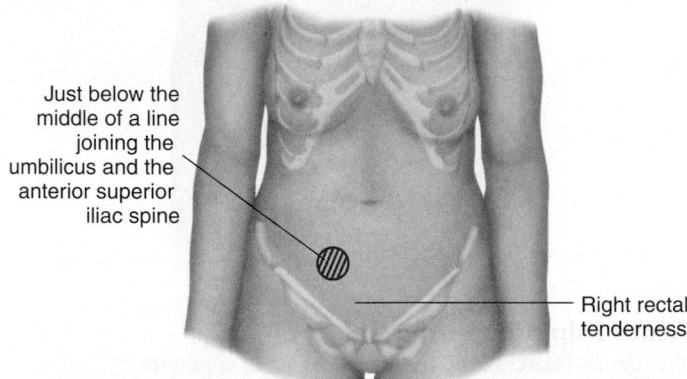

Just below the middle of a line joining the umbilicus and the anterior superior iliac spine

Right rectal tenderness

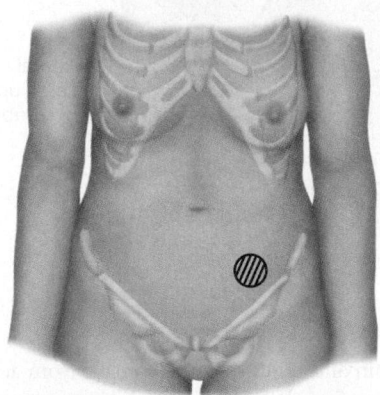

Acute Appendicitis[11]

Right lower quadrant signs are typical of acute appendicitis but may be absent early in the course. The typical area of tenderness is illustrated. Explore other portions of the right lower quadrant as well as the right flank.

Acute Diverticulitis

Acute diverticulitis most often involves the sigmoid colon and then resembles a left-sided appendicitis.

TABLE 16-12   **Liver Enlargement: Apparent and Real**

A palpable liver does not necessarily indicate hepatomegaly (an enlarged liver), but more often results from a change in consistency—from the normal softness to an abnormal firmness or hardness, as in cirrhosis. Clinical estimates of liver size should be based on both percussion and palpation, although even these techniques are far from perfect.[15]

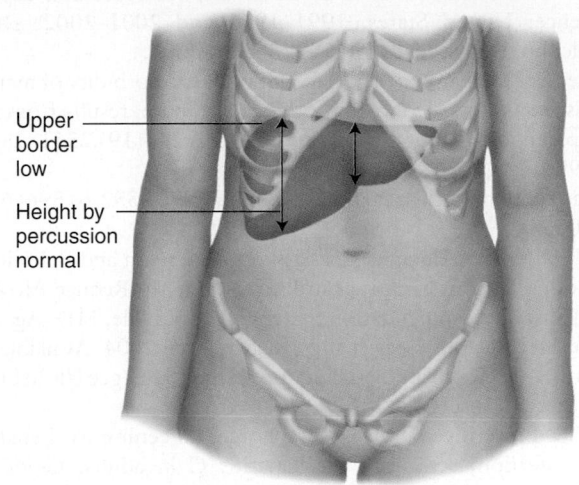

Downward Displacement of the Liver by a Low Diaphragm

This finding is common when the diaphragm is low (e.g., in COPD). The liver edge may be readily palpable well below the costal margin. Percussion, however, reveals a low upper edge also, and the vertical span of the liver is normal.

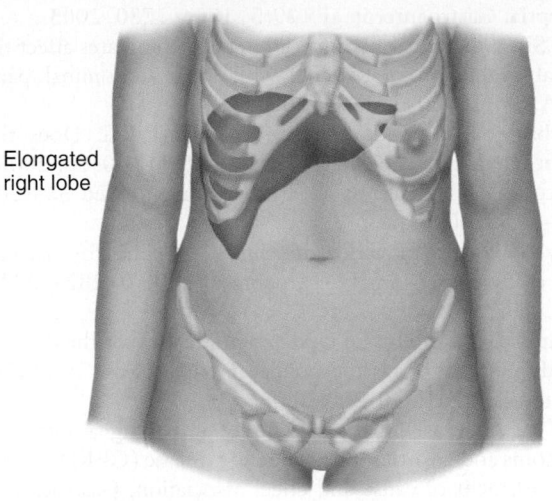

Normal Variations in Liver Shape

In some people, especially those with a lanky build, the liver tends to be elongated so that its right lobe is easily palpable as it projects downward toward the iliac crest. Such an elongation, sometimes called *Riedel lobe,* represents a variation in shape, not an increase in liver volume or size. Examiners can only estimate the upper and lower borders of an organ with three dimensions and differing shapes. Some error is unavoidable.

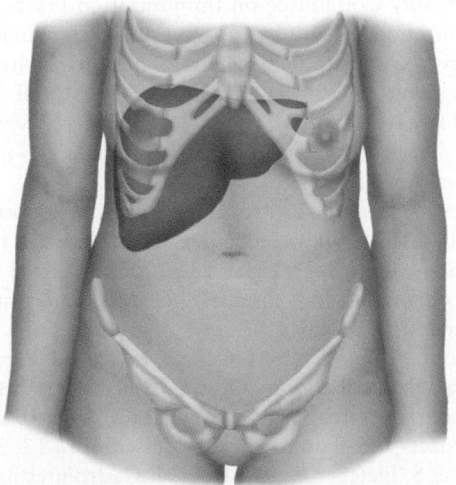

Smooth Large Liver

Cirrhosis may produce an enlarged liver with a firm, *nontender* edge. The liver is not always enlarged in this condition, however, and many other diseases may produce similar findings. An enlarged liver with a smooth, *tender* edge suggests inflammation, as in hepatitis, or venous congestion, as in right-sided heart failure.

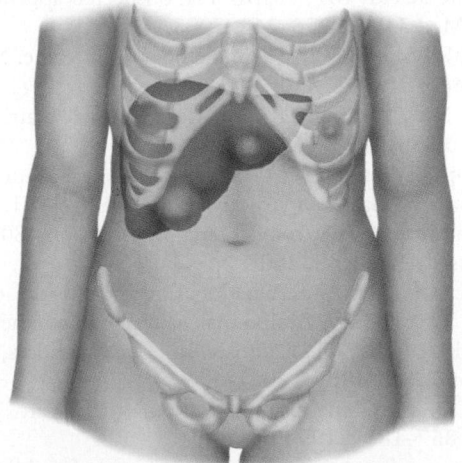

Irregular Large Liver

An enlarged liver that is firm or hard and has an irregular edge or surface suggests malignancy. There may be one or more nodules. The liver may or may not be tender.

BIBLIOGRAPHY

CITATIONS

1. Talley NJ, Vakil NB, Moayyedi P, et al. American Gastroenterological Association technical review on the evaluation of dyspepsia. Gastroenterology 129(5):1756–1780, 2005.

2. Ranji SR, Goldman LE, Simel DL, et al. Do opiates affect the clinical evaluation of patients with acute abdominal pain? JAMA 296(14):1764–1774, 2006.

3. Trowbridge RL, Rutkowshi NK, Shojania KG. Does this patient have acute cholecystitis? JAMA 289(1):80–86, 2003.

4. Whitcomb DC. Acute pancreatitis. N Engl J Med 354(20): 2142–2150, 2006.

5. Talley NJ, Vakil N. Practice guidelines: guidelines for management of dyspepsia. Am J Gastroenterol 100(10):2324–2337, 2005.

6. DeVault KR, Castell DO. Updated guidelines for the diagnosis and treatment of gastroesophageal reflux disease. Am J Gastroenterol 100(1):190–200, 2005.

7. Vaezi MF, Hicks DM, Abelson TI, et al. Laryngeal signs and symptoms and gastroesophageal reflux disease (GERD): a critical assessment of cause and effect association. Gastroenterol Hepatol 1(5):333–344, 2003.

8. Talley NJ. American Gastroenterological Association medical position statement: evaluation of dyspepsia. Gastroenterology 129(5):1753–1755, 2005.

9. Shaheen N, Ransohoff DF. Gastroesophageal reflux, Barrett esophagus, and esophageal cancer. Scientific review. JAMA 287(15):1972–1981, 2002.

10. Moayyedi P, Talley NJ, Fennerty MB, et al. Can the clinical history distinguish between organic and functional dyspepsia? JAMA 295(13):1566–1576, 2006.

11. Paulson EK, Kalady MF, Pappas TN. Suspected appendicitis. N Engl J Med 348(3):236–242, 2003.

12. Horwitz BJ, Fisher RS. The irritable bowel syndrome. N Engl J Med 344(24):1846–1850, 2001.

13. Theilman NM, Guerrant RL. Acute infectious diarrhea. N Engl J Med 350(1):38–46, 2004.

14. Longstreth GF, Thompson WG, Chey WD, et al. Functional bowel disorders. Gastroenterology 130(5):1480–1491, 2006. Available at: http://www.romecriteria.org/ pdfs/p1480FBDs.pdf. Accessed October 5, 2007.

15. McGee S. Chapter 47, Palpation and percussion of the abdomen; Chapter 48, Abdominal pain and tenderness. In: Evidence-Based Physical Diagnosis. St. Louis: Saunders, 2007, pp. 553–555, 572–582.

16. Naylor CD. Physical examination of the liver. JAMA 271(23):1857–1859, 1994.

17. U.S. Preventive Services Task Force. Screening for abdominal aortic aneurysm: recommendation statement. Ann Intern Med 142(3):198–202, 2005.

18. Birkmeyer JD, Upchurch GR. Evidence-based screening and management of abdominal aortic aneurysm (editorial). Ann Intern Med 146(10):749–750, 2007.

19. Lederle FA, Simel DL. Does this patient have abdominal aortic aneurysm? JAMA 281(1):77–82, 1999.

20. Grover SA, Barkun AN, Sackett DL. Does this patient have splenomegaly? JAMA 270(18):2218–2221, 1993.

21. Williams JW, Simel DL. Does this patient have ascites? How to divine fluid in the abdomen. JAMA 267(19):2645–2648, 1992.

22. Grant BF, Dawson DA, Stinson FS, et al. The 12-month prevalence and trends in DSM-IV alcohol abuse and dependence: United States, 1991–1992 and 2001–2002. Drug Alcohol Dependence 74(3):223–234, 2004.

23. Regier DA, Farmer ME, Rae DS, et al. Comorbidity of mental disorders with alcohol and other drug abuse: results from the Epidemiologic Catchment Study. JAMA 264(19):2511–2518, 1990.

24. Saitz R. Unhealthy alcohol use. N Engl J Med 352(6):596–607, 2005.

25. U.S. Preventive Services Task Force. Screening and Behavioral Counseling Interventions in Primary Care to Reduce Alcohol Misuse: Recommendation Statement. Rockville, MD: Agency for Healthcare Research and Quality, April 2004. Available at: http://www.ahrq.gov/clinic/pocketgd1011/gcp10s2c.htm. Accessed April 13, 2011.

26. U.S. Preventive Services Task Force. Screening for hepatitis B infection; screening for hepatitis C in adults. Guide to Clinical Preventive Services, 2006. Available at: http://www.uspreventiveservicestaskforce.org/uspstf/uspshepb.htm. Accessed April 13, 2011

27. Fiore AF, Wasley A, Bell BP. Recommendations of the Advisory Committee on Immunization Practices: prevention of hepatitis A through active or passive immunization. MMWR Morb Mortal Wkly Rep 55(RR07):1–23, 2006. Available at: http://www.cdc.gov/mmwr/preview/mmwrhtml/rr5507a1.htm. Accessed April 13, 2011

28. Mast E, Weinbaum CM, Fiore AE, et al. Recommendations of the Advisory Committee on Immunization Practices. Part II: Immunization of adults. A comprehensive immunization strategy to eliminate transmission of hepatitis B virus infection in the United States. MMWR Morb Mortal Wkly Rep 55(RR16):1–25, 2006. Available at: http://www.cdc.gov/mmwr/preview/mmwrhtml/rr5516a1.htm?s_cid=rr5516a1_e. Accessed April 13, 2011

29. Centers for Disease Control and Prevention. National Center for HIV/AIDS, Viral Hepatitis, STD, and TB Prevention. Hepatitis C Fact Sheet. May 24, 2005. Available at: http://www.cdc.gov/ncidod/diseases/hepatitis/c/fact.htm. Accessed April 13, 2011.

30. American Cancer Society. Cancer Facts and Figures 2010. Atlanta: National Home Office. Available at: http://www.cancer.org/Research/CancerFactsFigures/CancerFactsFigures/cancer-facts-and-figures-2010. Accessed April 13, 2011.

31. Winawer S, Fletcher R, Rex D, et al. Gastrointestinal Consortium Panel. Colorectal cancer screening and surveillance: clinical guidelines and rationale. Update based on new evidence. Gastroenterology 124(2):544–560, 2003.

32. Winawer S, Zauber A, Fletcher RH, et al. Guidelines for colonoscopy surveillance after polypectomy: a consensus update by the US Multi-Society Task Force on Colorectal Cancer and the American Cancer Society. Gastroenterology 130(6):1872–1885, 2006.

33. Collins JF, Leiberman DA, Dirbom TE, et al. Accuracy of screening for fecal occult blood on a single stool sample obtained by digital rectal examination: a comparison with recommended sampling practice. Ann Intern Med 142(2):81–85, 2005.

34. Boolchand V, Olds G, Singh J, et al. Colorectal screening after polypectomy: a national survey study of primary care physicians. Ann Intern Med 145(9):654–659, 2006.

35. American Cancer Society. What are the risk factors for colorectal cancer? Available at: http://www.cancer.org/Cancer/ColonandRectumCancer/DetailedGuide/colorectal-cancer-prevention. Accessed April 13, 2011.

36. American Cancer Society. Can colorectal polyps and cancer be found early? Available at: http://www.cancer.org/Cancer/ColonandRectumCancer/OverviewGuide/colorectal-cancer-overview-detection Accessed April 13, 2011.

37. Schatzkin A, Lanza E, Corle D, et al. Lack of effect of a low-fat, high-fiber diet on the recurrence of colorectal adenomas. N Engl J Med 342(16):1149–1155, 2000.

38. Alberts DS, Martinez ME, Roe DJ, et al. Lack of effect of a high-fiber cereal supplement on the recurrence of colorectal adenomas. N Engl J Med 342(16):1156–1162, 2000.

39. U.S. Preventive Services Task Force. Routine aspirin or non-steroidal anti-inflammatory drugs for the primary prevention of colorectal cancer: U.S. Preventive Services Task Force Recommendation Statement. Ann Intern Med 146(5):361–364, 2007.

40. Drossman DA. The functional gastrointestinal disorders and the Rome III process. Gastroenterology 130(5):1377–1390, 2007.

ADDITIONAL REFERENCES

Examination of the Abdomen

Fink HA, Lederle FA, Roth CS. The accuracy of physical examination to detect abdominal aortic aneurysm. Arch Intern Med 160(6):833–836, 2000.

Kim LG, Scott AP, Ashton HA, et al. A sustained mortality benefit from screening for abdominal aortic aneurysm. Ann Intern Med 146(10):696–706, 2007.

McGee SR. Percussion and physical diagnosis: separating myth from science. Dis Mon 41(10):641–688, 1995.

Silen W, Cope Z. Cope's Early Diagnosis of the Acute Abdomen, 21st ed. Oxford, UK, and New York: Oxford University Press, 2005.

Sleisenger MH, Feldman M, Griedman LS, et al (eds). Sleisenger and Fortran's Gastrointestinal and Liver Disease: Pathophysiology, Diagnosis, Management, 8th ed. Philadelphia: WB Saunders, 2006.

Turnbull JM. Is listening for abdominal bruits useful in the evaluation of hypertension? JAMA 274(16):1299–1301, 1995.

Yamamoto W, Kono H, Maekawa H, et al. The relationship between abdominal pain regions and specific diseases: an epidemiologic approach to clinical practice. J Epidemiol 7(1):27–32, 1997.

Examination of the Liver

Meidl EJ, Ende J. Evaluation of liver size by physical examination. J Gen Intern Med 8(11):635–637, 1993.

Zoli M, Magliotti D, Drimaldi M, et al. Physical examination of the liver: is it still worth it? Am J Gastroenterol 90(9):1428–1432, 1995.

Examination of the Spleen

Barkun ANB, Camus M, Green L, et al. The bedside assessment of splenic enlargement. Am J Med 91(5):512–518, 1991.

Barkun AN, Camus M, Meagher T, et al. Splenic enlargement and Traube's space: how useful is percussion? Am J Med 87(5):562–566, 1989.

Tamayo SG, Rickman LS, Matthews WC, et al. Examiner dependence on physical diagnostic tests of splenomegaly: a prospective study with multiple observers. J Gen Intern Med 8(2):69–75, 1993.

Gastrointestinal Conditions

American Gastroenterological Association. American Gastroenterological Association Medical Position Statement: guidelines on constipation. Gastroenterology 119(6):1761–1778, 2000.

Bak E, Raman G, Chung M, et al. Effectiveness of management strategies for renal artery stenosis: a systematic review. Ann Intern Med 145(12):901–912, 2006.

Castronovo A, Bradway C. Urinary incontinence (UI) in older adults admitted to acute care. In: Capezuti E, Zwicker D, Mezey M, Fulmer T (eds). Evidence-Based Geriatric Nursing Protocols for Best Practice, 3rd ed. New York: Springer Publishing Company, 2008, pp. 309–336.

Craig AS, Schaffner W. Prevention of hepatitis A with the hepatitis A vaccine. N Engl J Med 350(5):476–480, 2004.

Lembo A, Camilleri M. Chronic constipation. N Engl J Med 349(14):1360–1368, 2003.

Mertz HR. Irritable bowel syndrome. N Engl J Med 349(22):2136–2146, 2003.

Ouslander JG. Management of the overactive bladder. N Engl J Med 350(8):786–799, 2004.

Shaheen N, Ransohoff DF. Gastroesophageal reflux, Barrett esophagus, and esophageal cancer: clinical applications. JAMA 287(15):1982–1986, 2002.

Thielman NM, Guerrant RL. Acute infectious diarrhea. N Engl J Med 350(1):38–47, 2004.

The Breasts and Axillae

LEARNING OBJECTIVES

The student will:

1. Identify the structures and function of the breasts and axillae.
2. Perform an accurate health history of the breasts and axillae.
3. Describe the physical examination techniques performed to evaluate the breasts and axillae.
4. Demonstrate how to perform a clinical breast examination.
5. Document a complete breast and axilla assessment utilizing information from the health history and the physical examination.
6. Determine the measures for prevention or early detection of breast cancer.

Breasts are present in both men and women. Until puberty, the male and female breasts are similar. The female breast tissue enlarges with the release of estrogen and progesterone and produces milk for nutrition of the newborn.

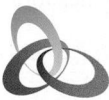 ## ANATOMY AND PHYSIOLOGY

THE FEMALE BREAST

The female breast lies against the anterior thoracic wall, extending from the clavicle down to the 6th rib, and from the sternum across to the midaxillary line. Its surface area is generally rectangular rather than round. The breast overlies the pectoralis major and, at its inferior margin, the serratus anterior.

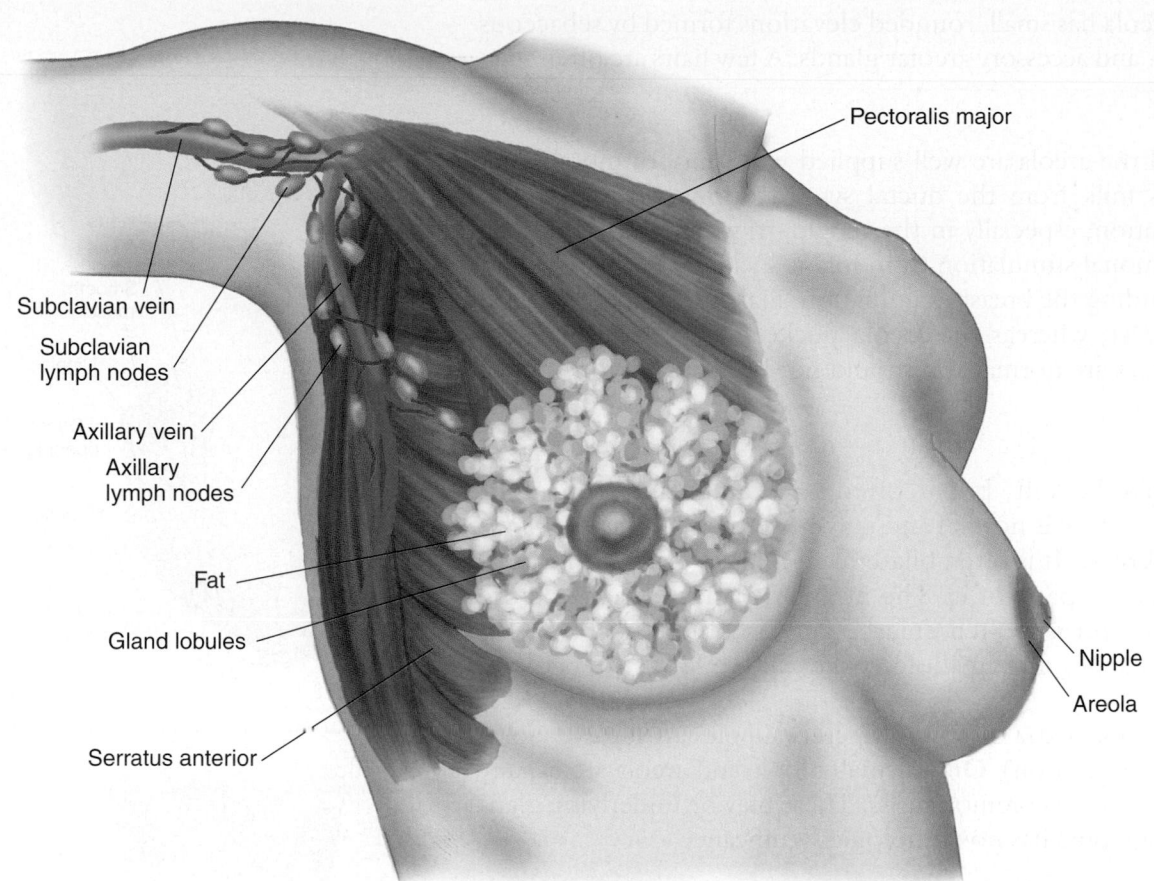

The breast is hormonally sensitive tissue, responsive to the changes of monthly cycles and aging. At the tip of the breast is an area called, the areola and at the center is the nipple. About 15 to 20 lactiferous ducts empty into a depression at the top of the nipple. Each duct leads from the alveoli within the breast called lobules, where the milk is secreted. Along their length, the duct widens into areas that form reservoirs where milk can be stored. These ducts and lobules form the *glandular tissue*. *Fibrous connective tissue* provides structural support in the form of fibrous bands or suspensory ligaments connected to both the skin and the underlying fascia. *Adipose tissue*, or fat, surrounds the breast, predominantly in the superficial and peripheral areas. The proportions of these components vary with age, the general state of nutrition, pregnancy, exogenous hormone use, and other factors.

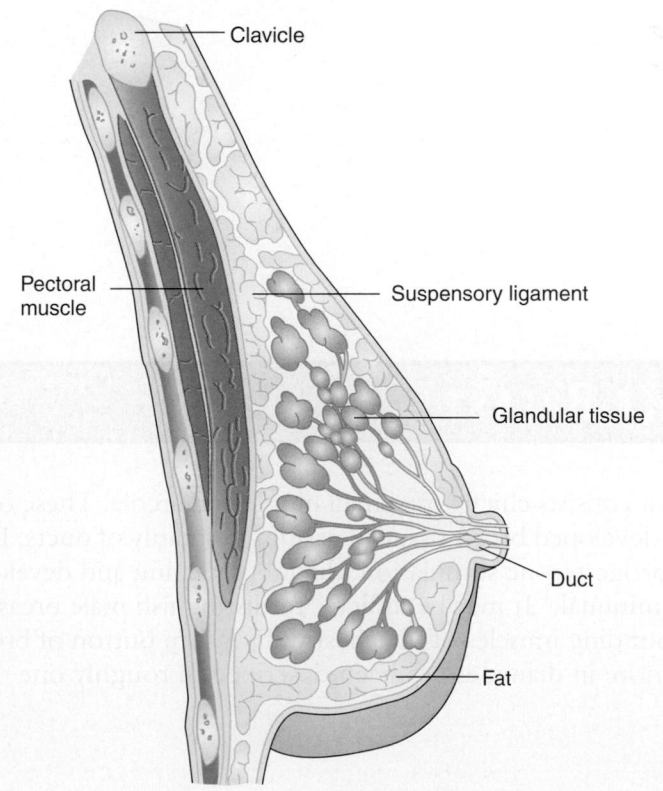

The surface of the areola has small, rounded elevations formed by sebaceous glands, sweat glands, and accessory areolar glands. A few hairs are often seen on the areola.

Both the nipple and the areola are well supplied with smooth muscle that contracts to express milk from the ductal system during breast-feeding. Rich sensory innervation, especially in the nipple, triggers "milk letdown" following neurohormonal stimulation from infant sucking. Tactile stimulation of the area, including the breast examination, makes the nipple smaller, firmer, and more erect, whereas the areola puckers and wrinkles. These smooth muscle reflexes are normal and should not be mistaken for signs of breast disease.

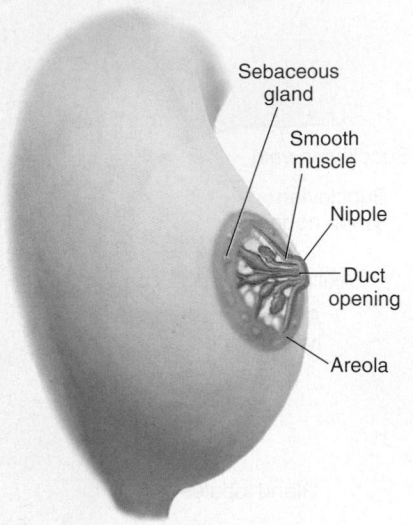

The adult breast may be soft, but it often feels granular, nodular, or lumpy. This uneven texture is normal and may be termed *physiologic nodularity* or fibrocystic breast. It is often bilateral. It may be evident throughout the breast or only in parts of it. The nodularity may increase before menses—a time when breasts often enlarge and become tender or even painful. For breast changes during adolescence go to p. 812.

Occasionally, one or more extra or supernumerary nipples are located along the "milk line," (see illustration). Only a small nipple and areola are usually present, often mistaken for a common mole. There may be underlying glandular tissue. An extra nipple has no pathologic significance.

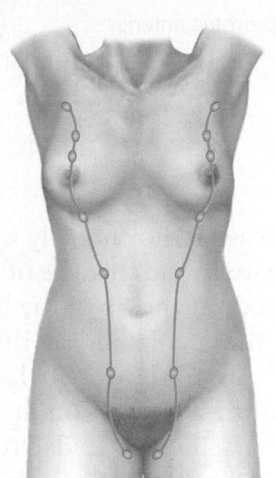

THE MALE BREAST

The male breast consists chiefly of a small nipple and areola. These overlie a thin disc of undeveloped breast tissue consisting primarily of ducts. Lacking estrogen and progesterone stimulation, ductal branching and development of lobules are minimal.[1] It may be difficult to distinguish male breast tissue from the surrounding muscles of the chest wall. A firm button of breast tissue, 2 cm or more in diameter has been described in roughly one of three adult men.

LYMPHATICS

Lymphatics from most of the breast drain toward the axilla. Of the axillary lymph nodes, the *central nodes* are palpable most frequently. They lie along the chest wall, usually high in the axilla and midway between the anterior and posterior axillary folds. Into them drain channels from three other groups of lymph nodes, which are seldom palpable:

- *Pectoral nodes—anterior,* located along the lower border of the pectoralis major inside the anterior axillary fold. These nodes drain the anterior chest wall and much of the breast.

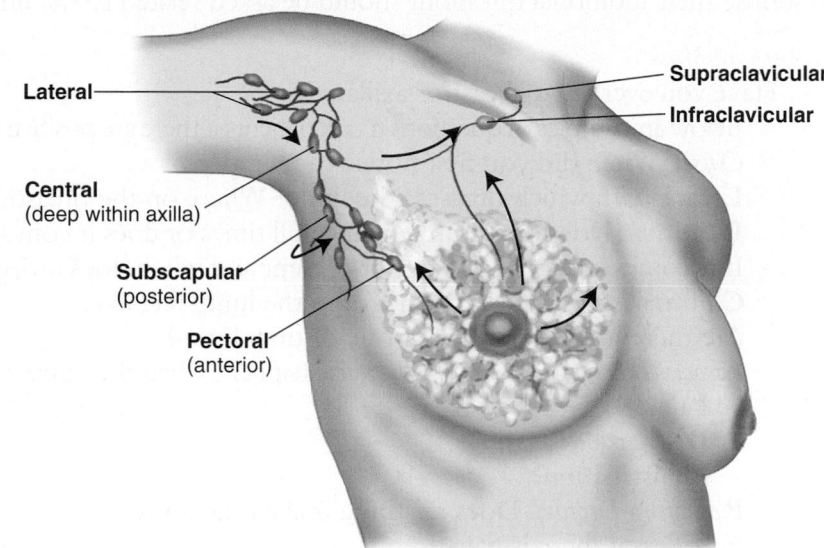

- *Subscapular nodes—posterior,* located along the lateral border of the scapula; palpated deep in the posterior axillary fold. They drain the posterior chest wall and a portion of the arm.

- *Lateral nodes*—located *along the upper humerus.* They drain most of the arm.

ARROWS INDICATE DIRECTION OF LYMPH FLOW

Lymph drains from the central axillary nodes to the *infraclavicular* and *supraclavicular* nodes.

Not all the lymphatics of the breast drain into the axilla. Malignant cells from a breast cancer may spread directly to the infraclavicular nodes or into deep channels within the chest.

 **THE HEALTH HISTORY**

COMMON OR CONCERNING SYMPTOMS

- Breast lump or mass
- Breast pain or discomfort
- Change in shape
- Nipple discharge
- Edema
- Rashes
- Scaling
- Dimpling
- Retraction

During the nursing assessment of the breast examination, begin with an open-ended question, such as:

"Have you noticed any changes in your breast?"

If the patient does not have any comments, then more specific questions are necessary as they may trigger a memory, reveal another area that the patient thought was "nothing" or not worth mentioning, or because during the breast assessment the patient may be too embarrassed to ask or answer questions related to this system. In addition, if the patient does have a positive response then additional questions should be asked related to the finding.

Lump or Mass

Have you ever felt a breast or axillary lump?

Below are samples of questions to ask patients if there are positive findings:

O*nset:* When did you first notice the lump?

L*ocation:* In which breast is the lump? Where on the breast?

D*uration:* Does the lump remain at all times or does it come and go? If it comes and goes, when is it present and when does it disappear?

C*haratistic Symptoms:* What does the lump feel like? Are there multiple lumps or one distinct lump?

A*ssociated Manifestations:* What else happens when the lump is present:
Pain?
Discharge?
Menstruation?

R*elieving Factors:* Does anything make it go away? Hurt less if there is pain?

T*reatment:* Have you done anything about the lump to make it disappear? Have you spoken to a health care provider?

Lumps may be physiologic or pathologic, ranging from cysts and fibroadenomas to breast cancer. See Table 17-1, p. 514, Common Breast Masses, and Table 17-2, p. 515, Visible Signs of Breast Cancer.

Pain or Discomfort

O*nset:* Do you ever have breast pain/discomfort? When do you have pain/discomfort?

L*ocation:* Where do you have pain/discomfort?

D*uration:* Does it come and go or is it constant?

C*haracteristic Symptoms:* Describe the pain/discomfort.

A*ssociated Manifestations:* What else happens with the pain/discomfort?

R*elieving Factors:* What have you done to make the pain/discomfort feel better?

T*reatment:* Have you done anything to treat the pain?

There are many questions related to the breast and use of the OLD CART mnemonic insures all areas of questioning are covered. Additional examples of questions continue for a variety of findings.

Change in Shape

Have you noticed any change in the *shape* of your breast?

When did you notice a change in the shape?

Where is the change? Which breast?

When did this occur?

What else happened at this time?

Can you associate anything else with this?

How are you coping with/treating this?

Discharge

Have you ever had *nipple discharge*?

When does the discharge occur?

In which breast does it occur, or is it both?

How long does the discharge last?

What is the color of the discharge? Consistency? Amount? Is there an odor?

What is associated with the discharge?

How do you deal with this?

Galactorrhea, or the inappropriate discharge of milk-containing fluid, is abnormal if it occurs 6 or more months after childbirth or cessation of breast-feeding.

Edema

Have you noticed any breast *edema*?

When does the edema occur?

Where does it occur? Which breast? Which quadrant?

How long does it last?

Is it painful?

What is the color of the breast?

What else occurs?

What do you do to relieve the swelling?

Rashes or Scaling

Have you noticed any *rashes*? *Scaling*? (Scaling consists of thin flakes of keratinized epithelium.)

When did this begin?

Where did this begin?

How long has it been going on?

Besides the rash/scaling of the skin, what else is happening?

Does it hurt?

What do you do to relieve the rash/scaling?

Dimpling

Have you noticed *dimpling* (small indents) of the breast tissue?

When did this begin?

In which breast did this begin?

How long has it been going on? Is it constant?

Are there any other symptoms occurring at this time?

Do you associate anything with this?

Are you treating this?

Retraction

Have you ever had nipple *retraction*?

When did the retraction occur?

Which nipple is retracted?

How long does it occur for? Does it evert at any time? When?

What happens when the nipple retracts?

Does anything else occur during the retraction?

Do you do anything to protract the nipple?

Nipple retraction is when the nipple is pulled inward. This is not an issue if the breast has had an inverted nipple since birth; however, it is noteworthy if this is a change as it could be an indicator of breast cancer or adhesions below the skin surface.

History

What medications (hormone replacement therapy [HRT], oral contraceptives [OC],) are you currently taking?

When did you begin taking the medication?
What is the medication name and dosage?
Are you having any side effects?
What other medications have you taken in the past?
　When did you take them and when did you stop?
　For how long did you take them?
　Why did you stop?
　Were there any side effects?
Pregnancies
　When were you pregnant?
　How many live births? Abortions? Miscarriages?
　How old were you at the delivery of your first baby?
　Did you breast feed your child(ren)? For how long?
Menstrual history
　How old were you at menarche?
　How old were you at menopause?
　How many days in your cycle?
Previous history of breast cancer and/or reproductive cancer
　When did you have breast cancer and/or reproductive cancer?
　In which breast did you have cancer? Or where was the reproductive
　　cancer?
　How did you find the cancer? Was there a lump?
　How was it treated?
　Who was on your health care team?
Previous breast biopsy
　Have you ever had a breast biospsy? If yes:
　　When? Where?
　　Results?
Breast self-examination (BSE)
　How often do you perform BSE?
　When do you perform BSE?
　What technique do you use?
　Have you ever palpated a lump or found any changes?
Clinical breast examination (CBE)
　When was your last examination by a health care provider?
　What were the results?
Mammogram or MRI
　When was your last mammogram or MRI?
　What were the results?
　What testing site do you utilize?
　Has the site changed? Did you transfer previous mammograms or
　　MRI results to this site?

Family History

Do you have a family history of breast cancer? genetic information or
　testing)?
　Do you have a family history of reproductive cancer? (eg ovarian)

If yes: who in the family has had any of the above? (sisters, mother, daughters, maternal aunts, maternal grandmother)?

Have you had BRCA testing?

Lifestyle Habits

How much alcohol do you use?

What do you do for physical activity?

 # PHYSICAL EXAMINATION

THE FEMALE BREAST

The clinical breast examination (CBE) is an important component of women's health care: it enhances detection of breast cancers that mammography may miss and provides an opportunity to demonstrate techniques for self-examination to the patient. Clinical investigation has shown, however, that variations in nurses' experience and technique affect the value of the clinical breast examination. Nurses are advised to adopt a more standardized approach, especially for palpation, and to use a systemic and thorough search pattern, varying palpation pressure, and a circular motion with the fingerpads.[2] These techniques will be discussed in more detail in the following pages. Inspection is routinely recommended, but its value in breast cancer detection is less well studied.

As you begin the examination of the breasts, be aware that women and girls may feel apprehensive. Be reassuring and adopt a courteous and gentle approach. Before you begin, let the patient know that you are about to examine her breasts. This may be a good time to ask if she has noticed any lumps, other problems or if she performs BSE. All women should be familiar with the look and feel of their breasts to detect any changes. A woman who chooses to do BSE should receive instructions.

A comprehensive inspection initially requires full exposure of the chest, but later in the examination, cover one breast while you are palpating the other. Because breasts tend to swell and become more nodular before menses as a result of increasing estrogen stimulation, the best time for examination is 5 to 7 days *after* the onset of menstruation. Nodules appearing prior to menstruation should be reevaluated 5 to 7 days after the onset of menses.

Inspection

Inspect the breasts and nipples with the patient in the sitting position and disrobed to the waist. A thorough examination of the breast includes careful inspection for skin changes, symmetry, contours, and retraction in four views—arms at sides, arms over head, arms pressed against hips, and leaning forward. When examining an adolescent girl, assess her breast development according to Tanner's sex maturity ratings described on p. 812.

Risk factors for breast cancer include previous breast cancer, an affected mother or sister, biopsy showing atypical hyperplasia, increasing age, early menarche, late menopause, late or no pregnancies, and previous radiation to the chest wall. See table on Breast Cancer in Women: Factors That Increase Relative Risk, p. 508.

See Patient Instructions for the Breast Self-Examination, pp. 505–506.

Arms at Sides. Note the clinical features listed below.

- The *appearance of the skin*, including:

  - Color

    Redness in a light complexion or deeper pigmentation in a dark skin woman may be from local infection or inflammatory carcinoma.

  - Thickening of the skin and unusually prominent pores, which may accompany lymphatic obstruction

    Thickening and prominent pores suggest breast cancer.

- The *size and symmetry of the breasts.* Some difference in the size of the breasts, including the areolae, is common and is usually normal, as shown in the photograph below.

- The *contour of the breasts.* Look for changes such as masses, dimpling, or flattening. Compare one side with the other.

  Flattening of the normally convex breast suggests cancer. See Table 17-2, Visible Signs of Breast Cancer (p. 515).

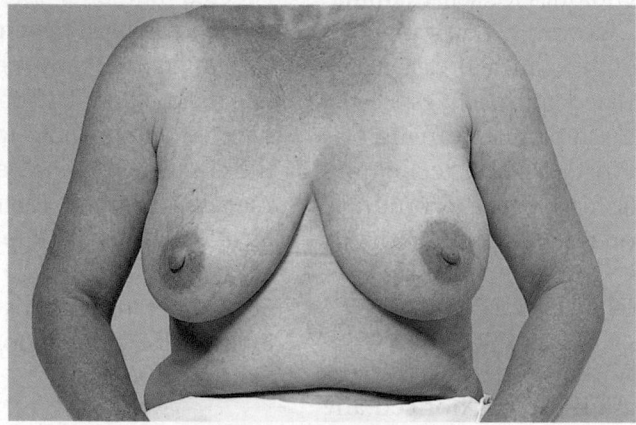

ARMS AT SIDES

- The *characteristics of the nipples,* including *size and shape, direction* in which they point, any *rashes* or *ulceration*, or any *discharge*

  Asymmetry of directions in which nipples point suggests an underlying cancer. Rash or ulceration in Paget disease of the breast[3] (see p. 515)

Occasionally, the shape of the nipple is *inverted,* or depressed below the areolar surface. It may be enveloped by folds of areolar skin, as illustrated. Long-standing inversion is usually a normal variant of no clinical consequence, except for possible difficulty when breast-feeding.

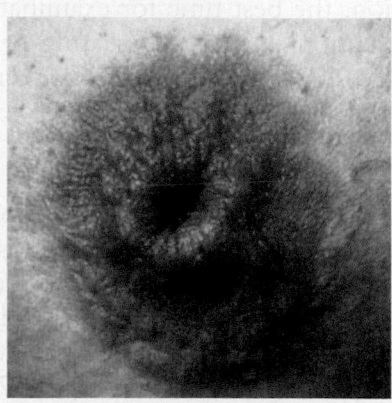

Recent or fixed flattening or depression of the nipple suggests nipple retraction. A retracted nipple may also be broadened and thickened, suggesting an underlying cancer.

Arms Over Head; Hands Pressed Against Hips; Leaning Forward.

To bring out dimpling or retraction that may otherwise be invisible, ask the patient to raise her arms over her head, and then press her hands against her hips to contract the pectoral muscles. Inspect the breast contours carefully in each position. If the breasts are large or pendulous, it may be useful to have the patient stand and lean forward, supported by the back of the chair.

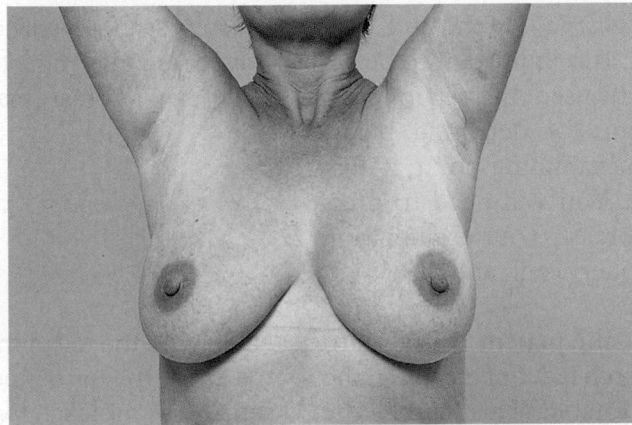

ARMS OVER HEAD

Dimpling or retraction of the breasts in these positions suggests an underlying cancer. When a cancer or its associated fibrous strands are attached to both the skin and the fascia overlying the pectoral muscles, pectoral contraction can draw the skin inward, causing dimpling.

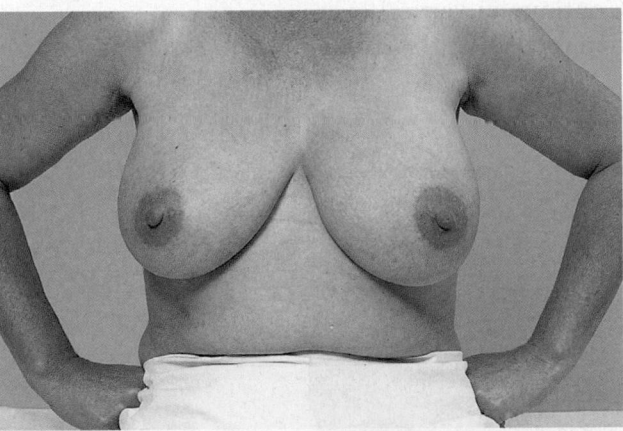

HANDS PRESSED AGAINST HIPS

Occasionally, these signs may be associated with benign lesions such as posttraumatic fat necrosis or mammary duct ectasia, but they must always be further evaluated.

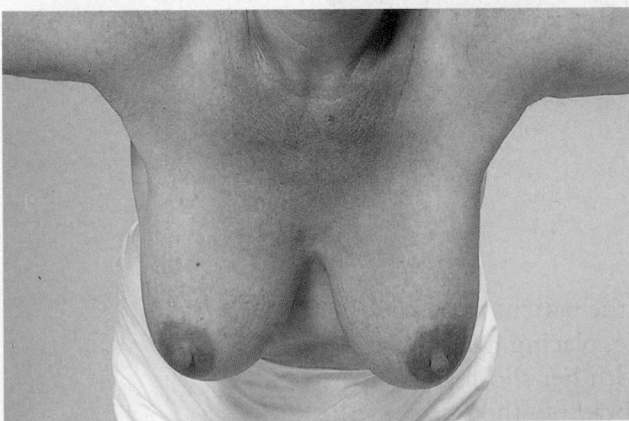

LEANING FORWARD

This position may reveal an asymmetry of the breast or nipple not otherwise visible. Retraction of the nipple and areola suggests an underlying cancer. See Table 17-2, Visible Signs of Breast Cancer (p. 515).

Palpation

The Breast.   Palpation is best performed when the breast tissue is flattened. The patient should be supine. Plan to palpate a rectangular area
extending from the clavicle to the inframammary fold or lower bra line, and
from the midsternal line to the posterior axillary line and well into the axilla
for the tail of the breast.

A thorough examination will take time. Use the *fingerpads* of the 2nd, 3rd,
and 4th fingers, keeping the fingers slightly flexed. It is important to be *systematic*. Although a circular or wedge pattern can be used, the *vertical strip
pattern* is currently the best validated technique for detecting breast
masses.[2] Palpate in *small, concentric circles* at each examining point, if possible applying light, medium, and deep pressure. You will need to press
more firmly to reach the deeper tissues of a large breast. Your examination
should cover the entire breast, including the periphery, tail, and axilla.

- To examine *the lateral portion of the breast,* ask the patient to roll onto
  the opposite hip, placing her hand on her forehead but keeping the
  shoulders pressed against the bed or examining table. This flattens the
  lateral breast tissue. Begin palpation in the axilla, moving in a straight
  line down to the bra line, and then move the fingers medially and palpate
  in a vertical strip up the chest to the clavicle. Continue in vertical overlapping strips until you reach the nipple, and then reposition the patient
  to flatten the medial portion of the breast.

When pressing deeply on the
breast, you may mistake a normal
rib for a hard breast mass.

Nodules in the tail of the breast in
the axilla (the tail of Spence) are
sometimes mistaken for enlarged
axillary lymph nodes.

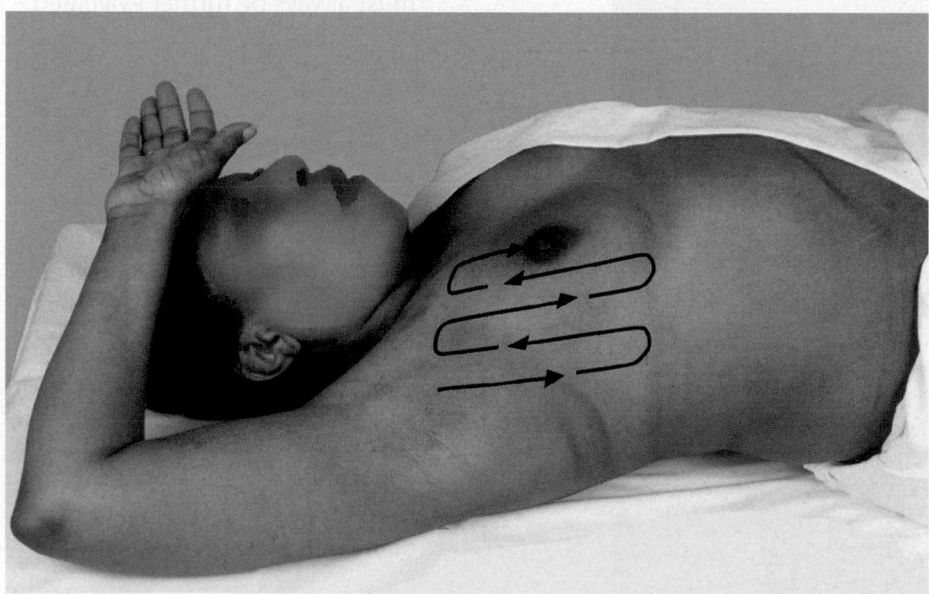

- To examine *the medial portion of the breast,* ask the patient to lie with her
  shoulders flat against the bed or examining table, placing her hand at her
  neck and lifting up her elbow until it is even with her shoulder. Palpate
  in a straight line down from the nipple to the bra line, then back to the
  clavicle, continuing in vertical overlapping strips to the midsternum.

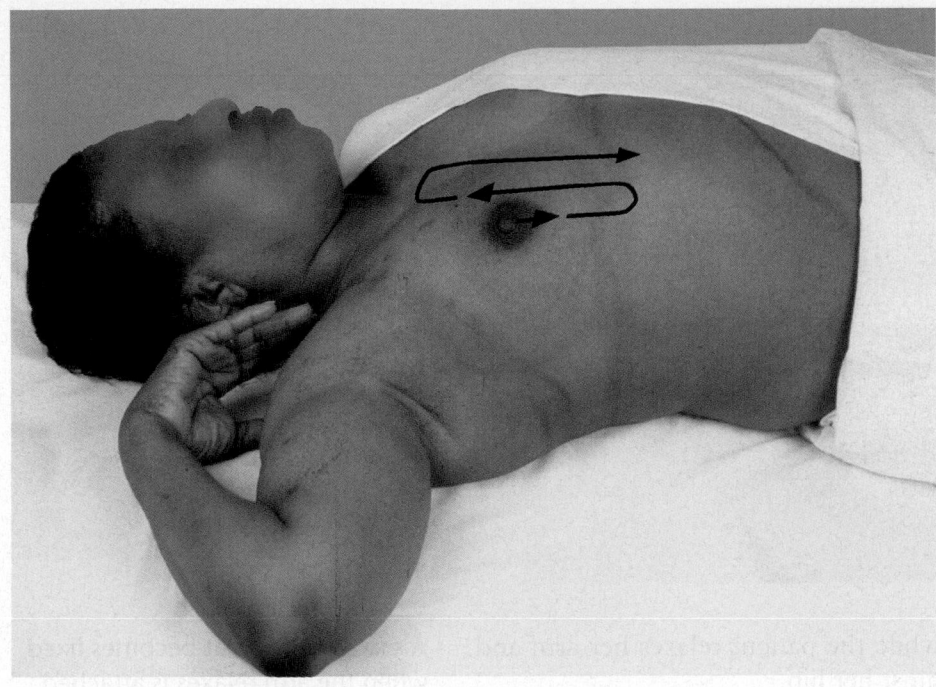

Examine the breast tissue carefully for:

- *Consistency* of the tissues. Normal consistency varies widely, depending in part on the relative proportions of firmer glandular tissue and soft fat. Physiologic nodularity may be present, increasing before menses. There may be a firm transverse ridge of compressed tissue along the lower margin of the breast, especially in large breasts. This is the normal inframammary ridge, not a tumor.

- *Tenderness,* as in premenstrual fullness

- *Nodules.* Palpate carefully for any lump or mass that is different from the rest of the breast tissue. This is sometimes called a dominant mass and may reflect a pathologic change that requires evaluation by mammogram, MRI, aspiration, or biopsy. Document the characteristics of any nodule:

    Location—which breast, the quadrant or clock site, centimeters from the nipple
    Size—in centimeters
    Shape—round or cystic, disc-like, or irregular in contour
    Consistency—soft, firm, or hard
    Delineation—well circumscribed or not
    Tenderness—tender or nontender
    Mobility—in relation to the skin, pectoral fascia, and chest wall. Gently move the breast near the mass and watch for dimpling.

Tender cords suggest *mammary duct ectasia,* a benign but sometimes painful condition of dilated ducts with surrounding inflammation, sometimes with associated masses.

See Table 17-1, Common Breast Masses (p. 514).

Hard, irregular, poorly circumscribed nodules, fixed to the skin or underlying tissues, strongly suggest breast cancer.

Cysts, inflamed areas; some cancers may be tender.

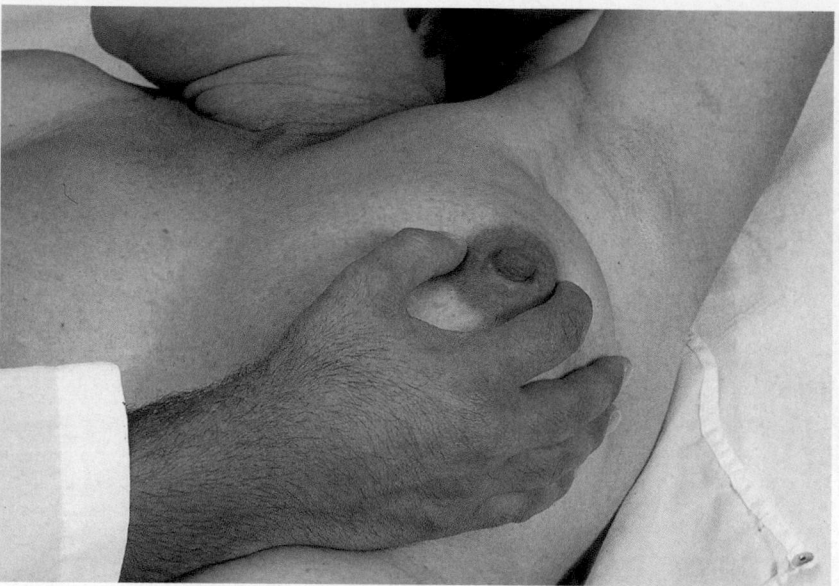

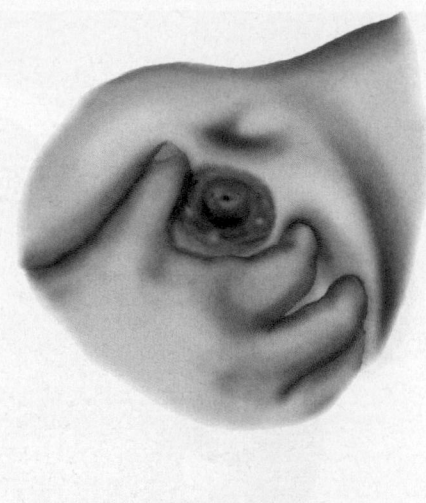

- Next, try to move the mass itself while the patient relaxes her arm and then while she presses her hand against her hip.

A mobile mass that becomes fixed when the arm relaxes is attached to the ribs and intercostal muscles; if fixed when the hand is pressed against the hip, it is attached to the pectoral fascia.

If a lump is detected, documentation of the breast assessment is acceptable in either of two forms:

1. Divide the breast into four quadrants with a horizontal line and a vertical line crossing at the nipple, the center point.

2. The breast is the face of a clock with 12 o'clock at the top, 6 o'clock at the bottom.

If an area needs to be specifically identified (e.g., to determine the exact site of a lump), the distance in centimeters from the nipple in the respective quadrant is charted. The area that extends laterally across the exterior fold is the tail of Spence.

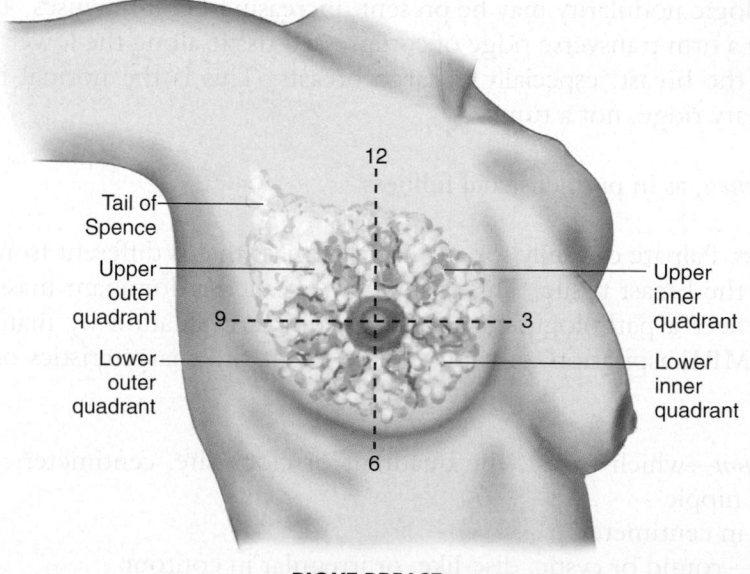

RIGHT BREAST

The Nipple. Palpate each nipple, noting its elasticity.

Thickening of the nipple and loss of elasticity suggest an underlying breast cancer.

THE MALE BREAST

Examination of the male breast may be brief but is important. *Inspect the nipple and areola* for nodules, swelling, or ulceration. *Palpate the areola and breast tissue* for nodules. If the breast appears enlarged, distinguish between the soft fatty enlargement of obesity and the firm disc of glandular enlargement, called *gynecomastia*.

Gynecomastia arises from an imbalance of estrogens and androgens, sometimes medication related. A hard, irregular, eccentric, or ulcerating nodule suggests breast cancer.

Male breast cancer constitutes only 1% of breast cancer cases, peaking in frequency around age 71.[4,5]

THE AXILLAE

Although the axillae may be examined with the patient lying down, a sitting position is preferable.

Inspection

Inspect the skin of each axilla, noting evidence of:

- Rash

Deodorant and other rashes

- Infection

Sweat gland infection (*hidradenitis suppurativa*)

- Unusual pigmentation

Deeply pigmented, velvety axillary skin suggests *acanthosis nigricans*—one form is associated with internal malignancy.

Palpation

To examine the left axilla, ask the patient to relax with the left arm down. Help by supporting the left wrist or hand with your left hand. Wearing a glove, cup together the fingers of your right hand and reach as high as you can toward the apex of the axilla. Warn the patient that this may feel uncomfortable. Your fingers should lie directly behind the pectoral muscles, pointing toward the midclavicle. Now press your fingers in toward the chest wall and slide them downward, trying to feel the central nodes against the chest wall. Of the axillary nodes, these are the most often palpable. One or more soft, small (<1 cm), nontender nodes are frequently felt.

Enlarged axillary nodes are from an infection of the hand or arm, recent immunizations or skin tests in the arm, or part of a generalized lymphadenopathy. Check the epitrochlear nodes and other groups of lymph nodes.

Nodes that are large (≥1 cm) and firm or hard, matted together, or fixed to the skin or to underlying tissues suggest malignant involvement.

Use your left hand to examine the right axilla.

If the central nodes feel large, hard, or tender, or if there is a suspicious lesion in the drainage areas for the axillary nodes, feel for the other groups of axillary lymph nodes:

- *Pectoral nodes*—grasp the anterior axillary fold between your thumb and fingers, and with your fingers, palpate inside the border of the pectoral muscle.

- *Lateral nodes*—from high in the axilla, feel along the upper humerus.

- *Subscapular nodes*—step behind the patient and, with your fingers, feel inside the muscle of the posterior axillary fold.

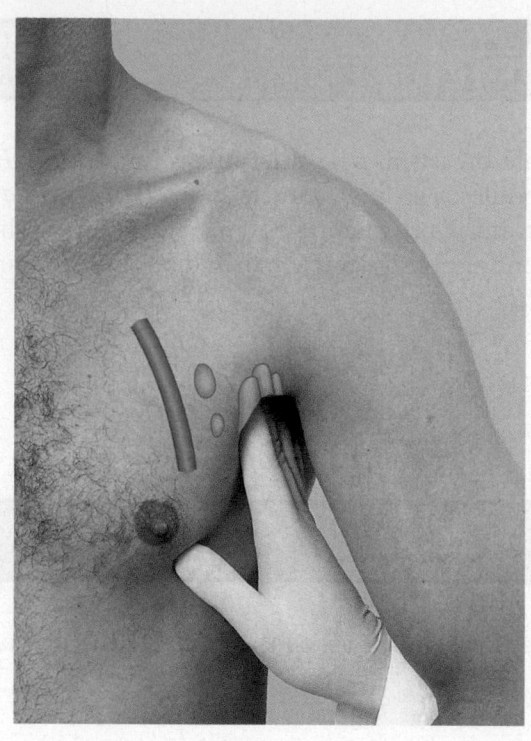

Also, feel for infraclavicular nodes and reexamine the supraclavicular nodes.

SPECIAL TECHNIQUES

Assessment of Spontaneous Nipple Discharge.   If there is a history of spontaneous nipple discharge, try to determine its origin by compressing the areola with your index finger, placed in radial positions around the nipple. Watch for discharge appearing through one of the duct openings on the nipple's surface. Note the color, consistency, and quantity of any discharge and the exact location where it appears.

Milky discharge unrelated to a prior pregnancy and lactation is *nonpuerperal galactorrhea.* Causes include *hypothyroidism,* pituitary *prolactinoma,* and drugs that are dopamine agonists, including many psychotropic agents and phenothiazines.

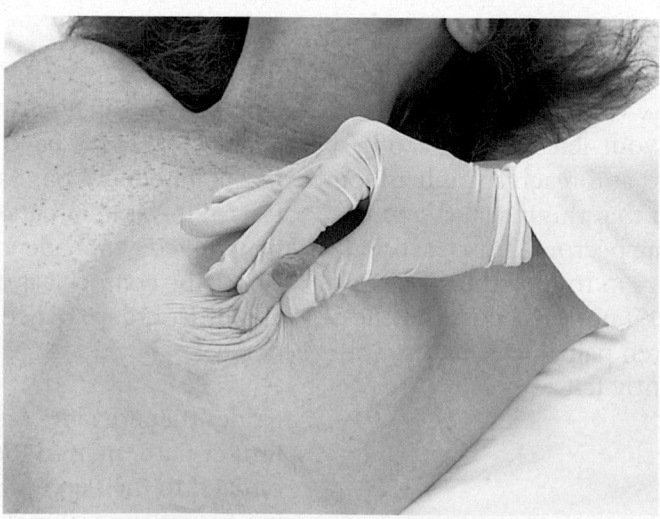

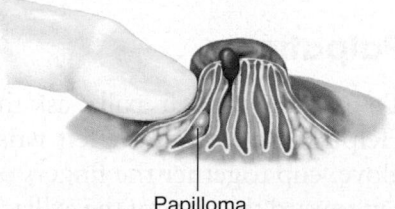

Papilloma

Spontaneous unilateral bloody discharge from one or two ducts warrants further evaluation for intraductal *papilloma,* as shown; ductal carcinoma in situ; or Paget disease of the breast. Clear, serous, green, black, or nonbloody discharges that are multiductal usually require only reassurance.[1]

Examination of the Mastectomy or Breast Augmentation Patient. The woman with a mastectomy warrants special care on examination. Inspect the mastectomy scar and axilla carefully for any masses or unusual nodularity. Note any change in color or signs of inflammation. Lymphedema may be present in the axilla and upper arm from impaired lymph drainage after surgery. Palpate gently along the scar—these tissues may be unusually sensitive. Use a circular motion with two or three fingers. Pay special attention to the upper outer quadrant and axilla, as 50% of breast lumps are found in the upper outer quadrant. Note any enlargement of the lymph nodes or signs of inflammation or infection.

Masses, nodularity, and change in color or inflammation, especially in the incision line, suggest recurrence of breast cancer.

It is especially important to carefully palpate the breast tissue and incision lines of women with breast augmentation or reconstruction.

Self Awareness and Instructions for the Breast Self-Examination. If a woman chooses to perform SBE, the nurse should take the opportunity to teach her the technique. Breast masses can be detected by women examining their own breasts. Although BSE has not been shown to reduce breast cancer mortality, BSE is inexpensive and may promote stronger health awareness and more active self-care. For early detection of breast cancer, the BSE is an option for women and is most useful when coupled with regular breast examination by an experienced clinician and mammography or MRI. The BSE is best timed just after menses, when hormonal stimulation of breast tissue is low.

BREAST AWARENESS AND SELF EXAMINATION INSTRUCTIONS

Lying Supine

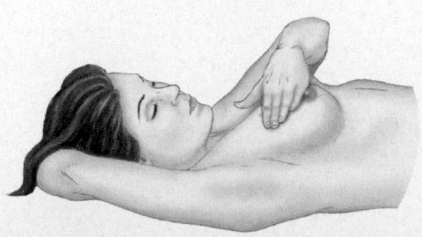
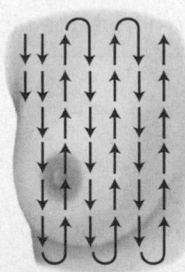

- Lie down and place your right arm behind your head. The exam is done while lying down, not standing up.
- Use the finger pads of the 3 middle fingers on your left hand to feel for lumps in the right breast. Use overlapping dime-sized circular motions of the finger pads to feel the breast tissue.
- Use 3 different levels of pressure to feel all the breast tissue. Light pressure is needed to feel the tissue closest to the skin;

medium pressure to feel a little deeper; and firm pressure to feel the tissue closest to the chest and ribs. If you are not sure how hard to press, talk with your health care provider.
- Move in an up and down pattern. Be sure to check the entire breast.
- Repeat the exam on your left breast, putting your left arm behind your head and using the finger pads of your right hand to do the exam.

(continued)

BREAST AWARENESS AND SELF EXAMINATION INSTRUCTIONS (continued)

Standing

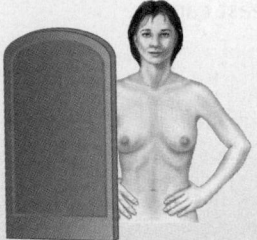

- Stand in front of a mirror with your hands pressing firmly on your hips, look for any changes of: size, shape, contour, dimpling, redness or scaliness of the nipple or breast skin.
- Examine each underarm while sitting up or standing and with your arm only slightly raised so you can easily feel in this area.

Adapted from the American Cancer Society. Available at: http://www.cancer.org/Cancer/BreastCancer/DetailedGuide/breast-cancer-detection. Accessed April 17, 2011.

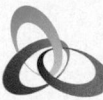

RECORDING YOUR FINDINGS

Recording the Physical Examination—Breasts and Axillae

"Breasts symmetric, color tan without pigment changes and smooth bilaterally; no masses, dimpling, lumps, edema, or thickening; nipples everted, equal in size, point outward; no discharge, rashes, or ulcerations."

OR

"Breasts pendulous with diffuse fibrocystic changes. Single firm 1 × 1 cm mass, mobile and nontender, with overlying peau d'orange appearance in right breast, upper outer quadrant at 11 o'clock, 2 cm from the nipple."

Suggests possible breast cancer

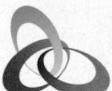

HEALTH PROMOTION AND COUNSELING

Important Topics for Health Promotion and Counseling

- Palpable masses of the breast
- Assessing risk of breast cancer
- Breast cancer screening

Overview

Women may experience a wide range of changes in breast tissue and sensation, from cyclic swelling and nodularity to a distinct lump or mass. The examination of the breast provides a meaningful opportunity for the nurse to explore concerns important to women's health—what to do if a lump or mass is detected, risk factors for breast cancer, and measures such as BSE, the CBE by a health care provider, mammography, and MRI. Women will frequently seek information during the clinical encounter. Men can also have breast cancer. If any noted changes or lumps are detected, men should also see their health care provider.

Palpable Masses of the Breast and Breast Symptoms. Breast cancer occurs in up to 4% of women with breast complaints, in approximately 5% of women reporting a nipple discharge, and in up to 11% of women specifically complaining of a breast lump or mass.[1,2] Breast masses show marked variation in etiology, from fibroadenomas and cysts seen in younger women, to abscess or mastitis, to primary breast cancer. On initial assessment, the woman's age and physical characteristics of the mass provide clues about its etiology. All breast masses require careful assessment. Nurses are the advocates and help navigate the complex health care system. Nurses assist patients to follow up for accurate diagnosis and treatment.

Assessing Risk of Breast Cancer. Women are increasingly interested in information about breast cancer. Nurses are urged to be familiar with the literature detailing the epidemiology of and risk factors for breast cancer that supports recommendations for screening. Key facts and figures are presented here, but further reading will enhance your counseling of patients.

Breast cancer is the second leading cause of cancer death in women, with highest mortality rates in women 35 years or younger and older than 75 years. There are several trends of note.[4]

● *Declines in new cases of invasive breast cancer.* The number of new cases of invasive breast cancer has been falling since 2000, explained by two main factors: decreased mammography screening, which leads to underdiagnosis or delayed diagnosis rather than a true decrease in disease incidence, and decreased use of HRT.[6]

● *Earlier and more advanced breast cancer in African-American women.*

Breast cancer is the most commonly diagnosed cancer among African American women. Breast cancer incidence rates increased rapidly among African American women during the 1980s. This coincided with increased detection with the use of mammography. Incidence rates stabilized among African American women aged 50 and older during 1994–2007, while rates decreased by 0.6% per year from 1991–2007 among women under age 50.[7]

The 5-year relative survival rate for breast cancer diagnosed in 1999–2006 among African American women was 78%, compared to 90% among white women. This disparity relates to the cancer detection at later stages. Only about 51% of African American women are diagnosed at a local stage and 61% of white women are diagnosed at this point. A number of factors contribute to the later diagnosis: fewer African American woman receiving mammograms, longer time periods between mammograms or follow up to health care providers and there has also been data that suggests the tumors are more aggressive in African American women.[3]

Assessing Risk Factors for Breast Cancer. Both *modifiable* and *nonmodifiable risk factors* for breast cancer have been identified, as listed in the table on the next page. Many risk factors cannot be readily altered, such as gender, age, family history, race, genetics, personal history of breast cancer, age at first full-term pregnancy, early menarche, late menopause, and breast density.[4] Others can be modified, although these tend to confer lower relative risk: postmenopausal obesity, use of estrogen-progesterone combination HRT, alcohol use, and physical inactivity. The table below from the American Cancer Society report "Breast Cancer Facts and Figures 2009–2010."[4] summarizes the strengths of current risk factors. Readers are encouraged to review the excellent discussions of individual risk factors presented in this report.

● **Breast Cancer in Women: Factors That Increase Relative Risk**

Relative Risk	Factor
>4.0	• Female • Age (65+ versus <65 years, although risk increases across all ages until age 80) • Certain inherited genetic mutations for breast cancer (BRCA1 and/or BRCA2) • Two or more first-degree relatives with breast cancer diagnosed at an early age • Personal history of breast cancer • High breast tissue density • Biopsy-confirmed atypical hyperplasia
2.1–4.0	• One first-degree relative with breast cancer • High-dose radiation to chest • High bone density (postmenopausal)
1.1–2.0 Factors that affect circulating hormones	• Late age at first full-term pregnancy (>30 years) • Early menarche (<12 years) • Late menopause (>55 years) • No full-term pregnancies • Never breast-fed a child • Recent oral contraceptive use • Recent and long-term use of hormone replacement therapy • Obesity (postmenopausal)
Other factors	• Personal history of endometrium, ovary, or colon cancer • Alcohol consumption • Height (tall) • High socioeconomic status • Jewish heritage

(Source: American Cancer Society. Breast Cancer Facts & Figures 2009-2010. Atlanta: American Cancer Society, Inc. Available at: http://www.cancer.org/acs/groups/content/@nho/documents/document/f861009final90809pdf.pdf, Accessed April 17, 2011.

Selected Risk Factors That Affect Screening Decisions

BRCA1 and 2 Mutations. It is important to begin evaluating a woman's risk for breast cancer even in her 20s. Women of all ages should be asked if there is a family history of breast or ovarian cancer, or both, on both the maternal and paternal sides. Approximately 5% to 10% of women have genetic risk of BRCA1 or BRCA2 gene mutation. These genes are autosomal dominant. Women with BRCA1 mutations and BRCA2 mutations have an estimated 57% and 49% risk of developing breast cancer by age 70, respectively.[4] To identify women who should be referred for possible genetic testing, two strategies are recommended, detailed in the table below.[9]

CRITERIA FOR IDENTIFYING WOMEN AT RISK FOR BRCA1 OR 2 MUTATION

- Using the risk calculator at http://astor.som.jhmi.edu/brcapro/, determine that the risk for a BRCA1 or 2 mutation is at least 10%.
- Establish one of the following risk factors:
  - First-degree relative with a known BRCA1 or 2 mutation
  - ≥2 relatives with a diagnosis of breast cancer before age 50, and ≥1 is a first-degree relative
  - ≥3 relatives with a diagnosis of breast cancer, and ≥1 occurred before age 50
  - ≥2 relatives with a diagnosis of ovarian cancer
  - ≥1 relative with a diagnosis of breast cancer, and ≥1 relative has a diagnosis of ovarian cancer

(Source: Fletcher SW, Elmore JG. Mammographic screening for breast cancer. N Engl J Med 348[14]:1672–1680, 2003.)

Benign Breast Disorders. Mammograms are resulting in increasing numbers of breast biopsies, and clinicians should now understand the effects of benign breast disease on risk for later breast cancer.[1,10] Within a decade of starting annual screening, 20% of women have had a breast biopsy.[11] Breast lesions are believed to evolve in somewhat linear fashion from usual ductal hyperplasia, or unfolded lobules, to atypical hyperplasia, to the pathologic stages of ductal carcinoma in situ (DCIS) and invasive cancer. These disorders are now classified by degree of cellular proliferation on biopsy and degree of risk for breast cancer. Women with atypia are more likely to have strong family history of breast cancer (approximately 28% vs. 20%). Their risk increases when atypia is diagnosed at younger ages. Currently studies show no increased risk for women with *nonproliferative* findings and no family history of breast cancer.

● Risk of Breast Cancer and Histology of Benign Breast Lesions[1,10]

- *No increased risk,* relative risk approximately 1.3

  Nonproliferative changes: including cysts and ductal *ectasia,* mild *hyperplasia,* simple *fibroadenoma, mastitis, granuloma,* diabetic mastopathy

- *Small increased risk,* or relative risk 1.5–2.0

  Proliferative without atypia: including usual ductal hyperplasia, complex fibroadenoma, papilloma

- *Moderate increased risk,* or relative risk >2.0 to approximately 4.2

  Proliferative with atypia: including atypical ductal hyperplasia and atypical lobular hyperplasia

---

Breast Density.   Mammographic breast density has been identified as "the most undervalued and underused risk factor" in studies of breast cancer.[12] It is a strong independent risk factor even after adjusting for the effects of other risk factors, and it has the important attribute of "being present in the tissue from which the cancer arises."[13] Stromal and epithelial tissues appear radiologically light and dense, reflecting higher proportions of stromal and glandular tissue and increased ductal and atypical ductal hyperplasia. A proposed mechanism is proliferation of breast epithelial cells and stromal fibrosis in response to growth factors induced by circulating sex hormones.

An analysis of studies quantifying breast density found that women with radiologic density in more than 60% to 75% of the breast are at four to six times greater risk of breast cancer than women with no breast density.[12] Breast density may account for up to 30% of the risk for breast cancer and has a strong inherited component.[14] It is not yet known if breast density is associated with the increased risk of breast cancer seen in women with elevated blood levels of estrogen, free estradiol, and testosterone, which metabolizes to estrone and estradiol.[1,15]

Breast density affects the sensitivity and specificity of mammograms, dropping from 88% and 96% in women with predominantly fatty breast tissue to 62% and 89% in women with breasts that are extremely dense, respectively.[12] Sensitivity and specificity appear lowest in younger women taking HRT, leading authors to recommend that mammography reports include statements about breast density that might influence decisions about use of HRT.

Recommendations for Breast Cancer Screening and Chemoprevention

Individualized and BRCA1 and BRCA2 Screening.   Discussions about risk factors for breast cancer can begin at any age. Screen all women regardless of age for general risk of breast cancer and risk of BRCA1 and 2 inheritance, using the methods noted above. Also assess family history of ovarian cancer.

Mammography
Women 40 to 50 Years.   Use of *mammography* in asymptomatic women in this age group has been controversial because of lower sensitivity

and specificity, possibly related to breast density; increasing risk of false positives and subsequent biopsy; difficulty individualizing risks and benefits; and variation in individual values and preferences. Over the past several years, there have been some differing opinions among the professional groups over the best recommendations, The American Cancer Society endorses mammography annually for women in their 40s. The U.S. Preventive Health Services Task Force recommends biennial screening mammography for women aged 50 to 74 years.

A review for the American College of Physicians supports individualized discussion of risks and benefits in this age group. *Shared decision making* is especially important for this age group given the varying risks and benefits.[9,16]

Women 50 Years or Older. Screening mammography reduces breast cancer mortality in women 50 to 74 years.[4] Mammography detects 80% to 90% of breast cancers in asymptomatic women and has a specificity of 90%. Screening should continue for women older than 74 years, taking life expectancy and health status into account. (See Chapter 24, The Older Adult, p. 869). Inform women of the increased likelihood of recall for return examinations because of unclear findings and that abnormal findings may lead to biopsy.[17] Digital mammography shows promise for even greater accuracy, especially for younger women and women with dense breasts.[18]

Clinical Breast Examination. The American Cancer Society recommends performing the *clinical breast examination* every 3 years in women 20 to 40 years, and annually after 40 years. Other professional groups find evidence of benefit insufficient to support a definitive recommendation.[4] CBE sensitivity and specificity are 54% and 94%, respectively, and depend on the technique of the examiner.[2] CBE has not been clearly shown to decrease mortality and should be performed in conjunction with mammography.

Breast Self-Examination. The American Cancer Society no longer recommends monthly BSE. Although BSE does not improve detection of breast cancer, it does promote patient self-awareness, and a nurse should instruct women interested in using BSE in proper technique. Monthly BSE 5 to 7 days after the onset of menses can be taught to women as early as their 20s. (See Patient Instructions for the BSE, on pp. 505–506.)

Magnetic Resonance Imaging (MRI). Some recent studies have investigated use of *breast MRI* in women at high risk for breast cancer, younger women, women with dense breasts, and the contralateral breast of women with newly diagnosed breast cancer. In these groups, breast MRI has helped improve detection of multicentric or contralateral breast cancer prior to management decisions about breast-conserving strategies or initiation of treatment regimens.[19–21] However, cost is high and specificity is 70% to 90%, resulting in more false positives, recalls, and biopsies.[4,9,17] Expertise in reading MRIs and MRI-guided biopsy, an important adjunct to use of breast MRI, is not widely available. Finally, breast MRI has not been evaluated for screening in the general population. Currently the American Cancer Society recommends breast MRI for women at high lifetime risk, or risk of 20% or more.[4] Women at moderately increased lifetime risk, or risk of 15% to 20%, are encouraged to discuss benefits and drawbacks with their providers. Criteria for classifying risk are given next.

● Criteria for Classifying Breast Cancer Risk and Referrals for Breast MRI

High Risk, or 20%–25%	Moderate Risk, or 15%–20%
• Known BRCA1 or 2 mutation • Known first-degree relative, including father or brother, with BRCA1 or 2 mutation, but woman not tested • Lifetime risk 20%–25% using assessment tools • History of chest radiation between ages 10 and 30 • Has high-risk genetic syndrome or first-degree relative with high-risk syndrome	• History of breast cancer, ductal or lobular carcinoma in situ, atypical ductal or lobular hyperplasia • Extremely dense breasts or unevenly dense breasts on mammograms

(Source: American Cancer Society. Breast Cancer Facts and Figures 2009–2010. p 16. Available at: http://www.cancer.org/acs/groups/content@nho/documents/document/f861009final90809pdf.pdf. Accessed June 20, 2011.)

Chemoprevention. The U.S. Preventive Services Task Force recommends discussion of chemoprevention with estrogen-receptor modulators in women at high risk for breast cancer and at low risk for adverse effects, but it recommends against routine use for primary prevention in women at low or average risk. The Task Force found substantial evidence that these modulators reduce the incidence of estrogen-receptor–positive breast cancer.[4,22–24] Clinicians are urged to review the literature on risks and benefits of these agents for women at high risk for developing breast cancer within 5 years. The Task Force notes that the balance of benefit and harm is more favorable for women in their 40s or 50s at increased risk and without predisposition to thromboembolic events, and for women in their 50s without a uterus. Further, key studies use the Gail model cutoff of 1.66 as high risk; however, the revised Gail model addresses prevention of invasive and noninvasive cancers, but it does not discriminate between risks of estrogen-receptor–positive versus estrogen-receptor–negative cancers.[25,26] *Prophylactic bilateral mastectomy* is also advised in women at very high genetic risk.

Counseling Women about Breast Cancer

The Challenges of Communicating Risks and Benefits. As breast cancer screening and prevention options become more complex, nurses should consider how best to express statistics on risks and benefits in terms that patients can easily understand. Framing, or the effect of presenting the same information in terms of either increased benefit or decreased harm, is one of several ways of presenting data that can compromise informed consent. Elmore recommends, for example, that instead of reporting a Gail model risk of diagnosis of breast cancer in 5 years as 1.1%, explaining that only 11 out of 1000 women would get such a diagnosis is easier for patients to grasp.[11] Likewise, for patients absolute risk might be preferable to relative risk. Instead of stating that 379 of 6061 women with nonproliferative breast disease developed breast cancer, compared with an expected number of 298, giving a relative risk of 1.27, it is clearer to use absolute risk. In 100 women followed for 15 years, 6 in 100 with nonproliferative disease developed breast cancer, compared with 5 in the general population.

Web Sites for Breast Cancer Information.   Encourage female patients to pursue breast cancer–related information from recommended reputable sources to help them make informed choices during shared decision making.[17]

BREAST CANCER WEB SITES

Calculation of the risk of a breast cancer diagnosis and death at the level of individual women:

http://bcra.nci.nih.gov/brc/start.htm (Gail model)

http://astor.som.jhmi.edu/brcapro (Gail Model, Claus Model, and a model that predicts the probability of carrying a *BRCA1* or *BRCA2* mutation)

http://www.komen.org/BreastCancer/BreastSelfAwareness.html? ecid=vanityurl:28

http://www.breastselfexam.ca

National Guidelines for Breast Cancer Screening

http://www.guidelines.gov

Randomized Clinical Trials of New Modalities in Breast Cancer Screening

http://www.clinicaltrials.gov

Support Groups

http://www.cancer.org/Treatment/SupportProgramsServices/

Acknowledgement

kellyrooneyfoundation.org

TABLE
17-1

Common Breast Masses

The three most common kinds of breast masses are *fibroadenoma* (a benign tumor), *cysts*, and *breast cancer*. The clinical characteristics of these masses are listed below. However, any breast mass should be carefully evaluated and usually warrants further investigation by ultrasound, aspiration, mammography, or biopsy. The masses depicted below are large for purposes of illustration. Ideally, breast cancer should be identified early, when the mass is small. *Fibrocystic changes,* not illustrated, are also commonly palpable as nodular, rope-like densities in women ages 25–50. They may be tender or painful. They are considered benign and are not viewed as a risk factor for breast cancer.

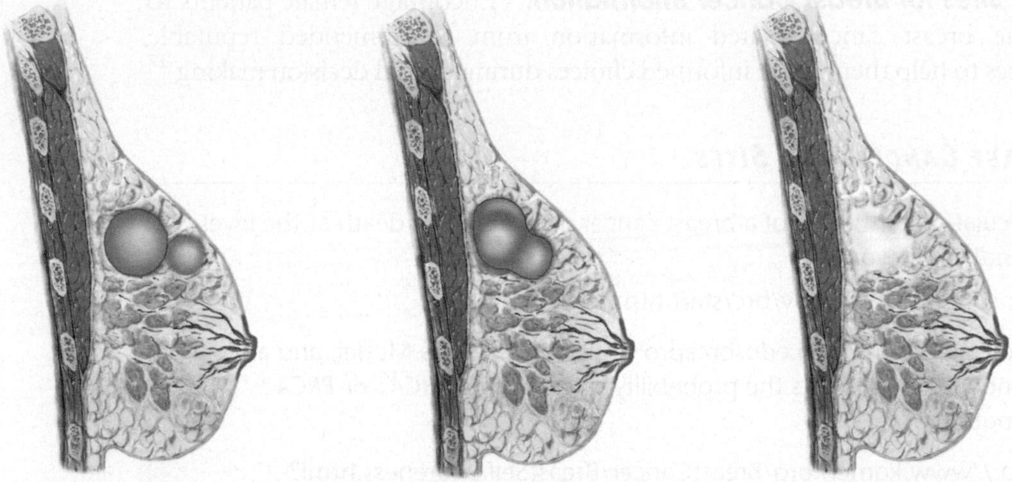

	Fibroadenoma	Cysts	Cancer
Usual Age	15–25, usually puberty and young adulthood, but up to age 55	30–50, regress after menopause except with estrogen therapy	30–90, most common over age 50
Number	Usually single, may be multiple	Single or multiple	Usually single, although may coexist with other nodules
Shape	Round, disc-like, or lobular	Round	Irregular or stellate
Consistency	May be soft, usually firm	Soft to firm, usually elastic	Firm or hard
Delineation	Well delineated	Well delineated	Not clearly delineated from surrounding tissues
Mobility	Very mobile	Mobile	May be fixed to skin or underlying tissues
Tenderness	Usually nontender	Often tender	Usually nontender
Retraction Signs	Absent	Absent	May be present

Visible Signs of Breast Cancer

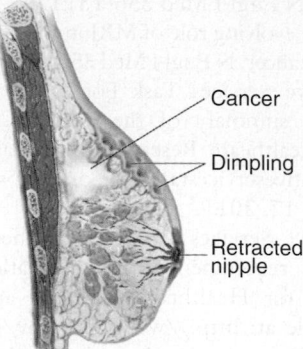

Cancer

Dimpling

Retracted nipple

Retraction Signs

As breast cancer advances, it causes fibrosis (scar tissue). Shortening of this tissue produces *dimpling, changes in contour,* and *retraction or deviation of the nipple.* Other causes of retraction include fat necrosis and mammary duct ectasia.

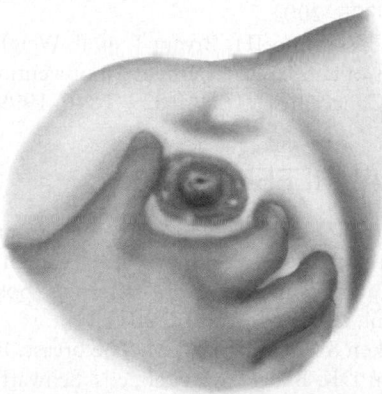

Skin Dimpling

Look for this sign with the patient's arm at rest, during special positioning, and on moving or compressing the breast, as illustrated here.

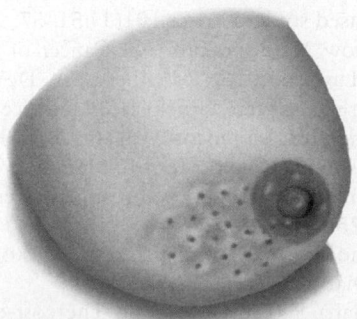

Edema of the Skin

Edema of the skin is produced by lymphatic blockade. It appears as thickened skin with enlarged pores—the so-called *peau d'orange* (orange peel) *sign.* It is often seen first in the lower portion of the breast or areola.

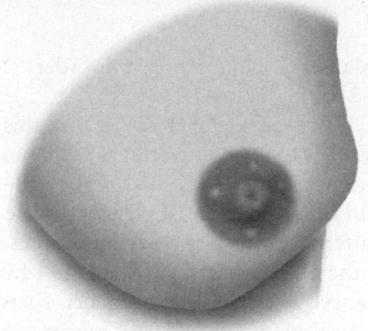

Abnormal Contours

Look for any variation in the normal convexity of each breast, and compare one side with the other. Special positioning may again be useful. Shown here is marked flattening of the lower outer quadrant of the left breast.

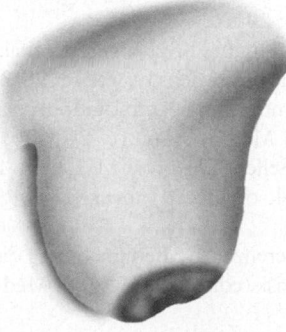

Nipple Retraction and Deviation

A retracted nipple is flattened or pulled inward, as illustrated here. It may also be broadened, and feels thickened. When involvement is radially asymmetric, the nipple may deviate or point in a different direction from its normal counterpart, typically toward the underlying cancer.

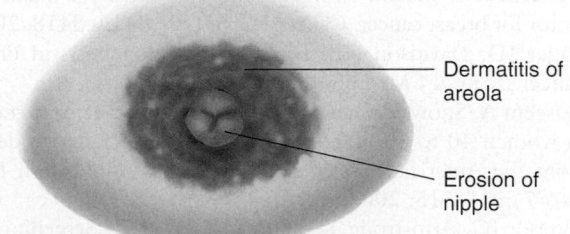

Dermatitis of areola

Erosion of nipple

Paget Disease of the Nipple

This uncommon form of breast cancer usually starts as a scaly, eczema-like lesion that may weep, crust, or erode. A breast mass may be present. Suspect Paget disease in any persisting dermatitis of the nipple and areola. Can present with invasive breast cancer or ductal carcinoma in situ.[3]

BIBLIOGRAPHY

CITATIONS

1. Santen RJ, Mansel R. Benign breast disorders. N Engl J Med 353(3):275–285, 2005.
2. Barton MB, Harris R, Fletcher SW. Does this patient have breast cancer? The screening clinical breast examination: should it be done? How? JAMA 282(13):1270–1280, 1999.
3. Chen CY, Sun LM, Anderson BO. Paget disease of the breast: changing patterns of incidence, clinical presentation, and treatment in the U.S. Cancer 197(7):1448–1458, 2006.
4. American Cancer Society. Breast Cancer Facts and Figures 2009–2010. Available at: http://www.cancer.org/downloads/STT/BCFF-Final.pdf. Accessed April 17, 2011.
5. Fentiman IS. Male breast cancer. Lancet 367(9510):595–604, 2006.
6. Ravdin PM, Cronin KA, Howlader N, et al. The decrease in breast-cancer incidence in 2003 in the United States. N Engl J Med 356(16):1670–1674, 2007.
7. Altekruse SF, Kosary CL, Krapcho M, et al., eds. SEER Cancer Statistics Review, 1975–2007. Bethesda, MD: National Cancer Institute; 2010.
8. del Carmen MG, Hughes KS, Halpern E, et al. Racial differences in mammographic breast density. Cancer 98(3):590–596, 2003.
9. Fletcher SW, Elmore JG. Mammographic screening for breast cancer. N Engl J Med 348(14):1672–1680, 2003.
10. Hartmann LC, Sellers TA, Frost MH, et al. Benign breast disease and the risk of breast cancer. N Engl J Med 353(3):229–237, 2005.
11. Elmore JG, Gigerenzer G. Benign breast disease: the risks of communicating risk (editorial). N Engl J Med 353(3):297–298, 2005.
12. Carney PA, Migloiretti DL, Yankaskas, et al. Individual and combined effects of age, breast density, and hormone replacement therapy use on the accuracy of screening mammography. Ann Intern Med 138(3):168–175, 2003.
13. Boyd NF, Lockwood GA, Byng JW, et al. Mammographic densities and breast cancer risk. Cancer Epidemiol Biomarkers Prevent 7(12):1133–1144, 1998.
14. Vachon CM, Sellers TA, Carlson EE, et al. Strong evidence of a genetic determinant for mammographic density, a major risk factor for breast cancer. Cancer Res 67(17):8412–8418, 2007.
15. Yager JD, Davidson NE. Estrogen carcinogenesis in breast cancer. N Engl J Med 354(3):270–282, 2006.
16. Qaseem A, Snow V, Sherif K, et al. Screening mammography in women 40 to 49 years of age: a clinical practice guideline from the American College of Physicians. Ann Intern Med 146(7):511–515, 2007.
17. Elmore JG, Armstrong K, Lehman CD, et al. Screening for breast cancer. JAMA 293(10):1245–1256, 2005.
18. Pisano ED, Gatsonis C, Hendrick E, et al. Diagnostic performance of digital versus film mammography for breast-cancer screening. N Engl J Med 353(17):1773–1783, 2005.
19. Kreige M, Brekelmans CTM, Boetes C, et al. Efficacy of MRI and mammography for breast-cancer screening in women with a familial or genetic predisposition. N Engl J Med 351(5):427–437, 2004.
20. Lehman CD, Gatsonis C, Kuhl CK, et al. MRI evaluation of the contralateral breast in women with recently diagnosed breast cancer. N Engl J Med 356(13):1295–1303, 2007.
21. Smith RA. The evolving role of MRI in the detection and evaluation of breast cancer. N Engl J Med 356(13):1362–1363, 2007.
22. U.S. Preventive Services Task Force. Chemoprevention of breast cancer: summary of the evidence. Rockville, MD: Agency for Healthcare Research and Quality. Available at: www.uspreventiveservicestaskforce.org/uspstf/uspsbrpv.htm Accessed April 17, 2011.
23. U.S. Preventive Services Task Force. Chemoprevention of breast cancer: recommendations and rationale. Rockville, MD: Agency for Healthcare Research and Quality, July 2002. Available at: http://www.ahrq.gov/clinic/3rduspstf/breastchemo/breastchemorr.htm. Accessed April 17, 2011.
24. Vogel VG, Constantino JP, Wickerham DL, et al. Effects of tamoxifen vs raloxifene on the risk of developing invasive breast cancer and other disease outcomes. The NSABP study of tamoxifen and raloxifene (STAR) P-2 trial. JAMA 295(23):2727–2741, 2006.
25. Gail MH, Costantino JP. Validating and improving models for projecting the absolute risk of breast cancer. J Natl Cancer Inst 93(5):334–335, 2001.
26. Gail MH, Costantino JH, Bryant J, et al. Weighing the risks and benefits of tamoxifen treatment for preventing breast cancer. J Natl Cancer Inst 91(21):1829–1846, 1999.

ADDITIONAL REFERENCES

American Geriatrics Society Clinical Practice Committee. Position statement: breast cancer screening in older women. Available at: http://www.americangeriatrics.org/products/positionpapers/brstcncr.shtml. Accessed April 17, 2011.

Bland KI, Beenken SW, Copeland EM. The breast. In: Brunicardi FC, Andersen DK, Billiar TM, et al., eds. Schwartz's Principles of Surgery, 8th ed. New York: McGraw-Hill Medical, 2005.

Chlebowski RT, Hentrix SL, Langer RD, et al. Influence of estrogen plus progestin on breast cancer and mammography in healthy postmenopausal women: the Women's Health Initiative randomized trial. JAMA 289(24):3243–3253, 2003.

Giordano SH, Cohen DS, Buzdar AU. Breast carcinoma in men: a population-based study. Cancer 101(1):51–57, 2004.

Harris JR, Morrow M, Bonadonna G. Cancer of the breast. In: DeVita VT, Lawrence TS, Rosenberg SA. DeVita, Hellman, and Rosenberg's Cancer: Principles & Practice of Oncology, 8th ed. Philadelphia: Lippincott Williams & Wilkins, 2008.

Jones BA, Patterson EA, Calvocoressi L. Mammography screening in African American women: evaluating the research. Cancer 97(Suppl.1):258–272, 2003.

Kudva YC, Reynolds CA, O'Brien T, et al. Mastopathy and diabetes. Curr Diab Rep 3(1):56–59, 2003.

Mandalblatt J, Saha S, Teusch S, et al. The cost-effectiveness of screening mammography beyond age 65 years: a systematic review for the U.S. Preventive Services Task Force. Ann Intern Med 139(10):835–842, 2003.

Robson M, Offit K. Clinical practice: management of an inherited predisposition to breast cancer. N Engl J Med 357(2):154–162, 2007.

The Musculoskeletal System

LEARNING OBJECTIVES

The student will:

1. Describe the structure and functions of the bones, muscles, and joints.
2. Identify the key landmarks of each joint.
3. Obtain an accurate history of the musculoskeletal system.
4. Appropriately prepare and position the patient for the musculoskeletal examination.
5. Describe the equipment necessary to perform a musculoskeletal examination.
6. Inspect and palpate the joints, bones, and muscles.
7. Describe the range of motion of the major joints.
8. Assess muscle strength using the muscle strength grading scale.
9. Correctly document the findings of the musculoskeletal assessment.
10. Discuss risk factors for osteoporosis.
11. Discuss risk factors for falls.
12. Discuss risk reduction and health promotion strategies to reduce musculoskeletal injuries and disease.

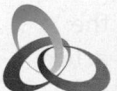

ASSESSING THE MUSCULOSKELETAL SYSTEM

Overview

Musculoskeletal complaints and disorders are leading causes of health care visits in clinical practice. Since the musculoskeletal system is enervated by the neurologic system, examinations of the two systems are closely aligned. Indeed, these systems may be examined at the same time. Careful questioning during the history and acute observations will help the nurse distinguish the cause of the patient's symptoms.

Because of the specialized nature of the musculoskeletal assessment, the organization of this chapter is a unique departure from other regional examination chapters in this book. Assessment of joints requires both visualization and thorough knowledge of surface landmarks and underlying anatomy. To help students pair their knowledge of joint structure and function with related methods of examination, the Anatomy and Physiology and Physical Examination for each joint *are combined*. The format of the chapter is as follows:

CHAPTER ORGANIZATION

- **Joint Structure and Function**
- **The Health History**
- **Examination of Specific Joints: Anatomy and Physiology and Physical Examination**
  - To promote a systematic approach to examining the joints, the chapter follows a "head-to-toe" sequence, beginning with the jaw and joints of the upper extremities, then proceeding to the spine, hip, and joints of the lower extremities.
  - Sequence: *temporomandibular joint, shoulder, elbow, wrist and hand, spine, hip, knee and lower leg, ankle and foot*
  - For each joint there are subsections on **Joint Overview, Bony Structures and Joints, Muscle Groups and Additional Structures,** and **Physical Examination.**
    - **Joint Overview** presents the distinguishing anatomic and functional characteristics of each joint.
    - **Physical Examination** presents the fundamental steps for examining that joint—**inspection, palpation** of bony landmarks and soft-tissue structures, assessment of **range of motion** (the arc of measurable joint movement in a single plane), and **maneuvers** to test the joint's function and stability.
    - Muscle strength
- **Health Promotion**

Joint Structure and Function

It is helpful to begin by reviewing some anatomic terminology.

- *Articular structures* include the joint capsule and articular cartilage, the synovium and synovial fluid, intra-articular ligaments, and juxta-articular bone.

  Articular disease typically involves swelling and tenderness of the entire joint and limits both active and passive range of motion.

- *Extra-articular structures* include periarticular ligaments, tendons, bursae, muscle, fascia, bone, nerve, and overlying skin.

  Extra-articular disease typically involves selected regions of the joint and types of movement.

- *Ligaments* are rope-like bundles of collagen fibrils that connect bone to bone.

- *Tendons* are collagen fibers connecting muscle to bone. Another type of collagen matrix forms the *cartilage* that overlies bony surfaces.

- *Bursae* are pouches of synovial fluid that cushion the movement of tendons and muscles over bone or other joint structures.

To understand joint function, study the various types of joints and how they articulate, or interconnect, and the role of bursae in easing joint movement.

Types of Joint Articulation

There are three primary types of joint articulation—synovial, cartilaginous, and fibrous—allowing varying degrees of joint movement.

● **Joints**		
Type of Joint	**Extent of Movement**	**Example**
Synovial	Freely movable	Knee, shoulder
Cartilaginous	Slightly movable	Vertebral bodies of the spine
Fibrous	Immovable	Skull sutures

Synovial Joints. The bones do not touch each other, and the joint articulations are *freely movable*. The bones are covered by *articular cartilage* and separated by a *synovial cavity* that cushions joint movement, as shown. A *synovial membrane* lines the synovial cavity and secretes a small amount of viscous lubricating fluid—the *synovial fluid*. The membrane is attached at the margins of the articular cartilage and pouched or folded to accommodate joint movement. Surrounding the synovial membrane is a fibrous *joint capsule*, which is strengthened by ligaments extending from bone to bone.

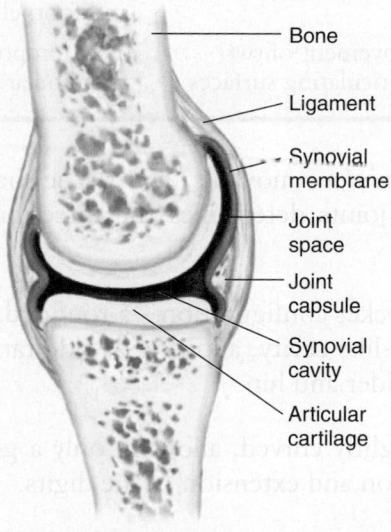

Bone
Ligament
Synovial membrane
Joint space
Joint capsule
Synovial cavity
Articular cartilage

SYNOVIAL

Cartilaginous Joints. These joints, such as those between vertebrae and the symphysis pubis, are *slightly movable*. Fibrocartilaginous discs separate the bony surfaces. At the center of each disc is the *nucleus pulposus*, fibrocartilaginous material that serves as a cushion or shock absorber between bony surfaces.

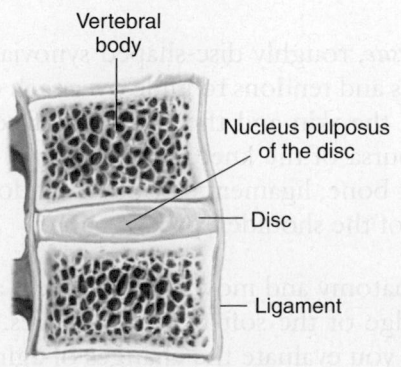

Vertebral body
Nucleus pulposus of the disc
Disc
Ligament

CARTILAGINOUS

Fibrous Joints. In these joints, such as the sutures of the skull, intervening layers of fibrous tissue or cartilage hold the bones together. The bones are almost in direct contact, which allows *no appreciable movement.*

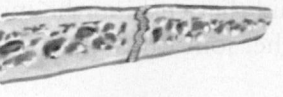

FIBROUS

Structure of Synovial Joints

As you learn about the examination of the musculoskeletal system, think about how the anatomy of the joint relates to its movement.

Type of Joint	Articular Shape	Movement	Example
● Synovial Joints			
Spheroidal (ball and socket)	Convex surface in concave cavity	Wide-ranging flexion, extension, abduction, adduction, rotation, circumduction	Shoulder, hip
Hinge	Flat, planar	Motion in one plane; flexion, extension	Interphalangeal joints of hand and foot; elbow
Condylar	Convex or concave	Movement of two articulating surfaces	Knee; temporomandibular joint

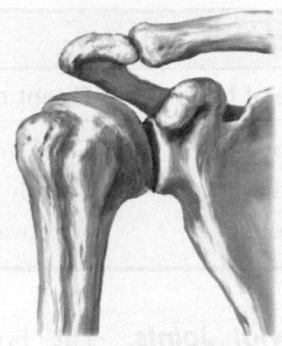

SPHEROIDAL JOINT (BALL AND SOCKET)

Many of the joints examined are *synovial,* or movable, *joints.* The shape of the articulating surfaces of synovial joints determines the direction and extent of joint motion.

- *Spheroidal joints* have a ball-and-socket configuration—a rounded, convex surface articulating with a cup-like cavity, allowing a wide range of rotatory movement, as in the shoulder and hip.

- *Hinge joints* are flat, planar, or slightly curved, allowing only a gliding motion in a single plane, as in flexion and extension of the digits.

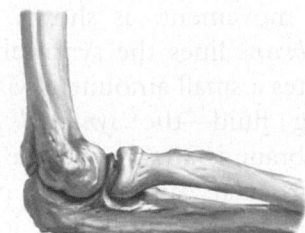

HINGE JOINT

- In *condylar joints,* such as the knee, the articulating surfaces are convex or concave, termed condyles. One articulating surface is convex and the matching surface is concave.

Bursae. Easing joint action are *bursae,* roughly disc-shaped synovial sacs that allow adjacent muscles or muscles and tendons to glide over each other during movement. They lie between the skin and the convex surface of a bone or joint (as in the prepatellar bursa of the knee, p. 568), or in areas where tendons or muscles rub against bone, ligaments, or other tendons or muscles (as in the subacromial bursa of the shoulder, p. 532).

Knowledge of the underlying joint anatomy and movement will help assess joints subjected to trauma. Knowledge of the soft-tissue structures, ligaments, tendons, and bursae will help you evaluate the changes of aging, as well as arthritis.

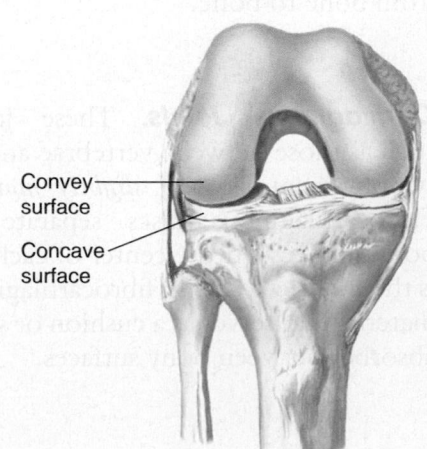

Convey surface

Concave surface

CONDYLAR JOINT

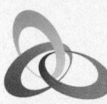

THE HEALTH HISTORY

COMMON OR CONCERNING SYMPTOMS

- Joint pain
- Joint pain associated with systemic symptoms, such as fever, chills, rash, weakness, and weight loss
- Low back pain
- Neck pain
- Bone pain
- Muscle pain or cramps
- Muscle weakness

Begin the history with a broad open-ended question:

"Do you have any pain in your joints, bones, or muscles?"

Joint pain is one of the leading complaints of patients seeking health care. Joint pain may also be *extra-articular*, involving bones, muscles, and tissues around the joint such as tendons, ligaments, bursae, or overlying skin.

May be due to sprains from stretching or tearing of ligaments, muscle or tendon strain, bursitis, or tendinitis

Generalized "aches and pains" are called *myalgias* if they occur in muscles, and *arthralgias* if there is pain in a joint but no evidence of arthritis.

The "OLD CART" mnemonic may be used to obtain more information.

Onset: When did the pain begin?
  Was the onset rapid or insidious?
  Did the pain follow an injury? Describe the injury.
Location: Where is the pain located? Point to the site.
  Is the pain in one joint or multiple joints (or multiple muscles)?

Pain in one joint suggests trauma, monoarticular arthritis, possible tendinitis, or bursitis. Lateral hip pain near the greater trochanter suggests *trochanteric bursitis.*

  Does the pain migrate from joint to joint?
  Does the pain radiate (e.g., down a limb)?
Duration: How long have you had the pain?
  Does the pain come and go or is it constant?
  Is it worse at a particular time of day or night?

Migratory pattern of spread in *rheumatic fever* or *gonococcal arthritis*; progressive additive pattern with symmetric involvement in *rheumatoid arthritis*

Characteristic Symptoms: Describe the pain. Is it sharp, dull, achy, or shooting?
Associated Manifestations: Do you have any other symptoms such as bruising, warmth, swelling, stiffness, deformity such as nodules, fever, chills, rash, muscle weakness, numbness, tingling, or burning?
  Is your motion limited?
  Does the limitation affect activities, such as walking, rising from a chair, or holding objects?

Extra-articular pain in inflammation of bursae (*bursitis*), tendons (*tendinitis*), or tendon sheaths (*tenosynovitis*); also *sprains* from stretching or tearing of ligaments

Relieving/Exacerbating Factors: Does anything relieve the pain or make it worse, such as a heating pad or cool compress?

Treatment: Have you taken any medication or tried other treatments to relieve the pain?

Low Back Pain.   Low back pain is the second most common reason for office visits. Using open-ended questions gives a clearer picture of the problem, especially the location of the pain.

See Table 18-1, Low Back Pain, p. 584.

Approximately 85% of patients have *idiopathic low back pain* without a precise underlying cause (this term is preferred to "sprain" or "strain").[1]

Determine if the pain is *on the midline,* over the vertebrae, or *off the midline.*

Midline back pain, suggests musculoligamentous injury, disc herniation, vertebral collapse, spinal cord metastases, or rarely *epidural abscess.* Pain off the midline, suggests sacroiliitis, trochanteric bursitis, sciatica, or hip arthritis.

Is there radiation into the leg? If yes, is there any associated numbness or paresthesias?

Radicular gluteal and posterior leg pain in the S1 distribution in *sciatica* that increases with cough or Valsalva manuver. Leg pain that resolves with rest and/or lumbar forward flexion suggests *spinal stenosis.*

What about associated bladder or bowel dysfunction?

Elicit any *"red flags" for serious underlying systemic disease:* age older than 50 years, history of cancer, unexplained weight loss, pain lasting more than 1 month or not responding to treatment, pain at night or increased by rest, history of intravenous drug use, or presence of infection.[2,3]

Suspect *Cauda equina syndrome* from S2–4 midline disc or tumor if bowel or bladder dysfunction (usually urinary retention and overflow incontinence)[2]

In cases of low back pain plus a red flag, there is a 10% probability of serious systemic disease.[2,3]

Neck Pain.   Neck pain is also common. Although usually self-limited, it is important to ask about radiation into the arm, arm or leg weakness or paresthesias, or change in bladder or bowel function. Be sure to elicit symptoms related to the "red flags" listed above. Persisting pain after blunt trauma or a motor vehicle accident warrants further evaluation.[4]

See Table 18-2, Pains in the Neck, p. 585.

Radicular pain from spinal nerve compression, most commonly C7 followed by C6. Unlike low back pain, usually from foraminal impingement from degenerative joint changes (70% to 75%) rather than disc herniation (20% to 25%)[5,6]

EXAMINATION OF JOINTS: ANATOMY AND PHYSIOLOGY AND PHYSICAL EXAMINATION

Important Areas of Examination for Each of the Major Joints

- Inspection for joint symmetry, alignment, bony deformities
- Inspection and palpation of surrounding tissues for skin changes, nodules, muscle atrophy, crepitus
- Range of motion and maneuvers to test joint function and stability, and integrity of ligaments, tendons, bursae, especially if pain or trauma
- Assessment of inflammation or arthritis, especially swelling, warmth, tenderness, redness
- Assessment of muscle strength

During the interview the patient's ability to carry out normal activities of daily living was evaluated. Keep these abilities in mind during the physical examination.

The detail needed for examination of the musculoskeletal system varies widely. This section presents examination techniques for both comprehensive and targeted assessment of joint function. Patients with extensive or severe musculoskeletal problems will require more time. A briefer survey for those without musculoskeletal symptoms is outlined in Chapter 7 (see p. 108).

In the general survey of the patient, general appearance, body proportions, and ease of movement have been assessed. The examination should be systematic. It should include inspection, palpation of bony landmarks as well as related joint and soft-tissue structures, assessment of range of motion, muscle strength, and *special maneuvers* to test specific movements. Recall that the anatomic shape of each joint determines its range of motion. There are two phases to *range of motion*: *active* (by the patient) and *passive* (by the examiner).

EQUIPMENT

- Tape measure
- Goniometer
- Skin marking pen

TIPS FOR SUCCESSFUL EXAMINATION OF THE MUSCULOSKELETAL SYSTEM

- During inspection, look for *symmetry* of involvement. Is there a symmetric change in joints on both sides of the body, or is the change only in one or two joints?

Acute involvement of only one joint suggests trauma, septic arthritis, gout. *Rheumatoid arthritis* typically involves several joints, symmetrically distributed.[8-10]

(continued)

TIPS FOR SUCCESSFUL EXAMINATION OF THE MUSCULOSKELETAL SYSTEM (continued)

Note any *joint deformities* or *malalignment of bones.*	*Dupuytren contracture* (p. 590), bowlegs or knock-knees.
• Use inspection and palpation to assess the *surrounding tissues,* noting skin changes, subcutaneous nodules, and muscle atrophy. Note any *crepitus,* an audible or palpable crunching during movement of tendons or ligaments over bone. This may occur in normal joints but is more significant when associated with symptoms or signs.	Subcutaneous nodules in *rheumatoid arthritis* or *rheumatic fever;* effusions in trauma; crepitus over inflamed joints, in *osteoarthritis,* or in inflamed tendon sheaths
• Test range of motion and maneuvers (described for each joint) to demonstrate *limitations in range of motion* or joint instability from excess mobility of joint ligaments, called *ligamentous laxity.*	Decreased range of motion in arthritis, inflammation of tissues around a joint, fibrosis in or around a joint, or bony fixation (*ankylosis*). Ligamentous laxity of the anterior cruciate ligament (ACL) in knee trauma.
• Finally, test *muscle strength* to aid in the assessment of joint function.	Muscle atrophy or weakness in *rheumatoid arthritis.*
Be especially alert to *signs of inflammation and arthritis.*	
• *Swelling.* Palpable swelling may involve (1) the synovial membrane, which can feel boggy or doughy; (2) effusion from excess synovial fluid within the joint space; or (3) soft-tissue structures such as bursae, tendons, and tendon sheaths.	Palpable bogginess or doughiness of the synovial membrane indicates *synovitis,* which is often accompanied by effusion. Palpable joint fluid in effusion, tenderness over the tendon sheaths in *tendinitis*
• *Warmth.* Use the backs of your fingers to compare the involved joint with its unaffected contralateral joint, or with nearby tissues if both joints are involved.	Arthritis, tendinitis, bursitis, *osteomyelitis*
• *Tenderness.* Try to identify the specific anatomic structure that is tender. Trauma may also cause tenderness.	Tenderness and warmth over a thickened synovium suggest arthritis or infection.
• *Redness.* Redness of the overlying skin is the *least* common sign of inflammation near the joints.	Redness over a tender joint suggests septic or gouty arthritis, or possibly *rheumatoid arthritis.*

Examination of the muscles includes muscle bulk, muscle tone and muscle strength.

Muscle Bulk.   *Begin the exam by* inspecting the size and contours of muscles. Do the muscles look flat or concave, suggesting atrophy? If so, is the process unilateral or bilateral? Is it proximal or distal?

When looking for atrophy, pay particular attention to the hands, shoulders, and thighs. The thenar and hypothenar eminences should be full and convex, and the spaces between the metacarpals, where the dorsal interosseous

Muscular *atrophy* refers to a loss of muscle bulk, or wasting. It results from diseases of the peripheral nervous system such as diabetic neuropathy, as well as diseases of the muscles themselves. *Hypertrophy* is an increase

muscles lie, should be full or only slightly depressed. Atrophy of hand muscles may occur with normal aging, however, as shown on the right below.

in bulk with proportionate strength, whereas increased bulk with diminished strength is called *pseudohypertrophy* (seen in the *Duchenne form of muscular dystrophy*)

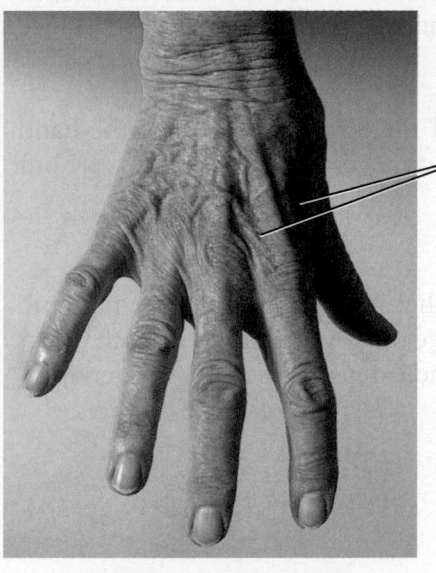

Flattening of the thenar and hypothenar eminences and furrowing between the metacarpals suggest atrophy. Localized atrophy of the thenar and hypothenar eminences in median and ulnar nerve damage, respectively.

Hand of a 44-year-old woman   Hand of an 84-year-old woman

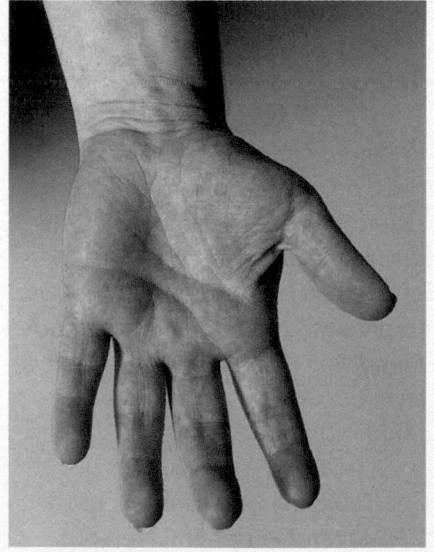

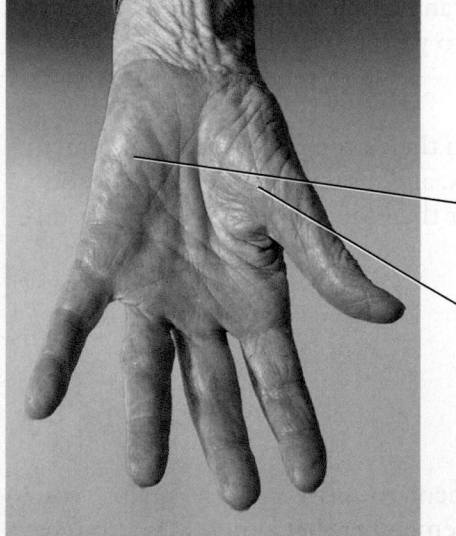

Other causes of muscular atrophy include motor neuron diseases, any disease that affects the peripheral motor system projecting from the spinal cord, rheumatoid arthritis, and protein-calorie malnutrition.

Hand of a 44-year-old woman   Hand of an 84-year-old woman

Be alert for fasciculations in atrophic muscles. If absent, tap on the muscle with a reflex hammer to try to stimulate them.

Fasciculations with atrophy and muscle weakness suggest disease of the peripheral motor unit.

Muscle Tone. When a normal muscle with an intact nerve supply is relaxed voluntarily, it maintains a slight residual tension known as muscle tone. This can be assessed best by feeling the muscle's resistance to passive stretch. Persuade the patient to relax. Take one hand with yours and, while

Decreased resistance suggests disease of the peripheral nervous system, cerebellar disease, or the acute stages of spinal cord injury.

supporting the elbow, flex and extend the patient's fingers, wrist, and elbow, and put the shoulder through a moderate range of motion. With practice, these actions can be combined into a single smooth movement. On each side, note muscle tone—the resistance offered to your movements. Tense patients may show increased resistance. The feel of normal resistance is learned with repeated practice.

See Table 20-13, Disorders of Muscle Tone (p. 680).

If you suspect decreased resistance, hold the forearm and shake the hand loosely back and forth. Normally the hand moves back and forth freely but is not completely floppy.

Marked floppiness indicates muscle *hypotonia* or *flaccidity*, usually from a disorder of the peripheral motor system.

If resistance is increased, determine whether it varies as you move the limb or whether it persists throughout the range of movement and in both directions, for example, during both flexion and extension. Feel for any jerkiness in the resistance.

Spasticity is increased resistance that worsens at the extremes of range. Spasticity, seen in central corticospinal tract diseases, is rate dependent, increasing with rapid movement. *Rigidity* is increased resistance throughout the range of movement and in both directions (not rate dependent).

To assess muscle tone in the legs, support the patient's thigh with one hand, grasp the foot with the other, and flex and extend the patient's knee and ankle on each side. Note the resistance to your movements.

Muscle Strength.

People vary widely in their strength, and the assessment should allow for such variables as age, sex, and muscular training. A person's dominant side is usually slightly stronger than the other side. Keep this difference in mind when comparing sides.

Impaired strength is called weakness, or *paresis*. Absence of strength is called paralysis, or *plegia*. *Hemiparesis* refers to weakness of one half of the body; *hemiplegia* to paralysis of one half of the body. *Paraplegia* means paralysis of the legs; *quadriplegia*, paralysis of all four limbs.

Test muscle strength by asking the patient to move actively against your resistance or to resist your movement. Remember that a muscle is strongest when shortest, and weakest when longest.

See Table 20-11, Disorders of the Central and Peripheral Nervous Systems (pp. 676–677).

If the muscles are too weak to overcome resistance, test them against gravity alone or with gravity eliminated. When the forearm rests in a pronated position, for example, dorsiflexion at the wrist can be tested against gravity alone. When the forearm is midway between pronation and supination, extension at the wrist can be tested with gravity eliminated. Finally, if the patient fails to move the body part, watch or feel for weak muscular contraction.

SCALE FOR GRADING MUSCLE STRENGTH

Muscle strength is graded on a 0 to 5 scale:

0—No muscular contraction detected
1—A barely detectable flicker or trace of contraction
2—Active movement of the body part with gravity eliminated
3—Active movement against gravity
4—Active movement against gravity and some resistance
5—Active movement against full resistance without evident fatigue. This is
   normal muscle strength.

When documenting muscle strength, indicate the scale used (e.g., muscle strength 3 out of 5 or 3/5).

Methods for testing the major muscle groups are described below. The spinal root innervations and the muscles affected are shown in parentheses.

If the person has painful joints, move the person gently. Patients may move more comfortably by themselves. Let them show you how they manage. If joint trauma is present, ask the nurse practitioner or physician about an x-ray before attempting movement.

TEMPOROMANDIBULAR JOINT

Overview, Bony Structures, and Joints

The temporomandibular joint (TMJ) is the most active joint in the body, opening and closing up to 2000 times a day. It is formed by the fossa and articular tubercle of the temporal bone and the condyle of the mandible. It lies midway between the external acoustic meatus and the zygomatic arch.

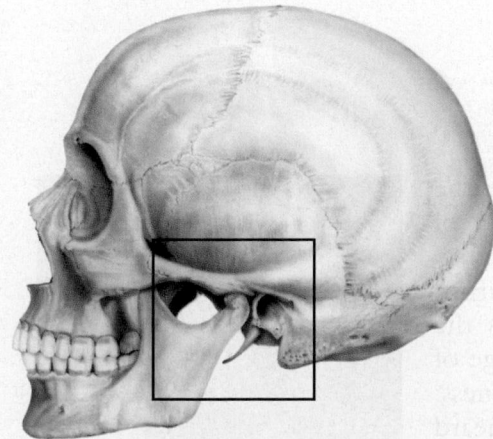

A fibrocartilaginous disc cushions the action of the condyle of the mandible against the synovial membrane and capsule of the articulating surfaces of the temporal bone. Hence, it is a condylar synovial joint.

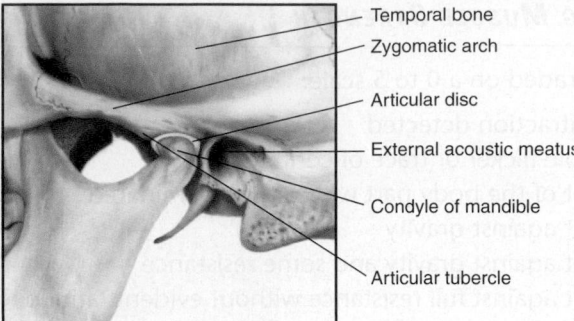

Temporal bone
Zygomatic arch
Articular disc
External acoustic meatus
Condyle of mandible
Articular tubercle

Muscle Groups and Additional Structures

The principal muscles opening the mouth are the *external pterygoids.* Closing the mouth are the muscles innervated by cranial nerve V, the trigeminal nerve (see p. 617)— the *masseter,* the *temporalis,* and the *internal pterygoids.*

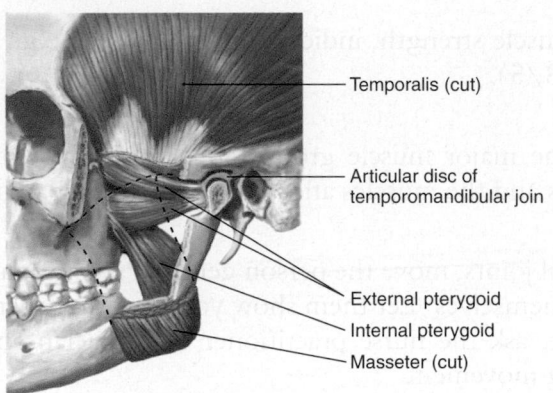

Temporalis (cut)
Articular disc of temporomandibular join
External pterygoid
Internal pterygoid
Masseter (cut)

Physical Examination

Inspection and Palpation. Inspect the face for symmetry. Inspect the TMJ for swelling or redness. Swelling may appear as a rounded bulge approximately 1/2 cm anterior to the external auditory meatus.

Facial asymmetry associated with *TMJ syndrome.* Typical features are unilateral chronic pain with chewing, jaw clenching, or teeth grinding, often associated with stress (may also present as headache). Pain with chewing also in *trigeminal neuralgia, temporal arteritis*

Swelling, tenderness, and decreased range of motion in inflammation or arthritis

To locate and palpate the joint, place the tips of your index fingers just in front of the tragus of each ear and ask the patient to open his or her mouth. The fingertips should drop into the joint spaces as the mouth opens. Check for smooth range of motion; note any swelling or tenderness. Snapping or clicking may be felt or heard in normal people.

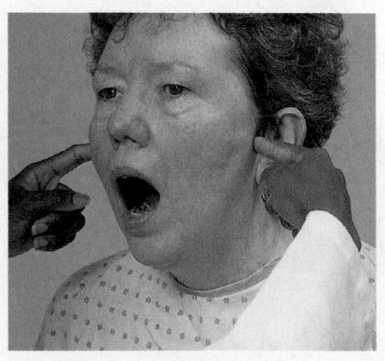

Dislocation of the TMJ may be seen in trauma.

Palpable crepitus or clicking in poor occlusion, meniscus injury, or synovial swelling from trauma

Palpate the muscles of mastication:

- The *masseters,* externally at the angle of the mandible

- The *temporal muscles,* externally during clenching and relaxation of the jaw

Pain and tenderness on palpation in *TMJ syndrome*

Range of Motion and Maneuvers. The temporomandibular joint has glide and hinge motions in its upper and lower portions, respectively. Grinding or chewing consists primarily of gliding movements in the upper compartments.

Range of motion is three-fold: ask the patient to demonstrate opening and closing, protrusion and retraction (by jutting the jaw forward), and lateral, or side-to-side, motion. Normally as the mouth is opened wide, three fingers can be inserted between incisors. During normal protrusion of the jaw, the bottom teeth can be placed in front of the upper teeth.

Muscle Strength. If the patient complains of difficulty chewing or jaw weakness, test muscle strength by asking him or her to perform the range-of-motion maneuvers, projection, lateral, and opening of mouth, against your resistance.

THE SHOULDER

Overview

The glenohumeral joint of the shoulder is distinguished by wide-ranging movement in all directions. This joint is largely uninhibited by bony structures. The humeral head contacts less than one third of the surface area of the glenoid fossa and virtually dangles from the scapula, attached by the joint capsule, the intra-articular capsular ligaments, the glenoid labrum, and a meshwork of muscles and tendons.

The shoulder derives its mobility from a complex interconnected structure of four joints, three large bones, and three principal muscle groups, often referred to as the *shoulder girdle.*

Bony Structures

The bony structures of the shoulder include the humerus, the clavicle, and the scapula. The scapula is anchored to the axial skeleton only by the sternoclavicular joint and inserting muscles, often called the *scapulothoracic articulation* because it is not a true joint.

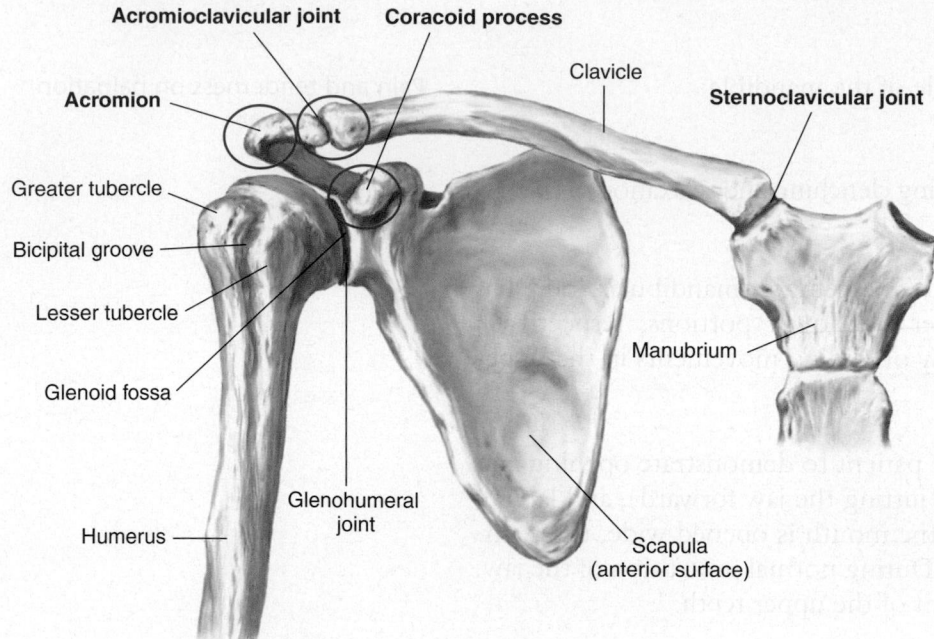

Acromioclavicular joint   Coracoid process

Clavicle

Acromion   Sternoclavicular joint

Greater tubercle

Bicipital groove

Lesser tubercle

Manubrium

Glenoid fossa

Glenohumeral
joint

Humerus

Scapula
(anterior surface)

IMPORTANT BONES OF THE SHOULDER

Identify the *manubrium*, the *sternoclavicular joint*, and the *clavicle*. Also identify the *tip of the acromion*, the *greater tubercle of the humerus*, and the *coracoid process*, which are important landmarks for shoulder anatomy.

Joints

Three different joints articulate at the shoulder:

● The *glenohumeral joint*. In this joint, the head of the humerus articulates with the shallow glenoid fossa of the scapula. This joint is deeply situated and not normally palpable. It is a ball-and-socket joint, allowing the arm its wide arc of movement—flexion, extension, abduction (movement away from the trunk), adduction (movement toward the trunk), rotation, and circumduction.

● The *sternoclavicular joint*. The convex medial end of the clavicle articulates with the concave hollow in the upper sternum.

● The *acromioclavicular joint*. The lateral end of the clavicle articulates with the acromion process of the scapula.

Muscle Groups

Three groups of muscles attach at the shoulder:

The Scapulohumeral Group. This group extends from the scapula to the humerus and includes the muscles inserting directly on the humerus, known as *"SITS muscles"* of the *rotator cuff*:

- *Supraspinatus*—runs above the glenohumeral joint; inserts on the greater tubercle

- *Infraspinatus* and *teres minor*—cross the glenohumeral joint posteriorly; insert on the greater tubercle

- *Subscapularis* (not illustrated)—originates on the anterior surface of the scapula and crosses the joint anteriorly; inserts on the lesser tubercle

The scapulohumeral group rotates the shoulder laterally (the *rotator cuff*) and depresses and rotates the head of the humerus. (See pp. 536–538 for discussion of rotator cuff injuries.)

The Axioscapular Group. This group attaches the trunk to the scapula and includes the trapezius, rhomboids, serratus anterior, and levator scapulae. These muscles rotate the scapula.

The Axiohumeral Group. This group attaches the trunk to the humerus and includes the pectoralis major and minor and the latissimus dorsi. These muscles produce internal rotation of the shoulder.

The biceps and triceps, which connect the scapula to the bones of the forearm, are also involved in shoulder movement, particularly abduction.

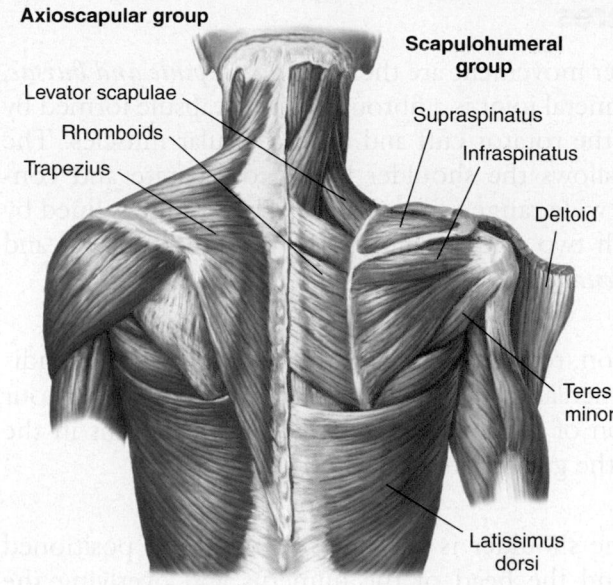

Axioscapular group

Levator scapulae
Rhomboids
Trapezius

Scapulohumeral group
Supraspinatus
Infraspinatus
Deltoid
Teres minor
Latissimus dorsi

Posterior view

Axioscapular group (pulls shoulder backward)
Scapulohumeral group (rotates shoulder laterally; includes rotator cuff)

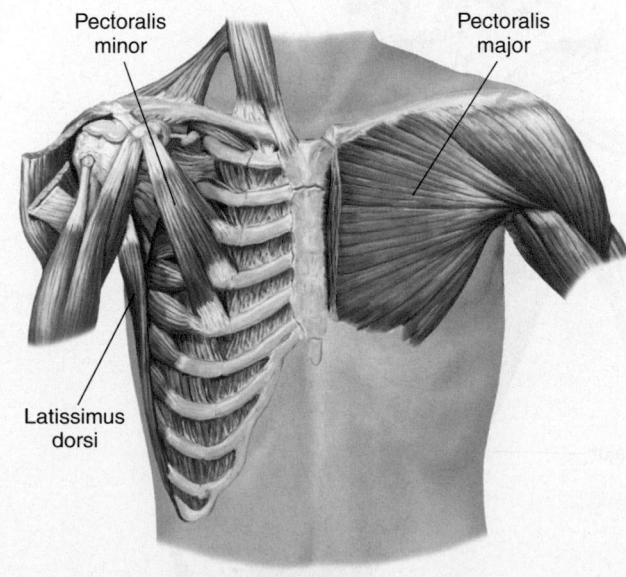

Pectoralis minor
Pectoralis major
Latissimus dorsi

Anterior view

Axiohumeral group (rotates shoulder internally)

Additional Structures

Also important to shoulder movement are the *articular capsule and bursae.* Surrounding the glenohumeral joint is a fibrous articular capsule formed by the tendon insertions of the rotator cuff and other capsular muscles. The loose fit of the capsule allows the shoulder bones to separate and contributes to the shoulder's wide range of movement. The capsule is lined by a synovial membrane with two outpouchings—the *subscapular bursa* and the *synovial sheath of the tendon of the long head of the biceps.*

To locate the biceps tendon, rotate your arm externally and find the tendinous cord that runs just medial to the greater tubercle. Roll it under your fingers. This is the tendon of the long head of the biceps. It runs in the bicipital groove between the greater and lesser tubercles.

The principal bursa of the shoulder is the *subacromial bursa,* positioned between the acromion and the head of the humerus and overlying the supraspinatus tendon. Abduction of the shoulder compresses this bursa. Normally, the supraspinatus tendon and the subacromial bursa are not palpable. However, if the bursal surfaces are inflamed (subacromial bursitis), there may be tenderness just below the tip of the acromion, pain with abduction and rotation, and loss of smooth movement.

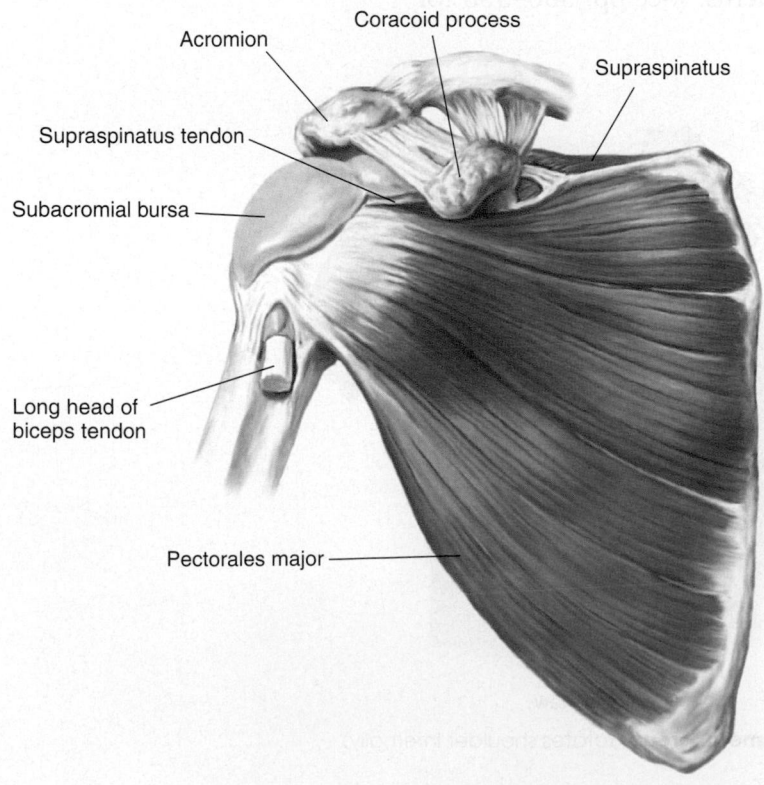

ANTERIOR VIEW OF THE SHOULDER

Physical Examination

Inspection. Observe the shoulder and shoulder girdle anteriorly, and inspect the scapulae and related muscles posteriorly.

Note any swelling, deformity, muscle atrophy or fasciculations (fine tremors of the muscles), or abnormal positioning.

Survey the entire upper extremity for color change, skin alteration, or unusual bony contours.

Palpation. Begin by palpating the bony landmarks of the shoulder; then palpate any area of pain.

- Beginning medially, at the *sternoclavicular joint,* trace the clavicle laterally with your fingers.

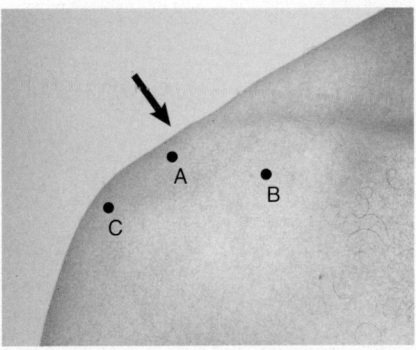

- Now, from behind, follow the bony spine of the scapula laterally and upward until it becomes the acromion (**A**), the summit of the shoulder. Its upper surface is rough and slightly convex. Identify the anterior tip of the acromion.

- With your index finger on top of the acromion, just behind its tip, press medially with your thumb to find the slightly elevated ridge that marks the distal end of the clavicle at the *acromioclavicular joint* (shown by the arrow). Move your thumb medially and down a short step to the next bony prominence, the *coracoid process* (**B**) of the scapula.

- Now, with your thumb on the coracoid process, allow your fingers to fall on and grasp the lateral aspect of the humerus to palpate the *greater tubercle* (**C**), where the SITS muscles insert.

Range of Motion and Maneuvers

Range of Motion. The six motions of the shoulder girdle are flexion, extension, abduction, adduction, and internal and external rotation.

Standing in front of the patient, watch for smooth fluid movement as the patient performs the motions listed in the table on page 534. Note the specific muscles responsible for each motion and clear, simple instructions that prompt the requested patient response.

Scoliosis may cause elevation of one shoulder. With *anterior dislocation of the shoulder,* the rounded lateral aspect of the shoulder appears flattened.[11,12]

Atrophy of supraspinatus and infraspinatus over posterior scapula with increased prominence of scapular spine within 2 to 3 weeks of *rotator cuff tear*

See Table 18-4, Painful Shoulders (p. 588).

Restricted range of motion in *bursitis, capsulitis, rotator cuff tears* or *sprains,* or *tendinitis*

Shoulder Movement	Principal Muscles Affecting Movement	Patient Instructions
Flexion	Anterior deltoid, pectoralis major (clavicular head), coracobrachialis, biceps brachii (short head)	*"Raise your arms in front of you and overhead."*
Extension	Latissimus dorsi, teres major, posterior deltoid, triceps brachii (long head)	*"Raise your arms behind you."*
Abduction	Supraspinatus, middle deltoid, serratus anterior (via upward rotation of the scapula)	*"Raise your arms out to the side and overhead."* Note that to test *pure glenohumeral motion*, the patient should raise the arms to shoulder level at 90°, with palms facing down. To test *scapulothoracic motion*, the patient should turn the palms up and raise the arms an additional 60°. The final 30° tests combined glenohumeral and scapulothoracic motion.

(continued)

Shoulder Movement	Principal Muscles Affecting Movement	Patient Instructions
Adduction	Pectoralis major, coracobrachialis, latissimus dorsi, teres major, subscapularis	*"Cross your arm in front of your body."*
Internal Rotation	Subscapularis, anterior deltoid, pectoralis major, teres major, latissimus dorsi	*"Place one hand behind your back and touch your shoulder blade."* Identify the highest midline spinous process the patient is able to reach.
External Rotation	Infraspinatus, teres minor, posterior deltoid	*"Raise your arm to shoulder level; bend your elbow and rotate your forearm toward the ceiling."* or *"Place one hand behind your neck or head as if you are brushing your hair."*

Maneuvers.   The examination of the shoulder often requires selective evaluation of specific motions and structures. There are more than 20 different maneuvers for testing shoulder function, not all well studied.[13] Common recommended maneuvers, with evidence when available, are described on pp. 536–538. Using these maneuvers will take practice with supervision, but you will find them helpful in identifying shoulder pathology.

Note that the most common cause of shoulder pain involves the rotator cuff, usually involving the supraspinatus tendon with later possible progression posteriorly and anteriorly. Compression of the rotator cuff muscles and tendons between the head of the humerus and the acromion cause "impingement signs" during frequently performed maneuvers such as Neer's, Hawkins, and the dropped-arm tests. However, the best predictors of rotator cuff tear are supraspinatus weakness on abduction, infraspinatus weakness during external rotation, and a positive impingement sign.[13,14]

Age 60 years or older and a positive dropped-arm test are the individual findings most likely to identify a rotator cuff tear.

● Maneuvers for Examining the Shoulder

Structure	Technique	
Acromioclavicular Joint	Palpate and compare both joints for swelling or tenderness. Adduct the patient's arm across the chest, sometimes called the *"crossover test."*	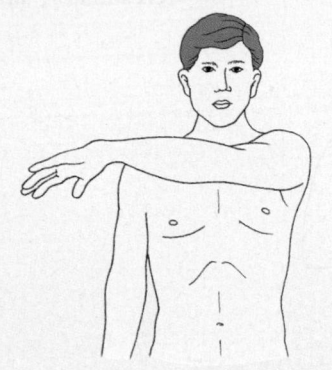

See Table 18-4, Painful Shoulders (p. 588). Localized tenderness or pain with *adduction* suggests inflammation or arthritis of the acromioclavicular joint. But sensitivity and specificity of tenderness is ~95% and 10%; of adduction, ~80% and 50%, respectively.

Overall Shoulder Rotation	Ask the patient to touch the opposite scapula using the two motions shown below (the Apley scratch test).	

Difficulty with these motions suggests rotator cuff disorder.

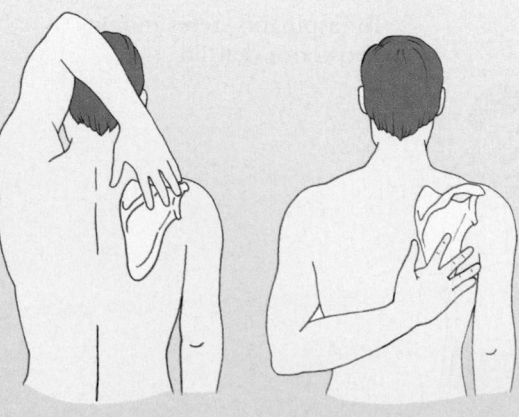

Tests abduction and external rotation   Tests adduction and internal rotation

(continued)

● Maneuvers for Examining the Shoulder (continued)

Structure	Technique	
Rotator Cuff	Test the *"drop-arm" sign.* Ask the patient to fully abduct the arm to shoulder level (or up to 90°) and lower it slowly. (Note that abduction above shoulder level, from 90° to 120°, reflects action of the deltoid muscle.) 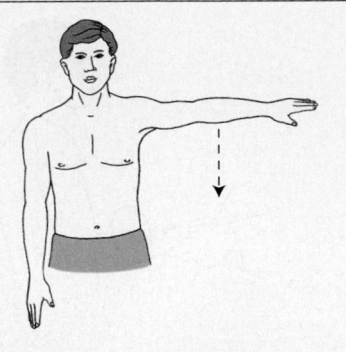	If the patient cannot hold the arm fully abducted at shoulder level, the test is *positive,* indicating a *rotator cuff tear* (LR, 5.0).[13]
Muscle Strength Tests	Test *supraspinatus strength* (sometimes called the "empty can test"). Elevate the arms to 90° and internally rotate the arms with the thumbs pointing down, as if emptying a can. Ask the patient to resist as you place downward pressure on the arms. 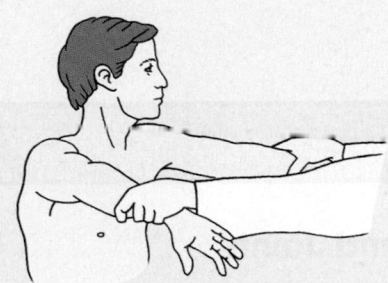	Weakness during this maneuver is a *positive test* indicating possible *rotator cuff tear.*
	Test *infraspinatus strength.* Ask the patient to place arms at the side and flex the elbows to 90° with the thumbs turned up. Provide resistance as the patient presses the forearms outward. 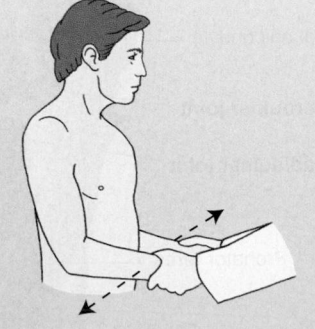	Weakness during this maneuver is a *positive test* indicating possible *rotator cuff tear* or *bicipital tendinitis.*

(continued)

● **Maneuvers for Examining the Shoulder** (continued)

Structure	Technique	
	Test *forearm supination*. Flex the patient's forearm to 90° at the elbow and pronate the patient's wrist. Provide resistance when the patient supinates the forearm.	Pain during this maneuver is a *positive test* indicating inflammation of the long head of the biceps tendon and possible *rotator cuff tear*.

THE ELBOW

Overview, Bony Structures, and Joints

The elbow helps position the hand in space and stabilizes the lever action of the forearm. The elbow joint is formed by the humerus and the two bones of the forearm, the radius, and the ulna. Identify the medial and lateral epicondyles of the humerus and the olecranon process of the ulna.

These bones have three articulations: the *humeroulnar joint*, the *radiohumeral joint*, and the *radioulnar joint*. All three share a large common articular cavity and an extensive synovial lining.

Muscle Groups and Additional Structures

Muscles traversing the elbow include the *biceps* and *brachioradialis* (flexion), the *triceps* (extension), the *pronator teres* (pronation), and the *supinator* (supination).

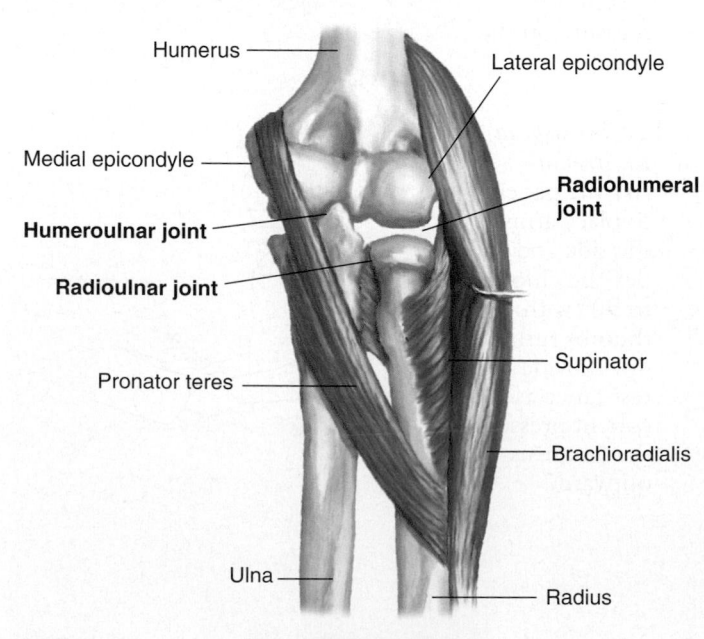

LEFT ANTERIOR ELBOW

Note the location of the *olecranon bursa* between the olecranon process and the skin. The bursa is not normally palpable but swells and becomes tender when inflamed. The *ulnar nerve* runs posteriorly in the ulnar groove between the medial epicondyle and the olecranon process. On the ventral forearm, the *median nerve* is just medial to the brachial artery.

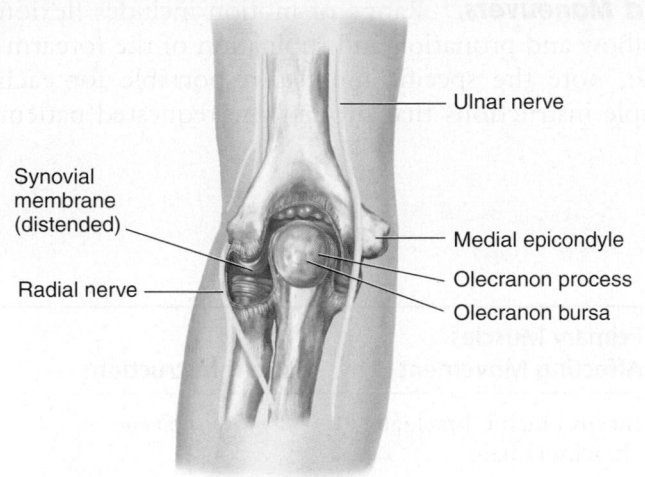

Ulnar nerve

Synovial membrane (distended)

Medial epicondyle

Olecranon process

Radial nerve

Olecranon bursa

LEFT POSTERIOR ELBOW

Physical Examination

Inspection. Support the patient's forearm with your opposite hand so the elbow is flexed to about 70°. Identify the medial and lateral epicondyles and the olecranon process of the ulna. Inspect the contours of the elbow, including the extensor surface of the ulna and the olecranon process. Note any nodules or swelling.

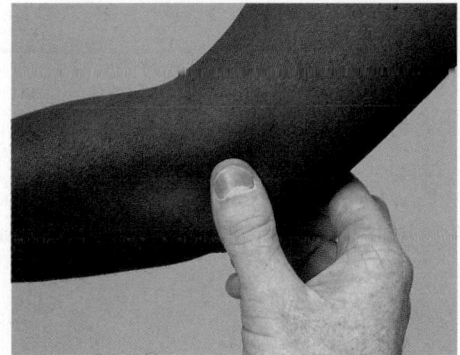

Swelling over the olecranon process in olecranon bursitis; inflammation or synovial fluid in arthritis

Palpation. Palpate the olecranon process and press over the epicondyles for tenderness. Note any displacement of the olecranon.

Tenderness distal to the epicondyle in *lateral epicondylitis* (tennis elbow) and less commonly in *medial epicondylitis* (pitcher's or golfer's elbow)

The olecranon is displaced posteriorly in *posterior dislocation of the elbow* and *supracondylar fracture.*

Palpate the grooves between the epicondyles and the olecranon, noting any tenderness, swelling, or thickening. The synovium is most accessible to examination between the olecranon and the epicondyles. (Normally neither synovium nor bursa is palpable.) The sensitive ulnar nerve can be felt posteriorly between the olecranon process and the medial epicondyle.

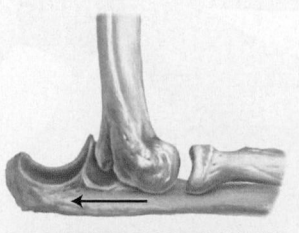

POSTERIOR DISLOCATION OF THE ELBOW

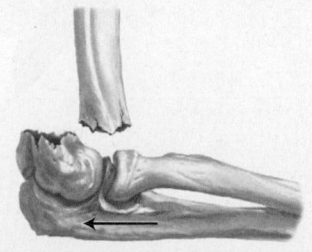

SUPRACONDYLAR FRACTURE OF THE ELBOW

Range of Motion and Maneuvers. Range of motion includes flexion and extension at the elbow and pronation and supination of the forearm. In the following table, note the specific muscles responsible for each motion and clear, simple instructions that prompt the requested patient response.

Full elbow extension makes intra-articular effusion or hemarthrosis unlikely.

Elbow Movement	Primary Muscles Affecting Movement	Patient Instructions
Flexion	Biceps brachii, brachialis, brachioradialis	*"Bend your elbow."*
Extension	Triceps brachii, anconeus	*"Straighten your elbow."*
Supination	Biceps brachii, supinator	*"Turn your palms up, as if carrying a bowl of soup."*
Pronation	Pronator teres, pronator quadratus	*"Turn your palms down."*

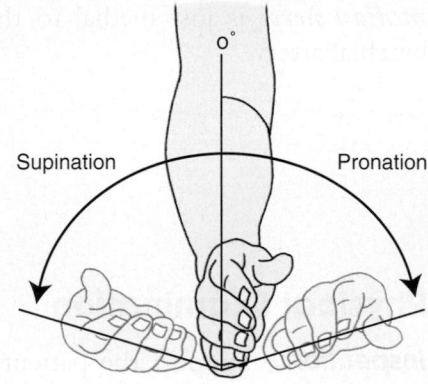

Muscle Strength Tests. *Test flexion* (C5, C6—biceps) *and extension* (C6, C7, C8—triceps) *at the elbow* by having the patient pull and push against your hand.

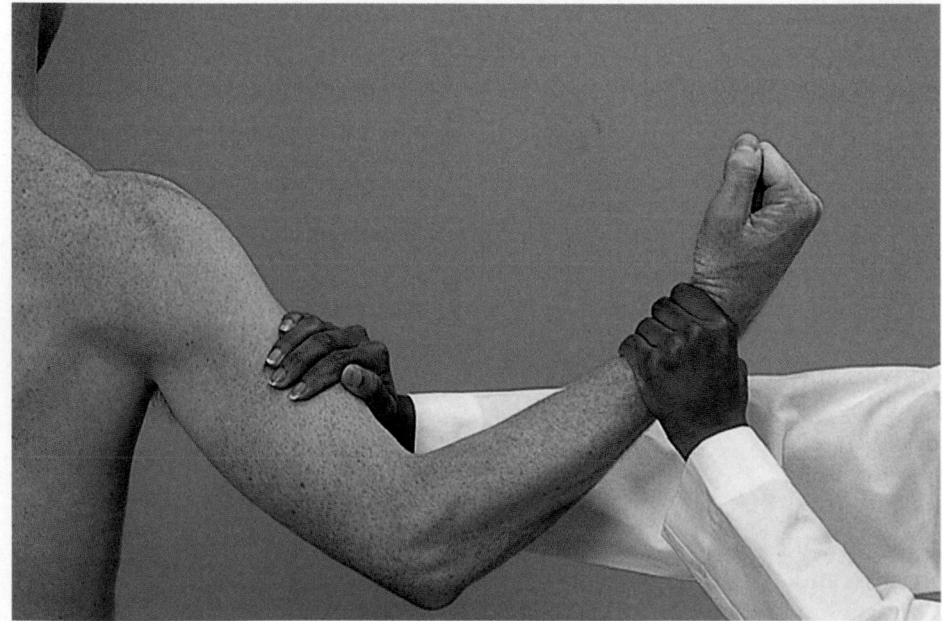

FLEXION AT ELBOW

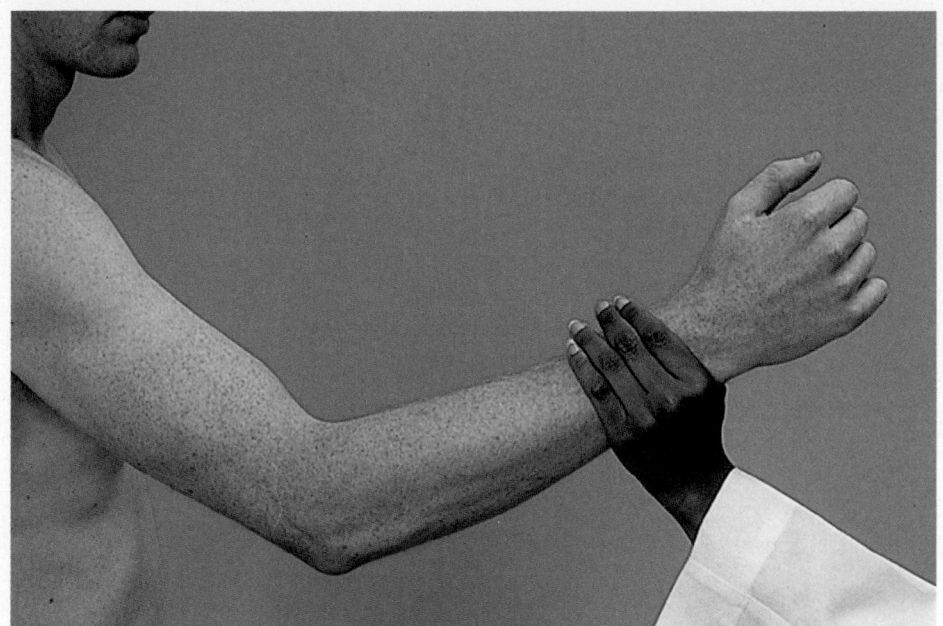

EXTENSION AT ELBOW

THE WRIST AND HANDS

Overview

The wrist and hands form a complex unit of small, highly active joints used almost continuously during waking hours. There is little protection from overlying soft tissue, increasing vulnerability to trauma and disability.

Bony Structures

The wrist includes the distal radius and ulna and eight small carpal bones. At the wrist, identify the bony tips of the radius and the ulna.

The carpal bones lie distal to the wrist joint within each hand. Identify the carpal bones, each of the five metacarpals, and the proximal, middle, and distal phalanges. Note that the thumb lacks a middle phalanx.

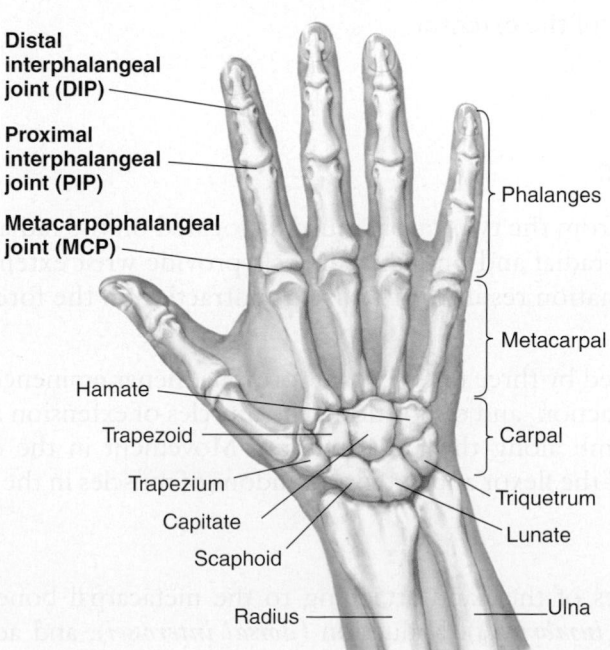

Distal interphalangeal joint (DIP)

Proximal interphalangeal joint (PIP)

Metacarpophalangeal joint (MCP)

Phalanges

Metacarpal

Hamate

Trapezoid

Carpal

Trapezium

Triquetrum

Capitate

Lunate

Scaphoid

Radius

Ulna

Joints

The numerous joints of the wrist and hand lend unusual dexterity to the hands.

- *Wrist joints.* The wrist joints include the *radiocarpal* or *wrist joint*, the *distal radioulnar joint*, and the *intercarpal joints.* The joint capsule, articular disc, and synovial membrane of the wrist join the radius to the ulna and to the proximal carpal bones. On the dorsum of the wrist, locate the groove of the *radiocarpal joint,* which provides most of the flexion and extension at the wrist because the ulna does not articulate directly with the carpal bones.

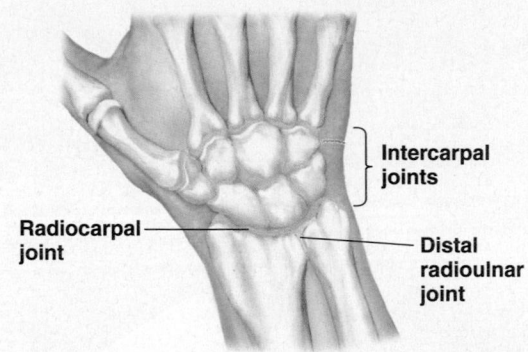

Intercarpal joints

Radiocarpal joint

Distal radioulnar joint

- *Hand joints.* The joints of the hand include the *metacarpophalangeal joints* (MCPs), the *proximal interphalangeal joints* (PIPs), and the *distal interphalangeal joints* (DIPs). Flex the hand and find the groove marking the MCP joint of each finger. It is distal to the knuckle and is best felt on either side of the extensor tendon.

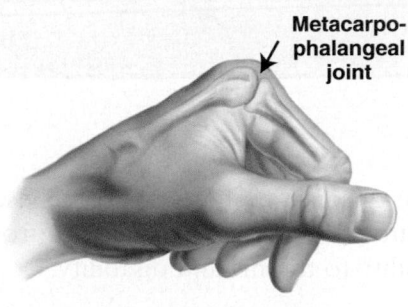

Metacarpophalangeal joint

Muscle Groups

Wrist flexion arises from the two carpal muscles, located on the radial and ulnar surfaces. Two radial and one ulnar muscle provide wrist extension. Supination and pronation result from muscle contraction in the forearm.

The thumb is powered by three muscles that form the thenar eminence and provide flexion, abduction, and opposition. The muscles of extension are at the base of the thumb along the radial margin. Movement in the digits depends on action of the flexor and extensor tendons of muscles in the forearm and wrist.

The intrinsic muscles of the hand attaching to the metacarpal bones are involved in flexion (*lumbricals*), abduction (*dorsal interossei*), and adduction (*palmar interossei*) of the fingers.

Additional Structures

Soft-tissue structures, especially tendons and tendon sheaths, are especially important to movement of the wrist and hand. Six extensor tendons and two flexor tendons pass across the wrist and hand to insert on the fingers. Through much of their course these tendons travel in tunnel-like sheaths, generally palpable only when swollen or inflamed.

Understanding the structures in the *carpal tunnel* is important. It is a channel beneath the palmar surface of the wrist and proximal hand. The channel contains the sheath and flexor tendons of the forearm muscles and the *median nerve*.

Holding the tendons and tendon sheath in place is a transverse ligament, the *flexor retinaculum*. The median nerve lies between the flexor retinaculum and the tendon sheath. It provides sensation to the palm and the palmar surface of most of the thumb, the second and third digits, and half of the fourth digit. It also innervates the thumb muscles of flexion, abduction, and opposition.

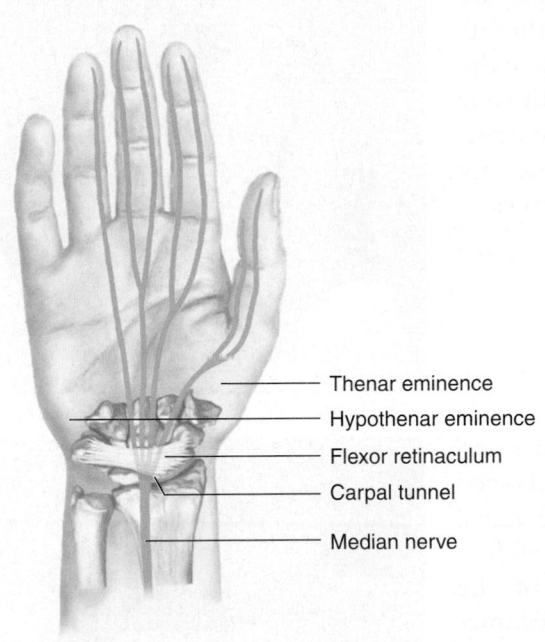

— Thenar eminence
— Hypothenar eminence
— Flexor retinaculum
— Carpal tunnel
— Median nerve

Physical Examination

Inspection.   Observe the position of the hands in motion to see if movements are smooth and natural. At rest, the fingers should be slightly flexed and aligned almost in parallel.

Inspect the palmar and dorsal surfaces of the wrist and hand carefully for swelling over the joints.

Note any deformities of the wrist, hand, or finger bones, as well as any angulation from radial or ulnar deviation.

Guarded movement suggests injury. Poor finger alignment is seen in flexor tendon damage.

Diffuse swelling in arthritis or infection; local swelling from cystic ganglion. See Table 18-5, Arthritis in the Hands (p. 589), and Table 18-6, Swellings and Deformities of the Hands (p. 590).

In *osteoarthritis,* Heberden nodes at the DIP joints, Bouchard nodes at the PIP joints. In *rheumatoid arthritis,* symmetric deformity in the PIP, MCP, and wrist joints, with ulnar deviation

Observe the contours of the palm, namely, the thenar and hypothenar eminences.

Thenar atrophy in median nerve compression from *carpal tunnel syndrome*; hypothenar atrophy in *ulnar nerve compression*.

Note any thickening of the flexor tendons or flexion contractures in the fingers.

Flexion contractures in the ring, 5th, and 3rd fingers, or *Dupuytren contractures*, arise from thickening of the palmar fascia (see p. 590).

Palpation. At the wrist, palpate the distal radius and ulna on the lateral and medial surfaces. Palpate the groove of each wrist joint with your thumbs on the dorsum of the wrist, your fingers beneath it. Note any swelling, bogginess, or tenderness.

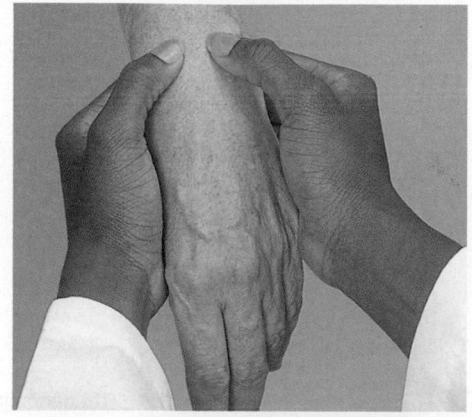

Tenderness over the distal radius in *Colles fracture.* Any tenderness or bony step-offs are suspicious for fracture.

Swelling and/or tenderness suggest *rheumatoid arthritis* if bilateral and of several weeks' duration.

Palpate the radial styloid bone and the *anatomic snuffbox*, a hollowed depression just distal to the radial styloid process formed by the abductor and extensor muscles of the thumb. The "snuffbox" becomes more visible with lateral extension of the thumb away from the hand.

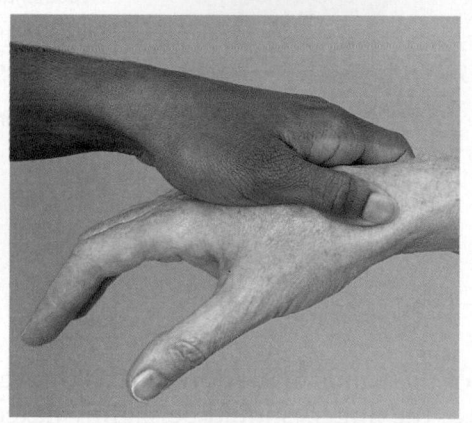

Tenderness over the "snuffbox" in *scaphoid fracture,* the most common injury of the carpal bones. Poor blood supply puts the scaphoid bone at risk for *avascular necrosis.*

Palpate the eight carpal bones lying distal to the wrist joint, and then each of the five metacarpals and the proximal, middle, and distal phalanges.

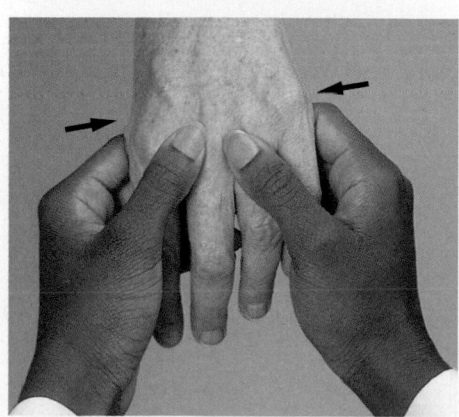

Synovitis in the MCPs is painful with this pressure—a point to remember when shaking hands.

Palpate any other area where you suspect an abnormality.

The MCPs are often boggy or tender in *rheumatoid arthritis* (but rarely involved in osteoarthritis). Pain with compression also in *post-traumatic arthritis*.

Compress the MCP joints by squeezing the hand from each side between the thumb and fingers. Alternatively, use your thumb to palpate each MCP joint just distal to and on each side of the knuckle as your index finger feels the head of the metacarpal in the palm. Note any swelling, bogginess, or tenderness.

Now examine the fingers and thumb. Palpate the medial and lateral aspects of each PIP joint between your thumb and index finger, again checking for swelling, bogginess, bony enlargement, or tenderness.

PIP changes seen in *rheumatoid arthritis*, Bouchard nodes in *osteoarthritis*. Pain at the base of the thumb in first *carpometacarpal arthritis*.

Hard dorsolateral nodules on the DIP joints, or *Heberden nodes*, common in osteoarthritis

Using the same techniques, examine the DIP joints.

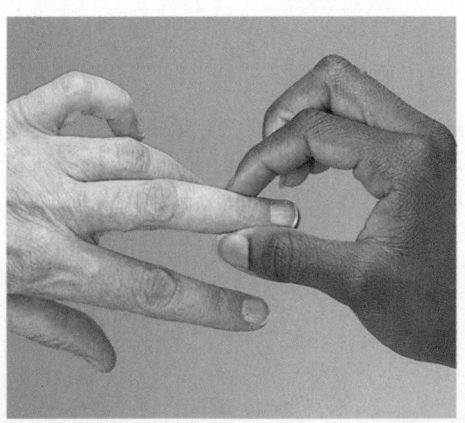

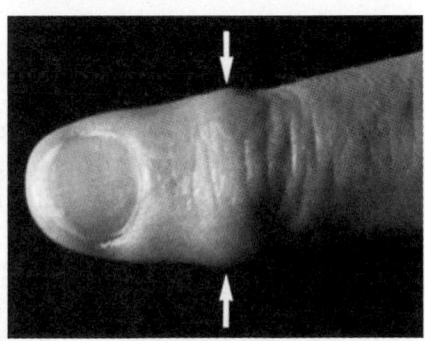

HEBERDEN NODES

In any area of swelling or inflammation, palpate along the tendons inserting on the thumb and fingers.

Wrists: Range of Motion and Maneuvers

Range of Motion. Refer to the table on page 546 for specific muscles responsible for each movement and clear, simple instructions that prompt the patient to properly follow your directions.

Conditions that impair range of motion include *arthritis, tenosynovitis, Dupuytren contracture*. See Table 18-6, Swellings and Deformities of the Hands (p. 590).

Wrist Movement	Primary Muscles Affecting Movement	Patient Instructions
Flexion	Flexor carpi radialis, flexor carpi ulnaris	*"With palms down, point your fingers toward the floor."*
Extension	Extensor carpi ulnaris, extensor carpi radialis longus, extensor carpi radialis brevis	*"With palms down, point your fingers toward the ceiling."*
Adduction (radial deviation)	Flexor carpi ulnaris	*"With palms down, bring your fingers toward the midline."*
Abduction (ulnar deviation)	Flexor carpi radialis	*"With palms down, bring your fingers away from the midline."*

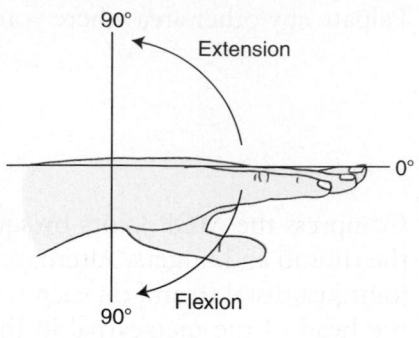

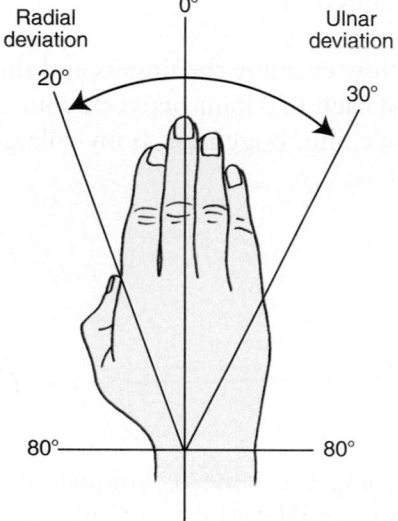

Muscle Strength Tests. *Test extension at the wrist* (C6, C7, C8, radial nerve—extensor carpi radialis longus and brevis) by asking the patient to make a fist and resist your pulling it down.

Weakness of extension is seen in peripheral nerve disease such as radial nerve damage and in central nervous system disease producing hemiplegia, as in *stroke* or *multiple sclerosis.*

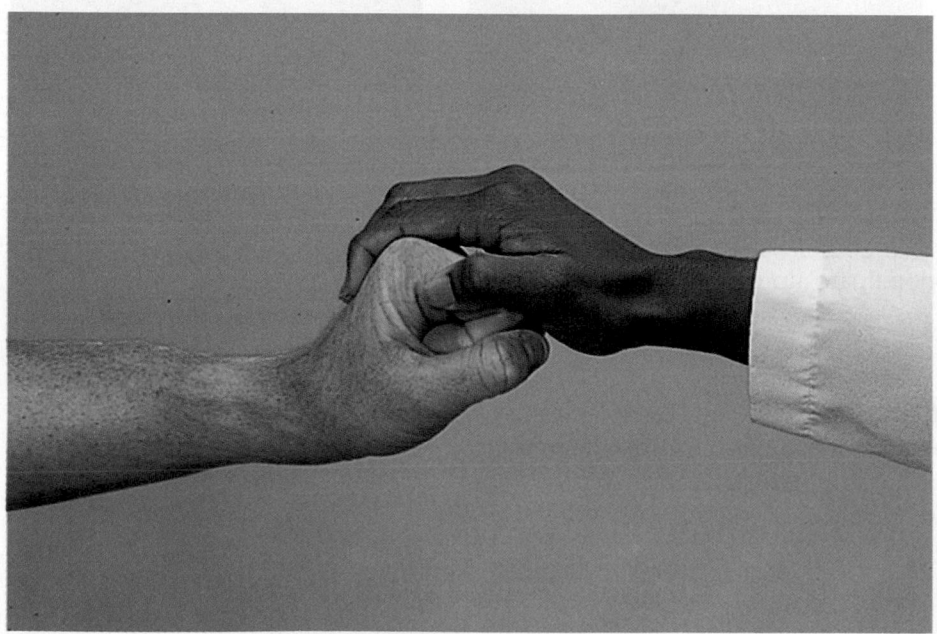

EXTENSION AT WRIST

Test the grip (C7, C8, T1). Ask the patient to squeeze two of your fingers as hard as possible and not let them go. (To avoid getting hurt by hard squeezes, place your own middle finger on top of your index finger.) You should normally have difficulty removing your fingers from the patient's grip. Testing both grips simultaneously with arms extended or in the lap facilitates comparison.

A weak grip in cervical radiculopathy, *de Quervain tenosynovitis, carpal tunnel syndrome,* arthritis, epicondylitis

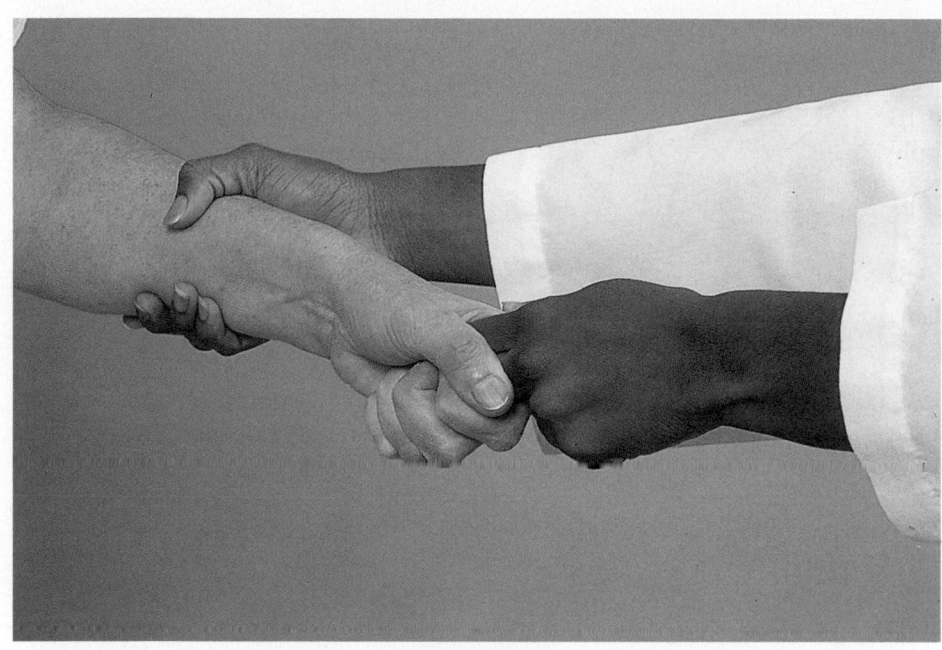

TEST OF GRIP

Maneuvers. Several maneuvers useful for assessing common office complaints relating to the wrist are listed below. For complaints of dropping objects, inability to twist lids off jars, aching at the wrist or even the forearm, and numbness of the first three digits, use the tests on the next page for assessing *carpal tunnel syndrome.* Note the distribution of the median, radial, and ulnar nerve innervations of the wrist and hand on the next page.

Onset of *carpal tunnel syndrome* often related to repetitive motion with wrists flexed (as in keyboard use, mail sorting), pregnancy, rheumatoid arthritis, diabetes, hypothyroidism

Thenar atrophy may also be present.

Decreased sensation in the median nerve distribution in *carpal tunnel syndrome*

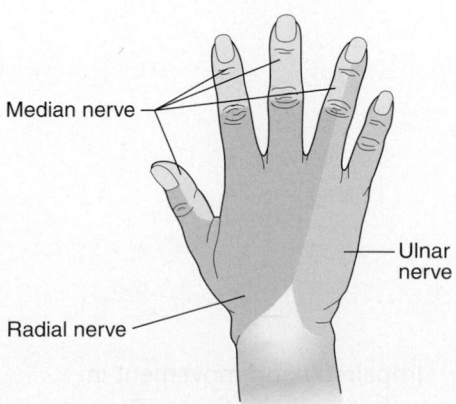

Median nerve

Ulnar nerve

Radial nerve

DORSAL SURFACE

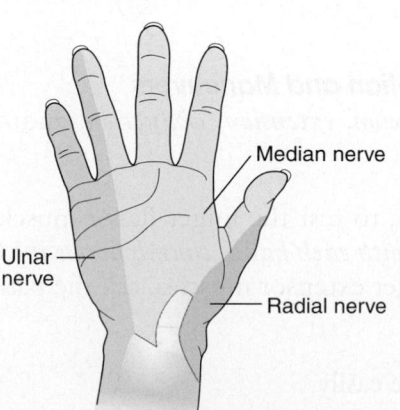

Median nerve

Ulnar nerve

Radial nerve

VOLAR SURFACE

If carpal tunnel syndrome is suspected, test sensation of:

- The index finger—median nerve

- The 5th finger—ulnar nerve

- Dorsal web space of the thumb and index finger—radial nerve

CARPAL TUNNEL—THUMB ABDUCTION, TINEL'S TEST, AND PHALEN'S TEST.[15-17] Test *thumb abduction* by asking the patient to raise the thumb straight up as you apply downward resistance.

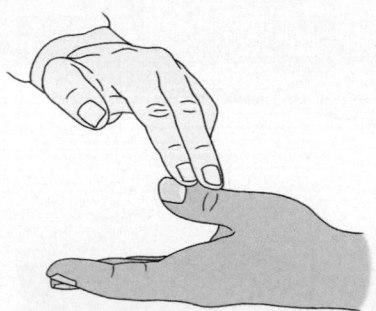

Weakness on thumb abduction is a *positive test*—the abductor pollicis longus is innervated only by the median nerve. Weak thumb abduction and decreased sensation indicate carpal tunnel disease.[17]

Test *Tinel's sign* for median nerve compression by tapping lightly over the course of the median nerve in the carpal tunnel as shown.

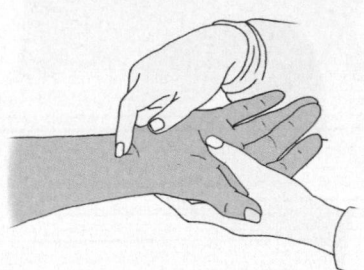

Aching and numbness in the median nerve distribution is a *positive test.*

Test *Phalen's sign* for median nerve compression by asking the patient to hold the wrists in flexion for 60 seconds. Alternatively, ask the patient to press the backs of both hands together to form right angles. These maneuvers compress the median nerve.

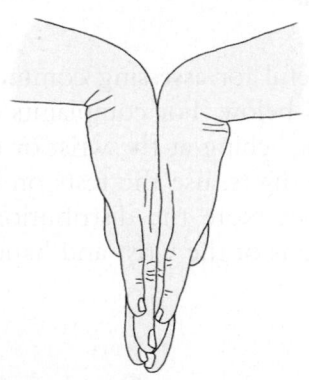

Numbness and tingling in the median nerve distribution within 60 seconds is a *positive test.*

Fingers and Thumbs: Range of Motion and Maneuvers

Range of Motion. Assess *flexion, extension, abduction,* and *adduction* of the fingers.

- *Flexion and extension.* For *flexion,* to test the finger flexor muscles, ask the patient to *"Make a tight fist with each hand, thumb across the knuckles."* For *extension,* to test the finger extensor muscles, ask the patient to *"Extend and spread the fingers."*

The fingers should open and close easily.

Impaired hand movement in arthritis, trigger finger, Dupuytren contracture

● *Abduction and adduction.* Ask the patient to spread the fingers apart (abduction from dorsal interossei) and back together (adduction from palmar interossei). Check for smooth, coordinated movement.

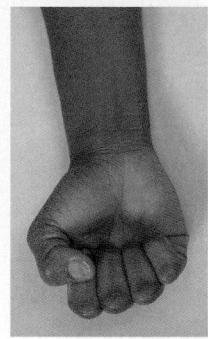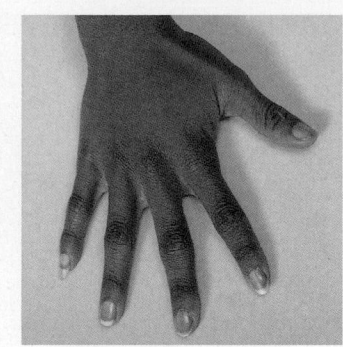

Thumbs. At the *thumb,* assess *flexion, extension, abduction, adduction,* and *opposition.* Each of these movements is powered by a related muscle of the thumb. Ask the patient to move the thumb across the palm and touch the base of the 5th finger to test *flexion,* and then to move the thumb back across the palm and away from the fingers to test *extension.*

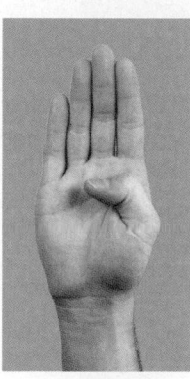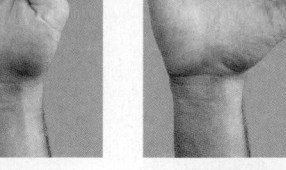

FLEXION   **EXTENSION**

Next, ask the patient to place the fingers and thumb in the neutral position with the palm up; then have the patient move the thumb anteriorly away from the palm to assess abduction and back down for adduction. To test opposition, or movements of the thumb across the palm, ask the patient to touch the thumb to each of the other fingertips.

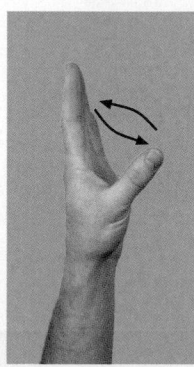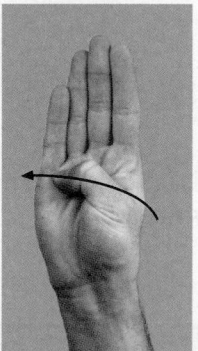

**ABDUCTION AND   OPPOSITION
ADDUCTION**

Finger Muscle Strength Tests. *Test finger abduction* (C8, T1, ulnar nerve). Position the patient's hand with palm down and fingers spread. Instructing the patient not to let you move the fingers, try to force them together.

Weak finger abduction in ulnar nerve disorders

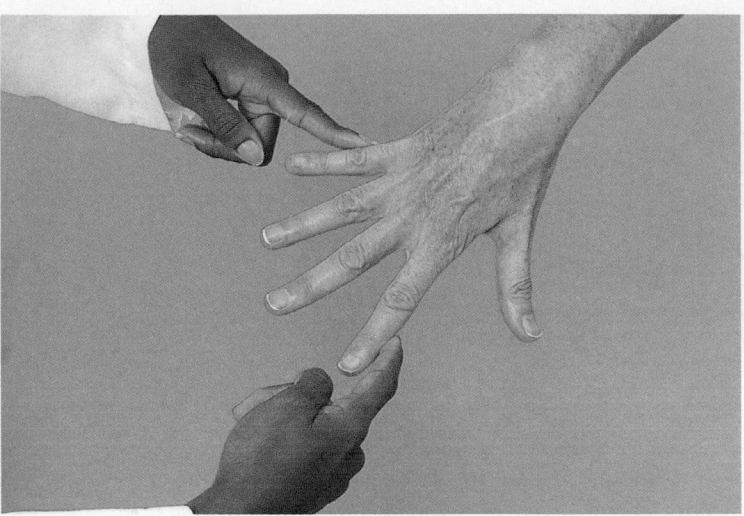

FINGER ABDUCTION

Test opposition of the thumb (C8, T1, median nerve). The patient should try to touch the tip of the little finger with the thumb, against your resistance.

Weak opposition of the thumb in median nerve disorders such as *carpal tunnel syndrome*

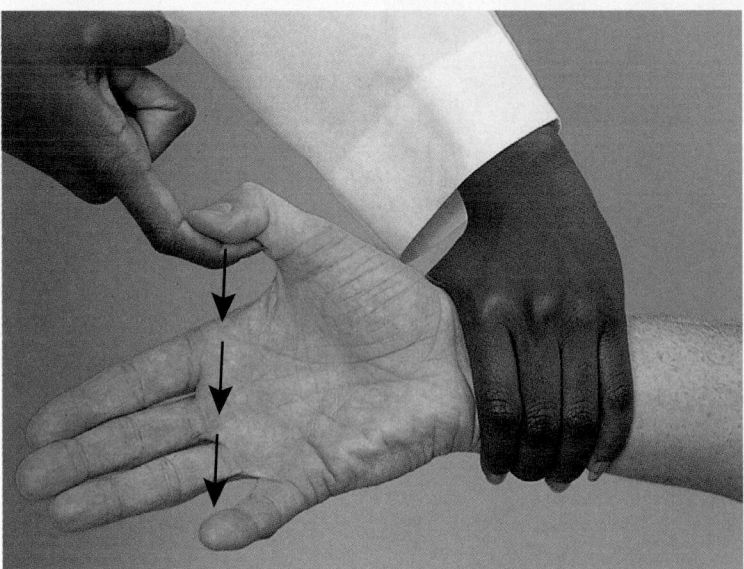

OPPOSITION OF THE THUMB

THE SPINE

Overview

The vertebral column, or spine, is the central supporting structure of the trunk and back. Note the *concave curves* of the cervical and lumbar spine and the *convex curves* of the thoracic and sacrococcygeal spine. These curves help distribute upper body weight to the pelvis and lower extremities and cushion the concussive impact of walking or running.

The complex mechanics of the back reflect the coordinated action of:

- The vertebrae and intervertebral discs

- An interconnecting system of ligaments between anterior vertebrae and posterior vertebrae, ligaments between the spinous processes, and ligaments between the lamina of two adjacent vertebrae

- Large superficial muscles, deeper intrinsic muscles, and muscles of the abdominal wall

Bony Structures

The vertebral column contains 24 vertebrae stacked on the sacrum and coccyx. A typical vertebra contains sites for joint articulations, weight bearing, and muscle attachments, as well as foramina for the spinal nerve roots and peripheral nerves. Anteriorly, the *vertebral body* supports weight bearing. The posterior *vertebral arch* encloses the spinal cord. Review the location of the vertebral processes and foramina, with particular attention to:

- The *spinous process* projecting posteriorly in the midline and the two transverse processes at the junction of the *pedicle* and the *lamina*. Muscles attach at these processes.

- The *articular processes*—two on each side of the vertebra, one facing up and one facing down, at the junction of the pedicles and laminae, often called *articular facets*.

- The *vertebral foramen*, which encloses the spinal cord, the *intervertebral foramen*, formed by the inferior and superior articulating process of adjacent vertebrae, creating a channel for the spinal nerve roots; and in the cervical vertebrae, the *transverse foramen* for the vertebral artery.

REPRESENTATIVE CERVICAL AND LUMBAR VERTEBRAE

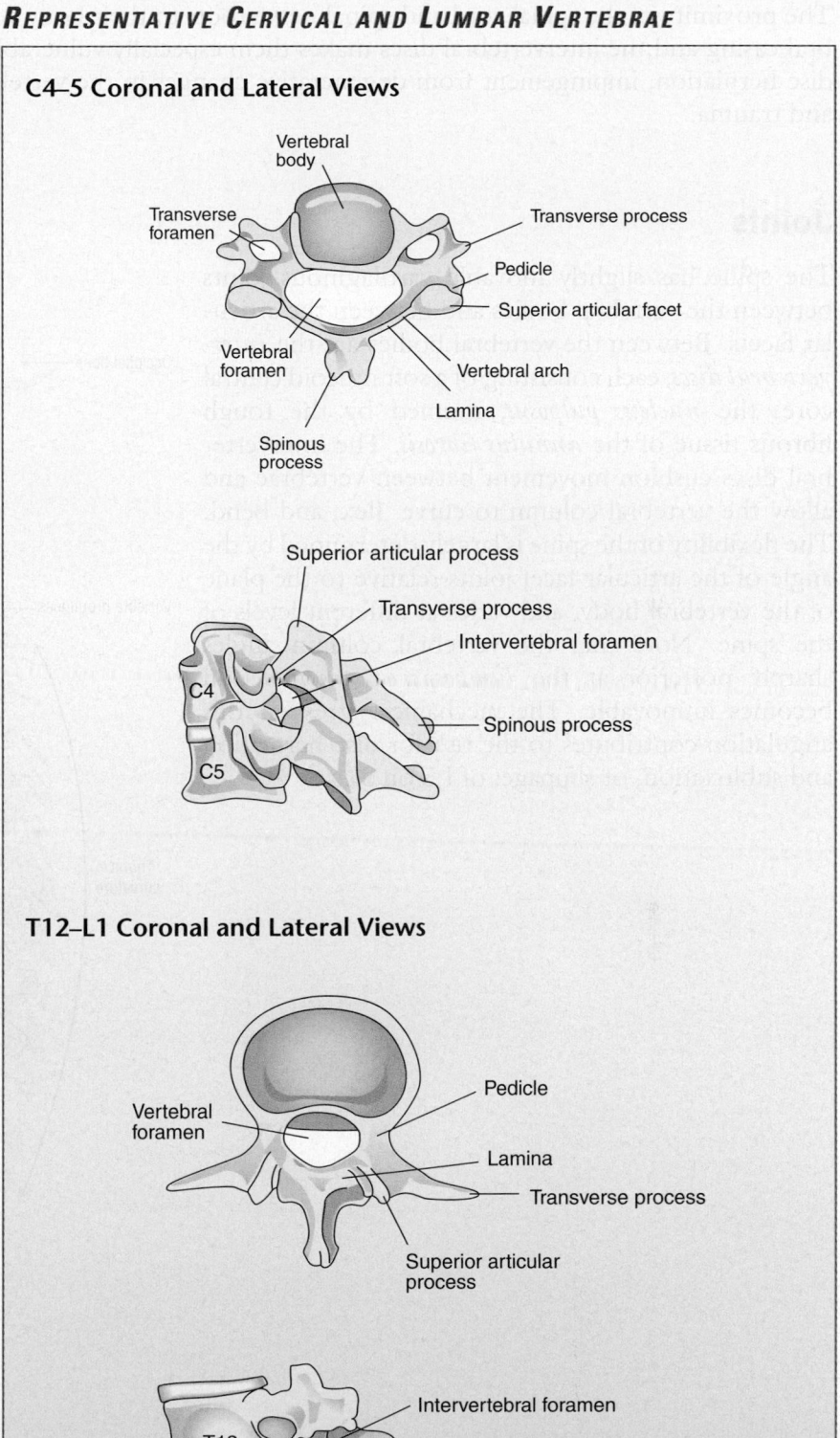

C4–5 Coronal and Lateral Views

T12–L1 Coronal and Lateral Views

The proximity of the spinal cord and spinal nerve roots to their bony vertebral casing and the intervertebral discs makes them especially vulnerable to disc herniation, impingement from degenerative changes in the vertebrae, and trauma.

Joints

The spine has slightly movable cartilaginous joints between the vertebral bodies and between the articular facets. Between the vertebral bodies are the *intervertebral discs,* each consisting of a soft mucoid central core, the *nucleus pulposus,* rimmed by the tough fibrous tissue of the *annulus fibrosis.* The intervertebral discs cushion movement between vertebrae and allow the vertebral column to curve, flex, and bend. The flexibility of the spine is largely determined by the angle of the articular facet joints relative to the plane of the vertebral body, and varies at different levels of the spine. Note that the vertebral column angles sharply posterior at the *lumbosacral junction* and becomes immovable. The mechanical stress at this angulation contributes to the risk for disc herniation and subluxation, or slippage, of L5 on S1.

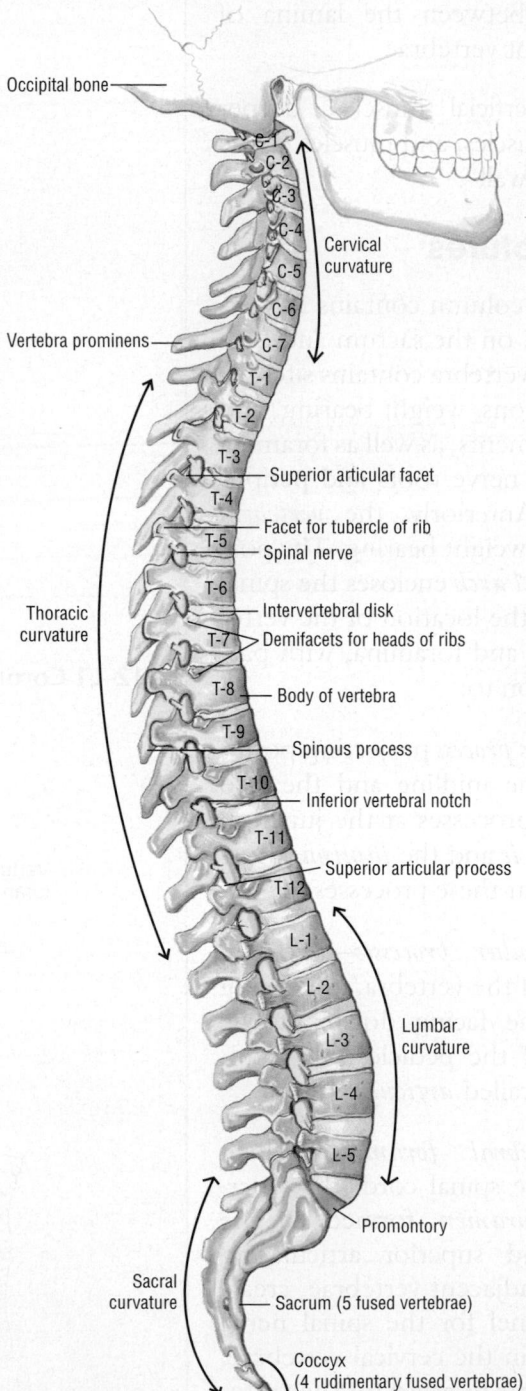

Occipital bone

C-1
C-2
C-3
C-4
C-5
C-6

Cervical curvature

Vertebra prominens — C-7

T-1
T-2
T-3 — Superior articular facet
T-4
T-5 — Facet for tubercle of rib
Spinal nerve
T-6
Intervertebral disk
Thoracic curvature
T-7 — Demifacets for heads of ribs
T-8 — Body of vertebra
T-9
T-10 — Spinous process
Inferior vertebral notch
T-11
Superior articular process
T-12

L-1
L-2
L-3 — Lumbar curvature
L-4
L-5

Promontory

Sacral curvature
Sacrum (5 fused vertebrae)

Coccyx (4 rudimentary fused vertebrae)

Muscle Groups

The *trapezius* and *latissimus dorsi* form the large outer layer of muscles attaching to each side of the spine. They overlie two deeper muscle layers—a layer attaching to the head, neck, and spinous processes (*splenius capitis*, *splenius cervicis*, and *sacrospinalis*) and a layer of smaller intrinsic muscles between vertebrae. Muscles attaching to the anterior surface of the vertebrae, including the *psoas* muscle and muscles of the abdominal wall, assist with flexion.

Muscles moving the neck and lower vertebral column are summarized in the table on pp. 557–558.

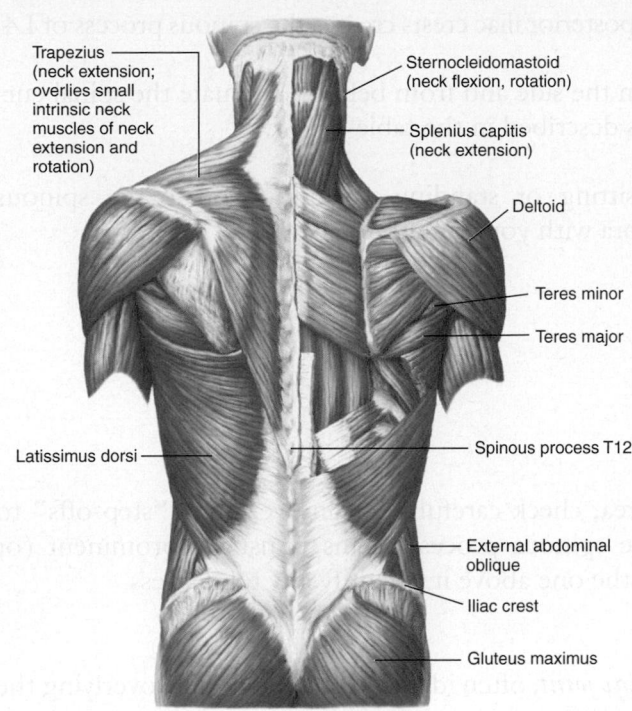

Physical Examination

Inspection.   Begin by observing the patient's posture, including the position of both the neck and trunk, when entering the room.

Assess the patient for erect position of the head; smooth, coordinated neck movement; and ease of gait.

Drape or gown the patient to expose the entire back for complete inspection. If possible, the patient should be upright in the natural standing position—with feet together and arms hanging at the sides. The head should be midline in the same plane as the sacrum, and the shoulders and pelvis should be level.

Viewing the patient from behind, identify the following landmarks:

● Spinous processes of C7 and T1 are usually more prominent with forward neck flexion

● Paravertebral muscles on either side of the midline

● Iliac crests

● Posterior superior iliac spines, usually marked by skin dimples

Neck stiffness signals arthritis, muscle strain, or other underlying pathology that should be pursued.

Lateral deviation and rotation of the head suggest *torticollis*, from contraction of the sternocleidomastoid muscle.

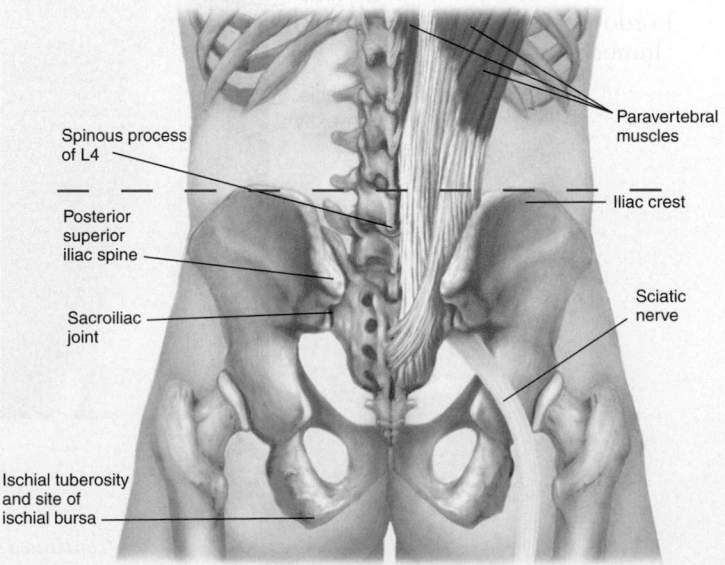

A line drawn above the posterior iliac crests crosses the spinous process of L4.

Inspect the patient from the side and from behind. Evaluate the spinal curvatures and the features described in the table below.

Palpation. From a sitting or standing position, palpate the spinous processes of each vertebra with your thumb.

Tenderness suggests fracture or dislocation if preceded by trauma; if no trauma, suspect underlying infection or arthritis.

Tenderness in arthritis, especially at the facet joints between C5 and C6

In the lower lumbar area, check carefully for any vertebral "step-offs" to determine whether one spinous process seems unusually prominent (or recessed) in relation to the one above it. Identify any tenderness.

Forward slippage of one vertebra may compress the spinal cord. Vertebral tenderness is suspicious for fracture or infection.

Palpate over the *sacroiliac joint*, often identified by the dimple overlying the posterior superior iliac spine.

Tenderness over the sacroiliac joint in sacroiliitis[18]

● Inspection of the Spine

View of Patient	Focus of Inspection	
From the side	Cervical, thoracic, and lumbar curves Kyphosis—increased thoracic curvature Lordosis—increased lumbar curvature	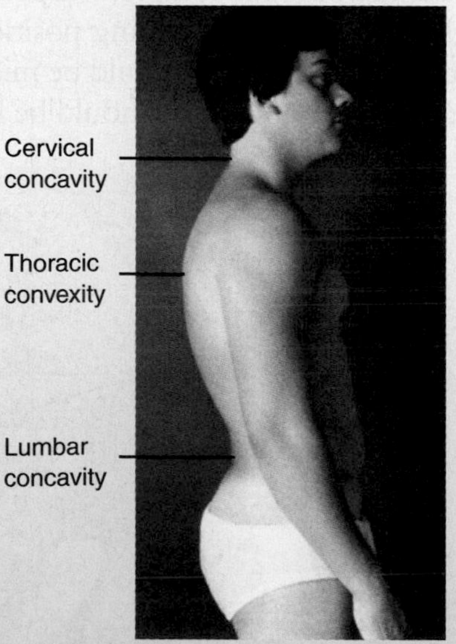 Cervical concavity Thoracic convexity Lumbar concavity	Increased *thoracic kyphosis* often occurs with aging. In children a correctable structural deformity should be pursued.

(continued)

● Inspection of the Spine (continued)

View of Patient	Focus of Inspection	
From behind	Upright spinal column (an imaginary line should fall from C7 through the gluteal cleft) Alignment of the shoulders, the iliac crests, and the skin creases below the buttocks (gluteal folds) Scoliosis—lateral curvature of the spine If scoliosis is suspected, perform the Adam's bend test and use a scoliometer to test for the degree of scoliosis. See further discussion in Chapter 23, Assessing Children.	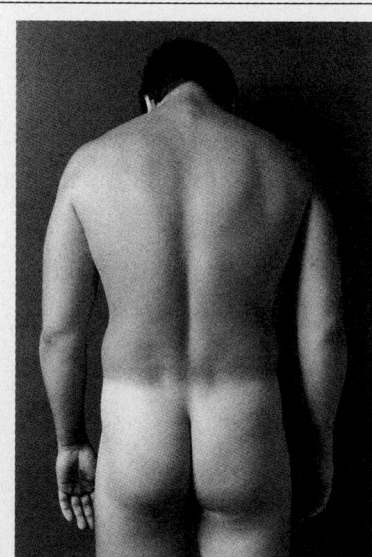 In *scoliosis,* there is lateral and compensatory curvature of the spine to bring the head back to midline. Scoliosis often becomes evident during adolescence. *Unequal shoulder heights* are seen in scoliosis. *Unequal heights of the iliac crests,* or *pelvic tilt,* suggest unequal lengths of the legs and disappear when a block is placed under the short leg and foot. Scoliosis and hip abduction or adduction may also cause a pelvic tilt. "Listing" of the trunk to one side is seen with a herniated lumbar disc.
	Skin markings, tags, or masses	Birthmarks, port-wine stains, hairy patches, and lipomas often overlie bony defects such as *spina bifida.* Café-au-lait spots (discolored patches of skin), skin tags, and fibrous tumors in *neurofibromatosis*

Inspect and palpate the *paravertebral muscles* for tenderness and spasm. Muscles in spasm feel firm and knotted and may be visible.

With the hip flexed and the patient lying on the opposite side, palpate the *sciatic nerve,* the largest nerve in the body, consisting of nerve roots from L4, L5,

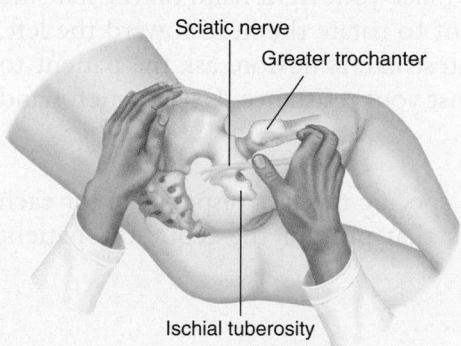

Sciatic nerve
Greater trochanter
Ischial tuberosity

Spasm occurs in degenerative and inflammatory processes of muscles, prolonged contraction from abnormal posture, or anxiety.

Sciatic nerve tenderness suggests a herniated disc or mass lesion impinging on the contributing nerve roots.

S1, S2, and S3. The nerve lies midway between the greater trochanter and the ischial tuberosity as it leaves the pelvis through the sciatic notch.

Herniated intervertebral discs, most common at L5–S1 or L4–L5, may produce tenderness of the spinous processes, the intervertebral joints, the paravertebral muscles, the sacrosciatic notch, and the sciatic nerve.

Palpate for tenderness in any other areas that are suggested by the patient's symptoms.

Rheumatoid arthritis may also cause tenderness of the intervertebral joints.

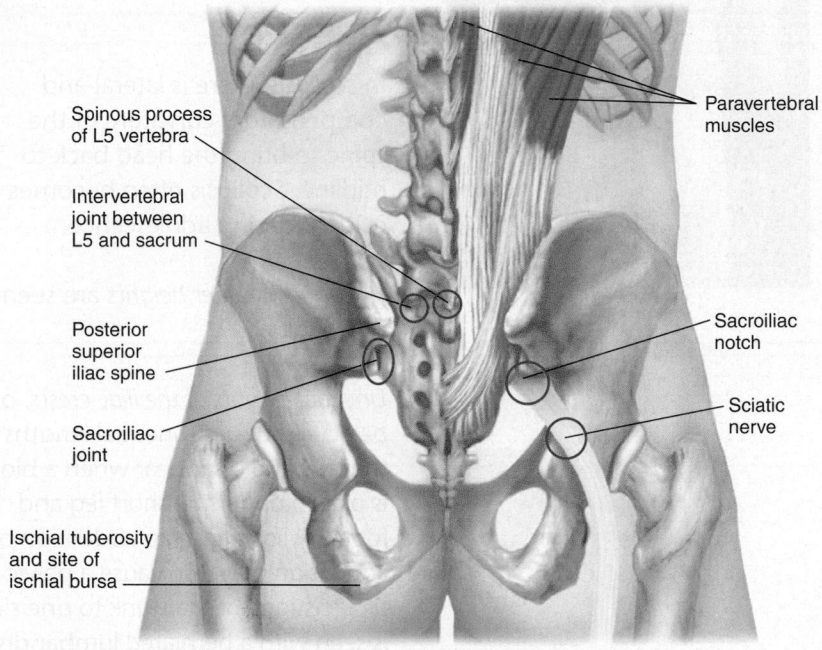

- Spinous process of L5 vertebra
- Intervertebral joint between L5 and sacrum
- Posterior superior iliac spine
- Sacroiliac joint
- Ischial tuberosity and site of ischial bursa
- Paravertebral muscles
- Sacroiliac notch
- Sciatic nerve

Remember that tenderness in the costovertebral angles may signify kidney infection rather than a musculoskeletal problem.

See Table 18-1, Low Back Pain (p. 584).

Range of Motion and Maneuvers

Range of Motion: Neck.   The neck is the most mobile portion of the spine, remarkable for its seven fragile vertebrae supporting the 10- to 15-pound head. *Flexion* and *extension* occur primarily between the skull and C1, the atlas; *rotation* at C1–C2; the axis, and *lateral bending* at C2–C7.

Limitations in range of motion can arise from stiffness from arthritis, pain from trauma, or muscle spasm such as *torticollis*.

Muscle Strength Test.   Muscle strength of the neck may be tested with range of motion by the examiner placing a hand to resist the motion of the patient. For example, to test rotation, place your right hand on the left side of the patient's face and ask the patient to rotate the head toward the left, and then return to midline; then, to test lateral flexion, ask the patient to touch the left ear to the shoulder against your resistance. Use your left hand for the opposite side.

In the table following page, note the specific muscles responsible for each motion and clear, simple instructions that prompt the requested patient response.

Neck, shoulder, or arm pain or numbness may indicate cervical cord or nerve root compression. See Table 18-2, Pains in the Neck (p. 585).

Neck Movement	Primary Muscles Affecting Movement	Patient Instructions
Flexion	Sternocleidomastoid, scalene, prevertebral muscles	*"Bring your chin to your chest."*
Extension	Splenius capitis and cervicis, small intrinsic neck muscles	*"Look up at the ceiling."*
Rotation	Sternocleidomastoid, small intrinsic neck muscles	*"Look over one shoulder, and then the other."*
Lateral Bending	Scalenes and small intrinsic neck muscles	*"Bring your ear to your shoulder."*

If the patient has tenderness, loss of sensation, muscle weakness or impaired movement, perform careful neurologic testing of the neck and upper extremities.

Tenderness at C1–C2 in *rheumatoid arthritis* suggests possible risk for subluxation and high cervical cord compression.

Range of Motion: Spinal Column. Now assess range of motion in the spinal column. In the table below, note the specific muscles responsible for each motion and clear, simple instructions that prompt the requested patient response.

Back Movement	Primary Muscles Affecting Movement	Patient Instructions
Flexion	Psoas major, psoas minor, quadratus lumborum; abdominal muscles attaching to the anterior vertebrae, such as the internal and external obliques and rectus abdominis	*"Bend forward and try to touch your toes."* Note the smoothness and symmetry of movement, the range of motion, and the curve in the lumbar area. As flexion proceeds, the lumbar concavity should flatten out.

Deformity of the thorax on forward bending in *scoliosis*

To measure flexion of the spine, mark the spine at the lumbosacral junction, then 10 cm above and 5 cm below this point. A 4-cm increase between the two upper marks is normal; the distance between the lower two marks should be unchanged.

10+ cm

5 cm

Normally increased by up to 4 cm

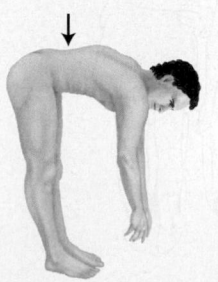

Persistence of lumbar lordosis suggests muscle spasm or *ankylosing spondylitis*.

(continued)

Back Movement	Primary Muscles Affecting Movement	Patient Instructions	
Extension	Deep intrinsic muscles of the back, such as the erector spinae and transversospinalis groups	*"Bend back as far as possible."*	Decreased *spinal mobility* in *osteoarthritis* and *ankylosing spondylitis*,[18,19] among other conditions
		Support the patient by placing your hand on the posterior superior iliac spine, with your fingers pointing toward the midline.	
Rotation	Abdominal muscles, intrinsic muscles of the back	*"Rotate from side to side."*	
		Stabilize the patient's pelvis by placing one hand on the patient's hip and the other on the opposite shoulder. Then rotate the trunk by pulling the shoulder and then the hip posteriorly. Repeat these maneuvers for the opposite side.	
Lateral Bending	Abdominal muscles, intrinsic muscles of the back	*"Bend to the side from the waist."*	
		Stabilize the patient's pelvis by placing your hand on the patient's hip. Repeat for the opposite side.	

Muscle Strength Test. Assessment of **muscle strength** of the spinal column may also be performed during the range-of-motion assessment by having the patient flex, extend, and flex laterally against resistance.

Pain or tenderness with these maneuvers, particularly with radiation into the leg, warrants careful neurologic testing of the lower extremities and referral to an advanced practitioner or physician.

Underlying cord or nerve root compression should be considered. Note that arthritis or infection in the hip, rectum, or pelvis may cause symptoms in the lumbar spine. See Table 18-1, p. 584, Low Back Pain

THE HIP

Overview

The hip joint is deeply embedded in the pelvis and is notable for its strength, stability, and wide range of motion. The stability of the hip joint, so essential for weight bearing, arises from the deep fit of the head of the femur into the *acetabulum*, its strong fibrous articular capsule, and the powerful muscles crossing the joint and inserting below the femoral head, providing leverage for movement of the femur.

Bony Structures and Joints

The hip joint lies below the middle third of the inguinal ligament but in a deeper plane. It is a ball-and-socket joint—note how the rounded head of the femur articulates with the cup-like cavity of the acetabulum. Because of its overlying muscles and depth, it is not readily palpable. Review the bones of the pelvis—the *acetabulum*, the *ilium*, and the *ischium*—and the connection inferiorly at the *symphysis pubis* and posteriorly with the sacroiliac bone.

On the *anterior surface of the hip,* locate the following bony landmarks:

- The iliac crest at the level of L4

- The iliac tubercle

- The anterior superior iliac spine

- The greater trochanter

- The pubic symphysis

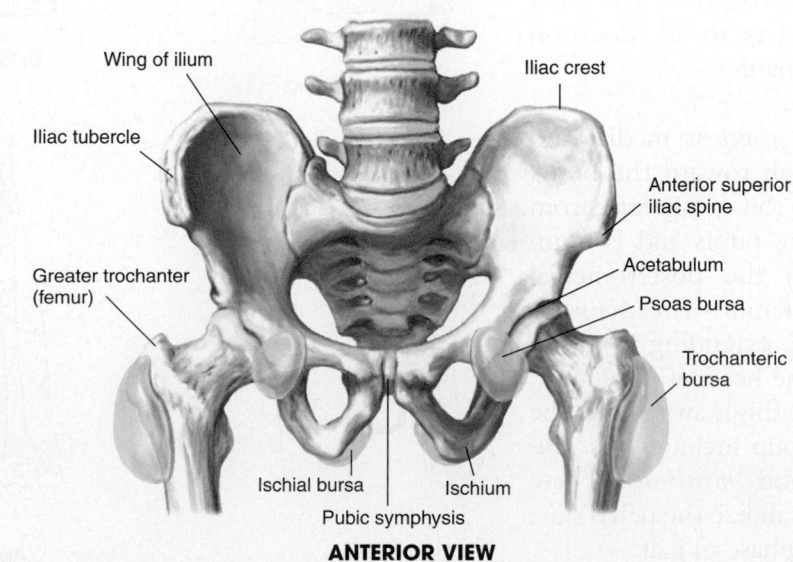

Wing of ilium

Iliac crest

Iliac tubercle

Anterior superior iliac spine

Greater trochanter (femur)

Acetabulum

Psoas bursa

Trochanteric bursa

Ischial bursa

Ischium

Pubic symphysis

ANTERIOR VIEW

On the *posterior surface of the hip,* locate the following:

- The posterior superior iliac spine
- The greater trochanter
- The ischial tuberosity
- The sacroiliac joint

Note that an imaginary line between the posterior superior iliac spines crosses the joint at S2.

Muscle Groups

Four powerful muscle groups move the hip. Picture these groups as you examine patients, and remember that to move the femur or any bone in a given direction, the proximal and distal muscle insertions must **extend across the joint line.**

The *flexor group* lies anteriorly and flexes the thigh. The primary hip flexor is the *iliopsoas,* extending from above the iliac crest to the lesser trochanter. The *extensor group* lies posteriorly and extends the thigh. The *gluteus maximus* is the primary extensor of the hip. It forms a band crossing from its origin along the medial pelvis to its insertion below the trochanter.

The *adductor group* is medial and swings the thigh toward the body. The muscles in this group arise from the rami of the pubis and ischium and insert on the posteromedial aspect of the femur. The *abductor group* is lateral, extending from the iliac crest to the head of the femur, and moves the thigh away from the body. This group includes the *gluteus medius* and *minimus.* These muscles help stabilize the pelvis during the stance phase of gait.

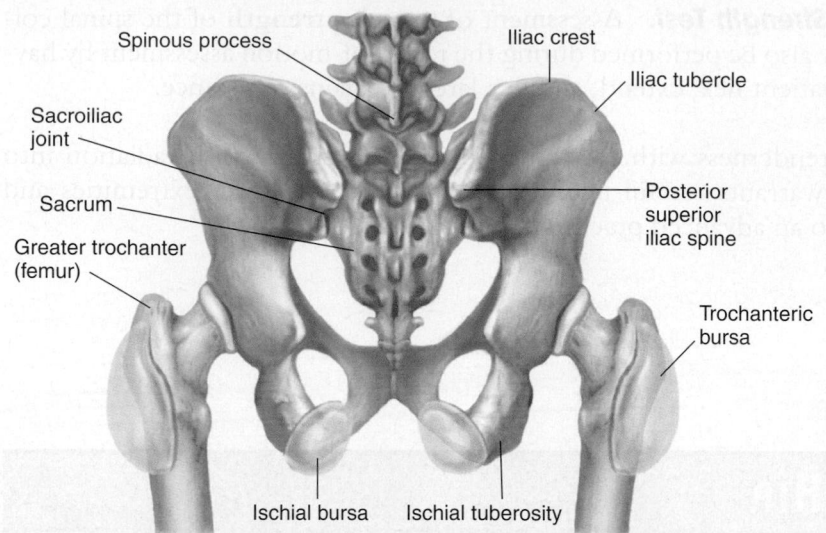

POSTERIOR VIEW

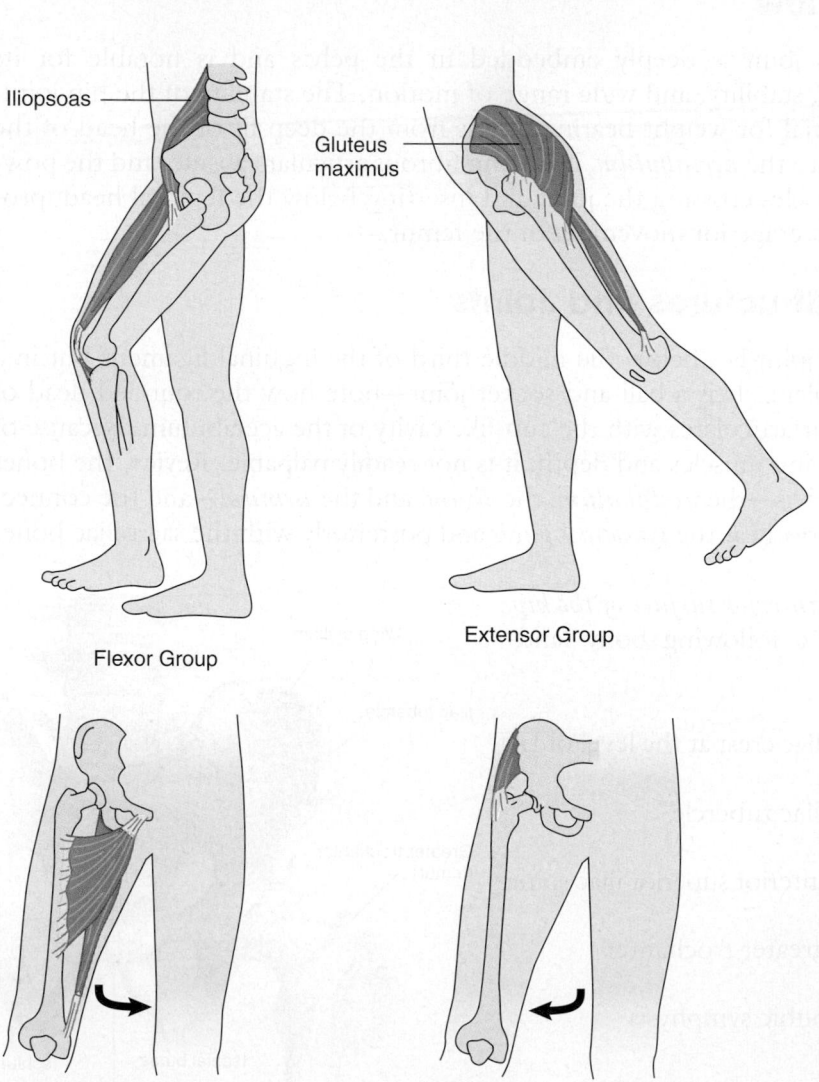

Flexor Group

Extensor Group

Adductor Group

Abductor Group

Additional Structures

A strong, dense articular capsule, extending from the acetabulum to the femoral neck, encases and strengthens the hip joint, reinforced by three overlying ligaments and lined with synovial membrane. There are three principal bursae at the hip. Anterior to the joint is the *psoas* (also termed *iliopectineal* or *iliopsoas*) *bursa*, overlying the articular capsule and the psoas muscle. Find the bony prominence lateral to the hip joint—the *greater trochanter* of the femur. The large multilocular *trochanteric bursa* lies on its posterior surface. The *ischial* (or *ischiogluteal*) *bursa*—not always present—lies under the *ischial tuberosity*, on which a person sits. Note its proximity to the sciatic nerve, as shown on p. 556.

Physical Examination

Inspection. Inspection of the hip begins with careful observation of the patient's gait on entering the room. Observe the two phases of gait:

- *Stance*—when the foot is on the ground and bears weight (60% of the walking cycle)

Most problems appear during the weight-bearing stance phase.

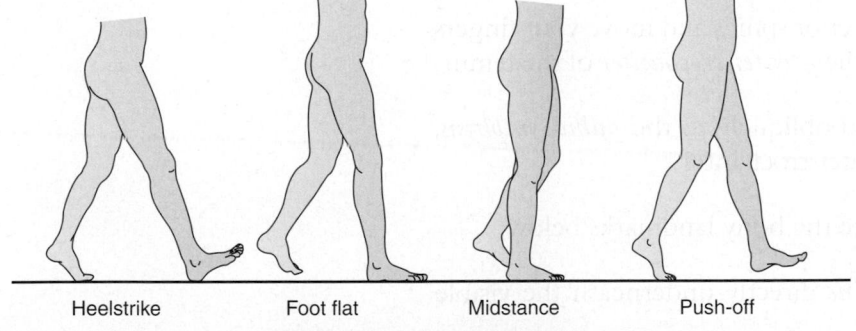

Heelstrike   Foot flat   Midstance   Push-off

THE STANCE PHASE OF GAIT

- *Swing*—when the foot moves forward and does not bear weight (40% of the cycle)

Observe the gait for the width of the base, the shift of the pelvis, and flexion of the knee. The width of the base should be 2 to 4 inches from heel to heel. Normal gait has a smooth, continuous rhythm, achieved in part by contraction of the abductors of the weight-bearing limb. Abductor contraction stabilizes the pelvis and helps maintain balance, raising the opposite hip. The knee should be flexed throughout the stance phase, except when the heel strikes the ground to counteract motion at the ankle. The ankle should dorsiflex so the foot does not drag the ground during the swing phase.

A wide base suggests cerebellar disease or foot problems.

Hip dislocation, arthritis, or abductor weakness can cause the pelvis to drop on the opposite side, producing a waddling gait.

Lack of knee flexion interrupts the smooth pattern of gait.

Lack of dorsiflexion may be due to footdrop. The patient will compensate by lifting the knee higher when walking.

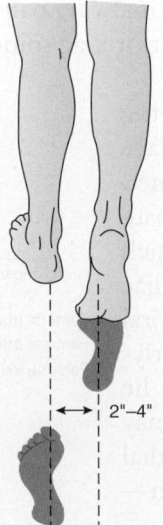

2"–4"

Observe the lumbar portion of the spine for slight lordosis and, with the patient supine, assess the length of the legs for symmetry. (To measure leg length, see Special Techniques, pp. 576–577).

Inspect the anterior and posterior surfaces of the hip for any areas of muscle atrophy or bruising.

Loss of lordosis may reflect *paravertebral spasm*; excess lordosis suggests a *flexion deformity* of the hip.

Changes in leg length are seen in abduction or adduction deformities and scoliosis. Leg shortening and external rotation suggest *hip fracture*.

Palpation

Bony Landmarks. Palpate the surface landmarks of the hip, identified on pp. 559–560. On the *anterior aspect* of the hips, palpate the key structures listed below.

● Identify the *iliac crest* at the upper margin of the pelvis at the level of L4.

● Follow the downward anterior curve and locate the *iliac tubercle*, marking the widest point of the crest, and continue tracking downward to the *anterior superior iliac spine*.

● Place your thumbs on the anterior superior spines and move your fingers downward from the iliac tubercles to the *greater trochanter* of the femur.

● Then move your thumbs medially and obliquely to the *pubic symphysis*, which lies at the same level as the greater trochanter.

On the *posterior aspect* of the hips, palpate the bony landmarks below.

● Palpate the *posterior superior iliac spine* directly underneath the visible dimples just above the buttocks.

● Placing your left thumb and index finger over the posterior superior iliac spine, next locate the *greater trochanter* laterally with your fingers at the level of the gluteal fold, and place your thumb medially on the *ischial tuberosity*. The *sacroiliac joint* is not always palpable. Note that an imaginary line along the posterior superior iliac spines crosses the joint at S2.

Inguinal Structures. With the patient supine, ask the patient to place the heel of the leg being examined on the opposite knee. Then palpate along the *inguinal ligament*, which extends from the anterior superior iliac spine to the pubic tubercle. The femoral nerve, artery, and vein bisect the overlying inguinal ligament; lymph nodes lie medially. The mnemonic **NAVEL** may help you remember the lateral-to-medial sequence of **N**erve—**A**rtery—**V**ein—**E**mpty space—**L**ymph node.

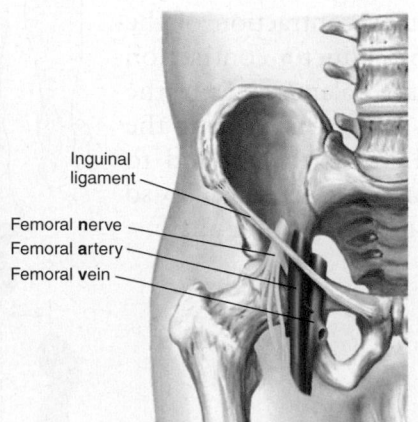

Inguinal ligament
Femoral nerve
Femoral artery
Femoral vein

Bulges along the ligament may suggest an *inguinal hernia* or, on occasion, an *aneurysm*.

Enlarged lymph nodes suggest infection in the lower extremity or pelvis.

Tenderness in the groin area may be from *synovitis* of the hip joint, *bursitis*, or possibly *psoas abscess*.

Range of Motion and Maneuvers

Range of Motion.   Now assess hip range of motion, referring to the table below for specific muscles responsible for each movement and clear, simple instructions that prompt the patient to properly follow your directions.

Hip Movement	Primary Muscles Affecting Movement	Patient Instructions
Flexion	Iliopsoas	*"Bend your knee to your chest and pull it against your abdomen."*
Extension (actually hyperextension)	Gluteus maximus	*"Lie face down, and then bend your knee and lift it up."* *"Or "Lying flat, move your lower leg away from the midline and down over the side of the table."*
Abduction	Gluteus medius and minimus	*"Lying flat, move your lower leg away from the midline."*
Adduction	Adductor brevis, adductor longus, adductor magnus, pectineus, gracilis	*"Lying flat, bend your knee and move your lower leg toward the midline."*
External Rotation	Internal and external obturators, quadratus femoris, superior and inferior gemelli	*"Lying flat, bend your knee and turn your lower leg and foot across the midline."*
Internal Rotation	Gluteus medius and minimus	*"Lying flat, bend your knee and turn your lower leg and foot away from the midline."*

Before performing range of motion on patients who have had hip replacement surgery, ascertain whether they have hip motion limitations. To prevent hip dislocation, patients may be limited to a 90° flexion, and should avoid adduction beyond the midline and internal rotation.

Maneuvers.   Often the examiner must assist the patient with hip range of motion. Further detail is provided below for knee flexion, abduction, adduction, and external and internal rotation.

- *Flexion.* With the patient supine, place your hand under the patient's lumbar spine. Ask the patient to bend each knee in turn up to the chest and pull it firmly against the abdomen. Note that the hip can flex further when the knee is flexed. When the back touches your hand, indicating normal flattening of the lumbar lordosis, further flexion must arise from the hip joint itself.

In *flexion deformity of the hip,* as the opposite hip is flexed (with the thigh against the chest), the affected hip does not allow full leg extension, and the affected thigh appears flexed. See picture on right, p. 564.

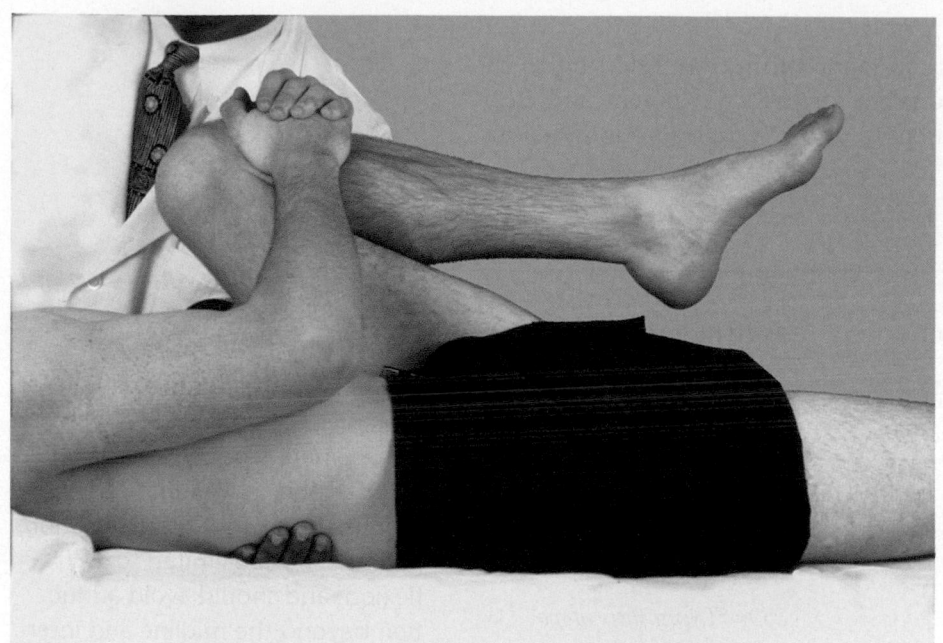
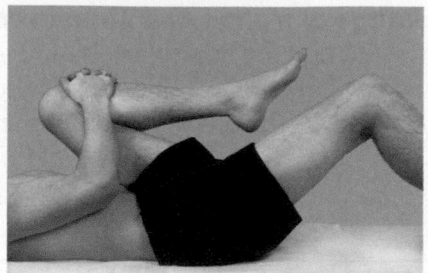

HIP FLEXION AND FLATTENING OF LUMBAR LORDOSIS

As the thigh is held against the abdomen, observe the degree of flexion at the hip and knee. Normally the anterior portion of the thigh can almost touch the chest wall. Note whether the opposite thigh remains fully extended, resting on the table.

Muscle Strength Test. *Test muscle strength during flexion at the hip* (L2, L3, L4—iliopsoas) by placing your hand on the patient's thigh and asking the patient to raise the leg against your hand.

Flexion deformity may be masked by an increase, rather than flattening, in lumbar lordosis and an anterior pelvic tilt.

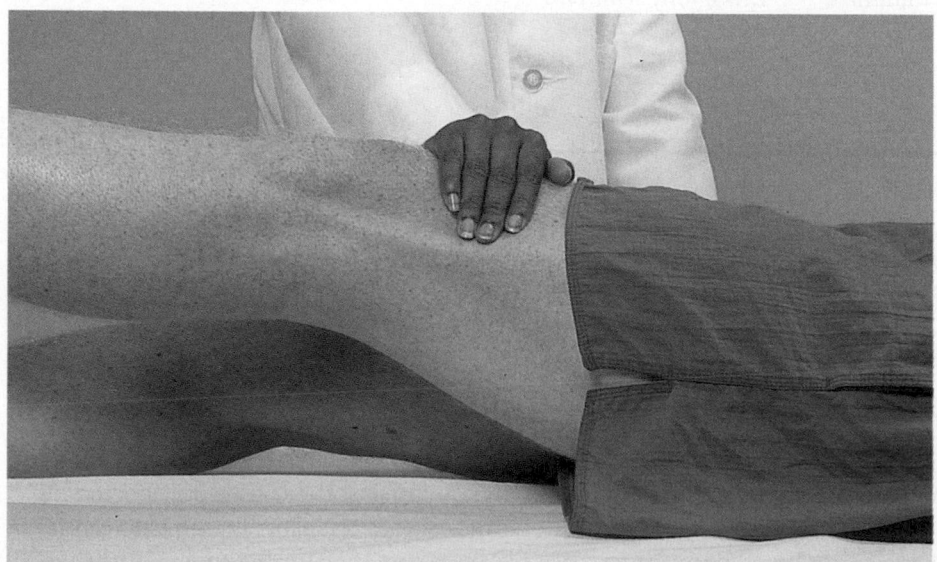

FLEXION OF THE HIP

- *Extension.* With the patient lying face down, extend the thigh toward you in a posterior direction. Alternatively, carefully position the supine patient near the edge of the table and extend the leg posteriorly.

Muscle Strength Test. *Test muscle strength during extension at the hips* (S1—gluteus maximus) by having the supine patient push the posterior thigh down against your hand.

- *Abduction.* Stabilize the pelvis by pressing down on the opposite anterior superior iliac spine with one hand. With the other hand, grasp the ankle and abduct the extended leg until you feel the iliac spine move. This movement marks the limit of hip abduction.

Restricted abduction is common in hip *osteoarthritis.*

Alternatively, stand at the foot of the table, grasp both ankles, and spread them maximally, abducting both extended legs at the hips. This method provides easy comparison of two sides when movements are restricted, but it is impractical when range of motion is full.

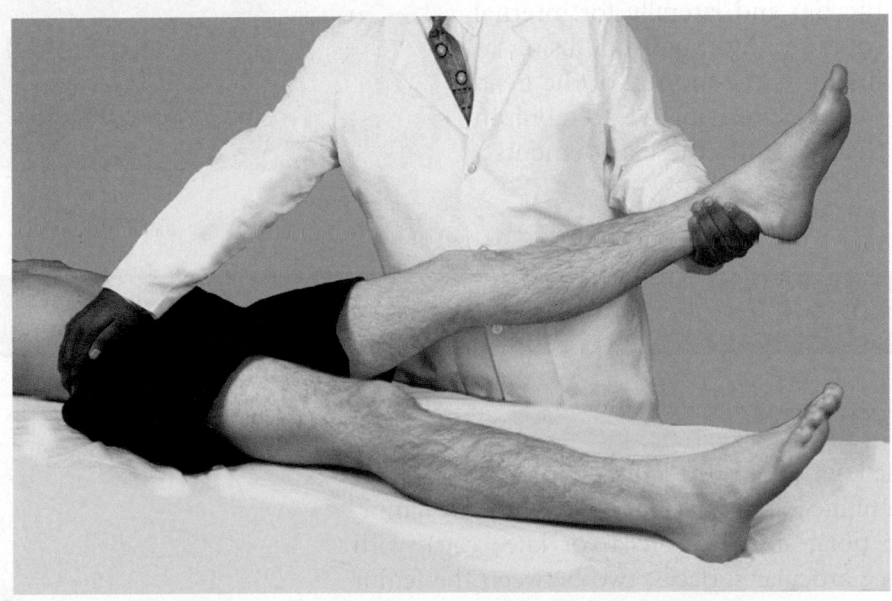

Test muscle strength during abduction at the hips (L4, L5, S1—gluteus medius and minimus) By placing your hands firmly on the bed outside the patient's knees. Ask the patient to spread both legs against your hands.

- *Adduction.* With the patient supine, stabilize the pelvis, hold one ankle, and move the leg medially across the body and over the opposite extremity.

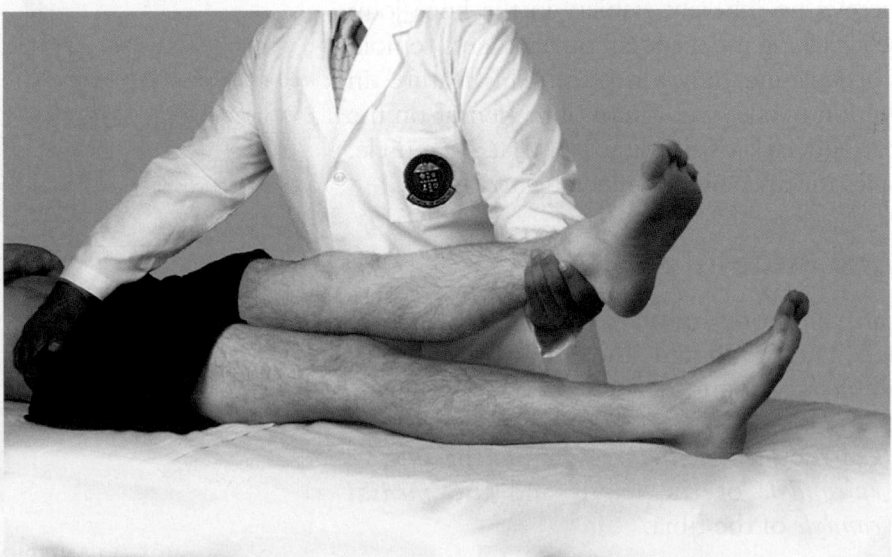

Test muscle strength during adduction at the hips (L2, L3, L4—adductors) by placing your hands firmly on the bed between the patient's knees. Ask the patient to bring both legs together.

Symmetric weakness of the proximal muscles suggests a *myopathy* or muscle disorder; symmetric weakness of distal muscles suggests a *polyneuropathy,* or disorder of peripheral nerves.

- *External and internal rotation.* Flex the leg to 90° at hip and knee, stabilize the thigh with one hand, grasp the ankle with the other, and swing the lower leg— medially for external rotation at the hip and laterally for internal rotation. Although confusing at first, it is the motion of the head of the femur in the acetabulum that identifies these movements.

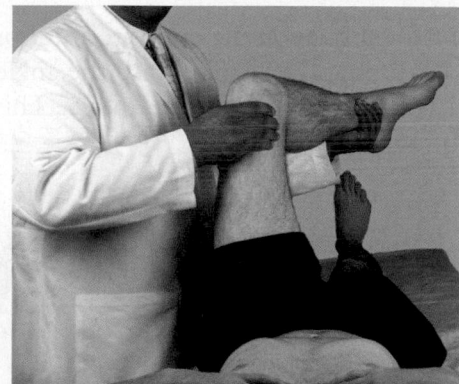

Restrictions of internal and external rotation are sensitive indicators of hip disease such as arthritis.[20]

THE KNEE

Overview

The knee joint is the largest joint in the body. It is a hinge joint involving three bones: the femur, the tibia, and the patella (or knee cap), with three articular surfaces, two between the femur and the tibia and one between the femur and the patella. Note how the two rounded condyles of the femur rest on the relatively flat tibial plateau. There is no inherent stability in the knee joint itself, making it dependent on ligaments to hold its articulating bones in place. This feature, in addition to the lever action of the femur on the tibia and lack of padding from fat or muscle, makes the knee highly vulnerable to injury.

Bony Structures

Learn the bony landmarks in and around the knee. These will guide the examination of this complicated joint.

- On the *medial surface,* identify the *medial epicondyle* of the femur and the *medial condyle* of the tibia.

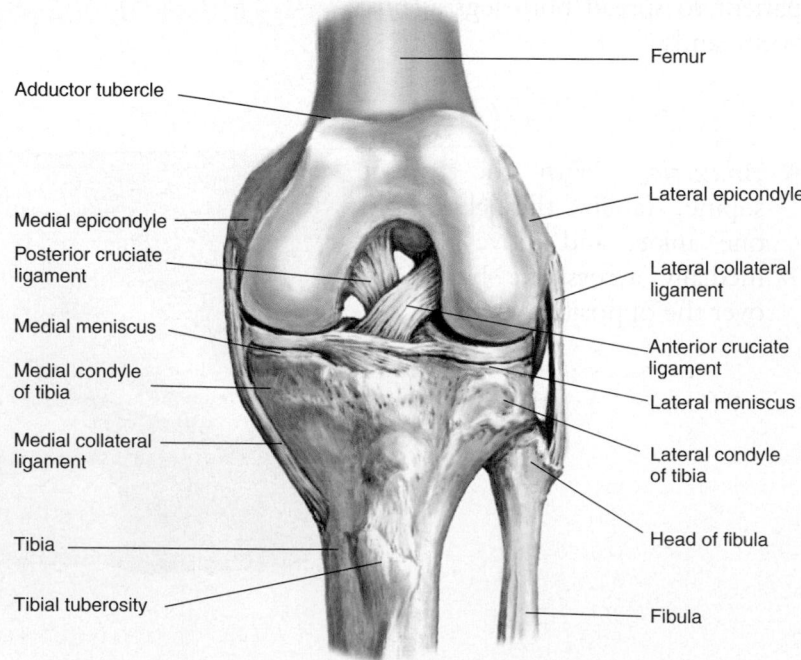

ANTERIOR ASPECT OF THE KNEE

Labels: Adductor tubercle; Medial epicondyle; Posterior cruciate ligament; Medial meniscus; Medial condyle of tibia; Medial collateral ligament; Tibia; Tibial tuberosity; Femur; Lateral epicondyle; Lateral collateral ligament; Anterior cruciate ligament; Lateral meniscus; Lateral condyle of tibia; Head of fibula; Fibula

- On the *anterior surface*, identify the patella, which rests on the anterior articulating surface of the femur midway between the epicondyles, embedded in the tendon of the quadriceps muscle. This tendon continues below the knee joint as the *patellar tendon*, which inserts distally on the *tibial tuberosity*.

- On the *lateral surface*, find the *lateral epicondyle* of the femur and the *lateral condyle* of the tibia.

Joints

Two condylar *tibiofemoral joints* are formed by the convex curves of the medial and lateral condyles of the femur as they articulate with the concave condyles of the tibia. The third articular surface is the *patellofemoral joint*. The patella slides on the groove of the anterior aspect of the distal femur, called the *trochlear groove*, during flexion and extension of the knee.

Muscle Groups

Powerful muscles move and support the knee. The *quadriceps femoris* extends the leg, covering the anterior, medial, and lateral aspects of the thigh. The *hamstring muscles* lie on the posterior aspect of the thigh and flex the knee.

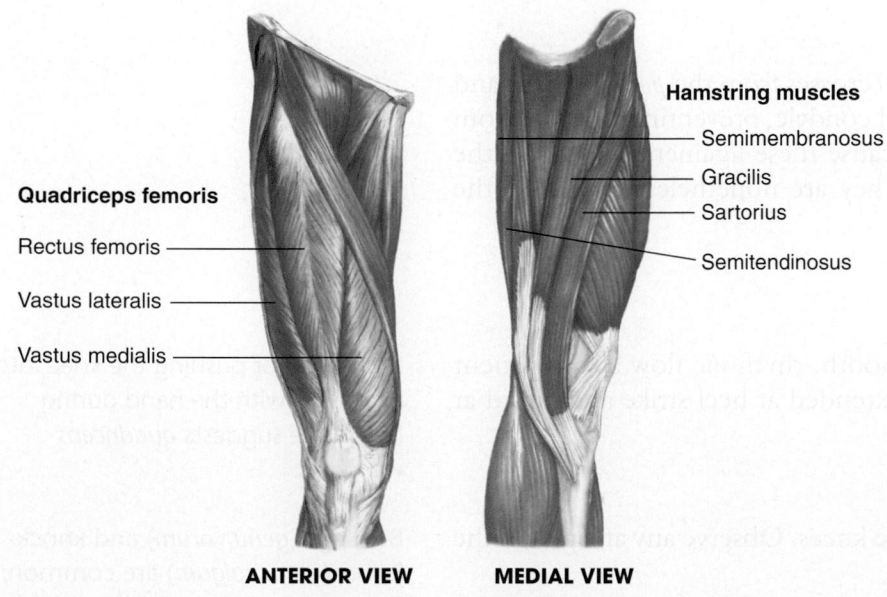

Quadriceps femoris

Rectus femoris

Vastus lateralis

Vastus medialis

Hamstring muscles

Semimembranosus

Gracilis

Sartorius

Semitendinosus

ANTERIOR VIEW   **MEDIAL VIEW**

Additional Structures

The menisci and two important pairs of ligaments, the collaterals and the cruciates, are crucial to stability of the knee. Identify these structures on the illustrations on p. 566 and below.

- The *medial and lateral menisci* cushion the action of the femur on the tibia. These crescent-shaped fibrocartilaginous discs add a cup-like surface to the otherwise flat tibial plateau.

- The *medial collateral ligament (MCL)*, not easily palpable, is a broad, flat ligament connecting the medial femoral epicondyle to the medial condyle of the tibia. The medial portion of the MCL also attaches to the medial meniscus.

- The *lateral collateral ligament (LCL)* connects the lateral femoral epicondyle and the head of the fibula. The MCL and LCL provide medial and lateral stability to the knee joint.

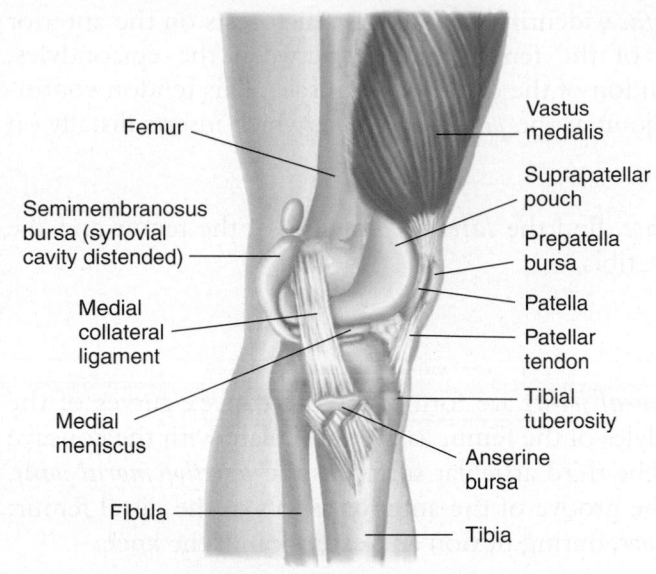

LEFT KNEE—MEDIAL VIEW

- The *anterior cruciate ligament (ACL)* crosses obliquely from the anterior medial tibia to the lateral femoral condyle, preventing the tibia from sliding forward on the femur.

- The *posterior cruciate ligament (PCL)* crosses from the *posterior* tibia and lateral meniscus to the medial femoral condyle, preventing the tibia from slipping backward on the femur. Because these ligaments lie within the knee joint, they are not palpable. They are nonetheless crucial to the anteroposterior stability of the knee.

Physical Examination

Inspection. Observe the gait for a smooth, rhythmic flow as the patient enters the room. The knee should be extended at heel strike and flexed at all other phases of swing and stance.

Stumbling or pushing the knee into extension with the hand during heel strike suggests *quadriceps weakness.*

Check the alignment and contours of the knees. Observe any atrophy of the quadriceps muscles.

Bowlegs (*genu varum*) and knock-knees (*genu valgum*) are common; flexion contracture (inability to extend fully) in limb paralysis

Look for loss of the normal hollows around the patella, a sign of swelling in the knee joint and suprapatellar pouch; note any other swelling in or around the knee.

Swelling over the patella suggests *prepatellar bursitis.* Swelling over the tibial tubercle suggests *infrapatellar* or, if more medial, *anserine bursitis.*

Palpation.   Ask the patient to sit on the edge of the examining table with the knees in flexion. In this position, bony landmarks are more visible, and the muscles, tendons, and ligaments are more relaxed, making them easier to palpate.

Pay special attention to any areas of tenderness. Pain is a common complaint in knee problems, and localizing the structure causing pain is important for accurate evaluation.

The Tibiofemoral Joint.
Palpate the *tibiofemoral joint*. Facing the knee, place your thumbs in the soft-tissue depressions on either side of the *patellar tendon*. Identify the groove of the tibiofemoral joint. Note that the patella lies just above this joint line. As you press your thumbs downward, feel the edge of the tibial plateau. Follow it medially, then laterally, until you are stopped by the converging femur and tibia. By moving your thumbs upward toward the midline to the top of the patella, you can follow the articulating surface of the femur and identify the margins of the joint.

Note any irregular bony ridges along the joint margins.

Osteoarthritis if tender bony ridges along the joint margins, genu varum deformity, and stiffness 30 minutes or less (likelihood ratios: 11.8, 3.4, and 3.0, respectively).[21-24] Crepitus may also be present.

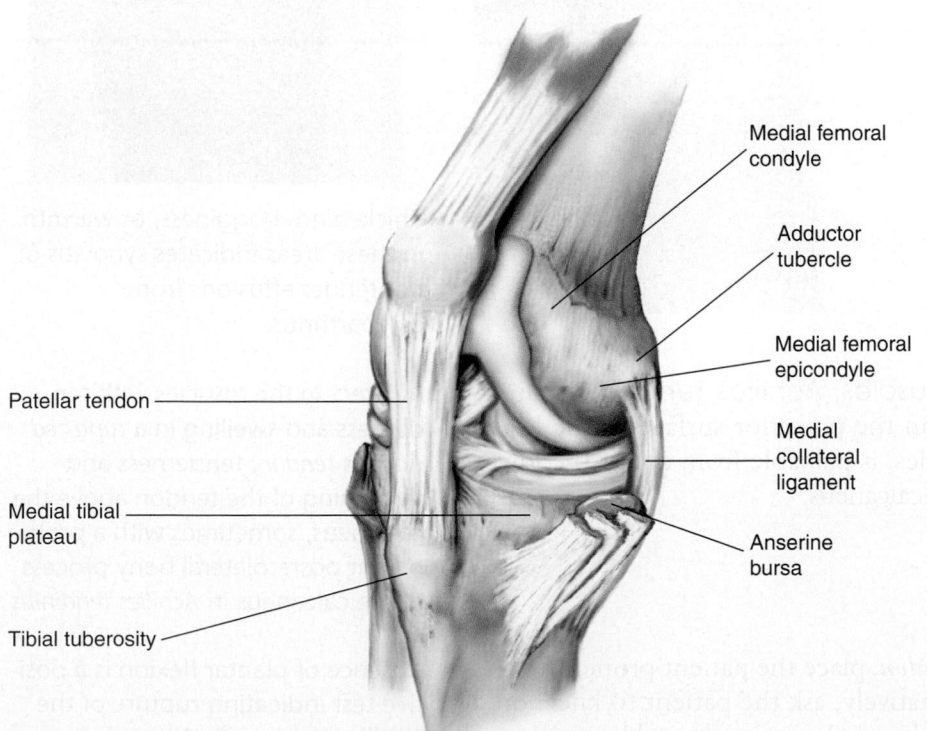

Medial femoral condyle

Adductor tubercle

Medial femoral epicondyle

Medial collateral ligament

Anserine bursa

Patellar tendon

Medial tibial plateau

Tibial tuberosity

Now locate the *patella* and trace the *patellar tendon* distally until you palpate the *tibial tuberosity*. Ask the patient to extend the leg to make sure the patellar tendon is intact.

Tenderness over the tendon or inability to extend the leg suggests a partial or complete tear of the patellar tendon.

With the patient supine and the knee extended, compress the patella against the underlying femur. Ask the patient to tighten the quadriceps as the patella moves distally in the trochlear groove. Check for a smooth sliding motion (the *patellofemoral grinding test*).

Pain and crepitus suggest roughening of the patellar undersurface that articulates with the femur. Similar pain may occur with climbing stairs or getting up from a chair.

Pain with compression and with patellar movement during quadriceps contraction suggests *chondromalacia,* or degenerative patella (the *patellofemoral syndrome*).

The Suprapatellar Pouch, Prepatellar Bursa, and Anserine Bursa. Try to palpate any thickening or swelling in the *suprapatellar pouch* and along the margins of the patella. Start 10 cm above the superior border of the patella, well above the pouch, and feel the soft tissues between your thumb and fingers. Move your hand distally in progressive steps, trying to identify the pouch. Continue your palpation along the sides of the patella. Note any tenderness or warmth greater than in the surrounding tissues.

Swelling above and adjacent to the patella suggests synovial thickening or effusion in the knee joint.

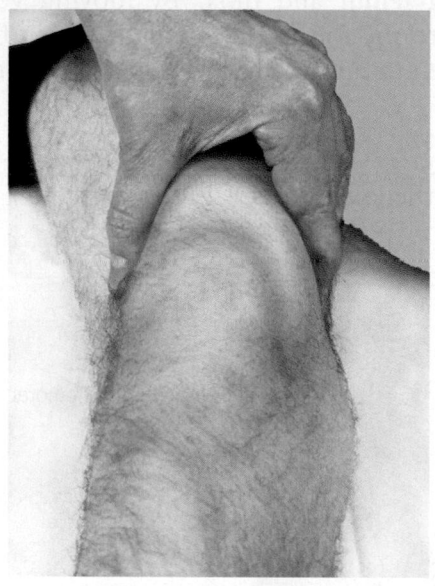

Thickening, bogginess, or warmth in these areas indicates synovitis or nontender effusions from osteoarthritis.

Gastrocnemius and Soleus Muscles, Achilles Tendon. Palpate the *gastrocnemius* and *soleus muscles* on the posterior surface of the lower leg. Their common tendon, the Achilles, is palpable from about the lower third of the calf to its insertion on the calcaneus.

A defect in the muscles with tenderness and swelling in a *ruptured Achilles tendon;* tenderness and thickening of the tendon above the calcaneus, sometimes with a protuberant posterolateral bony process of the calcaneus in *Achilles tendinitis*

To test the integrity of the *Achilles tendon,* place the patient prone with the knee and ankle flexed at 90°, or alternatively, ask the patient to kneel on a chair. Squeeze the calf and watch for plantar flexion at the ankle.

Absence of plantar flexion is a positive test indicating rupture of the Achilles tendon. Sudden severe pain "like a gunshot wound," an ecchymosis from the calf into the heel, and a flat-footed gait with absence of "toe-off" may also be present.

Range of Motion and Maneuvers

Range of Motion.   Now assess knee range of motion, referring to the table below for specific muscles responsible for each movement and clear, simple instructions that prompt the patient to properly follow your directions. Be sure to examine both knees and compare findings.

Knee Movement	Primary Muscles Affecting Movement	Patient Instructions
Flexion	Hamstring group: biceps femoris, semitendinosus, and semimembranosus	*"Bend or flex your knee."* Or *"Squat down to the floor."*
Extension	Quadriceps: rectus femoris, vastus medialis, lateralis, and intermedius	*"Straighten your leg."* Or *"After you squat down to the floor, stand up."*
Internal Rotation	Sartorius, gracilis, semitendinosus, semimembranosus	*"While sitting, swing your lower leg toward the midline."*
External Rotation	Biceps femoris	*"While sitting, swing your lower leg away from the midline."*

Crepitus with flexion and extension in osteoarthritis[22,23]

Muscle Strength Test.   *Test muscle strength during extension at the knee* (L2, L3, L4—quadriceps). Support the knee in flexion and ask the patient to straighten the leg against your hand. The quadriceps is the strongest muscle in the body, so expect a forceful response.

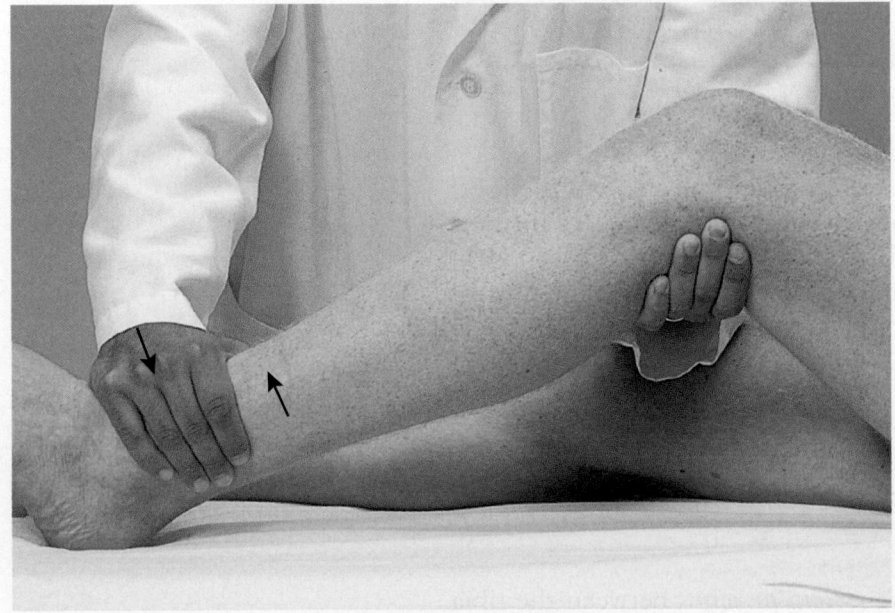

EXTENSION AT THE KNEE

Test flexion at the knee (L4, L5, S1, S2—hamstrings) as shown below. Place the patient's leg so that the knee is flexed with the foot resting on the bed. Tell the patient to keep the foot down as you try to straighten the leg.

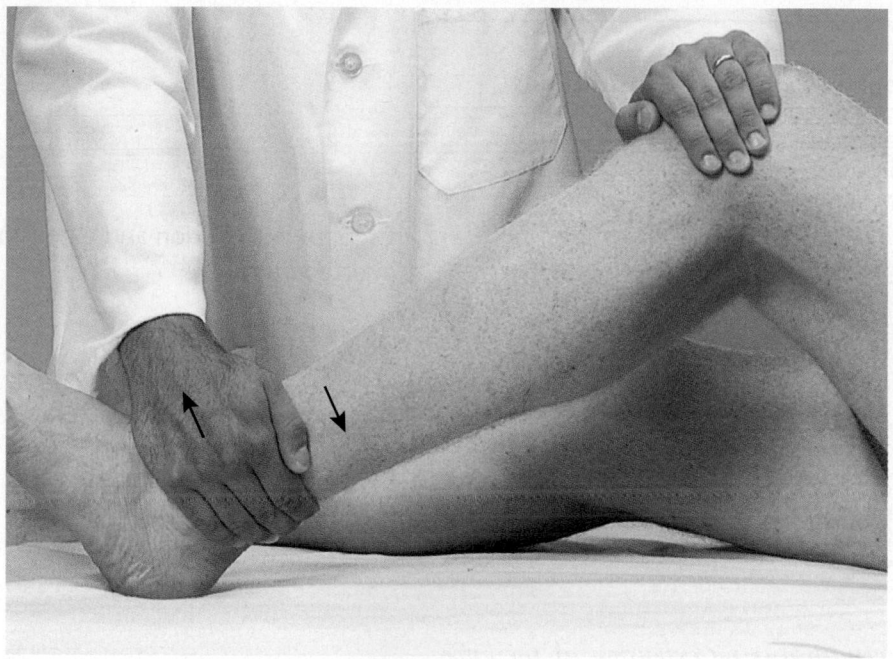

FLEXION AT THE KNEE

THE ANKLE AND FOOT

Overview

The total weight of the body is transmitted through the ankle to the foot. The ankle and foot must balance the body and absorb the impact of the heel strike and gait. Despite thick padding along the toes, sole, and heel and stabilizing ligaments at the ankles, the ankle and foot are frequent sites of sprain and bony injury.

Bony Structures and Joints

The ankle is a hinge joint formed by the *tibia*, the *fibula*, and the *talus*. The tibia and fibula act as a mortise, stabilizing the joint while bracing the talus like an inverted cup.

The principal joints of the ankle are the *tibiotalar joint*, between the tibia and the talus, and the *subtalar (talocalcaneal) joint*.

Note the principal landmarks of the ankle: the *medial malleolus,* the bony prominence at the distal end of the tibia, and the *lateral malleolus,* at the distal end of the fibula. Lodged under the talus and jutting posteriorly is the *calcaneus,* or heel.

An imaginary line, the *longitudinal arch,* spans the foot, extending from the calcaneus of the hind foot along the tarsal bones of the midfoot (see cuneiforms, navicular, and cuboid bones below) to the forefoot metatarsals and toes. The *heads of the metatarsals* are palpable in the ball of the foot. In the forefoot, identify the *metatarsophalangeal joints,* proximal to the webs of the toes, and the *proximal and distal interphalangeal joints* of the toes.

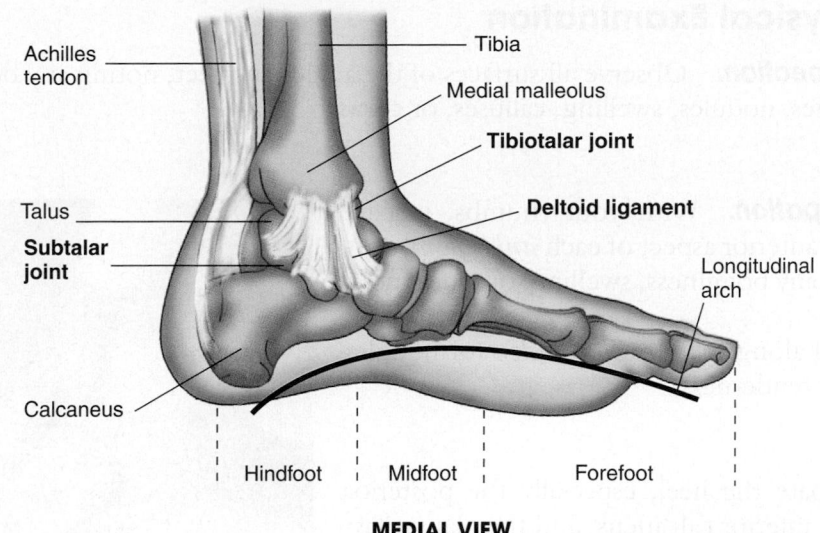

MEDIAL VIEW

Muscle Groups and Additional Structures

Movement at the ankle joint is limited to dorsiflexion and plantar flexion. *Plantar flexion* is powered by the gastrocnemius, the posterior tibial muscle, and the toe flexors. Their tendons run behind the malleoli. The *dorsiflexors* include the anterior tibial muscle and the toe extensors. They lie prominently on the anterior surface, or dorsum, of the ankle, anterior to the malleoli.

Ligaments extend from each malleolus onto the foot.

- Medially, the triangle-shaped *deltoid ligament* fans out from the inferior surface of the medial malleolus to the talus and proximal tarsal bones, protecting against stress from eversion (ankle bowing inward).

- Laterally, the three ligaments are less substantial, with higher risk for injury: the *anterior talofibular ligament*—most at risk in injury from inversion (ankle bows outward) injuries; the *calcaneofibular ligament*; and the *posterior talofibular ligament.* The strong Achilles tendon attaches the gastrocnemius and soleus muscles to the posterior calcaneus. The plantar fascia inserts on the medial tubercle of the calcaneus.

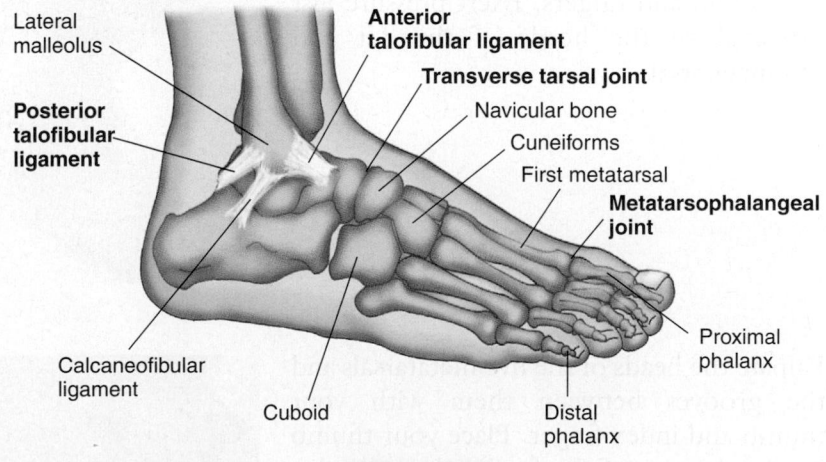

LATERAL VIEW

Physical Examination

Inspection.   Observe all surfaces of the ankles and feet, noting any deformities, nodules, swelling, calluses, or corns.

See Table 18-7, p. 591, Abnormalities of the Feet and Table 18-8, p. 592, Abnormalities of the Toes and Soles

Palpation.   With your thumbs, palpate the anterior aspect of each *ankle joint,* noting any bogginess, swelling, or tenderness.

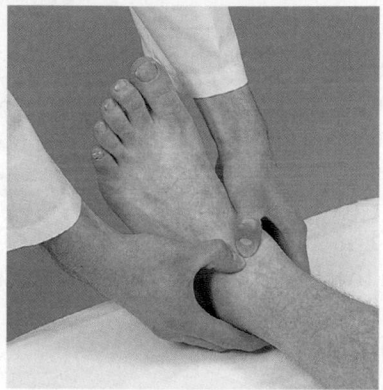

Localized tenderness in arthritis, ligamentous injury, or infection of the ankle

Feel along the *Achilles tendon* for nodules and tenderness.

Rheumatoid nodules; tenderness in Achilles tendinitis, bursitis, or partial tear from trauma

Palpate the heel, especially the posterior and inferior calcaneus, and the plantar fascia for tenderness.

Bone spurs may be present on the calcaneus. Focal heel pain on palpation of the plantar fascia suggests *plantar fasciitis;* seen in prolonged standing or heel-strike exercise, also in *rheumatoid arthritis, gout.*[27,28]

Palpate for tenderness over the medial and lateral malleolus, especially in cases of trauma.

After trauma, inability to bear weight after 4 steps and tenderness over the posterior aspects of either malleolus, especially the medial malleolus, is suspicious for ankle fracture.[29]

Palpate the *metatarsophalangeal joints* for tenderness. Compress the forefoot between the thumb and fingers. Exert pressure just proximal to the heads of the 1st and 5th metatarsals.

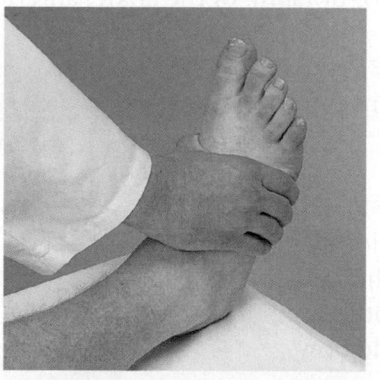

Tenderness on compression is an early sign of *rheumatoid arthritis.* Acute inflammation of the first metatarsophalangeal joint in *gout*

Palpate the heads of the five metatarsals and the grooves between them with your thumb and index finger. Place your thumb on the dorsum of the foot and your index finger on the plantar surface.

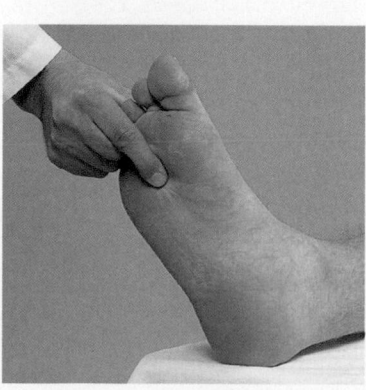

Pain and tenderness, called *metatarsalgia,* in trauma, arthritis, vascular compromise

Range of Motion and Maneuvers

Range of Motion. Assess flexion and extension at the tibiotalar (ankle) joint. In the foot, assess inversion and eversion at the subtalar and transverse tarsal joints.

Ankle and Foot Movement	Primary Muscles Affecting Movement	Patient Instructions
Ankle Flexion (plantar flexion)	Gastrocnemius, soleus, plantaris, tibialis posterior	*"Point your foot toward the floor."*
Ankle Extension (dorsiflexion)	Tibialis anterior, extensor digitorum longus, and extensor hallucis longus	*"Point your foot toward the ceiling."*
Inversion	Tibialis posterior and anterior	*"Bend your heel inward."*
Eversion	Peroneus longus and brevis	*"Bend your heel outward."*

Passive Range of Motion Maneuvers

● *The Ankle (Tibiotalar) Joint.* Dorsiflex and plantar flex the foot at the ankle.

Pain during movements of the ankle and the foot helps to localize possible arthritis.

Muscle Strength Test. *Test muscle strength during dorsiflexion* (mainly L4, L5—tibialis anterior) and *plantar flexion* (mainly S1—gastrocnemius, soleus) at the ankle by asking the patient to pull up and push down against your hand.

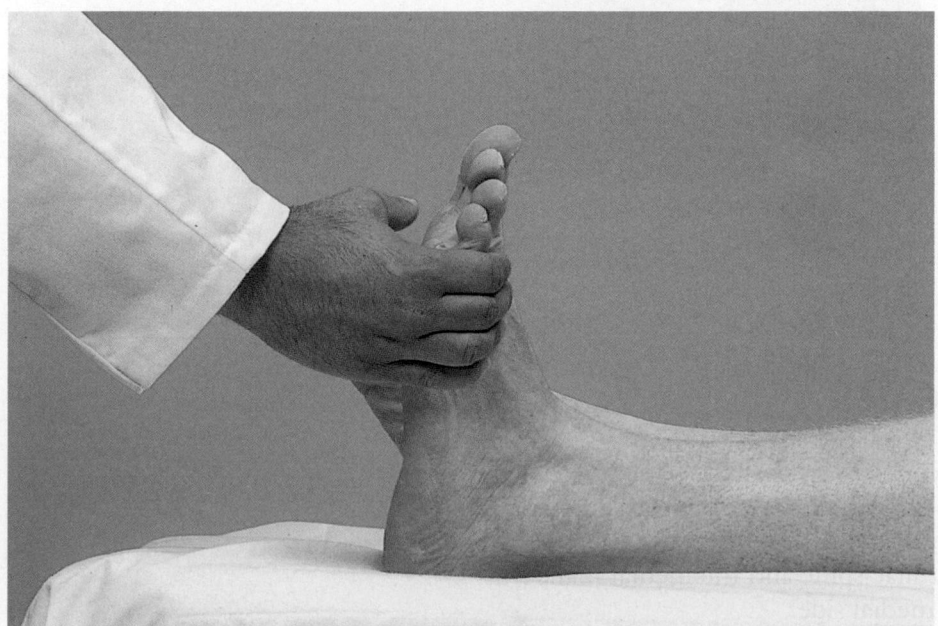

DORSIFLEXION AT THE ANKLE

● *The Subtalar (Talocalcaneal) Joint.* Stabilize the ankle with one hand, grasp the heel with the other, and invert and evert the foot.

An arthritic joint is frequently painful when moved in any direction, whereas a ligamentous sprain produces maximal pain when the ligament is stretched. For example, in a common form of sprained ankle, inversion and plantar flexion of the foot cause pain, whereas eversion and plantar flexion are relatively pain free.

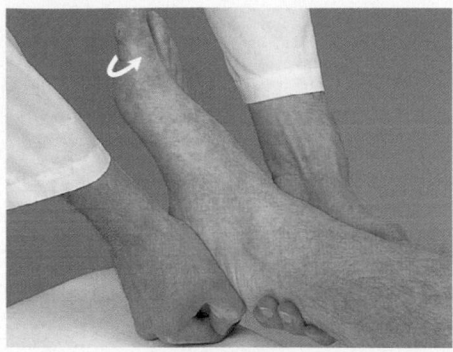
INVERSION

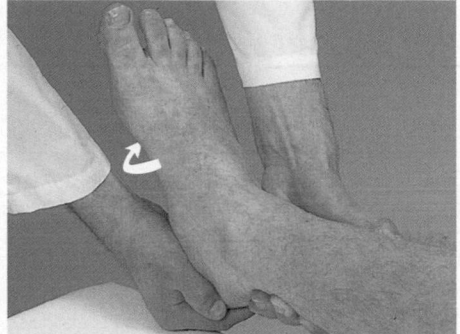
EVERSION

● *The Transverse Tarsal Joint.* Stabilize the heel and invert and evert the forefoot.

● *The Metatarsophalangeal Joints.* Flex the toes in relation to the feet.

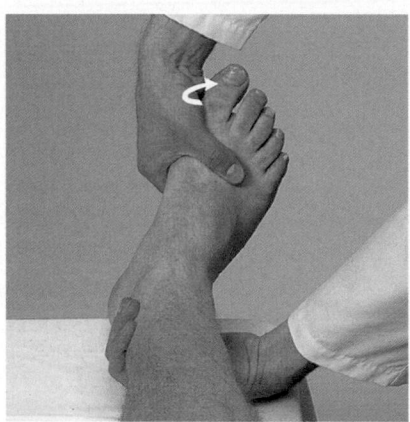
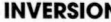
INVERSION

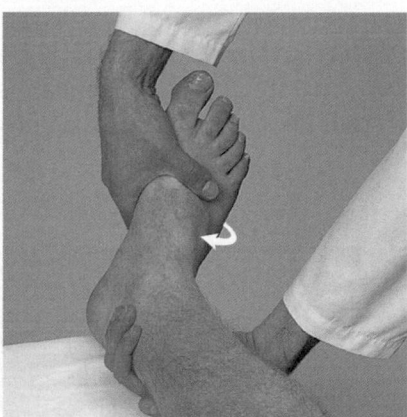
EVERSION

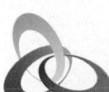 **SPECIAL TECHNIQUES**

Measuring the Length of Legs. If you suspect that the patient's legs are unequal in length, measure them. Get the patient relaxed in the supine position and symmetrically aligned with legs extended. With a tape, measure the distance between the anterior superior iliac spine and the medial malleolus. The tape should cross the knee on its medial side.

Unequal leg length may explain a scoliosis.

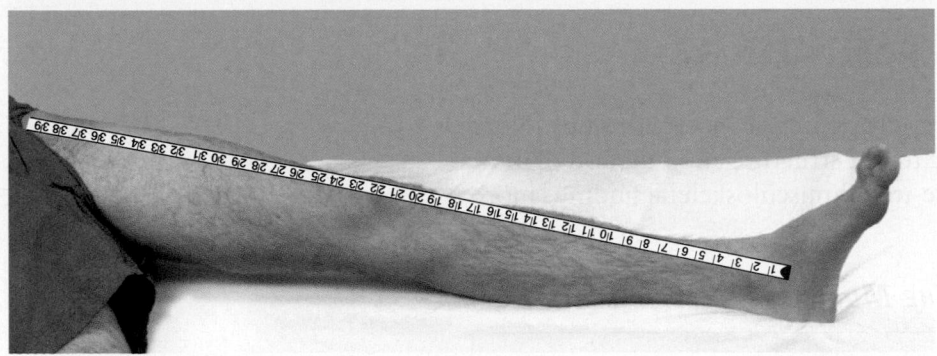

Describing Limited Motion of a Joint. Although measurement of motion is seldom necessary, limitations can be described in degrees. Pocket goniometers are available for this purpose. In the two examples shown below, the red lines indicate the limited range of the patient's movement, and the black lines suggest the normal range.

Observations may be described in several ways.

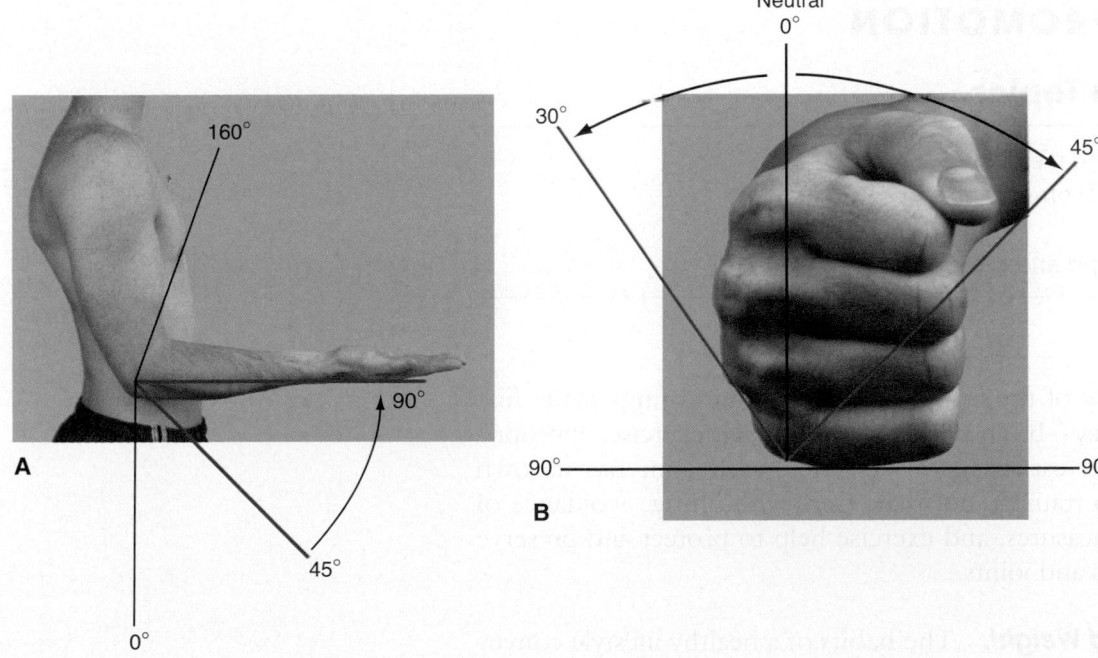

A. The elbow flexes from 45° to 90°

    -or-

The elbow flexion limited to 45° to 90°

B. Supination at elbow limited to 30°

Pronation at elbow limited to 45°

RECORDING YOUR FINDINGS

The examples below contain phrases appropriate for most write-ups. Note that use of the anatomic terms specific to the structure and function of individual joint problems makes your write-up of musculoskeletal findings more meaningful and informative.

RECORDING THE EXAMINATION—THE MUSCULOSKELETAL SYSTEM

"FROM (Full range of motion) in all joints with muscle strength 5/5. No swelling or deformity."
OR
"FROM in all joints. Heberden nodes noted at the DIP joints of hand, Bouchard nodes at PIP joints; muscle strength 4/5. Pain 2/10 with flexion, extension, and rotation of both hips; muscle strength 5/5. FROM in the knees, with moderate crepitus; strength 5/5. Hallux valgus bilaterally at the first metatarsophalangeal joints."

Suggests *osteoarthritis*

HEALTH PROMOTION

Health Promotion Topics

- Nutrition, exercise, and weight
- Low back: lifting and biomechanics
- Falls: prevention
- Osteoporosis: screening and prevention

Maintaining the integrity of the musculoskeletal system brings many features of daily life into play—balanced nutrition, regular exercise, appropriate weight. As described earlier in this chapter, each joint has its own specific vulnerabilities to trauma and wear. Care with lifting, avoidance of falls, household safety measures, and exercise help to protect and preserve well-functioning muscles and joints.

Nutrition, Exercise, and Weight. The habits of a healthy lifestyle convey direct benefit to the skeleton. Good nutrition supplies calcium needed for bone mineralization and bone density. Exercise appears to maintain and possibly increase bone mass, in addition to improving outlook and management of stress. Weight appropriate to height and body frame reduces excess mechanical wear on weight-bearing joints such as hips and knees. Regular physical activity has been shown to help prevent osteoporosis, obesity, cardiovascular disease, hypertension, and type 2 diabetes, and may reduce all-cause morbidity and lengthen life span.[30] Even modest activity, such as walking or bicycling 30 minutes each day, benefits health. Twenty to 30% of adult Americans report sedentary lifestyles and may benefit from routine counseling, although evidence linking counseling to behavior change is still preliminary.

Low Back: Lifting and Biomechanics.   One of the most vulnerable parts of the skeleton is the low back, especially L5–S1, where the sacral vertebrae take a sharp posterior angle. From 60% to 80% of the population experiences *low back pain* at least once in a lifetime.[31] Usually symptoms are short lived, but 30% to 60% of people experience recurrences when onset is work related. Exercises to strengthen the low back, especially in flexion and extension, and risk factor modification are often recommended (although studies have not demonstrated a consistent benefit for these interventions).[2,32,33] Alternatively, fitness exercises appear equally effective. Education on lifting strategies, posture, and the biomechanics of injury is prudent for people doing repetitive lifting such as: nurses, heavy-machinery operators, and construction workers. For occupational back pain, increasing graded physical activity and behavioral counseling show promise in improving functional status and return to work.[34] Such programs focus on improvements in function and do not make pain relief a condition for resuming work.

Preventing Falls.   Among elderly people in the United States, *falls* exact a heavy toll in morbidity and mortality. They are the leading cause of nonfatal injuries and account for a dramatic rise in death rates after 65 years, increasing from approximately 5/100,000 in the general population to 10/100,000 between the ages of 65 and 74 years, to approximately 147/100,000 after age 85 years.[35] Nine out of 10 hip fractures in older Americans are the result of a fall. For those living independently before a hip fracture, 15 to 25 percent will still be in long-term care institutions a year after their fracture.[36]

Risk factors are both cognitive and physiologic, including unstable gait, imbalanced posture, reduced strength, previous fall, impaired mobility, medications, incontinence, hypertension, cognitive loss as in dementia, altered mental status, deficits in vision and proprioception, and osteoporosis.[37] Poor lighting, stairs, chairs at awkward heights, slippery or irregular surfaces, and ill-fitting shoes are environmental dangers that can often be corrected. Nurses should work with patients and families to help modify such risks whenever possible. Home health assessments have proven useful in reducing environmental hazards, as have exercise programs to improve patient balance and strength. Fall-risk assessment tools, such as the Morse, Hendrich II, St. Thomas, or Spartanburg, are helpful for identifying persons at risk for falling. (See Chapter 24, The Older Adult, pp. 870–871.)

Osteoporosis: Screening and Prevention.   Osteoporosis is a major threat to U.S. public health.[36,40–41]

- By 2012 twelve million Americans older than 50 years are expected to have osteoporosis; 1 in 2 postmenopausal women and 1 in 5 older men are at risk for an osteoporotic fracture.

- Osteoporosis can occur at any age, and 42% of those at risk are men. Prevalence in U.S. white women increases from 15% at ages 50 to 59 years to 70% in women older than 80 years. Prevalence in African-American women older than 50 years is 12%, and in Mexican-American women, 18%.

- One of every two women and one in four men older than 50 years will have a fracture related to osteoporosis. Approximately one third of fractures occur in younger women.

- Twenty percent of patients with osteoporotic hip fractures die within 1 year.

The National Institutes of Health define osteoporosis as a "skeletal disorder characterized by compromised bone strength predisposing a person to an increased risk of fracture."[40] *Bone strength* reflects both *bone density* and *bone quality. Bone density* is determined by the interaction of bone mass (highest in the second decade), new bone formation, and bone resorption or loss. *Bone quality* refers to "architecture, turnover, damage accumulation from microfractures, and mineralization." Osteoporosis typically arises from bone loss during aging, but reduced bone mass from suboptimal bone growth in childhood and adolescence can also cause osteoporosis.

There is no direct measurement of bone strength. Bone mineral density, which accounts for approximately 70% of bone strength, is used as a proxy measure.[40] The World Health Organization uses bone density to define osteopenia and osteoporosis:

- *Osteopenia* is bone density 1.0–2.5 standard deviations below the mean for young adult white women (T score between –2.5 and –1.0).

- *Osteoporosis* is bone density 2.5 or more standard deviations below the mean for young adult white women (T score less than –2.5).

Z scores for age-matched controls are more useful for young people, because they allow comparison with those of similar age, height, and weight. Bone density is measured at the hip, femoral neck, Ward's triangle at the femoral neck, greater trochanter, and total hip, which includes all the measurements. A 10% drop in bone density, equivalent to 1.0 standard deviation, is associated with a 20% increase in risk for fracture.

The U.S. Preventive Services Task Force recommends routine bone density screening for women 65 years or older and for younger women with risk factors.[41] The relative fracture risk is higher in those with osteoporosis; however, almost half of all fragility fractures occur in the osteopenic group, which is larger.[42]

RISK FACTORS FOR OSTEOPOROSIS[38,42]

- Postmenopausal status in white and Asian women
- Age older than 50 years
- Weight less than 70 kg
- Family history of fracture in a first-degree relative
- History of fracture
- Higher intakes of alcohol
- Women with delayed menarche or early menopause
- Current smokers
- Low levels of 25-hydroxyvitamin D
- Use of corticosteroids for more than 2 months
- Inflammatory disorders of the musculoskeletal, pulmonary, or gastrointestinal systems, including celiac sprue, chronic renal disease, organ transplantation, hypogonadism, anorexia nervosa
- Sedentary lifestyle or extended bed rest

Basic screening questions for older women include the following:

- Have you ever had a fracture?

- Did either parent or a sibling ever have a fracture?

- Do you smoke?

- What is your weight?

- Have you ever taken estrogen replacement therapy?[40]

Screening should be expanded to younger women and men with risk factors. Low body weight is the single best predictor of low bone density, and bone density at the femoral neck is the best predictor of subsequent hip fracture.[41,43] Falls increase risk of fracture, so assess the risk factors for falls: impaired cognition, vision, or gait; neuromuscular deficits; and medications affecting balance.

The therapeutic uses of available agents and options for preventing and treating osteoporosis are briefly summarized here:[44,45]

- Adequate **calcium intake** at all ages is necessary to prevent osteoporosis. By the time teens finish their growth spurt 90% of adult bone mass is established. Fewer than 1 in 10 girls and 1 in 4 boys ages 9 to 13 are at or above their adequate calcium intake.[46] For the older person increased calcium intake reduces age-related hyperparathyroidism and increases mineralization of newly formed bone. The nurse should assess the calcium intake with the history.

● For the older person, **increased calcium** intake reduces age-related hyperparathyroidism and increases mineralization of newly formed bone.

● Recommended Calcium Intakes	
Age	mg/day
Birth to 6 months	210
6 months to 1 year	270
1–3 years	500
4–8 years	800
9–13 years	1300
14–18 years	1300
19–30 years	1000
31–50 years	1000
51–70 years	1200
70 years and older	1200
Pregnant or Lactating	
14–18 years	1300
19–50 years	1000

● Up to two thirds of patients with hip fractures are deficient in **vitamin D,** essential for calcium absorption and muscle strength.[44] Vitamin D is synthesized in the skin through exposure to sunlight. Many people obtain enough vitamin D naturally, by receiving 15 minutes of sunlight each day. Studies show that vitamin D production decreases in the elderly, in people who are housebound, and for most people during the winter. They may need vitamin D supplements to achieve the recommended daily intake of 400 to 600 IU (International Units). Food sources of vitamin D include egg yolks, saltwater fish, and liver.[47]

● **Antiresorptive agents** inhibit osteoclast activity and slow bone remodeling, allowing better mineralization of bone matrix and stabilization of the trabecular microarchitecture. These agents include bisphosphonates, selective estrogen-receptor modulators (SERMs), calcitonin, and postmenopausal estrogen, now in question because of associated risks of breast cancer and vascular problems.

● **Anabolic agents** such as parathyroid hormone stimulate bone formation by acting primarily on osteoblasts but require subcutaneous administration and monitoring for hypercalcemia. They are reserved for moderate to severe cases of osteoporosis.

- **Regular exercise** that includes weight-bearing and resistance training can increase bone density and muscle strength but has not yet been shown to reduce fracture risk.[40] Multidisciplinary programs to improve strength, balance, and home and medication safety can help prevent falls.

- Alcohol prevents absorption of calcium. Women should limit alcohol to one drink per day and men to two drinks per day.

- Limit caffeine in the diet. Caffeine causes increased calcium excretion.

Despite the benefits of estrogen on bone density, three recent trials have shown increased risk of stroke for women taking hormone replacement therapy and failure to reduce risk of coronary heart disease; two of the trials found an increased risk of breast cancer.[48-50] The U.S. Preventive Services Task Force now recommends against routine use of estrogen and progestin for the prevention of chronic conditions in postmenopausal women.[51] Despite public interest, natural estrogens, including plant-derived phyto-estrogens, have not been shown to reduce fracture risk.[40]

TABLE
18-1
Low Back Pain[52]

Patterns	Possible Causes	Physical Signs
Mechanical Low Back Pain Aching pain in the lumbosacral area; may radiate into lower leg, especially along L5 (lateral leg) or S1 (posterior leg) dermatomes. Refers to anatomic or functional abnormality in absence of neoplastic, infectious, or inflammatory disease.[2] Usually acute (<3 months), idiopathic, benign, and self-limiting; represents 97% of symptomatic low back pain. Commonly work-related and occurring in patients 30–50 years. Risk factors include heavy lifting, poor conditioning, obesity.	Often arises from muscle and ligament injuries (~70%) or age-related intervertebral disc or facet disease (~4%).[2] Causes also include herniated disc (~4%), spinal stenosis (~3%), compression fractures (~4%), and spondylolisthesis (2%).	Paraspinal muscle or facet tenderness, pain with back movement, loss of normal lumbar lordosis, but no motor or sensory loss or reflex abnormalities. In osteoporosis, check for thoracic kyphosis, percussion tenderness over a spinous process, or fractures in the thoracic spine or hip.
Sciatica (Radicular Low Back Pain) Shooting pain below the knee, commonly into the lateral leg (L5) or posterior calf (S1); typically accompanies low back pain. Patients report associated paresthesias and weakness. Bending, sneezing, coughing, straining during bowel movements often worsen pain.[1]	Sciatic pain very sensitive, ~95%, and specific, ~88%, for disc herniation. Usually from herniated intervertebral disc with compression or traction of nerve root(s) in people 50 years or older. Involves L5 and S1 roots in ~95% of disc herniations.[2] Root or spinal cord compression from neoplastic conditions in fewer than 1% of cases. Tumor or midline disc herniation in bowel or bladder dysfunction, leg weakness from cauda equina syndrome (S2–4).	Disc herniation most likely if calf wasting, weak ankle dorsiflexion, absent ankle jerk, positive crossed straight-leg raise (pain in affected leg when healthy leg tested); negative straight-leg raise makes diagnosis highly unlikely. Ipsilateral straight-leg raise sensitive, ~65%–98%, but not specific, ~10%–60%.[53]
Chronic Back Stiffness	*Ankylosing spondylitis*, an inflammatory polyarthritis, most common in men younger than 40 years.[18]	
Pain Referred from the Abdomen or Pelvis Usually a deep, aching pain; the level varies with the source. Accounts for approximately 1% of low back pain.	Peptic ulcer, pancreatitis, pancreatic cancer, chronic prostatitis, endometriosis, dissecting aortic aneurysm, retroperitoneal tumor, and other causes.	Variable with the source. Local vertebral tenderness may be present. Spinal movements are not painful and range of motion is not affected. Look for signs of the primary disorder.

TABLE
18-2

Pains in the Neck

Patterns	Possible Causes	Physical Signs
Mechanical Neck Pain Aching pain in the cervical paraspinal muscles and ligaments with associated muscle spasm, with associated stiffness and tightness in the upper back and shoulder, lasting up to 6 weeks. No associated radiation, paresthesias, or weakness. Headache may be present.	Mechanism poorly understood, possibly sustained muscle contraction. Associated with poor posture, stress, poor sleep, poor head position during activities such as computer use, watching television, driving.	Local muscle tenderness, pain on movement. No neurologic deficits. Possible trigger points in *fibromyalgia*. *Torticollis* if prolonged abnormal neck posture and muscle spasm.
Mechanical Neck Pain—Whiplash[5] Also mechanical neck pain with aching paracervical pain and stiffness, often beginning the day after injury. Occipital headache, dizziness, malaise, and fatigue may be present. Chronic whiplash syndrome if symptoms last more than 6 months, present in 20%–40% of injuries.	Musculoligamental sprain or strain from forced hyperflexion–hyperextension injury to the neck, as in rear-end collisions.	Localized paracervical tenderness, decreased neck range of motion, perceived weakness of the upper extremities. Causes of cervical cord compression such as fracture, herniation, head injury, or altered consciousness are excluded.
Cervical Radiculopathy—from nerve root compression[5,6] Sharp burning or tingling pain in the neck and one arm, with associated paresthesias and weakness. Sensory symptoms often in myotomal pattern, deep in muscle, rather than dermatomal pattern.	Dysfunction of cervical spinal nerve, nerve roots, or both from foraminal encroachment of the spinal nerve (~75%), herniated cervical disc (~25%). Rarely from tumor, syrinx, multiple sclerosis. Mechanisms may involve hypoxia of the nerve root and dorsal ganglion, release of inflammatory mediators.	C7 nerve root affected most often (45%–60%), with weakness in triceps and finger flexors and extensors. C6 nerve root involvement also common, with weakness in biceps, brachioradialis, wrist extensors.
Cervical Myelopathy—from cervical cord compression[5] Neck pain with bilateral weakness and paresthesias in both upper and lower extremities, often with urinary frequency. Hand clumsiness, palmar paresthesias, and gait changes may be subtle. Neck flexion often exacerbates symptoms.	Usually from cervical *spondylosis,* defined as cervical degenerative disc disease from spurs, protrusion of ligamentum flavum, and/or disc herniation (~80%); also from cervical stenosis from osteophytes, ossification of ligamentum flavum. Large central or paracentral disc herniation may also compress cord.	Hyperreflexia; clonus at the wrist, knee, or ankle; extensor plantar reflexes (positive Babinski signs); and gait disturbances. May also see *Lhermitte's sign:* neck flexion with resulting sensation of electrical shock radiating down the spine. Confirmation of cervical myelopathy warrants neck immobilization and neurosurgical evaluation.

TABLE
18-3

Patterns of Pain In and Around the Joints

Problem	Process	Common Locations	Pattern of Spread	Onset	Progression and Duration
Rheumatoid Arthritis[8–10,54]	Chronic inflammation of *synovial membranes* with secondary erosion of adjacent cartilage and bone, and damage to ligaments and tendons	Hands (proximal interphalangeal and metacarpophalangeal joints), feet (metatarsophalangeal joints), wrists, knees, elbows, ankles	Symmetrically additive: progresses to other joints while persisting in the initial ones	Usually insidious	Often chronic, with remissions and exacerbations
Osteoarthritis (*degenerative joint disease*)[19]	Degeneration and progressive loss of *cartilage* within the joints, damage to underlying bone, and formation of new bone at the margins of the cartilage	Knees, hips, hands (distal, sometimes proximal interphalangeal joints), cervical and lumbar spine, and wrists (first carpometacarpal joint); also joints previously injured or diseased	Additive; however, only one joint may be involved.	Usually insidious	Slowly progressive, with temporary exacerbations after periods of overuse
Gouty Arthritis[7] *Acute Gout*	An inflammatory reaction to microcrystals of sodium urate	Base of the big toe (the first metatarsophalangeal joint), the instep or dorsa of feet, the ankles, knees, and elbows	Early attacks usually confined to one joint	Sudden, often at night, often after injury, surgery, fasting, or excessive food or alcohol intake	Occasional isolated attacks lasting days up to 2 weeks; they may get more frequent and severe, with persisting symptoms.
Fibromyalgia Syndrome[55–57]	Widespread musculoskeletal pain and tender points. May accompany other diseases. Mechanisms unclear	"All over," but especially in the neck, shoulders, hands, low back, and knees	Usually insidious	Variable	Chronic, with "ups and downs"

The vagueness of these characteristics is in itself a clue to the fibromyalgia syndrome.

Associated Symptoms

Swelling	Redness, Warmth, and Tenderness	Stiffness	Limitation of Motion	Generalized Symptoms
Frequent swelling of synovial tissue in joints or tendon sheaths; also subcutaneous nodules	Tender, often warm, but seldom red	Prominent, often for an hour or more in the mornings, also after inactivity	Often develops	Weakness, fatigue, weight loss, and low fever are common.
Small effusions in the joints may be present, especially in the knees; also bony enlargement	Possibly tender, seldom warm, and rarely red	Frequent but brief (usually 5–10 min), in the morning and after inactivity	Often develops	Usually absent
Present, within and around the involved joint	Exquisitely tender, hot, and red	Not evident	Motion is limited primarily by pain.	Fever may be present.
None	Multiple specific and symmetric tender "trigger points," often not recognized until the examination	Present, especially in the morning	Absent, though stiffness is greater at the extremes of movement	A disturbance of sleep, usually associated with morning fatigue

TABLE 18-4	**Painful Shoulders**[11,23,58]

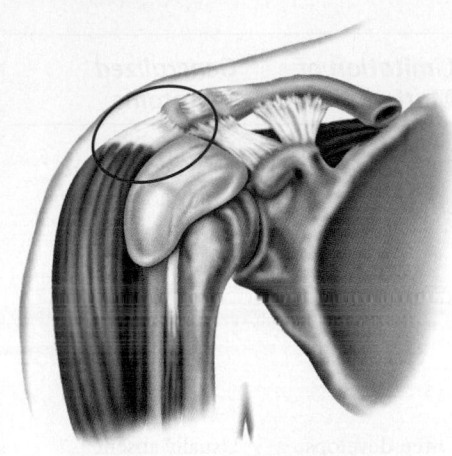

Rotator Cuff Tendinitis

Repeated shoulder motion, as in throwing or swimming, can cause edema and hemorrhage followed by inflammation, most commonly involving the supraspinatus tendon. Acute, recurrent, or chronic pain may result, often aggravated by activity. Patients report sharp catches of pain, grating, and weakness when lifting the arm overhead. When the supraspinatus tendon is involved, tenderness is maximal just below the tip of the acromion. Patients are typically athletically active.

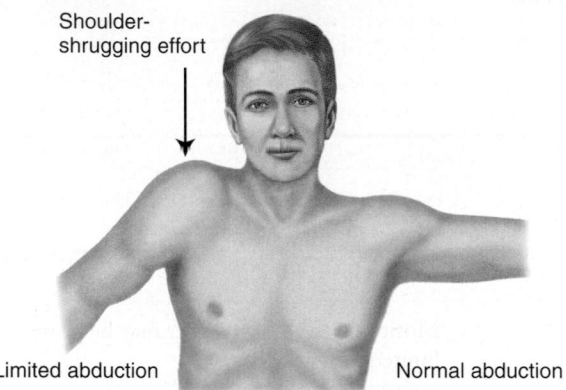

Shoulder-shrugging effort

Limited abduction   Normal abduction

Rotator Cuff Tears

When the arm is raised in forward flexion, the rotator cuff may impinge against the undersurface of the acromion and the coracoacromial ligament. Injury from a fall or repeated impingement may weaken the rotator cuff, causing a partial or complete tear, usually after age 40. Weakness, atrophy of the supraspinatus and infraspinatus muscles, pain, and tenderness may ensue. In a complete tear of the supraspinatus tendon (illustrated), active abduction and forward flexion at the glenohumeral joint are severely impaired, producing a characteristic shrugging of the shoulder and a positive "drop arm" test (see p. 537).

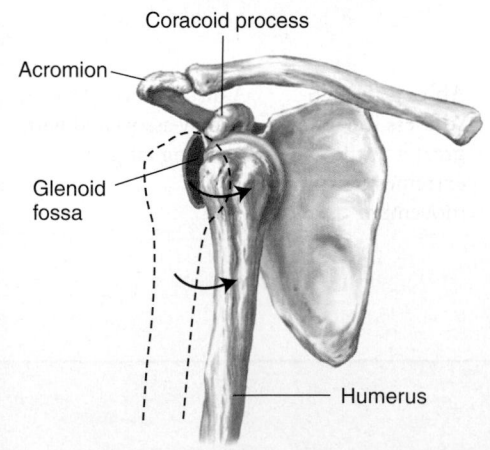

Coracoid process

Acromion

Glenoid fossa

Humerus

Anterior Dislocation of the Humerus[11,12,60]

Shoulder instability from anterior dislocation of the humerus usually results from a fall or forceful throwing motion, then becomes recurrent. The shoulder seems to "slip out of the joint" when the arm is abducted and externally rotated, causing a *positive apprehension sign* for anterior instability when the examiner places the arm in this position. Any shoulder movement may cause pain, and patients hold the arm in a neutral position. The rounded lateral aspect of the shoulder appears flattened. Dislocations may also be inferior, posterior (relatively rare), and multidirectional.

TABLE
18-5

Arthritis in the Hands

Acute Rheumatoid Arthritis

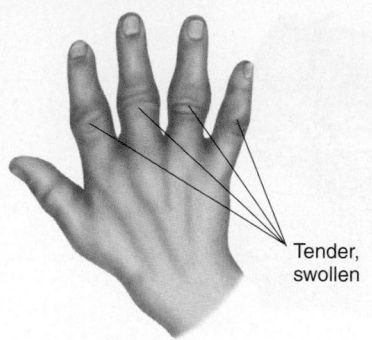

Tender,
swollen

Tender, painful, stiff joints in *rheumatoid arthritis*, usually with *symmetric* involvement on both sides of the body. The proximal interphalangeal, metacarpophalangeal, and wrist joints are the most frequently affected. Note the fusiform or spindle-shaped swelling of the proximal interphalangeal joints in acute disease.

Chronic Rheumatoid Arthritis

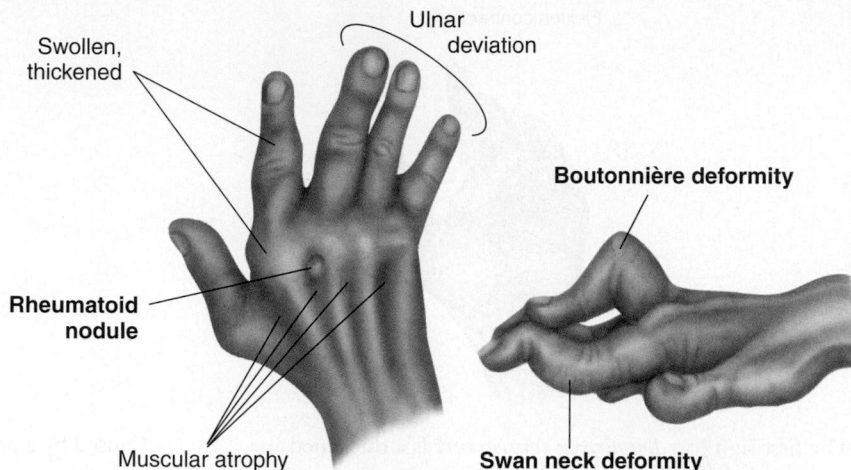

Swollen,
thickened

Ulnar
deviation

Boutonnière deformity

**Rheumatoid
nodule**

Muscular atrophy

Swan neck deformity

In chronic disease, note the swelling and thickening of the metacarpophalangeal and proximal interphalangeal joints. Range of motion becomes limited, and fingers may deviate toward the ulnar side. The interosseous muscles atrophy. The fingers may show *"swan neck" deformities* (hyperextension of the proximal interphalangeal joints with fixed flexion of the distal interphalangeal joints). Less common is a *boutonnière deformity* (persistent flexion of the proximal interphalangeal joint with hyperextension of the distal interphalangeal joint). Rheumatoid nodules are seen in the acute or the chronic stage.

Osteoarthritis (*Degenerative Joint Disease*)

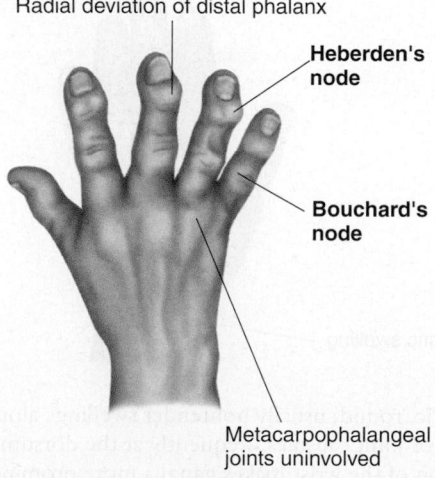

Radial deviation of distal phalanx

**Heberden's
node**

**Bouchard's
node**

Metacarpophalangeal
joints uninvolved

Heberden nodes on the dorsolateral aspects of the distal interphalangeal joints from bony overgrowth of osteoarthritis. Usually hard and painless, they affect the middle-aged or elderly; often associated with arthritic changes in other joints. Flexion and deviation deformities may develop. *Bouchard nodes* on the proximal interphalangeal joints are less common. The metacarpophalangeal joints are spared.

Chronic Tophaceous Gout

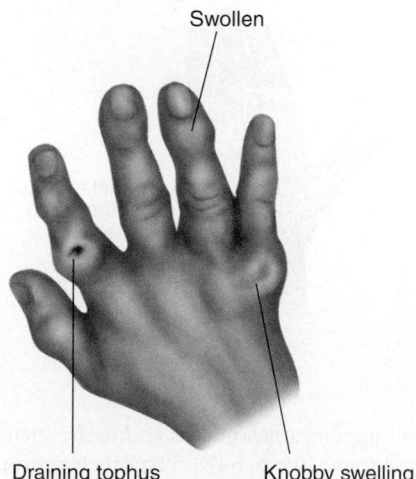

Swollen

Draining tophus

Knobby swelling

The deformities of long-standing chronic tophaceous gout can mimic rheumatoid arthritis and osteoarthritis. Joint involvement is usually not as symmetric as in rheumatoid arthritis. Acute inflammation may be present. Knobby swellings around the joints ulcerate and discharge white chalk-like urates.

TABLE
18-6

Swellings and Deformities of the Hands

Dupuytren Contracture

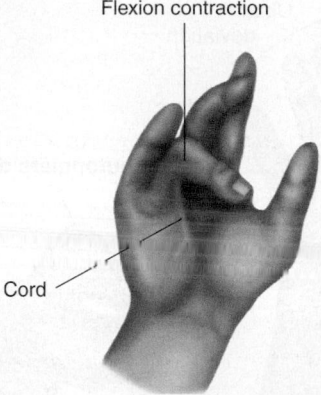

Flexion contraction

Cord

The first sign of a *Dupuytren contracture* is a thickened plaque overlying the flexor tendon of the ring finger and possibly the little finger at the level of the distal palmar crease. Subsequently, the skin in this area puckers, and a thickened fibrotic cord develops between palm and finger. Flexion contracture of the fingers may gradually ensue.

Trigger Finger

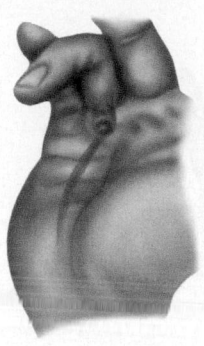

Caused by a painless nodule in a flexor tendon in the palm, near the metacarpal head. The nodule is too big to enter easily into the tendon sheath during extension of the fingers from a flexed position. With extra effort or assistance, the finger extends and flexes with a palpable and audible snap as the nodule pops into the tendon sheath. Watch, listen, and palpate the nodule as the patient flexes and extends the fingers.

Thenar Atrophy

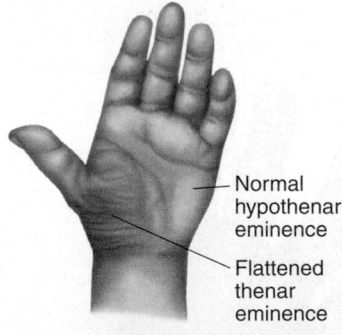

Normal hypothenar eminence

Flattened thenar eminence

Thenar atrophy suggests a *median nerve disorder* such as *carpal tunnel syndrome* (see p. 548). Hypothenar atrophy suggests an *ulnar nerve disorder*.

Ganglion

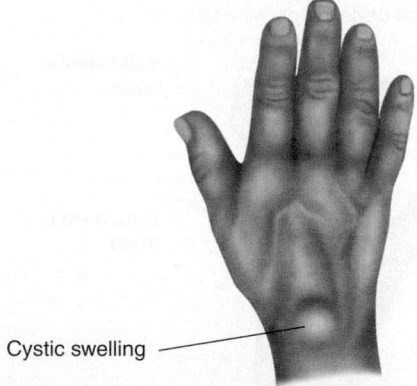

Cystic swelling

Ganglia are cystic, round, usually nontender swellings along tendon sheaths or joint capsules, frequently at the dorsum of the wrist. Flexion of the wrist makes ganglia more prominent; extension tends to obscure them. Ganglia may also develop elsewhere on the hands, wrists, ankles, and feet.

TABLE
18-7

Abnormalities of the Feet

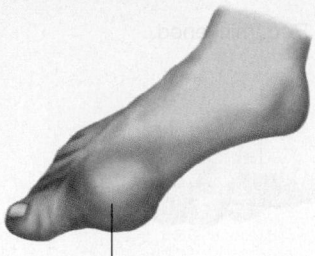

Hot, red, tender, swollen

Acute Gouty Arthritis

The metatarsophalangeal joint of the great toe may be the first joint involved in *acute gouty arthritis*. It is characterized by a very painful and tender, hot, dusky red swelling that extends beyond the margin of the joint. It is easily mistaken for a cellulitis. Acute gout may also involve the dorsum of the foot.

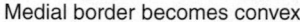

Medial border becomes convex

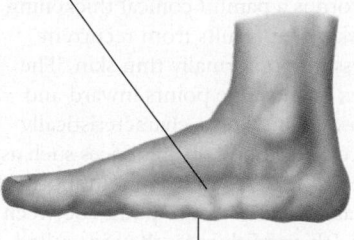

Sole touches floor

Flat Feet

Signs of *flat feet* may be apparent only when the patient stands, or they may become permanent. The longitudinal arch flattens so that the sole approaches or touches the floor. The normal concavity on the medial side of the foot becomes convex. Tenderness may be present from the medial malleolus down along the medial-plantar surface of the foot. Swelling may develop anterior to the malleoli. Inspect the shoes for excess wear on the inner sides of the soles and heels.

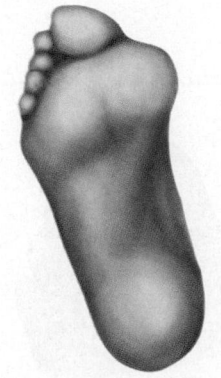

Hallux Valgus

In *hallux valgus,* the great toe is abnormally abducted in relationship to the first metatarsal, which itself is deviated medially. The head of the first metatarsal may enlarge on its medial side, and a bursa may form at the pressure point. This bursa may become inflamed.

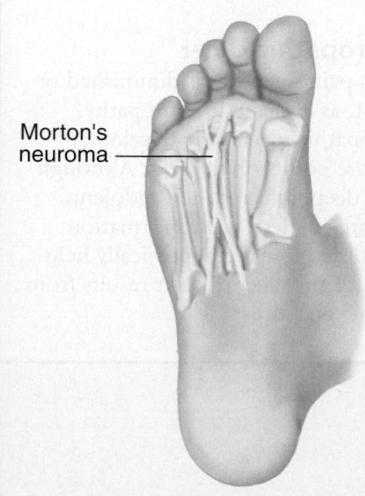

Morton's neuroma

Morton Neuroma

Tenderness over the plantar surface, 3rd and 4th metatarsal heads, from probable entrapment of the medial and lateral plantar nerves. Symptoms include hyperesthesia, numbness, aching, and burning from the metatarsal heads into the 3rd and 4th toes.

TABLE
18-8

Abnormalities of the Toes and Soles

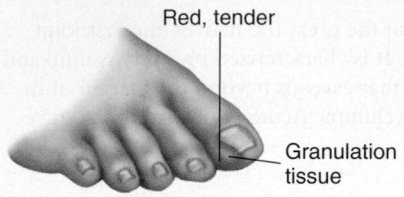

Red, tender

Granulation tissue

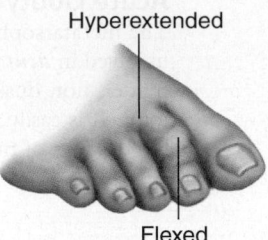

Hyperextended

Flexed

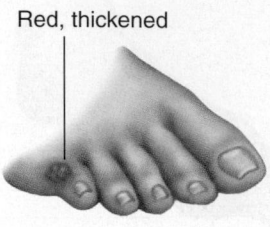

Red, thickened

Ingrown Toenail

The sharp edge of a toenail may dig into and injure the lateral nail fold, resulting in inflammation and infection. A tender, reddened, overhanging nail fold, sometimes with granulation tissue and purulent discharge, results. The great toe is most often affected.

Hammer Toe

Most commonly involving the second toe, a hammer toe is characterized by hyperextension at the metatarsophalangeal joint with flexion at the proximal interphalangeal joint. A corn frequently develops at the pressure point over the proximal interphalangeal joint.

Corn

A corn is a painful conical thickening of skin that results from recurrent pressure on normally thin skin. The apex of the cone points inward and causes pain. Corns characteristically occur over bony prominences such as the 5th toe. When located in moist areas such as pressure points between the 4th and 5th toes, they are called soft corns.

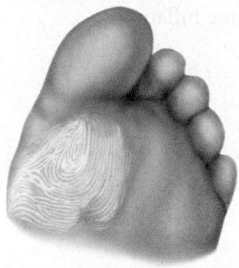

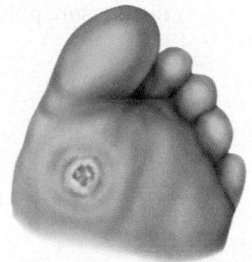

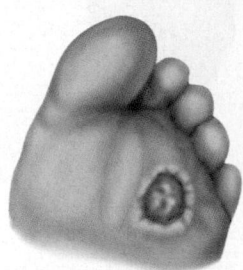

Callus

Like a corn, a callus is an area of greatly thickened skin that develops in a region of recurrent pressure. Unlike a corn, a callus involves skin that is normally thick, such as the sole, and is usually painless. If a callus is painful, suspect an underlying plantar wart.

Plantar Wart

A plantar wart is a common wart, *verruca vulgaris,* located in the thickened skin of the sole. It may look like a callus or even be covered by one. Look for the characteristic small dark spots that give a stippled appearance to a wart. Normal skin lines stop at the wart's edge.

Neuropathic Ulcer

When pain sensation is diminished or absent, as in diabetic neuropathy, neuropathic ulcers may develop at pressure points on the feet. Although often deep, infected, and indolent, they are painless. Callus formation about the ulcer is diagnostically helpful. Like the ulcer itself, it results from chronic pressure.

BIBLIOGRAPHY

CITATIONS

1. Deyo RA. Diagnostic evaluation of LBP: reaching a specific diagnosis is often impossible. Arch Intern Med 162(13):1444–1447, 2002.

2. Deyo RA, Weinstein JN. Low back pain. N Engl J Med 344(5):363–370, 2001.

3. Lurie JD, Gerber PD, Sox HC. A pain in the back. N Engl J Med 343(10):723–726, 2000.

4. Hoffman JR, Mower WR, Wolfson AB, et al. Validity of a set of clinical criteria to rule out injury to the cervical spine in patients with blunt trauma. N Engl J Med 343(2):94–99, 2000.

5. Devereaux MW. Neck and low back pain. Med Clin North Am 87(3):643–662, 2003.

6. Carette S, Fehlings MG. Cervical radiculopathy. N Engl J Med 353(4):392–399, 2005.

7. Terkeltaub RA. Gout. N Engl J Med 249(17):1647–1655, 2003.

8. Arnett FC, Edworthy SM, Bloch DA, et al. The American Rheumatism Association 1987 revised criteria for the classification of rheumatoid arthritis. Arthritis Rheum 31:315–324, 1988.

9. Goldring SR. A 55-year-old woman with rheumatoid arthritis. JAMA 283(4):524–529, 2000.

10. Lee DM, Weinblatt ME. Rheumatoid arthritis. Lancet 358:903–911, 2001.

11. Woodward TW, Best TM. The painful shoulder. Part II. Acute and chronic disorders. Am Fam Phys 61(11):3291–3300, 2000.

12. Liume JJ, Verhagen AP, Meidema HS, et al. Does this patient have an instability of the shoulder or a labrum lesion? The rational clinical examination. JAMA 292:1989–1999, 2004.

13. McGee S. Examination of the musculoskeletal system: the shoulder. In: Evidence-based Physical Diagnosis, 2nd ed. St. Louis: Saunders, 2007:628–638.

14. Murrell GA. Diagnosis of rotator cuff tears. Lancet 357:769–770, 2001.

15. D'Arcy CA, McGee S. Does this patient have carpal tunnel syndrome? The rational clinical examination. JAMA 283(23):3110–3117, 2000.

16. Griffin LY, ed. Hand and wrist. In: Essentials of Musculoskeletal Care 3. Rosemont, IL: American Academy of Orthopedic Surgeons, 2005:297–299, 321–327.

17. Katz JN, Simmons BP. Carpal tunnel syndrome. N Engl J Med 346(23):1807–1811, 2002.

18. Haywood KL, Garratt AM, Jordan K, et al. Spinal mobility in ankylosing spondylitis: reliability, validity and responsiveness. Rheumatology 43(6):750–757, 2004.

19. Laine C, Goldmann D, eds. In the clinic: osteoarthritis. Ann Intern Med 147(3):ITC8-1–ITC8-16, 2007.

20. Steultjens MPM, Dekker J, van Baar ME, et al. Range of joint motion and disability in patients with osteoarthritis of the knee or hip. Rheumatology 39(9):955–961, 2000.

21. McGee S. Examination of the musculoskeletal system: the knee. In: Evidence-based Physical Diagnosis, 2nd ed. St. Louis: Saunders, 2007:638–652.

22. Altman R, Asch E, Bloch D, et al. Development of criteria for the classification and reporting of osteoarthritis: classification of osteoarthritis of the knee. Arthritis Rheum 29(8):1039–1049, 1986.

23. Cibere J, Bellamy N, Thorne A, et al. Reliability of the knee examination in osteoarthritis. Arthritis Rheum 50(2):458–468, 2004.

24. Felson DT. Osteoarthritis of the knee. N Engl J Med 354(8):841–848, 2006.

25. Solomon DH, Simel DL, Bates DW, et al. Does this patient have a torn meniscus or ligament of the knee? Value of the physical examination. The rational physical examination. JAMA 286(13):1610–1620, 2001.

26. Jackson JL, O'Malley PG, Kroenke K. Evaluation of acute knee pain in primary care. Ann Intern Med 139(7):575–588, 2003.

27. Young CC, Rutherford DS, Niedfeldt MW. Treatment of plantar fasciitis. Am Fam Phys 63:467–474, 477–478, 2001.

28. Buchbinder R. Plantar fasciitis. N Engl J Med 350(21):2159–2166, 2004.

29. Stiell IG, Greenberg GH, McKnight RD, et al. Decision rules for the use of radiography in acute ankle injuries: refinement and prospective validation. JAMA 269(9):1127–1132, 1993.

30. U.S. Preventive Services Task Force. Behavioral counseling in primary care to promote physical activity: recommendations and rationale. Rockville, MD: Agency for Healthcare Research and Quality, July 2002. Available at: http://www.uspreventiveservicestaskforce.org/uspstf/uspsphys.htm. Accessed April 28, 2011.

31. U.S. Preventive Services Task Force. Counseling to prevent low back pain. In: Guide to Clinical Preventive Services, 2nd ed. Baltimore: Williams & Wilkins, 1996:600–709.

32. U.S. Preventive Services Task Force. Primary care interventions to prevent low back pain in adults: recommendation statement. Rockville, MD: Agency for Healthcare Research and Quality, February 2004. Available at: http://www.uspreventiveservicestaskforce.org/uspstf/uspsback.htm. Accessed April 28, 2011.

33. Caragee EJ. Persistent low back pain. N Engl J Med 352(18):1891–1898, 2005.

34. Staal JB, Hlobil H, Twoisk JWR, et al. Graded activity for low back pain in occupational health care. Ann Intern Med 140(2):77–84, 2004.

35. U.S. Preventive Services Task Force. Counseling to prevent household and recreational injuries. In: Guide to Clinical Preventive Services, 2nd ed. Baltimore: Williams & Wilkins, 1996:659–686.

36. National Institutes of Health Osteoporosis and Related Bone Disease National Resource Center. Osteoporosis overview: facts and figures. Available at: http://www.niams.nih.gov/Health_Info/Bone/Osteoporosis/Fracture/prevent_falls.asp Accessed April 28, 2011.

37. Robey-Williams C. Rush KL. Bendyk H, et al. Spartanburg Fall Risk Assessment Tool: A simple three-step process. Applied Nursing Research 20: 86–93, 2007.

38. NIH Consensus Development Panel on Osteoporosis Prevention, Diagnosis, and Therapy. Osteoporosis prevention, diagnosis, and therapy. JAMA 285(6):785–795, 2001.

39. Green CJ. Postmenopausal osteoporosis. N Engl J Med 353(6): 595–603, 2005.

40. Kuehn BM. Evidence-based guidelines needed for osteoporosis screening and treatment. JAMA 294(1):34, 2005.

41. U.S. Preventive Services Task Force. Screening for osteoporosis: recommendations and rationale. Rockville, MD: Agency for Healthcare Research and Quality, January 2011. Available at: http://www.uspreventiveservicestaskforce.org/uspstf/uspsoste.htm. Accessed April 28, 2011.

42. Raisz LG. Screening for osteoporosis. N Engl J Med 353(2): 164–171, 2005.

43. Margolis KL, Ensrud KE, Schreiner PJ, et al. Body size and risk for clinical fractures in older women. Ann Intern Med 133(2):123–127, 2000.

44. Rosen CJ. Postmenopausal osteoporosis. N Engl J Med 353 (6):595–603, 2005.

45. Benton M, White A. Osteoporosis: recommendations for resistance exercise and supplementation with calcium and vitamin D to promote bone health. J Community Health Nurs 23(4):201–211, 2006.

46. National Institute of Child Health & Human Development. Tweens* and teens need calcium now more than ever! Available at: www.nichd.nih.gov/milk. Accessed April 28, 2011.

47. National Institutes of Health. Osteoporosis and related bone diseases—National Resource Center. Available at: www.niams.nih.gov/bone. Accessed April 28, 2011.

48. Hulley S, Grady D, Bush T, et al. Randomized trial of estrogen plus progestin for secondary prevention of coronary heart disease in postmenopausal women. Heart and Estrogen/Progestin Replacement Study (HERS) Research Group. JAMA 280(7):605–613, 1998.

49. Writing Group for the Women's Health Initiative Investigators. Risks and benefits of estrogen plus progestin in healthy postmenopausal women: principal results from the Women's Health Initiative randomized controlled trial. JAMA 288:321–333, 2002.

50. Women's Health Initiative Steering Committee. Effects of conjugated equine estrogen in postmenopausal women with hysterectomy: the Women's Health Initiative randomized controlled trial. JAMA 291:1701–1712, 2004.

51. U.S. Preventive Services Task Force. Hormone replacement therapy for primary prevention of chronic conditions: recommendations and rationale. Rockville, MD: Agency for Healthcare Research and Quality, May 2005. Available at: http://www.uspreventiveservicestaskforce.org/uspstf/uspspmho.htm. Accessed April 28, 2011.

52. Chou R, Qaseem A, Sonow V, et al. Diagnosis and treatment of low back pain: a joint clinical practice guideline from the American College of Physicians and the American Pain Society. Ann Intern Med 147(7):478–491, 2007.

53. McGee S. Disorders of the nerve roots, plexi, and peripheral nerves. In: Evidence-based Physical Diagnosis, 2nd ed. St. Louis: Saunders, 2007:777–788.

54. Davis BT, Pasternak MS. Case 19-2007: a 19-year-old college student with fever and joint pain. N Engl J Med 356(25): 2631–2637, 2007.

55. Goldenberg DL, Burckhardt C, Crofford L. Management of fibromyalgia syndrome. JAMA 292(19):2388–2395, 2004.

56. Levanthal LJ. Management of bromyalgia. Ann Intern Med 131(11):850–858, 1999.

57. Wolfe F, Smythe HA, Yunus MB, et al. The American College of Rheumatology 1990 criteria for the classification of fibromyalgia. Report of the Multicenter Criteria Committee. Arthritis Rheum 33(2):160–172, 1990.

58. Griffin LY, ed. Shoulder. In: Essentials of Musculoskeletal Care 3. Rosemont, IL: American Academy of Orthopedic Surgeons 2005:155–211, 321.

ADDITIONAL REFERENCES

Centers for Disease Control (CDC). Preventing falls among older adults. Available at: http://www.cdc.gov/ncipc/duip/preventadultfalls.htm.

Chou R, Huffman AH. Nonpharmacologic therapies for acute and chronic low back pain: a review of the evidence for an American Pain Society/American College of Physicians Clinical Practice Guideline. Ann Intern Med 147(7):492–504, 2007.

Clegg DO, Reda DJ, Harria CL. Glucosamine, chondroitin sulfate, and the two in combination for painful knee osteoarthritis. N Engl J Med 354(8):795–808, 2006.

Fransen M, Nairn L, Winstanley J, et al. Physical activity for osteoarthritis management: a randomized controlled clinical trial evaluating hydrotherapy or Tai Chi classes. Arthritis Rheum 57(3):407–414, 2007.

Godfrey J, Rosen C. Toward optimal health: advances in diagnosis and preventive strategies to promote bone health in women. J Womens Health 17(9):1425–1430, 2008.

Lane NE. Osteoarthritis of the hip. N Engl J Med 357(14): 1413–1421, 2007.

Matsen FA. Rotator-cuff failure. N Engl J Med 358(20):2138–2147, 2008.

Moyad M. Vitamin D: a rapid review. Reprinted with permission from Urol Nurs 28(5), 343–349, 384, 2008. Dermatol Nurs 21(1):25–30, 55, 2009.

National Osteoporosis Foundation. Available at: www.nof.org.

Reiser L, Schlenk E. Clinical use of physical activity measures. J Am Acad Nurse Practitioners 21(2):87–94, 2009.

Sharma S, Hoelscher D, Kelder S, et al. Psychosocial, environmental and behavioral factors associated with bone health in middle-school girls. Health Educ Res 24(2):173–184, 2009.

Stolee P, Poss J, Cook R, et al. Risk factors for hip fracture in older home care clients. J Gerontol Series A Biol Sci Med Sci 64(3):403–410, 2009.

U.S. Preventive Services Task Force. Screening for osteoporosis in postmenopausal women. Available at: http://www.ahrq.gov/CLINIC/USPSTF/uspsoste.htm.

CHAPTER 19

Mental Status

LEARNING OBJECTIVES

The student will:

1. Describe the multiple areas assessed in the mental status examination.
2. Determine the symptoms and behaviors for mental health screening.
3. Obtain an accurate mental status history for a patient.
4. Perform a mini-mental status examination
5. Identify the screening and health promotion and counseling tools for depression, suicide and dementia.
6. Correctly document the findings of the mental status assessment.

As nurses, we are uniquely poised to screen, detect, investigate, and encourage health-promoting behaviors. Empathic listening and close observation open a unique vista on the patient's outlook, concerns, and habits. Nevertheless, nurses often miss clues of mental illness and harmful dysfunctional behaviors in patients. This chapter introduces common symptoms and behaviors encountered in routine patient interactions, concepts guiding history taking related to mental health, priorities for mental health promotion and counseling, and the formal elements of the *mental status examination* that should be conducted when behavioral problems are suspicious indicators of mental health disorders.

Health and human behavior are intimately linked, as amply noted in the Health Promotion and Counseling sections throughout this book. Government statistics, advisories of the Surgeon General, reports from the U.S. Preventive Services Task Force and the Centers for Disease Control and Prevention, and position statements from leading professional societies all attest to the importance of maintaining and promoting the mental and physical health of our patients. Despite the prevalence of mental disorders, detection is difficult and recognition and treatment rates are low. The prevalence of mental disorders in the U.S. population is 30%,[1] yet only approximately 20% of affected patients receive treatment. Even for patients who obtain care, evidence suggests that adherence to treatment guidelines in primary care offices is less than 50%.[2]

It is especially important for nurses to learn how to assess for both mental and physical changes. Often patients have more than one mental disorder, with symptoms that mirror medical illnesses. The astute assessment and documentation of findings are crucial to formulate the best plan for each individual patient. The patient with depression or anxiety may also be dealing with substance abuse, and someone with substance abuse may have depression or anxiety. Further, it is increasingly important for nurses to recognize that "difficult patients" are frequently those with multiple unexplained symptoms and underlying psychiatric conditions that are amenable to therapy. Patient health, function, and quality of life are at risk without adequate assessment and treatment.

SYMPTOMS AND BEHAVIOR

Patient Symptoms: What Do They Mean? For beginning nurses, the challenge is to sort out the array of symptoms encountered. Symptoms may be psychological, relating to mood or anxiety, or *physical*, relating to a body sensation such as pain, fatigue, or palpitations. In the mental health literature, such physical symptoms are often termed *somatic*. Studies reveal that physical symptoms prompt more than 50% of U.S. office visits.[3] Approximately 5% of these symptoms are acute, triggering immediate evaluation. Another 70% to 75% are minor or self-limited and resolve in 6 weeks. Nevertheless, approximately 25% of patients have persisting and recurrent symptoms that elude assessment through the history and physical examination and fail to improve. Overall, 30% of symptoms are *medically unexplained*. Some of them involve single complaints that appear to persist longer than others—for example, back pain, headache, or musculoskeletal complaints. Others occur in clusters presenting as *functional syndromes*, such as: irritable bowel syndrome, fibromyalgia, chronic fatigue, temporomandibular joint disorder, or multiple chemical sensitivity.

A *physical symptom* can be explained physically or medically or can be unexplained; a *somato-form symptom* lacks an adequate medical or physical explanation.

Unexplained Symptoms. Two thirds of patients with depression, for example, present with physical complaints, and half report multiple unexplained physical or somatic symptoms.[4] Further, the functional syndromes have been shown to "frequently co-occur and share key symptoms and selected objective abnormalities."[5] Failure to recognize the admixture of physical symptoms and functional syndromes with common mental health disorders—anxiety, depression, unexplained or somato-form physical symptoms, and substance abuse—adds to loss of the patient's quality of life and impaired treatment outcomes. Often these patients are "high users" of the health care system and have significant disability.

Patient Identifiers for Selective Mental Health Screening. Unexplained conditions lasting beyond 6 weeks are increasingly recognized as common chronic disorders that should prompt screening for depression, anxiety, or both. Because screening all patients is time-consuming and expensive, experts recommend a two-tier approach: brief screening questions with high sensitivity and specificity for patients at risk, followed by a referral for a more detailed investigation when indicated.

Chronic pain may be a spectrum disorder in patients with anxiety, depression, or somatic symptoms. See Chapter 7, General Survey, Vital Signs, and Pain, pp. 119–121.

PATIENT IDENTIFIERS FOR MENTAL HEALTH SCREENING[3,4]

- Medically unexplained physical symptoms—more than half have a depressive or anxiety disorder
- Multiple physical or somatic symptoms or "high symptom count"
- High severity of the presenting somatic symptom
- Chronic pain
- Symptoms for more than 6 weeks
- Rating as a "difficult encounter" with a patient
- Recent stress
- Low self-rating of health
- High use of health care services
- Substance abuse

HIGH-YIELD SCREENING QUESTIONS FOR PATIENTS—BUT FOLLOW-UP SYSTEMS FOR DIAGNOSIS AND TREATMENT NEEDED...

Depression[6–8]
- Over the past 2 weeks, have you felt down, depressed, or hopeless?
- Over the past 2 weeks, have you felt little interest or pleasure in doing things (anhedonia)?

Anxiety
- Anxiety disorders include: generalized anxiety disorder, social phobia, panic disorder, posttraumatic stress disorder, and acute stress disorder.
- Panic Disorder: In the past 4 weeks, have you had an anxiety attack—suddenly feeling fear or panic?[9]

Alcohol and Substance Abuse
- CAGE questions adapted for alcohol and drug abuse—see Chapter 4, Health History, p. 68.

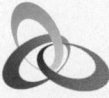 # THE HEALTH HISTORY

COMMON OR CONCERNING SYMPTOMS

- Changes in attention, mood, or speech
- Changes in insight, orientation, or memory
- Delirium or dementia

Overview. As with the General Survey, your assessment of mental status begins with the patient's first words. As you gather the health history, you will quickly discern the patient's level of *alertness* and *orientation, mood, attention,* and *memory*. As the history unfolds, you will learn about the patient's *insight* and *judgment,* as well as any *recurring or unusual thoughts or perceptions*. For some, you will need to supplement your interview with specific questions and a more formal evaluation of mental status. Just as symptoms, blood pressure, and valvular murmurs help to distinguish, health from disease in the cardiovascular system, specific components of mental function illuminate specific concerns and conditions.

Many of the terms pertinent to the mental health history and the mental status examination are familiar to you from social conversation. Take the time to learn their precise meanings in the context of formal evaluation of mental status, as detailed in the next table.

Attention, Mood, Speech; Insight, Orientation, Memory. Much of the information about the patient's *mental status* becomes evident during the interview. As you talk with the patient and listen to the patient's story, assess *level of consciousness; general appearance; mood,* including depression or mania; and *ability to pay attention, remember, understand,* and *speak*. By placing the patient's vocabulary and general amount of information in the context of the cultural and educational background, you can often make a rough estimate of intelligence but not necessarily health history. Likewise, the patient's responses to illness and life circumstances often tell you about the degree of *insight and judgment*. If you suspect a problem in orientation and memory, you can ask, "Let's see, your last clinic appointment was when . . . ?" "And the date today?" The more you can integrate your exploration of mental status into a sensitive patient history, the less it will seem like an interrogation.

See Table 20-9, Disorders of Speech, p. 674.

● Terminology: The Mental Status Examination

Level of consciousness	Alertness or state of awareness of the environment
Attention	The ability to focus or concentrate over time on one task or activity—an inattentive or distractible person with impaired consciousness has difficulty giving a history or responding to questions.
Memory	The process of registering or recording information, tested by asking for immediate repetition of material, followed by storage or retention of information. *Recent or short-term memory* covers minutes, hours, or days; *remote or long-term memory* refers to intervals of years.
Orientation	Awareness of personal identity, place, and time; requires both memory and attention
Perceptions	Sensory awareness of objects in the environment and their interrelationships (external stimuli); also refers to internal stimuli such as dreams or hallucinations

(continued)

● **Terminology: The Mental Status Examination** (continued)

Thought processes	The logic, coherence, and relevance of the patient's thought as it leads to selected goals, or *how* people think
Thought content	*What* the patient thinks about, including level of insight and judgment
Insight	Awareness that symptoms or disturbed behaviors are normal or abnormal; for example, distinguishing between daydreams and hallucinations that seem real
Judgment	Process of comparing and evaluating alternatives when deciding on a course of action; reflects values that may or may not be based on reality and social conventions or norms
Affect	An observable, usually episodic, feeling or tone expressed through voice, facial expression, and demeanor
Mood	A more sustained emotion that may color a person's view of the world (mood is to affect as climate is to weather)
Language	A complex symbolic system for expressing, receiving, and comprehending words; as with consciousness, attention, and memory, language is essential for assessing other mental functions.
Higher cognitive functions	Assessed by vocabulary, amount of information, abstract thinking, calculations, and construction of objects that have two or three dimensions

Delirium or Dementia. All patients with documented or suspected brain lesions, psychiatric symptoms, or reports from family members of vague or changed behavioral symptoms need further systematic assessment. Patients may have subtle behavioral changes, difficulty taking medications properly, problems attending to household chores or paying bills, or loss of interest in their usual activities. Other patients may have changes related to the hospitalization or medications and behave strangely after surgery or during an acute illness. Each problem should be identified as expeditiously as possible. The nurse may assess the change in the patient and will be the advocate and detective, determining when the change occurred and what was new in the treatment. Prompt assessment alleviates unexpected changes in the patient.

See Table 24-2, Delirium and Dementia, p. 876.

May be signs of depression or dementia

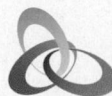

PHYSICAL EXAMINATION

EQUIPMENT

Pencil
Paper
Mini-mental status examination tool

Important Areas of the Mental Status Examination

- Appearance and behavior
- Speech and language
- Mood
- Thoughts and perceptions
- Cognition, including memory, attention, information and vocabulary, calculations, abstract thinking, and constructional ability

The interplay between mental disorders and physical health is challenging and complex. Mental disorders often take the form of somatic complaints, and physical illnesses provoke behavioral and emotional responses. Changes in mental status may be related to disease processes or medications. Personality factors, psychodynamics, or the patient's personal experiences can complicate assessments of mental status. These areas can be explored during the interview. By integrating and correlating your observations and findings from the history and examination, including the mental status examination, you will come to understand the patient as a whole, molded by life experiences, family, and culture.

The nervous system, mental status, and brain structure and function are intimately intertwined. The assessment of mental status is an integral component of the assessment of the nervous system, and the first segment of the nervous system write-up. With practice, you will learn to describe the patient's mood, speech, behavior, and cognition and relate these findings to your examination of the cranial nerves, motor and sensory systems, and reflexes.

Novice nurses may feel reluctant to perform mental status examinations, wondering if it will upset patients or invade their privacy. Such concerns are understandable. An insensitive examination may alarm a patient, and even a skillful examination may bring to conscious awareness a deficit that the patient is trying to ignore. Discuss concerns with your instructor or other experienced nurses. Remember that patients appreciate an understanding listener.

The mental status examination consists of the following components:

- Appearance and behavior

- Speech and language

- Mood

- Thoughts and perceptions

- Cognitive function, including memory, attention, information and vocabulary, calculations, abstract thinking, and constructional ability

The format that follows should help to organize your observations, but it is not intended as a step-by-step guide. When a full examination is indicated, be flexible in approach but thorough in what is covered. In some situations, however, sequence is important. If, during the initial interview, the patient's consciousness, attention, comprehension of words, or ability to speak seems impaired, assess this attribute promptly. Such a patient cannot give a reliable history, and cannot be tested for most other mental functions.

Appearance and Behavior

Utilize all the relevant observations made throughout the course of the history and examination. Include these areas:

Level of Consciousness. Is the patient awake and alert? Does the patient seem to understand the questions and respond appropriately and reasonably quickly, or is there a tendency to lose track of the topic and fall silent or even asleep?

See the table on Level of Consciousness (Arousal), Chapter 20, The Neurological System, p. 652.

If the patient does not respond to your questions, escalate the stimulus in steps:

- Speak to the patient by name and in a loud voice.

Lethargic patients are drowsy but open their eyes and look at you, respond to questions, and then fall asleep.

- Shake the patient gently, as if awakening a sleeper.

Obtunded patients open their eyes and look at you, but respond slowly and are somewhat confused.

If there is no response to these stimuli, promptly assess the patient for stupor or coma—severe reductions in level of consciousness.

Stuporous patients are unaware of surroundings and are totally or almost totally immobile and unresponsive, even to painful stimuli.

Comatose patients are unconscious and do not respond to painful stimuli or voice and do not open their eyes.

Posture and Motor Behavior. Does the patient lie in bed, or prefer to walk around? Note body posture and the patient's ability to relax. Observe the pace, range, and character of movements. Do they seem to be under voluntary control? Are certain parts immobile? Do posture and motor activity change with topics under discussion or with activities or people around the patient?

Tense posture, restlessness, and fidgeting of anxiety; crying, pacing, and hand wringing of *agitated depression*; hopeless, slumped posture and slowed movements of *depression*; singing, dancing, and expansive movements of a *manic episode*

Dress, Grooming, and Personal Hygiene. How is the patient dressed? Is clothing clean, pressed, and properly fastened? How does it compare with clothing worn by people of comparable age and social group? Note the patient's hair, nails, teeth, skin, and, if present, beard. How are they groomed? How do the person's grooming and hygiene compare with those of other people of comparable age, lifestyle, and socioeconomic group? Compare one side of the body with the other.

Grooming and personal hygiene may deteriorate in *depression*, *schizophrenia*, and *dementia*. Excessive fastidiousness may be seen with *obsessive–compulsive disorder*. One-sided neglect may result from a lesion in the opposite parietal cortex, usually the nondominant side.

Facial Expression. Observe the face, both at rest and when the patient interacts with others. Watch for variations in expression with topics under discussion. Are they appropriate? Or is the face relatively immobile throughout?

Expressions of anxiety, depression, apathy, anger, elation; facial immobility in *parkinsonism*

Manner, Affect, and Relationship to People and Things. Using your observations of facial expressions, voice, and body movements, assess the patient's *affect,* or external expression of the inner emotional state. Does it vary appropriately with topics under discussion, or is the affect labile, blunted, or flat? Does it seem inappropriate or extreme at certain points? If so, how? Note the patient's openness, approachability, and reactions to others and to the surroundings. Does the patient seem to hear or see things that you do not or seem to be conversing with someone who is not there?

Anger, hostility, suspiciousness, or evasiveness of patients with *paranoia*. Elation and euphoria of *mania*. Flat affect and remoteness of *schizophrenia*. Apathy (dulled affect with detachment and indifference) of *dementia*. Anxiety, depression

Speech and Language

Throughout the interview, note the characteristics of the patient's speech, including the following:

Quantity. Is the patient talkative or relatively silent? Are comments spontaneous or only responsive to direct questions?

Rate. Is speech fast or slow?

Loudness. Is speech loud or soft?

Slow speech of *depression*; accelerated, rapid, loud speech in *mania*

Articulation of Words. Are the words spoken clearly and distinctly? Is there a nasal quality to the speech?

Dysarthria refers to defective articulation. *Aphasia* refers to a disorder of language. See Table 20-9, Disorders of Speech, p. 674.

Fluency. This involves the rate, flow, and melody of speech and the content and use of words. Be alert for abnormalities of spontaneous speech such as:

● Hesitancies and gaps in the flow and rhythm of words

These abnormalities suggest *aphasia*. The patient may have so much difficulty in talking or in understanding others that you may not be able to obtain a history. You may also falsely suspect a psychotic disorder.

● Disturbed inflections, such as a monotone

● Circumlocutions, in which phrases or sentences are substituted for a word the person cannot think of, such as "what you write with" for "pen"

● Paraphasias, in which words are malformed ("I write with a den"), wrong ("I write with a bar"), or invented ("I write with a dar")

If the patient's speech lacks meaning or fluency, proceed with further testing as outlined in the following table.

● Testing for Aphasia	
Word Comprehension	Ask the patient to follow a one-stage command, such as "Point to your nose." Try a two-stage command: "Point to your mouth, then your knee."
Repetition	Ask the patient to repeat a phrase of one-syllable words (the most difficult repetition task): "No ifs, ands, or buts."
Naming	Ask the patient to name the parts of a watch.
Reading Comprehension	Ask the patient to read a paragraph aloud.
Writing	Ask the patient to write a sentence.

These tests help you determine the kind of aphasia the patient may have. Remember that deficiencies in vision, hearing, intelligence, and education may also affect performance. Two common kinds of aphasia—Wernicke and Broca—are compared in Table 20-9, Disorders of Speech, p. 674.

A person who can write a correct sentence does not have aphasia.

Mood

Assess mood during the interview by exploring the patient's perceptions of his or her mood. Find out about the patient's usual mood level and how it has varied with life events. "How did you feel about that?", for example, or, more generally, "How is your overall mood?" The reports of relatives and friends may be of great value.

Moods include sadness and deep melancholy; contentment, joy, euphoria, and elation; anger and rage; anxiety and worry; and detachment and indifference.

What has the patient's mood been like? How intense has it been? Has it been labile or fairly unchanging? How long has it lasted? Is it appropriate to the patient's circumstances? In case of depression, have there also been episodes of an elevated mood, suggesting a bipolar disorder?

If you suspect depression, assess its depth and any associated risk of suicide. The following series of questions is useful, proceeding as far as the patient's positive answers warrant:

- Do you get pretty discouraged (or depressed or blue)?

- How low do you feel?

- What do you see for yourself in the future?

- Do you ever feel that life isn't worth living? Or that you would just as soon be dead?

- Have you ever thought of doing away with yourself?

- How did (do) you think you would do it?

- Do you have the means to carry out a suicide?

- What do you think would happen after you were dead?

Asking about suicidal thoughts does not implant the idea in the patient's mind, and it may be the only way to get the information. Although you may feel uneasy about direct questions, most patients discuss their thoughts and feelings freely, sometimes with considerable relief. By open discussion, you demonstrate your interest and concern for a possibly life-threatening problem.

Thought and Perceptions

Thought Processes. Assess the logic, relevance, organization, and coherence of the patient's thought processes as revealed in the patient's words and speech throughout the interview. Does speech progress logically toward a goal? Here you use speech as a window into the patient's mind. Listen for patterns of speech that suggest disorders of thought processes. A few examples of variations in thought processes are:

- Flight of ideas: An almost continuous flow of accelerated speech in which a person changes abruptly from topic to topic. Changes are usually based on understandable associations, plays on words, or distracting stimuli, but the ideas do not progress to sensible conversation.

  Most frequently noted in *manic episodes*

- Incoherence: Speech that is largely incomprehensible because of illogic, lack of meaningful connections, abrupt changes in topic, or disordered grammar or word use. Shifts in meaning occur within clauses. Flight of ideas, when severe, may produce incoherence.

  Observed in severe psychotic disturbances (usually *schizophrenia*)

- Confabulation: Fabrication of facts or events in response to questions, to fill in the gaps in an impaired memory

  Seen in Korsakoff syndrome from alcoholism

Thought Content. Assess information relevant to thought content during the interview. Follow appropriate leads as they occur rather than using stereotyped lists of specific questions. For example, "You mentioned a few minutes ago that a neighbor was responsible for your entire illness. Can you tell me more about that?" Or, in another situation, "What do you think about at times like these?"

You may need to make more specific inquiries. If so, phrase them in tactful and accepting terms. "When people are upset like this, sometimes they can't keep certain thoughts out of their minds," or ". . . things seem unreal. Have you experienced anything like this?"

Perceptions. Inquire about false perceptions in a manner similar to that used for thought content. For example, "When you heard the voice speaking to you, what did it say? How did it make you feel?" Or, "After you've been drinking a lot, do you ever see things that aren't really there?" Or, "Sometimes after major surgery like this, people hear peculiar or frightening things. Have you experienced anything like that?" In these ways, find out about abnormal perceptions.

Insight and Judgment. These attributes are usually best assessed during the interview.

Insight. Some of the first interview questions to the patient often yield important information about insight: "What brings you to the hospital?" "What seems to be the trouble?" "What do you think is wrong?" More specifically, note whether the patient is aware that a particular mood, thought, or perception is abnormal or part of an illness.

> Patients with psychotic disorders often lack insight into their illness. Denial of impairment may accompany some neurologic disorders.

Judgment. Assess judgment by noting the patient's responses to family situations, jobs, use of money, and interpersonal conflicts. "How do you plan to get the help you'll need after leaving the hospital?" "How are you going to manage if you lose your job?" "If your husband starts to abuse you again, what will you do?" "Who will attend to your financial affairs while you are in the nursing home?"

> Judgment may be poor in delirium, dementia, mental retardation, and psychotic states. Anxiety, mood disorders, intelligence, education, income, and cultural values also influence judgment.

Note whether decisions and actions are based on reality or, for example, on impulse, wish fulfillment, or disordered thought content. What values seem to underlie the patient's decisions and behavior? Allowing for cultural variations, how do these compare with mature adult standards? Because judgment reflects maturity, it may be variable and unpredictable during adolescence.

> Disorientation occurs especially when memory or attention is impaired, as in delirium.

Cognitive Functions

Orientation. By skillful questioning, the patient's orientation can be determined in the context of the interview. For example, ask naturally for specific dates and times, the patient's address and telephone number, the names of family members, or the route taken to the hospital. At times—when rechecking the status of a patient with delirium, for example—simple, direct questions may be indicated. When choosing the questions to ask, be sure you know the correct answer. Otherwise, the person may answer appropriately; however, it may or may not be correct.

"Can you tell me what time it is now . . . and what day it is?" In either of these ways, determine the patient's orientation for the following:

● *Time*—the time of day, day of the week, month, season, date and year, duration of hospitalization

● *Place*—the patient's residence, the names of the hospital, city, and state

● *Person*—the patient's own name, and the names of relatives and professional personnel

Attention. These tests of attention are commonly used:

Number List.   Explain that you would like to test the patient's ability to concentrate, perhaps adding that this can be difficult when people are in pain, or ill, or feverish. Recite a series of numbers, starting with two at a time and speaking each number clearly at a rate of about one per second. Ask the patient to repeat the numbers back to you. If this repetition is accurate, try a series of three numbers, then four, as long as the patient responds correctly. Jot down the numbers as you say them to ensure your own accuracy. If the patient makes a mistake, try once more with another series of the same length. Stop after a second failure in a single series.

In choosing numbers you may use street numbers, zip codes, telephone numbers, and other numerical sequences that are familiar to you, but avoid consecutive numbers, easily recognized dates, and sequences that possibly are familiar to the patient.

Now, starting again with a series of two, ask the patient to repeat the numbers to you backward.

Normally, a person should be able to repeat correctly at least five numbers forward and four backward.

Serial 7s.   Instruct the patient, "Starting from a hundred, subtract 7, and keep subtracting 7. . . ." Note the effort required and the speed and accuracy of the responses. After 5 correct answers, the patient has a positive serial 7 response. Writing down the answers helps you keep up with the arithmetic. Normally, a person can complete serial 7s in 1½ minutes, with fewer than four errors. If the patient cannot do serial 7s, try 3s or counting backward.

Spelling Backward.   This can substitute for serial 7s. Say a five-letter word, spell it (e.g., W-O-R-L-D), and ask the patient to spell it backward.

Causes of poor performance include *delirium, dementia, mental retardation,* and performance anxiety.

Poor performance may result from delirium, the late stage of dementia, mental retardation, loss of calculating ability, anxiety, or depression. Also consider the possibility of limited education.

Remote Memory. Inquire about birthdays, anniversaries, social security number, names of schools attended, jobs held, or past historical events such as wars relevant to the patient's past.

Remote memory may be impaired in the late stage of *dementia*.

Recent Memory. This could involve the events of the day. Ask questions with answers you can check against other sources so you can see if the patient is confabulating (making up facts to compensate for a defective memory). These might include the day's weather, today's appointment time, and medications or laboratory tests taken during the day. (Asking what the patient had for breakfast may be a waste of time unless you can check the accuracy of the answer.)

Recent memory is impaired in *dementia* and *delirium*. *Amnestic disorders* impair memory or new learning ability significantly and reduce a person's social or occupational functioning, but they do not have the global features of delirium or dementia. Anxiety, depression, and mental retardation may also impair recent memory.

New Learning Ability. Give the patient three or four words such as "table, flower, green, and hamburger." Ask the patient to repeat them so that you know that the information has been heard and registered. This step, like number list, tests registration and immediate recall. Then proceed to other parts of the examination. After about 3 to 5 minutes, ask the patient to repeat the words. Note the accuracy of the response, awareness of whether it is correct, and any tendency to confabulate. Normally, a person should be able to remember the words.

Higher Cognitive Functions

Information and Vocabulary. Information and vocabulary, when observed clinically, provide a rough estimate of a person's intelligence. Assess them during the interview. Ask a student, for example, about favorite courses, or inquire about work, hobbies, reading, favorite television programs, or current events. Explore such topics first with simple questions, then with more difficult ones. Note the person's grasp of information, the complexity of the ideas expressed, and the vocabulary used.

If considered in the context of cultural and educational background, information and vocabulary are fairly good indicators of intelligence. They are relatively unaffected by any but the most severe psychiatric disorders, and may be helpful for distinguishing mentally retarded adults (whose information and vocabulary are limited) from those with mild or moderate *dementia* (whose information and vocabulary are fairly well preserved).

More directly, you can ask about specific facts such as:

The name of the president, vice president, or governor
The names of the last four or five presidents
The names of five large cities in the country

Calculating Ability. Test the patient's ability to do arithmetic calculations, starting at the rote level with simple addition ("What is 4 + 3? . . . 8 + 7?") and multiplication ("What is 5 × 6? . . . 9 × 7?"). The task can be made more difficult by using two-digit numbers ("15 + 12" or "25 × 6") or longer, written examples.

Poor performance may be a useful sign of dementia or may accompany *aphasia,* but it must be assessed in terms of the patient's intelligence and education.

Alternatively, pose practical and functionally important questions, such as "If something costs 78 cents and you give the clerk one dollar, how much should you get back?"

Abstract Thinking. Test the capacity to think abstractly in two ways.

Proverbs. Ask the patient what people mean when they use some of the following proverbs:

People who live in glass houses should not throw stones.
Don't count your chickens before they're hatched.
A rolling stone gathers no moss.
The squeaking wheel gets the grease.

Note the relevance of the answers and their degree of concreteness or abstractness. For example, "Don't throw stones at glass or it will break" is concrete, whereas "Someone who repeatedly does something (e.g., is late) should not criticize someone else for the same thing" is abstract. Average patients should give abstract or semiabstract responses.

Similarities. Ask the patient to tell you how the following are alike:

An orange and an apple   A church and a theater
A cat and a mouse   A piano and a violin
A child and a dwarf   Wood and coal

Note the accuracy and relevance of the answers and their degree of concreteness or abstractness. For example, "A cat and a mouse are both animals" is abstract, "They both have tails" is concrete, and "A cat chases a mouse" is not relevant.

Constructional Ability. The task here is to copy figures of increasing complexity onto a piece of blank unlined paper. Show each figure one at a time and ask the patient to copy it as well as possible.

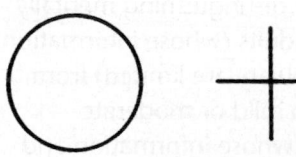 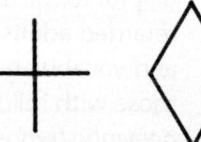 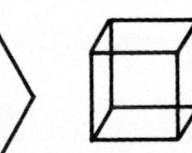 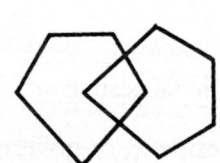

In another approach, ask the patient to draw a clock face complete with numbers and hands. The example below is rated excellent.

If vision and motor ability are intact, poor constructional ability suggests dementia or parietal lobe damage. Mental retardation may also impair performance.

Concrete responses are often given by people with mental retardation, *delirium,* or *dementia* but may also be a function of limited education, culture, or exposure. Patients with *schizophrenia* may respond concretely or with personal, bizarre interpretations.

The three diamonds below are rated poor, fair, and good (but not excellent).[10]

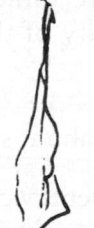 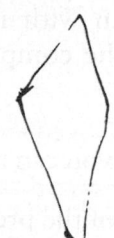 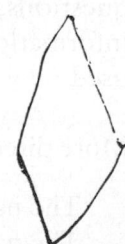

These three clocks are poor, fair, and good.[10]

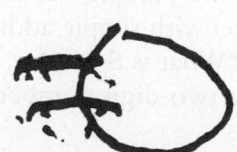 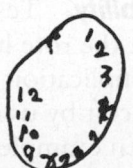 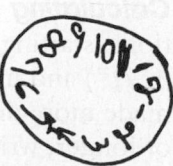

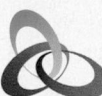

SPECIAL TECHNIQUES

Mini-Mental State Examination (MMSE). This brief test is useful in screening for cognitive dysfunction or dementia and following their course over time. For more detailed information regarding the MMSE, contact the Publisher, Psychological Assessment Resources, Inc., 16204 North Florida Avenue, Lutz, Florida 33549. Below are some sample questions.

MMSE Sample Items

Orientation to Time
  "What is the date?"

Registration
  "Listen carefully; I am going to say three words. You say them back after I stop. Ready? Here they are . . .
  APPLE (pause), PENNY (pause), TABLE (pause). Now repeat those words back to me." [Repeat up to five times, but score only the first trial.]

Naming
  "What is this?" [Point to a pencil or pen.]

Reading
  "Please read this and do what it says." [Show examinee the words on the stimulus form.]

  CLOSE YOUR EYES

(Reproduced by special permission of the Publisher, Psychological Assessment Resources, Inc., 16204 North Florida Avenue, Lutz, Florida 33549, from the Mini Mental State Examination, by Marshal Folstein and Susan Folstein, Copyright 1975, 1998, 2001 by Mini Mental LLC, Inc. Published 2001 by Psychological Assessment Resources, Inc. Further reproduction is prohibited without permission of PAR, Inc. The MMSE can be purchased from PAR, Inc. by calling (813) 968-3003.)

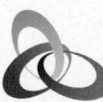

RECORDING YOUR FINDINGS

Recording Behavior and Mental Status

*"**Mental Status:** Alert, well groomed, cheerful. Speech fluent, words clear. Thought processes coherent, insight intact. O×3 (Oriented to person, place, and time). Serial 7s accurate; recent and remote memory intact. Calculations intact."*
OR
*"**Mental Status:** Appears sad, fatigued; clothes wrinkled. Speech slow, words mumbled. Thought processes coherent but insight into current life reverses limited. O×2 (person, and place). Digit span, serial 7s, and calculations accurate but responses delayed. Clock drawing appropriate."*

Suggests depression

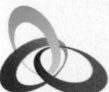

HEALTH PROMOTION AND COUNSELING

Important Topics for Health Promotion and Counseling

- Screening for depression
- Screening for suicide
- Screening for alcohol and substance abuse
- Screening for dementia

"Tools need to be age appropriate.

The burden of suffering that mental disorders impose is great. They affect approximately 58 million Americans 18 years or older.[11] This number represents roughly one in four adults in a given year. Serious mental illness affects approximately 6% of the population. Most people with one mental illness, or 45%, meet criteria for two or more other mental disorders. Illness severity is strongly linked to comorbidity. For the general population, focus health promotion and counseling on depression, suicide risk, and dementia, three important conditions often overlooked. Also screen routinely for addiction to alcohol or drugs.

See Chapter 4, Health History, p. 75.

Depression. *Major depression* is a common medical illness and frequently coexists with other mental disorders, notably anxiety disorders and substance abuse. Lifetime prevalence is high, 16%, with an annual prevalence of 6.7%, or almost 15 million adults.[1,11] Depression is twice as likely in women as in men; the prevalence of postpartum depression is 10% to 15%. Depression frequently accompanies serious medical illnesses, including diabetes, heart disease, cancer, stroke, dementia, and HIV/AIDS; outcomes and costs of care for these illnesses improve when depression is treated. Primary care providers often miss signs of early depression such as low self-esteem, loss of pleasure in daily activities (*anhedonia*), sleep disorders, and difficulty concentrating or making decisions. Watch carefully for depressive symptoms, especially in patients who are young, female, single, divorced or separated, seriously or chronically ill, or bereaved. Those with a prior history or family history of depression are also at risk.

The U.S. Preventive Services Task Force recommends screening in clinical settings that can provide accurate diagnosis, treatment, and follow-up.[12,13] Screening tools suitable for the office are readily available. All positive screening results warrant more formal diagnostic evaluation. Failure to diagnose depression can have fatal consequences—suicide rates among patients with major depression are eight times higher than in the general population.

See screening questions on pp. 67–68 and review screening tools readily available for office practice.[8,14-15]

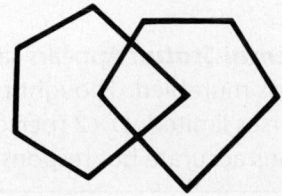

Suicide. Preventing suicide is a national public health initiative. Suicide now ranks as the 11th leading cause of death in the United States.

Clues to pending suicide are variable and subtle. More than half of patients completing suicide have visited their physicians in the prior month, and 10% to 40% in the prior week.[16] Two thirds of suicides occur on the first attempt. Powerful risk factors have been identified: more than 90% of people who die by suicide have depression or other mental disorders, or they are substance abusers. Other risk factors are prior suicide attempts; delusional or psychotic thinking; family history of suicide, mental disorders, or substance abuse; family violence, including physical or sexual abuse; firearms in the home; and incarceration. Pursue any clinical suspicion of suicide by asking patients directly about suicidal ideation and plans. Refer at-risk patients immediately for psychiatric care. Currently, given the low incidence of suicide, nurses are urged to intensify targeted rather than general screening.

See Chapter 24, The Older Adult, pp. 840–882; Table 24-1, Minimum Geriatric Competencies, p. 875; and Table 24-2, Delirium and Dementia, p. 876.

Alcohol and Substance Abuse. As detailed throughout this chapter, the interactions and comorbidity of alcohol and substance abuse with mental disorders and suicide are both extensive and profound. Alcohol, tobacco, and illicit drugs account for more illness, deaths, and disabilities than any other preventable condition. Lifetime prevalence of alcohol and illicit drug use in the United States is 13% for alcohol and 3% for drugs. An estimated 3% are dependent on or abuse illicit drugs; of these cases, 60% involve marijuana.[17] Because screening for alcohol and drug use is part of *every* patient history, information on screening is found in Chapter 4, The Health History.

See Chapter 4, The Health History—Alcohol and Illicit Drugs, pp. 67–68. See also Chapter 16, The Gastrointestinal and Renal Systmes—Screening for Alcohol Abuse, pp. 467–468.

BIBLIOGRAPHY

CITATIONS

1. U.S. Department of Health and Human Services. Mental Health: A Report of the Surgeon General—Executive Summary. Rockville, MD: U.S. Department of Health and Human Services, Substance Abuse and Mental Health Services Administration, Center for Mental Health Services, National Institutes of Health, National Institute of Mental Health, 1999. Available at: www.surgeongeneral.gov/library/mental health/chapter2/sec2_1.html. Accessed April 27, 2011.
2. Hepner KA, Rowe M, Rost K, et al. The effect of adherence to practice guidelines on depression outcomes. Ann Intern Med 147(5):320–329, 2007.
3. Kroenke K. Patients presenting with somatic complaints: epidemiology, psychiatric comorbidity, and management. Int J Methods Psychiatr Res 12(1):34–43, 2003.
4. Kroenke K. The interface between physical and psychological symptoms. Primary Care Companion. J Clin Psychiatry 5(Suppl. 7):11–18, 2003.
5. Aaron LA, Buchwald D. A review of the evidence for overlap among unexplained clinical conditions. Ann Intern Med 134(9):868–881, 2001.
6. Staab JP, Datto CJ, Weinreig RM, et al. Detection and diagnosis of psychiatric disorders in primary medical care settings. Med Clin N Am 85(3):579–596, 2001.
7. U.S. Preventive Services Task Force. Screening for depression: recommendations and rationale. Ann Intern Med 136(10): 760–764, 2002.
8. Whooley MA, Avins AL, Miranda J, et al. Case-finding instruments for depression: two questions are as good as many. J Gen Intern Med 12(7):439–445, 1997.
9. Lowe B, Grafe K, Zipfel S, et al. Detecting panic disorder in medical and psychosomatic outpatients: comparative validation of the Hospital Anxiety and Depression Scale, the Patient Health Questionnaire, a screening question, and physicians' diagnosis. J Psychosom Res 55(6):515–519, 2003.
10. Strub RL, Black FW. The Mental Status Examination in Neurology, 2nd ed. Philadelphia: F.A. Davis, 1985.
11. National Institutes of Mental Health. The numbers count: mental disorders in America. Available at: http://www.nimh.nih. gov/ health /publications/ the-numbers-count-mental-disorders-in-america.shtml. Accessed April 28, 2011.
12. U.S. Preventive Services Task Force. Screening for depression in adults: recommendations and rationale. Ann Intern Med 136(10):760–764, 2002. Available at: http://www.ahrq.gov/ clinic/3rduspstf/depression/depressrr.htm. Accessed April 28, 2011.

13. U.S. Preventive Services Task Force. Screening for depression in adults: summary of the evidence. Ann Intern Med 136(10):765–776, 2002. Available at: http://www.ahrq.gov/clinic/3rduspstf/depression/depsum1.htm. Accessed April 28, 2011.

14. Williams JW, Noel H, Cordes JA, et al. Is this patient clinically depressed? JAMA 287(9):1160–1170, 2002.

15. Beck AT, Steer RA. Internal consistencies of the original and revised Beck Depression Inventory. J Clin Psychol 40(6):1365–1367, 1984.

16. U.S. Preventive Services Task Force. Screening for suicide risk in adults: recommendations and rationale. May 2004. Available at: http://www.ahrq.gov/clinic/3rduspstf/suicide/suiciderr.htm. Accessed April 28, 2011.

17. U.S. Preventive Services Task Force. Screening for illicit drug use: recommendation statement. January 2008. Available at: http://www.ahrq.gov/clinic/uspstf08/druguse/drugrs.htm#clinical. Accessed April 28, 2011.

ADDITIONAL REFERENCES

American Psychiatric Association. Diagnostic and Statistical Manual of Mental Disorders, 4th ed. Washington, DC: American Psychiatric Association, 2000.

Antai-Otong D. Managing geriatric psychiatric emergencies: delirium and dementia. Nurs Clin North Am 38(1):123–135, 2003.

Coffey CE, Cummings JL. American Psychiatric Press Textbook of Geriatric Neuropsychiatry, 2nd ed. Washington, DC: American Psychiatric Press, 2000.

Cottler LB, Campbell W, Krishna VAS, et al. Predictors of high rates of suicidal ideation among drug users. J Nerv Ment Dis 193(7):431–437, 2005.

Fancher T, Kravitz R. In the clinic: depression. Ann Intern Med 146(9):ITC5-1–ITC5-16, 2007.

Folstein M, Folstein SE, McHugh PR. "Mini-mental state": a practical method for grading the cognitive state of patients for the clinician. J Psych Res 12(3):189–198, 1975.

Haas LJ, Leiser JP, Magill MK. Management of the difficult patient. Am Fam Phys 72(10):2063–2068, 2005.

Hales RE, Yudofsky SC, eds. Essentials of Clinical Psychiatry, 2nd ed. Washington, DC: American Psychiatric Press, 2004.

Hull SK, Broquet K. How to manage difficult patient encounters. Family Practice Management, June 2007. Available at: www.aafp.org/fpm. Accessed April 28, 2011.

Khan AK, Khan A, Harezlak JH, et al. Somatic symptoms in primary care. Psychosomatics 11(6):471–478, 2003.

Luoma JB, Martin CE, Pearson JL. Contact with mental health and primary care providers before suicide: a review of the evidence. Am J Psychiatry 159(6):909–916, 2002.

Manchikanti L, Giordano J, Boswell MV, et al. Psychological factors as predictors of opioid abuse and illicit drug use in chronic pain patients. J Opioid Manag 3(2):89–100, 2007.

National Center for Health Statistics. Fast stats A to Z: self-inflicted injury/suicide. Available at: http://www.cdc.gov/nchs/fastats/suicide.htm. Accessed January 26, 2008.

Sadock BJ, Sadock VA, Kaplan HI, eds. Kaplan & Sadock's Comprehensive Textbook of Psychiatry, 8th ed. Philadelphia: Lippincott Williams & Wilkins, 2005.

Schiffer RB, Rao SM, Fogel BS, eds. Neuropsychiatry. Philadelphia: Lippincott Williams & Wilkins, 2002.

Silber MH. Chronic insomnia. N Engl J Med 353(8):803–810, 2005.

Weisner C, Mertens J, Parthasarathy S, et al. Integrating primary medical care with addiction treatment: a randomized controlled trial. JAMA 286(14):1715–1723, 2001.

The Nervous System

LEARNING OBJECTIVES

The student will:

1. Describe the structure and function of the nervous system.
2. Obtain an accurate history of the neurologic system.
3. Identify the cranial nerves and the motor and sensory functions.
4. Perform a screening neurologic examination.
5. Assess level of consciousness utilizing the Glasgow Coma Scale.
6. Document the finding of the nervous system examination.
7. Discuss risk reduction and health promotion strategies to reduce strokes.

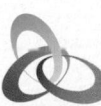

ANATOMY AND PHYSIOLOGY

Central Nervous System

The Brain. The brain has four regions: the cerebrum, the diencephalon, the brainstem, and the cerebellum. The cerebral hemispheres contain the greatest mass of brain tissue. Each hemisphere is subdivided into frontal, parietal, temporal, and occipital lobes, as shown.

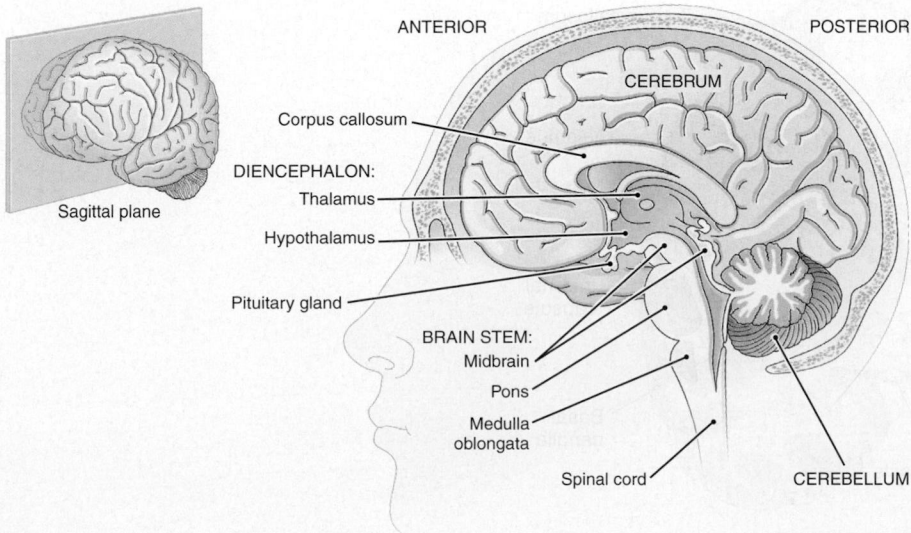

ANTERIOR   POSTERIOR

CEREBRUM

Corpus callosum

DIENCEPHALON:
    Thalamus
    Hypothalamus

Pituitary gland

Sagittal plane

BRAIN STEM:
    Midbrain
    Pons
    Medulla oblongata

Spinal cord   CEREBELLUM

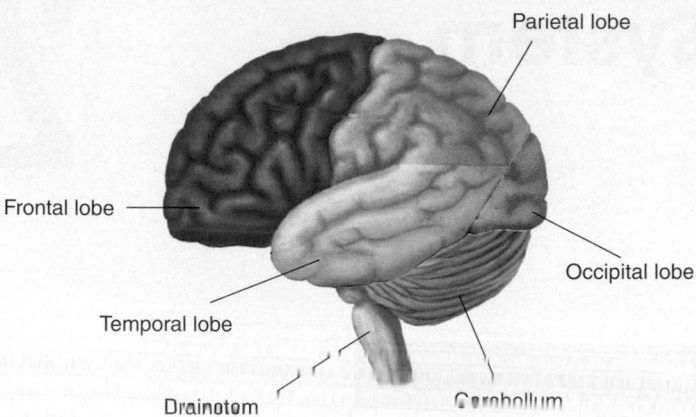

LEFT LATERAL VIEW OF THE BRAIN

The brain is a vast network of interconnecting *neurons* (nerve cells). These consist of cell bodies and their *axons*—single long fibers that conduct impulses to other parts of the nervous system.

Brain tissue may be gray or white. *Gray matter* consists of aggregations of neuronal cell bodies. It rims the surfaces of the cerebral hemispheres, forming the cerebral cortex. *White matter* consists of neuronal axons that are coated with myelin. The myelin sheaths, which create the white color, allow nerve impulses to travel more rapidly.

Deep in the brain lie additional clusters of gray matter. These include the *basal ganglia*, which affect movement, and the thalamus and the hypothalamus, structures in the diencephalon. The *thalamus* processes sensory impulses and relays them to the cerebral cortex. The *hypothalamus* maintains homeostasis and regulates temperature, heart rate, and blood pressure. The hypothalamus affects the endocrine system and governs emotional behaviors such as anger and sexual drive. Hormones secreted in the hypothalamus act directly on the pituitary gland.

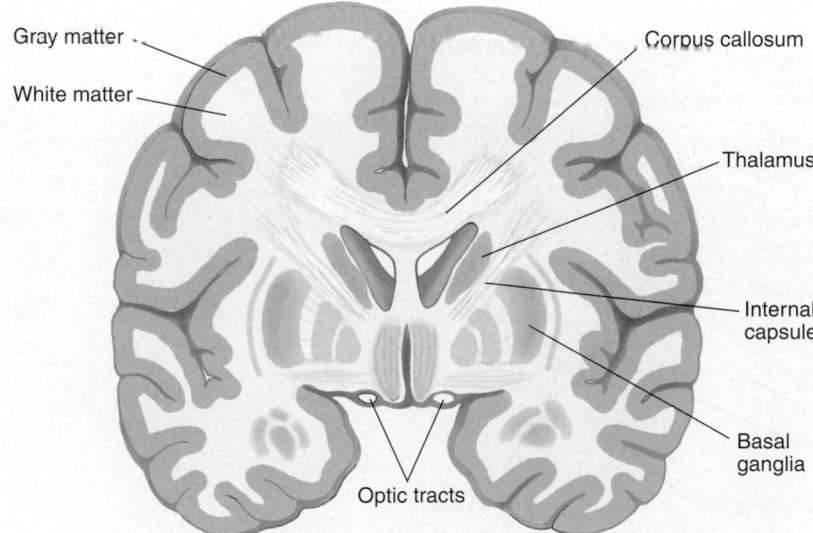

CORONAL SECTION OF THE BRAIN

In contrast, note the *internal capsule,* a white-matter structure where myelinated fibers converge from all parts of the cerebral cortex and descend into the brainstem. The *brainstem,* which connects the upper part of the brain with the spinal cord, has three sections: the midbrain, the pons, and the medulla.

Consciousness depends on the interaction between intact cerebral hemispheres and an important structure in the diencephalon and upper brainstem, the *reticular activating (arousal) system.*

The *cerebellum,* which lies at the base of the brain, coordinates all movement and helps maintain the body upright in space.

The Spinal Cord. Below the medulla, the central nervous system extends itself as the elongated *spinal cord,* encased within the bony vertebral column and terminating at the first or second lumbar vertebra. The cord provides a series of segmental relays with the periphery, serving as a conduit for information flow to and from the brain. The motor and sensory nerve pathways relay neural signals that enter and exit the cord through posterior and anterior nerve roots through the spinal and peripheral nerves.

The spinal cord is divided into five segments: cervical, from C1 to C8; thoracic, from T1 to T12; lumbar, from L1 to L5; sacral, from S1 to S5; and coccygeal.

Note that the spinal cord is not as long as the vertebral canal. The lumbar and sacral roots travel the longest intraspinal distance and fan out like a horse's tail at L1 to L2, giving rise to the term *cauda equina.* To avoid injury to the spinal cord, most lumbar punctures are performed at the L3–4 or L4–5 vertebral interspaces.[1,2]

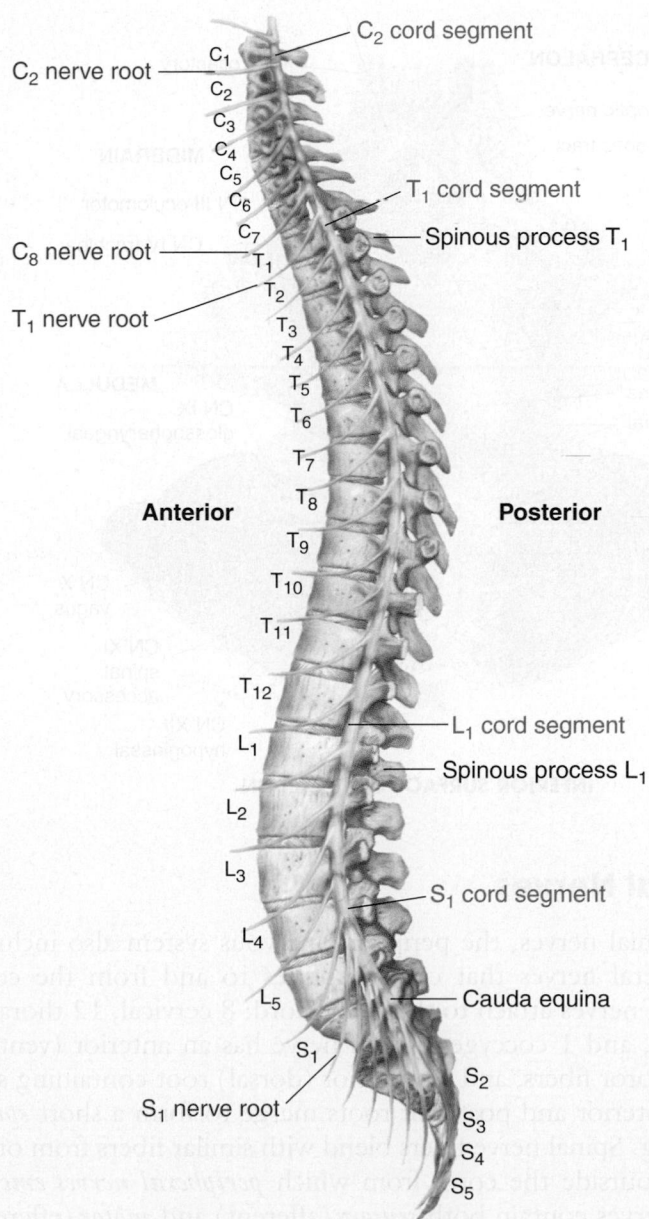

THE SPINAL CORD, LATERAL VIEW

Peripheral Nervous System

The Cranial Nerves. Twelve pairs of special nerves called *cranial nerves* emerge from within the skull or *cranium*. Cranial nerves III through XII arise from the diencephalon and the brainstem, as illustrated. Cranial nerves I and II are actually fiber tracts emerging from the brain. Some cranial nerves are limited to general motor or sensory functions, whereas others are specialized, producing smell, vision, or hearing (I, II, VIII).

Functions of the cranial nerves (CNs) most relevant to physical examination are summarized on the next pages.

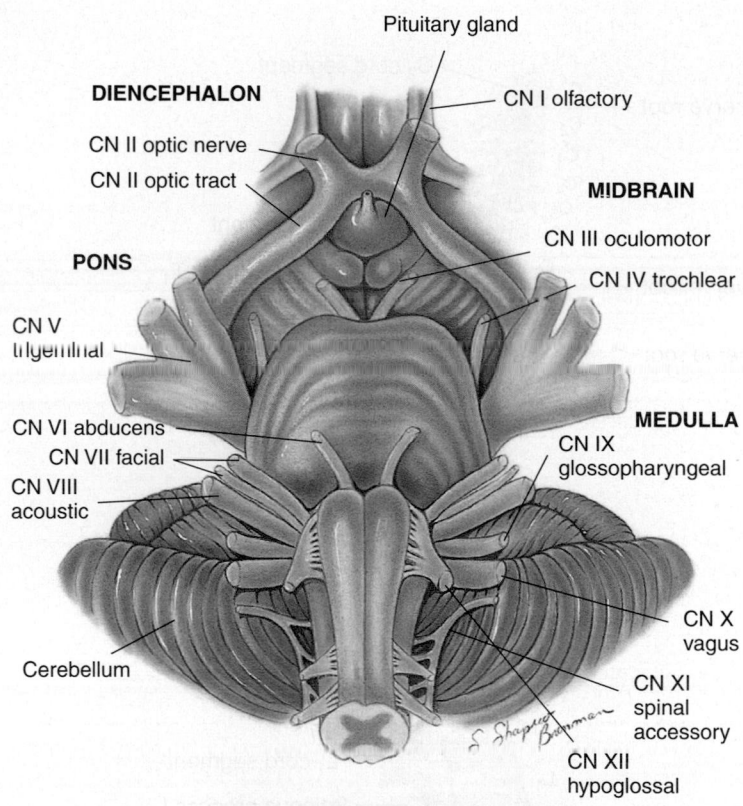

Pituitary gland

DIENCEPHALON

CN I olfactory

CN II optic nerve

CN II optic tract

MIDBRAIN

PONS

CN III oculomotor

CN IV trochlear

CN V trigeminal

CN VI abducens

MEDULLA

CN VII facial

CN IX glossopharyngeal

CN VIII acoustic

CN X vagus

Cerebellum

CN XI spinal accessory

CN XII hypoglossal

INFERIOR SURFACE OF THE BRAIN

The Peripheral Nerves

In addition to cranial nerves, the peripheral nervous system also includes spinal and peripheral nerves that carry impulses to and from the cord. Thirty-one pairs of nerves attach to the spinal cord: 8 cervical, 12 thoracic, 5 lumbar, 5 sacral, and 1 coccygeal. Each nerve has an anterior (ventral) root containing motor fibers, and a posterior (dorsal) root containing sensory fibers. The anterior and posterior roots merge to form a short *spinal nerve*, <5 mm long. Spinal nerve fibers blend with similar fibers from other levels in plexuses outside the cord, from which *peripheral nerves emerge*. Most peripheral nerves contain both *sensory* (afferent) and *motor* (efferent) fibers.

● Cranial Nerves

No.	Name	Function	Type of Impulse
I	**Olfactory**	Sense of smell	Sensory
II	**Optic**	Vision	Sensory
III	**Oculomotor**	Pupillary constriction, opening the eye (lid elevation), and most extraocular movements	Motor
IV	**Trochlear**	Downward, internal rotation of the eye	Motor
V	**Trigeminal**	*Motor*—temporal and masseter muscles (jaw clenching), lateral pterygoids (lateral jaw movement) *Sensory*—facial. The nerve has three divisions: (1) ophthalmic, (2) maxillary, and (3) mandibular.	Both (motor, sensory)

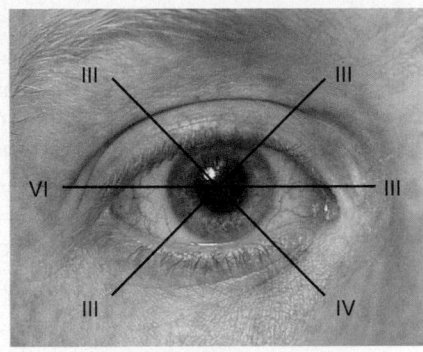

RIGHT EYE (CN III, IV, VI)

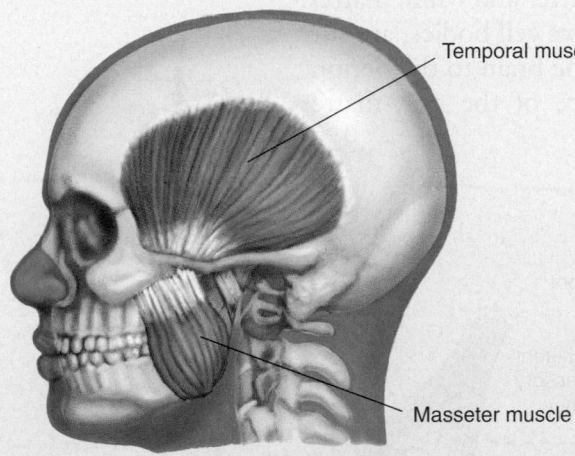

Temporal muscle

Masseter muscle

CN V—MOTOR

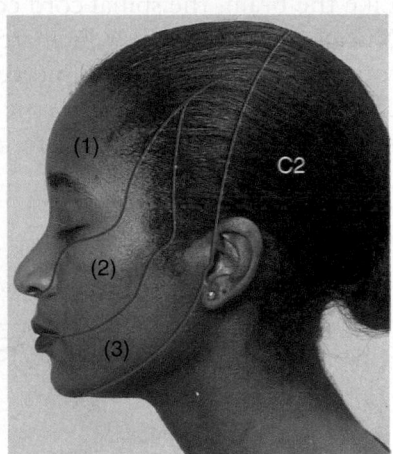

CN V—SENSORY

No.	Name	Function	Type of Impulse
VI	**Abducens**	Lateral deviation of the eye	Motor
VII	**Facial**	*Motor*—facial movements, including those of facial expression, closing the eye, and closing the mouth *Sensory*—taste for salty, sweet, sour, and bitter substances on the anterior two thirds of the tongue	Both (motor, sensory)
VIII	**Acoustic**	Hearing (cochlear division) and balance (vestibular division)	Sensory

(continued)

● **Cranial Nerves** (continued)

No.	Name	Function	Type of Impulse
IX	**Glossopharyngeal**	*Motor*—pharynx *Sensory*—posterior portions of the eardrum and ear canal, the pharynx, and the posterior tongue, including taste (salty, sweet, sour, bitter)	Both (motor, sensory)
X	**Vagus**	*Motor*—palate, pharynx, and larynx *Sensory*—pharynx and larynx	Both (motor, sensory)
XI	**Spinal accessory**	*Motor*—the sternomastoid and upper portion of the trapezius	Motor
XII	**Hypoglossal**	*Motor*—tongue	Motor

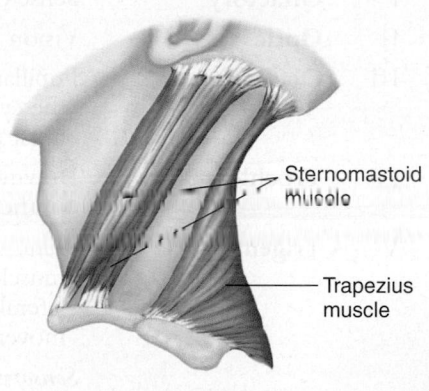

Sternomastoid muscle

Trapezius muscle

CN XI—MOTOR

Like the brain, the spinal cord contains both gray matter and white matter. Nuclei of gray matter, which are aggregations of nerve cell bodies, are surrounded by white tracts of nerve fibers connecting the brain to the peripheral nervous system. Note the butterfly appearance of the gray-matter nuclei, with anterior and posterior horns.

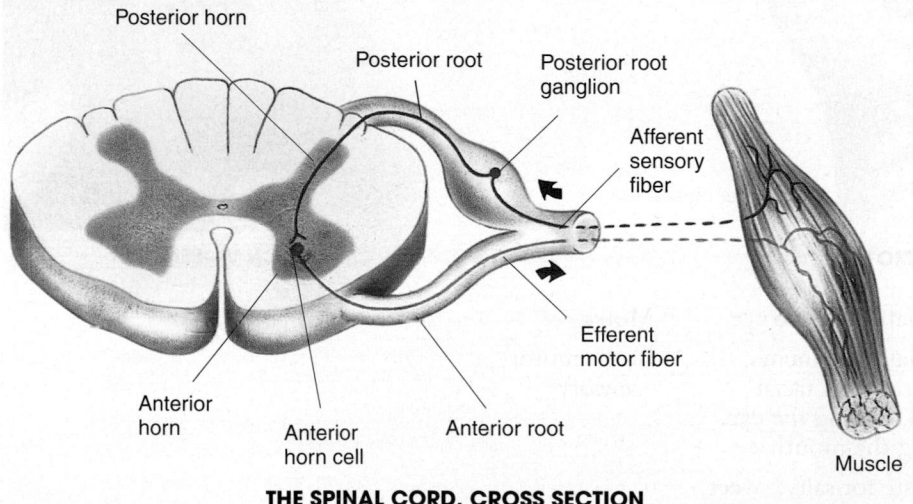

Posterior horn

Posterior root

Posterior root ganglion

Afferent sensory fiber

Anterior horn

Anterior horn cell

Anterior root

Efferent motor fiber

Muscle

THE SPINAL CORD, CROSS SECTION

Motor Pathways

Motor pathways are complex avenues, extending from upper motor neurons through long white-matter tracts, to synapses with lower motor neurons, and into the periphery through peripheral nerve structures. Nerve cell bodies or *upper motor neurons* lie in the motor strip of the cerebral cortex and in several brainstem nuclei; their axons synapse with motor nuclei in the brainstem (for cranial nerves) and in the spinal cord (for peripheral nerves). *Lower motor neurons* have cell bodies in the spinal cord, termed anterior horn cells; their axons transmit impulses through the anterior roots and spinal nerves into peripheral nerves, terminating at the neuromuscular junction.

THE PRINCIPAL MOTOR PATHWAYS

- The **corticospinal (pyramidal) tract.** The corticospinal tracts mediate voluntary movement and integrate skilled, complicated, or delicate movements by stimulating selected muscular actions and inhibiting others. They also carry impulses that inhibit *muscle tone,* the slight tension maintained by normal muscle even when it is relaxed. The corticospinal tracts originate in the motor cortex of the brain. Motor fibers travel down into the lower medulla, where they form an anatomic structure resembling a pyramid. There, most of these fibers cross to the opposite or *contralateral* side of the medulla, continue downward, and synapse with anterior horn cells or with intermediate neurons. Tracts synapsing in the brainstem with motor nuclei of the cranial nerves are termed *corticobulbar.*
- The **basal ganglia system.** This exceedingly complex system includes motor pathways between the cerebral cortex, basal ganglia, brainstem, and spinal cord. It helps to maintain muscle tone and to control body movements, especially gross automatic movements such as walking.
- The **cerebellar system.** The cerebellum receives both sensory and motor input and coordinates motor activity, maintains equilibrium, and helps to control posture.

Three kinds of motor pathways impinge on the anterior horn cells: the corticospinal tract, the basal ganglia system, and the cerebellar system. Additional pathways originating in the brainstem mediate flexor and extensor tone in limb movement and posture, most notably in coma (see Table 20-1, p. 662).

All of these higher motor pathways affect movement only through the lower motor neuron systems—sometimes called the "final common pathway." Any movement, whether initiated voluntarily in the cortex, "automatically" in the basal ganglia, or reflexively in the sensory receptors, must ultimately be translated into action via the anterior horn cells. A lesion in any of these areas will affect movement or reflex activity.

When the corticospinal tract is damaged or destroyed, its functions are reduced or lost below the level of injury. *When upper motor neuron systems are damaged above the crossover of its tracts in the medulla, motor impairment develops on the opposite or contralateral side. In damage below the crossover, motor impairment occurs on the same or ipsilateral side of the body.* The affected limb becomes weak or paralyzed, and skilled, complicated, or delicate movements are performed especially poorly when compared with gross movements.

In upper motor neuron lesions, muscle tone is increased and deep tendon reflexes are exaggerated. Damage to the lower motor neuron systems causes ipsilateral weakness and paralysis, but in this case, muscle tone and reflexes are decreased or absent.

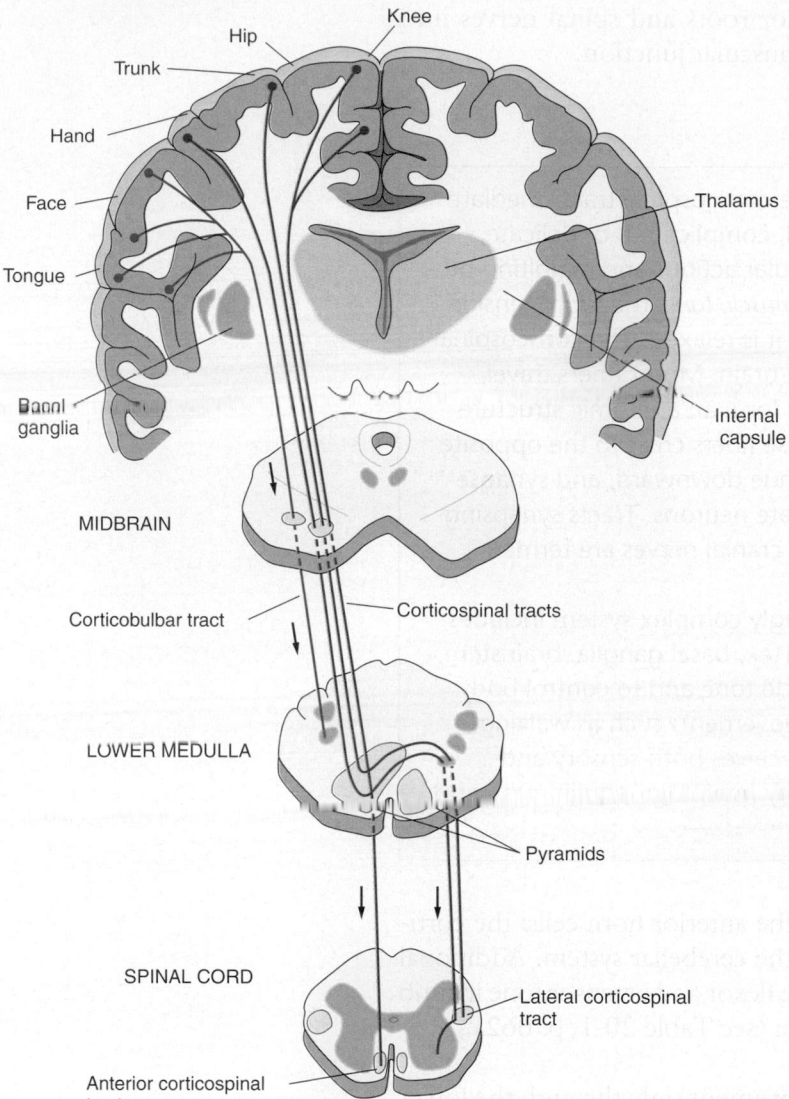

Trunk

Hip

Knee

Hand

Face

Tongue

Basal
ganglia

Thalamus

Internal
capsule

MIDBRAIN

Corticobulbar tract

Corticospinal tracts

LOWER MEDULLA

Pyramids

SPINAL CORD

Lateral corticospinal
tract

Anterior corticospinal
tract

MOTOR PATHWAYS: CORTICOSPINAL AND CORTICOBULBAR TRACTS

Disease of the basal ganglia system or cerebellar system does not cause paralysis but can be disabling. Damage to the basal ganglia system produces changes in muscle tone (most often an increase), disturbances in posture and gait, a slowness or lack of spontaneous and automatic movements termed *bradykinesia,* and various involuntary movements. Cerebellar damage impairs coordination, gait, and equilibrium and decreases muscle tone.

Sensory Pathways

Sensory impulses not only participate in reflex activity, as previously described, but also give rise to conscious sensation, calibrate body position in space, and help regulate internal autonomic functions like blood pressure, heart rate, and respiration.

A complex system of sensory receptors relays impulses from skin, mucous membranes, muscles, tendons, and viscera. Sensory fibers registering sensations such as pain, temperature, position, and touch pass through the peripheral nerves and posterior roots and enter the spinal cord. Once inside the cord, sensory impulses reach the sensory cortex of the brain via one of the two pathways: the spinothalamic tracts or the posterior columns.

Within one or two spinal segments from their entry into the cord, fibers conducting the sensations of *pain* and *temperature* pass into the posterior horn of the spinal cord and synapse with secondary sensory neurons. Fibers conducting *crude touch*—a sensation perceived as light touch but without accurate localization—also pass into the posterior horn and synapse with secondary neurons. The secondary neurons then cross to the opposite side and pass upward in the *spinothalamic tract* into the thalamus.

Fibers conducting the sensations of *position* and *vibration* pass directly into the *posterior columns* of the cord and travel upward to the medulla, together with fibers transmitting *fine touch*—touch that is accurately localized and finely discriminating. These fibers synapse in the medulla with secondary sensory neurons. Fibers projecting from secondary neurons cross to the opposite side at the medullary level and continue on to the thalamus.

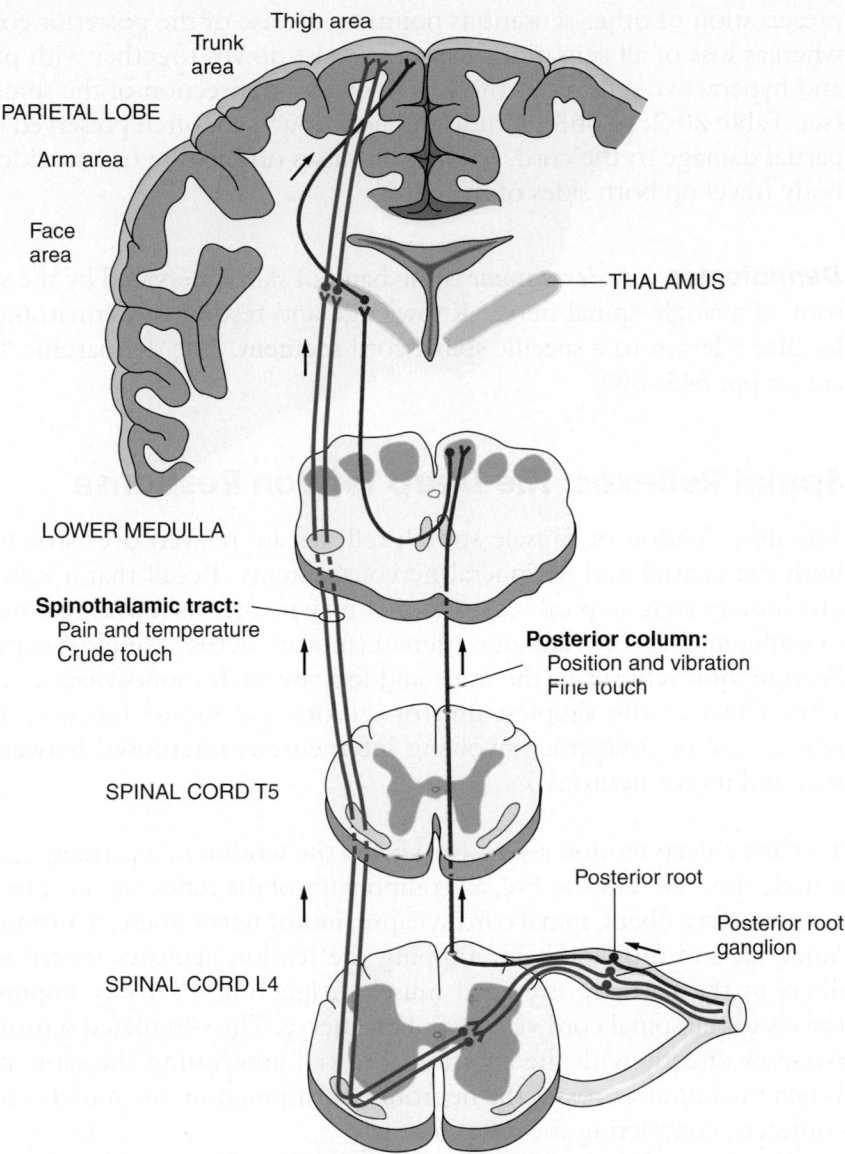

SENSORY PATHWAYS: SPINOTHALAMIC TRACT AND POSTERIOR COLUMNS

At the *thalamic level,* the general quality of sensation is perceived (e.g., pain, cold, pleasant, unpleasant), but fine distinctions are not made. For full perception, a third group of sensory neurons sends impulses from the thalamus to the *sensory cortex* of the brain. Here stimuli are localized and higher-order discriminations are made.

Lesions at different points in the sensory pathways produce different kinds of sensory loss. Patterns of sensory loss, together with their associated motor findings, help identify where the causative lesions might be. A lesion in the sensory cortex may not impair the perception of pain, touch, and position, for example, but does impair finer discrimination. A person so affected cannot appreciate the size, shape, or texture of an object by feeling it and therefore cannot identify it. Loss of position and vibration sense with preservation of other sensations points to disease of the posterior columns, whereas loss of all sensations from the waist down, together with paralysis and hyperactive reflexes in the legs, indicates transection of the spinal cord (see Table 20-2; p. 663). Crude and light touch are often preserved despite partial damage to the cord, because impulses originating on one side of the body travel up both sides of the cord.

Dermatomes. A *dermatome* is the band of skin innervated by the sensory root of a single spinal nerve. Knowledge and testing of dermatomes help localize a lesion to a specific spinal cord segment. The dermatome "maps" are on pp. 643–644.

Spinal Reflexes: The Deep Tendon Response

The deep tendon or muscle stretch reflexes are relayed over structures of both the central and peripheral nervous systems. Recall that a *reflex* is an involuntary stereotypical response that may involve as few as two neurons, one afferent (sensory) and one efferent (motor), across a single synapse. The deep tendon reflexes in the arms and legs are such monosynaptic reflexes. They illustrate the simplest unit of sensory and motor function. (Other reflexes are polysynaptic, involving interneurons interposed between sensory and motor neurons.)

To elicit a deep tendon reflex, briskly tap the tendon of a partially stretched muscle. For the reflex to fire, all components of the reflex arc must be intact: sensory nerve fibers, spinal cord synapse, motor nerve fibers, neuromuscular junction, and muscle fibers. Tapping the tendon activates special sensory fibers in the partially stretched muscle, triggering a sensory impulse that travels to the spinal cord via a peripheral nerve. The stimulated sensory fiber synapses directly with the anterior horn cell innervating the same muscle. When the impulse crosses the neuromuscular junction, the muscle suddenly contracts, completing the reflex arc.

Because each deep tendon reflex involves specific spinal segments, together with their sensory and motor fibers, an abnormal reflex can help locate a pathologic lesion. Learn the segmental levels of the deep tendon reflexes. They can be remembered by their numerical sequence in ascending order from ankle to triceps: S1–L2, 3, 4–C5, 6, 7.

● Deep Tendon Reflexes

Ankle reflex (Achilles)	Sacral 1 primarily
Knee reflex (patellar)	Lumbar 2, 3, 4
Supinator (brachioradialis) reflex	Cervical 5, 6
Biceps reflex	Cervical 5, 6
Triceps reflex	Cervical 6, 7

Reflexes may be initiated by stimulating skin as well as muscle. Stroking the skin of the abdomen near the umbilicus, for example, produces a localized muscular twitch associated with the T10 level. These superficial (cutaneous) reflexes and their corresponding spinal segments include the following:

● Cutaneous Stimulation Reflexes	
Abdominal reflexes—upper	Thoracic 8, 9, 10
—lower	Thoracic 10, 11, 12
Plantar responses (Babinski)	Lumbar 5, sacral 1
Anal reflex	Sacral 2, 3, 4

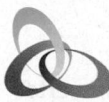

THE HEALTH HISTORY

COMMON OR CONCERNING SYMPTOMS

- Headache
- Dizziness or vertigo
- Generalized, proximal, or distal weakness
- Numbness, abnormal or loss of sensations
- Loss of consciousness, syncope, or near syncope
- Seizures
- Tremors or involuntary movements

Two of the most common symptoms in neurologic disorders are *headache* and *dizziness*. Review the health history pertinent to headaches.

See Table 10-1, p. 205, Primary Headaches, and Table 10-2, pp. 206-207, Secondary Headaches.

Headache. For headache, ask about onset, location, duration, severity and any associated symptoms such as visual changes, weakness, or loss of sensation. Ask if the headache is affected by coughing, sneezing, or sudden movement of the head, which can increase intracranial pressure.

Subarachnoid hemorrhage may present as "the worst headache of my life."[3,4] Severe headache in *meningitis.*[5] Dull headache affected by the actions listed, especially in the same location, in mass lesions such as *brain* tumor or *abscess*

Dizziness or Vertigo. The complaint of *dizziness* can have many meanings. You will need to elicit exactly what the patient has experienced.

Light-headedness in palpitations, near syncope from vasovagal stimulation, low blood pressure, febrile illness, and others. Vertigo in inner-ear conditions, brainstem tumor. See Table 12-1, p 277, Dizziness and Vertigo.

Formulating subjective questions is important to differentiate whether the patient is experiencing dizziness or vertigo. Begin with an open-ended question: "Tell me about the dizziness." When eliciting additional information regarding a sign or symptom, utilize the "OLD CART" mnemonic to focus on specific questions so that the sequence of events will become clearer.

Onset: When did this feeling of "dizziness" begin?

Location: Does it seem to occur on one side of the head or the other?

Duration: How often does the dizziness occur?

How long does it last?

Does it go away?

Does it come and go?

Characteristic Symptoms: What does it feel like?

Is the room spinning?

Are you spinning?

Is the room rotating?

Are you light-headed?

Do you feel faint?

Associated Manifestations: Does anything else occur when you feel dizzy?

Do you have double vision (diplopia)?

Do you feel nauseous?

Do you experience difficulty forming words (dysarthria)?

Are there times when you have difficulty with balance or walking (ataxia)?

Have you taken any new medications? Prescribed? Over the counter?

Relieving Factors: Does anything make the dizziness go away? Decrease? What makes it feel better?

Treatment: Have you taken any medications to relieve the dizziness?

Have you utilized any therapies to help treat the dizziness? Aromatherapy? Chiropractor? Acupuncture? Any others?

Have you talked to your health care provider previously about the dizziness?

Diplopia, dysarthria, ataxia in vertebrobasilar transient ischemic attack (TIA) or stroke.[6] See Table 20-3, pp. 664–665, Types of Stroke.

Weakness. What about any associated *weakness*, either generalized or in the face or a part of the body? Weakness is another common symptom and requires careful attention to detail. Probe for exactly what it means to the patient. Explore whether there is *paralysis*, or inability to move a part or side of the body.

Weakness or paralysis in *transient ischemic attack* or *stroke*[7]

Focal weakness may arise from ischemic, vascular, or mass lesions in the central nervous system; also from peripheral nervous system disorders, neuromuscular disorders, or diseases in the muscles themselves.

Onset: When did the weakness begin?

Did it start slowly or suddenly?

Location: What areas of the body are involved?

Does the weakness affect one or both sides?

What movements are affected?

Duration: Has it progressed? How so?

How long does it last?

Does it go away?

Does it come and go?

For weakness without light-headedness, try to distinguish between *proximal* and *distal weakness*.

Bilateral proximal weakness in myopathy. Bilateral, predominantly

Characteristic Symptoms

    If assessing for proximal weakness:

        Are you able to reach something on a high shelf?

        Do you have difficulty getting out of a chair?

        How does it feel when you brush your hair?

        Are you able to walk up steps? How many?

        Does the weakness increase with repeated effort?

        Does it improve with rest?

    If assessing for distal weakness in the arms:

        Have you noticed any changes in hand movements?

        Do you have any difficulty opening jars or cans?

        Has it become more cumbersome to use scissors, screwdrivers, or pliers?

    If assessing for distal weakness in the legs:

        Have you noticed yourself tripping?

Associated Manifestations: Are there any sensations you experience when the weakness occurs?

    Have you noticed that there are some activities that you are not able to participate in any longer? Or need assistance completing?

    Do you experience any other symptoms when the weakness occurs:

        Nausea/vomiting?

        Headaches?

        Double vision?

        Difficulty swallowing?

        Slurred speech?

        Rash?

    Have you recently changed medications?

Relieving Factors: Does anything relieve the weakness?

    What makes the weakness better:

        Rest?

        Caffeine?

        Exercise?

    Have you noticed you are sleeping or resting more?

Treatment: Have you taken any medications to relieve the weakness?

    Have you talked to your health care provider previously about the weakness?

Loss of Sensation.   Find out if the patient has had any *loss of sensation*. Ask if there has been any *numbness*, but clarify its meaning and location. Has there been loss of sensation, difficulty moving a limb, or altered sensations such as tingling or pins and needles? There may be peculiar sensations without an obvious stimulus, called *paresthesias*. These occur commonly when an arm or leg "goes to sleep" following compression of a nerve, and may be described as tingling, prickling, or feelings of warmth, coldness, or pressure. *Dysesthesias* are distorted sensations in response to a stimulus and may last longer than the stimulus itself. For example, a person may perceive a light touch or pinprick as a burning or tingling sensation that is irritating or unpleasant. *Pain* may arise from neurologic causes but is usually reported with symptoms of other body systems, such as the head and neck or the musculoskeletal system.

distal weakness in polyneuropathy. Weakness made worse with repeated effort and improved with rest suggests *myasthenia gravis*.[8]

Loss of sensation, paresthesias, and dysesthesias in central lesions in the brain and spinal cord, as well as disorders of peripheral sensory roots and nerves; paresthesias in the hands and around the mouth in hyperventilation. Burning pain in painful sensory neuropathy[9]

See Table 18-1, p. 584, Low Back Pain, and Table 18-2, p. 585, Pains in the Neck.

Have you noticed any change in sensation?

> **O**nset: When did this begin?
> **L**ocation: What part(s) of the body experience this change/loss in sensation?
> **D**uration: How long does it last? Is it continuous? Does it come and go?
> **C**haracteristic Symptoms: Describe what it feels like (pins and needles, goes to sleep, tingling, prickling, pressure, warmth, cold, burning, irritating).
> **A**ssociated Manifestations: Have you noticed any other changes (vision changes, difficulty eating)?
> **R**elieving Factors: Does anything make it feel better?
> **T**reatment: What treatments or medications have you tried? What were the results?

Loss of Consciousness (Fainting).

"Have you ever fainted or passed out?" leads the discussion to any *loss of consciousness*. Begin by exploring what the patient means by loss of consciousness. Did the patient black out completely, or could voices be heard throughout the episode, indicating some consciousness? Be sure to use descriptive terms carefully and precisely. *Syncope* is the sudden but temporary loss of consciousness and postural tone that occurs with decreased blood flow to the brain, commonly described as *fainting*. Symptoms of feeling faint, light-headed, or weak, but without actual loss of consciousness, are called *near syncope* or *presyncope*.

See Table 20-4, pp. 666–667, Syncope and Similar Disorders.

Get as complete and unbiased a description of the event as possible.

> What brought on the episode?
> Were there any warning symptoms?
> Was the patient standing, sitting, or lying down when the episode began?
> How long did it last?
> Could voices be heard while passing out and coming to?
> How rapidly did the patient recover?
> In retrospect, were onset and offset slow or fast?

Young people with emotional stress and warning symptoms of flushing, warmth, or nausea may have *vasodepressor (or vasovagal) syncope* of slow onset, slow offset. *Cardiac syncope* from arrhythmias, more common in older patients, often with sudden onset, sudden offset[10]

Also ask if anyone observed the episode.

> If so, what did the patient look like before losing consciousness, during the episode, and afterward?
> Was there any seizure-like movement of the arms or legs?
> Any incontinence of the bladder or bowel?
> Any drowsiness or impaired memory after the episode ended?

Tonic–clonic motor activity, bladder or bowel incontinence, and *postictal state* suggest a generalized *seizure*. Unlike syncope, injury such as tongue biting or bruising of limbs may occur.[11]

Seizures.

A *seizure* is a paroxysmal disorder caused by sudden excessive electrical discharge in the cerebral cortex or its underlying structures. Seizures can be of several types.[11] Depending on the type, there may or may

See Table 20-5, pp. 668–669, Seizure Disorders.

not be loss of consciousness. With some types of seizures, there may be abnormal feelings, thought processes, and sensations, including smells, as well as abnormal movements. Asking "Have you ever had any seizures or 'spells'?" . . . "Any fits or convulsions?" can open the discussion.

Onset: At what age did the seizures begin?
  When was the last seizure?
  Has there been a change in frequency?
Location: Do you lose consciousness when you have a seizure?
  Does it affect your entire body?
Duration: How often do the seizures occur?
  How long do the seizures last?
Characteristic Symptoms: What are the precipitating circumstances or warnings prior to a seizure?
  What are the behaviors and feelings that occur during the seizure?
  What occurs after the seizure? How do you feel?
Associated Manifestations: What is causing the seizures?
  Is there a history of a head injury or other condition that may be related to the seizures?
Relieving Factors: What can be done to relieve the actual seizure?
  What is instrumental in relieving the symptoms associated with the actual seizure or postseizure period?
Treatment: What medications are currently being administered?
  What has been used previously?
  Who is monitoring your medications and condition?

Tremors.   *Tremors* and other *involuntary movements* occur with or without additional neurologic manifestations. Ask about any trembling, shakiness, or body movements that the patient seems unable to control.

See Table 20-6, pp. 670–671, Tremors and Involuntary Movements. Tremor, rigidity, and bradykinesia in Parkinson disease[12,13]

Distinct from these symptoms is an almost indescribable *restlessness of the legs* that typically develops at rest and is accompanied by an urge to move about. Walking gives relief.

The common but often overlooked *restless legs syndrome,* is usually benign[14]

PHYSICAL EXAMINATION

Assessment of the nervous system calls for many complex skills of examination and clinical reasoning. You have already learned the principles and techniques for assessing mental status, a critical component of the nervous system examination. As you saw in Chapter 19, Behavior and Mental Status, often the patient's mental status offers clues about delirium, memory disorders, and other neurologic conditions. As you study this chapter, let three important questions guide the approach to this challenging clinical area:

● Is the mental status intact?

● Are right-sided and left-sided examination findings symmetric?

- If the findings are asymmetric or otherwise abnormal, does the lesion lie in the *central nervous system*, consisting of the brain and spinal cord, or in the *peripheral nervous system*, consisting of the 12 pairs of cranial nerves and the spinal and peripheral nerves?

Patient symptoms or signs point to the affected area of the nervous system.

EQUIPMENT

Cranial Nerve Examination
Penlight
Snellen chart
Newspaper or hand-held news print
Ophthalmoscope
Cotton swab
Tongue blades
Gloves
Scents for olfactory (e.g., vanilla, cinnamon, coffee, lemon juice, or soap)
Tuning fork

Sensory Examination
Objects to feel (e.g., coin, paper clip)
Tuning fork
Hot and cold water in test tubes/glass
Cotton swab

Reflexes
Reflex hammer
Tongue blade

IMPORTANT AREAS OF EXAMINATION

- Mental status—see Chapter 19, Behavior and Mental Status
- Cranial nerves I through XII
- Motor system: coordination, gait, and stance
- Sensory system: pain and temperature, position and vibration, light touch, discrimination
- Deep tendon, abdominal, and plantar reflexes

In this section, the techniques for a practical and reasonably comprehensive examination of the nervous system will be discussed. It is important to master the techniques for a thorough examination. Be active in your learning and ask your instructors to review your skills.

The detail of an appropriate neurologic examination varies widely. In healthy people, the examination will be relatively brief. When abnormal findings are detected, the examination will become more comprehensive. Be aware that neurologists may use many other techniques in specific situations.

For efficiency, integrate the neurologic assessment with other parts of the examination. Survey the patient's mental status and speech during the interview, even though further testing may be necessary during the neurologic evaluation. Some of the cranial nerves are examined with the head and neck. Inspect the arms and legs for neurologic abnormalities while observing the peripheral vascular and musculoskeletal systems. Chapter 6 provides an outline of an integrated approach. Think about and describe your findings, however, in terms of the nervous system as a unit.

GUIDELINES FOR A SCREENING NEUROLOGIC EXAMINATION FROM THE AMERICAN ACADEMY OF NEUROLOGY

Students should be able to perform a brief screening neurologic examination that is sufficient to detect significant neurologic disease even in patients with no neurologic complaints. Although the exact sequence of such screening may vary, it should contain at least some assessment of mental status, cranial nerves, strength, gait, coordination, sensation, and reflexes. One example of a screening examination is given here.

Mental Status—level of alertness, appropriateness of responses, orientation to date and place

Cranial Nerves
- Visual acuity
- Pupillary light reflex
- Eye movements
- Hearing
- Facial strength—smile, eye closure

Motor System
- Strength—shoulder abduction, elbow extension, wrist extension, finger abduction, hip flexion, knee flexion, ankle dorsiflexion
- Gait—casual, tandem
- Coordination—fine finger movements, finger-to-nose

Sensory System—one modality at toes—can be light touch, pain/temperature, or proprioception

Reflexes
- Deep tendon reflexes—biceps, patellar, Achilles
- Plantar responses

Note: If there is reason to suspect neurologic disease based on the patient's history or the results of any components of the screening examination, a more complete neurologic examination may be necessary.
(Source: Adapted from the American Academy of Neurology. Available at: http://www.aan.com/globals/axon/assets/2770.pdf. Accessed April 27. 2011.)

Whether conducting a comprehensive or screening examination, organize your thinking into five categories: (1) mental status, speech, and language; (2) cranial nerves; (3) the motor system; (4) the sensory system; and (5) reflexes. If the findings are abnormal, begin to group them into patterns of central or peripheral disorders.

The Cranial Nerves

Overview. The examination of the cranial nerves (abbreviated as CN) can be summarized as follows.

● Summary: Cranial Nerves I–XII	
I	Smell
II	Visual acuity, visual fields, and ocular fundi
II, III	Pupillary reactions
III, IV, VI	Extraocular movements
V	Corneal reflexes, facial sensation, and jaw movements
VII	Facial movements
VIII	Hearing
IX, X	Swallowing and rise of the palate, gag reflex
V, VII, X, XII	Voice and speech
XI	Shoulder and neck movements
XII	Tongue symmetry and position

Cranial Nerve I—Olfactory. Test the *sense of smell* by presenting the patient with familiar and nonirritating odors. First be sure that each nasal passage is open by compressing one side of the nose and asking the patient to sniff through the other. The patient should then close both eyes. Occlude one nostril and test smell in the other with such substances as: cloves, coffee, soap, or vanilla. (Avoid noxious triggers like ammonia that might stimulate CN V.) Ask if the patient smells anything and, if so, what. Test the other side. A person normally perceives odor on each side and can often identify it.

Loss of smell may occur in sinus conditions, head trauma, smoking, aging, he use of cocaine or in *Parkinson disease*

Cranial Nerve II—Optic. Test *visual acuity* (see pp. 211–212).

Inspect the *optic fundi* with your ophthalmoscope, paying special attention to the optic discs (see pp. 230–232).

Disc pallor in optic atrophy; disc bulging in papilledema (see p. 231)

Test the visual fields by confrontation (see pp. 222–223). Occasionally—in stroke patients, for example—patients will complain of partial loss of vision, and testing of both eyes reveals a *visual field defect*, or abnormality in peripheral vision, such as *homonymous hemianopsia*. Testing one eye would not confirm the finding.

See Table 11-1 p. 236, Visual Field Defects. Prechiasmal, or anterior defects, in *glaucoma, retinal emboli, optic neuritis* (visual acuity poor). Bitemporal hemianopsias from defects at the optic chiasm, usually from *pituitary tumor.* Homonymous hemianopsias or quadrantanopsia in postchiasmal lesions, usually in the *parietal lobe,* with associated findings of stroke (visual acuity normal)[15]

Cranial Nerves II and III—Optic and Oculomotor.
Inspect the size and shape of the pupils, and compare one side with the other. *Anisocoria*, or a difference of >0.4 mm in the diameter of one pupil compared to the other, is seen in up to 38% of healthy individuals. Test the *pupillary reactions to light*.

See Table 11-5 p. 240, Pupillary Abnormalities. Minimal constriction in the larger pupil if there is an abnormality of the pupillary *constrictor* muscle from an iris disorder or *CN III palsy* with parasympathetic denervation, ptosis, and ophthalmoplegia (eyes not aligned). Sluggish reaction of dilation of one pupil may indicate a cranial bleed or brain tumor. Pupils constrict to light in *Horner syndrome*, but due to sympathetic degeneration, the affected pupil remains small (miosis) due to abnormal pupillary *dilator* muscle.[15]

Also check the *near response* or accommodation (p. 216), which tests pupillary constriction (pupillary constrictor muscle), convergence (medial rectus muscles), and accommodation of the lens (ciliary muscle).

Cranial Nerves III, IV, and VI—Oculomotor, Trochlear, and Abducens.
Test the *extraocular movements* in the six cardinal directions of gaze, and look for loss of conjugate movements in any of the six directions, which causes *diplopia*. Ask the patient which direction makes the diplopia worse and inspect the eye closely for asymmetric deviation of movement. Determine if the diplopia is *monocular* or *binocular* by asking the patient to cover one eye, or perform the cover-uncover test (see Table 11-7, p. 242).

See Table 11-7, Dysconjugate Gaze, p. 242. Monocular diplopia in local problems with glasses or contact lenses; cataracts; astigmatism; ptosis. Binocular diplopia In *CN III, IV, VI neuropathy* (40% of patients), eye muscle disease from *myasthenia gravis, trauma, thyroid ophthalmopathy, internuclear ophthalmoplegia*[15]

Check convergence of the eyes. Identify any *nystagmus*, an involuntary jerking movement of the eyes with quick and slow components. Note the direction of gaze in which it appears, the plane of the nystagmus (horizontal, vertical, rotary, or mixed), and the direction of the quick and slow components (see p. 228). *Nystagmus is named for the direction of the quick component.*

See Table 20-7, p, 672, Nystagmus). Nystagmus in *cerebellar disease*, especially with gait ataxia and dysarthria (increases with retinal fixation) and *vestibular disorders* (decreases with retinal fixation)

Ask the patient to focus on a distant object and observe if the nystagmus increases or decreases.

Look for *ptosis* (drooping of the upper eyelids). A slight difference in the width of the palpebral fissures may be a normal variation in approximately one third of all people.

Ptosis in *3rd nerve palsy* (CN III), *Horner syndrome* (ptosis, meiosis, anhidrosis), *myasthenia gravis*

Cranial Nerve V—Trigeminal
Motor. While palpating the temporal and masseter muscles in turn, ask the patient to clench the teeth. Note the strength of muscle contraction. Ask the patient to move the jaw side to side.

Difficulty clenching the jaw or moving it to the opposite side in masseter and lateral

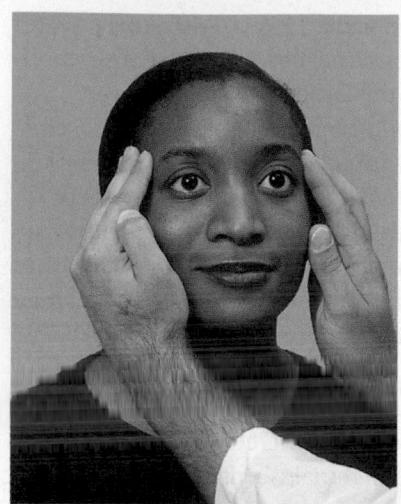

PALPATING TEMPORAL MUSCLES

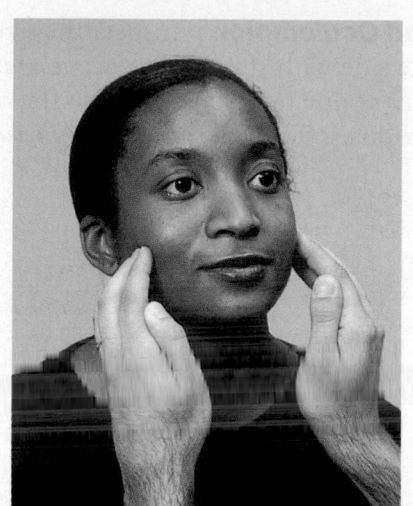

PALPATING MASSETER MUSCLES

pterygoid muscle weakness, respectively

Unilateral weakness in CN V lesions in the pons; bilateral weakness in cerebral hemispheric disease because of bilateral cortical innervation

Central nervous system patterns from stroke include facial and body sensory loss on the same side but from contralateral cortical or thalamic lesion; ipsilateral face but contralateral body sensory loss in brainstem lesions

Isolated facial sensory loss in peripheral nerve disorders like *trigeminal neuralgia*

Sensory. After explaining what will be done and demonstrating what sharp and dull feels like, test the forehead, cheeks, and jaw on each side for *pain sensation*. Suggested areas are indicated by the circles. The patient's eyes should be closed. Use a sharp object, such as a sharp wood splinter by breaking or twisting a cotton swab for the sharp sensation and the end of a cotton swab as a dull stimulus. Ask the patient to report whether it is "sharp" or "dull" and to compare sides.

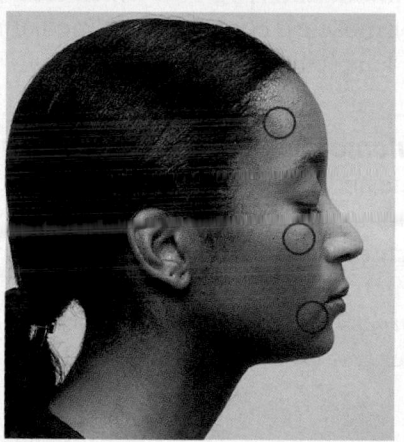

If you find an abnormality, confirm it by testing *temperature sensation*. Two test tubes, filled with hot and ice-cold water, are the traditional stimuli. A tuning fork may also be used. It usually feels cool. If you are near running water, the fork is easily made colder or warm. Dry it before use. Touch the skin and ask the patient to identify "hot" or "cold."

Then test for *light touch,* using a fine wisp of cotton. Ask the patient to respond whenever you touch the skin.

Corneal Reflex. Test the *corneal reflex.* Ask the patient to look up and away from you. Approaching from the other side, out of the patient's line of vision, and avoiding the eyelashes, touch the cornea (not just the conjunctiva) lightly with a fine wisp of cotton. If the patient is apprehensive, however, first touching the conjunctiva may allay fear.

Look for blinking of the eyes, the normal reaction to this stimulus. The sensory limb of this reflex is carried in CN V, and the motor response, in CN VII. Use of contact lenses frequently diminishes or abolishes this reflex and therefore it is not utilized as frequently.

Absent blinking from CN V or VII lesion. Absent blinking and sensorineural hearing loss in *acoustic neuroma*

Cranial Nerve VII—Facial. Inspect the face, both at rest and during conversation with the patient. Note any asymmetry (e.g., of the nasolabial folds), and observe any tics or other abnormal movements.

Ask the patient to:

1. Raise both eyebrows.

2. Frown.

3. Close both eyes tightly so that you cannot open them. Test muscular strength by trying to open them, as illustrated.

4. Show both upper and lower teeth.

5. Smile.

6. Puff out both cheeks.

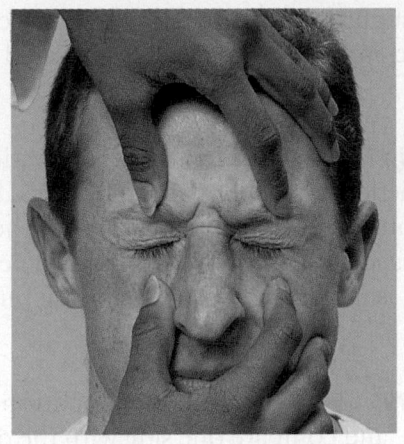

Flattening of the nasolabial fold and drooping of the lower eyelid suggest facial weakness.

A peripheral injury to CN VII, as in *Bell palsy,* affects both the upper and lower face; a central lesion affects mainly the lower face. Loss of taste, hyperacusis, increased or decreased tearing also in *Bell palsy.* See Table 20-8, p. 673, Types of Facial Paralysis.

In unilateral facial paralysis, the mouth droops on the paralyzed side when the patient smiles or grimaces.

Cranial Nerve VIII—Acoustic. Assess hearing with the whispered voice test. If hearing loss is present, determine if the loss is *conductive,* from impaired "air through ear" transmission, or *sensorineural,* from damage to the cochlear branch of CN VIII. Test for (1) *air and bone conduction,* using the Rinne test, and (2) *lateralization,* using the Weber test.

See techniques for Weber and Rinne test and Table 12-4, p. 281, Patterns of Hearing Loss. The whispered voice test is both sensitive (>90%) and specific (>80%) when assessing presence or absence of hearing loss.[15] Excess cerumen, otosclerosis, *otitis media* in conductive hearing loss; *presbycusis* from aging, most commonly in sensorineural hearing loss

Specific tests of the vestibular function of CN VIII are rarely included in the usual neurologic examination.

Vertigo with hearing loss and nystagmus in *Ménière disease*—see Table 12-1, p. 277, Dizziness and Vertigo, and Table 20-7, p. 672, Nystagmus.

Cranial Nerves IX and X—Glossopharyngeal and Vagus. Listen to the patient's *voice.* Is it hoarse, or does it have a nasal quality?

Hoarseness in vocal cord paralysis; nasal voice in paralysis of the palate

Is there difficulty in swallowing?

Pharyngeal or palatal weakness

Ask the patient to say "ah" or to yawn as you watch the *movements of the soft palate and the pharynx.* The soft palate normally rises symmetrically, the uvula remains in the midline, and each side of the posterior pharynx

The palate fails to rise with a bilateral lesion of the vagus nerve. In unilateral paralysis, one side of the

moves medially, like a curtain. The slightly curved uvula seen occasionally as a normal variation should not be mistaken for a uvula deviated by a lesion of CN X.

palate fails to rise and, together with the uvula, is pulled toward the normal side (see p. 273).

Warn the patient when testing the *gag reflex*, which consists of elevation of the tongue and soft palate and constriction of the pharyngeal muscles. Stimulate the back of the throat lightly on each side in turn and note the gag reflex. It may be symmetrically diminished or absent in some normal people. If a patient is healthy and swallowing is intact, then checking a gag reflex is not necessary.

Unilateral absence of this reflex suggests a lesion of CN IX, perhaps CN X.

Cranial Nerve XI—Spinal Accessory. From behind, look for atrophy or fasciculations in the trapezius muscles, and compare one side with the other. Fasciculations are fine flickering irregular movements in small groups of muscle fibers. Ask the patient to shrug both shoulders upward against your hands. Note the strength and contraction of the trapezii.

Trapezius weakness with atrophy and fasciculations indicates a peripheral nerve disorder. In trapezius muscle paralysis, the shoulder droops, and the scapula is displaced downward and laterally.

Ask the patient to turn the head to each side against your hand. Observe the contraction of the opposite sternomastoid and note the force of the movement against your hand.

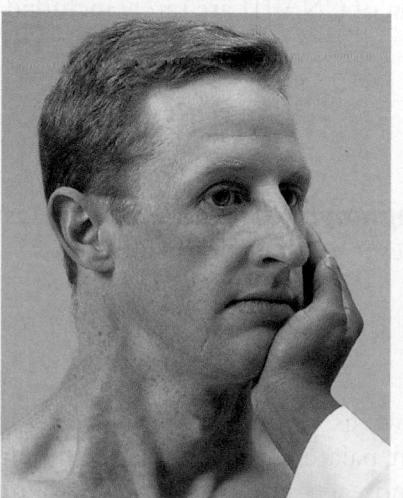

A supine patient with bilateral weakness of the sternomastoids has difficulty raising the head off the pillow.

Cranial Nerve XII—Hypoglossal. Listen to the articulation of the patient's words. This depends on cranial nerves V, VII, and X as well as XII. Inspect the patient's tongue as it lies on the floor of the mouth. Look for any atrophy or *fasciculations*. Some coarser restless movements are often seen in a normal tongue. Then, with the patient's tongue

For poor articulation, or *dysarthria*, see Table 20-9, p. 674, Disorders of Speech. Tongue atrophy and fasciculations in *amyotrophic lateral sclerosis, polio*

In a unilateral cortical lesion, the protruded tongue deviates transiently in a direction away from the

protruded, look for asymmetry, atrophy, or deviation from the midline. Ask the patient to move the tongue from side to side, and note the symmetry of the movement. In ambiguous cases, ask the patient to push the tongue against the inside of each cheek in turn as you palpate externally for strength.

side of the cortical lesion, toward the side of weakness.

The Motor System

Coordination. Coordination of muscle movement requires that four areas of the nervous system function in an integrated way:

- The motor system, for muscle strength

- The cerebellar system (also part of the motor system), for rhythmic movement and steady posture

- The vestibular system, for balance and for coordinating eye, head, and body movements

- The sensory system, for position sense

To assess coordination, observe the patient's performance in:

- Rapid alternating movements

- Point-to-point movements

- Gait and other related body movements

- Standing in specified ways

In cerebellar disease look for nystagmus, dysarthria, hypotonia, and ataxia.

Rapid Alternating Movements

ARMS. Show the patient how to strike one hand on the thigh, raise the hand, turn it over, and then strike the back of the hand down on the same place. Both hands can be assessed at the same time.

Observe the speed, rhythm, and smoothness of the movements. Repeat with the other hand. The nondominant hand often performs somewhat less well.

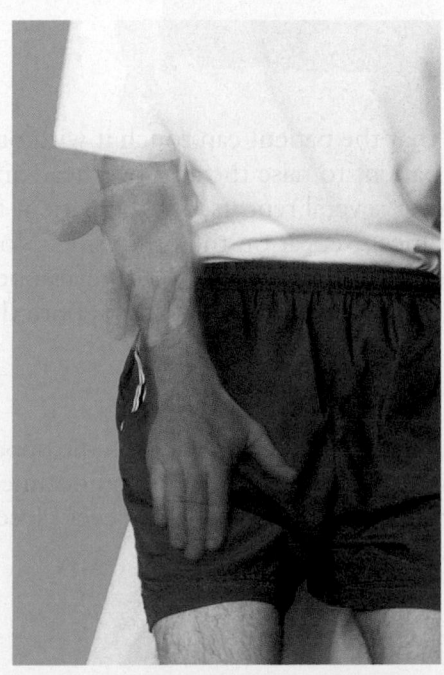

In cerebellar disease, one movement cannot be followed quickly by its opposite and movements are slow, irregular, and clumsy. This abnormality is called *dysdiadochokinesis.* Upper motor neuron weakness and basal ganglia disease may also impair rapid alternating movements, but not in the same manner.

Show the patient how to tap the distal joint of the thumb with the tip of the index finger, again as rapidly as possible. Again, observe the speed, rhythm, and smoothness of the movements. The nondominant side often performs less well.

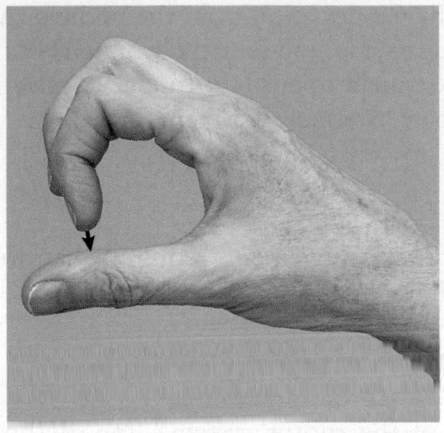

LEGS. Ask the patient to tap your hand as quickly as possible with the ball of each foot in turn. Note any slowness or awkwardness. The feet normally perform less well than the hands.

Point-to-Point Movements

ARMS—FINGER-TO-NOSE TEST. Ask the patient to touch your index finger and then his or her nose alternately several times. Move your finger about so that the patient has to alter directions and extend the arm fully to reach it. Observe the accuracy and smoothness of movements and watch for any tremor. Normally the patient's movements are smooth and accurate.

In cerebellar disease, movements are clumsy, unsteady, and inappropriately varying in their speed, force, and direction. The finger may initially overshoot its mark, but finally reaches it fairly well, termed *dysmetria*. An *intention tremor* may appear toward the end of the movement (see p. 670).

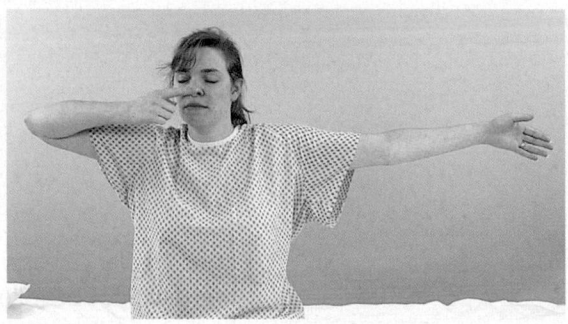

Now hold your finger in one place so that the patient can touch it with one arm and finger outstretched. Ask the patient to raise the arm overhead and lower it again to touch your finger. After several repeats, ask the patient to close both eyes and try several more times. Repeat on the other side. Normally a person can touch the examiner's finger successfully with eyes open or closed. These maneuvers test position sense and the functions of both the labyrinth and the cerebellum.

Cerebellar disease causes incoordination that worsens with eyes closed. If present, this suggests loss of position sense. Repetitive and consistent deviation to one side, referred to as *past pointing*, worse with the eyes closed, suggests cerebellar or vestibular disease.

LEGS—HEEL-TO-SHIN TEST. Ask the patient to place one heel on the opposite knee, and then run it down the shin to the big toe. Note the smoothness and accuracy of the movements. Repetition with the patient's eyes closed tests for position sense. Repeat on the other side.

In cerebellar disease, the heel may overshoot the knee and then oscillate from side to side down the shin. When position sense is lost, the heel is lifted too high and the patient tries to look. With eyes closed, performance is poor.

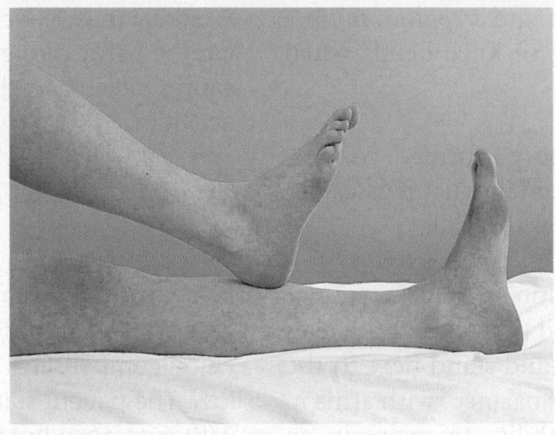

Gait. Ask the patient to:

- *Walk across the room* or down the hall, then turn, and come back. Observe posture, balance, swinging of the arms, and movements of the legs. Normally balance is easy, the arms swing at the sides, and turns are accomplished smoothly.

- *Walk heel-to-toe* in a straight line—a pattern called *tandem walking*.

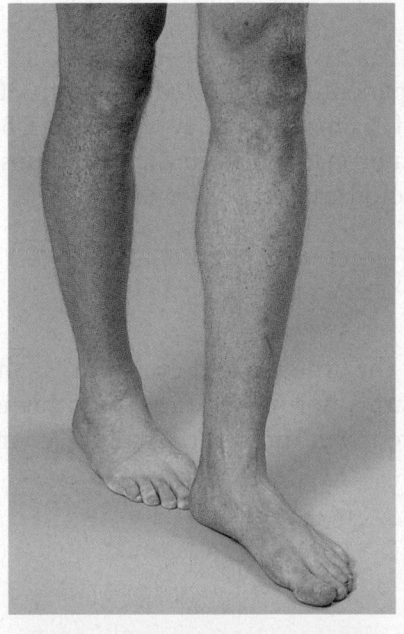

- *Walk on the toes*, then *on the heels*—sensitive tests, respectively, for plantar flexion and dorsiflexion of the ankles, as well as for balance.

- *Hop in place* on each foot in turn (if the patient is not too ill). Hopping involves the proximal muscles of the legs as well as the distal ones and requires both good position sense and normal cerebellar function.

- *Do a shallow knee bend*, first on one leg, then on the other. Support the patient's elbow if you think the patient is in danger of falling.

Abnormalities of gait increase risk of falls.

A gait that lacks coordination, with reeling and instability, is called *ataxic*. Ataxia may be due to cerebellar disease, loss of position sense, or intoxication. See Table 20-10, p. 675, Abnormalities of Gait and Posture.

Tandem walking may reveal an ataxia not previously obvious.

Walking on toes and heels may reveal distal muscular weakness in the legs. Inability to heel-walk is a sensitive test for corticospinal tract damage.

Difficulty with hopping may be due to weakness, lack of position sense, or cerebellar dysfunction.

Difficulty here suggests proximal weakness (extensors of the hip), weakness of the quadriceps (the extensor of the knee), or both.

- *Rising from a sitting position* without arm support and *stepping up* on a sturdy stool are more suitable tests than hopping or knee bends when patients are old or less robust.

Proximal muscle weakness involving the pelvic girdle and legs causes difficulty with both of these activities.

Stance. The following two tests can often be performed concurrently. They differ only in the patient's arm position and in what is assessed. In each case, stand close enough to the patient to prevent a fall.

THE ROMBERG TEST. This is mainly a test of position sense. The patient should first stand with feet together and eyes open and then close both eyes for 30 to 60 seconds without support. The nurse should stand in as in the patient without touching him or her, in case of loss of balance, with arms in front and back of the patient. Note the patient's ability to maintain an upright posture. Normally only minimal swaying occurs.

In ataxia from dorsal column disease and loss of position sense, vision compensates for the sensory loss. The patient stands fairly well with eyes open but loses balance when they are closed, a *positive Romberg sign*. In *cerebellar ataxia*, the patient has difficulty standing with feet together whether the eyes are open or closed.

TEST FOR PRONATOR DRIFT. The patient should stand for 20 to 30 seconds with both arms straight forward, palms up, and eyes closed. A person who cannot stand may be tested for a pronator drift in the sitting position. In either case, a normal person can hold this arm position well.

Pronator drift is the pronation of one forearm. It is both sensitive and specific for a corticospinal tract lesion originating in the contralateral hemisphere. Downward drift of the arm with flexion of fingers and elbow may also occur.[16]

Now, instructing the patient to keep the arms up and eyes shut, as shown, *tap the arms briskly downward*. The arms normally return smoothly to the horizontal position. This response requires muscular strength, coordination, and a good sense of position.

A sideward or upward drift, sometimes with searching, writhing movements of the hands, suggests loss of position sense—the patient may not recognize the displacement and, if told to correct it, does so poorly. In cerebellar incoordination, the arm returns to its original position but overshoots and bounces.

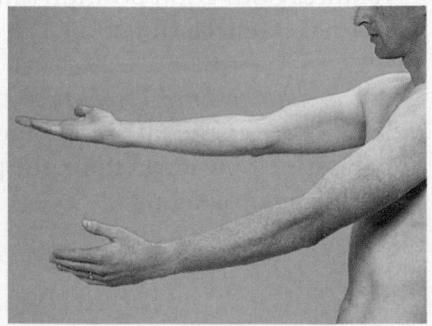

The Sensory System

To evaluate the sensory system, test the following:

- Pain and temperature (spinothalamic tracts)

- Position and vibration (posterior columns)

- Light touch (both spinothalamic and posterior)

- Discriminative sensations, which depend on some of the above sensations but also involve the cortex

When abnormal findings are detected, correlate them with motor and reflex activity. Assess the patient carefully as the following questions are considered:

> Is the underlying lesion central or peripheral?
> Is the sensory loss bilateral or unilateral?
> Does it have a pattern suggesting a dermatomal distribution, a polyneuropathy, or a spinal cord syndrome?
> Is there a loss of pain and temperature sensation? Intact touch and vibration?

See Table 20-11, pp. 676–678, Disorders of the Central and Peripheral Nervous Systems.

See textbooks in Additional References, p. 682, for discussion of *spinal cord syndromes* with crossed sensory findings, both ipsilateral and contralateral to the cord injury.

Patterns of Testing. Because sensory testing quickly fatigues many patients, producing unreliable results, conduct the examination as efficiently as possible. Pay special attention to those areas (1) where there are symptoms such as numbness or pain, (2) where there are motor or reflex abnormalities that suggest a lesion of the spinal cord or peripheral nervous system, and (3) where there are abnormal findings, such as absent or excessive sweating, atrophic skin, or cutaneous ulceration. Repeat testing at another time is often required to confirm abnormalities.

Meticulous sensory mapping helps to establish the level of a spinal cord lesion and to determine whether a more peripheral lesion is in a nerve root, a major peripheral nerve, or one of its branches.

The following patterns of testing help you to identify sensory deficits accurately and efficiently.

- *Compare symmetric areas* on the two sides of the body, including the arms, legs, and trunk.

Hemisensory loss from a lesion in the spinal cord or higher pathways

- When testing pain, temperature, and touch sensation, also *compare the distal with the proximal areas* of the extremities. Further, scatter the stimuli to sample most of the dermatomes and major peripheral nerves (see pp. 694–695). One suggested pattern includes both shoulders (C4), the inner and outer aspects of the forearms (C6 and T1), the thumbs and little fingers (C6 and C8), the fronts of both thighs (L2), the medial and

Symmetric distal sensory loss suggests a *polyneuropathy*. This finding may be missed unless the distal and proximal areas are compared.

lateral aspects of both calves (L4 and L5), the little toes (S1), and the medial aspect of each buttock (S3).

● When testing vibration and position sensation, first test the fingers and toes. If these are normal, it is safe to assume that more proximal areas will also be normal.

● *Vary the pace of your testing*. This is important so that the patient does not merely respond to the repetitive rhythm.

● When sensory loss or hypersensitivity is detected, map out the affected area in detail. Stimulate first at a point of reduced sensation, and move by progressive steps until the patient detects the change. An example is shown on the right.

By identifying the distribution of sensory abnormalities and the kinds of sensations affected, you can infer where the causative lesion might be. Any motor deficit or reflex abnormality also helps in this localizing process.

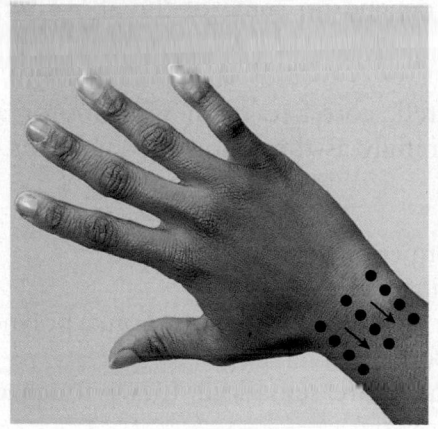

Here all sensation in the hand is lost. Repetitive testing in a proximal direction reveals a gradual change to normal sensation at the wrist. This pattern fits neither a peripheral nerve nor a dermatome (see pp. 643–644). If bilateral, it suggests the "glove and stocking" sensory loss of a *polyneuropathy*, often seen in *alcoholism* or *diabetes*.

Before each of the following tests, show the patient what is planned and what the response should be. Unless otherwise specified, the patient's eyes should be closed during actual testing.

Pain. Use a broken tongue blade/cotton swab or other suitable tool. Occasionally, substitute the blunt end for the point.

Demonstrate "This is sharp and this is dull" by touching the patient. Ask the patient to close his or her eyes and to differentiate between sharp and dull. Apply the lightest pressure needed for the stimulus to feel sharp, and do not draw blood.

Analgesia refers to absence of pain sensation, *hypalgesia* to decreased sensitivity to pain, and *hyperalgesia* to increased sensitivity.

Temperature. Testing is often omitted if pain sensation is normal, but include it if there is any question. Use two test tubes, filled with hot and cold water, or a tuning fork heated or cooled by water. Touch the skin and ask the patient to identify "hot" or "cold."

Light Touch. With a fine wisp of cotton, touch the skin lightly, avoiding pressure. Ask the patient to respond whenever a touch is felt, and to compare one area with another. Calloused skin is relatively insensitive and should be avoided.

Anesthesia is absence of touch sensation, *hypesthesia* is decreased sensitivity, and *hyperesthesia* is increased sensitivity.

Vibration. Use a relatively low-pitched tuning fork of 128 Hz. Tap it on the heel of your hand and place it firmly over a distal interphalangeal joint of the patient's finger, and test over the interphalangeal joint of the big toe.

Vibration sense is often the first sensation to be lost in a peripheral neuropathy. Common causes

Ask what the patient feels. If you are uncertain whether it is pressure or vibration, ask the patient to tell you when the vibration stops, and then touch the fork to stop it. If vibration sense is impaired, proceed to more proximal bony prominences (e.g., wrist, elbow, medial malleolus, patella, anterior superior iliac spine, spinous processes, and clavicles).

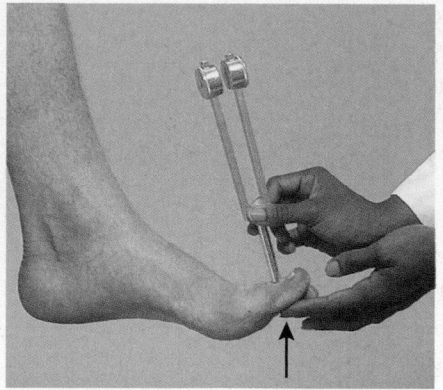

include *diabetes* or *alcoholism*. Vibration sense is also lost in posterior column disease, as in *tertiary syphilis* or *vitamin B$_{12}$ deficiency*.

Testing vibration sense in the trunk may be useful in estimating the level of a cord lesion.

Proprioception (Position). Grasp the patient's big toe, *holding it by its sides* between the thumb and index finger, and then pull it away from the other toes. (These precautions prevent extraneous tactile stimuli from revealing position changes that might not otherwise be detected.) Demonstrate "up" and "down" as you move the patient's toe clearly upward and downward. Then, with the patient's eyes closed, ask for a response of "up" or "down" when moving the large toe in a small arc.

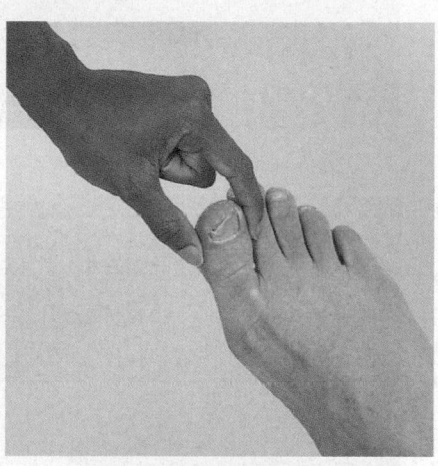

Loss of position sense, like loss of vibration sense, in *tabes dorsalis*, *multiple sclerosis*, or B$_{12}$ *deficiency* from posterior column disease; and in peripheral neuropathy from diabetes

Repeat several times on each side, avoiding simple alternation of the stimuli. If position sense is impaired, move proximally to test it at the ankle joint. In a similar fashion, test position in the fingers, moving proximally if indicated to the metacarpophalangeal joints, wrist, and elbow.

When touch and position sense are normal or only slightly impaired, a disproportionate decrease in or loss of discriminative sensations suggests disease of the sensory cortex. Stereognosis, number identification, and two-point discrimination are also impaired in posterior column disease.

Discriminative Sensations. Several additional techniques test the ability of the sensory cortex to correlate, analyze, and interpret sensations. Because discriminative sensations depend on touch and position sense, they are useful only when these sensations are either intact or only slightly impaired.

Screen a patient with *stereognosis,* and proceed to other methods if indicated. The patient's eyes should be closed during all these tests.

● *Stereognosis.* Stereognosis refers to the ability to identify an object by feeling it. Place in the patient's hand a familiar object such as a coin, paper clip, key, pencil, or cotton ball, and ask the patient to tell you what it is.

Astereognosis refers to the inability to recognize objects placed in the hand.

Normally a patient will manipulate it skillfully and identify it correctly within 5 seconds. Asking the patient to distinguish "heads" from "tails" on a coin is a sensitive test of stereognosis.

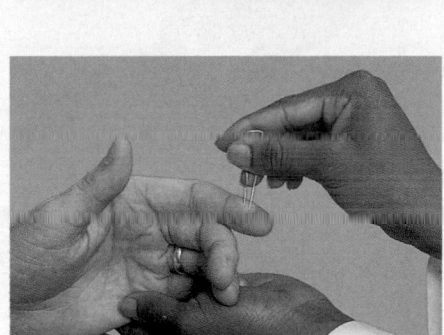

● *Number identification (graphesthesia)*. When motor impairment, arthritis, or other conditions prevent the patient from manipulating an object well enough to identify it, test the ability to identify numbers. With the blunt end of a pen or pencil, draw a large number in the patient's palm. A normal person can identify most such numbers.

The inability to recognize numbers, like astereognosis, suggests a lesion in the sensory cortex.

● *Two-point discrimination*. Using the two ends of an opened paper clip, touch a finger pad in two places simultaneously. Alternate the double stimulus irregularly with a one-point touch. Be careful not to cause pain.

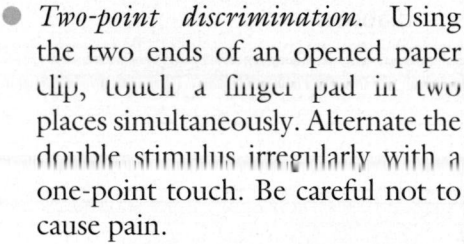

Find the minimal distance at which the patient can discriminate one from two points (normally <5 mm on the fingerpads). This test may be used on other parts of the body, but normal distances vary widely from one body region to another.

Lesions of the sensory cortex increase the distance between two recognizable points.

● *Point localization*. Briefly touch a point on the patient's skin. Then ask the patient to open both eyes and point to the place touched. Normally a person can do so accurately. This test, together with the test for extinction, is especially useful on the trunk and the legs.

Lesions of the sensory cortex impair the ability to localize points accurately.

● *Extinction*. Simultaneously stimulate corresponding areas on both sides of the body. Ask where the patient feels your touch. Normally both stimuli are felt.

With lesions of the sensory cortex, only one stimulus may be recognized. The stimulus on the side opposite the damaged cortex is extinguished.

Dermatomes. Knowledge of dermatomes helps you localize neurologic lesions to a specific level of the spinal cord, particularly in spinal cord injury. *A dermatome is the band of skin innervated by the sensory root of a single spinal nerve.* Dermatome patterns are mapped in the next two figures,

In spinal cord injury, the sensory level may be several segments *lower* than the spinal lesion, for reasons that are not well

using the international standard recommended by the American Spinal Injury Association.[17] Dermatome levels are more variable than these diagrams suggest. They overlap at their upper and lower margins and also slightly across the midline.

understood. Tapping for the level of vertebral pain may be helpful.[15]

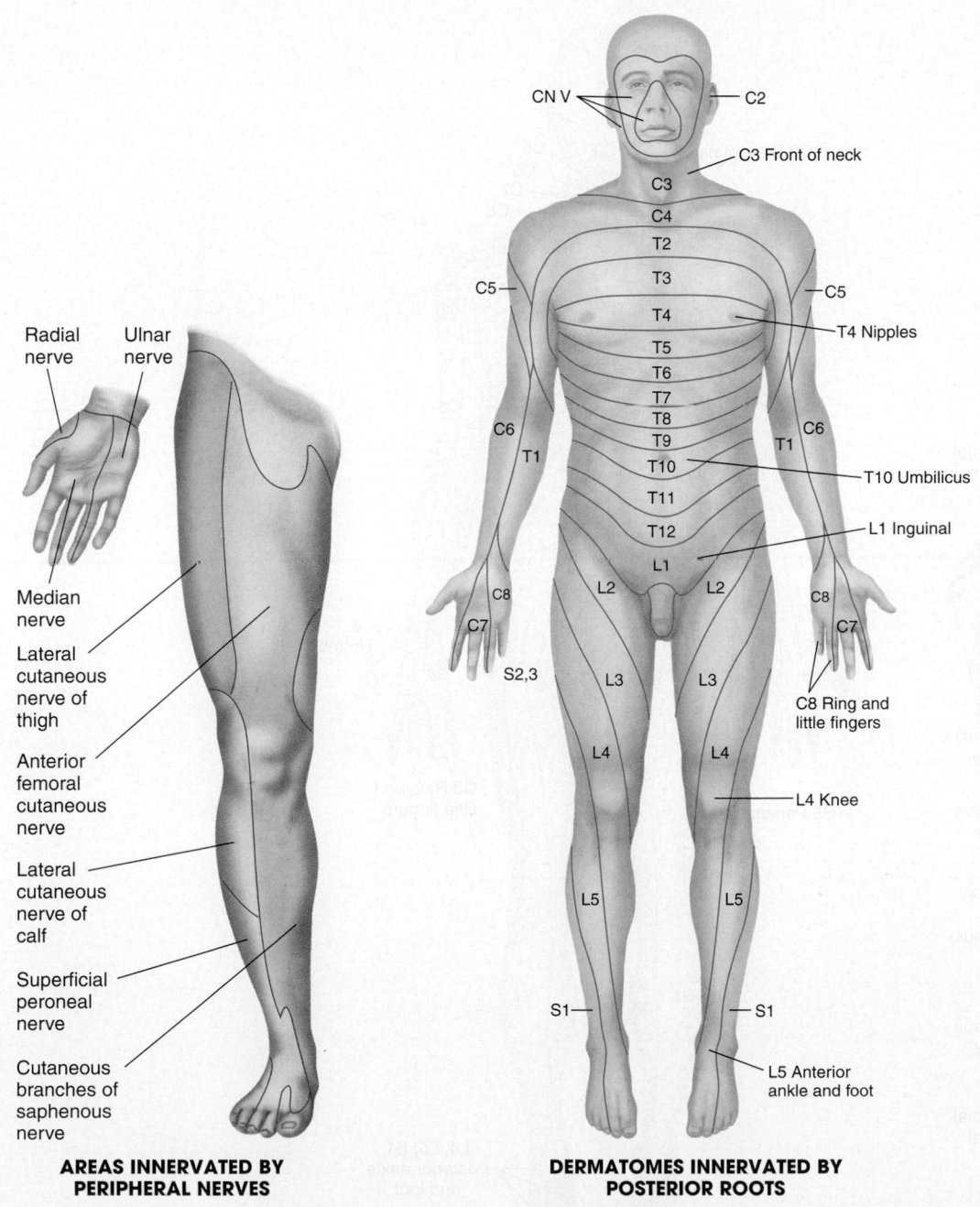

AREAS INNERVATED BY PERIPHERAL NERVES

DERMATOMES INNERVATED BY POSTERIOR ROOTS

Do not try to memorize all the dermatomes. Instead, focus on learning selected dermatomes such as those specifically named on the diagrams. The distribution of a few key peripheral nerves is shown in the inserts on the left.

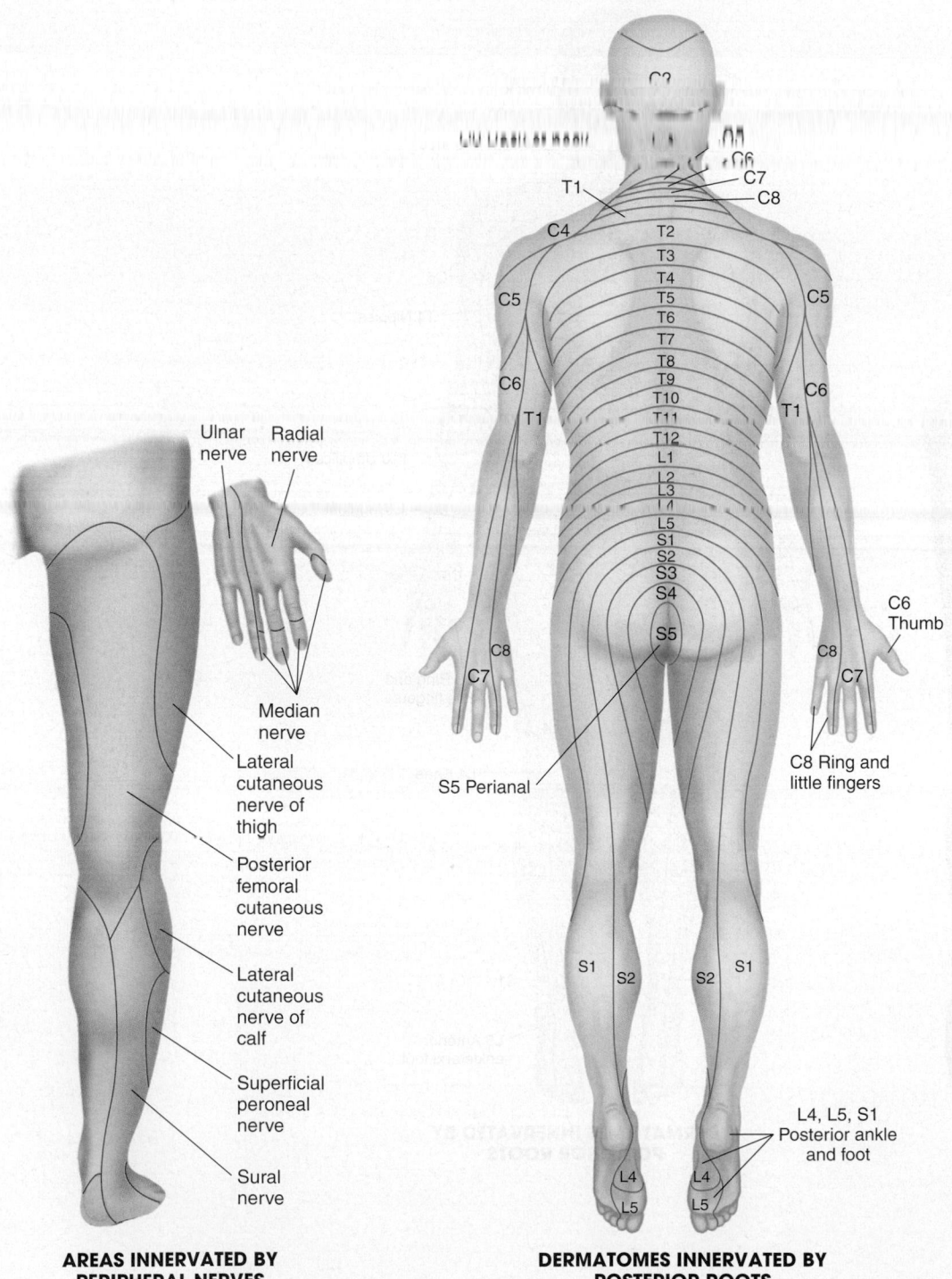

AREAS INNERVATED BY PERIPHERAL NERVES

DERMATOMES INNERVATED BY POSTERIOR ROOTS

Deep Tendon Reflexes

Eliciting the *deep tendon reflexes* involves a series of examiner skills. Be sure to select a properly weighted reflex hammer. Learn when to use either the pointed or the flat end of the hammer. For example, the pointed end is useful for striking small areas, such as your finger as it overlies the biceps tendon. Now test the reflexes as follows:

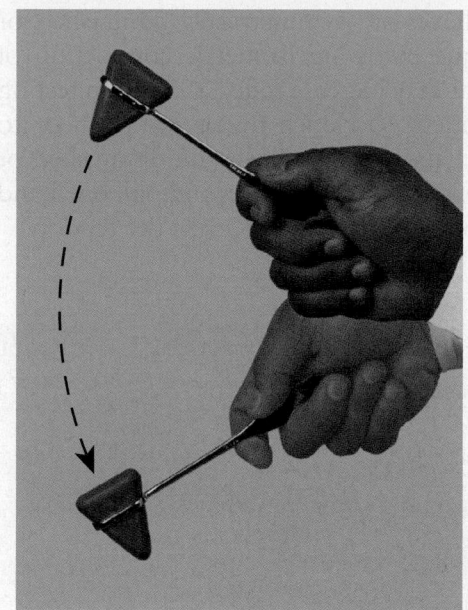

- Encourage the patient to relax, then position the limbs properly and symmetrically.

- Hold the reflex hammer loosely between your thumb and index finger so that it swings freely in an arc within the limits set by your palm and other fingers.

- With your wrist relaxed, strike the tendon briskly using a rapid wrist movement. Your strike should be quick and direct, not glancing.

- Note the speed, force, and amplitude of the reflex response and grade the response using the scale below. Always compare the response of one side with the other. Reflexes are usually graded on a 0 to 4+ scale.[18]

Hyperactive reflexes (hyperreflexia) in central nervous system lesions along the descending corticospinal tract. Look for associated upper motor neuron findings of weakness, spasticity, or a positive Babinski sign.

● Scale for Grading Reflexes	
4+	Very brisk, hyperactive, with *clonus* (rhythmic oscillations between flexion and extension)
3+	Brisker than average; possibly but not necessarily indicative of disease
2+	Average; normal
1+	Somewhat diminished; low normal
0	No response

Hypoactive or *absent reflexes (hyporeflexia)* in diseases of spinal nerve roots, spinal nerves, plexuses, or peripheral nerves. Look for associated findings of lower motor unit disease, namely, weakness, atrophy, and fasciculations.[15]

Reflex response depends partly on the force of your stimulus. Use no more force than you need to provoke a definite response. Differences between sides are usually easier to assess than symmetric changes. Symmetrically diminished or even absent reflexes may be found in normal people.

Reinforcement. If the patient's reflexes are symmetrically diminished or absent, use *reinforcement*, a technique involving isometric contraction of other muscles for up to 10 seconds that may increase reflex activity. In testing arm reflexes, for example, ask the patient to clench his or her teeth or to squeeze one thigh with the opposite hand. If leg reflexes are diminished or absent, reinforce them by asking the patient to lock fingers and pull one hand against the other. Tell the patient to pull just before you strike the tendon.

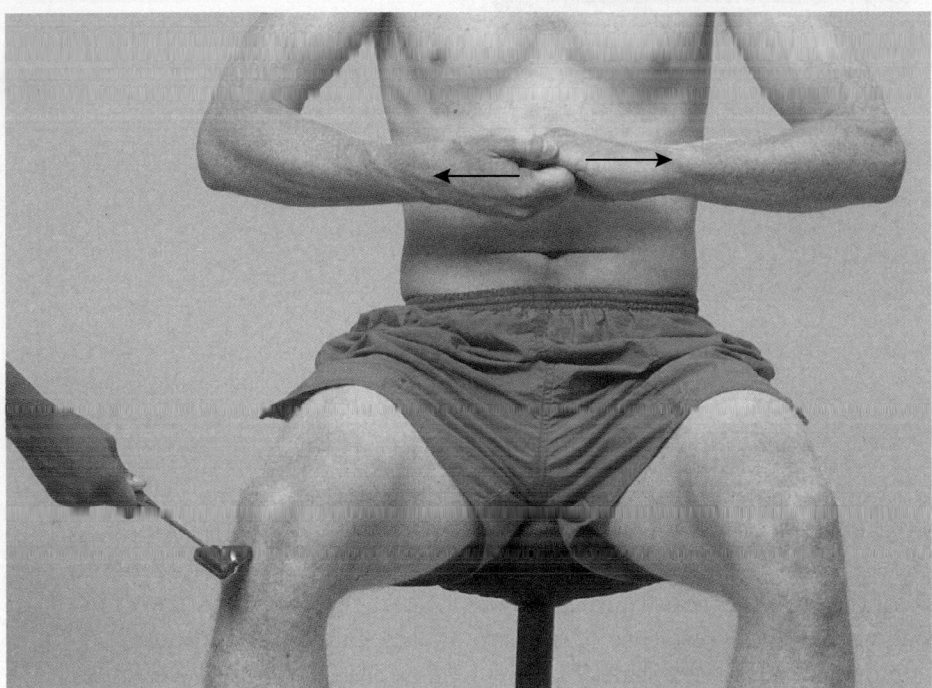

REINFORCEMENT OF KNEE REFLEX

The Biceps Reflex (C5, C6). The patient's arm should be partially flexed at the elbow with palm down and fully relaxed. Support the arm on your arm or the patient's leg. Place your thumb or finger firmly on the biceps tendon. Strike with the reflex hammer so that the blow is aimed directly through your digit toward the biceps tendon.

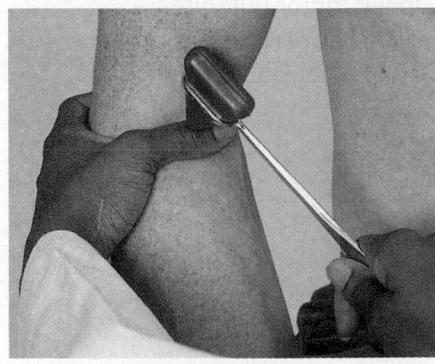

PATIENT SITTING

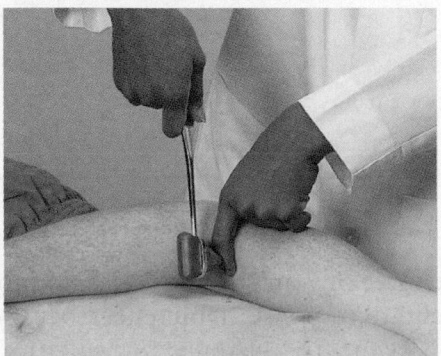

PATIENT LYING DOWN

Observe flexion at the elbow, and watch for and feel the contraction of the biceps muscle.

The Triceps Reflex (C6, C7).   The patient may be sitting or supine. Flex the patient's arm at the elbow, with palm toward the body, and pull it slightly across the chest. Strike the triceps tendon above the elbow. Use a direct blow from directly behind it. Watch for contraction of the triceps muscle and extension at the elbow.

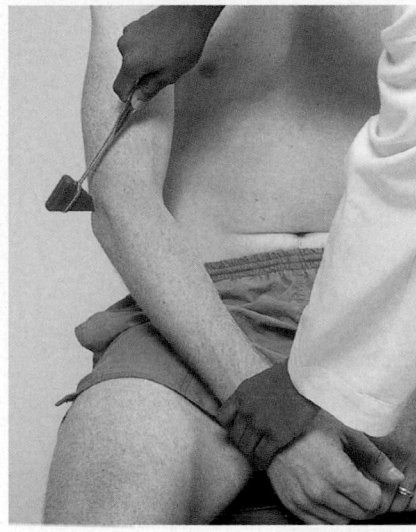
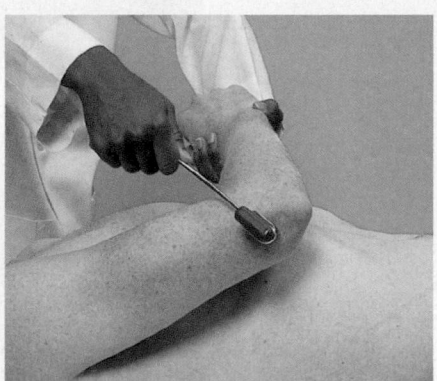

If you have difficulty getting the patient to relax, try supporting the upper arm as illustrated on the right. Ask the patient to let the arm go limp, as if it were "hung up to dry." Then strike the triceps tendon.

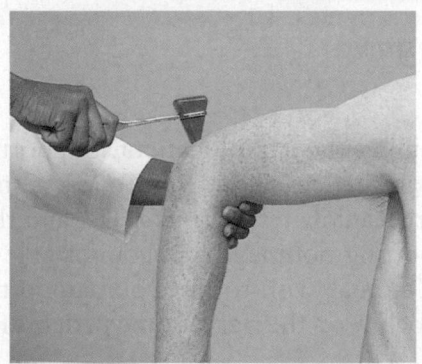

The Supinator or Brachioradialis Reflex (C5, C6).   The patient's hand should rest on the abdomen or the lap, with the forearm partly pronated. Strike the radius with the point or flat edge of the reflex hammer, about 1 to 2 inches above the wrist. Watch for flexion and supination of the forearm.

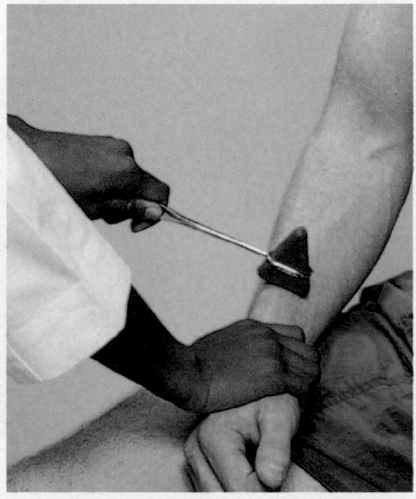

The Knee Reflex (Patellar Reflex) (L2, L3, L4). The patient may be either sitting or lying down as long as the knee is flexed. Briskly tap the patellar tendon just below the patella. Note contraction of the quadriceps with extension at the knee. A hand on the patient's anterior thigh lets you feel this reflex.

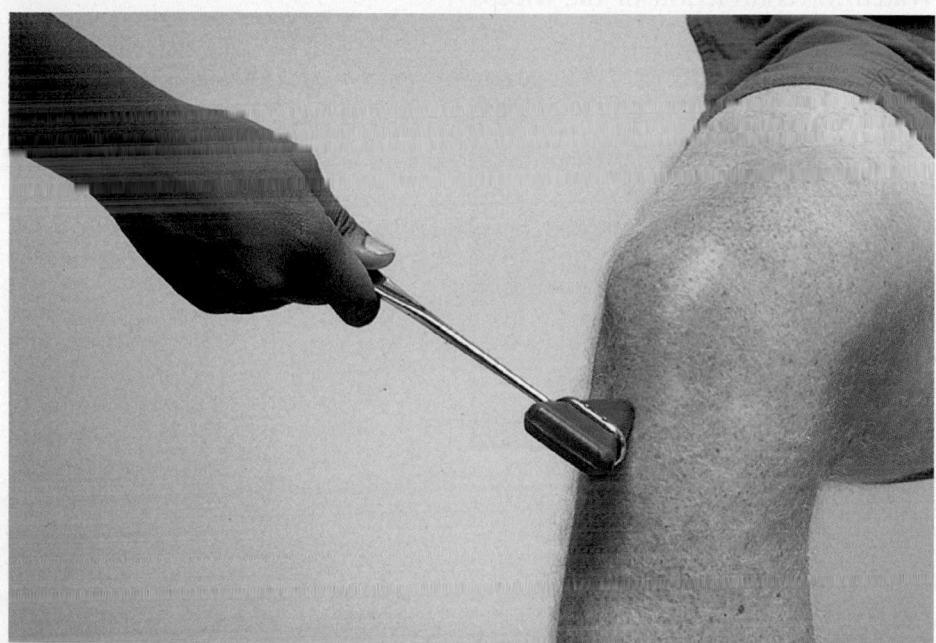

PATIENT SITTING

Two methods are useful when examining the supine patient. Supporting both knees at once, as shown below on the left, allows you to assess small differences between knee reflexes by repeatedly testing one reflex and then the other. Sometimes, however, supporting both legs is uncomfortable for both the examiner and the patient. You may wish to rest your supporting arm under the patient's leg, as shown below on the right. Some patients find it easier to relax with this method.

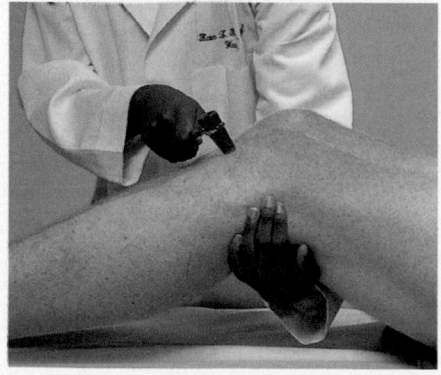

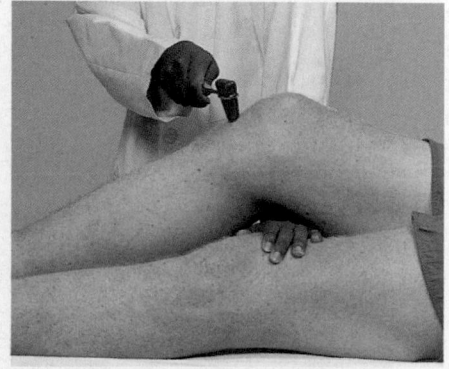

The Ankle Reflex (Achilles Reflex) (primarily S1).   If the patient is sitting, dorsiflex the foot at the ankle. Persuade the patient to relax. Strike the Achilles tendon. Watch and feel for plantar flexion at the ankle. Note also the speed of relaxation after muscular contraction.

The slowed relaxation phase of reflexes in *hypothyroidism* is often easily seen and felt in the ankle reflex.

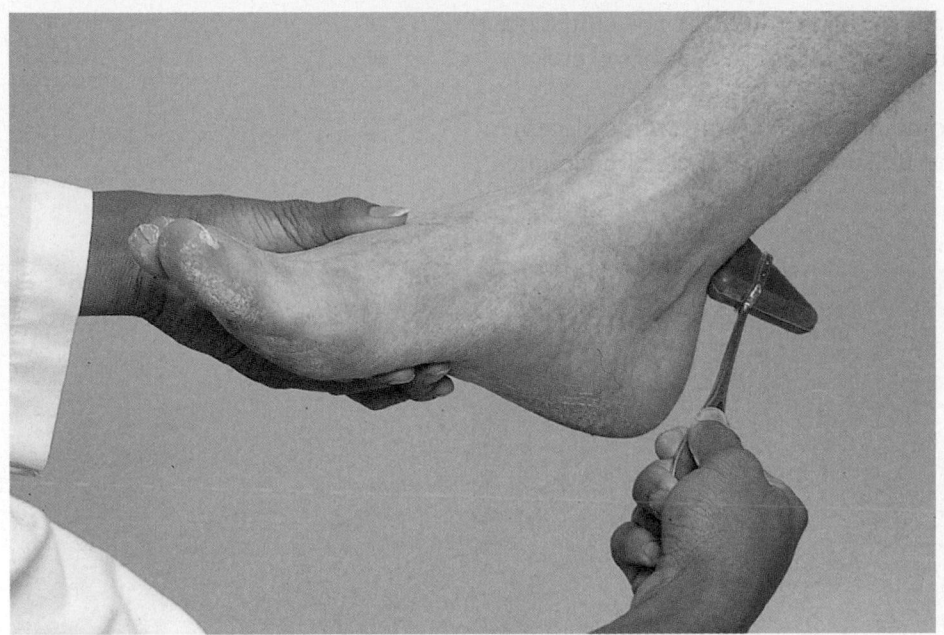

PATIENT SITTING

When the patient is lying down, flex one leg at both hip and knee and rotate it externally so that the lower leg rests across the opposite shin. Then dorsiflex the foot at the ankle and strike the Achilles tendon.

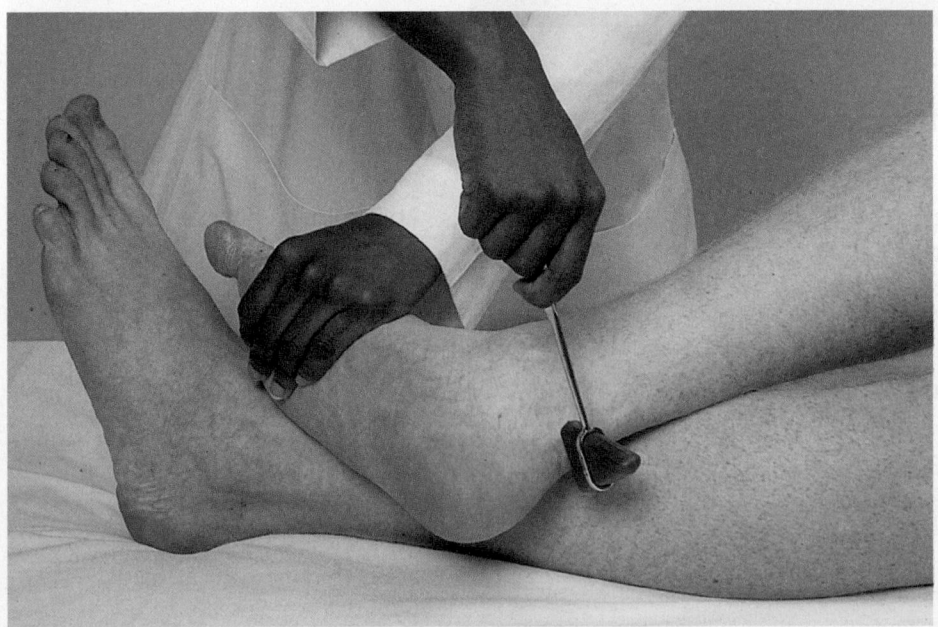

PATIENT LYING DOWN

Clonus. If the reflexes seem hyperactive, test for *ankle clonus.* Support the knee in a partly flexed position. With your other hand, dorsiflex and plantar flex the foot a few times while encouraging the patient to relax, and then sharply dorsiflex the foot and maintain it in dorsiflexion. Look and feel for rhythmic oscillations between dorsiflexion and plantar flexion. In most normal people, the ankle does not react to this stimulus. A few clonic beats may be seen and felt, especially when the patient is tense or has exercised.

Clonus may also be elicited at other joints. A sharp downward displacement of the patella, for example, may elicit patellar clonus in the extended knee.

Sustained clonus indicates central nervous system disease. The ankle plantar flexes and dorsiflexes repetitively and rhythmically.

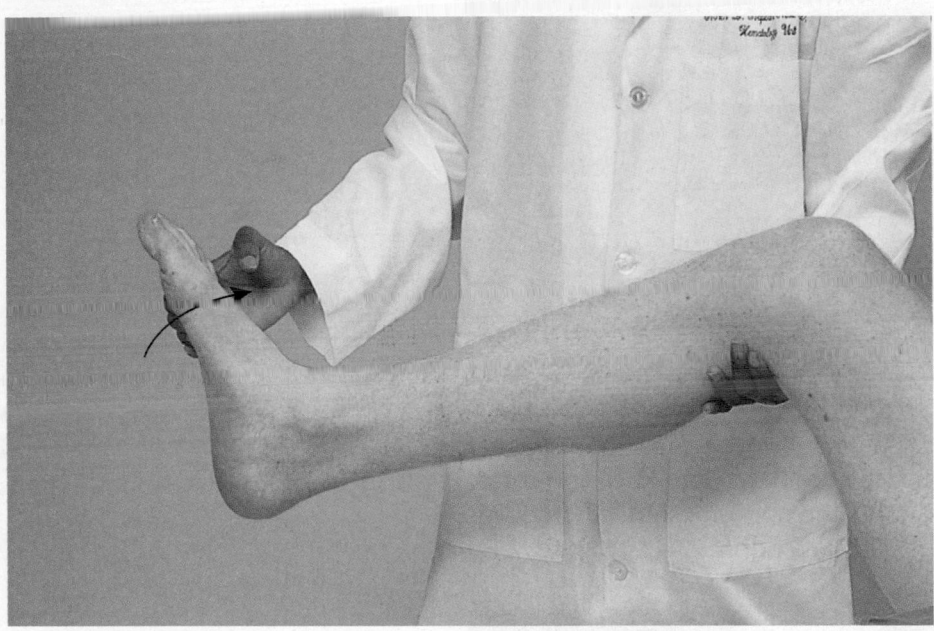

Cutaneous Stimulation Reflexes (Superficial Reflexes)

The Abdominal Reflexes. Test the abdominal reflexes by lightly but briskly stroking each side of the abdomen, above (T8, T9, T10) and below (T10, T11, T12) the umbilicus, in the directions illustrated. Use a key, the wooden end of a cotton-tipped applicator, or a tongue blade twisted and split longitudinally. Note the contraction of the abdominal muscles and deviation of the umbilicus toward the stimulus. Obesity may mask an abdominal reflex. In this situ-

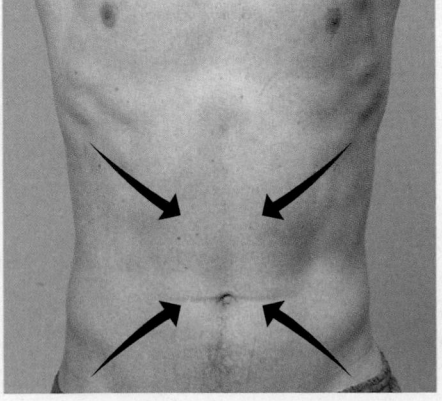

Abdominal reflexes may be absent in both central and peripheral nerve disorders.

ation, use your finger to retract the patient's umbilicus away from the side to be stimulated. Feel with your retracting finger for the muscular contraction.

The Plantar Response (L5, S1). With the end of a tongue blade, stroke from the heel moving up toward the small toe to the ball of the foot, curving medially across the ball. Use the lightest stimulus that will provoke a response, but be increasingly firm if necessary. The normal response is a downward contraction of the toes, called the plantar response.

Dorsiflexion of the big toe and "fanning" of other toes is a *positive Babinski response* from a central nervous system lesion in the corticospinal tract; also seen in unconscious states from drug or alcohol intoxication or the postictal period following a seizure.

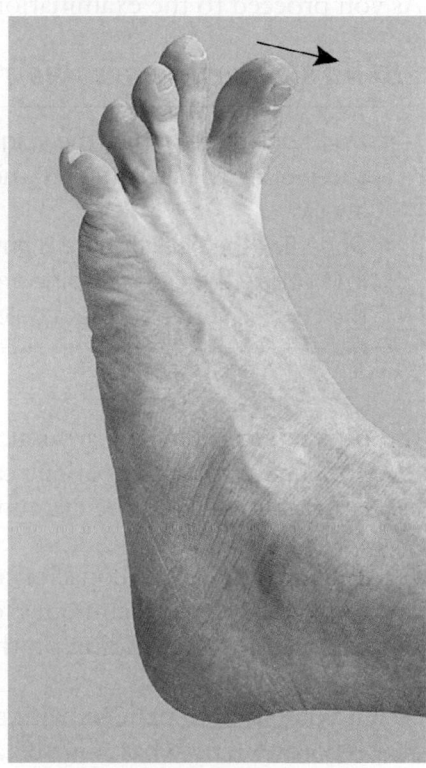

Some patients withdraw from this stimulus by flexing the hip and the knee. Hold the ankle, if necessary, to complete your observation. It is sometimes difficult to distinguish withdrawal from a Babinski response.

A marked Babinski response is occasionally accompanied by reflex flexion at hip and knee.

 **ABBREVIATED NEUROLOGIC ASSESSMENT**

Assessment for Comatose Patient

Comatose Patient. Coma signals a potentially life-threatening event affecting the two hemispheres, the brainstem, or both. The usual sequence of history, physical examination, and laboratory evaluation does not apply. Instead, you must:

- First assess the ABCs (airway, breathing, and circulation)

- Establish the patient's level of consciousness

See Table 20-2, p. 663, Metabolic and Structural Coma.

● Examine the patient neurologically. Look for focal or asymmetric findings, and determine whether impaired consciousness arises from a metabolic or a structural cause.

Interview the relatives, friends, or witnesses to establish the speed of onset and duration of unconsciousness. The warning symptoms, precipitating factors, or previous episodes; and the prior appearance and behavior of the patient is helpful. Any history of past medical and psychiatric illnesses is also useful.

As you proceed to the examination, remember two cardinal DON'Ts:

"DON'T'S" WHEN ASSESSING THE COMATOSE PATIENT

- *Don't* dilate the pupils, the single most important clue to the underlying cause of coma (structural vs. metabolic), and pupillary response will be invalid.
- *Don't* flex the neck if there is any question of trauma to the head or neck. Immobilize the cervical spine and get an x-ray first to rule out fractures of the cervical vertebrae that could compress and damage the spinal cord.

Level of Consciousness. Level of consciousness primarily reflects the patient's capacity for arousal, or wakefulness. It is determined by the level of activity that the patient can be aroused to perform in response to escalating stimuli from the examiner.

Five clinical levels of consciousness are described in the table below, together with related techniques for examination. Increase your stimuli in a stepwise manner, depending on the patient's response.

When you examine patients with an altered level of consciousness, describe and record exactly what you see and hear. Imprecise use of terms such as lethargy, obtundation, stupor, or coma may mislead other examiners.

● Level of Consciousness (Arousal): Techniques and Patient Response

Level	Technique	Abnormal Response
Alertness	Speak to the patient in a normal tone of voice. An alert patient opens the eyes, looks at you, and responds fully and appropriately to stimuli (arousal intact).	
Lethargy	Speak to the patient in a loud voice. For example, call the patient's name or ask, "How are you?"	A lethargic patient appears drowsy but opens the eyes and looks at you, responds to questions, and then falls asleep.
Obtundation	Shake the patient gently as if awakening a sleeper.	An obtunded patient opens the eyes and looks at you, but responds slowly and is somewhat confused. Alertness and interest in the environment are decreased.

(continued)

● Level of Consciousness (Arousal): Techniques and Patient Response (continued)

Level	Technique	Abnormal Response
Stupor	Apply a painful stimulus. For example, pinch a tendon, rub the sternum, or roll a pencil across a nail bed. (No stronger stimuli needed!)	A stuporous patient arouses from sleep only after painful stimuli. Verbal responses are slow or even absent. The patient lapses into an unresponsive state when the stimulus ceases. There is minimal awareness of self or the environment.
Coma	Apply repeated painful stimuli.	A comatose patient remains unarousable with eyes closed. There is no evident response to inner need or external stimuli.

The Glasgow Coma Scale.   Because imprecise terms may mislead other examiners, the Glasgow Coma Scale, a standardized tool for objective assessment of patients, should be used. There is a numeric value assigned to three different components: eye opening, motor response, and verbal response. Each area receives a score and the scores are then added together to determine the level of brain function.

● Using the Glasgow Coma Scale

The points associated with the Glasgow Coma Scale are determined to assess levels of consciousness and coma. Points are allotted for each of the 3 areas: eye opening, verbal response and motor responses per the grid below:

Eye Opening	Points		Motor Response (arms)	Points
Spontaneous	4		Follows verbal command	6
To verbal stimuli	3		Localizes pain	5
To pain stimuli	2		Withdraws from pain	4
No response	1		Flexion (decorticate)	3
			Extension (decerebrate)	2
Verbal Response	**Points**		No response	1
Oriented	5		Total Score:	3–15
Confused	4			
Inappropriate words	3			
Incomprehensive	2			
No response	1			

A score of 15 is a fully alert and functioning person, and a score of 7 or below denotes a coma state. A score of 3 is the lowest possible score and denotes "no response" in any of the 3 areas assessed.

Neurologic Evaluation

RESPIRATIONS. Observe the rate, rhythm, and pattern of respirations. Because neural structures that govern breathing in the cortex and brainstem overlap those that govern consciousness, abnormalities of respiration often occur in coma.

See Table 20-2, p. 663, Metabolic and Structural Coma, and Table 7-1, p. 127, Abnormalities in Rate and Rhythm of Breathing.

PUPILS. Observe the size and equality of the pupils and test their reaction to light. The presence or absence of the light reaction is one of the most important signs distinguishing structural from metabolic causes of coma. The light reaction often remains intact in metabolic coma.

See Table 20-12, p. 679, Pupils in Comatose Patients.

Structural lesions from stroke, bleeding, abscess, or tumor mass may lead to asymmetric pupils and loss of light reaction.

OCULAR MOVEMENT. Observe the position of the eyes and eyelids at rest. Check for horizontal deviation of the eyes to one side (*gaze preference*). When the oculomotor pathways are intact, the eyes look straight ahead.

In structural hemispheric lesions, the eyes "look at the lesion" in the affected hemisphere.

In irritative lesions from epilepsy or early cerebral hemorrhage, the eyes "look away" from the affected hemisphere.

OCULOCEPHALIC REFLEX (DOLL'S EYE MOVEMENTS). This reflex helps to assess brainstem function in a comatose patient. Holding open the upper eyelids so that you can see the eyes, turn the head quickly, first to one side and then to the other. (Make sure the patient has no neck injury before performing this test.)

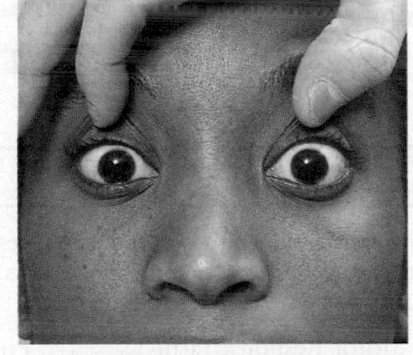

In a comatose patient with absence of doll's eye movements, shown below, the ability to move both eyes to one side is lost, suggesting a lesion of the midbrain or pons.

In a comatose patient with an intact brainstem, as the head is turned, the eyes move toward the opposite side (the doll's eye movements). In the adjacent photo, for example, the patient's head has been turned to the right; her eyes have moved to the left. Her eyes still seem to gaze at the camera. The doll's eye movements are intact.

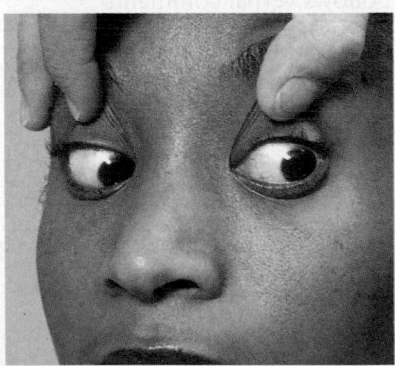

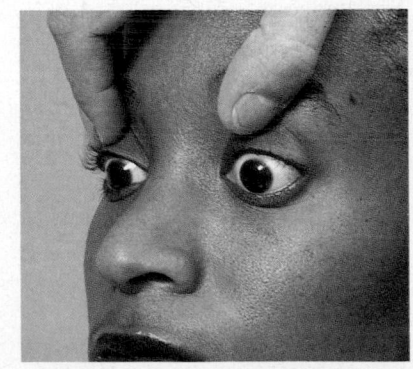

POSTURE AND MUSCLE TONE. Observe the patient's posture. If there is no spontaneous movement, you may need to apply a painful stimulus (see p. 653). Classify the resulting pattern of movement as:

See Table 20-1, p. 662, Abnormal Postures in Comatose Patients.

- *Normal–avoidant*—the patient pushes the stimulus away or withdraws.

- *Stereotypic*—the stimulus evokes abnormal postural responses of the trunk and extremities.

- *Flaccid paralysis or no response*

Test muscle tone by grasping each forearm near the wrist and raising it to a vertical position. Note the position of the hand, which is usually only slightly flexed at the wrist.

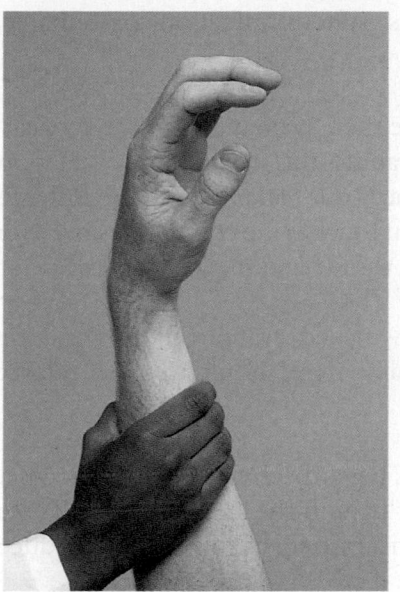

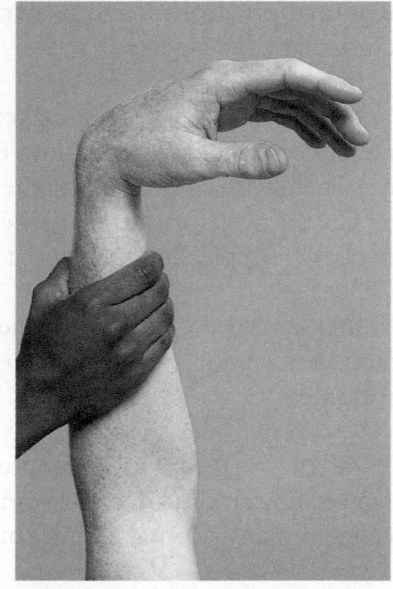

The hemiplegia of sudden cerebral accidents is usually flaccid at first. The limp hand drops to form a right angle with the wrist.

Then lower the arm to about 12 or 18 inches off the bed and drop it. Watch how it falls. A normal arm drops somewhat slowly.

A flaccid arm drops rapidly, like a flail.

Support the patient's flexed knees. Then extend one leg at a time at the knee and let it fall (see below). Compare the speed with which each leg falls.

In *acute hemiplegia*, the flaccid leg falls more rapidly.

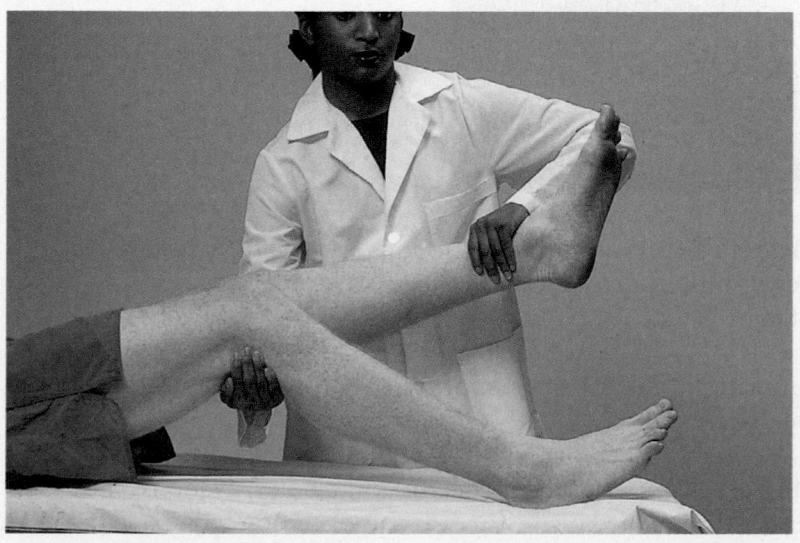

Flex both legs so that the heels rest on the bed and then release them. The normal leg returns slowly to its original extended position.

In acute hemiplegia, the flaccid leg falls rapidly into extension, with external rotation at the hip.

SPECIAL TECHNIQUES

Meningeal Signs. Testing for these signs is important if meningeal inflammation from central nervous system infection or subarachnoid hemorrhage is suspected.

Neck Mobility. First make sure there is no injury to the cervical vertebrae or cervical cord. (In settings of trauma, this may require evaluation by x-ray.) Then, with the patient supine, place your hands behind the patient's head and flex the neck forward, until the chin touches the chest if possible. Normally the neck is supple, and the patient can easily bend the head and neck forward.

Neck stiffness and resistance to flexion in 90% of patients with acute bacterial meningitis and in 20% to 05% with subarachnoid hemorrhage.[15] Also in arthritis and neck injury

Brudzinski Sign. As the neck is flexed, watch the hips and knees in reaction to your maneuver. Normally they should remain relaxed and motionless.

Flexion of the hips and knees is a *positive Brudzinski sign* and suggests meningeal inflammation.

Kernig Sign. Flex the patient's leg at both the hip and the knee, and then straighten the knee. Discomfort behind the knee during full extension occurs in many normal people, but this maneuver should not produce pain.

Pain and increased resistance to extending the knee are *positive Kernig signs*. When bilateral, it suggests meningeal irritation.

Compression of a lumbosacral nerve root may also cause resistance, together with pain in the low back and the posterior thigh. Only one leg is usually involved.

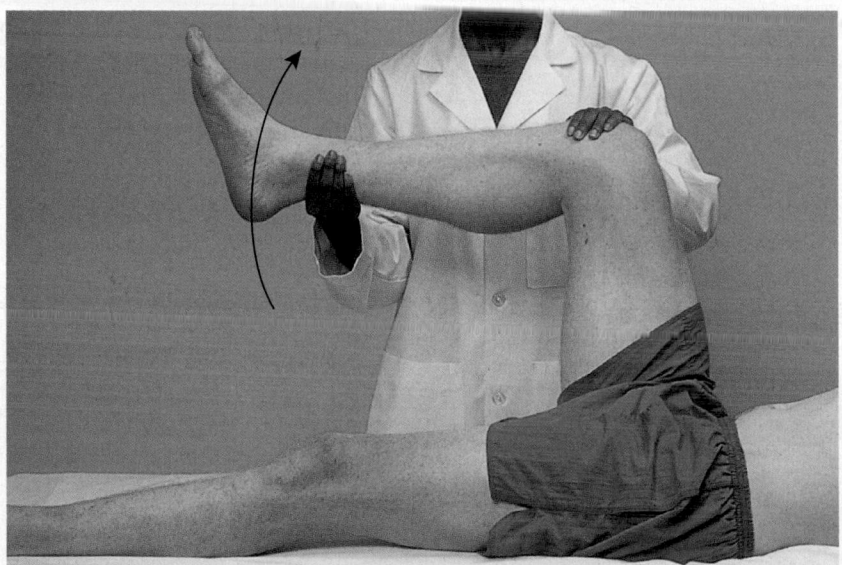

Further Examination. As you complete the neurologic examination, check for facial asymmetry and asymmetries in motor, sensory, and reflex function. Test for meningeal signs if indicated.

Meningitis, subarachnoid hemorrhage[3]

As you proceed to the general physical examination look for signs in other body systems that may support neurological diseases.

Alcohol, liver failure, uremia

Look for abnormalities of the skin, including color, moisture, evidence of bleeding disorders, needle marks, and other lesions.

Jaundice, cyanosis, cherry red color of carbon monoxide poisoning

Examine the scalp and skull for signs of trauma.

Bruises, lacerations, swelling

Examine the fundi carefully.

Papilledema, hypertensive retinopathy

Check to make sure the corneal reflexes are intact. (Remember that use of contact lenses may abolish these reflexes.)

Reflex loss in coma and lesions affecting CN V or CN VII

Inspect the ears and nose, and examine the mouth and throat.

Blood or cerebrospinal fluid in the nose or the ears suggests a skull fracture; otitis media suggests a possible brain abscess.

Be sure to evaluate the heart, lungs, and abdomen.

Tongue injury suggests a seizure.

RECORDING YOUR FINDINGS

Recording the Examination—The Nervous System

> "**Mental Status:** Alert, relaxed, and cooperative. Thought process coherent. Ox3 (person, place, and time). Detailed cognitive testing deferred. **Cranial Nerves:** I—not tested; II through XII intact. **Motor:** Cerebellar—Rapid alternating movements (RAMs), finger-to-nose, heel-to-shin intact bilaterally. Gait rhythmic, with smooth alternating arm swing and stable base. Romberg—maintains balance with eyes closed. No pronator drift. **Sensory:** Sharp/dull, light touch, position, and vibration intact bilaterally. **Reflexes** (biceps, triceps, brachioradialis, knee, ankle): 2+ and symmetric with bilateral plantar responses."
>
> **OR**
>
> "**Mental Status:** Patient alert and tries to answer questions but has difficulty finding words. **Cranial Nerves:** I—not tested; II—visual acuity intact, visual fields full; III, IV, VI—extraocular movements intact; V motor—temporal and masseter strength intact; VII motor—prominent right facial droop and flattening of right nasolabial fold, left facial movements intact, sensory—taste not tested; VIII—hearing intact bilaterally to whispered voice; IX, X—gag intact; XI—strength of sternomastoid and trapezius muscles 5/5; XII—tongue midline. **Motor:** increased tone and spasticity. Gait—unable to test. Cerebellar—unable to test on right due to right arm and leg weakness; RAMs, Finger → Nose, Heel → Shin intact on left, unable to perform on the right. Romberg—unable to test due to right leg weakness. Right pronator drift present. **Sensory:** decreased sensation to sharp over right face, arm, and leg; intact on the left. Stereognosis and two-point discrimination not tested. **Reflexes** (can record in two ways):

Suggests left hemispheric cerebrovascular accident in distribution of the left middle cerebral artery, with right-sided hemiparesis

	Biceps	Triceps	Brach	Knee	Ankle	Plantar
RT	4+	4+	4+	4+	4+	↑
LT	2+	2+	2+	2+	1+	↓

OR

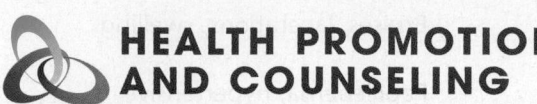

HEALTH PROMOTION AND COUNSELING

Important Topics for Health Promotion and Counseling

- Preventing stroke or transient ischemic attack (TIA)
- Reducing risk of peripheral neuropathy

Preventing Stroke and Transient Ischemic Attack (TIA). Stroke from cerebrovascular disease is the third leading cause of death in the United States and the leading cause of long-term disability in the workforce and general population.

- *Stroke* is a sudden neurologic deficit caused by cerebrovascular ischemia (80% to 85%) or hemorrhage (15% to 20%).[19,20]

- *TIA* is a sudden focal neurologic deficit defined in the past as lasting <24 hours, but more recently defined as lasting <1 hour and without underlying structural defects.[21–23] A TIA is an important harbinger of stroke—in the first 3 months after a TIA, 15% of patients will progress to stroke, especially those with diabetes, age older than 60 years, or changes in speech or motor function.[23] Risk of stroke is highest in the first 30 days after a TIA.

STROKE AT A GLANCE

Key Facts for Prevention and Patient Education[19]

- Stroke is the third leading cause of U.S. deaths after heart disease and cancer and affects more than 5,700,000 people.
- Stroke incidence and mortality are disproportionately higher in African-Americans compared to whites:
  - *Incidence, black vs. white, ages 45 to 84 years:* 6.6 vs. 3.6 per 1000 (men); 4.9 vs. 2.3 per 1000 (women)
  - *Mortality, black vs. white, ages 45 to 84 years:* 73.9 vs. 48.1 (men); 64.9 vs. 47.4 (women)
- Crude cumulative incidence of stroke is disproportionately higher in Mexican-Americans compared to non-Hispanic whites: 16.8 vs. 13.6 per 1000.
- One-year mortality after TIA is approximately 25%.
- Public awareness of stroke warning signs is high, but only 17% would call 911 if they thought someone was having a stroke.
- Stroke outcomes markedly improve if therapy is given within 3 hours of onset of symptoms; however, the median emergency-room arrival time from onset of symptoms is 3 to 6 hours.
- Physician awareness of warning signs, risk factors, and prevention remains insufficient.

Symptoms and signs of stroke depend on the vascular territory affected in the brain. The most common cause of ischemic symptoms and signs is occlusion of the *middle cerebral artery*, which causes visual field cuts and contralateral hemiparesis and sensory deficits. In the left hemisphere, occlusion of the middle cerebral artery often produces *aphasia*, and if the right hemisphere is affected the result is the person has a decreased attention to what is happening on the opposite side of the body.

See Table 20-3, pp. 664–665, Types of Stroke.

Table 20-9, p. 674, Disorders of Speech, for discussion of *aphasia*.

Stroke Warning Signs. The American Heart Association and the American Stroke Association urge patients to seek immediate care for any of the following critical warning signs:

● Sudden numbness or weakness of the face, arm, or leg

● Sudden confusion or trouble speaking or understanding

● Sudden trouble walking, dizziness, or loss of balance or coordination

● Sudden trouble seeing in one or both eyes

● Sudden severe headache

Teach these warning signs of "stroke attack" or "brain attack" to your patients, especially those with risk factors.

Stroke Risk Factors—Primary Prevention.

Primary prevention targets *modifiable risk factors for ischemic stroke*, namely, hypertension, smoking, hyperlipidemia, diabetes, excess weight, lack of exercise, and heavy alcohol use. Careful management of atrial fibrillation and asymptomatic carotid artery disease reduces disease-specific risk of stroke. To prevent hemorrhagic stroke from intracerebral hemorrhage, control of hypertension is key. Rupture of saccular aneurysms in the circle of Willis is the most common cause of hemorrhagic stroke from subarachnoid hemorrhage—risk factors are smoking, hypertension, alcohol abuse, and family history in a first-degree relative.

In Chapter 7, see Blood Pressure Classification in Adults, p. 117.

Stroke Risk Factors—Secondary Prevention.

Once a patient has experienced an ischemic stroke or TIA, focus on addressing any secondary risk factors, depending on the etiology. Causes of ischemic stroke are atherosclerotic large vessel disease, cardiac emboli secondary to atrial fibrillation or cardiac defect, small vessel lacunar disease, other/unusual causes, and idiopathic (no mechanism identified). Note that younger patients are most likely to have strokes that are cryptogenic or from other or unusual causes such as collagen vascular disease, arterial dissection, fibromuscular dysplasia, or cocaine and illicit drug use. Learn the indications for preventive therapy with aspirin or coumadin.[24]

See Table 20-3, pp. 664–665, Types of Stroke, for further discussion of lacunar and other types of stroke.

● Stroke Risk Factors—Primary Prevention for Ischemic Stoke

Behavioral Risk Factors

- **Hypertension**
  Hypertension is the leading determinant of risk for both ischemic and hemorrhagic stroke. Patients with blood pressure <120/80 have half the lifetime risk of stroke compared to those with hypertension.[19] Optimal blood pressure control is especially important for African-Americans because of their higher risk of stroke.[26]

- **Smoking**
  Heavy *smoking*, or smoking more than 40 cigarettes a day, doubles the risk of stroke compared to light smoking, or smoking fewer than 10 cigarettes a day. It takes 5 years for ex-smokers to drop to the same risk level as nonsmokers.

- **Hyperlipidemia**
  Growing evidence from cardiovascular studies using statin agents shows that reducing *hyperlipidemia* lowers stroke risk by 25%.[27,28]

- **Diabetes**
  Diabetes increases risk of ischemic stroke, hypertension, and hyperlipidemia. Guidelines recommend tight control to prevent the microvascular complications of diabetes, but studies do not yet consistently show that improved glucose control reduces risk of stroke. Noteworthy is the United Kingdom Prospective Diabetes Study, in which patients with hypertension and type 2 diabetes and aggressive blood pressure control had a 44% reduction in the risk of fatal and nonfatal stroke.[24,29]

- **Weight**
  Obesity doubles risk of stroke.

- **Exercise**
  As with other conditions like coronary heart disease, hypertension, and diabetes, moderate *exercise*, namely, 30 minutes of brisk walking or its equivalent on most days, reduces risk of stroke.[19] Evidence of a consistent "dose-response" benefit between amount of physical activity and stroke risk is still inconclusive.[29]

- **Alcohol use**
  Heavy alcohol use has a "direct dose-dependent effect on the risk of hemorrhagic stroke" and appears to increase risk of ischemic stroke through the interaction of its effects on hypertension, hypercoagulable states, cardiac arrhythmias, and reductions in cerebral blood flow.[24]

Disease-Specific Risk Factors

- **Atrial fibrillation**
  Atrial fibrillation increases risk of stroke 5- and 17-fold, respectively, compared to controls.[24] Risk reductions for ischemic stroke with warfarin therapy at international normalized ratio (INR) values of 2 to 3 and with aspirin therapy are 68% and 20%, respectively, but individual risk levels vary. When considering antithrombotic therapy, experts recommend individual risk stratification into high-, moderate-, and low-risk groups to balance risk of stroke against risk of bleeding. Improved risk assessment tools using community-based scoring systems are now emerging.[30-32] Patients with atrial fibrillation at highest risk for stroke are those with additional risk factors: prior TIA

(continued)

● **Stroke Risk Factors—Primary Prevention for Ischemic Stoke** (continued)

or stroke, hypertension, diabetes, poor left ventricular function, rheumatic mitral valve disease, and female gender if older than 75 years.

Disease-Specific Risk Factors

● Carotid artery disease

The prevalence of *carotid artery disease* from atherosclerotic disease of the extracranial carotid arteries in the U.S. population older than 65 years is 1%.[33] Carotid endarterectomy in asymptomatic patients with more than 60% carotid stenosis reduces stroke risk over 5 years from 11% to 5%, even with a perioperative stroke or death rate of 3%.[33,34] No single risk factor or risk assessment tool currently identifies people with clinically significant high-risk carotid disease. In 2007 the U.S. Preventive Services Task Force recommended against screening in the general population because of risks of false positives using carotid ultrasound for screening, risk of stroke using angiography, and the need for surgical risk of endarterectomy to be <3%.[35]

Reducing Risk of Peripheral Neuropathies. Diabetes is the most common cause of peripheral neuropathy, present in 10% of patients at diagnosis and rising to 50% within 5 years.[36] Diabetes causes several types of neuropathy, including a slowly progressive *distal symmetric sensorimotor polyneuropathy*, the "stocking" of the "stocking-glove" changes and the most common of the diabetic neuropathies; *autonomic dysfunction* leading to erectile dysfunction, orthostatic hypotension, and gastroparesis; *mononeuritis multiplex*, causing patchy sensory and motor deficits in at least two separate nerve areas; and *diabetic amyotrophy*, causing thigh pain and proximal lower extremity weakness, initially unilateral. Counsel patients to achieve optimal glycemic control. When HgA1C is ≤7.4%, onset of diabetic neuropathy drops by 50% to 60%.[37]

Abnormal Postures in Comatose Patients

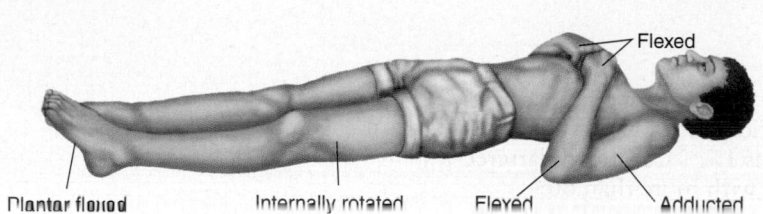

Flexed
Plantar flexed   Internally rotated   Flexed   Adducted

Decorticate Rigidity
(Abnormal Flexor Response)

In *decorticate rigidity*, the upper arms are flexed tight to the sides with elbows, wrists, and fingers flexed. The legs are extended and internally rotated. The feet are plantar flexed. This posture implies a destructive lesion of the corticospinal tracts within or very near the cerebral hemispheres. When unilateral, this is the posture of chronic spastic hemiplegia.

Hemiplegia (Early)

Sudden unilateral brain damage involving the corticospinal tract may produce a *hemiplegia* (one-sided paralysis), which early in its course is flaccid. Spasticity will develop later. The paralyzed arm and leg are slack. They fall loosely and without tone when raised and dropped to the bed. Spontaneous movements or responses to noxious stimuli are limited to the opposite side. The leg may lie externally rotated. One side of the lower face may be paralyzed, and that cheek puffs out on expiration. Both eyes may be turned away from the paralyzed side.

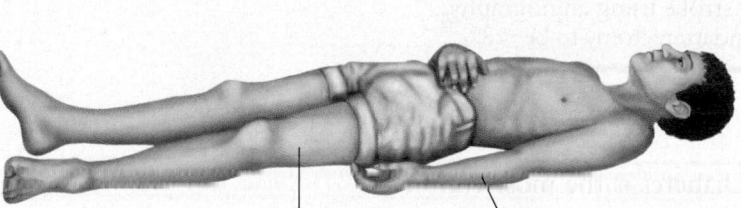

Externally rotated   Flaccid

Decerebrate Rigidity
(Abnormal Extensor Response)

In *decerebrate rigidity*, the jaws are clenched and the neck is extended. The arms are adducted and stiffly extended at the elbows, with forearms pronated, wrists and fingers flexed. The legs are stiffly *extended at the knees*, with the feet plantar flexed. This posture may occur spontaneously or only in response to external stimuli such as light, noise, or pain. It is caused by a lesion in the diencephalon, midbrain, or pons, although severe metabolic disorders such as hypoxia or hypoglycemia may also produce it.

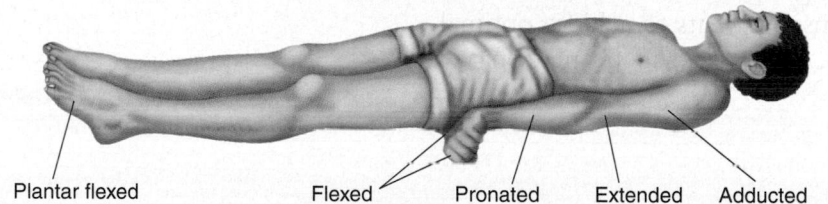

Plantar flexed   Flexed   Pronated   Extended   Adducted

TABLE
20-2
Metabolic and Structural Coma

Although there are many causes of coma, most can be classified as either *structural* or *metabolic*. Findings vary widely in individual patients; the features listed are general guidelines rather than strict diagnostic criteria. Remember that psychiatric disorders may mimic coma.

	Toxic–Metabolic	Structural
Pathophysiology	Arousal centers poisoned or critical substrates depleted	Lesion destroys or compresses brainstem arousal areas, either directly or secondary to more distant expanding mass lesions.
Clinical Features		
• Respiratory pattern	If regular, may be normal or hyperventilation. If irregular, usually Cheyne-Stokes	Irregular, especially Cheyne-Stokes or ataxic breathing. Also with selected stereotypical patterns like "apneustic" respiration (peak inspiratory arrest) or central hyperventilation
• Pupillary size and reaction	Equal, reactive to light. If *pinpoint* from opiates or cholinergics, you may need a magnifying glass to see the reaction.	Unequal or unreactive to light (fixed) *Midposition, fixed*—suggests midbrain compression
	May be unreactive if *fixed and dilated* from anticholinergics or hypothermia	*Dilated, fixed*—suggests *compression* of CN III from herniation
• Level of consciousness	Changes *after* pupils change	Changes *before* pupils change
Examples of Cause	Uremia, hyperglycemia	Epidural, subdural, or intracerebral hemorrhage
	Alcohol, drugs, liver failure	
	Hypothyroidism, hypoglycemia	Cerebral infarct or embolus
	Anoxia, ischemia	Tumor, abscess
	Meningitis, encephalitis	Brainstem infarct, tumor, or hemorrhage
	Hyperthermia, hypothermia	Cerebellar infarct, hemorrhage, tumor, or abscess

TABLE
20-3

Types of Stroke

Assessing patients with stroke involves three fundamental questions based on a careful history and detailed physical examination: *What brain area and related vascular territory explain the patient's findings? Is the stroke ischemic or hemorrhagic? If ischemic, is the mechanism thrombus or embolus?* Stroke is a medical emergency, and timing is of the essence. Answers to these questions are critical to patient outcomes and use of antithrombotic therapies in acute ischemic stroke.

In *acute ischemic stroke*, ischemic brain injury begins with a central core of very low perfusion and often irreversible cell death. This core is surrounded by an *ischemic penumbra* of metabolically disturbed cells that are still potentially viable, depending on restoration of blood flow and duration of ischemia. Because most irreversible damage occurs in the first 3 to 6 hours after onset of symptoms, therapies targeted to the 3-hour window achieve the best outcomes, with recovery in up to 50% of patients in some studies.[20]

Clinical Features and Vascular Territories of Stroke

Clinical Finding	Vascular Territory	Additional Comments
Contralateral leg weakness	*Anterior circulation*—anterior cerebral artery (ACA)	Includes stem of circle of Willis connecting internal carotid artery to ACA, and the segment distal to ACA and its anterior choroidal branch
Contralateral face, arm > leg weakness, sensory loss, vision field cut, aphasia (left MCA) or neglect, apraxia (right MCA)	*Anterior circulation*—middle cerebral artery (MCA)	Largest vascular bed for stroke
Contralateral motor or sensory deficit without cortical signs	*Subcortical circulation*—lenticulostriate deep penetrating branches of MCA	Small vessel subcortical *lacunar infarcts* in internal capsule, thalamus, or brainstem. Four common syndromes: pure motor hemiparesis; pure sensory hemianesthesia; ataxic hemiparesis; clumsy hand–dysarthria syndrome
Contralateral field cut	*Posterior circulation*—posterior cerebral artery (PCA)	Includes paired vertebral and basilar artery, paired posterior cerebral arteries. Bilateral PCA infarction causes cortical blindness but preserved pupillary light reaction.
Dysphagia, dysarthria, tongue/palate deviation and/or ataxia with crossed sensory/motor deficits (= ipsilateral face with contralateral body)	*Posterior circulation*—brainstem, vertebral, or basilar artery branches	
Oculomotor deficits and/or ataxia with crossed sensory/motor deficits	*Posterior circulation*—basilar artery	Complete basilar artery occlusion—"locked-in syndrome" with intact consciousness but with inability to speak and quadriplegia

*Learn to differentiate cortical from subcortical involvement. *Subcortical or lacunar syndromes* do not affect higher cognitive function, language, or visual fields.
(Source: Adapted from American College of Physicians. Stroke, in Neurology. Medical Knowledge Self-Assessment Program (MKSAP) 14. Philadelphia: American College of Physicians, 2006. pp. 52–68.)

(table continues on page 665)

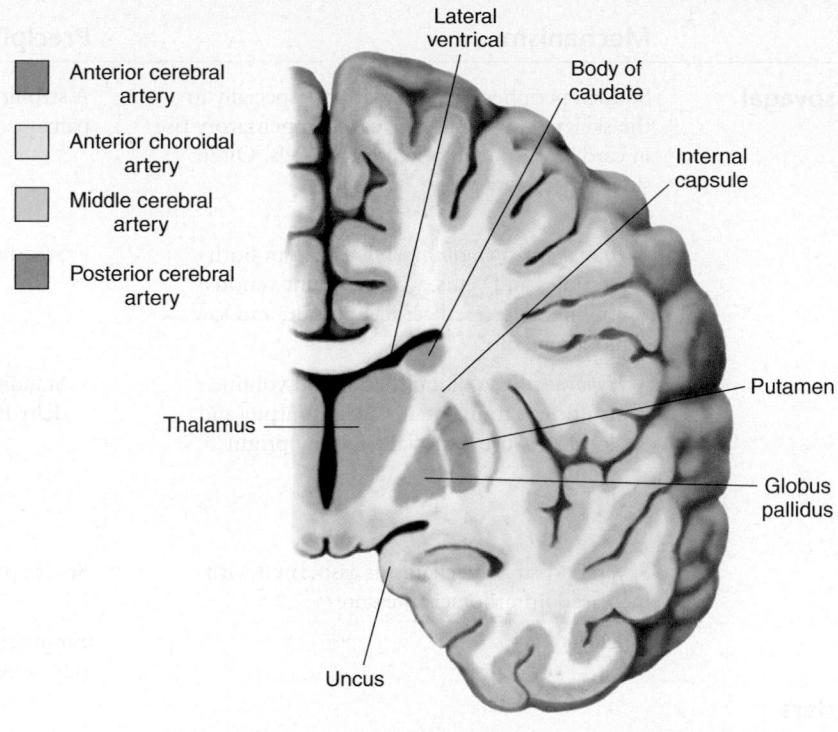

Lateral ventrical

Body of caudate

Internal capsule

Anterior cerebral artery

Anterior choroidal artery

Middle cerebral artery

Posterior cerebral artery

Putamen

Thalamus

Globus pallidus

Uncus

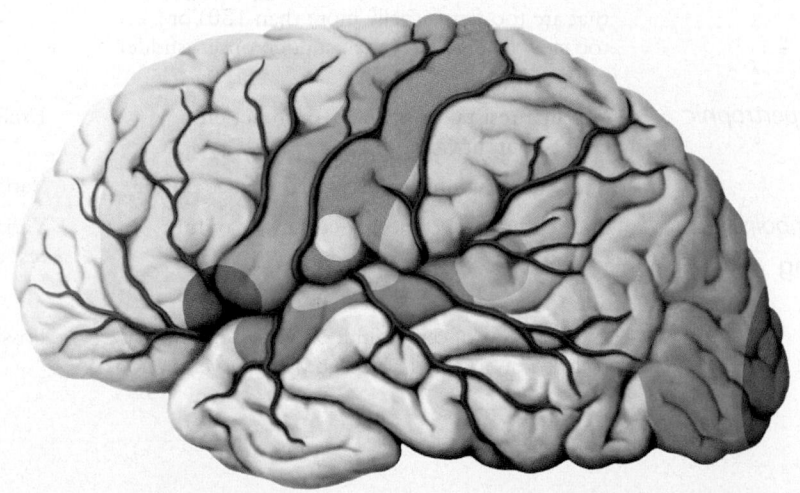

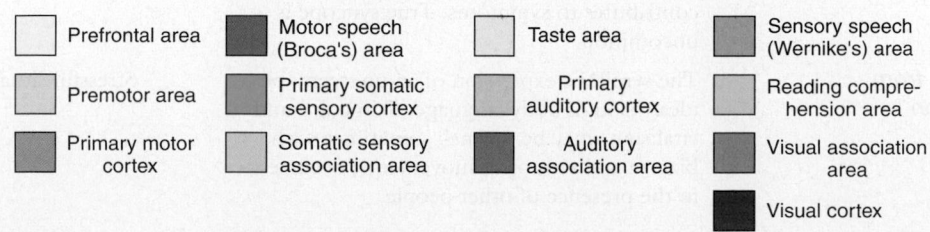

Prefrontal area

Premotor area

Primary motor cortex

Motor speech (Broca's) area

Primary somatic sensory cortex

Somatic sensory association area

Taste area

Primary auditory cortex

Auditory association area

Sensory speech (Wernike's) area

Reading comprehension area

Visual association area

Visual cortex

Syncope and Similar Disorders[38,39]

Problem	Mechanism	Precipitating Factors
Vasodepressor or Vasovagal Syncope *(the common faint)*	Sudden peripheral vasodilatation, especially in the skeletal muscles, without a compensatory rise in cardiac output. Blood pressure falls. Often slow onset, slow offset	A strong emotion such as fear or pain
Postural *(orthostatic)* **Hypotension**	• *Inadequate vasoconstrictor reflexes* in both arterioles and veins, with resultant venous pooling, decreased cardiac output, and low blood pressure	• Standing up
	• *Hypovolemia,* a diminished blood volume insufficient to maintain cardiac output and blood pressure, especially in the upright position	• Standing up after hemorrhage or dehydration
Cough Syncope	Several possible mechanisms associated with increased intrathoracic pressure	Severe paroxysm of coughing
Micturition Syncope	Unclear	Emptying the bladder after getting out of bed to void
Cardiovascular Disorders		
Arrhythmias	Decreased cardiac output secondary to rhythms that are too fast (usually more than 180) or too slow (<35–40). Often sudden onset, sudden offset	A sudden change in rhythm
Aortic Stenosis and Hypertrophic Cardiomyopathy	Vascular resistance falls with exercise, but cardiac output cannot rise.	Exercise
Myocardial Infarction	Sudden arrhythmia or decreased cardiac output	Variable
Massive Pulmonary Embolism	Sudden hypoxia or decreased cardiac output	Variable, including prolonged bed rest and clotting disorders
Disorders Resembling Syncope		
Hypocapnia due to Hyperventilation	Constriction of cerebral blood vessels secondary to hypocapnia that is induced by hyperventilation	Possibly a stressful situation
Hypoglycemia	Insufficient glucose to maintain cerebral metabolism; secretion of epinephrine contributes to symptoms. True syncope is uncommon.	Variable, including fasting
Hysterical Fainting from Conversion Reaction	The symbolic expression of an unacceptable idea through body language. Skin color and vital signs may be normal; sometimes with bizarre and purposive movements; occurrence in the presence of other people.	Stressful situation

Predisposing Factors	Prodromal Manifestations	Postural Associations	Recovery
Fatigue, hunger, a hot humid environment	Restlessness, weakness, pallor, nausea, salivation, sweating, yawning	Usually occurs when standing, possibly when sitting	Prompt return of consciousness when lying down, but pallor, weakness, nausea, and slight confusion may persist for a time.
• Peripheral neuropathies and disorders affecting the autonomic nervous system; drugs such as antihypertensives and vasodilators; prolonged bed rest	• Often none	• Occurs soon after the person stands up	• Prompt return to normal when lying down
• Bleeding from the GI tract or trauma, potent diuretics, vomiting, diarrhea, polyuria	• Light-headedness and palpitations (tachycardia) on standing up	• Usually occurs soon after the person stands up	• Improvement on lying down
Chronic bronchitis in a muscular man	Often none except for cough	May occur in any position	Prompt return to normal
Nocturia, usually in elderly or adult men	Often none	Standing to void	Prompt return to normal
Heart disease and old age decrease tolerance of abnormal rhythms.	Often none	May occur in any position	Prompt return to normal unless brain damage has resulted
Cardiac disorders	Often none. Onset is sudden.	Occurs with or after exercise	Usually a prompt return to normal
Coronary artery disease	Often none	May occur in any position	Variable
Deep vein thrombosis	Often none	May occur in any position	Variable
A predisposition to anxiety attacks and hyperventilation	Dyspnea, palpitations, chest discomfort, numbness and tingling of the hands and around the mouth lasting for several minutes. Consciousness is often maintained.	May occur in any position	Slow improvement as hyperventilation ceases
Insulin therapy and a variety of metabolic disorders	Sweating, tremor, palpitations, hunger, headache, confusion, abnormal behavior, coma	May occur in any position	Variable, depending on severity and treatment
Hysterical personality traits	Variable	A slump to the floor, often from a standing position without injury	Variable, may be prolonged, often with fluctuating responsiveness

TABLE
20-5

Seizure Disorders[11]

Partial Seizures

Partial seizures start with focal manifestations. They are further divided into *simple partial seizures,* which do not impair consciousness, and *complex partial seizures,* which do. *Partial seizures may become generalized.* Partial seizures of all kinds usually indicate a structural lesion in the cerebral cortex, such as a scar, tumor, or infarction. The quality of such seizures helps the clinician to localize the causative lesion in the brain.

Problem	Clinical Manifestations	Postictal (*postseizure*) State
Partial Seizures		
Simple Partial Seizures		
• With motor symptoms		
Jacksonian	Tonic and then clonic movements that start unilaterally in the hand, foot, or face and spread to other body parts on the same side	Normal consciousness
Other motor	Turning of the head and eyes to one side, or tonic and clonic movements of an arm or leg without the jacksonian spread	Normal consciousness
• With sensory symptoms	Numbness, tingling; simple visual, auditory, or olfactory hallucinations such as flashing lights, buzzing, or odors	Normal consciousness
• With autonomic symptoms	A "funny feeling" in the epigastrium, nausea, pallor, flushing, light-headedness	Normal consciousness
• With psychiatric symptoms	Anxiety or fear; feelings of familiarity (déjà vu) or unreality; dreamy states; fear or rage; flashback experiences; more complex hallucinations	Normal consciousness
Complex Partial Seizures	The seizure may or may not start with the autonomic or psychic symptoms outlined above. Consciousness is impaired, and the person appears confused. Automatisms include automatic motor behaviors such as chewing, smacking the lips, walking about, and unbuttoning clothes; also more complicated and skilled behaviors such as driving a car.	The patient may remember initial autonomic or psychic symptoms (which are then termed an *aura*), but is amnesic for the rest of the seizure. Temporary confusion and headache may occur.
Partial Seizures That Become Generalized	Partial seizures that become generalized resemble tonic–clonic seizures. Unfortunately, the patient may not recall the focal onset, and observers may overlook it.	Two attributes indicate a partial seizure that has become generalized: (1) the recollection of an *aura* and (2) a *unilateral* neurologic deficit during the postictal period.

(Source: Commission on Classification and Terminology of the International League Against Epilepsy. Proposal for revised classification of epilepsies and epileptic syndromes. Epilepsia 30:389–399, 1989. See also International League against Epilepsy. A proposed diagnostic scheme for people with epileptic seizures and with epilepsy: report of the ILAE Task Force on Classification and Terminology. Available at: http://www.ilae-epilepsy.org/Visitors/Centre/ctf/overview.cfm#2. Accessed June 29, 2011.)

(*table continues on page 669*)

Generalized Seizures and Pseudoseizures

Generalized seizures begin with bilateral body movements, impairment of consciousness, or both. They suggest a widespread, bilateral cortical disturbance that may be either hereditary or acquired. When generalized seizures of the tonic–clonic (grand mal) variety start in childhood or young adulthood, they are often hereditary. When tonic–clonic seizures begin after age 30, suspect either a partial seizure that has become generalized or a general seizure caused by a toxic or metabolic disorder. Toxic and metabolic causes include withdrawal from alcohol or other sedative drugs, uremia, hypoglycemia, hyperglycemia, hyponatremia, and bacterial meningitis.

Problem	Clinical Manifestations	Postictal (*postseizure*) State
Generalized Seizures		
Tonic–Clonic Convulsion (grand mal) *	The person loses consciousness suddenly, sometimes with a cry, and the body stiffens into tonic extensor rigidity. Breathing stops, and the person becomes cyanotic. A clonic phase of rhythmic muscular contraction follows. Breathing resumes and is often noisy, with excessive salivation. Injury, tongue biting, and urinary incontinence may occur.	Confusion, drowsiness, fatigue, headache, muscular aching, and sometimes the temporary persistence of bilateral neurologic deficits such as hyperactive reflexes and Babinski responses. The person has amnesia for the seizure and recalls no aura.
Absence	A sudden brief lapse of consciousness, with momentary blinking, staring, or movements of the lips and hands but no falling. Two subtypes are recognized. *Petit mal absences* last <10 sec and stop abruptly. *Atypical absences* may last more than 10 sec.	No aura recalled. In petit mal absences, a prompt return to normal; in atypical absences, some postictal confusion
Atonic Seizure, or Drop Attack	Sudden loss of consciousness with falling but no movements. Injury may occur.	Either a prompt return to normal or a brief period of confusion
Myoclonus	Sudden, brief, rapid jerks, involving the trunk or limbs. Associated with a variety of disorders	Variable
Pseudoseizures		
May mimic seizures but are due to a conversion reaction (a psychological disorder)	The movements may have personally symbolic significance and often do not follow a neuroanatomic pattern. Injury is uncommon.	Variable

Febrile convulsions that resemble brief tonic–clonic seizures may occur in infants and young children. They are usually benign but occasionally may be the first manifestation of a seizure disorder.

TABLE
20-6

Tremors and Involuntary Movements[12,13]

Tremors: Tremors are relatively rhythmic oscillatory movements, which may be roughly subdivided into three groups: resting (or static) tremors, postural tremors, and intention tremors.

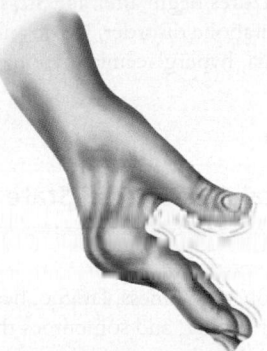

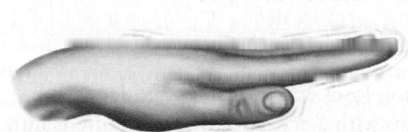

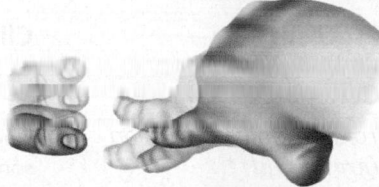

Resting (Static) Tremors

These tremors are most prominent at rest, and may decrease or disappear with voluntary movement. Illustrated is the common, relatively slow, fine, pill-rolling tremor of parkinsonism, about 5 per second.

Postural (Action) Tremors

These tremors appear when the affected part is actively maintaining a posture. Examples include the fine rapid tremor of hyperthyroidism, the tremors of anxiety and fatigue, and benign essential (and sometimes familial) tremor. Tremor may worsen somewhat with intention.

Intention Tremors

Intention tremors, absent at rest, appear with activity and often get worse as the target is neared. Causes include disorders of cerebellar pathways, as in multiple sclerosis.

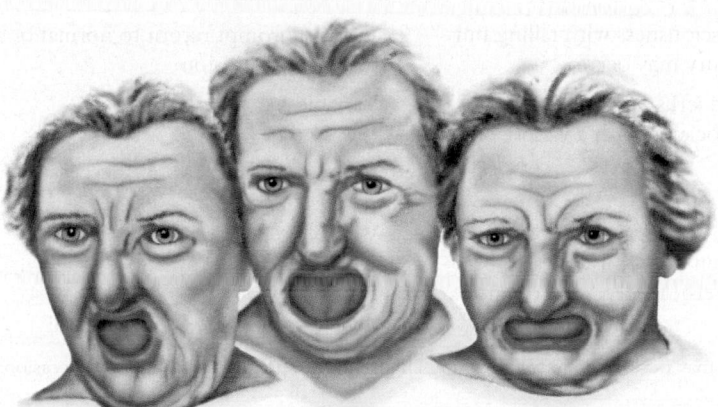

Oral–Facial Dyskinesias

Oral–facial dyskinesias are rhythmic, repetitive, bizarre movements that chiefly involve the face, mouth, jaw, and tongue: grimacing, pursing of the lips, protrusions of the tongue, opening and closing of the mouth, and deviations of the jaw. The limbs and trunk are involved less often. These movements may be a late complication of psychotropic drugs such as phenothiazines, termed *tardive* (late) dyskinesias. They also occur in long-standing psychoses, in some elderly individuals, and in some edentulous persons (without teeth).

(table continues on page 671)

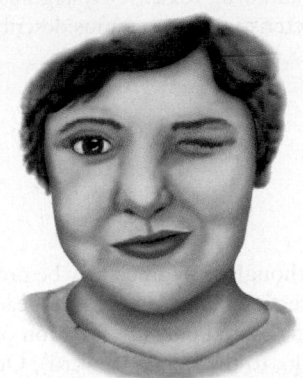

Tics

Tics are brief, repetitive, stereotyped, coordinated movements occurring at irregular intervals. Examples include repetitive winking, grimacing, and shoulder shrugging. Causes include Tourette syndrome and drugs such as phenothiazines and amphetamines.

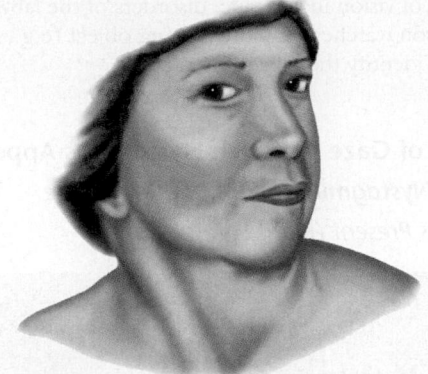

Dystonia

Dystonic movements are similar to athetoid movements, but often involve larger portions of the body, including the trunk. Grotesque, twisted postures may result. Causes include drugs such as phenothiazines, primary torsion dystonia, and as illustrated, spasmodic torticollis.

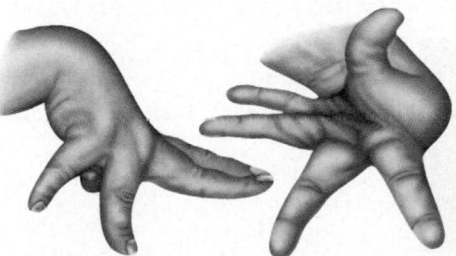

Athetosis

Athetoid movements are slower and more twisting and writhing than choreiform movements, and have a larger amplitude. They most commonly involve the face and the distal extremities. Athetosis is often associated with spasticity. Causes include cerebral palsy.

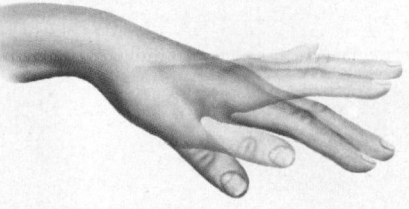

Chorea

Choreiform movements are brief, rapid, jerky, irregular, and unpredictable. They occur at rest or interrupt normal coordinated movements. Unlike tics, they seldom repeat themselves. The face, head, lower arms, and hands are often involved. Causes include Sydenham chorea (with rheumatic fever) and Huntington disease.

TABLE
20-7

Nystagmus

Nystagmus is a rhythmic oscillation of the eyes, analogous to a tremor in other parts of the body. Its causes are multiple, including impairment of vision in early life, disorders of the labyrinth and the cerebellar system, and drug toxicity. Nystagmus occurs normally when a person watches a rapidly moving object (e.g., a passing train). Study the characteristics of nystagmus described in this table to correctly identify the type of nystagmus.

Direction of Gaze in Which Nystagmus Appears

Example: Nystagmus on Right Lateral Gaze

Nystagmus Present (Right Lateral Gaze)

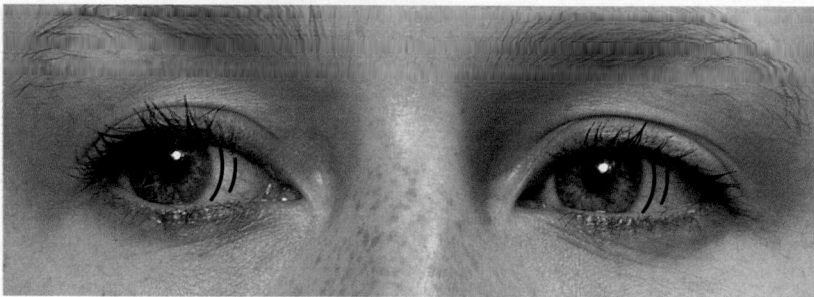

Although nystagmus may be present in all directions of gaze, it may appear or become accentuated only on deviation of the eyes (e.g., to the side or upward). On extreme lateral gaze, the normal person may show a few beats resembling nystagmus. Avoid making assessments in such extreme positions, and *observe for nystagmus only within the field of full binocular vision.*

Nystagmus Not Present (Left Lateral Gaze)

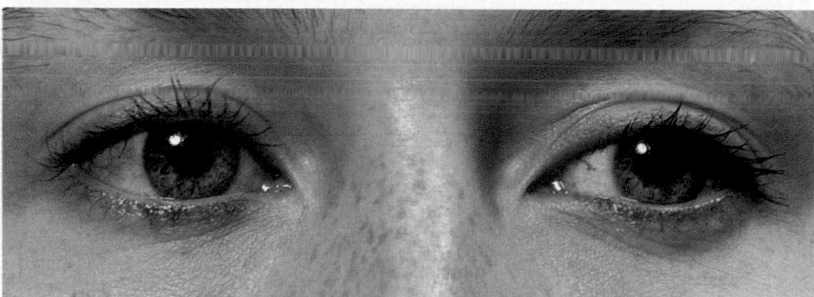

Direction of the Quick and Slow Components

Example: Left-Beating Nystagmus—a Quick Jerk to the Left in Each Eye, Then a Slow Drift to the Right

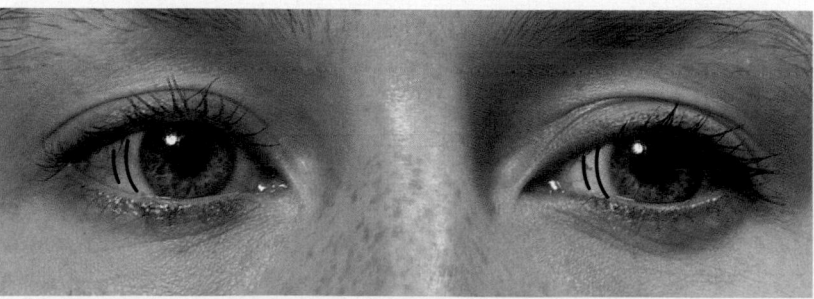

Nystagmus usually has both slow and fast movements, but *is defined by its fast phase.* For example, if the eyes jerk quickly to the patient's left and drift back slowly to the right, the patient is said to have *left-beating nystagmus.* Occasionally, nystagmus consists only of coarse oscillations without quick and slow components. It is then said to be *pendular.*

Types of Facial Paralysis

Facial weakness or paralysis may result either (1) from a peripheral lesion of CN VII, the facial nerve, anywhere from its origin in the pons to its periphery in the face, or (2) from a central lesion involving the upper motor neuron system between the cortex and the pons. A peripheral lesion of CN VII, exemplified here by a Bell palsy, is compared with a central lesion, exemplified by a left hemispheric cerebrovascular accident. These can be distinguished by their different effects on the upper part of the face.

The lower part of the face normally is controlled by upper motor neurons located on only one side of the cortex—the opposite side. *Left-sided damage to these pathways, as in a stroke, paralyzes the right lower face.* The upper face, however, is controlled by pathways from both sides of the cortex. Even though the upper motor neurons on the left are destroyed, others on the right remain, and the right upper face continues to function fairly well.

CN VII—Peripheral Lesion

Peripheral nerve damage to CN VII paralyzes the entire right side of the face, including the forehead.

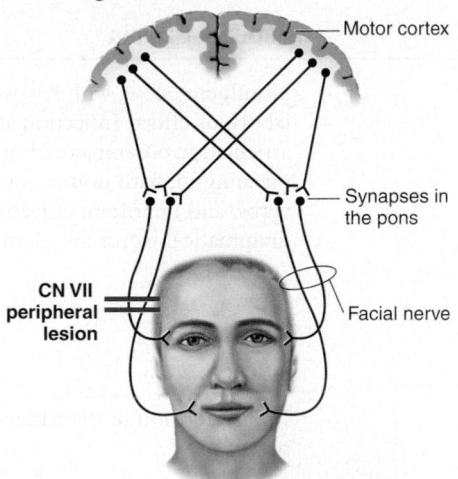

Motor cortex

Synapses in the pons

CN VII peripheral lesion

Facial nerve

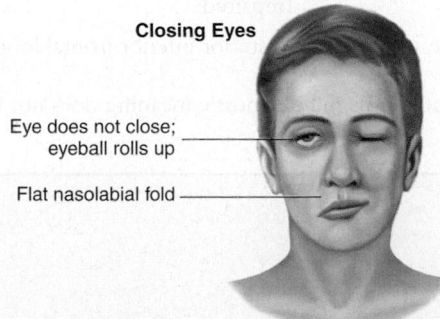

Closing Eyes

Eye does not close; eyeball rolls up

Flat nasolabial fold

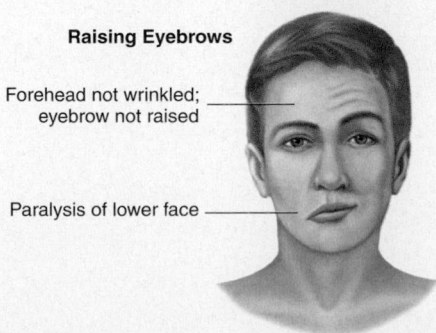

Raising Eyebrows

Forehead not wrinkled; eyebrow not raised

Paralysis of lower face

CN VII—Central Lesion

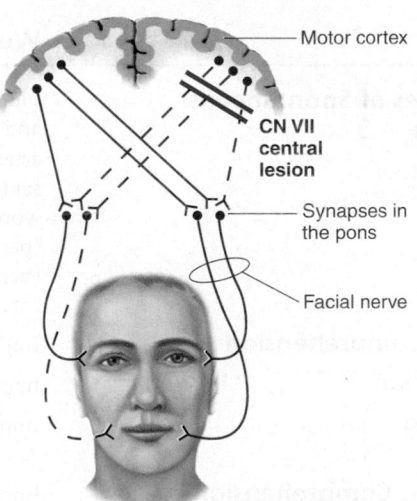

Motor cortex

CN VII central lesion

Synapses in the pons

Facial nerve

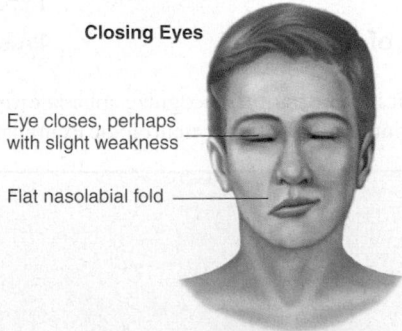

Closing Eyes

Eye closes, perhaps with slight weakness

Flat nasolabial fold

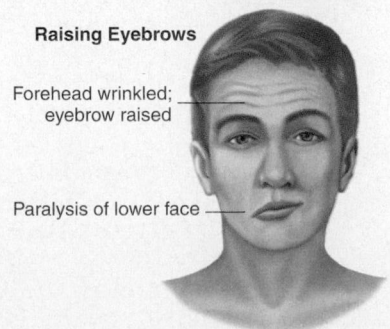

Raising Eyebrows

Forehead wrinkled; eyebrow raised

Paralysis of lower face

TABLE
20-9

Disorders of Speech

Disorders of speech fall into three groups: those affecting (1) the voice, (2) the articulation of words, and (3) the production and comprehension of language.

Aphonia refers to a loss of voice that accompanies disease affecting the larynx or its nerve supply. *Dysphonia* refers to less severe impairment in the volume, quality, or pitch of the voice. For example, a person may be hoarse or only able to speak in a whisper. Causes include laryngitis, laryngeal tumors, and a unilateral vocal cord paralysis (cranial nerve X).

Dysarthria refers to a defect in the muscular control of the speech apparatus (lips, tongue, palate, or pharynx). Words may be nasal, slurred, or indistinct, but the central symbolic aspect of language remains intact. Causes include motor lesions of the central or peripheral nervous system, parkinsonism, and cerebellar disease.

Aphasia refers to a disorder in producing or understanding language. It is often caused by lesions in the dominant cerebral hemisphere, usually the left.

Compared below are two common types of aphasia: (1) Wernicke, a fluent (receptive) aphasia, and (2) Broca, a nonfluent (or expressive) aphasia. There are other less common kinds of aphasia, which are distinguished by differing responses on the specific tests listed. Neurologic consultation is usually indicated.

	Wernicke Aphasia	Broca Aphasia
Qualities of Spontaneous Speech	Fluent; often rapid, voluble, and effortless. Inflection and articulation are good, but sentences lack meaning and words are malformed (paraphasias) or invented (neologisms). Speech may be totally incomprehensible.	Nonfluent; slow, with few words and laborious effort. Inflection and articulation are impaired but words are meaningful, with nouns, transitive verbs, and important adjectives. Small grammatical words are often dropped.
Word Comprehension	Impaired	Fair to good
Repetition	Impaired	Impaired
Naming	Impaired	Impaired, though the patient recognizes objects
Reading Comprehension	Impaired	Fair to good
Writing	Impaired	Impaired
Location of Lesion	Posterior superior temporal lobe	Posterior inferior frontal lobe

Although it is important to recognize aphasia early in the encounter with a patient, its full diagnostic meaning does not become clear until integrated with the neurologic examination.

TABLE
20-10

Abnormalities of Gait and Posture

Spastic Hemiparesis

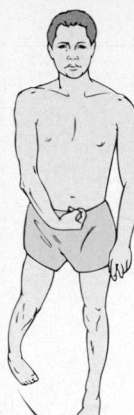

Seen in corticospinal tract lesion in stroke, causing poor control of flexor muscles during swing phase. Affected arm is flexed, immobile, and held close to the side, with elbow, wrists, and interphalangeal joints flexed. Affected leg extensors spastic; ankle plantar flexed and inverted. Patients may drag toe, circle leg stiffly outward and forward (*circumduction*), or lean trunk to contralateral side to clear affected leg during walking.[15]

Scissors Gait

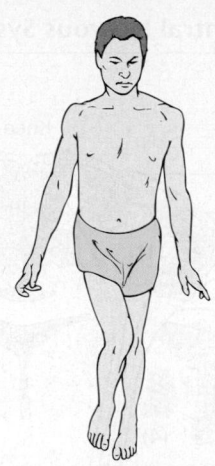

Seen in spinal cord disease causing bilateral lower extremity spasticity, including adductor spasm, and abnormal proprioception. Gait is stiff. Patients advance each leg slowly, and the thighs tend to cross forward on each other at each step. Steps are short. Patients appear to be walking through water.

Steppage Gait

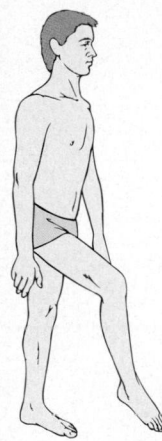

Seen in foot drop, usually secondary to peripheral motor unit disease. Patients either drag the feet or lift them high, with knees flexed, and bring them down with a slap onto the floor, thus appearing to be walking up stairs. They cannot walk on their heels. The steppage gait may involve one or both legs. Tibialis anterior and toe extensors are weak.

Parkinsonian Gait

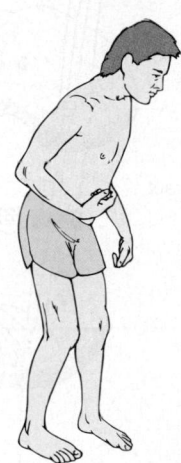

Seen in the basal ganglia defects of Parkinson disease. Posture is stooped, with flexion of head, arms, hips, and knees. Patients are slow getting started. Steps are short and shuffling, with involuntary hastening (*festination*). Arm swings are decreased, and patients turn around stiffly—"all in one piece." Postural control is poor (*retropulsion*).

Cerebellar Ataxia

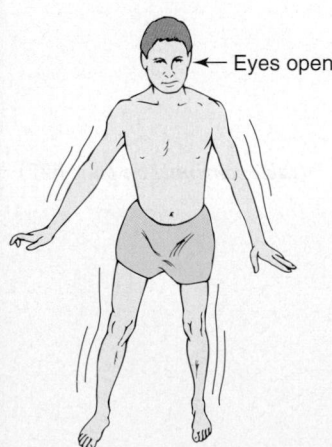

← Eyes opened

Seen in disease of the cerebellum or associated tracts. Gait is staggering, unsteady, and wide based, with exaggerated difficulty on turns. Patients cannot stand steadily with feet together, whether eyes are open or closed. Other cerebellar signs are present such as dysmetria, nystagmus, and intention tremor.

Sensory Ataxia

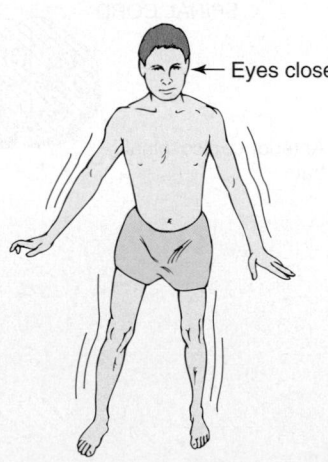

← Eyes closed

Seen in loss of position sense in the legs (with polyneuropathy or posterior column damage). Gait is unsteady and wide based (with feet wide apart). Patients throw their feet forward and outward and bring them down, first on the heels and then on the toes, with a double tapping sound. They watch the ground for guidance when walking. With eyes closed, they cannot stand steadily with feet together (positive Romberg sign), and the staggering gait worsens.

TABLE
20-11

Disorders of the Central and Peripheral Nervous Systems

Central Nervous System Disorders

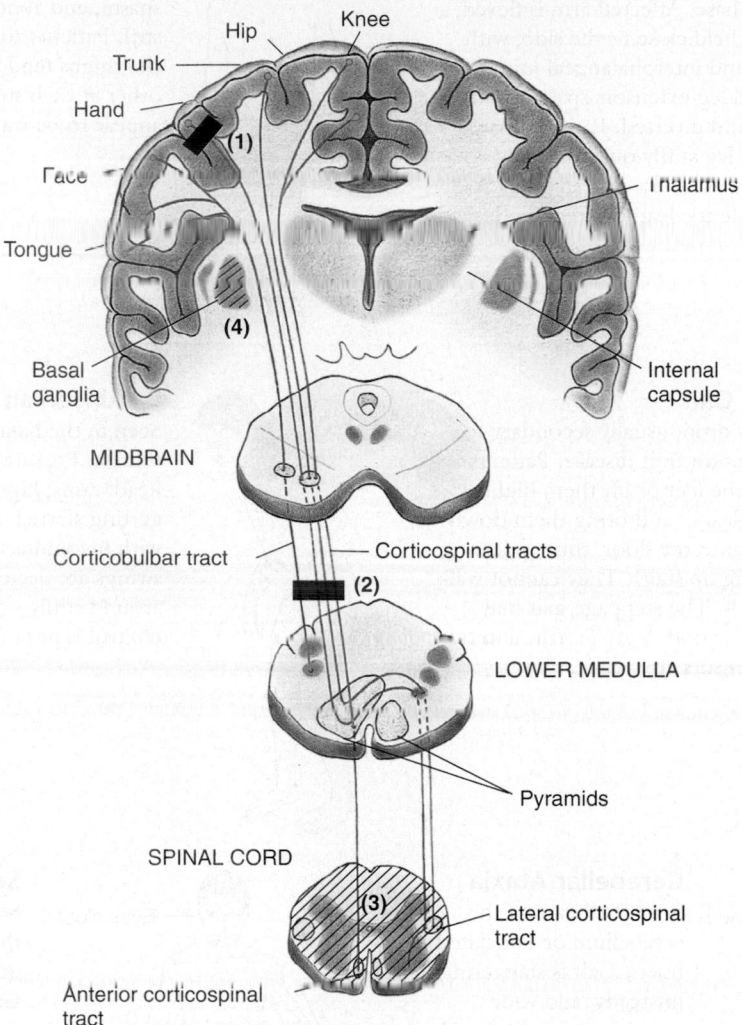

Hip
Knee
Trunk
Hand
Face
Tongue

(1)

Thalamus

Basal
ganglia

(4)

Internal
capsule

MIDBRAIN

Corticobulbar tract

Corticospinal tracts

(2)

LOWER MEDULLA

Pyramids

SPINAL CORD

(3)

Lateral corticospinal
tract

Anterior corticospinal
tract

(table continues on page 677)

Central Nervous System Disorders

Location of Lesion	Typical Findings			
	Motor	*Sensory*	*Deep Tendon Reflexes*	*Examples of Cause*
Cerebral Cortex (1)	Chronic contralateral corticospinal-type weakness and spasticity. Flexion is stronger than extension in the arm, plantar flexion is stronger than dorsiflexion in the foot, and the leg is externally rotated at the hip.	Contralateral sensory loss in the limbs and trunk on the same side as the motor deficits	↑	Cortical stroke
Brainstem (2)	Weakness and spasticity as above, plus cranial nerve deficits such as diplopia (from weakness of the extraocular muscles) and dysarthria	Variable; no typical sensory findings	↑	Brainstem stroke, acoustic neuroma
Spinal Cord (3)	Weakness and spasticity as above, but often affecting both sides (when cord damage is bilateral), causing paraplegia or quadriplegia depending on the level of injury	Dermatomal sensory deficit on the trunk bilaterally at the level of the lesion, and sensory loss from tract damage below the level of the lesion	↑	Trauma, causing cord compression
Subcortical Gray Matter: Basal Ganglia (4)	Slowness of movement (bradykinesia), rigidity, and tremor	Sensation not affected	Normal or ↓	Parkinsonism
Cerebellar (not illustrated)	Hypotonia, ataxia, and other abnormal movements, including nystagmus, dysdiadochokinesis, and dysmetria	Sensation not affected	Normal or ↓	Cerebellar stroke, brain tumor

(table continues on page 678)

Peripheral Nervous System Disorders

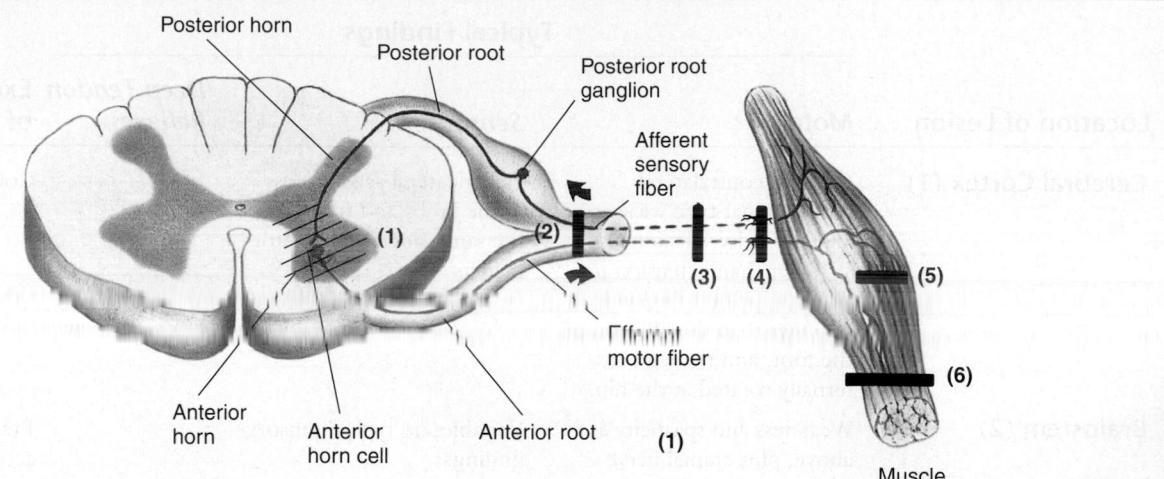

Posterior horn

Posterior root

Posterior root ganglion

Afferent sensory fiber

Anterior horn

Anterior horn cell

Anterior root

Efferent motor fiber

Muscle

(1) (2) (3) (4) (5) (6)

Typical Findings

Location of Lesion	Motor	Sensory	Deep Tendon Reflexes	Examples of Cause
Anterior Horn Cell (1)	Weakness and atrophy in a segmental or focal pattern; fasciculations	Weakness and atrophy in a segmental or focal pattern; fasciculations	↓	Polio, amyotrophic lateral sclerosis
Spinal Roots and Nerves (2)	Weakness and atrophy in a root-innervated pattern; sometimes with fasciculations	Weakness and atrophy in a root-innervated pattern; sometimes with fasciculations	↓	Herniated cervical or lumbar disc
Peripheral Nerve—Mononeuropathy (3)	Weakness and atrophy in a peripheral nerve distribution; sometimes with fasciculations	Weakness and atrophy in a peripheral nerve distribution; sometimes with fasciculations	↓	Trauma
Peripheral Nerve—Polyneuropathy (4)	Weakness and atrophy more distal than proximal; sometimes with fasciculations	Weakness and atrophy more distal than proximal; sometimes with fasciculations	↓	Peripheral polyneuropathy of alcoholism, diabetes
Neuromuscular Junction (5)	Fatigability more than weakness	Fatigability more than weakness	Normal	Myasthenia gravis
Muscle (6)	Weakness usually more proximal than distal; fasciculations rare	Weakness usually more proximal than distal; fasciculations rare	Normal or ↓	Muscular dystrophy

TABLE
20-12

Pupils in Comatose Patients

Pupillary size, equality, and light reactions help in assessing the cause of coma and in determining the region of the brain that is impaired. Remember that unrelated pupillary abnormalities, including miotic drops for glaucoma or mydriatic drops for a better view of the ocular fundi, may have preceded the coma.

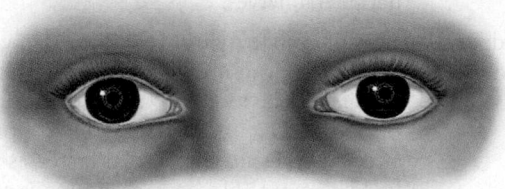

Small or Pinpoint Pupils

Bilaterally small pupils (1–2.5 mm) suggest (1) damage to the sympathetic pathways in the hypothalamus or (2) metabolic encephalopathy (a diffuse failure of cerebral function that has many causes, including drugs). Light reactions are usually normal.

Pinpoint pupils (<1 mm) suggest (1) a hemorrhage in the pons or (2) the effects of morphine, heroin, or other narcotics. The light reactions may be seen with a magnifying glass.

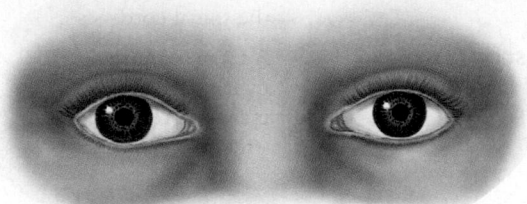

Midposition Fixed Pupils

Pupils that are in the *midposition or slightly dilated* (4–6 mm) and are *fixed to light* suggest structural damage in the midbrain.

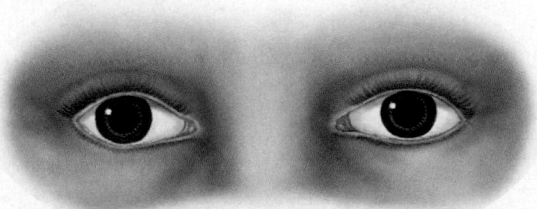

Large Pupils

Bilaterally fixed and dilated pupils may be due to severe anoxia and its sympathomimetic effects, as seen after cardiac arrest. They may also result from atropine-like agents, phenothiazines, or tricyclic antidepressants.

Bilaterally large reactive pupils may be due to cocaine, amphetamine, LSD, or other sympathetic nervous system agonists.

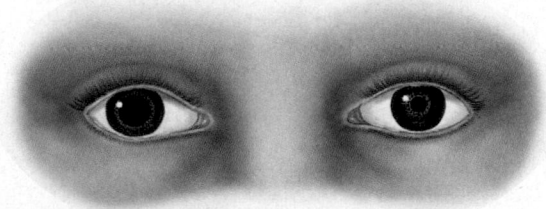

One Large Pupil

A pupil that is *fixed and dilated* warns of herniation of the temporal lobe, causing compression of the oculomotor nerve and midbrain.

TABLE
20-13

Disorders of Muscle Tone

	Spasticity	Rigidity	Flaccidity	Paratonia
Location of Lesion	Upper motor neuron of the corticospinal tract at any point from the cortex to the spinal cord	Basal ganglia system	Lower motor neuron system at any point from the anterior horn cell to the peripheral nerves	Both hemispheres, usually in the frontal lobes
Description	A form of muscular hypertonicity with increased resistance to stretch	Condition of hardness, stiffness, or inflexibility	Loss of muscle tone (*hypotonia*), causing the limb to be loose or floppy. The affected limbs may be hyperextensible or even flail-like. Flaccid muscles are also weak.	Sudden changes in tone with passive range of motion. Sudden loss of tone that increases the ease of motion is called *mitgehen* (moving with). Sudden increase in tone making motion more difficult is called *gegenhalten* (holding against).
Common Cause	Stroke, especially late or chronic stage	Parkinsonism	Guillain-Barré syndrome; also initial phase of spinal cord injury (spinal shock) or stroke	Dementia

BIBLIOGRAPHY

CITATIONS

1. Mental Health: A report from the surgeon general. www.surgeongeneral.gov/library/**mental**health/chapter2/sec2_1.html

2. Straus SE, Thorpe KE, Holroyd-Leduc J. How do I perform a lumbar puncture and analyze the results to diagnose bacterial meningitis? JAMA 296(16):2012–2022, 2006.

3. Ellenby MS, Tegtmeyer K, Lai S, et al. Lumbar puncture. N Engl J Med 355(13):e12, 2006.

4. Suarez JI, Tarr RW, Selman WR. Aneurysmal subarachnoid hemorrhage. N Engl J Med 354(4):387–396, 2006.

5. Brisman JL, Song JK, Newell DW. Cerebral aneurysms. N Engl J Med 355(9):928–939, 2006.

6. Van de Beek D, de Gans J, Spanjaard L, et al. Clinical features and prognostic factors in adults with bacterial meningitis. N Engl Med 351(18):1849–1859, 2004.

7. Savitz SI, Caplan LR. Vertebrobasilar disease. N Engl J Med 352(25):2618–2626, 2005.

8. Johnston SC. Transient ischemic attack. N Engl J Med 347(21):1687–1692, 2002.

9. Scherer K, Bedlack RS, Simel DL. Does this patient have myasthenia gravis? JAMA 293(15):1906–1914, 2005.

10. Mendell JR, Sahenk Z. Painful sensory neuropathy. N Engl J Med 348(13):1243–1255, 2003.

11. Kapoor WN. Syncope. N Engl J Med 343(25):1856–1862, 2000.

12. Browne TR, Holmes GL. Epilepsy. N Engl J Med 344(15):1145–1151, 2001.

13. Rao G, Fisch L, Srinivasan S, et al. Does this patient have Parkinson disease? JAMA 289(3):347–353, 2003.

14. Louis ED. Essential tremor. N Engl J Med 345(12):887–891, 2001.

15. Earley CJ. Restless legs syndrome. N Engl J Med 348(21):2103–2109, 2003.

16. McGee S. Evidence-Based Physical Diagnosis, 2nd ed. St. Louis: Saunders, 2005. See especially Visual field defects, pp. 663–670; The pupils, pp. 203–233; Nerves of the eye muscles (III, IV, and VI): approach to diplopia, pp. 671–689; Coordination and cerebellar testing, pp. 793–800; Miscellaneous cranial nerves, pp. 690–706; Hearing, pp. 242–249; Stance and gait, pp. 57–74; Examination of the sensory system, pp. 736–753; Examination of the reflexes, pp. 754–771; Disorders of the nerve roots, plexi, and peripheral nerves, pp. 772–792; and Meninges, pp. 277–282.

17. Teitelbaum JS, Eliasziw M, Garner M. Tests of motor function in patients suspected of having mild unilateral cerebral lesions. Can J Neurol Sci 29(4):337–344, 2002.

18. Maynard FM, Bracken MB, Creasey G, et al. International standards for neurological and functional classification of spinal cord injury. Journal of Spinal Cord Medicine;26 Suppl 1:S50-6, 2003. Available at http://www.ncbi.nlm.nih.gov/pubmed/16296564Accessed May 1, 2011.

19. Hallett M. NINDS myotatic reflex scale. Neurology 43(12):2723, 1993.

20. American Heart Association. Heart Disease and Stroke Statistics—2007 Update. Available at: http://www.americanheart.org/downloadable/heart/1166712318459HS_StatsInsideText.pdf. Accessed May 1, 2011.

21. Van der Worp HB, van Gijn J. Acute ischemic stroke. N Engl J Med 357(6):572–570, 2007.

22. Kidwell CS, Warach S. Acute ischemic cerebrovascular syndrome: diagnostic criteria. Stroke 34(12):2995–2998, 2003.

23. Albers GW, Caplan LR, Easton JD, et al. Transient ischemic attack: proposal for a new definition. N Engl J Med 347(21):1713–1716, 2002.

24. Johnston SC, Gress DR, Browner WS, et al. Short-term prognosis after emergency department diagnosis of TIA. JAMA 284(22):2901–2906, 2000.

25. Straus SE, Majumdar SR, McAlister FA. New evidence for stroke prevention: scientific review. JAMA 288(11):1388–1395, 2002.

26. American College of Physicians. Stroke in Neurology: Medical Knowledge Self-Assessment Program (MKSAP) 14. Philadelphia: American College of Physicians, 2006:52–68.

27. Douglas JG, Bakris GL, Epstein M, et al. Management of high blood pressure in African Americans: consensus statement of the Hypertension in African Americans Working Group of the International Society on Hypertension in Blacks. Arch Intern Med 163(5):525–541, 2003.

28. Corvol JC, Bouzamondo A, Sirol M, et al. Differential effects of lipid-lowering therapies on stroke prevention: a meta-analysis of randomized trials. Arch Intern Med 163(6):669–676, 2003.

29. Collins R, Armitage J, Parish S, et al. Effects of cholesterol lowering with simvastatin on stroke and other major vascular events in 20,536 people with cerebrovascular disease or other high-risk conditions. Lancet 363(9411):757–767, 2004.

30. Gorelick PB, Sacco RL, Smith DB, et al. Prevention of a first stroke: a review of the guidelines and a multidisciplinary consensus statement from the National Stroke Association. JAMA 281(12):1112–1120, 1999.

31. Waldo AL. Stroke prevention after atrial fibrillation. JAMA 290(8):1093–1094, 2003.

32. Wang TJ, Massaro JM, Levy D, et al. A risk score for predicting stroke or death in individuals with new-onset atrial fibrillation in the community. The Framingham Heart Study. JAMA 290(8):1049–1056, 2003.

33. Hart RG. Atrial fibrillation and stroke prevention. JAMA 349(11):1015–1016, 2003.

34. Wolff T, Guirgulis-Blake J, Miller T, et al. Screening for carotid artery stenosis: an update of the evidence for the U.S. Preventive Services Task Force. Ann Intern Med 147(12):860–870, 2007.

35. Halliday I, Mansfield A, Marro J, et al. Prevention of disabling and fatal strokes by successful carotid endarterectomy in patients without recent neurological symptoms: randomized controlled trial. Lancet 363(9420):1491–1502, 2004.

36. U.S. Preventive Services Task Force. Screening for Carotid Artery Stenosis. Rockville, MD: Agency for Healthcare Research and Quality, December 2007. Available at: http://www.uspreventiveservicestaskforce.org/uspstf/uspsacas.htm. Accessed May 1, 2011.

37. Boulton AJ, Vinik AT, Arezzo JC, et al. Diabetic neuropathies: a statement by the American Diabetes Association. Diabetes Care 28(4):956–962, 2005.

38. Martin CL, Albers J, Herman WH, et al. Neuropathy among the Diabetes Control and Complications Trial Cohort 8 years after trial completion. Diabetes Care 29(2):340–344, 2006.

39. Grubb BP. Neurocardiogenic syncope. N Engl J Med 352(10):1004–1010, 2004.

40. Soteriades ES, Evans JC, Larson MG, et al. Incidence and prognosis of syncope. N Engl J Med 347(12):878–885, 2002.

ADDITIONAL REFERENCES

Aids to the Examination of the Peripheral Nervous System. Medical Research Council Memorandum No. 45. London: Her Majesty's Stationery Office, 1976.

Booth CN, Boone RH, Tomlinson G, et al. Is this patient dead, vegetative, or severely neurologically impaired? JAMA 291(7):870–879, 2004.

Boyer EW, Shannon M. The serotonin syndrome. N Engl J Med 352(11):1112–1120, 2005.

Budson AE, Price BH. Memory dysfunction. N Engl J Med 352(7):692–699, 2005.

Campbell WW, DeJong RN, Haerer AF. DeJong's The Neurologic Examination, 6th ed. Philadelphia: Lippincott Williams & Wilkins, 2005.

Center for Disease Control and Prevention. Emergency Preparedness and Response. Glascow Coma Scale. Available at: http://www.bt.cdc.gov/masscasualties/gscale.asp. Accessed on July 7, 2011.

Chang BS, Lowenstein DH. Epilepsy. N Engl J Med 349(13):1257–1266, 2003.

Chimowitz MI. The accuracy of bedside neurological diagnoses. Ann Neurol 28(1):78–85, 1990.

Darouiche RO. Spinal epidural abscess. N Engl J Med 355(19):2012–2020, 2006.

Detsky ME, McDonald DR, Baerlocher MO, et al. Does this patient with headache have a migraine or need neuroimaging? JAMA 296(10):1272–1283, 2006.

Freeman R. Clinical practice: neurogenic orthostatic hypotension. N Engl J Med 358(6):615–624, 2008.

Gardner P. Prevention of meningococcal disease. N Engl J Med 355(14):1466–1473, 2006.

Gilden DH. Bell's palsy. N Engl J Med 351(13):1323–1331, 2004.

Gilman S, Manter JT, Gatz AJ, et al. Manter and Gatz's Essentials of Clinical Neuroanatomy and Neurophysiology, 10th ed. Philadelphia: FA Davis, 2003.

Gilron I, Watson PN, Cahill C, et al. Neuropathic pain: a practical guide for the clinician. CMAJ 175(3):265–275, 2006.

Griggs RC, Joynt RJ, eds. Baker and Joynt's Clinical Neurology on CD-ROM. Philadelphia: Lippincott Williams & Wilkins, 2003.

Jeha LE, Sila CA, Lederman RJ, et al. West Nile virus infection: a new acute paralytic illness. Neurology 61(1):55–59, 2003.

Katz JN. Carpal tunnel syndrome. N Engl J Med 346(23):1807–1812, 2002.

Lavan ZP. Stroke prevention through community action. J Community Nurs 19(3):4, 6, 8–10, 2005.

Louis ED. Essential tremor. N Engl J Med 345(12):887–891, 2001.

Magnetic Resonance Angiography in Relatives of Patients with Subarachnoid Hemorrhage Study Group. Risks and benefits of screening for intracranial aneurysms in first-degree relatives of patients with sporadic subarachnoid hemorrhage. N Engl J Med 341(18):1344–1350, 1999.

McGill M, Molyneaux L, Spencer R, et al. Possible sources of discrepancies in the use of the Semmes-Weinstein monofilament. Diabetes Care 22(4):598–602, 1999.

Mendell JR, Sahenk Z. Painful sensory neuropathy. N Engl J Med 348(13):1243–1294, 2003.

Nutt JG, Wooten GF. Clinical practice: diagnosis and initial management of Parkinson's disease. N Engl J Med 353(10):1021–1027, 2005.

Partanen J, Kiskanen L, Leghtinen J, et al. Natural history of peripheral neuropathic pain patients with non insulin dependent diabetes mellitus. N Engl J Med 333(2):89–94, 1995.

Plum F, Posner JB. Plum and Posner's Diagnosis of Stupor and Coma, 4th ed. Oxford, New York: Oxford University Press, 2007.

Ropper AH, Adams RD, Victor MV, et al. Adams and Victor's Principles of Neurology, 8th ed. New York: McGraw-Hill, 2005.

Rosenberg RN. Atlas of Clinical Neurology, 3rd ed. Philadelphia: Current Medicine Group, 2008.

Rowland LP, Merritt HH. Merritt's Neurology, 11th ed. Philadelphia: Lippincott Williams & Wilkins, 2005.

Saltzman CL, Rashid R, Hayes A, et al. 4.5 Gram monofilament sensation beneath both first metatarsal heads indicates protective foot sensation in diabetic patients. J Bone Joint Surg 86(4):717–723, 2004.

Tan MP, Parry SW. Vasovagal syncope in the older patient. J Am Coll Cardiol 51(6):599–606, 2008.

Tarsy D, Simon DK. Dystonia. N Engl J Med 355(8):818–829, 2006.

Teasdale G, Jennett B. Assessment of coma and impaired consciousness. Lancet 1974; 81–84.

Van de Beek D, de Gans J, Tunkel AR, et al. Community-acquired bacterial meningitis in adults. N Engl J Med 354(1):44–53, 2006.

Reproductive Systems

LEARNING OBJECTIVES

The student will:

1. Describe the anatomy and physiology of the female and male reproductive systems.
2. Conduct a focused interview to obtain patient history pertinent to the reproductive system.
3. Explain appropriate technique in inspecting and palpating external reproductive structures.
4. Discuss factors related to developmental, psychosocial, cultural, and environmental areas that affect the reproductive systems.
5. Differentiate between normal and abnormal findings in the reproductive system.
6. Accurately document subjective and objective data findings related to the reproductive system using the appropriate terminology.

The reproductive system is intimately intertwined with a person's self-concept, more so than any other body system. Cultural and religious beliefs and attitudes also influence a person's reproductive knowledge and health care. Sensitive care by all nurses is important. Although internal pelvic and rectal examinations are not within the role of the generalist nurse, it is important for the nurse to explain the anatomy and physiology of the reproductive systems, interview a patient for a thorough system history, and recognize normal and abnormal external genitalia. This knowledge will allow the nurse to educate patients about their reproductive systems in order to promote optimal health and function; assist with family planning; prevent the spread of sexually transmitted diseases; and promote early recognition of problems for referral to an advanced practice nurse or physician. It is not uncommon for a hospital or clinic patient, who has developed a relationship with the nurse, to feel more comfortable discussing intimate concerns with the nurse rather than family or the physician. For example, an adolescent may be uncomfortable discussing reproductive function with his parents. This chapter will provide the generalist nurse with the ability to carry out this role. The chapter is organized into the female reproductive system and the male reproductive system for ease of reading.

FEMALE REPRODUCTIVE SYSTEM

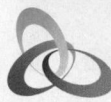 ## ANATOMY AND PHYSIOLOGY

The anatomy of the external female genitalia, or *vulva,* includes the *mons pubis,* a hair-covered fat pad overlying the symphysis pubis; the *labia majora,* rounded folds of adipose tissue; the *labia minora,* thinner pinkish-red folds that extend anteriorly to form the *prepuce;* and the *clitoris.* The *vestibule* is the boat-shaped fossa between the labia minora. In its posterior portion lies the vaginal opening, the *introitus,* which in virgins may be hidden by the *hymen.* The term *perineum,* as commonly used clinically, refers to the tissue between the introitus and the anus.

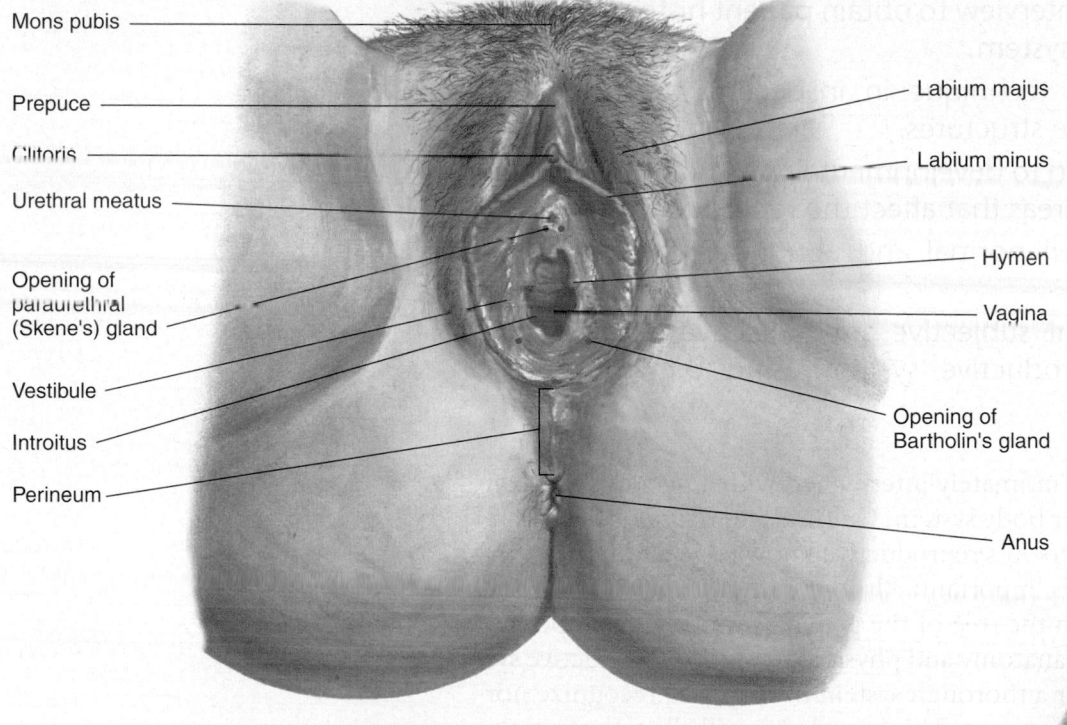

Mons pubis

Prepuce

Clitoris

Urethral meatus

Opening of paraurethral (Skene's) gland

Vestibule

Introitus

Perineum

Labium majus

Labium minus

Hymen

Vagina

Opening of Bartholin's gland

Anus

The *urethral meatus* opens into the vestibule between the clitoris and the vagina. Just posterior to it on either side lie the openings of the *para urethral* (Skene) *glands.*

The openings of *Bartholin glands* are located posteriorly on either side of the vaginal opening but are not usually visible. Bartholin glands themselves are situated more deeply. Both the Skene glands and the Bartholin glands provide lubrication during sexual intercourse.

The *vagina* is a musculomembranous tube extending upward and posteriorly between the urethra and the rectum. The vaginal mucosa lies in transverse folds, or rugae.

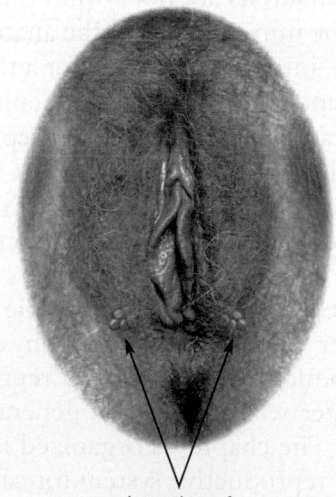

Location of Bartholin's glands

The vagina lies almost at a right angle to the *uterus*, a flattened fibromuscular structure shaped like an inverted pear. The uterus has two parts: the body, or *corpus*, and the cervix, both joined at the *isthmus*. The convex upper surface of the body is termed the uterine *fundus*. The distal cervix protrudes into the vagina, dividing the upper vagina into three recesses, the *anterior, posterior,* and *lateral fornices*.

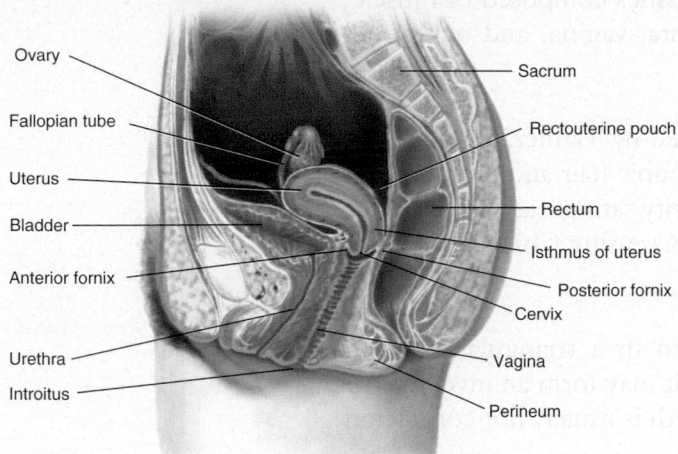

The vaginal surface of the cervix, the *ectocervix,* is seen easily with the help of a speculum. At its center is a round, oval, or slit-like depression, the *external os* of the cervix, which marks the opening into the endocervical canal. The ectocervix is covered by the plushy, red *columnar epithelium* surrounding the os, which resembles the lining of the endocervical canal, and a shiny pink *squamous epithelium* continuous with the vaginal lining. The *squamocolumnar junction* forms the boundary between these two types of epithelium. The squamocolumnar junction migrates toward the os, creating the *transformation zone*. This is the area at risk for later dysplasia and cancer, which is sampled by the Papanicolaou, or Pap smear.

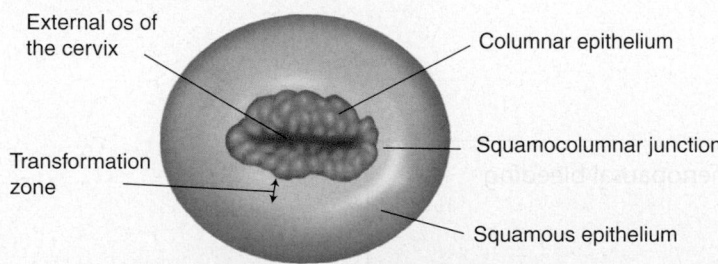

CERVICAL EPITHELIA AND TRANSFORMATION ZONE

A *fallopian tube* with a fan-like tip extends from each side of the uterus toward the ovary. The two ovaries are almond-shaped structures that vary considerably in size but average approximately 3.5 × 2 × 1.5 cm from adulthood through menopause. The ovaries are palpable on pelvic examination in roughly half of women during the reproductive years. Normally, fallopian tubes cannot be felt. The term *adnexa,* a plural Latin word meaning appendages, refers to the ovaries, tubes, and supporting tissues.

The ovaries have two primary functions: the production of ova and the secretion of hormones, including estrogen, progesterone, and testosterone. Increased hormonal secretions during puberty stimulate the growth of the uterus and its endometrial lining, enlargement of the vagina, and thickening of the vaginal epithelium. They also stimulate the development of secondary sex characteristics, including the breasts and pubic hair.

The pelvic organs are supported by a sling of tissues composed of muscle, ligaments, and fascia, through which the urethra, vagina, and rectum all pass.

Assessment of sexual maturity in girls, as classified by Tanner, depends not on internal examination, but on the growth of pubic hair and the development of breasts. Tanner's stages, or sexual maturity ratings, as they relate to pubic hair and breasts are shown in Chapter 23, Assessing Children: Infancy Through Adolescence, pp. 812, 816.

In most women, pubic hair spreads downward in a triangular pattern, pointing toward the vagina. In 10% of women, it may form an inverted triangle, pointing toward the umbilicus. This growth is usually not completed until the middle 20s or later.

Just before menarche, there is a physiologic increase in vaginal secretions—a normal change that sometimes worries a girl or her mother. As menses become established, increased secretions (*leukorrhea*) coincide with ovulation. They also accompany sexual arousal. These normal kinds of discharges must be differentiated from those of infectious processes.

Lymphatics.   Lymph from the vulva and lower vagina drains into the inguinal nodes. Lymph from the internal genitalia, including the upper vagina, flows into the pelvic and abdominal lymph nodes, which are not palpable.

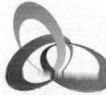 # THE HEALTH HISTORY

COMMON CONCERNS

- Menarche, menstruation, menopause, postmenopausal bleeding
- Dysmenorrhea
- Pregnancy
- Contraception
- Vulvovaginal symptoms
- Sexual preference and sexual response
- Sexually transmitted diseases

There are three parts to a woman's reproductive history: menstrual history, obstetric history, and sexual history. It is usually more comfortable for the patient if the nurse begins with the menstrual and obstetric history and saves the sexual history questions for last. However, if the woman comes to you with a sexual problem, it is appropriate to follow her lead with questions relating to the issue.

There are five phases of a woman's reproductive health: prepuberty (pre-menstruation), puberty (menarche), childbearing (menstruation), peri-menopausal, and menopausal. The nurse must incorporate the needs of each phase into the assessment process as appropriate for the individual.

When a woman reports a problem in the reproductive system, the "OLD CART" mnemonic may be used to elicit a full history of the problem. If no problem is reported, obtain a baseline reproductive history starting with the menstrual history.

Menstrual History

Menarche, Menstruation, Menopause. Learn to recognize patterns of menstrual flow, using the terms below.

THE MENSTRUAL HISTORY—HELPFUL DEFINITIONS

1. Menses—monthly flow of bloody fluid from the uterus.
   - *Menarche*—age at onset of menses
   - *Menopause*—absence of menses for 12 consecutive months, usually occurring between 48 and 55 years
   - *Perimenopause*—period of years during which a woman transitions to menopause
   - *Postmenopausal bleeding*—bleeding occurring 6 months or more after cessation of menses
   - *Amenorrhea*—absence of menses
   - *Dysmenorrhea*—pain with menses, often with bearing down, aching, or cramping sensation in the lower abdomen or pelvis
   - *Premenstrual syndrome (PMS)*—a cluster of emotional, behavioral, and physical symptoms occurring 5 days before menses for three consecutive cycles
   - *Abnormal uterine bleeding*—bleeding between menses; or infrequent, excessive, prolonged, or postmenopausal bleeding
2. Frequency—measured from the first day of one menses to the first day of the next menses. The interval between periods ranges roughly from 24 to 32 days.
3. Duration—number of days the flow lasts, usually 3 to 7 days.

Questions about *menarche, menstruation,* and *menopause* often give the nurse an opportunity to explore the patient's concerns and attitude toward her body. When talking with an adolescent girl, for example, opening questions might include: "How did you first learn about monthly periods? How did you feel when they started? Many girls worry when their periods aren't regular or come late. Has anything like that bothered you?" You can explain that girls in the United States usually begin to menstruate between the ages of 9 and 16 years, and often it takes 1 year or more before periods settle into a regular pattern. Age at menarche is variable, depending on genetic endowment, socioeconomic status, and nutrition.

For the menstrual history, ask the patient:

> How old were you when your menstrual periods began (age at *menarche*)?
> When did your last period start? If possible, the one before that?
> How often do you have periods?
> How long do they last?
>
> What color is the flow?
> How heavy is the flow?

The dates of previous periods can signal possible pregnancy or menstrual irregularities.

Unlike the normal dark red menstrual discharge, excessive flow tends to be bright red and may include "clots" (not true fibrin clots).

Flow can be assessed roughly by the number of pads or tampons used daily. Because women vary in their practices for sanitary measures, however, ask the patient whether she usually soaks a pad or tampon, spots it lightly, etc. Further, does she use more than one at a time? Does she have any bleeding between periods? Any bleeding after intercourse?

Up to 50% of women report *dysmenorrhea*, or pain with menses. Ask the patient:

> Do you have any discomfort or pain before or during your periods?
> If so, what is it like? How long does it last, and does it interfere with usual activities?
> Are there other associated symptoms?
> Dysmenorrhea may be *primary*, without an organic cause, or *secondary*, with an organic cause.

Primary dysmenorrhea results from increased prostaglandin production during the luteal phase of the menstrual cycle, when estrogen and progesterone levels decline.

Causes of *secondary dysmenorrhea* include endometriosis, adenomyosis (endometriosis in the muscular layers of the uterus), pelvic inflammatory disease, and endometrial polyps.

Premenstrual syndrome (PMS) includes emotional and behavioral symptoms such as depression, angry outbursts, irritability, anxiety, confusion, crying spells, sleep disturbance, poor concentration, and social withdrawal.[1] Ask about signs such as bloating and weight gain, swelling of the hands and feet, and generalized aches and pains. Criteria for diagnosis are symptoms and signs in the 5 days prior to menses for at least three consecutive cycles, cessation of symptoms and signs within 4 days after onset of menses, and interference with daily activities.

Amenorrhea refers to the absence of periods. Failure of periods to initiate is called *primary amenorrhea*, whereas the cessation of periods after they have been established is termed *secondary amenorrhea*. Pregnancy, lactation, and menopause are physiologic forms of the secondary type.

Other causes of *secondary amenorrhea* include low body weight from any cause, including malnutrition, anorexia nervosa, stress, chronic illness, or hypothalamic–pituitary–ovarian dysfunction.

Ask about any abnormal bleeding. The term *abnormal uterine bleeding* encompasses several patterns:

- *Polymenorrhea*, or intervals of fewer than 21 days between menses

- *Oligomenorrhea*, or infrequent bleeding

- *Menorrhagia*, or excessive flow

- *Metrorrhagia*, or intermenstrual bleeding

- Postcoital bleeding

Causes vary by age group and include pregnancy, cervical or vaginal infection, cancer, cervical or endometrial polyps or hyperplasia, fibroids, bleeding disorders, hormonal contraception or replacement therapy. *Postcoital bleeding* suggests cervical polyps or cancer, or in an older woman, atrophic vaginitis.

Menopause usually occurs between 48 and 55 years, following a period of fluctuation in pituitary secretion of follicle-stimulating hormone (FSH) and luteinizing hormone (LH) and ovarian function.[2] If the patient is *peri menopausal*, with onset of variable cycle length, ask about such vasomotor symptoms as hot flashes, flushing, and sweating. Sleep disturbances are also common. After menopause, there may be vaginal dryness and *dyspareunia*, or painful intercourse; hair loss; and mild hirsutism as the androgen-to-estrogen ratio increases. Urinary symptoms may also occur in the absence of infection because of atrophy of the urethra and urinary trigone.

Women may ask about many alternative compounds and botanicals for relief of menopause-related symptoms. Most have not been well studied or proved to be beneficial. Estrogen replacement relieves symptoms but increases risk of thrombosis.

Ask a middle-aged or older woman:

> Have you stopped menstruating? When?
> Did you have any symptoms at that time?
> Have you had any bleeding since?

Ask:

> How do (did) you feel about not having your period anymore?
> Has it affected your life in any way?
> Have you had any bleeding after menopause?

Postmenopausal bleeding in endometrial cancer, hormone replacement therapy, uterine and cervical polyps

Obstetric History

Pregnancy. Questions relating to pregnancy include:

Have you ever been pregnant? How many times?
What years did you give birth (or miscarry)?
How many living children do you have?
Have you ever had a miscarriage or an abortion? How many times?
Did you have any difficulties during pregnancy?
Follow-up includes the timing and circumstances of any abortion, whether spontaneous or induced.
How did you experience these losses?

The term *abortion* is used by health care providers to mean either a spontaneous or an induced termination of a pregnancy before the fetus is viable. *Miscarriage* is a lay term for the spontaneous loss of a pregnancy. Be sure to clarify whether an abortion is spontaneous or therapeutic (i.e., induced).

Obstetricians commonly record the pregnancy history using the "gravida-para" system.

THE GRAVIDA-PARA NOTATION

- G = gravida, or total number of pregnancies.
- P = para, or outcomes of pregnancies. After P, you will often see the notations F (full term), P (premature), A (abortion), and L (living child).

If amenorrhea suggests a *current pregnancy*, inquire about the history of intercourse and *common early symptoms:* tenderness, tingling, or increased size of the breasts; urinary frequency; nausea and vomiting; easy fatigability; and feelings that the baby is moving, usually noted at about 20 weeks. Be considerate of the patient's feelings about discussing these topics and explore them when the patient has special concerns.

Amenorrhea followed by heavy bleeding suggests a *threatened abortion* or *dysfunctional uterine bleeding* related to lack of ovulation.

Contraception. Inquire about methods of contraception used by the patient and her partner. Is the patient satisfied with the method chosen? Are there any questions about the options available?

Vulvovaginal Symptoms. The most common vulvovaginal symptoms are *vaginal discharge* and local *itching*. Use the "OLD CART" approach to obtain a thorough history. If the patient reports a discharge, inquire about its amount, color, consistency, and odor. Ask about any local *sores* or *lumps* in the vulvar area. Are they painful or not? Because patients vary in their understanding of anatomic terms, be prepared to try alternative phrasing such as "Any itching (or other symptoms) near your vagina? . . . between your legs? . . . where you urinate?"

See Table 21-1, Lesions of the Vulva, p. 711; and Table 21-2, Vaginal Discharge, p. 712.

Sexual Preference and Sexual Response. Review the Tips for Taking the Sexual History below. Using neutral and nonjudgmental questions, ask about your patient's relationship status. If they are living (or have lived) with someone, ask what their relationship is to that person, then follow up using the patient's language. (Loss of a partner can sometimes be determined by asking about who they have lived with in the past.) Direct questions about sexual orientation may be difficult to answer. Patients with same-sex partners (or who have been in same-sex relationships) may be more anxious or fearful during clinical encounters because of past experiences. A reassuring manner will help them express concerns about their sexual health and activity.

TIPS FOR TAKING THE SEXUAL HISTORY

- Explain why you are taking the sexual history.
- Note that you realize this information is highly personal, and encourage the patient to be open and direct.
- Relate that you gather this history on all your patients.
- Affirm that your conversation is confidential.

For example, you can begin with a general statement such as:

> "To provide good care I need to review your sexual health and see if you are at risk for any sexually transmitted diseases. I know this is a sensitive area. Any information you share is confidential."

Ask general questions such as:

Do you have sex with men, women or both?
How is sex for you?
Are you having any problems with sex?
Are you satisfied with your sex life as it is now?
Has there been any significant change in the last few years?
Are you satisfied with your ability to perform sexually?
How satisfied do you think your partner is?
Do you feel that your partner is satisfied with the frequency of sexual activity?
Has your partner ever hurt you during sex or forced you to have sex?
Are you comfortable with your partner's sexual practices?

If the patient has concerns about sexual activity, ask her to tell you about them. Direct questions help you assess each phase of the sexual response: desire, arousal, and orgasm:

Do you have an interest in (appetite for) sex?" inquires about the desire phase.

For the orgasmic phase:

Are you able to reach climax (reach an orgasm or "come")?
Is it important for you to reach climax?

For arousal:

Do you get sexually aroused?
Do you lubricate easily (get wet or slippery)?
Do you stay too dry?

Sexual dysfunction is classified by the phase of sexual response. A woman may lack desire, she may fail to become aroused and attain adequate vaginal lubrication, or, despite adequate arousal, she may be unable to reach orgasm. Causes may include lack of estrogen, medical illness, or psychiatric conditions.

Ask also about *dyspareunia* (pain or discomfort during intercourse). If present, try to localize the symptom. Is it near the outside, occurring at the start of intercourse, or does she feel it farther in, when her partner is pushing deeper? *Vaginismus* refers to an involuntary spasm of the muscles surrounding the vaginal orifice that makes penetration during intercourse painful or impossible.

Superficial pain suggests local inflammation, atrophic vaginitis, or inadequate lubrication; deeper pain may be from pelvic disorders or pressure on a normal ovary. The cause of *vaginismus* may be physical or psychological.

In addition to ascertaining the nature of a sexual problem, ask about its onset, severity (persistent or sporadic), setting, and factors, if any, that make it better or worse. What does the patient think is the cause of the problem, what has she tried to do about it, and what does she hope for? The setting of sexual dysfunction is an important but complicated topic, involving the patient's general health, medications and drugs, including use of alcohol; her partner's and her own knowledge of sexual practices and techniques; her attitudes, values, and fears; the relationship and communication between partners; and the setting in which sexual activity takes place.

More commonly, however, a sexual problem is related to situational or psychosocial factors.

Sexually Transmitted Diseases.

Local symptoms or findings on physical examination may raise the possibility of *sexually transmitted diseases (STDs)*. After establishing the usual attributes of any symptoms, identify sexual preference (male, female, or both). Inquire about sexual contacts and establish the number of sexual partners in the prior month. Ask if the patient has concerns about HIV infection, has been tested for HIV previously, desires HIV testing, or has current or past partners at risk. Also ask about oral and anal sex and, if indicated, about symptoms involving the mouth, throat, anus, and rectum. Review the past history of venereal disease, "Have you ever had herpes? . . . Any other problems such as gonorrhea? . . . Syphilis? . . . Pelvic infections?" What does the patient/partner use to prevent STDs? Continue with the more general questions suggested on pp. 74–76.

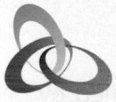 ## PHYSICAL EXAMINATION

Important Areas of Examination

> **External Examination**
> - Mons pubis
> - Labia majora and minora
> - Urethral meatus, clitoris
> - Vaginal introitus
> - Perineum

The generalist nurse may prepare a woman for or assist with an internal pelvic examination. In addition, the nurse may inspect the external genitalia during a procedure, such as urinary catheterization; during postpartum or postabortion care; while following up on a patient complaint; or while giving a complete bed bath. Therefore, the nurse must know the normal appearance of the external genitalia.

Approach to the Pelvic Examination. Many women feel anxious or uncomfortable before and during pelvic examinations. Some women have had painful, embarrassing, or even demeaning experiences during previous examinations, whereas others may be facing a pelvic examination for the first time. Some are fearful about what the clinician may find and how findings may affect their lives. Asking the patient's permission to perform the examination shows courtesy and respect.

A woman having her first pelvic examination may not know what to expect. Using three-dimensional models, showing her the equipment and letting her handle the speculum, and explaining each step in advance can help her learn about her body and be more comfortable. Careful and gentle technique is especially important in minimizing any pain or discomfort during the first pelvic examination.

The woman's response to the pelvic examination may reveal clues about her feelings about the examination and her sexuality. If she pulls away, adducts her thighs, or reacts negatively to the examination, you can gently comment, "I notice you are having some trouble relaxing. Is it just being here, or are you troubled by the examination? . . . Is anything worrying you?" Behaviors that seem to present an obstacle may lead to a better understanding of your patient's concerns. Adverse reactions may signal prior abuse and should be explored.

Indications for a pelvic examination during adolescence include menstrual abnormalities such as amenorrhea, excessive bleeding, or dysmenorrhea; unexplained abdominal pain; vaginal discharge; the prescription of contraceptives; bacteriologic and cytologic studies in a sexually active girl; and the patient's own desire for assessment.

See Chapter 23, Assessing Children: Infancy Through Adolescence, pp. 815–817.

● Tips for the Successful Pelvic Examination

The Patient	The Nurse
• Avoids intercourse, douching, or use of vaginal suppositories for 24 to 48 hours before examination	• Obtains permission; acts as chaperone
	• Explains each step of the examination in advance
• Empties bladder before examination	• Drapes patient from midabdomen to knees; depresses drape between knees to provide eye contact with patient
• Lies supine, with head and shoulders elevated, arms at sides or folded across chest to enhance eye contact and reduce tightening of abdominal muscles	• Warms speculum with tap water
	• Monitors comfort of the examination by watching the patient's face

---

Helping the patient to relax is essential for an adequate examination. Adopting the tips above will help ensure the patient's comfort. Raising the head of the examination table and supplying a mirror for the patient to observe the exam helps her understand the process.

Note all examiners should be accompanied by an appropriate chaperone.

Rape Victims. Regardless of age, *rape* merits special evaluation, usually requiring gynecologic consultation and documentation. Often there is a special rape kit, provided in many emergency departments that must be used to ensure a chain of custody for evidence. Specimens must be labeled carefully with name, date, and time. Additional information may be needed for further legal investigation.

Equipment. Be sure the examiner has a good light, a vaginal speculum of appropriate size, water soluble lubricant, and equipment for taking Papanicolaou smears, bacteriologic cultures and DNA probes, or other diagnostic tests.

Positioning the Patient. Drape the patient appropriately and then assist her into the lithotomy position. Help her to place one heel and then the other into the stirrups. She will be more comfortable with shoes or socks on than with bare feet. Then ask her to slide all the way down the examining table until her buttocks extend slightly beyond the edge. Her thighs should be flexed, abducted, and externally rotated at the hips. A pillow should support her head.

EXTERNAL EXAMINATION

Assess the Sexual Maturity of an Adolescent Patient. You can assess pubic hair during either the abdominal or the pelvic examination. Note its character and distribution, and rate it according to Tanner's stages, described on p. 816.

Delayed puberty is often familial or related to chronic illness. It may also arise from abnormalities in the hypothalamus, anterior pituitary gland, or ovaries.

Examine the External Genitalia. Warn the patient that you will be touching her genital area. Inspect the mons pubis, labia, and perineum. Separate the labia and inspect:

Excoriations or itchy, small, red maculopapules suggest *pediculosis pubis* (lice or "crabs"). Look for nits or lice at the bases of the pubic hairs.

● The labia minora

● The clitoris

Enlarged clitoris in masculinizing conditions

● The urethral meatus

● The vaginal opening, or introitus

Note any inflammation, ulceration, discharge, swelling, lacerations, bruising, or nodules.

Herpes simplex, Behçet disease, syphilitic chancre, epidermoid cyst. See Table 21-1, Lesions of the Vulva (p. 711).

Lacerations and/or bruising may indicate sexual abuse.

INTERNAL EXAMINATION

The internal pelvic examination consists of a visual examination of the vagina and cervix with a speculum that separates the walls of the vagina. The examiner can assess vaginal muscle tone as well as color, ulcerations, inflammation, discharge, or masses in the vagina or on the cervix. The Papanicolaou smear is obtained at this time also. The speculum holding open the vagina prevents contamination of the cervical specimen.

After the speculum is removed, the examiner will manually palpate the organs of the reproductive system. In the bimanual examination one hand is placed on the lower abdomen and two fingers of the other hand are inserted into the vagina. The cervix and uterus can be palpated for position, size, mobility, shape, regularity, masses, and tenderness. In slender, relaxed women the ovaries may be palpated for size, position, regularity, and tenderness. Normally the fallopian tubes cannot be felt unless infection or a tubal pregnancy exists. Some examiners may perform a rectal exam at this time.

RECORDING YOUR FINDINGS

Recording the Pelvic Examination—Female Genitalia

"No inguinal adenopathy. External genitalia without erythema, lesions, or masses."

OR

"Bilateral shotty inguinal adenopathy. External genitalia without erythema or lesions. Thin white vaginal homogeneous discharge with mild fishy odor present."

HEALTH PROMOTION AND COUNSELING

Important Topics for Health Promotion and Counseling

- Anatomy and physiology of the reproductive system and its changes from puberty to menopause
- Cervical cancer screening: Papanicolaou (Pap) smear and human papilloma virus (HPV) infection
- Early prenatal care
- Options for family planning
- Sexually transmitted diseases and HIV

Reproductive System Education.   An accurate understanding of the normal appearance and function of the reproductive system will enable the woman to take control of her reproductive health through family planning and disease prevention; to recognize pregnancy, problems, and maturational changes; and to seek appropriate care in a timely fashion. The use of three-dimensional models and charts is helpful to convey the structure and function of the system.

Changes in Menopause.   Inform the patient of the psychological and physiologic changes of menopause—mood shifts and changes in self-concept, vasomotor changes ("hot flashes"), accelerated bone loss, increases in total and low-density lipoprotein (LDL) cholesterol, and vulvovaginal atrophy leading to symptoms of vaginal drying, dysuria and, at times, dyspareunia. Refer the woman to her midwife or gynecologist for treatment options for symptoms causing discomfort.

Cervical Cancer Screening: the Pap Smear and HPV Infection.   Widespread screening by *Pap smear* has contributed to a significant decline in the incidence of and mortality from cervical cancer. The U.S. Preventive Services Task Force notes that "the goal of cytologic screening is to sample the transformation zone of the cervix, the area where physiologic transformation from columnar endocervical epithelium to squamous (ectocervical) epithelium takes place and where dysplasia and cancer arise."[4]

Risk factors for cervical cancer are both viral and behavioral. The most important risk factor is infection with the *high-risk strains of HPV*. Genital infection with HPV is the most common STD in the United States.[5] More than 50% of sexually active people contract the infection during their lifetime. Most genital HPV infections are transient and become HPV DNA-negative in 1 to 2 years. Persisting HPV is thought to induce precancerous and cancerous lesions, and HPVs cause virtually all cervical cancers.[6]

Other risk factors for cervical cancer include early sexual activity, multiple sexual partners, a history of STDs, failure to undergo screening by Pap smear, age, nutritional status, smoking, immune status, and genetic polymorphisms affecting the entry of HPV DNA into cervical cells.[4]

The American College of Obstetricians and Gynecologists, the American Cancer Society, and the U.S. Preventive Services Task Force periodically update recommendations related to screening frequency.[4,7–9]

The HPV Vaccine.   In 2007 the Centers for Disease Control and Prevention (CDC) recommended administering the *HPV vaccine* to girls and women 11 to 26 years old to reduce the risk of cervical cancer.[10] Studies have shown that the vaccine, which targets HPV types 6, 11, 16, and 18, is almost 100% effective in preventing HPV 16– and 18–related cervical intraepithelial neoplasia grade 2 or 3 and adenocarcinoma in situ in women with no prior exposure to these types.[6] The vaccine also reduces risk of anogenital diseases such as warts, intraepithelial neoplasia, and invasive anogenital cancers.[11] The vaccine is less effective in women already exposed to one of the four HPV types, and it does not treat existing HPV cervical infections, genital warts, precancers, or cancers.[12]

Early vaccination before onset of sexual activity is felt to confer the highest benefit. Approximate initiation of sexual activity in adolescent age groups is 8% before 13 years of age, 33% by ninth grade, and 66% by the end of high school.[13] HPV prevalence is 40% for girls 14 to 19 years old.[14] Cervical screening by Pap smear and genital examinations should continue after vaccination to detect changes from new or persisting infection from other oncogenic HPV types. The duration of immunity provided by the HPV vaccine is currently undetermined.

Early Prenatal Care. "In 2005 the U.S. fetal mortality rate was 6.22 fetal deaths of 20 weeks gestation or more per 1,000 live births and fetal deaths."[15] This translates into 25,894 fetal deaths in 2005, the latest available year from the National Center of Health Statistics. Early prenatal care and preparation for pregnancy, such as stopping alcohol use and smoking, weight loss in obese women, and taking folic acid and calcium supplements, lower the perimortality rate. Women who express a desire to become pregnant or who are at risk for pregnancy should have a gynecologic examination to identify possible problems before pregnancy and be counseled on how to best prepare for pregnancy. If the history indicates the woman may be pregnant, she should be encouraged to obtain prenatal care as soon as possible.

Options for Family Planning. It is important to counsel women, particularly adolescents, about the timing of ovulation in the menstrual cycle and how to plan or prevent pregnancy. Survey data indicate that more than half of U.S. pregnancies are unintended, accounting for a high proportion of the 800,000 teen pregnancies each year.[16] Clinicians should be familiar with the numerous options for contraception and their effectiveness. Take the time to understand the patient or couple's concerns and preferences and respect these preferences whenever possible. Continued use of a preferred method is superior to a more effective method that is abandoned. For teenagers, a confidential setting eases discussion of topics that may seem private and difficult to explore.

Sexually Transmitted Diseases and HIV Infection. U.S. rates of STDs are the highest in the industrialized world.[17] *Chlamydia trachomatis* is the most commonly reported STD in the United States and the most common STD in women.[18] Infection rates are highest in women 15 to 19 years old and second highest in women 20 to 24 years old. African-American women and American Indian/Alaska Native women have the highest infection rates. Most cases are undiagnosed. If untreated, 40% of women will develop pelvic inflammatory disease (PID) and 20% will become infertile. Detection, groups most affected, and consequences of underdiagnosis and treatment are similar for *gonorrhea*. Infection with *syphilis* is less common; African-American and Hispanic women are at highest risk. The U.S. Preventive Services Task Force strongly recommends:

- Routine screening for cervical *chlamydia* and gonorrhea of all sexually active and pregnant women 24 years old or younger and older women at increased risk.[19–20]

- Routine screening for *syphilis* of women at increased risk and of pregnant women.[20–21]

In the United States, *HIV and AIDS infection* rates are increasing fastest in women, who now account for 30% of cases.[21] Transmission in women is primarily heterosexual. Among infected women, 60% are African-American, 20% are Latina, and 20% are Caucasian. In 2006 the CDC published new guidelines recommending universal HIV testing for all people in the age range of 13 to 64 years, regardless of risk factors. The U.S. Preventive Services Task Force recommendation remains directed at screening those at high risk.[22]

Nurses should assess risk factors for STDs and HIV infection by taking a careful sexual history and counseling patients about spread of disease and how to reduce high-risk practices. Key to effective clinician counseling are respect, compassion, a nonjudgmental attitude, and use of open-ended and understandable questions like "Tell me about any new sex partners" and "Have you ever had anal sex, meaning 'penis in rectum/anus sex'?"[23] The CDC recommends interactive client-centered counseling, tailored to the person's specific risk factors and situation. Training in prevention counseling improves effectiveness. You can begin at the excellent Web sites recommended by the CDC such as http://effectiveinterventions.org or http://depts.washington.edu/nnptc/.

See Chapter 1, The Health History, pp. 74–76, on eliciting the sexual history, and , pp. 708–709, on risk factors for HIV infection.

MALE REPRODUCTIVE SYSTEM

ANATOMY AND PHYSIOLOGY

First review the anatomy of the male genitalia.

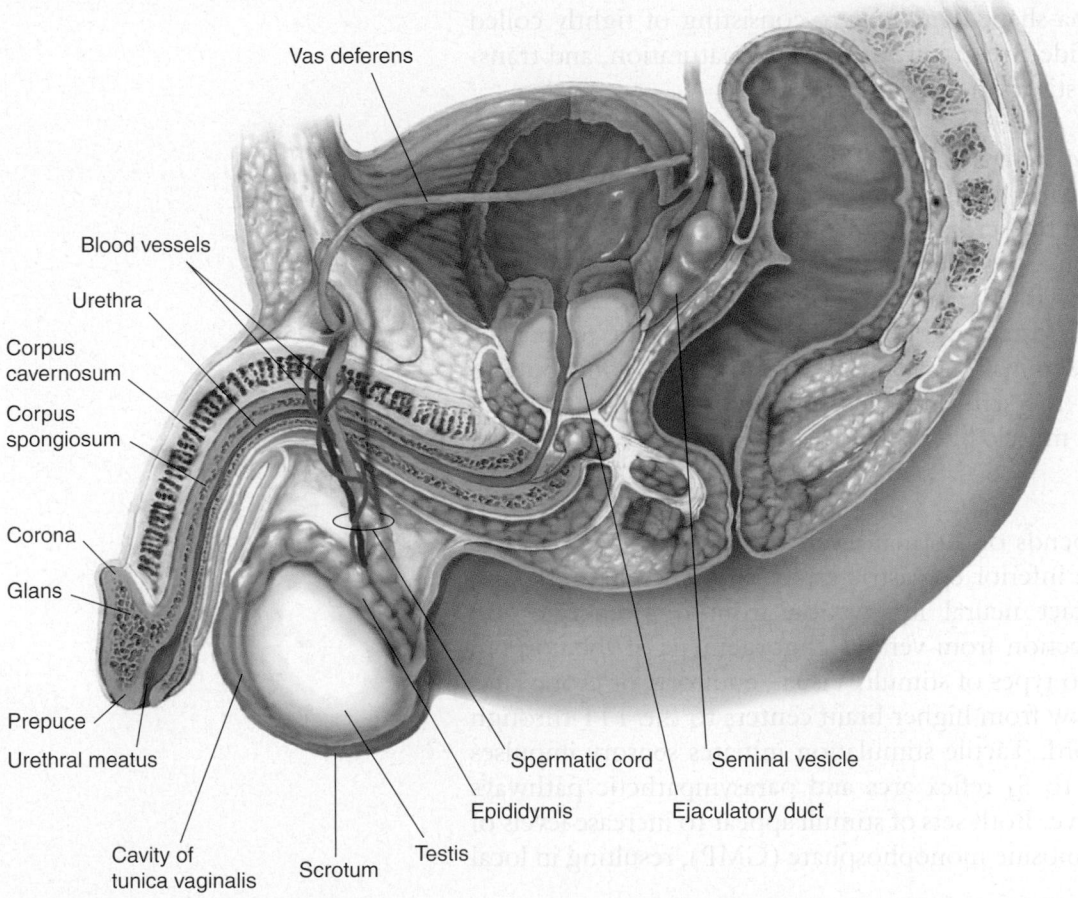

Vas deferens

Blood vessels

Urethra

Corpus cavernosum

Corpus spongiosum

Corona

Glans

Prepuce

Urethral meatus

Cavity of tunica vaginalis

Scrotum

Testis

Epididymis

Spermatic cord

Seminal vesicle

Ejaculatory duct

The *shaft of the penis* is formed by three columns of vascular erectile tissue: the *corpus spongiosum,* containing the urethra, and two *corpora cavernosa.* The corpus spongiosum forms the bulb of the penis, ending in the cone-shaped *glans* with its expanded base, or *corona.* In uncircumcised men, the glans is covered by a loose, hood-like fold of skin called the *prepuce* or *foreskin* where *smegma,* or secretions of the glans, may collect. The urethra is located ventrally in the shaft of the penis; urethral abnormalities may sometimes be felt there. The urethra opens into the vertical, slit-like *urethral meatus,* located somewhat ventrally at the tip of the glans.

The *testes* are ovoid, rubbery structures approximately 4.5 cm long, ranging in size from 3.5 cm to 5.5 cm. The left testis usually lies lower than the right. The testes produce spermatozoa and testosterone. Testosterone stimulates the pubertal growth of the male genitalia, prostate, and seminal vesicles. It also stimulates the development of masculine secondary sex characteristics, including facial hair, body hair, musculoskeletal growth, and enlargement of the larynx, with its associated low-pitched voice.

Surrounding or appended to the testes are several structures. The *scrotum* is a loose, wrinkled pouch divided into two compartments, each containing a testis or testicle. Covering the testis, except posteriorly, is the serous membrane of the *tunica vaginalis*. On the posterolateral surface of each testis is the softer, comma-shaped *epididymis*, consisting of tightly coiled spermatic ducts that provide a reservoir for storage, maturation, and transport of sperm from the testis to the *vas deferens*.

During ejaculation, the *vas deferens*, a cord-like structure, transports sperm from the tail of the epididymis along a somewhat circular route to the urethra. The *vas* ascends from the scrotal sac into the pelvic cavity through the external inguinal ring, then loops over the ureter to the prostate behind the bladder. There it merges with the *seminal vesicle* to form the *ejaculatory duct*, which traverses the prostate and empties into the urethra. Secretions from the *vas deferens*, the seminal vesicles, and the prostate all contribute to the seminal fluid. Within the scrotum, each vas is closely associated with blood vessels, nerves, and muscle fibers. These structures make up the *spermatic cord*.

Male sexual function depends on normal levels of testosterone, adequate arterial blood flow to the inferior epigastric artery and its cremasteric and pubic branches, and intact neural innervation from α-adrenergic and cholinergic pathways. Erection from venous engorgement of the corpora cavernosa results from two types of stimuli. Visual, auditory, or erotic cues trigger sympathetic outflow from higher brain centers to the T11 through L2 levels of the spinal cord. Tactile stimulation initiates sensory impulses from the genitalia to S_2 to S_4 reflex arcs and parasympathetic pathways through the pudendal nerve. Both sets of stimuli appear to increase levels of nitric oxide and cyclic guanosine monophosphate (GMP), resulting in local vasodilation.

Lymphatics. *Lymphatics from the penile and scrotal surfaces drain into the inguinal nodes.* When an inflammatory or possibly malignant lesion *is found on these surfaces*, assess the inguinal nodes *for enlargement or tenderness. The lymphatics of the testes, however, drain into the abdomen, where enlarged nodes are clinically undetectable. See p. 404 for further discussion of the inguinal nodes.*

Anatomy of the Groin. Because hernias are relatively common, it is important to understand the anatomy of the groin. The basic landmarks are the anterior superior iliac spine, the pubic tubercle, and the inguinal ligament that runs between them.

The *inguinal canal*, which lies above and approximately parallel to the inguinal ligament, forms a tunnel for the vas deferens as it passes through the abdominal muscles. The exterior opening of the tunnel—the *external inguinal ring*—is a triangular, slit-like structure palpable just above and lateral to the pubic tubercle. The internal opening of the canal—or *internal inguinal ring*—is approximately 1 cm above the midpoint of the inguinal ligament. Neither canal nor internal ring is palpable through the abdominal wall. When loops of bowel force their way through weak areas of the inguinal canal, they produce *inguinal hernias*, as illustrated on p. 717.

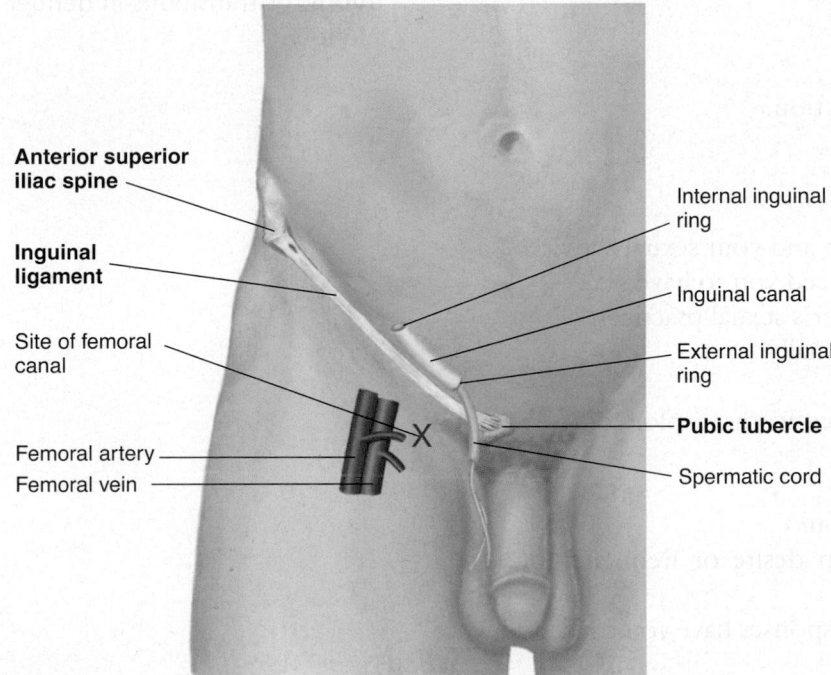

Another potential route for a herniating mass is the *femoral canal*. This lies below the inguinal ligament. Although you cannot see it, you can estimate its location by placing your right index finger, from below, on the right femoral artery. Your middle finger will then overlie the femoral vein; your ring finger, the femoral canal. Femoral hernias protrude here.

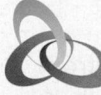 **THE HEALTH HISTORY**

COMMON OR CONCERNING SYMPTOMS

- Sexual preference and sexual response
- Penile discharge or lesions
- Scrotal pain, swelling, or lesions
- Problems with urination

Sexual Preference and Sexual Response. Review the Tips for Taking the Sexual History on p. 691. Use neutral nonjudgmental questions about sexual orientation such as "Are you in a relationship?" or "Tell me about your relationship. Do you prefer partners who are women, men, or both women and men?"

Approximately 1 in 10 patients may have same-sex, bisexual, or transgender partner preferences.[24] These patients often experience significant anxiety during clinical encounters, related to fears of clinician acceptance, coexisting mental health conditions, sparse information about complex issues of hormonal therapy, surgical alterations, or transitions in gender identity.[24]

Continue with questions about sexual function.

How is sex for you?
How is your current relationship?
Are you satisfied with your relationship and your sexual activity?
"Has your partner ever hurt you or forced you to have sex?"
"Are you comfortable with your partner's sexual practices?"
What about your ability to perform sexually?

If the patient expresses relational or sexual concerns, explore both their psychological and physiologic dimensions.

What does this relationship mean to you?
Have you experienced any changes in desire or frequency of sexual activity?
What is your view of the cause, what responses have you tried, and what are your hopes?
Direct questions help assess each phase of the sexual response.

To assess *libido*, or desire, ask:

Have you maintained interest in sex?

Lack of libido may arise from psychogenic causes such as depression, endocrine dysfunction, or side effects of medications.

For the *arousal phase*, ask:

Can you achieve and maintain an erection?

Explore the timing, severity, setting, and any other factors that may be contributing to problems.

Have any changes in the relationship with your partner or in your life circumstances coincided with onset of a problem?

Erectile dysfunction may be from psychogenic causes, especially if early morning erection is preserved; also from decreased testosterone, decreased blood flow in the hypogastric arterial system, or impaired neural innervation.

Are there circumstances when erection is normal? On awakening in the early morning or during the night? With other partners? With masturbation?

Other questions relate to the phase of *orgasm* and *ejaculation* of semen.

If ejaculation is premature, or early and out of control, ask:

About how long does intercourse last?
Do you climax too soon?
Do you feel you have control over climaxing?
Do you think your partner would like intercourse to last longer?

For reduced or absent ejaculation:

Do you find that you cannot have an orgasm even though you can have an erection?

Try to determine whether the problem involves the pleasurable sensation of orgasm, the ejaculation of seminal fluid, or both. Review the frequency and setting of the problem, medications, surgery, and neurologic symptoms.

Penile Discharge or Lesions.

To assess the possibility of genital infection from STDs, ask:

Have you had any discharge, leaking, or dripping from your penis or staining on your underwear?

If discharge is present, ask:

When did it start?
Is it continuous or intermittent?
How much discharge is there? A teaspoon? A tablespoon?
What color is the discharge?
Is the discharge thick or thin?
Have you had any sores or growths on the penis or scrotum? Or pain or swelling in the scrotum?
Have you had a fever, chills, rash, or any other symptoms?
Have you ever had these symptoms before? If yes, how were they treated?

Premature ejaculation is common, especially in young men. Less common is reduced or absent ejaculation affecting middle-aged or older men. Possible causes are medications, surgery, neurologic deficits, or lack of androgen. Lack of orgasm with ejaculation is usually psychogenic.

Penile discharge may accompany gonococcal (usually yellow) and nongonococcal urethritis (may be clear or white).

To assess further for STDs, ask:

> Have you ever been diagnosed with a sexually transmitted disease? Herpes? Gonorrhea? Syphilis?

Because STDs may involve other parts of the body, additional questions are often indicated. An introductory explanation may be useful: "Sexually transmitted diseases can involve any body opening where you have sex. It's important for you to tell me which openings you use." And further, as needed, "Do you have oral sex? Anal sex?" If the patient's answers are affirmative, ask about symptoms such as sore throat, diarrhea, rectal bleeding, anal itching or anal pain.

For the many patients without symptoms or known risk factors, it is wise to ask "Do you have any concerns about HIV infection?" as an important screening question and to continue with the more general questions suggested on pp. 74–76.

Scrotal Pain or Swelling. If the patient complains of pain or swelling in his scrotum, follow the "OLD CART" mnemonic to gather thorough information. A sudden onset of scrotal pain may indicate torsion of the testicle, which is an emergency. A painless lump may be cancer. Ask if he performs self-testicular examination and how often.

Inguinal Pain or Swelling. Inguinal pain or swelling may indicate an inguinal hernia. These hernias may be unilateral or bilateral. Ask the patient to point to the area of the pain and/or swelling and to describe it. "When did it begin? Is the pain continuous or intermittent? Achy or sharp? Does it occur with lifting heavy objects, standing, bending, or bearing down?"

Problems with Urination. The prostate gland wraps around the urethra. If the gland enlarges due to benign prostatic hyperplasia (BPH) or cancer, the patient may experience urinary symptoms. Men older than 70 years are at greatest risk. Therefore, the nurse should review the pattern of urination (see Chapter 16 Gastrointestinal and Renal Systems. Ask the patient:

> Do you have any difficulty starting or holding back the urine stream?
> Is the flow weak?
> How often do you urinate during the day? The night?
> Is there any pain or burning as urine is passed?
> Is there any blood in the urine or in your semen? Any pain with ejaculation?

See Table 21-3, Abnormalities of the Penis and Scrotum, p. 713, Table 21-4, Sexually Transmitted Diseases of Male Genitalia , p. 714, and Table 21-5, Abnormalities of the Testis, p. 715. In addition to STDs, many skin conditions affect the genitalia; likewise, some STDs have minimal symptoms or signs.

Infections from oral–penile transmission include gonorrhea, chlamydia, syphilis, and herpes. Symptomatic or asymptomatic proctitis may follow anal intercourse.

Hernia pain and swelling are more likely to occur when internal abdominal pressure increases (e.g., when lifting).

Do you have any discomfort or heaviness in the prostate area at the base of the penis?

Suggest possible prostatitis

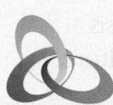 **PHYSICAL EXAMINATION**

The generalist nurse does not perform prostate examinations or examine the genitalia by palpation of the male patient. However, the nurse may inspect the genitalia during a bed bath, a procedure such as urinary catheterization, or postoperative follow-up care in the genitourinary system. The nurse should be able to recognize abnormal conditions found on inspection that require referral or treatment. For younger patients, review the Tanner sexual maturity ratings in Chapter 23, Assessing Children: Infancy to Adolescence p. 813–814.

Gloves should be worn. Occasionally male patients have erections during the examination or a procedure where the penis is touched. If this happens explain that this is a normal response, and finish your examination with an unruffled demeanor.

THE PENIS

Inspection

Inspect the penis, including:

See Table 21-3, Abnormalities of the Penis and Scrotum (p. 713).

- The *skin*

- The *prepuce* (foreskin). If present, retract the prepuce or ask the patient to retract it. This step is essential for the detection of many chancres and carcinomas. Smegma, a cheesy, whitish material, may accumulate normally under the foreskin.

Phimosis is a tight prepuce that cannot be retracted over the glans. *Paraphimosis* is a tight prepuce that, once retracted, cannot be returned. Edema ensues.

- The *glans.* Look for any ulcers, scars, nodules, or signs of inflammation.

Balanitis (inflammation of the glans); *balanoposthitis* (inflammation of the glans and prepuce)

Check the skin around the base of the penis for excoriations or inflammation. Look for nits or lice at the bases of the pubic hairs.

Pubic or genital excoriations suggest the possibility of lice (crabs) or sometimes scabies.

Note the location of the urethral meatus.

Hypospadias is a congenital, ventral displacement of the meatus on the penis Table 21-3, p. 713.

Inspect it for discharge. Normally there is none.

Profuse yellow discharge in *gonococcal urethritis*; scanty white or clear discharge in *nongonococcal urethritis*. Definitive diagnosis requires Gram stain and culture.

If you retracted the foreskin, replace it before proceeding on to examine the scrotum.

THE SCROTUM AND ITS CONTENTS

Inspection

Inspect the scrotum, including:

See Table 21-3, Abnormalities of the Penis and Scrotum (p. 713).

- The *skin*. Lift up the scrotum so that you can see its posterior surface.

Rashes, epidermoid cysts, rarely skin cancer

- The *scrotal contours*. Note any swelling, lumps, or veins.

A poorly developed scrotum on one or both sides suggests *cryptorchidism* (an undescended testicle). Common scrotal swellings include indirect *inguinal hernias*, *hydroceles*, and *scrotal edema*.

There may be dome shaped white or yellow papules or nodules formed by occluded follicles filled with keratin debris of desquamated follicular epithelium. Such *epidermoid cysts* are common, frequently multiple, and benign.

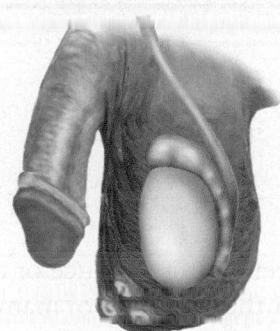

EPIDERMOID CYSTS

HERNIAS

Inspection

If the patient has complained of a bulge or pain in his lower abdomen, especially with lifting or straining, he should be examined for hernias. Standing is the preferred position, because the upright position causes gravity to accentuate the bulge. Inspect the inguinal and femoral areas for bulging and

A bulge that appears on straining suggests a *hernia*.

asymmetry. As you observe, ask the client to strain and bear down (the Valsalva maneuver) to increase intra-abdominal pressure, making it easier to observe a hernia. If a bulge is present, the patient should be referred to a physician or advanced practitioner for follow-up.

Absence of a bulge during inspection does not guarantee absence of a hernia, especially in an obese patient. If suspicious history findings have been reported, the patient should be referred to an advanced practitioner for further examination.

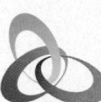

RECORDING YOUR FINDINGS

Recording the Physical Examination— Male Genitalia and Hernias

> "Circumcised male. No penile discharge or lesions. No scrotal swelling or discoloration. Testes descended bilaterally. No apparent inguinal or femoral hernias."

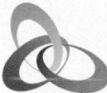

HEALTH PROMOTION AND COUNSELING

Important Topics for Health Promotion and Counseling

- Prevention of STDs and HIV
- Testicular self-examination
- Screening for prostate cancer

Prevention of Sexually Transmitted Diseases and HIV Infection. The case for aggressive clinician education, early detection during history taking and physical examination, and treatment for STDs and HIV is compelling. The growing burden of STDs affects the health of all segments of the population, but especially adolescents and young adults. The Institute of Medicine has documented that U.S. rates of STDs are the highest in the industrialized world.[25] In 2009 the CDC estimated 19 million new STD infections each year, with almost half in the age group 15 to 24 years.[26] Of the 1.5 million new cases reported in 2009, approximately 79% were infections from Chlamydia. The CDC notes that these figures represent "only a small proportion of the true national burden of STDs"—many cases are unreported, and viral infections such as human papillomavirus and genital herpes are not subject to requirements for mandatory reporting. Further, more than 1 million Americans are currently infected with HIV, with approximately 40,000 new infections annually. An estimated 25% of infected inhabitants in the United States are unaware of their infected status.[28] Hepatitis B and genital ulcers such as chancroid are also transmitted through sexual contact. The presence of any STD raises the need to investigate coinfection with HIV.

Nurses should master the skills of eliciting the sexual history and asking frank but tactful questions about sexual practices. Key information includes the patient's sexual orientation, the number of partners in the past month, and any history of past STDs Careful screening for alcohol and drug use, especially injection drugs, is also important. Counseling should be interactive and combine messages about general risk reduction relevant to the patient with education about specific actions for reducing the patient's risk (see also, pp. 607-608). Important topics include limiting the number of partners, using condoms, and establishing regular medical care for treatment of STDs and HIV. Men should seek prompt attention for any genital lesions or penile discharge.

In 2006 the CDC issued new recommendations advising universal HIV screening for all people 13 to 64 years, regardless of risk factors. The U.S. Preventive Services Task Force reviewed new evidence about screening in 2007 and continued to affirm screening targeted to those at increased risk and all pregnant women.[28] The Task Force recommends screening and counseling for the following groups: men with male sex partners; men and women having unprotected sex with multiple partners; past or present injection drug users; sex workers; individuals with past or present sex partners with a history of STDs, HIV infection, injection drug use, or bisexual practice; patients who received blood products between 1978 and 1985; and individuals requesting testing because they may be unwilling to disclose high-risk behaviors.

Testicular Self-Examination.   The incidence of testicular cancer is low, about 5 per 100,000 men, but it is the most common cancer of young men between the ages of 15 and 35. When detected early, testicular carcinoma has an excellent prognosis. Risk factors include cryptorchidism, which confers a high risk for testicular carcinoma in the undescended testicle; a history of carcinoma in the contralateral testicle; mumps orchitis; an inguinal hernia; or a hydrocele in childhood. Encourage men, especially young men, to perform monthly testicular self-examinations and to seek physician evaluation for the following findings: any painless lump, swelling, or enlargement in either testicle; pain or discomfort in a testicle or the scrotum; a feeling of heaviness or a sudden fluid collection in the scrotum; or a dull ache in the lower abdomen or the groin.[29]

Prostate Cancer.   Excluding skin cancer prostate cancer is the leading cancer diagnosed in U.S. men, and the second leading cause of death in men.[30] Although lifetime risk of diagnosis is high (approximately 17%), biologic risk and mortality are only approximately 3%. Age, ethnicity, and family history are the primary risk factors.

● ***Age.*** Risk of prostate cancer increases sharply with each advancing decade after 50 years. Probability of diagnosis rises by age group, from 2.4%

PATIENT INSTRUCTIONS FOR THE TESTICULAR SELF-EXAMINATION

This examination is best performed after a warm bath or shower. The heat relaxes the scrotum and makes it easier to find anything unusual.

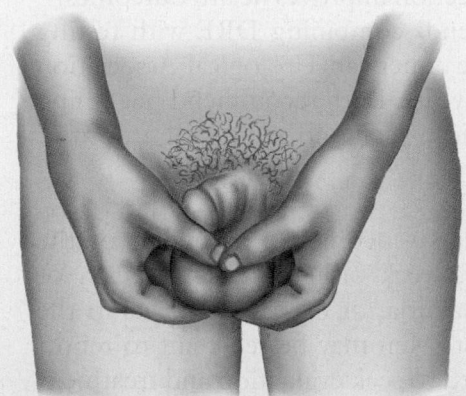

- Standing in front of a mirror, check for any swelling on the skin of the scrotum.
- Examine each testicle with both hands. Cup the index and middle fingers under the testicle and place the thumbs on top.
- Roll the testicle gently between the thumbs and fingers. One testicle may be larger than the other . . . that's normal, but be concerned about any lump or area of pain.
- Find the epididymis. This is a soft, tube-like structure at the back of the testicle that collects and carries sperm, not an abnormal lump.
- If you find any lump, do not wait. See your doctor. The lump may just be an infection, but if it is cancer, it will spread unless stopped by treatment.

(Source: Medline Plus. U.S. National Library of Medicine and National Institutes of Health. Medical Encyclopedia—Testicular self-examination. Available at: www.nlm.nih.gov/medlineplus/ency/article/003909.htm. Accessed May 20, 2011.)

in men 40 to 59 years, to 6.5% in men 60 to 69 years, to 12.5% in men 70 years and older.[30]

- **Ethnicity.** For undetermined reasons, incidence rates are significantly higher in African-American men than in Caucasian men: 232 cases per 100,000 compared with 146 cases per 100,000, even after adjustments for access to care.[30] Prostate cancer occurs at an earlier age and more advanced stage in African-American men.

- **Family history.** Approximately 15% of men diagnosed with prostate cancer have an affected first-degree relative.[32] One Scandinavian study of twins ascribed 42% of cases to inheritance.[33] Rare autosomal dominant alleles appear to contribute to early-onset prostate cancer, and several X-linked alleles are under investigation in families with onset at older ages.[34]

- **Diet.** A series of studies suggests an association between intake of dietary fat, especially saturated fats and fats from animal sources, and risk of prostate cancer. However, the evidence remains inconclusive.[32,34] Other possible influences include selenium, vitamins E and D, lycopene, and isoflavones.[35]

The optimal approach to prostate cancer *screening* remains controversial. The U.S. Preventive Services Task Force in 2008 found insufficient evidence to recommend for or against routine screening using *prostate-specific antigen (PSA) testing* or *digital rectal examination (DRE)*, primarily because of mixed evidence that early detection improves health outcomes.[36] The American Cancer Society recommends combining DRE with testing for PSA beginning at 50 years,while the American Urological Association recommends beginning screening at 40 years. Both recommend beginning screening at 40 years for African-American men and men with a positive family history.[30,37]

Men *with symptoms* of prostate disorders—incomplete emptying of the bladder, urinary frequency or urgency, weak or intermittent stream or straining to initiate flow, hematuria, nocturia, or even bony pains in the pelvis—should be referred to a urologist. Men may be reluctant to report such symptoms but should be encouraged to seek evaluation and treatment early.

TABLE
21-1

Lesions of the Vulva

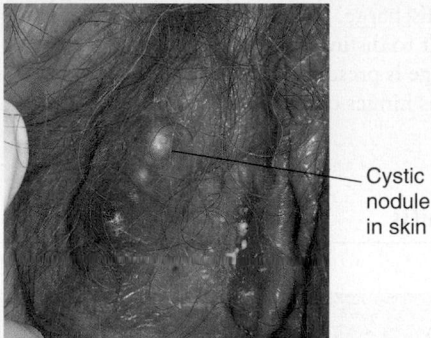

Cystic
nodule
in skin

Epidermoid Cyst

A small, firm, round cystic nodule in the labia suggests an epidermoid cyst. These are yellowish in color. Look for the dark punctum marking the blocked opening of the gland.

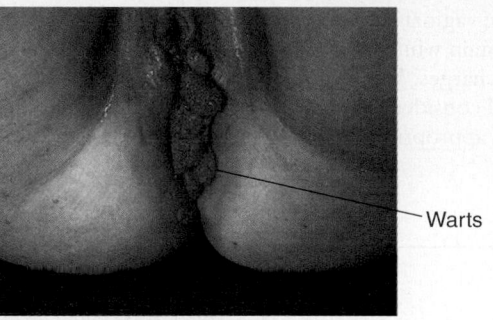

Warts

Venereal Wart (*Condyloma Acuminatum*)

Warty lesions on the labia and within the vestibule suggest condyloma acuminatum. They result from infection with *human papillomavirus.*

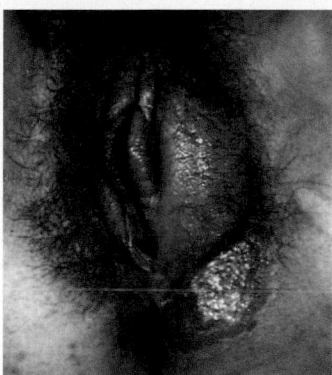

Syphilitic Chancre

A firm, painless ulcer suggests the chancre of primary syphilis. Because most chancres in women develop internally, they often go undetected.

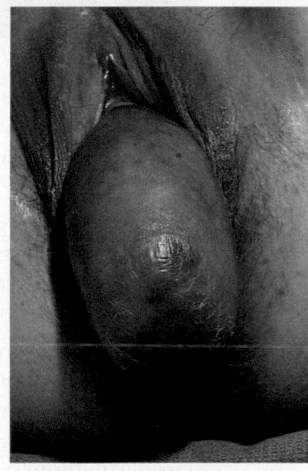

Uterine Prolapse

Uterine prolapse occurs when the uterus protrudes into the vagina.

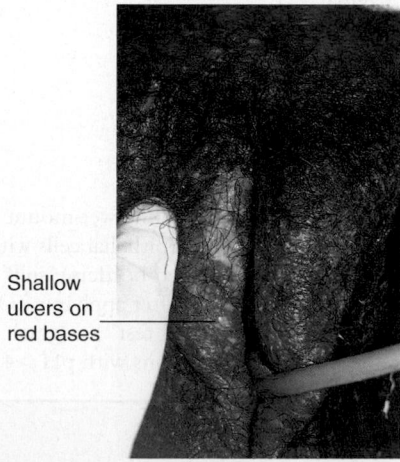

Shallow
ulcers on
red bases

Genital Herpes[38]

Shallow, small, painful ulcers on red bases suggest a herpes infection. Initial infection may be extensive, as shown. Recurrent infections usually are confined to a small local patch.

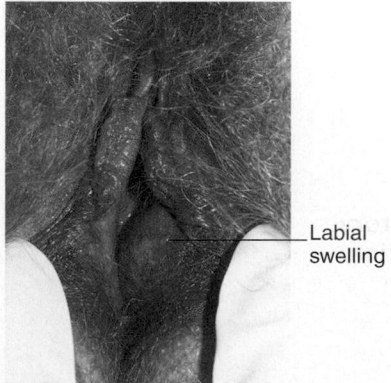

Labial
swelling

Bartholin Gland Infection

Causes of a Bartholin gland infection include trauma, gonococci anaerobes like bacteroides and peptostreptococci, and *Chlamydia trachomatis.* Acutely, it appears as a tense, hot, very tender abscess. Look for pus coming out of the duct or erythema around the duct opening. Chronically, a nontender cyst is felt. It may be large or small.

TABLE
21-2

Vaginal Discharge

The vaginal discharge from vaginitis must be distinguished from a physiologic discharge. The latter is clear or white and may contain white clumps of epithelial cells; it is not malodorous. It is also important to distinguish vaginal from cervical discharges. Use a large cotton swab to wipe off the cervix. If no cervical discharge is present in the os, suspect a vaginal origin and consider the causes below. Remember that diagnosis of cervicitis or vaginitis hinges on careful collection and analysis of the appropriate laboratory specimens.[39,40]

	Trichomonal Vaginitis	Candidal Vaginitis	Bacterial Vaginosis
Cause	*Trichomonas vaginalis*, a protozoan; often but not always acquired sexually	*Candida albicans*, a yeast (normal overgrowth of vaginal flora); many factors predispose, including antibiotic therapy	Bacterial overgrowth probably from anaerobic bacteria; may be transmitted sexually
Discharge	Yellowish green or gray, possibly frothy; often profuse and pooled in the vaginal fornix; may be malodorous	White and curdy; may be thin but typically thick, not as profuse as in trichomonal infection; not malodorous	Gray or white, thin, homogeneous, malodorous; coats the vaginal walls; usually not profuse, may be minimal
Other Symptoms	Pruritus (though not usually as severe as with *Candida* infection); pain on urination (from skin inflammation or possibly urethritis); dyspareunia	Pruritus; vaginal soreness; pain on urination (from skin inflammation); dyspareunia	Unpleasant fishy or musty genital odor
Vulva and Vaginal Mucosa	Vestibule and labia minora may be reddened. Vaginal mucosa may be diffusively reddened, with small red granular spots or petechiae in the posterior fornix. In mild cases, the mucosa looks normal.	The vulva and even the surrounding skin are often inflamed and sometimes swollen to a variable extent. Vaginal mucosa often reddened, with white, often tenacious patches of discharge. The mucosa may bleed when these patches are scraped off. In mild cases, the mucosa looks normal.	Vulva usually normal. Vaginal mucosa usually normal
Laboratory Evaluation	Scan saline wet mount for trichomonads	Scan potassium hydroxide (KOH) preparation for branching hyphae of *Candida*.	Scan saline wet mount for *clue cells* (epithelial cells with stippled borders); sniff for fishy odor after applying KOH ("whiff test"); vaginal secretions with pH >4.5

TABLE
21-3

Abnormalities of the Penis and Scrotum

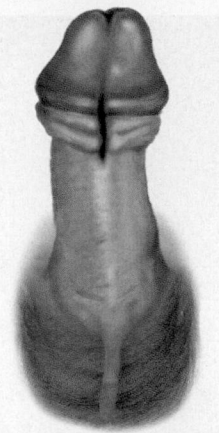

Hypospadias

A congenital displacement of the urethral meatus to the inferior surface of the penis. A groove extends from the actual urethral meatus to its normal location on the tip of the glans.

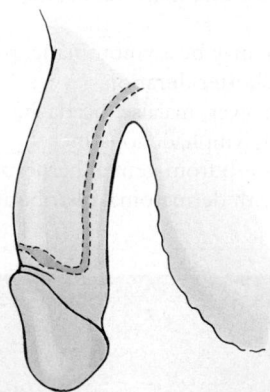

Epispadias

The urethral meatus is located on the top of the glans (dorsal side). This condition is a congenital defect and occurs rarely.

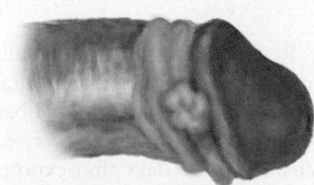

Carcinoma of the Penis

An indurated nodule or ulcer that is usually nontender. Limited almost completely to men who are not circumcised, it may be masked by the prepuce. Any persistent penile sore is suspicious.

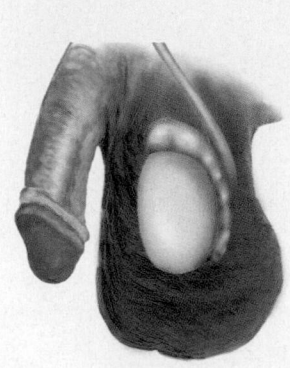

Scrotal Edema

Pitting edema may make the scrotal skin taut; seen in congestive heart failure or nephrotic syndrome.

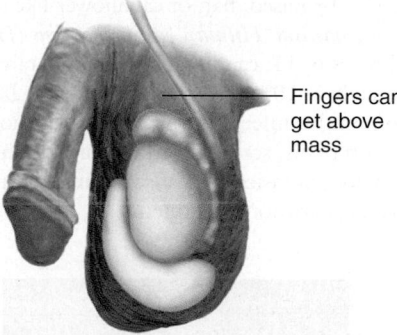

Fingers can get above mass

Hydrocele

A nontender, fluid-filled mass within the tunica vaginalis. It transilluminates, and the examining fingers can get above the mass within the scrotum.

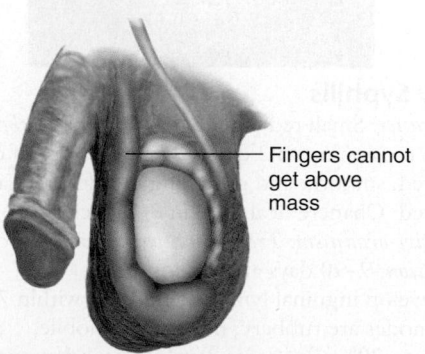

Fingers cannot get above mass

Scrotal Hernia

Usually an *indirect inguinal hernia* that comes through the external inguinal ring, so the examining fingers cannot get above it within the scrotum.

TABLE 21-4	Sexually Transmitted Diseases of Male Genitalia

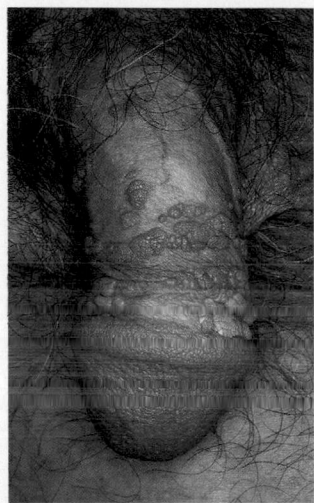

Genital Warts (condylomata acuminata)

- *Appearance:* Single or multiple papules or plaques of variable shapes; may be round, acuminate (or pointed), or thin and slender. May be raised, flat, or cauliflower-like (verrucous).
- *Causative organism: Human papillomavirus (HPV),* usually from subtypes 6, 11; carcinogenic subtypes rare, approximately 5–10% of all anogenital warts. *Incubation:* weeks to months; infected contact may have no visible warts.
- Can arise on penis, scrotum, groin, thighs, anus; usually asymptomatic, occasionally cause itching and pain.
- May disappear without treatment.

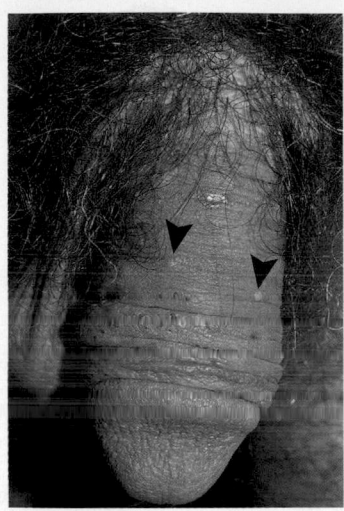

Genital Herpes Simplex

- *Appearance:* Small scattered or grouped vesicles, 1–3 mm in size, on glans or shaft of penis. Appear as erosions if vesicular membrane breaks.
- *Causative organism:* Usually *herpes simplex virus 2* (90%), a double-stranded DNA virus. *Incubation:* 2–7 days after exposure.
- Primary episode may be asymptomatic; recurrence usually less painful, of shorter duration.
- Associated with fever, malaise, headache, arthralgias; local pain and edema, lymphadenopathy.
- Need to distinguish from genital herpes zoster (usually in older patients with dermatomal distribution); candidiasis.

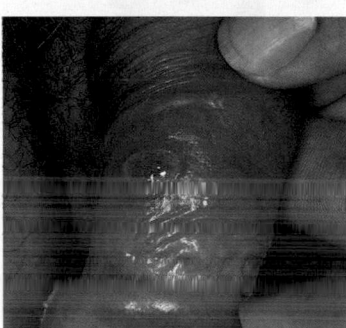

Primary Syphilis

- *Appearance:* Small red papule that becomes a *chancre,* or *painless* erosion up to 2 cm in diameter. Base of chancre is clean, red, smooth, and glistening; borders are raised and indurated. Chancre heals within 3–8 weeks.
- *Causative organism: Treponema pallidum,* a spirochete. *Incubation:* 9–90 days after exposure.
- May develop inguinal lymphadenopathy within 7 days; lymph nodes are rubbery, nontender, mobile.
- Twenty to 30% of patients develop secondary syphilis while chancre still present (suggests coinfection with HIV).
- Distinguish from genital herpes simplex; chancroid; granuloma inguinale from *Klebsiella granulomatis* (rare in U.S.; four variants, so difficult to identify).

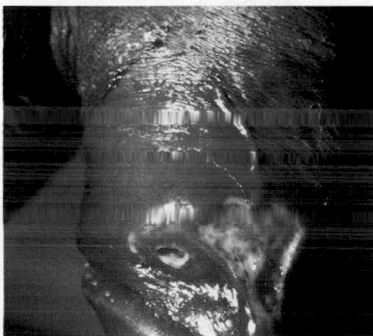

Chancroid

- *Appearance:* Red papule or pustule initially, then forms a *painful* deep ulcer with ragged nonindurated margins; contains necrotic exudate, has a friable base.
- *Causative organism: Haemophilus ducreyi,* an anaerobic bacillus. *Incubation:* 3–7 days after exposure.
- Painful inguinal adenopathy; suppurative buboes in 25% of patients.
- Need to distinguish from primary syphilis; genital herpes simplex; lymphogranuloma venereum, granuloma inguinale from *Klebsiella granulomatis* (both rare in U.S.).

TABLE
21-5

Abnormalities of the Testis

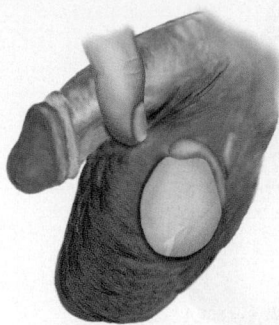

Cryptorchidism

The testis is atrophied and may lie in the inguinal canal or the abdomen, resulting in an unfilled scrotum. As above, there is no palpable left testis or epididymis. Cryptorchidism markedly raises the risk for testicular cancer.

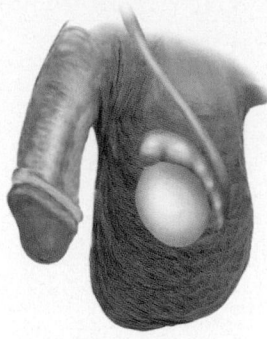

Small Testis

In adults, testicular length is usually ≤3.5 cm. Small, firm testes in *Klinefelter syndrome,* usually ≤2 cm. Small, soft testes suggesting atrophy are seen in cirrhosis, myotonic dystrophy, use of estrogens, and hypopituitarism; may also follow orchitis.

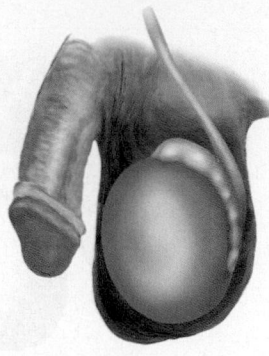

Acute Orchitis

The testis is acutely inflamed, painful, tender, and swollen. It may be difficult to distinguish from the epididymis. The scrotum may be reddened. Seen in mumps and other viral infections; usually unilateral.

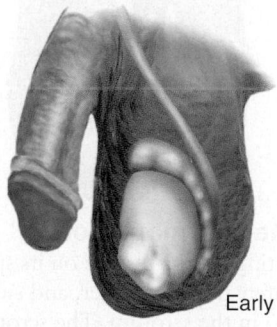

Early

Tumor of the Testis

Usually appears as a painless nodule. Any nodule within the testis warrants investigation for malignancy.

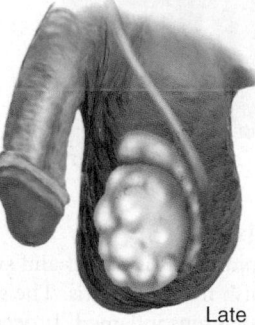

Late

As a testicular neoplasm grows and spreads, it may seem to replace the entire organ. The testicle characteristically feels heavier than normal.

TABLE
21-6

Abnormalities of the Epididymis and Spermatic Cord

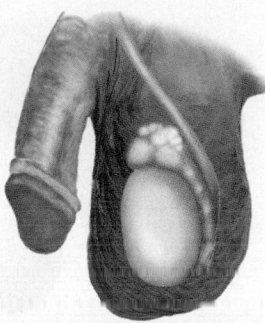

Spermatocele and Cyst of the Epididymis

A painless, movable cystic mass just above the testis suggests a spermatocele or an epididymal cyst. Both transilluminate. The former contains sperm, and the latter does not, but they are clinically indistinguishable.

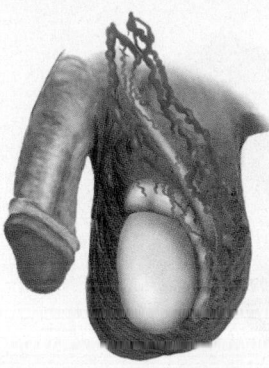

Varicocele of the Spermatic Cord

Varicocele refers to varicose veins of the spermatic cord, usually found on the left. It feels like a soft "bag of worms" separate from the testis, and slowly collapses when the scrotum is elevated in the supine patient. Infertility may be associated.

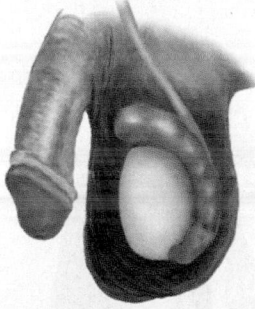

Acute Epididymitis

An acutely inflamed epididymis is tender and swollen and may be difficult to distinguish from the testis. The scrotum may be reddened and the vas deferens inflamed. It occurs chiefly in adults. Coexisting urinary tract infection or prostatitis supports the diagnosis.

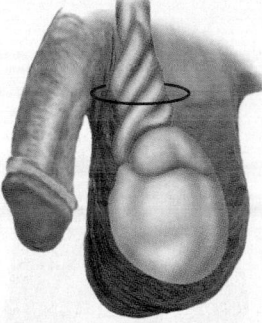

Torsion of the Spermatic Cord

Torsion, or twisting, of the testicle on its spermatic cord produces an acutely painful, tender, and swollen organ that is retracted upward in the scrotum. The scrotum becomes red and edematous. There is no associated urinary infection. Torsion, most common in adolescents, is a surgical emergency because of obstructed circulation.

TABLE
21-7

Course, Presentation, and Differentiation of Hernias in the Groin

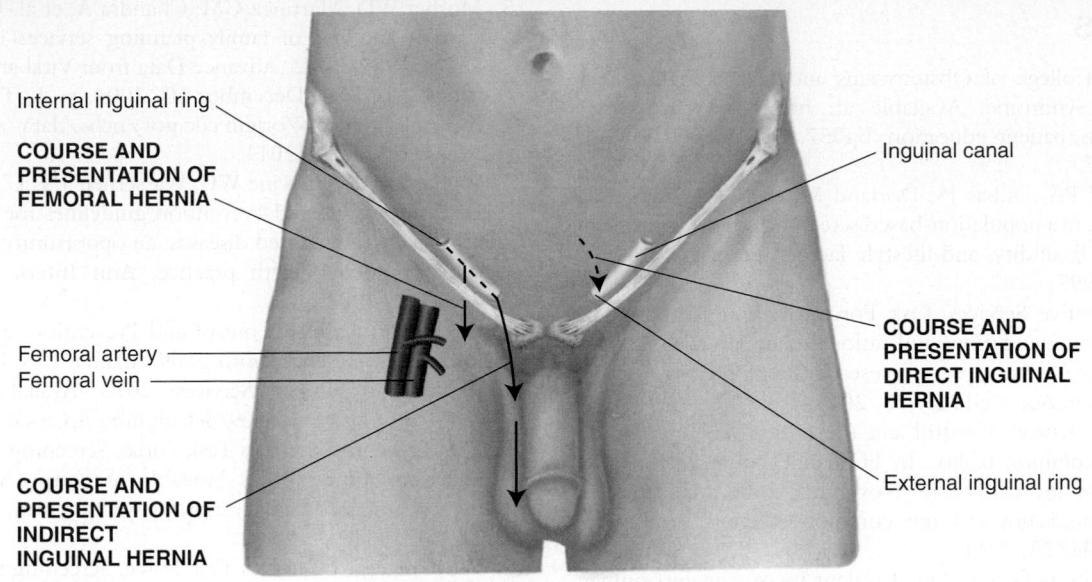

Internal inguinal ring

COURSE AND PRESENTATION OF FEMORAL HERNIA

Inguinal canal

Femoral artery
Femoral vein

COURSE AND PRESENTATION OF DIRECT INGUINAL HERNIA

COURSE AND PRESENTATION OF INDIRECT INGUINAL HERNIA

External inguinal ring

Inguinal Hernias

	Indirect	*Direct*	**Femoral Hernias**
	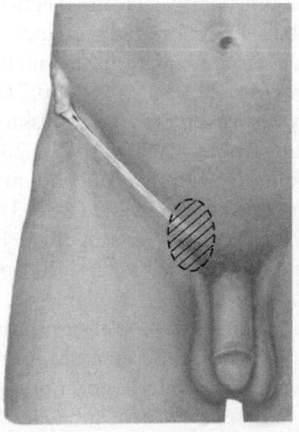	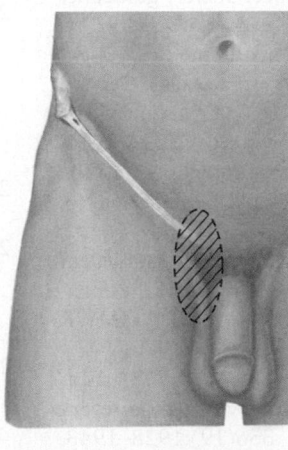	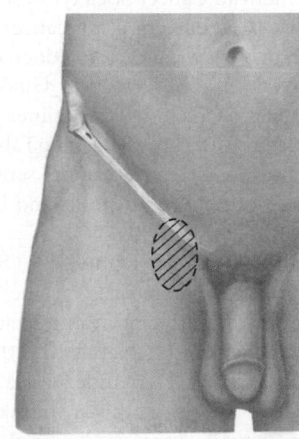
Frequency, Age, and Sex	Most common, all ages, both sexes. Often in children; may be in adults	Less common. Usually in men older than 40; rare in women	Least common. More common in women than in men
Point of Origin	Above inguinal ligament, near its midpoint (the internal inguinal ring)	Above inguinal ligament, close to the pubic tubercle (near the external inguinal ring)	Below the inguinal ligament; appears more lateral than an inguinal hernia. Can be hard to differentiate from lymph nodes
Course	Often into the scrotum	Rarely into the scrotum	Never into the scrotum
(Examining finger in inguinal canal during straining)	The hernia comes down the inguinal canal and touches the fingertip.	The hernia bulges anteriorly and pushes the side of the finger forward.	The inguinal canal is empty.

BIBLIOGRAPHY

CITATIONS

1. American College of Obstetricians and Gynecologists. Premenstrual syndrome. Available at: http://www.acog.org/publications/patient_education/bp057.cfm. Accessed November 2, 2007.

2. van Noord PA, Dubas JS, Dorland M, et al. Age at natural menopause in a population-based screening cohort: the role of menarche, fecundity, and lifestyle factors. Fertil Steril 68(1): 95–102, 1997.

3. U.S. Preventive Services Task Force. Screening for cervical cancer: recommendations and rationale. January 2003. Available at: http://www.uspreventiveservicestaskforce.org/uspstf/ uspscerv.htm. Accessed May 23, 2011.

4. Centers for Disease Control and Prevention. HPV, common infection, common reality. In Human Papillomavirus: HPV Information for Clinicians. November 2006. Available at: http://www.cdc.gov/std/hpv/common-infection/Bro-br.pdf. Accessed May 23, 2011.

5. Future II Study Group. Quadrivalent vaccine against human papillomavirus to prevent high-grade cervical infections. New Engl J Med 356(19):1915–1927, 2007.

6. American College of Obstetricians and Gynecologists. ACOG Practice Bulletin 109, December 2009: cervical cytology screening. Obstet Gynecol 114:1409–1420, 2009.

7. American Cancer Society. American Cancer Society guidelines for early detection of cancer–cervical cancer. Available at: http://www.cancer.org/docroot/PED/content/PED_2_3X _ACS_Cancer_Detection_Guidelines_36.asp. See also: Cervical cancer screening guidelines. Available at: http://www. cdc.gov/std/hpv/ScreeningTables.pdf. Accessed May 23, 2011.

8. Sawaya G. Cervical-cancer screening–new guidelines and the balance between benefits and harms. N Engl J Med 361(26): 2503–2505, 2009.

9. Markowitz LE, Dunne EF, Saraiya M, et al. Quadrivalent human papillomavirus vaccine: recommendations of the Advisory Committee on Immunization Practices (ACIP). MMWR 56(RR-2):1–24, March 12, 2007.

10. Garland SM, Hernandez-Avila M, Wheller CM, et al. Quadrivalent vaccine against human papillomavirus to prevent anogenital diseases. N Engl J Med 356(19):1928–1943, 2007.

11. Hildsheim A, Herrero R, Wacholder S, et al. Effect of human papillomavirus 16/18 L1 viruslike particle vaccine among young women with preexisting infection: a randomized trial. JAMA 298(7):743–752, 2007.

12. Steinbrook R. The potential of human papillomavirus vaccines: perspective. N Engl J Med 354(11):1109–1112, 2007.

13. Dunne EF, Unger ER, Sternberg M, et al. Prevalence of HPV infection among females in the United States. JAMA 297(8):810–813, 2007.

14. MacDorman M, Kirmeyer S. The challenge of fetal mortality. NCHS Data Brief No. 16, April 2009. Available at: http:// www.cdc.gov/nchs/data/databriefs/db16.htm. Accessed May 23, 2011.

15. Mosher WD, Martinez GM, Chandra A, et al. Use of contraception and use of family planning services in the United States: 1982–2002. Advance Data from Vital and Health Statistics, No. 350, December 10, 2004, p. 1, Table 9, p. 21. Available at: http://origin.cdc.gov/nchs/data/ad/ad350.pdf. Accessed May 23, 2011.

16. Workowski KA, Levine WC, Wasserheit JN. U.S. Centers for Disease Control and Prevention guidelines for the treatment of sexually transmitted diseases: an opportunity to unify clinical and public health practice. Ann Intern Med 137(4): 255–262, 2002.

17. Centers for Disease Control and Prevention. Sexually Transmitted Disease Surveillance 2009. Atlanta: U.S. Department of Health and Human Services; 2010. Available at: http:// www.cdc.gov/std/stats09/default.htm, Accessed May 21, 2022.

18. U.S. Preventive Services Task Force. Screening for chlamydial infection. June 2007. Available at: http://www.uspreven tiveservicestaskforce.org/uspstf/uspschlm.htm. Accessed May 23, 2011.

19. U.S. Preventive Services Task Force. Screening for gonorrhea. May 2005. Available at: http://www.uspreventiveservicestask force.org/uspstf/uspsgono.htm. Accessed May 23, 2011.

20. U.S. Preventative Health Services Task Force. Screening for Syphilis Infection. July 2004. Available at: http://www.uspre ventiveservicestaskforce.org/uspstf/uspssyph.htm. Accessed May 23, 2011.

21. U.S. Preventative Health Services Task Force. Screening for Syphilis Infection in Pregnancy: Evidence for the Reaffirmation Recommendation Statement. May 2009. first published Ann Intern Med 2009;150:710–16. Available at: http:// www.uspreventiveservicestaskforce.org/uspstf09/syphilis/ syphpgart.htm. Accessed May 23, 2011.

22. Levine AM. Evaluation and management of HIV-infected women. Ann Intern Med 136(3):228–242, 2002.

23. U.S. Preventive Services Task Force. Screening for human immunodeficiency virus infection. July 2005, with amendment April 2007. Available at: http://www.uspreventiveser vicestaskforce.org/uspstf/uspshivi.htm. Accessed May 23, 2011.

24. Workowski KA, Berman SM. Centers for Disease Control and Prevention. Clinical prevention guidance. Sexually transmitted diseases treatment guidelines 2006. MMWR 55(RR-11): 2–5, August 4, 2006.

25. Johnson, R. Interview with Gary Gates of The Williams Institute. About.com Gay Life. Available at: http://gaylife.about.com/ od/index/a/garygates.htm. Accessed May 24, 2011.

26. Institute of Medicine. Committee on Prevention and Control of Sexually Transmitted Diseases. The Hidden Epidemic: Confronting Sexually Transmitted Diseases. Washington, DC: National Academy Press, 1997:1–432.

27. Centers for Disease Control and Prevention. Sexually Transmitted Disease Surveillance 2009. Atlanta: U.S. Department of Health and Human Services; 2010. Available at: http:// www.cdc.gov/std/stats09/default.htm, Accessed May 21, 2022.

28. U.S. Preventive Services Task Force. Screening for HIV recommendation statement. Release date July 2005; amended April 2007. Available at: http://www.uspreventiveservices taskforce.org/uspstf/uspshivi.htm. Accessed May 21, 2011.

29. National Cancer Institute. Cancer facts. Available at: http://www.cancer.gov/cancertopics/factsheet/Sites-Types/testicular. Accessed May 21, 2011.

30. American Cancer Society. Cancer facts and figures 2007. Available at: http://www.cancer.org/Research/CancerFacts Figures/CancerFactsFigures/cancer-facts-and-figures-2010. Accessed May 21, 2011.

31. National Cancer Institute. Prostate cancer: prevention. Risk factors for prostate cancer development. Available at: http://www.cancer.gov/cancertopics/pdq/prevention/prostate/HealthProfessional/page3. Accessed May 22, 2011.

32. Lichtenstein P, Holm NV, Verkasalo PK, et al. Environmental and heritable factors in the causation of cancer—analyses of cohorts of twins from Sweden, Denmark, and Finland. N Engl J Med 343(2):78–85, 2000.

33. Nelson WG, DeMarzo AM, Isaacs WB. Prostate cancer. N Engl J Med 349(4):366–381, 2003.

34. National Cancer Institute. Opportunities for prevention. Available at: http://www.cancer.gov/cancertopics/pdq/prevention/prostate/HealthProfessional/page4. Accessed May 22, 2011.

35. U.S. Preventive Services Task Force. Screening for prostate cancer: recommendation and rationale. Available at: http://www.uspreventiveservicestaskforce.org/uspstf08/prostate/prostaters.htm. Accessed May 21, 2011.

36. American Urological Association. Policy Statements: Early Detection of Prostate Cancer, 2009. Available at: http://www.auanet.org/content/guidelines-and-quality-care/policy-statements/e/early-detection-of-prostate-cancer.cfm. Accessed May 22, 2011.

37. Kimberlin DW, Rouse DJ. Genital herpes. N Engl J Med 350(19):1970–1977, 2004.

38. Anderson MR, Klink K, Cohrssen A. Evaluation of vaginal complaints. JAMA 291(11):1368–1379, 2004.

39. Eckhert LO. Acute vulvovaginitis. N Engl J Med 355(12):1244–1252, 2006.

ADDITIONAL REFERENCES

Alvarez-Blasco F, Botella-Carretero JI, San Millan JL, et al. Prevalence and characteristics of the polycystic ovary syndrome in overweight and obese women. Arch Intern Med 166:2081–2086, 2006.

Anderson MR, Klink K, Cohrsson A. Evaluation of vaginal complaints. JAMA 291(11):368–379, 2004.

Collaborative Group on Epidemiological Studies of Ovarian Cancer, Beral V, Doll R, et al. Ovarian cancer and oral contraceptives: collaborative reanalysis of data from 45 epidemiological studies including 23,257 women with ovarian cancer and 87,303 controls. Lancet 371(9609):303–314, 2008.

Datta SD, Sternberg M, Johnson RE, et al. Gonorrhea and chlamydia in the United States among persons 14 to 39 years of age, 1999 to 2002. Ann Intern Med 147(2):89–96, 2007.

Future II Study Group. Quadrivalent vaccine against human papillomavirus to prevent high-grade cervical lesions. N Engl J Med 356(19):1915–1927, 2007.

Gupta R, Warren T, Wald A. Genital herpes. Lancet 370(9605):2127–2137, 2007.

Hwang LY, Shafer MA, Pollack LM, et al. Sexual behaviors after universal screening of sexually transmitted infections in healthy young women. Obstet Gynecol 109(1):105–113, 2007.

Mayrand MH, Duarte-Franco E, Rodriques I, et al. Human papillomavirus DNA versus Papanicolaou screening tests for cervical cancer. N Engl J Med 357(16):1579–1588, 2007.

Nelson HD. Menopause. Lancet 371(9614):760–770, 2008.

Peipert JF. Genital chlamydial infections. N Engl J Med 349(25):2424–2430, 2003.

Reif S, Whetten K, Thielman N. Association of race and gender with use of antiretroviral therapy among HIV-infected individuals in the Southeastern United States. South Med J 100(8):775–781, 2007.

Simon V, Ho DD, Abdool Karim Q. HIV/AIDS epidemiology, pathogenesis, prevention, and treatment. Lancet 368(9534):489–504, 2006.

Sirovich BE, Welch HG. Cervical cancer screening among women without a cervix. JAMA 291(24):2990–2993, 2004.

Putting It All Together

LEARNING OBJECTIVES

The student will:

1. Identify the components of the physical examination.
2. Identify the best approach for the physical examination based on individual patient needs.
3. Create an appropriate environment to ensure an accurate physical examination.
4. Demonstrate a head-to-toe physical examination.

Health assessment is the combination of both the interview history and the physical examination. Throughout the book, learning has focused on individual systems. Chapters are structured for nurses to first ask questions to elicit the subjective information and then utilize the techniques of inspection, palpation, percussion, and auscultation to identify the objective information. Learning each system in depth is important. Equally important is the integration of all systems into a complete physical examination, as well as the ability to critically evaluate the individual patient and decide which system(s) to focus on during the patient visit.

Assessments are performed on every patient in every setting. Generally, a complete assessment is performed on new patients or new admissions to a healthcare agency. The patient may be a healthy individual arriving at the clinic for a school physical or an ill patient admitted to the hospital.

A focused assessment targets specific body systems. The decision to limit the number of systems assessed may be based on history findings, timing, severity of illness, pain, or limited access to the patient. The nurse caring for a patient who arrives with a chief complaint of a painful arm will focus on the following systems: musculoskeletal, cardiovascular, peripheral vascular, and neurologic. Based on the information obtained in the health history, systems may be excluded from the examination. If the pain was caused by an injury to the arm that did not impact the heart and there is no cardiac history, cardiac examination may be eliminated, but musculoskeletal, neurologic, and peripheral vascular systems would still be important to evaluate.

Initially, the complete examination may seem cumbersome and time-consuming. The student may wonder how to condense all the information and skills into an orchestrated, consistent examination. At the same time, the student wants to exude confidence and demonstrate comprehension of the examination.

This will take time but also, most importantly, practice. During lab sessions it is important to utilize the time with your partner and guidance of your instructor to ensure proper technique and positioning for the examination. After lab sessions it is imperative to take additional time for repeat practice. Repetition is necessary to refine skills and coordinate the techniques into a thorough examination.

Generally, a complete assessment is performed in a head-to-toe sequence comparing side to side (bilaterally) for symmetry. Prior to trying the head-to-toe examination, review the systems and plot the best flow for the examination. Some systems overlap and can be interwoven during the examination. This limits the number of times patients need to change position from sitting to lying to standing, which can be difficult for patients who have pain, dyspnea, or limited range of motion. Multiple choices when organizing the examination and continued practice will assist you to gain proficiency and find the best flow. For example, some nurses cover the musculoskeletal examination, including range of motion, toward the beginning of the exam, while others prefer to wait until after assessing the core components (cardiac, pulmonary, abdomen). Determining the most efficient format for the physical examination is the initial step.

Now it is time to prepare for the actual examination. The equipment should be assembled prior to the start of the exam.

EQUIPMENT

Sphygmomanometer
Stethoscope
Thermometer
Watch with a second hand
Stadiometer
Scale
Paper and pen or computer
Mini-mental status examination tool

Examination gloves
Snellen chart or "E" card
Rosenbaum, Jaeger, or near-vision card
Index card
Penlight or flashlight
Ophthalmoscope
Tuning fork (512 Hz)

(continued)

EQUIPMENT (continued)

Otoscope
Speculums
Sense of smell (e.g., mint, coffee, or alcohol swab if other scents
    not available)
Tangential light
Cup of water
Tongue depressors

2×2 gauze pads (for use during tongue examination)
Q-tips, paper clips, or other disposable objects for testing two-point
    discrimination
Cotton for testing the sense of light touch
Two test tubes (optional) for testing temperature sensation
Ruler and/or flexible tape measure, preferable in centimeters

Doppler
Reflex hammer
Draw sheet or drape

During the examination, remember to consider the patient's privacy. Use a sheet to cover parts of the body not being examined at the time. While examining the patient, explain procedures and findings throughout the entire exam. Letting the patient know what you are doing and your findings, such as blood pressure results, creates teaching/learning moments and develops a rapport with your patient.

Many students find it beneficial to make note cards, which can be used as cues for each system. Do not write too much or you might be distracted. As a new practitioner, your examination of the patient should take less than 1 hour from start to finish. Below is a basic guide for conducting a physical examination while minimizing the number of position changes for the patient. Another sequence may work better for you; this is acceptable as long as the exam proceeds in a logical flow, includes all the necessary components, and limits patient position changes. However, if an assessment is missed, it may be inserted at another convenient place in the exam. The more you practice and repeat the techniques, the less likely this is to occur. Now assess your demeanor, and take a breath before entering the room.

A SAMPLE OF THE SEQUENCING FOR A HEAD-TO-TOE ASSESSMENT
Physical Examination Overview

On entering the room the nurse should: wash his or her hands, introduce self and purpose and begin the assessment and examination.

A SAMPLE OF THE SEQUENCING FOR A HEAD-TO-TOE ASSESSMENT

Patient Seated
General Survey
- Assess the environment for:
  - a. Noise
  - b. Safety
  - c. Privacy
  - d. Lighting

- Assess the individual for:
  - a. Age—stated age versus apparent age
  - b. Emotional state—compare verbal description and nonverbal indicators
  - c. Developmental stage—compare with behavior
  - d. Cultural background
  - e. Health requirements and learning needs

*Mental Status**

This will be assessed throughout the history and examination beginning with the General Survey; this includes assessment obtained when speaking to the patient. Assess for:

- a. Level of consciousness
- b. Facial expressions
- c. Speech
- d. Thought processes and perception
- e. Mood
- f. Grooming and hygiene
- g. Posture, gait, and body movements

Body Measurements
- a. Height
- b. Weight
- c. Body mass index and ideal body weight

Vital Signs
- a. Temperature
- b. Pulse
- c. Respirations
- d. Blood pressure—arm at heart level
- e. Pain

Integument
Assess throughout the examination as you examine each part of the body.

- a. Inspect for color, lesions, scars, rashes, or any changes in the skin.
- b. Palpate for moisture, temperature, and texture.
- c. Palpate for skin turgor.
- d. Inspect the hair for color, distribution, and texture.

---

*If changes are noted, then a mini-mental status examination should be performed.

e. Inspect and palpate the nails for size, shape, color, texture, angle, refill, and any changes.

Head

a. Inspect the skull for size and shape.
b. Inspect the scalp for tenderness, lesions, and bumps.

Face

a. Inspect facial features for symmetry
b. Palpate temporal and masseter strength.
c. Assess temporomandibular joint for pain, crepitus, and swelling.

Cranial nerve VII, facial: symmetry of face—raise eyebrows, frown, close eyes, smile, puff out cheeks

d. Assess sensation to sharp and light on face—forehead, cheeks, and chin (Continue assessing arms and feet for sharp and light touch.)

Cranial Nerve V, trigeminal

Eyes

a. Acuity (if a hand held eye chart is available, otherwise do in the beginning before the patient is seated or hold this part until the patient is standing for other parts of the assessment)
b. Inspect:
   – Eyelids
   – Eyelashes
   – Eyebrows
   – Lacrimal apparatus
   – Conjunctiva
   – Sclera
   – Cornea
   – Lens
   – Pupils
      – Size
      – Shape
      – Direct light reaction
      – Consensual light reaction

Cranial nerve II, optic; cranial nerve III, occulomotor

Cranial Nerve II, optic

Cranial nerve III, occulomotor; cranial nerve IV, trochlear; cranial nerve VI, abducens

c. Test confrontation
d. Eye muscle examinations
   – Test six cardinal directions of gaze
   – Convergence
   – Near reaction (accommodation)
   – Cover–uncover test
e. Ophthalmoscope examination
   Inspect:
   – Optic disc for color, size, shape
   – Retina for color, abnormalities
   – Arteries and veins for changes

Ears

a. Inspect auricle, lobe, and tragus for position, shape, ulcers, lesions, or discharge.
b. Palpate auricle and tragus for tenderness or lumps.
c. Palpate mastoid firmly for tenderness.

    d. Otoscopic examination—inspect inner canal, tympanic membrane, and cone of light.

    e. Hearing acuity   Cranial nerve VIII, acoustic

        – Whisper test

        – Weber (512 Hz on top of head)

        – Rinne (512 Hz on mastoid bone and compare to air conduction)

Nose and Sinuses

    a. Inspect for symmetry, alignment, and deformity.

    b. Palpate for tenderness and patency.

    c. Palpate frontal and maxillary sinuses.

    d. Inspect mucous membrane, septum, and turbinates for inflammation, polyps, ulcers, and deviation.

    e. Sense of smell—have patient identify two different scents with eyes   Cranial nerve I, olfactory
closed.

Mouth and Pharynx

    a. Inspect lips, oral mucosa, gums, roof of mouth, and floor of mouth for color, lesions, and moisture.

    b. Inspect dentition for condition, number, and placement.

    c. Tongue

        – Inspect for size, shape, color, moisture, lesions, and texture.

        – Articulation of words   Cranial nerve XII, hypoglossal

        – Range of motion—assess at-rest, raised, protruding, and side-to-side movements.

        – Taste   Cranial nerve VII, facial; cranial nerve IX, glossopharyngeal

    d. Pharynx—inspect rise of palate and uvula.   Cranial nerve IX, glossopharyngeal; cranial nerve X, vagus

Neck

    a. Inspect anteriorly for symmetry, masses, enlarged lymph nodes, or deviation.

    b. Inspect trachea position.

    c. Palpate head, neck and subclavicular lymph nodes

    d. Test sternomastoid and upper trapezius muscle strength.   Cranial nerve XI, spinal accessory

    e. Test head and neck range of motion (flexion, extension, rotation, and lateral bends).

    f. Inspect thyroid.

    g. Palpate thyroid. (May be from front or back of patient)

The nurse will assess the following from the back of the patient:

    Assess the cervical spine (inspection, palpation)

    Assess for pain at the costovertebral angle (CVA tenderness)

Posterior Thorax

    a. Inspect shape, deformities, retractions, symmetry, and skin integrity.

    b. Palpate for tenderness, tactile fremitus, respiratory expansion

    c. Percuss lung sounds and diaphragmatic excursion

    d. Ascultate lung sounds

As the nurse returns to the front of the patient, some portions of the anterior thorax, cardiac and breast examinations can be performed sitting or lying down.

Anterior Thorax
(Can also be performed with patient lying down if preferred)

a. Inspect for shape, deformities, retractions, symmetry, and skin integrity.
b. Palpate for
   - Tenderness
   - Tactile fremitus
   - Respiratory expansion
c. Percuss sounds and diaphragmatic excursion.
d. Auscultate lung sounds.

Cardiac
Auscultate with the bell at the apical impulse while the patient is leaning forward)—listening for aortic stenosis/murmur.

Breasts
a. Inspect with
   - Arms at side
   - Hands pressed into hips
   - Arms raised over head

Axillary Nodes
a. Palpate axillary nodes (central, lateral, pectoral, subscapular)

Patient Lying Down
Cardiovascular
Head of bed or table should be elevated at a 30 degree angle.

a. Inspect carotid arteries for pulsations.
b. Palpate carotid arteries.
c. Auscultate carotids with the bell while patient holds breath.
d. Inspect external jugular vein.
e. Inspect precordium.
f. Auscultate heart with the diaphragm at the right sternal border (RSB) 2nd intercostal space (ICS), left sternal border (LSB) 2nd ICS, left sternal border 3rd ICS, left sternal border 4th ICS, left sternal border 5th ICS, and left midclavicular line (MCL) 5th ICS.
g. Auscultate heart with the bell at the right sternal border 2nd ICS, left sternal border 2nd ICS, left sternal border 3rd ICS, left sternal border 4th ICS, left sternal border 5th ICS, and left MCL 5th ICS.
h. Auscultate with the bell at the apical impulse while in the left lateral decubitus position (listening for mitral murmur, S_3, S_4).

If patient is being followed for cardiac issues, assess the heart sounds in both the supine and left lateral positions.

Breast Examination
a. Before examining the breast place the arm that is on the side of the breast being examined under the head and drape the opposite breast.
b. Examine the breast using the vertical pattern technique.

Abdomen
   a. Inspect for contour, pulsations, bulges, and skin integrity.
   b. Auscultate for bowel sounds and aortic pulsation.
   c. Abdominal reflex—lightly stroke inward in all quadrants.
   d. Lightly palpate all four quadrants noting masses, tenderness, and patient's expression.
   e. Deeply palpate all four quadrants noting masses, tenderness, and patient's expression.
   f. Palpate for the liver, kidneys, and spleen.

Peripheral Vascular
   a. Inspect arms and legs for color, swelling, hair distribution, and nail bed color.
   b. Palpate pulses
      – Radial
      – Brachial
         – At this time, palpate the epitrochlear lymph nodes.
      – Femoral
         – At this time palpate the remaining lymph nodes: inguinal lymph nodes (vertical then horizontal groups).
      – Posterior tibial
      – Dorsalis pedis
   c. Palpate for pitting edema in feet and legs.

Musculoskeletal (lower body)
   a. Inspect for deformity, swelling, nodules, redness, and muscle bulk.
   b. Palpate for tenderness, crepitus, swelling, and increased warmth.
   c. Palpate strength and range of motion
      – Hips (flexion, extension, abduction, adduction, internal and external rotation)
      – Knees (flexion and extension)
      – Ankles (dorsiflexion, plantarflexion, inversion, eversion)
      – Toes (flexion, extension, abduction, adduction)

Patient Seated
Musculoskeletal (upper body)
   a. Inspect for deformity, swelling, nodules, redness, and muscle bulk.
   b. Palpate for tenderness, crepitus, swelling, and increased warmth.
   c. Palpate strength and range of motion
      – Shoulders (flexion, extension, abduction, adduction, internal and external rotation)
      – Forearm (pronation, supination)
      – Elbow (flexion, extension)
      – Wrists (extension (dorsiflexion), flexion (palmar flexion), radial and, ulnar deviation)
      – Fingers (grip and flexion, extension, abduction, adduction)
      – Thumb (flexion, extension, opposition, abduction, adduction)

Neurologic—Motor
   a. Inspect body position, noting tremors.

b. Deep tendon reflexes
 - Biceps
 - Triceps
 - Brachioradialis
 - Patellar
 - Achilles

Neurologic—Sensory
(If not incorporated previously then complete now)

a. Pain and light touch—if the patient is unable to feel pain and light touch, then assess for vibration and temperature.

Patient Standing
Musculoskeletal—Spine
a. Inspect for deformity, symmetry, and skin integrity.
b. Palpate spinous processes.
c. Assess range of motion (flexion, extension, lateral bends, rotation).

Neurologic
a. Perform Romberg, gait, balance, and other appropriate neurologic screenings.

It is recommended that visual acuity be assessed at the beginning or at the end of the examination to alleviate the patient getting up another time.

Cranial nerve II, optic.

Visual Acuity. If a hand-held Snellen is available, then inserting visual acuity in the eye assessment is appropriate.

Continue to practice and refine your physical examination skills. The integration of the subjective and objective data guides the nurse in preparing the best nursing plan of care for the patient.

BIBLIOGRAPHY

Boulware LE, Marinopoulos S, Phillips KA, et al. Systematic review; the value of the periodic health evaluation. Ann Intern Med 146(4):289–300, 2007.

Hensrud DD. Clinical preventive medicine in primary care: background and practice. Rational and current preventive practice. Mayo Clin Proc 75(4):1165–1172, 2000.

Laine C, The annual physical examination: needless ritual or necessary routine? Ann Intern Med 136(9):701–702, 2002.

Oboler SK, Prochazka AV, Gonzales R, et al. Public expectations and attitudes for annual physical examinations and testing. Ann Intern Med 136(9):652–659, 2002.

Sackett DL. A primer on the precision and accuracy of the clinical examination. JAMA 267(19):2638–2644, 1992.

Special Lifespan 3

CHAPTER 23
Assessing Children: Infancy Through Adolescence

CHAPTER 24
Assessing Older Adults

Assessing Children: Infancy Through Adolescence

23

Peter G. Szilagyi, MD, MPH

The student will:

1. Gather a history on an infant, child and adolescent.
2. Perform a developmental assessment on infants, children and adolescents.
3. Utilize age appropriate techniques to perform a physical examination on infants, children and adolescents.
4. Analyze findings against age appropriate norms and standards.
5. Identify education topics for anticipatory guidance, health promotion and risk reduction.
6. Correctly document infant, child and adolescent assessment findings.

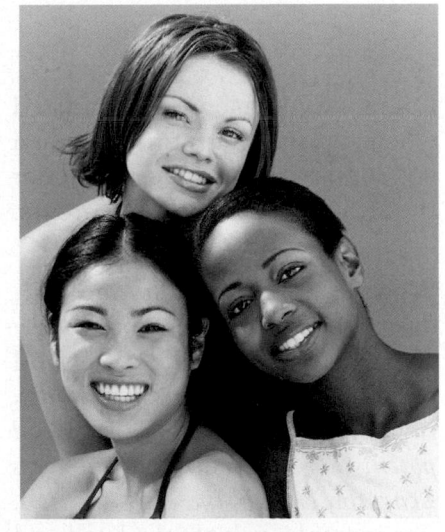

This chapter begins with general principles of development and key components of health promotion. It then includes sections on infants, young and school-aged children, and adolescents, with relevant discussions of development, history taking, health promotion and counseling, and physical examination for each. Many evidence-based citations are woven throughout the chapter as well.

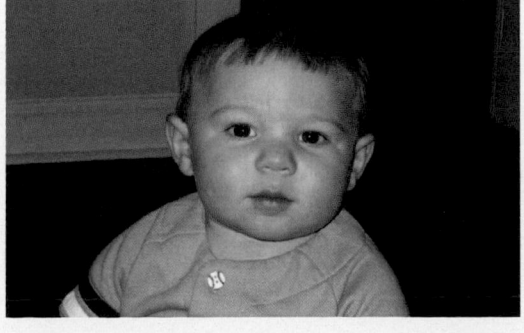

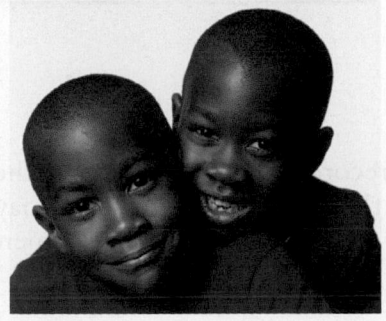

General Principles of Child Development
Health Promotion and Counseling: Key Components
Assessing the Infant
    Development
    The Health History
    Physical Examination
    Health Promotion and Counseling
Assessing Young and School-Aged Children
    Development
    The Health History
    Physical of Examination
    Health Promotion and Counseling
Assessing Adolescents
    Development: 11 to 20 Years
    The Health History
    Physical of Examination
    Health Promotion and Counseling
Recording Your Findings

Often, students are intimidated when approaching a tiny baby or a screaming child, especially under the critical eyes of anxious parents.

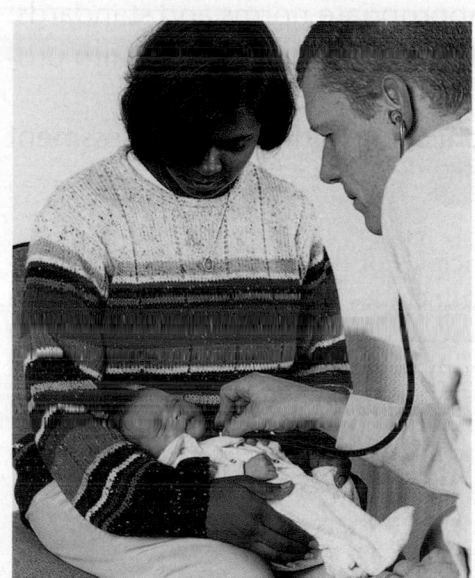

When examining infants and children, the sequence should vary according to the child's age and comfort level. *Perform potentially disturbing maneuvers early and potentially distressing maneuvers near the end of the examination.* For example, palpate the head and neck and auscultate the heart and lungs early, and examine the ears and mouth and palpate the abdomen near the end. If the child reports pain in one area, examine that part last.

The format of the pediatric medical record is the same as that of the adult record. Although the sequence of the physical examination may vary, convert your clinical findings back into the traditional documentation format.

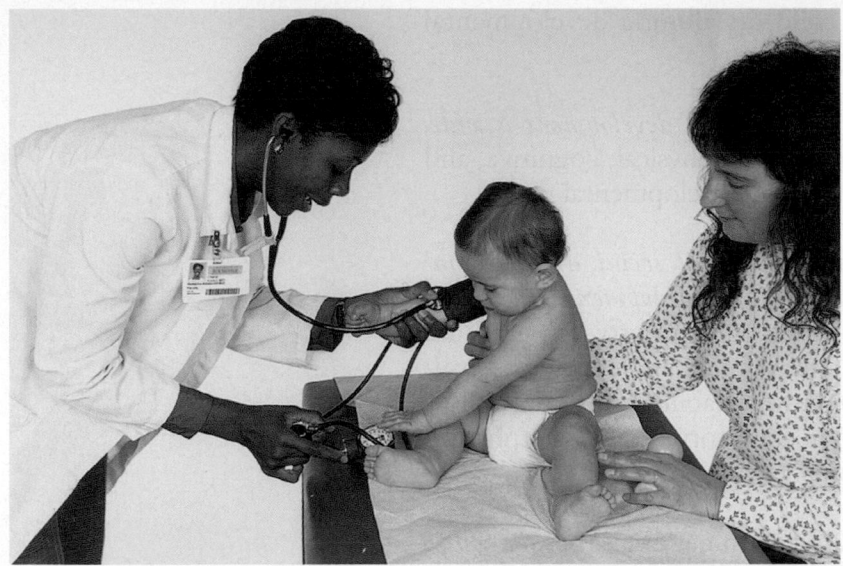

GENERAL PRINCIPLES OF CHILD DEVELOPMENT

Childhood is a period of remarkable physical, cognitive, and social growth—by far the greatest in a person's lifetime. Within a few short years, children physically increase 20-fold, acquire sophisticated language and reasoning, develop complex social interactions, and become mature adults. What a journey!

Understanding the normal physical, cognitive, and social development of children facilitates effective interviews and physical examinations, and helps nurses to distinguish normal and abnormal findings.

FOUR PRINCIPLES OF CHILD DEVELOPMENT[1]

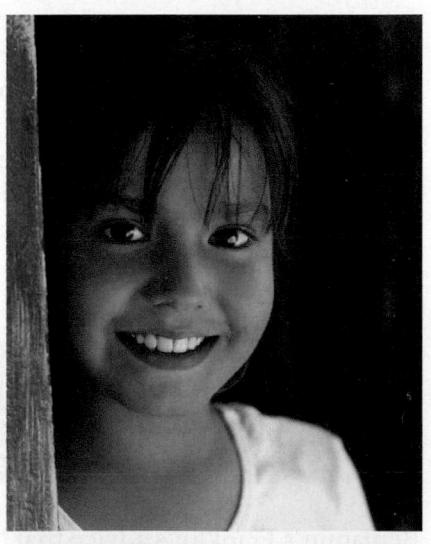

- Child development proceeds along a predictable pathway.
- The range of normal development is wide.
- Various physical, social, and environmental factors, as well as diseases, can affect child development and health.
- The child's developmental level affects how you conduct the history and physical examination.

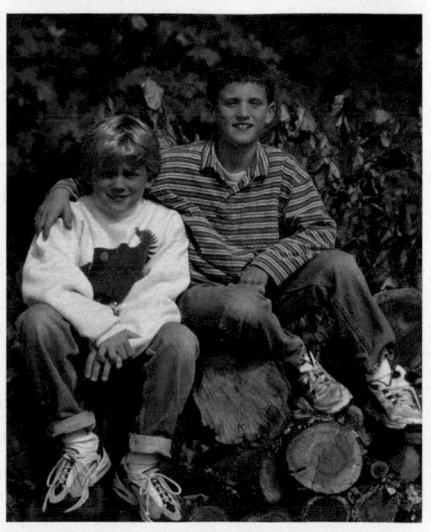

- The first principle of *child development* is that it *proceeds along a predictable pathway* governed by the maturing brain. You can measure age-specific milestones and characterize development as normal or abnormal according to the child's achievement of them. Once the child reaches a milestone, he or she proceeds to the next. Loss of milestones is concerning. Because physical examination takes place at one point in time, determine where the child fits along a developmental trajectory.

- The second principle is that the *range of normal development is wide*. Children mature at different rates. Each child's physical, cognitive, and social development should fall within a broad developmental range.

- The third principle recognizes that *various physical, social, and environmental factors, as well as diseases, can affect child development and health*. For example, chronic illnesses, child abuse, and poverty can all cause detectable physical abnormalities and alter the rate and course of development. Children with physical or cognitive disabilities may not follow the expected age-specific developmental trajectory. Tailor the physical examination to the child's developmental level.

- A fourth principle, specific to the pediatric examination, is that *the child's developmental level affects how you conduct the history and physical examination*. For example, interviewing a 5-year-old is fundamentally different from interviewing an adolescent. The physical examination of a curious toddler who is dismantling the examination room has little in common with that of a shy teenager. Both order and style differ from the examination of an adult. You must adjust your physical examination to the developmental level of the child while simultaneously attempting to ascertain that developmental level. An understanding of normal child development helps you achieve these tasks.

HEALTH PROMOTION AND COUNSELING: KEY COMPONENTS

Benjamin's Franklin's advice that "an ounce of prevention is worth a pound of cure" is particularly true for children and adolescents because prevention at a young age can result in improved health outcomes for decades. Pediatric clinicians dedicate substantial time to health supervision visits and health promotion activities.

Several national and international organizations have identified guidelines for health promotion for children.[2-5] Current concepts of health promotion include not only the detection and prevention of disease but also active promotion of the well-being of children and their families, spanning physical, cognitive, emotional, and social health.

Every interaction with a child and family is an opportunity for health promotion! From the interview to the physical examination, think about your interactions as opportunities for two things: the traditional detection of medical problems and the promotion of health. What a priceless gift!

Capitalize on your examination to offer age-appropriate guidance about the child's development. Provide suggestions about reading, conversing, playing music, and optimizing opportunities for gross and fine motor development. Advise parents about upcoming developmental stages and strategies to encourage their child's development. Remember, parents are the major agents of health promotion for children, and your advice is implemented through them.

The American Academy of Pediatrics (AAP) publishes guidelines for *health supervision visits* and key age-appropriate components of these visits (see www.aap.org). Remember that children and adolescents who have a chronic illness or high-risk family or environmental circumstances will probably require more frequent visits and more intensive health promotion. Key health promotion issues and strategies, tailored for specific age groups, are found throughout this chapter.

Integrate explanations of your physical findings with health promotion. For example, provide advice about expected maturational changes or how health behaviors can affect physical findings (e.g., exercise may reduce blood pressure and obesity). Be sure to demonstrate the relationship between healthy lifestyles and physical health.

Childhood immunizations are a mainstay for health promotion and have been heralded as the most significant medical achievement of public health worldwide. The childhood immunization schedule changes yearly, and updates are published widely and disseminated on Web sites of the Centers for Disease Control and Prevention (CDC) and the AAP.[6,7] To view the most current immunization schedule, go to the CDC's Web site: www.cdc.gov/vaccines.

Screening procedures are performed at certain ages. For all children, these include growth parameters and developmental screening at all ages, blood pressure after infancy, and vision and hearing screening at certain key ages. Screening procedures particularly recommended for high-risk patients include tests for lead poisoning, tuberculosis exposure, anemia, cholesterol, urinary tract infections, and sexually transmitted diseases. There is variation worldwide in recommendations for screening tests; the AAP recommendations are provided at www.aap.org.[2]

Anticipatory guidance is a major component of the pediatric visit. Key areas are shown on the next page and cover a broad range of topics, from purely "medical" to social and emotional health. All these factors affect children's health.

To achieve a healthier world, we *must* emphasize comprehensive and broadly defined health promotion during childhood. Our children's future depends on it.

Key Components of Pediatric Health Promotion

1. Age-appropriate developmental achievement of the child
   - Physical (maturation, growth, puberty)
   - Motor (gross and fine motor skills)
   - Cognitive (achievement of milestones, language, school performance)
   - Emotional (self-efficacy, self-esteem, independence, morality)
   - Social (social competence, self-responsibility, integration with family and community)
2. Health supervision visits
   - Periodic assessment of medical and oral health (per health supervision schedule)
   - Adjustment of frequency for children or families with special needs
3. Integration of physical examination findings with healthy lifestyles
4. Immunizations
5. Screening procedures
6. Anticipatory guidance[2]
   - Healthy habits
   - Nutrition and healthy eating
   - Safety and prevention of injury or illness
   - Sexual development and sexuality
   - Self-responsibility and efficacy
   - Family relationships (interactions, strengths, supports)
   - Community interactions
   - Emotional and mental health
   - Oral health
   - Prevention or recognition
   - Prevention of risky behaviors
   - School and vocation
   - Peer relationships
7. Partnership between health care provider and child, adolescent, and family

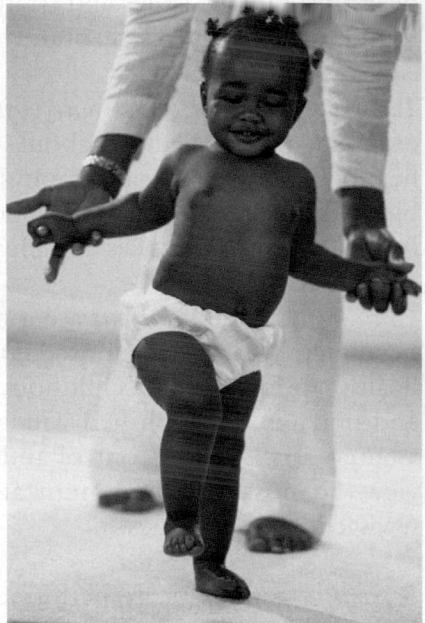

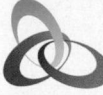 ## ASSESSING THE INFANT

DEVELOPMENT

Physical Development.[8]   Physical growth during infancy is faster than at any other age. By 1 year, the infant's birth weight should have tripled and height increased by 50%.

The figure on the next page shows the amazing developmental progression in infancy. Even newborns have surprising abilities, such as fixing upon and following human faces. Neurologic development progresses centrally to peripherally. Thus, newborns learn head control before trunk control and use of arms and legs before use of hands and fingers.

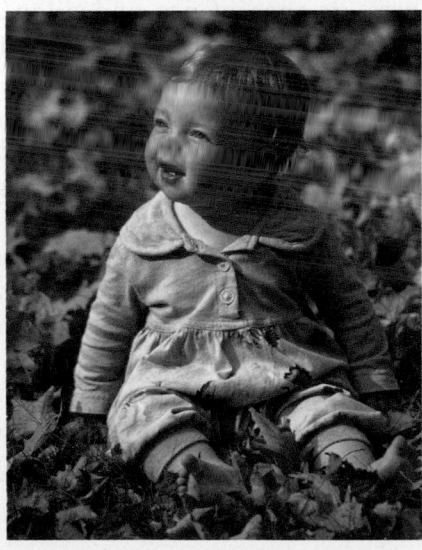

Developmental Milestones During Infancy[13]

	Birth	1m	2m	3m	4m	5m	6m	7m	8m	9m	10m	11m	12m

Physical	Fixes/follows			Rolls over			Sits		Pulls to stand		Stands		Walks
	Head control			Grasps rattle				Thumb-finger grasp			Crawls		
Cognitive/ Language	Responds to sounds	Squeals		Imitates speech sounds				Dada/Mama specific			2 words		3 words
Social/ Emotional	Smiles				Works for toy						Imitates activities		
	Regards face						Feeds self			Indicates wants			Uses spoon

Activity, exploration, and environmental manipulation contribute to learning. By 3 months, normal infants lift the head and clasp the hands. By 6 months, they roll over, reach for objects, turn to voices, and possibly sit with support. With increasing peripheral coordination, infants reach for objects, transfer them from hand to hand, crawl, stand by holding on, and play with objects by banging and grabbing. A 1-year-old may be standing and putting everything in the mouth.[9]

Cognitive and Language Development. Exploration fosters increased understanding of self and environment. Infants learn cause and effect (e.g., shaking a rattle produces sound), object permanence, and use of tools. By 9 months, they may recognize the examiner as a stranger deserving wary cooperation, seek comfort from parents during examinations, and actively manipulate reachable objects (e.g., equipment). Language development proceeds from cooing at 2 months, to babbling at 6 months, to saying 1 to 3 words by 1 year.[10]

Social and Emotional Development. Understanding of self and family also matures. Social tasks include bonding, attachment to caregivers, and trust that they will meet needs. Temperaments vary. Some infants are predictable, adaptable, and respond positively to new stimuli; others are less so and respond intensely or negatively. Because environment affects social development, observe the infant's interactions with caregivers.

THE HEALTH HISTORY

The health history is an important tool for assessing health, growth and development. After a full history is obtained, subsequent visits should ask about the child's health, growth, development, and health patterns as well as other changes (e.g., family life) since the previous visit.

Birth History

At the initial appointment ask the parent about the mother's pregnancy and the infant's birth.

Were there any problems during the pregnancy?
How close was the infant's birth to the due date?
Were there any problems during labor or birth?
Was the child born vaginally or by C-section?

Past History

Ask if the infant has any allergies.

Is he on any medications, including vitamins or fluoride drops?
Has he had any illnesses? Ask the parent to describe the illness, treatment, and outcome.

Family History

The family history may reveal hereditary disease patterns. Inquire about the age and health status of siblings, parents, grandparents, and aunts and uncles. A genogram is helpful to trace patterns emerging within a family.

Also inquire about *family structure*. Who lives in the house with the infant? What is their relationship to the infant?

Health Maintenance

● *Immunizations:* What immunizations has the infant had? Did he have any reaction to the "shots"?

● *Safety measures:* Inquire about the baby's position during sleep, use of car seats, and presence of smoke/carbon monoxide detectors in the house.

● *Risk factors:* The infant's environment may be affected by the parent's behaviors; therefore, inquire about:

Tobacco: Do you smoke? In the house? In the presence of the infant? Does anyone else in your house smoke?
Alcohol: Do you or your spouse drink alcoholic beverages? How much alcohol do you drink per sitting and per week?
Substance abuse: Do you or your spouse use marijuana, cocaine, heroin, or other recreational drugs?
Environmental hazards: Inquire about lead paint or other household hazards.

Conduct a Review of Systems, asking the parent about each system in turn.

Have you noted any problems with your infant's skin? Head or scalp? etc.

When the review is complete ask the parents if they have any concerns about their infant. Then move on to the infant's developmental status according to the infant's age. For example, ask the parents of a 6-month-old if he or she can sit alone. Inquire at what age the infant achieved each milestone.

Health Patterns

Complete the history by asking about the infant's health patterns.

- *Nutrition:* What does the infant drink? How many ounces at one time? Or how long does the infant nurse at each breast? How many times a day?

  Does the infant eat cereal or other foods?
  Does the infant have any problems during or after feedings?

- *Elimination:* Describe your infant's typical urination pattern and bowel pattern, including amount, consistency, and number.

- *Sleep:* Tell me about your infant's sleep pattern (including time of day the infant sleeps and hours of sleep).

- *Activity/play:* What amuses your infant? How do you play with your infant?

Approaching the Infant

Use developmentally appropriate methods such as *distraction* and *play* to examine the infant. Because infants pay attention to one thing at a time, it is relatively easy to bring the infant's attention to something other than the examination being performed. Distract the infant with a moving object, a flashing light, a game of peek-a-boo, or any sort of noise.

If you cannot distract the infant or make the awake infant attend to an object, your face, or a sound, consider a possible *visual* or *hearing deficit.*

TIPS FOR EXAMINING INFANTS

- Approach the infant gradually, using a toy or object for distraction.
- Perform much of the examination with the infant in the parent's lap.
- Speak softly to the infant or mimic the infant's sounds to attract attention.
- If the infant is cranky, make sure he or she is well fed before proceeding.
- Ask a parent about the infant's strengths to elicit useful developmental and parenting information.

General Guidelines

Start with the infant sitting or lying in the parent's lap. If the infant is tired, hungry, or ill, ask the parent to hold the baby against the parent's chest. Make sure appropriate toys, a blanket, or other familiar objects are nearby. A hungry infant may need to be fed first.

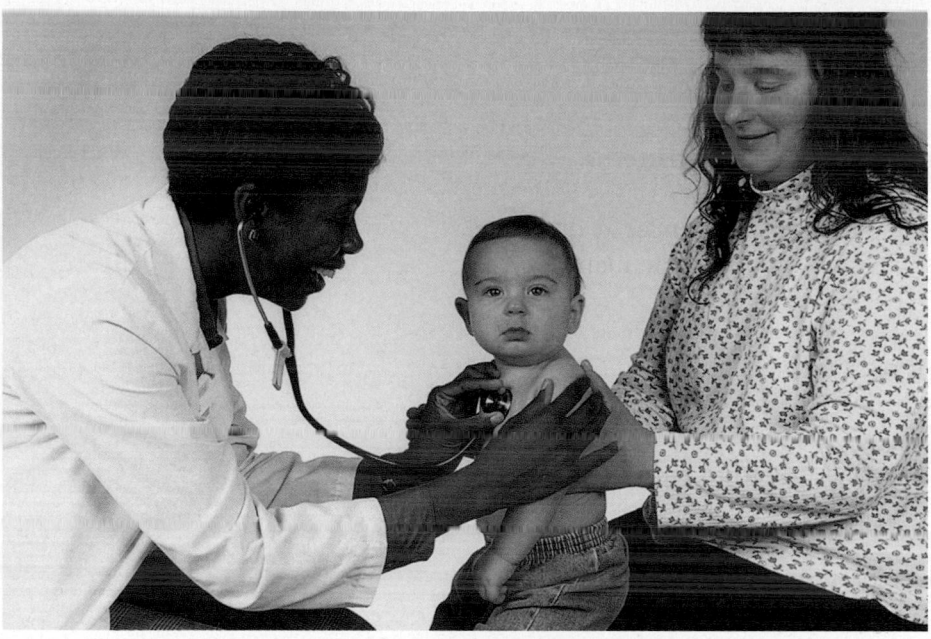

Observe parent–infant interactions. Watch the parent's affect when talking about the infant. Note the parent's manner of holding, moving, dressing, and comforting the infant. Assess and comment on positive interactions, such as the obvious pride in the mother's face above.

Observation of the infant's communication with the parent can reveal abnormalities such as *developmental delay, language delay, hearing deficits,* or *inadequate parental attachment.* Likewise, such observations may identify maladaptive nurturing patterns that may stem from *maternal depression* or *inadequate social support.*

Infants usually do not object to removal of their clothing. To keep yourself and your surroundings dry, it is wise to leave the diaper in place throughout the examination; remove it only to examine the genitals, rectum, lower spine, and hips.

Testing for Developmental Milestones

Because you will want to measure the infant's best performance, checking milestones is best at the end of the interview, just before the examination. This "fun and games" interlude also enhances cooperation during the examination. Experienced nurses can weave the developmental examination into the other parts of the examination. The table on p. 737 shows some key physical or motor, cognitive or language, and social–emotional milestones during the first year.

Many disorders cause delays in more than one milestone. For most children with developmental delay, the causes are unknown. Some known causes include *abnormality in embryonic development* (e.g., prenatal insult, chromosomal problem), *hereditary and genetic disorders* (e.g., inborn errors, genetic abnormalities), *environmental and social problems* (e.g., insufficient stimulation), *pregnancy or perinatal problems* (e.g., placental insufficiency, prematurity), and *childhood diseases* (e.g., infection, trauma, chronic illness).

One standard for measuring developmental milestones throughout infancy and childhood is the DENVER II Screening Test). It is designed to detect developmental delays in four domains of development from birth through 6 years: personal–social, fine motor–adaptive, language, and gross motor.

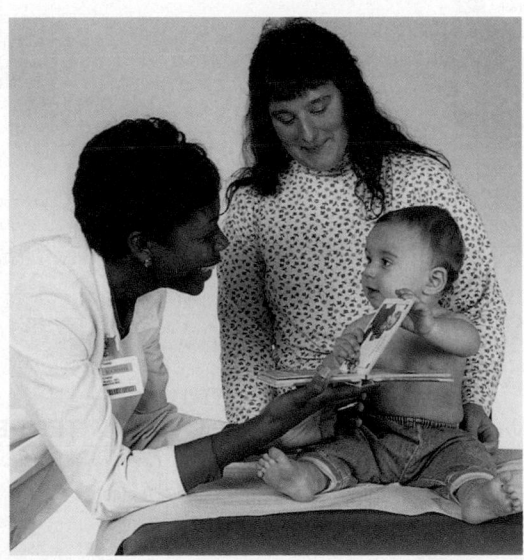

The DENVER II form is shown on the following two pages and includes instructions for recording specific observations. Each test item is represented on the form under the age by a bar, which indicates when 25%, 50%, 75%, and 90% of children attain the milestones depicted. The *DENVER II is a measure of developmental attainment only in the categories indicated. The DENVER II is not a measure of intelligence.*

The DENVER II is a highly specific screening test, so that normal children will test as normal. However, the DENVER II is not very sensitive. Many children with mild developmental delay score as normal. In particular, the language section is sparse and misses children with mild language delay. Although the DENVER II is useful, other, more sophisticated instruments are available to assess motor, language, and social development.

If a cooperative infant fails items on the DENVER II, developmental delay is possible, necessitating more precise testing and evaluation.

Use the DENVER II as an adjunct to a comprehensive developmental examination. Suspected delays from the general examination or DENVER II warrant further evaluation. For babies born prematurely, adjust expected developmental milestones for the gestational age up to approximately 12 months.

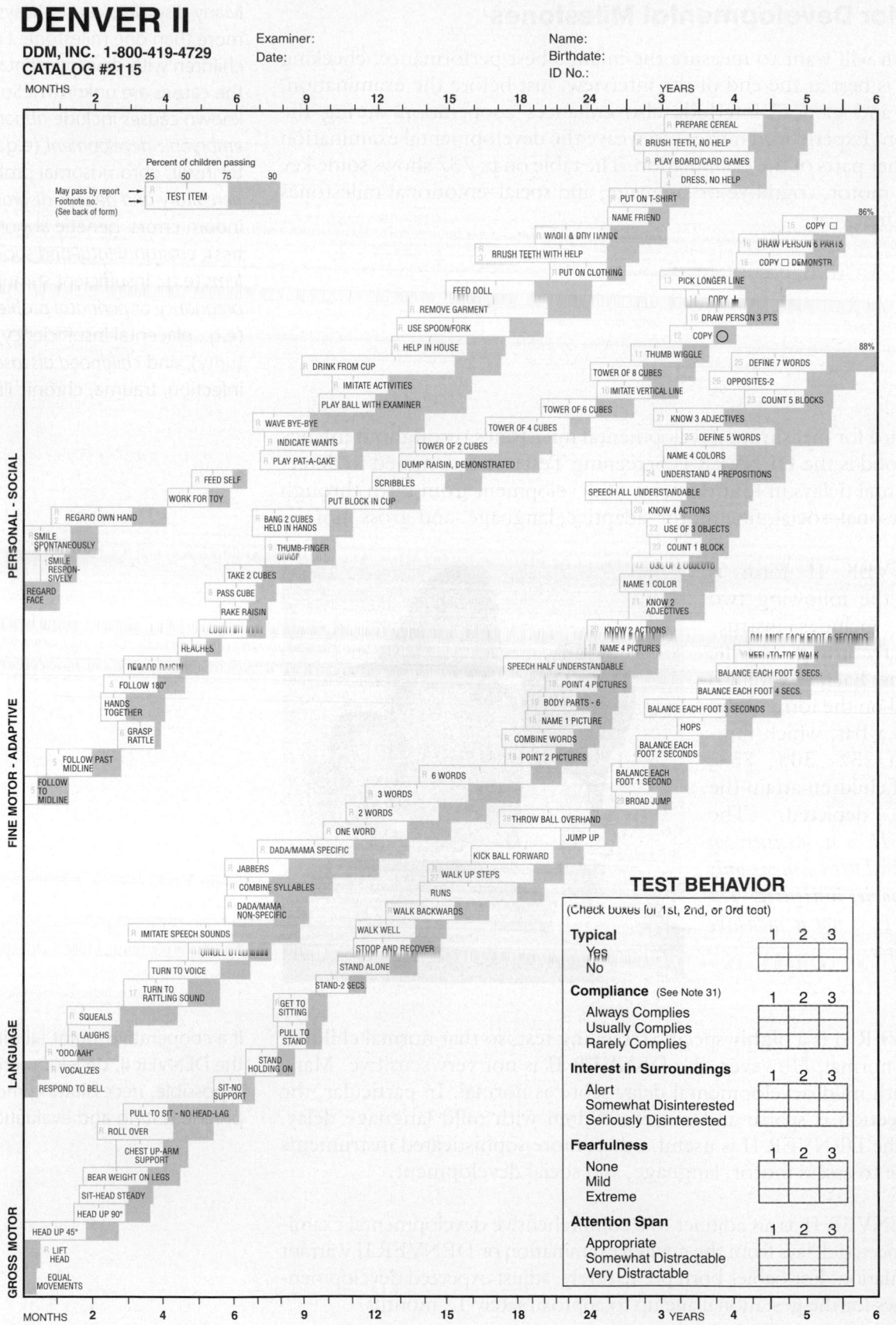

DENVER II

DDM, INC. 1-800-419-4729
CATALOG #2115

Examiner:
Date:

Name:
Birthdate:
ID No.:

©1969, 1989, 1990 W. K. Frankenburg and J. B. Dodds ©1978 W. K. Frankenburg and J. B. Dodds ©1978 W. K. Frankenburg ©2009 Wilhelmine R. Frankenburg

DIRECTIONS FOR ADMINISTRATION

1. Try to get child to smile by smiling, talking or waving. Do not touch him/her.
2. Child must stare at hand several seconds.
3. Parent may help guide toothbrush and put toothpaste on brush.
4. Child does not have to be able to tie shoes or button/zip in the back.
5. Move yarn slowly in an arc from one side to the other, about 8" above child's face.
6. Pass if child grasps rattle when it is touched to the backs or tips of fingers.
7. Pass if child tries to see where yarn went. Yarn should be dropped quickly from sight from tester's hand without arm movement.
8. Child must transfer cube from hand to hand without help of body, mouth, or table.
9. Pass if child picks up raisin with any part of thumb and finger.
10. Line can vary only 30 degrees or less from tester's line. /
11. Make a fist with thumb pointing upward and wiggle only the thumb. Pass if child imitates and does not move any fingers other than the thumb.

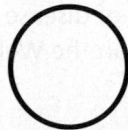      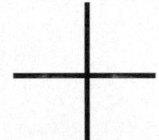   

12. Pass any enclosed form. Fail continuous round motions.
13. Which line is longer? (Not bigger.) Turn paper upside down and repeat. (pass 3 of 3 or 5 of 6)
14. Pass any lines crossing near midpoint.
15. Have child copy first. If failed, demonstrate.

When giving items 12, 14, and 15, do not name the forms. Do not demonstrate 12 and 14.

16. When scoring, each pair (2 arms, 2 legs, etc.) counts as one part.
17. Place one cube in cup and shake gently near child's ear, but out of sight. Repeat for other ear.
18. Point to picture and have child name it. (No credit is given for sounds only.)
    If less than 4 pictures are named correctly, have child point to picture as each is named by tester.

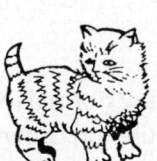   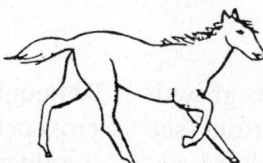   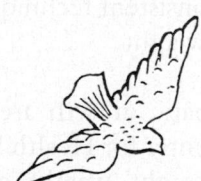   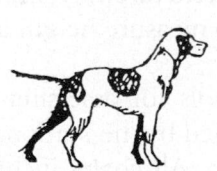   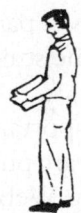

19. Using doll, tell child: Show me the nose, eyes, ears, mouth, hands, feet, tummy, hair. Pass 6 of 8.
20. Using pictures, ask child: Which one flies?...says meow?...talks?...barks?...gallops? Pass 2 of 5, 4 of 5.
21. Ask child: What do you do when you are cold?...tired?...hungry? Pass 2 of 3, 3 of 3.
22. Ask child: What do you do with a cup? What is a chair used for? What is a pencil used for?
    Action words must be included in answers.
23. Pass if child correctly places and says how many blocks are on paper. (1,5).
24. Tell child: Put block **on** table; **under** table; **in front of** me, **behind** me. Pass 4 of 4.
    (Do not help child by pointing, moving head or eyes.)
25. Ask child: What is a ball?...lake?...desk?...house?...banana?...curtain?...fence?...ceiling? Pass if defined in terms of use, shape, what it is made of, or general category (such as banana is fruit, not just yellow). Pass 5 of 8, 7 of 8.
26. Ask child: If a horse is big, a mouse is ___? If fire is hot, ice is ___? If the sun shines during the day, the moon shines during the ___? Pass 2 of 3.
27. Child may use wall or rail only, not person. May not crawl.
28. Child must throw ball overhand 3 feet to within arm's reach of tester.
29. Child must perform standing broad jump over width of test sheet (8 1/2 inches).
30. Tell child to walk forward, ⚬⚬⚬⚬⚬⚬⟶ heel within 1 inch of toe. Tester may demonstrate.
    Child must walk 4 consecutive steps.
31. In the second year, half of normal children are non-compliant.

OBSERVATIONS:

Denver Developmental Materials, Inc.
P.O. Box 371075
Denver, Colorado 80237-5075
Tele. #: (303) 355-4729
(800) 419-4729

Catalog #2115   **TO REORDER CALL: (800) 419-4729**

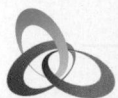

PHYSICAL EXAMINATION OF THE INFANT

General Survey and Vital Signs

Measurement of the infant's body size (length, weight, and head circumference) and assessment of vital signs (blood pressure, pulse, respiratory rate, and temperature) are critical. Tables on the accompanying Web site show norms for blood pressure, height, weight, body mass index (BMI), and head circumference. Compare vital signs or body proportions with age-specific norms, because they change dramatically as children grow. Pediatric nurses also assess pain regularly, using standardized pain scales.

Generally, measurement deviations beyond two standard deviations for age, or above the 95th percentile or below the 5th percentile, are indications for more detailed evaluation. These deviations may be the first and only indicators of disease (see examples on the Web site tables).

Somatic Growth. Measurement of growth is one of the most important indicators of infant health. Deviations may provide an early indication of an underlying problem. Compare growth parameters with respect to:

- Normal values for age and sex

- Prior readings on the same child, to assess trends

A common cause of an apparent deviation in somatic growth is *measurement error*, attributed partly to the challenge of measuring a squirming infant or child. Confirm abnormalities by repeat measurement.

Measure growth parameters carefully, using consistent technique and, optimally, the same scales to measure height and weight.

The most important tools for assessing somatic growth are the growth charts, which are published by the National Center for Health Statistics (see accompanying Web site). All charts include height, weight, and head circumference for age, with one set for children up to 36 months and a second set for 2 to 18 years. Charts plotting weight by length as well as BMI are also available. These growth charts have percentile lines indicating the percentage of normal children above and below the child's measurement by chronologic age. Special growth charts are available for use in infants born prematurely, to correct for this result.

Although many normal infants cross percentiles on growth charts, a sudden or significant change in growth may indicate systemic disease or malnutrition.

Length. For children younger than 2 years, measure body length by placing the child supine on a measuring board or in a measuring tray, as shown. Direct measurement of the infant using a tape measure is inaccurate unless an assistant holds the child still with hips and knees extended. Velocity growth curves are helpful in older children, especially those who are suspected of having endocrine disorders.

Reduced growth velocity, shown by a drop in height percentile on a growth curve, may signify a chronic condition. Comparison with normal standards is essential, because growth velocity normally is less during the second year than during the first year.

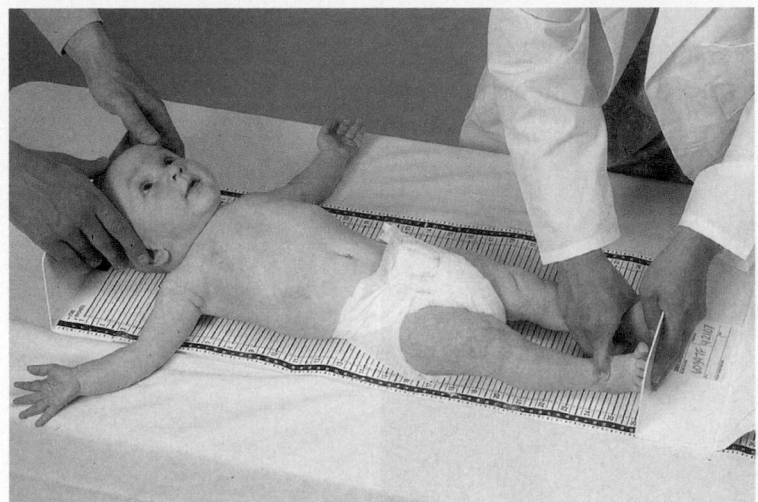

Chronic conditions causing reduced length or height include *neurologic, renal, cardiac,* and *endocrine disorders.*

Weight.   Weigh infants directly with an infant scale; this is more accurate than an indirect method based on weighing the parent and child together and subtracting the weight of the parent from the total weight. Infants should be clothed only in a dry diaper or weighed naked.

If the infant's weight is unexpectedly and significantly different than anticipated, redo the measurement to ensure accuracy.

Failure to thrive is inadequate weight gain for age. Common scenarios are:

● Growth <5th percentile for age
● Growth drop >2 quartiles in 6 months
● Weight for height <5th percentile

Causes include environmental or psychosocial factors and a variety of gastrointestinal, neurologic, cardiac, endocrine, renal, and other diseases.

Head Circumference.   The head circumference should be measured during the first 2 years of life, but measurement can be useful at any age to assess growth of the head. The head circumference in infants reflects the rate of growth of the cranium and the brain. Note position of tape in picture. Measuring the circumference of the head just above the ears produces the best results.

A small head size may be from *premature closure of the sutures* or *microcephaly.* Microcephaly may be familial or the result of various *chromosomal abnormalities, congenital infections, maternal metabolic disorders,* and *neurologic insults.*

An abnormally large head size (>97th percentile or 2 standard deviations above the mean) is *macrocephaly,* which may be from *hydrocephalus, subdural hematoma,* or rare causes like *brain tumor or inherited syndromes. Familial megaloencephaly* (large head) is a benign familial condition with normal brain growth.

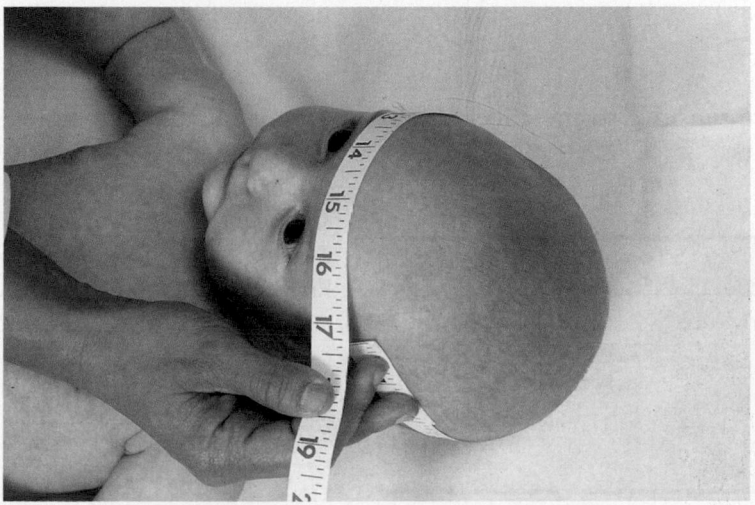

Vital Signs

Blood Pressure. Although obtaining accurate blood pressure readings in infants is challenging, this measurement is nevertheless important and should be performed at least once during infancy. You will need your skills in distraction or play, as shown in the accompanying photo.

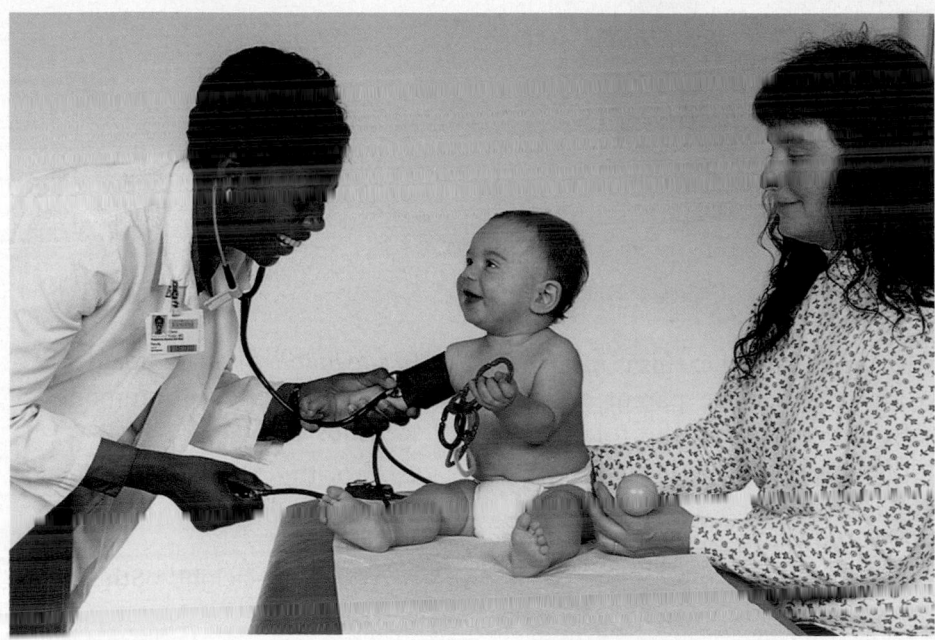

The most easily used measure of systolic blood pressure in infants is the *Doppler method*, which detects arterial blood flow vibrations, converts them to systolic blood pressure levels, and transmits them to a digital read-out device.

The systolic blood pressure gradually increases throughout childhood. For example, normal systolic pressure in males is about 70 mm Hg at birth, 85 mm Hg at 1 month, and 90 mm Hg at 6 months (see Web site: http://www.nhlbi.gov/guidelines/hypertension/child_tbl.htm).

Causes of *sustained hypertension* in infants include renal artery disease (stenosis, thrombosis), congenital renal malformations, and coarctation of the aorta.

Pulse. The heart rate of infants is more sensitive to the effects of illness, exercise, and emotion than that of adults.

A pulse rate that is too rapid to count (usually >180 to 200/min) usually indicates *paroxysmal supraventricular tachycardia*. See Table 23-1, Abnormalities in Heart Rhythm and Blood Pressure, p. 824.

● Heart Rates From Birth to 1 Year

Age	Average Heart Rate	Range
Birth–2 months	140	90–190
0–6 months	130	80–180
6–12 months	115	75–155

You may have trouble obtaining an accurate pulse rate in a squirming infant. The best strategy is to auscultate the heart or to palpate the femoral arteries in the inguinal area or the brachial arteries in the antecubital fossa.

Bradycardia may be from drug ingestion, hypoxia, intracranial or neurologic conditions, or, rarely, cardiac arrhythmia such as heart block.

Respiratory Rate.

As with heart rate, compared with that of adults, the respiratory rate in infants has a greater range and is more responsive to illness, exercise, and emotion. The rate of respirations per minute ranges between 30 and 60 in the newborn.

Extremely rapid and shallow respiratory rates are seen in newborns with *cyanotic cardiac disease* and right-to-left shunting, and metabolic acidosis.

The respiratory rate may vary considerably from moment to moment in the infant, with alternating periods of rapid and slow breathing. The sleeping respiratory rate is most reliable. Respiratory rates during active sleep compared with quiet sleep may be up to 10 breaths per minute faster. The respiratory pattern should be observed for at least 60 seconds. In infancy and early childhood, diaphragmatic breathing is predominant; thoracic excursion is minimal.

Fever can raise respiratory rates in infants by up to 10 respirations per minute for each degree centigrade of fever.

Commonly accepted cutoffs for defining *tachypnea* are:

- Birth to 2 months, >60/min

- 2 to 12 months, >50/min

Tachypnea and increased respiratory effort in an infant are signs of possible pneumonia.

Temperature.

Because fever is so common in children, obtain an accurate body temperature when you suspect infection, collagen vascular disease, or malignancy. The techniques for obtaining rectal, oral, temporal artery and auditory canal temperatures in adults are described on pp. 120 to 121.

Fever (>38.0°C or >100.0°F) in infants <2 to 3 months may be a sign of *serious infection* or disease. These infants should be evaluated promptly.

The technique for obtaining the *rectal temperature* is relatively simple. Place the infant prone, separate the buttocks with the thumb and forefinger on one hand, and with the other hand gently insert a well-lubricated rectal thermometer, to a depth of 1.3 to 2.5 cm (0.5 to 1 in.). Keep the thermometer in place for at least 2 minutes.

Body temperature in infants and children is less constant than in adults. The average rectal temperature is higher in infancy and early childhood, usually above 99.0°F (37.2°C) until after age 3 years. Body temperature may fluctuate as much as 3°F during a single day, approaching 101°F (38.3°C) in normal children, particularly in late afternoon and after vigorous activity.

Anxiety may elevate the body temperature of children. *Excessive bundling* of infants may elevate the skin temperature but not the core temperature.

Temperature instability in a newborn may result from sepsis, metabolic abnormality, or other serious conditions. Older infants rarely manifest temperature instability.

The Skin

Inspection. Carefully examine the infant's general color for cyanosis, paleness, ruddiness, or jaundice. To detect jaundice, apply pressure to blanch the skin of the normal pink or brown color. A yellowish color indicates jaundice.

Next examine the infant for normal and abnormal skin markings, such as birthmarks. Document their appearance and compare to the infant's last visit. See Table 23-2, Common Skin Rashes and Skin Findings in Newborns and Infants, p. 825 for examples.

- A dark or bluish pigmentation over the buttocks and lower lumbar regions is common in newborns of African, Asian, and Mediterranean descent. This is congenital dermal melanocytosis, formerly called Mongolian spots, result from pigmented cells in the deep layers of the skin; they become less noticeable with age and usually disappear during childhood. Document these pigmented areas to avoid later concern about bruising or abuse.

- A common *vascular marking* is the "salmon patch" (also known as *nevus simplex,* telangiectatic nevus, or capillary hemangioma). These flat, irregular, light pink patches (see p. 749) are most often seen on the nape of the neck ("stork bite"), upper eyelids, forehead, or upper lip ("angel kisses"). They are not true nevi, but result from distended capillaries. They almost all disappear by 1 year of age.

Central cyanosis in a baby or child of any age should raise suspicion of *congenital heart disease.* The best area to look for central cyanosis is the tongue and oral mucosa, not the nail beds or the extremities.

Pigmented light brown lesions (<1 to 2 cm at birth) are *café-au-lait spots.* Isolated lesions have no significance, but multiple lesions with smooth borders may suggest *neurofibromatosis.*

Midline hair tufts over the lumbosacral spine region suggest a *spinal cord defect.*

Jaundice that persists beyond 2 to 3 weeks should raise suspicions of *biliary obstruction* or *liver disease.*

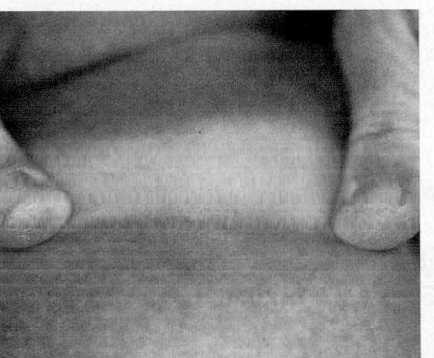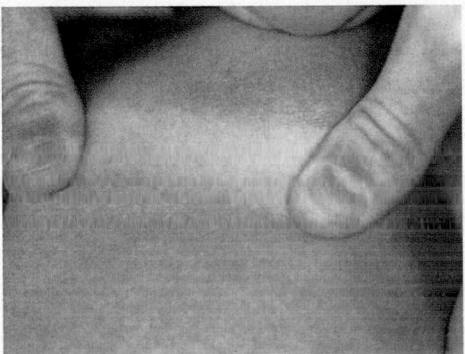

Pressing the red color from the skin allows better recognition of the yellow of jaundice. The infant on the left has no appreciable jaundice, while the infant on the right has a bilirubin level of 13 mg/dL (222 mmol/L). From Fletcher M. Physical Diagnosis in Neonatology. Philadelphia: Lippincott-Raven, 1998.

Palpation. Palpate the infant's skin to assess the degree of hydration, or *turgor.* Roll a fold of loosely adherent skin on the abdominal wall between your thumb and forefinger to determine its consistency. The skin in well-hydrated infants returns to its normal position immediately upon release. Delay in return is a phenomenon called "tenting" and usually occurs in children with significant *dehydration.*

Dehydration is a common problem in infants. Usual causes are insufficient intake or excess loss of fluids from diarrhea.

● Common Birthmarks

Finding	Description
Eyelid patch 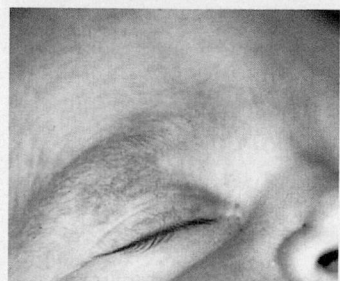	This birthmark fades, usually within the first year of life.
Salmon patch 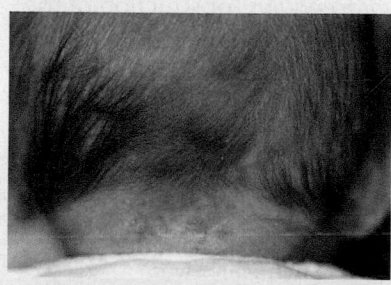	Also called the "stork bite," this splotchy pink mark fades with age.
Café-au-lait spots 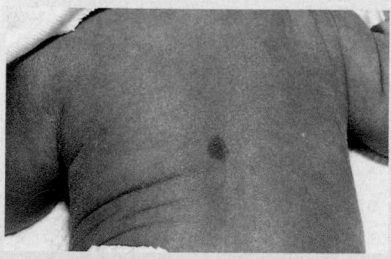	These light brown pigmented lesions usually have borders and are uniform. They are noted in more than 10% of black infants. *If more than five café-au-lait spots exist, consider the diagnosis of neurofibromatosis.*
Congenital dermal melanocytosis (Mongolian spots) 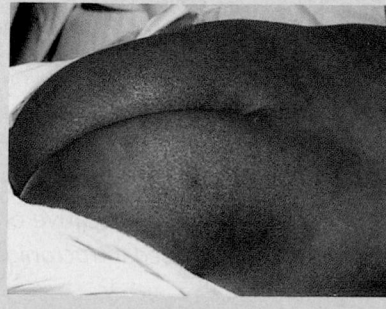	These are more common among dark-skinned babies. It is important to note them so that they are not mistaken for bruises or abuse.

The Head

A newborn's head accounts for one fourth of the body length and one third of the body weight; these proportions change, so that by adulthood, the head accounts for one eighth of the body length and about one tenth of the body weight.

Sutures and Fontanelles. Membranous tissue spaces called sutures separate the bones of the skull from one another. The areas where the major sutures intersect in the anterior and posterior portions of the skull are known as *fontanelles*. Examine the *sutures* and *fontanelles* carefully (see the figure below).

On palpation, the sutures feel like ridges and the fontanelles like soft concavities. The *anterior fontanelle* at birth measures 4 cm to 6 cm in diameter and usually closes between 4 and 26 months of age (90% between 7 and 19 months). The *posterior fontanelle* measures 1 cm to 2 cm at birth and usually closes by 2 months.

An enlarged posterior fontanelle may be present in *congenital hypothyroidism.*

A bulging, tense fontanelle is observed in infants with *increased intracranial pressure,* which may be caused by *central nervous system infections, neoplastic disease,* or *hydrocephalus* (obstruction of the circulation of cerebrospinal fluid within the ventricles of the brain; see Table 23-3, Abnormalities of the Head, p. 826.

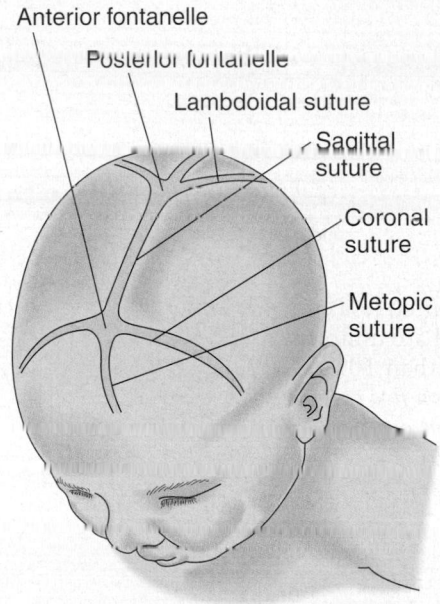

Anterior fontanelle
Posterior fontanelle
Lambdoidal suture
Sagittal suture
Coronal suture
Metopic suture

Carefully examine the fontanelle, because its fullness reflects *intracranial pressure.* Palpate the fontanelle while the baby is sitting quietly or being held upright. Experienced pediatric nurses often palpate the fontanelles at the beginning of the examination. In normal infants, the anterior fontanelle is soft and flat. Increased intracranial pressure produces a bulging, full anterior fontanelle and is seen when a baby cries, vomits, or has underlying pathology. Pulsations of the fontanelle reflect the peripheral pulse.

Inspect the scalp veins carefully to assess for dilatation.

A depressed anterior fontanelle may be a sign of *dehydration.*

Dilated scalp veins are indicative of long-standing *increased intracranial pressure.*

Skull Symmetry and Head Circumference.   Assess skull symmetry. Careful inspection of the skull from the front or back of the infant helps you assess its symmetry.

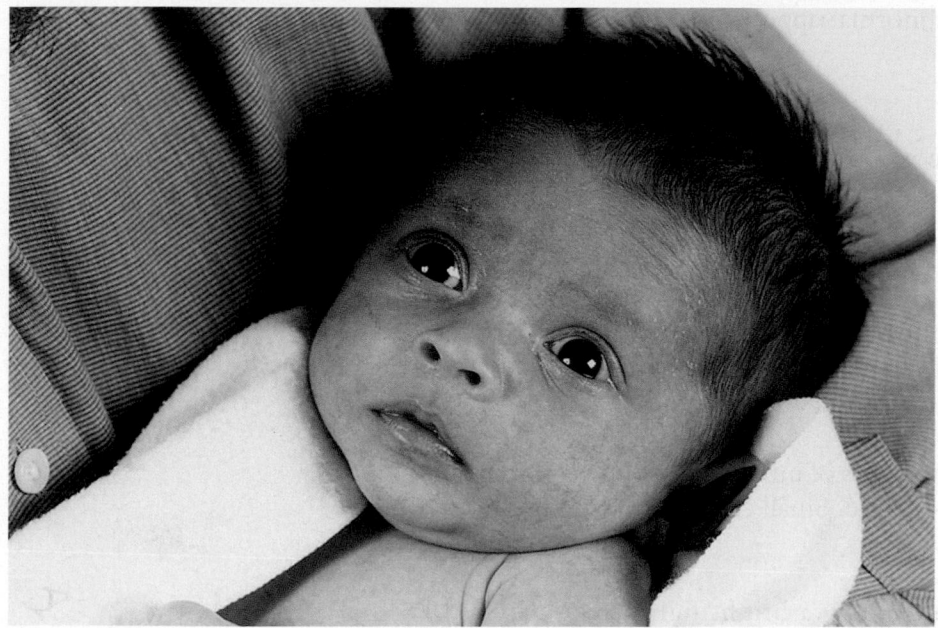

Look for asymmetric head swelling, which may be due to trauma from a fall or abuse.

Asymmetry of the cranial vault (*plagiocephaly*) occurs when an infant lies mostly on one side, resulting in a flattening of the parieto-occipital region on the dependent side and a prominence of the frontal region on the opposite side. It disappears as the baby becomes more active and spends less time in one position, and symmetry is almost always restored. Interestingly, the current trend to have newborns and infants sleep on their backs to reduce the risk for sudden infant death syndrome has resulted in more cases of plagiocephaly.

Plagiocephaly may also reflect pathology such as *torticollis* from injury to the sternocleidomastoid muscle at birth, or *lack of stimulation* of the infant.

Measure the head circumference (p. 745) to detect abnormally large head size (*macrocephaly*) or small head size (*microcephaly*), which may signify an underlying disorder affecting the brain. Palpate along the suture lines. A raised, bony ridge at a suture line suggests craniosynostosis.

Premature closure of cranial sutures causes *craniosynostosis* (p. 826), with an abnormally shaped skull. *Sagittal suture* synostosis causes a narrow head from lack of growth of the parietal bones.

Palpate the infant's skull with care. The cranial bones usually appear "soft" or pliable; they will normally become firmer with increasing age.

In *craniotabes,* the cranial bones feel springy. Craniotabes can result from increased intracranial pressure, as with *hydrocephaly,* metabolic disturbances such as *rickets,* and infection such as *congenital syphilis.*

Facial Symmetry.   Check the *face* of infants for symmetry. In utero positioning may result in transient facial asymmetries. If the head is flexed on the sternum, a shortened chin (*micrognathia*) may result.

Examine the face for an overall impression of the *facies*; it is helpful to compare with the face of the parents. An abnormal-appearing facies can identify specific syndromes.[11]

> Upslanting (Down syndrome)
> Downslanting (Noonan syndrome)
> Short (fetal alcohol effects)

The Eyes

Inspection.   Bright light causes infants to blink, so use subdued lighting. If you awaken the baby gently, turn down the lights, and support the baby in a sitting position, you will often find that the eyes open.

You will have to be clever to examine the eyes of infants and young children and use some tricks to get them to cooperate. Small colorful toys are useful as fixation devices in examining the eyes.

Newborns may look at your face and follow a bright light if you catch them during an alert period. By two months most infants can follow an object.

Examine infants for *eye movements*. Hold the baby upright, supporting the head. Rotate yourself with the baby slowly in one direction. This usually causes the baby's eyes to open, allowing you to examine the sclerae, pupils, irises, and extraocular movements. The baby's eyes gaze in the direction you are turning. When the rotation stops, the eyes look in the opposite direction, after a few nystagmoid movements.

Micrognathia may also be part of a syndrome, such as the *Pierre Robin syndrome*.

A child with abnormal shape or length of palpebral fissures: See Table 23-6, Diagnostic Facies in Infancy and Childhood, pp. 827–828.

Nystagmus (wandering or shaking eye movements) persisting after a few days after birth or persisting after the maneuver described on the left may indicate poor vision or *central nervous system disease*.

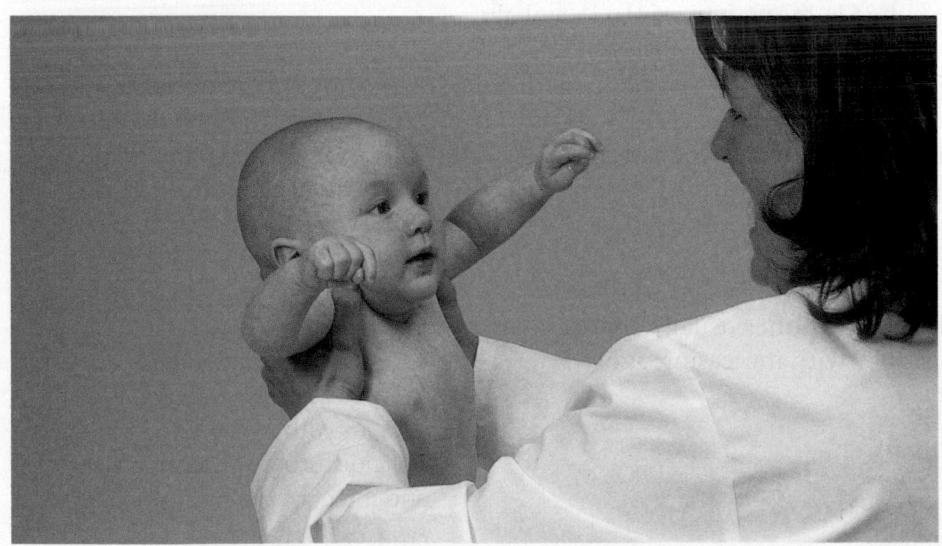

During the first few months of life, some infants have intermittent crossed eyes (*intermittent alternating convergent strabismus*, or *esotropia*) or laterally deviated eyes (*intermittent alternating divergent strabismus*, or *exotropia*).

Observe pupillary reactions by response to light or by covering each eye with your hand and then uncovering it. They should be equal in size and reaction to light.

Inspect the irises carefully for abnormalities.

Examine the *conjunctiva* for swelling or redness.

Visual acuity of infants cannot be measured. Visual reflexes can be used to indirectly assess vision: direct and consensual pupillary constriction in response to light, blinking in response to bright light (*optic blink reflex*), and blinking in response to quick movement of an object toward the eyes. During the first year of life, visual acuity sharpens as the ability to focus improves. Infants achieve the following visual milestones:

● **Visual Milestones of Infancy**[12]	
Birth	Blinks, may regard face
1 month	Fixes on objects
1½–2 months	Coordinated eye movements
3 months	Eyes converge, baby reaches
12 months	Acuity around 20/50

Ophthalmoscopic Examination. For the *ophthalmoscopic examination*, with the infant awake and eyes open, examine the red retinal reflex by setting the ophthalmoscope at 0 diopters and viewing the pupil from about 10 inches. Normally, a red or orange color is reflected from the fundus through the pupil.

If history or examination findings indicate the need for a thorough ophthalmologic examination, refer the infant to a pediatric ophthalmologist.

Alternating convergent or divergent *strabismus* persisting beyond 3 months, or persistent strabismus of any type, may indicate *ocular motor weakness* or another abnormality in the visual system.

Brushfield spots are a ring of white specks in the iris. Although sometimes present in normal children, these strongly suggest *Down syndrome.* See Table 23-7, Abnormalities of Eyes, Ears and Mouth, p. 830.

Persistent ocular discharge and tearing since birth may be from *dacryocystitis* or *nasolacrimal duct obstruction.*

Failure to progress along these visual developmental milestones may indicate *delayed visual maturation.*

Congenital glaucoma may cause cloudiness of the cornea. A dark light reflex can result from *cataracts, retinopathy of prematurity,* or other disorders. A white retinal reflex (*leukokoria*) is abnormal, and cataract, retinal detachment, chorioretinitis, or *retinoblastoma* should be suspected.

The Ears

The physical examination of the ears of infants is important because many abnormalities can be detected, including structural problems, otitis media, and hearing loss. The major goals are to determine the *position, shape,* and *features of the ear* and to detect abnormalities. Note ear position in relation to the eyes. An imaginary line drawn across the inner and outer canthi of the eyes should cross the pinna or auricle; if the pinna is below this line, then the infant has low-set ears. Draw this imaginary line across the face of the child on p. 756; note that it crosses the pinna.

Small, deformed, or low-set auricles may indicate associated *congenital defects,* especially renal disease.

A small skin tab, cleft, or pit found just forward of the tragus represents a remnant of the *first branchial cleft* and usually has no significance.

The infant's ear canal is directed downward from the outside; therefore, you may want to pull the auricle gently downward, not upward, for the best view of the eardrum. Once the tympanic membrane is visible, note that the light reflex is diffuse and does not become cone-shaped for several months.

● Signs That an Infant Can Hear	
Age	**Sign**
0–2 months	Startle response and blink to a sudden noise
	Calming down with soothing voice or music
2–3 months	Change in body movements in response to sound
	Change in facial expression to familiar sounds
3–4 months	Turning eyes and head to sound
6–7 months	Turning to listen to voices and conversation

Many children with *hearing deficits* are not diagnosed until as old as 2 years. Clues to hearing deficits include parental concern about hearing, delayed speech, and lack of developmental indicators of hearing.

The Nose and Sinuses

The most important component of the examination of the nose of infants is to test for patency of the nasal passages. You can do this by gently occluding each nostril alternately while holding the infant's mouth closed. This normally will not cause stress because most infants are nasal breathers. Indeed, some infants are *obligate nasal breathers* and have difficulty breathing through their mouths. Do not occlude both nares simultaneously—this will cause considerable distress!

The nasal passages in newborns may be obstructed in *choanal atresia.*

The Mouth and Pharynx

Use both inspection with a tongue blade and flashlight and palpation to inspect the mouth and pharynx. The newborn's mouth is edentulous, and the alveolar mucosa is smooth, with finely serrated borders. Occasionally, pearl-like retention cysts are seen along the alveolar ridges and are easily mistaken for teeth—they disappear within 1 or 2 months. Petechiae are commonly found on the soft palate after birth. Palpate the upper hard palate to make sure it is intact. *Epstein pearls,* tiny white or yellow, rounded mucous retention cysts, are located along the posterior midline of the hard palate. They disappear within months.

Rarely, *supernumerary teeth* are noted. These are usually dysmorphic and are shed within days but are removed to prevent aspiration.

Cysts may be noted on the tongue or mouth. Thyroglossal duct cysts

Infants produce little saliva during the first 3 months. Older infants produce lots of saliva and drool frequently.

Inspect the tongue. The frenulum varies, sometimes extending almost to the tip and other times being thick and short, limiting protrusion of the tongue (*ankyloglossia*, or *tongue tie*); these variations rarely interfere with speech or function.

Although unusual, a prominent, protruding tongue may signal congenital hypothyroidism or Down syndrome.

You will often see a whitish covering on the tongue. If this coating is from milk, it can be easily removed by scraping or wiping it away.

Oral candidiasis (thrush) is common in infants. The lesions are difficult to wipe away and have an erythematous raw base. See Table 23-7, Abnormalities of Eyes, Ears and Mouth, p. 830.

The pharynx of the infant is best seen while the baby is crying. You will likely have difficulty using a tongue blade because it produces a strong gag reflex. Do not expect to be able to visualize the tonsils.

Listen to the quality of the *infant's cry*. Normal infants have a lusty, strong cry. The following box lists some unusual types of infant cries.

Macroglossia is associated with several systemic conditions. If associated with hypoglycemia and omphalocele, the diagnosis is likely Beckwith-Wiedemann syndrome.

● Abnormal Infant Cries

Type	Possible Abnormality
Shrill or high-pitched	Increased intracranial pressure. Also in newborns born to narcotic-addicted mothers
Hoarse	Hypocalcemic tetany or congenital hypothyroidism
Continuous inspiratory and expiratory stridor	Upper airway obstruction from various lesions (e.g., a polyp or hemangioma), a relatively small larynx (*infantile laryngeal stridor*), or a delay in the development of the cartilage in the tracheal rings (*tracheomalacia*)
Absence of cry	Severe illness, vocal cord paralysis, or profound brain damage

There is a predictable pattern of tooth eruption and also wide variation. A rule of thumb is that a child will have one tooth for each month of age between 6 and 26 months, up to 20 primary teeth.

The Neck

Palpate the *lymph nodes of the neck* and assess for any additional masses such as *congenital cysts*. Because the necks of infants are short, it is best to palpate the neck while infants are lying supine, whereas older children are best examined while sitting. Check the position of the thyroid cartilage and trachea.

Preauricular cysts and sinuses are common, pinhole-size pits, usually located anterior to the helix of the ear. They are often bilateral and may occasionally be associated with *hearing deficits*.

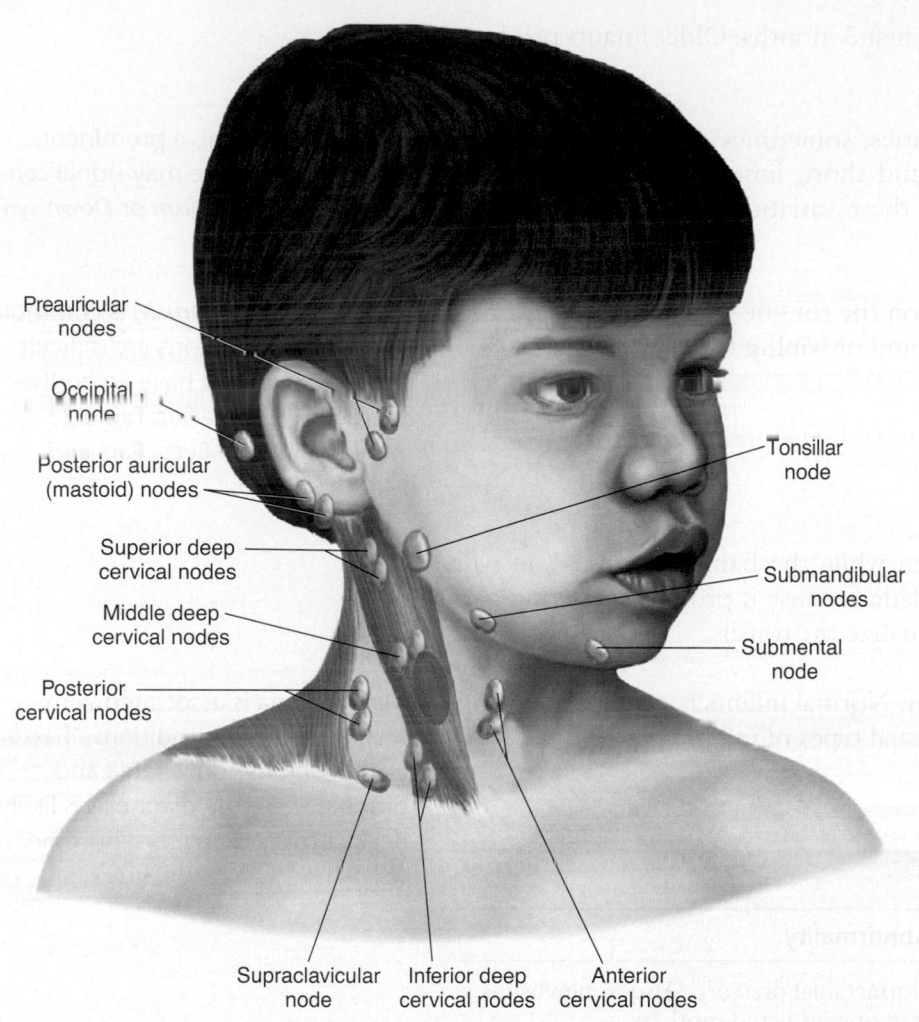

Preauricular
nodes

Occipital
node

Posterior auricular
(mastoid) nodes

Superior deep
cervical nodes

Middle deep
cervical nodes

Posterior
cervical nodes

Tonsillar
node

Submandibular
nodes

Submental
node

Supraclavicular
node

Inferior deep
cervical nodes

Anterior
cervical nodes

Palpate the *clavicles* and look for evidence of a fracture. If present, you may feel a break in the contour of the bone, tenderness, crepitus at the fracture site, and limited movement of the arm on the affected side.

The Thorax and Lungs

The infant's *thorax* is more rounded than that of older people. Also, the thin chest wall has little musculature; thus, lung and heart sounds are transmitted quite clearly. The bony and cartilaginous rib cage is soft and pliant. The tip of the xiphoid process often protrudes anteriorly, immediately beneath the skin.

Inspection.   Carefully *assess respirations* and *breathing patterns*.

Two types of chest wall abnormalities noted in childhood include *pectus excavatum,* or "funnel chest," and *pectus carinatum,* or "chicken breast deformity."

Apnea is cessation of breathing for more than 20 seconds. It is often accompanied by bradycardia and may indicate *respiratory disease, central nervous system disease,* or, rarely, a *cardiopulmonary condition.* Apnea may be a high-risk factor for *sudden infant death syndrome (SIDS).*

Do not rush to the stethoscope. Instead, observe the infant carefully as demonstrated on the next page. Inspection is easiest when infants are not crying; thus, work with the parents to settle the child. On observation, note general appearance, respiratory rate, color, nasal component of breathing, audible breath sounds, and work of breathing, as described below.

Because infants are obligate nasal breathers, observe their nose as they breathe. Look for *nasal flaring*. Observe breathing with the infant's mouth closed or during nursing or sucking on a bottle to assess for nasal patency. Listen to the sounds of breathing; note any *grunting, audible wheezing, or lack of breath sounds (obstruction)*.

Nasal flaring may be the result of *upper respiratory infections,* with subsequent obstruction of their small nares, but it may also be caused by pneumonia or other serious respiratory infections.

Observe two aspects of the infant's breathing: *audible breath sounds* and *work of breathing*. These are particularly relevant in assessing both upper and lower respiratory illness.

● **Observing Respiration—Before You Touch the Child!**

Type of Assessment	Specific Observable Pathology
General appearance	Inability to feed or smile Lack of consolability
Respiratory rate	Tachypnea (see Table 7 1, p. 124, Abnormalities of Rate and Rhythm of Breating).
Color	Pallor or cyanosis
Nasal component of breathing	Nasal flaring (enlargement of both nasal openings during inspiration)
Audible breath sounds	Grunting (repetitive, short expiratory sound) Wheezing (musical expiratory sound) Stridor (high-pitched, inspiratory noise) Obstruction (lack of breath sounds)

Work of breathing	Nasal flaring (excessive movement of nares)
	Grunting (expiratory noises)
	Retractions (chest indrawing):
	  Supraclavicular (soft tissue above clavicles)
	  Intercostal (indrawing of the skin between ribs)
	  Subcostal (just below the costal margin)
	Paradoxical (seesaw) breathing (abdomen moves outward while chest moves inward during inspiration)

Any of the abnormalities listed on the left should raise concern about underlying respiratory pathology.

Lower respiratory infections, defined as infections below the vocal cords, are common in infants and include *bronchiolitis* and *pneumonia*.

Acute stridor is a potentially serious condition; causes include laryngotracheobronchitis (croup), epiglottitis, bacterial tracheitis, foreign body, or a vascular ring.

In infants, abnormal work of breathing plus abnormal findings on auscultation are the best findings for ruling in *pneumonia*. The best sign for ruling *out* pneumonia is the absence of tachypnea.

In healthy infants, the ribs do not move much during quiet breathing. Any outward movement is produced by descent of the diaphragm, which compresses the abdominal contents and in turn shifts the lower ribs outward.

Asymmetric chest movement may indicate a space-occupying lesion. Pulmonary disease causes increased abdominal breathing and can result in *retractions (chest indrawing),* an indicator of pulmonary disease before 2 years of age. Chest indrawing is inward movement of the skin between the ribs during inspiration.

Obstructive respiratory disease in infants can result in the *Hoover sign,* or paradoxical (seesaw) breathing

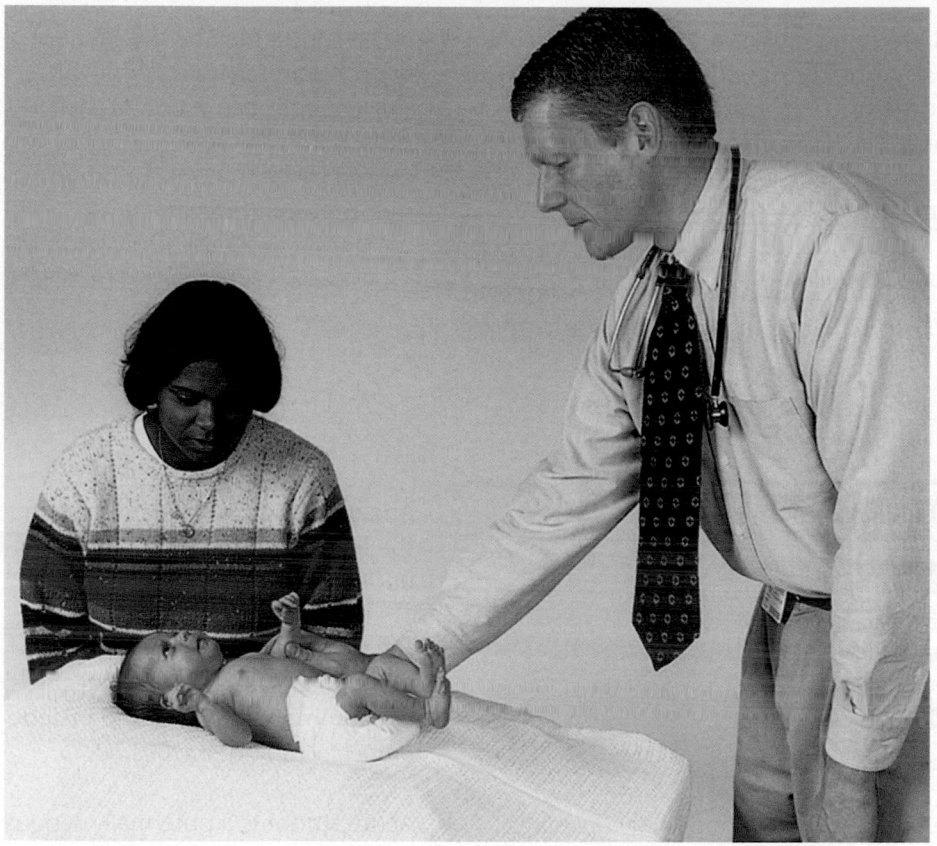

Palpation. Assess tactile fremitus by *palpation*. Place your hand on the chest when the infant cries or makes noise. Place your hand or fingertips over each side of the chest and feel for symmetry in the transmitted vibrations. Percussion is not helpful in infants except in extreme instances. The infant's chest is hyperresonant throughout, and it is difficult to detect abnormalities on percussion.

Because of the excellent transmission of sounds throughout the chest, any abnormalities of tactile fremitus or on percussion suggest severe pathology, such as a large *pneumonic consolidation.*

Auscultation. After performing these maneuvers, it is time for *auscultation*. Breath sounds are louder and harsher than those of adults because the stethoscope is closer to the origin of the sounds. Also, it is often difficult to distinguish transmitted upper airway sounds from sounds originating in the chest. The table that follows has some useful hints. Upper airway sounds tend to be loud, transmitted symmetrically throughout the chest, and loudest as you move your stethoscope toward the neck. They are usually inspiratory, coarse sounds. Lower airway sounds are loudest over the site of pathology, are often asymmetric, and often occur during expiration.

Biphasic sounds (wheezing) imply severe obstruction from intrathoracic airway narrowing or severe obstruction from extrathoracic airway narrowing.

Expiratory sounds usually arise from an intrathoracic source, while inspiratory sounds typically arise from an extrathoracic airway such as the trachea.

● Distinguishing Upper Airway From Lower Airway Sounds in Infants		
Technique	**Upper Airway**	**Lower Airway**
Compare sounds from nose/ stethoscope	Same sounds	Often different sounds
Listen to harshness of sounds	Harsh and loud	Variable
Note symmetry (left/right)	Symmetric	Often asymmetric
Compare sounds at different locations (higher or lower)	Sounds louder as stethoscope is moved up chest	Often sounds louder lower in chest toward abdomen
Inspiratory vs. expiratory	Almost always inspiratory	Often has expiratory phase

Diminished breath sounds in one side of the chest suggest unilateral lesions (e.g., *congenital diaphragmatic hernia*).

During expiration, the diameter of the intrathoracic airways decreases because radial forces from the surrounding lung do not "tether" the airways open as occurs during inspiration. Higher flow rates during inspiration produce turbulent flow, resulting in appreciable sounds.

The characteristics of the *breath sounds*, such as vesicular and bronchovesicular, and of the adventitious lung sounds, such as crackles, wheezes, and rhonchi, are the same as those for adults, except that they may be more difficult to distinguish in infants and often occur together. Wheezes and rhonchi are common in infants. *Wheezes*, often audible without the stethoscope, occur more frequently because of the smaller size of the tracheobronchial tree. *Rhonchi* reflect obstruction of larger airways, or bronchi. *Crackles* (rales) are discontinuous sounds (see p. 314), near the end of inspiration; they are usually caused by lung disorders, are far less likely to represent cardiac failure in infants than in adults, and tend to be harsher than in adults.

Wheezes in infants occur commonly from *asthma* or *bronchiolitis*.

Crackles (rales) can be heard with *pneumonia* and *bronchiolitis*.

The Heart

Inspection. Before examining the heart itself, observe the infant carefully for any cyanosis. It is important to detect *central cyanosis* because it is always abnormal and because many congenital cardiac abnormalities, as well as respiratory diseases, present with cyanosis.

Central cyanosis without acute respiratory symptoms suggests cardiac disease. See Table 23-9, Cyanosis in Children, p. 832 and Table 23-10, Congenital Heart Murmurs, pp. 833–834.

Recognizing minimal degrees of cyanosis requires care. Look at the tongue, or at the conjunctivae, instead of peering through the skin. A true strawberry pink is normal, whereas any hint of raspberry red suggests desaturation.

The distribution of the cyanosis should be evaluated. An oximetry reading will confirm desaturation.

Observe the infant for *general signs of health*. The infant's nutritional status, responsiveness, happiness, and irritability are all clues that may be useful in evaluating cardiac disease. Note that noncardiac findings can be present in infants with cardiac disease.

Tachypnea, tachycardia, and hepatomegaly in infants suggest *congestive heart failure*.

COMMON NONCARDIAC FINDINGS IN INFANTS WITH CARDIAC DISEASE

Poor feeding	Tachypnea	Poor overall appearance
Failure to thrive	Hepatomegaly	Weakness
Irritability	Clubbing	

Observe the respiratory rate and pattern to help distinguish the degree of illness and cardiac versus pulmonary diseases. An increase in respiratory effort is expected from pulmonary diseases, whereas in cardiac disease there may be tachypnea but not increased work of breathing until congestive heart failure becomes significant.

A diffuse bulge outward of the left side of the chest suggests long-standing *cardiomegaly*.

Palpation. The major branches of the aorta can be assessed by evaluation of the *peripheral pulses*. In neonates and infants, the brachial artery pulse in the antecubital fossa is easier to feel than the radial artery pulse at the wrist. Both temporal arteries should be felt just in front of the ear.

Feel the femoral pulses. They lie in the midline just below the inguinal crease, between the iliac crest and the symphysis pubis. Take your time and search for femoral pulses; they are difficult to detect in chubby, squirming infants. If the infant's thighs are flexed on the abdomen first, this may overcome the reflex flexion that occurs when you then extend the legs.

The absence or diminution of femoral pulses is indicative of *coarctation of the aorta*. If femoral pulses cannot be detected, measure blood pressures of the lower and upper extremities. If they are equal or lower in the legs, coarctation is likely to be present.

The dorsalis pedis and posterior tibial pulses (see figure) may be difficult to feel unless there is an abnormality involving aortic run-off. Normal pulses should have a sharp rise and should be firm and well localized.

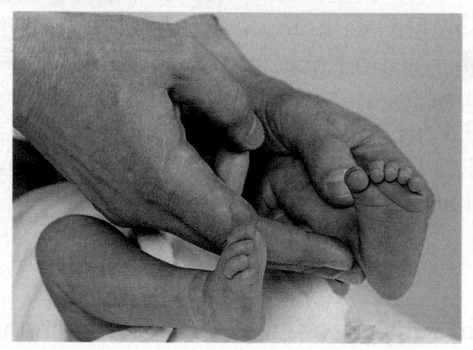

A weak or thready, difficult-to-feel pulse may reflect *myocardial dysfunction* and *congestive heart failure*, particularly if associated with an unusual degree of tachycardia.

As discussed on p. 746, carefully measure the *blood pressure* of infants and children as part of the cardiac examination.

The apical impulse is not always palpable in infants and is affected by respiratory patterns, a full stomach, and the infant's positioning. It is usually an interspace higher than in adults during the first few years of life because the heart lies more horizontally within the chest.

A *"rolling" heave* at the left sternal border suggests an *increase in right ventricular work*, whereas the same kind of motion closer to the apex suggests the same thing for the left ventricle.

Palpation of the chest wall will allow you to assess volume changes within the heart. For example, a hyperdynamic precordium reflects a big volume change.

Thrills are palpable when turbulence within the heart or great vessels is transmitted to the surface. Knowledge of the structures of the precordium helps pinpoint the origin of the thrill. Thrills are easiest to feel with your palm or the base of your fingers rather than your fingertips. Thrills have a somewhat rough, vibrating quality. The figure below shows locations of thrills from various cardiac abnormalities that occur in infants and children.

Visible and palpable chest pulsations suggest a hyperdynamic state from either increased metabolic rate or inefficient pumping as a result of an underlying cardiac effect.

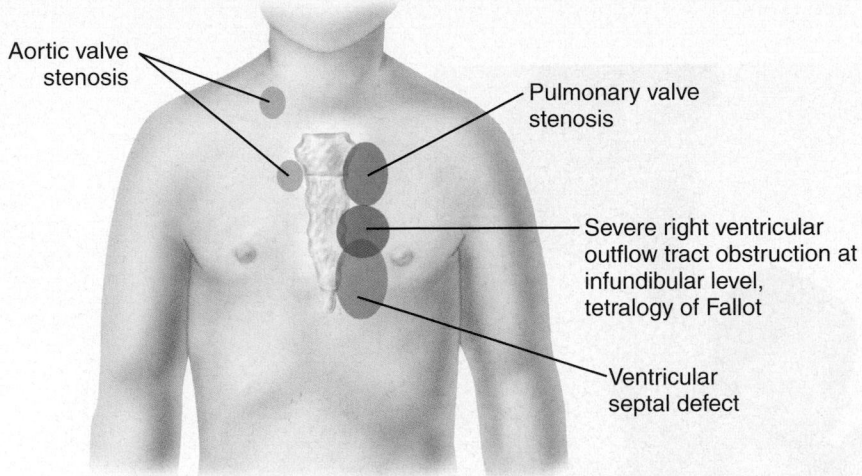

Aortic valve stenosis

Pulmonary valve stenosis

Severe right ventricular outflow tract obstruction at infundibular level, tetralogy of Fallot

Ventricular septal defect

LOCATION OF THRILLS IN INFANTS AND CHILDREN

Auscultation. The *heart rhythm can be evaluated* more easily in infants by listening to the heart than by feeling the peripheral pulses; in older children it can be done either way. Infants and children commonly have a normal sinus arrhythmia, with the heart rate increasing on inspiration and decreasing on expiration, sometimes quite abruptly. This normal finding can be identified by its repetitive nature, its correlation with respiration, and its involvement of several beats rather than a single beat.

The most common dysrhythmia in infants is *paroxysmal supraventricular tachycardia,* or *paroxysmal atrial tachycardia (PSVT, or PAT)*. It can occur at any age, including in utero. See Table 23-1, Abnormalities in Heart Rhythm and Blood Pressure, p. 824.

Many infants and some older children have premature atrial or ventricular beats that are often appreciated as "skipped" beats.

A split S2 is frequently heard at the base, but the two sounds should fuse into a single sound in deep expiration.

Distant heart tones suggest *pericardial effusion;* mushy, less distinct heart sounds suggest *myocardial dysfunction.*

In addition to trying to detect splitting of the S_2, listen for the intensity of A_2 and P_2. The aortic, or first component of the second sound at the base, is normally louder than the pulmonic, or second component.

A louder-than-normal pulmonic component, particularly when louder than the aortic sound, suggests *pulmonary hypertension.*

Persistent splitting of S_2 may indicate a right ventricular volume load such as *atrial septal defect, anomalies of pulmonary venous return,* or *chronic anemia.*

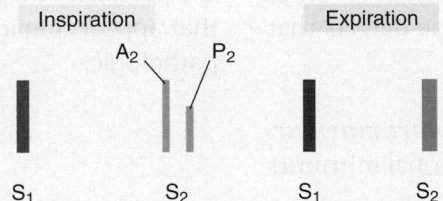

Inspiration

A_2 P_2

Expiration

S_1 S_2 S_1 S_2

A *third heart sound may be detected*. It is low-pitched, early diastolic sounds best heard at the lower left sternal border, or apex. These are frequently heard in children and are normal. They reflect rapid ventricular filling.

The third heart sound (S₃) should be differentiated from the higher-intensity third heart sound gallop, which is a sign of underlying pathology.

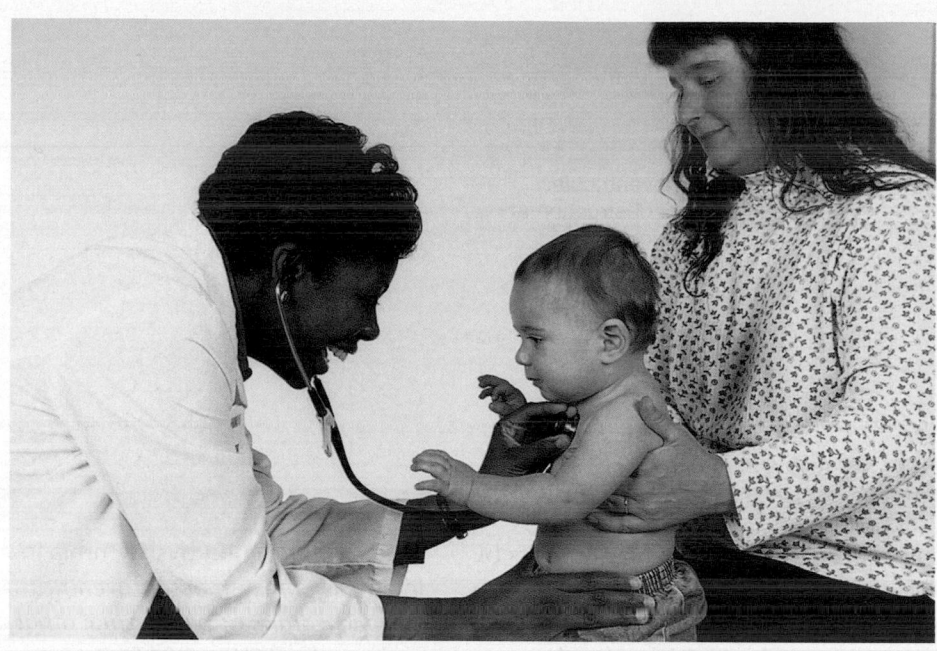

Fourth heart sounds (S4), which are not often heard in children, are low-frequency, late diastolic sounds, occurring just before the first heart sound.

Fourth heart sounds represent decreased ventricular compliance, suggesting *congestive heart failure*.

Heart Murmurs   One of the most challenging aspects of cardiac examination in children is the evaluation of *heart murmurs*. Characterize heart murmurs in infants and children by noting their specific location (e.g., left upper sternal border, not just left sternal border), timing, intensity, and quality.

See Table 23-10, Congenital Heart Murmurs, pp. 833-834.

An important rule of thumb is that, by definition, *benign murmurs in children have no associated abnormal findings*. Many (but not all) children with serious cardiac malformations have signs and symptoms other than a heart murmur obtainable on careful history or examination. Many have other noncardiac signs and symptoms, including evidence of genetic defects that may offer helpful diagnostic clues.

Any of the *noncardiac findings* that frequently accompany cardiac disease in children markedly raises the possibility that a murmur that appears benign is really pathologic.

Most children will have one or more *functional, or benign, heart murmurs* before reaching adulthood.[13] It is important to identify functional murmurs by their specific qualities rather than by their intensity.

PHYSIOLOGIC BASIS FOR SOME PATHOLOGIC HEART MURMURS

Change in Pulmonary Vascular Resistance

Heart murmurs that are dependent on a postnatal drop in pulmonary vascular resistance, allowing turbulent flow from the high-pressure systemic circuit to the lower-pressure pulmonary circuit, are not audible until such a drop has occurred. Therefore, except in premature infants, murmurs of a *ventricular septal defect* or *patent ductus arteriosus* are not expected in the first few days of life and usually become audible after a week to 10 days.

Obstructive Lesions

Obstructive lesions, such as *pulmonic and aortic stenosis,* are caused by normal blood flow through two small valves and, therefore, are not dependent on a drop in pulmonary vascular resistance and are audible at birth.

Pressure Gradient Differences

Murmurs of *atrioventricular valve regurgitation* are audible at birth because of the high pressure gradient between the ventricle and its atrium.

Changes Associated With Growth of Children

Some murmurs do not follow the rules above, but are audible due to alterations in normal blood flow and occur or change with growth. For example, even though it is an obstructive defect, *aortic stenosis* may not be audible until considerable growth has occurred and, indeed, is frequently not heard until adulthood, although a congenitally abnormal valve is responsible. Similarly, the pulmonary flow murmur of an *atrial septal defect* may not be heard for a year or more because right ventricular compliance gradually increases and the shunt becomes larger, eventually producing a murmur caused by too much blood flow across a normal pulmonic valve.

A newborn with a heart murmur and central cyanosis likely has congenital heart disease and requires urgent cardiac evaluation.

When a murmur in children is detected, note all of the qualities described in Chapter 14, The Cardiovascular System, to help you distinguish *pathologic murmurs* from the benign murmurs.

The Breasts

The breasts of the infant should be undeveloped and flush with the chest wall. Residual enlargement from maternal estrogen effect may be present for several months after birth.

In *premature thelarche,* breast development occurs, most often between 6 months and 2 years. Other signs of puberty or hormonal abnormalities are not present.

The Abdomen

Inspection.   *Inspect* the abdomen with the infant lying supine (and, optimally, asleep). The infant's abdomen is protuberant as a result of poorly developed abdominal musculature. Abdominal wall blood vessels and intestinal peristalsis are easily noticed.

Inspect the area around the umbilicus for redness or swelling. *Umbilical hernias* are detectable at a few weeks of age. Most disappear by 1 year, nearly all by 5 years.

Umbilical hernias in infants are caused by a defect in the abdominal wall and can be up to 6 cm in diameter and quite protuberant with intra-abdominal pressure.

In some normal infants, a *diastasis recti may be noticed*. This involves separation of the two rectus abdominis muscles, causing a midline ridge, most apparent when the infant contracts the abdominal muscles. A benign condition in most cases, it resolves during early childhood. Chronic abdominal distention may also predispose to this condition.

Auscultation. *Auscultation* of a quiet infant's abdomen is easy. Do not be surprised if you hear an orchestra of musical tinkling bowel sounds upon placement of your stethoscope on the infant's abdomen.

An increase in pitch or frequency of bowel sounds is heard with *gastroenteritis* or, rarely, with *intestinal obstruction*.

Percussion and Palpation. The infant's abdomen can be percussed as an adult's, but be prepared to note greater tympanitic sounds because of the infant's propensity to swallow air. Percussion is useful for determining the size of organs and abdominal masses.

A silent, tympanic, distended and tender abdomen suggests *peritonitis*.

It is easy to *palpate* an infant's abdomen because infants like being touched. A useful technique to relax the infant, shown here, is to hold the legs flexed at the knees and hips with one hand and palpate the abdomen with the other. A pacifier may be used to quiet the infant in this position.

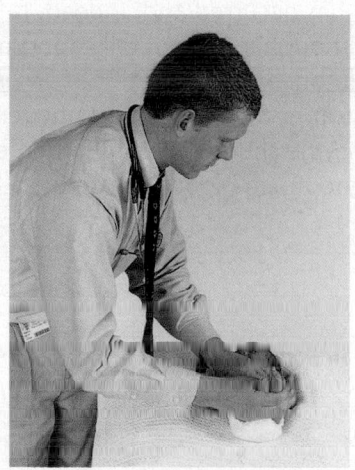

Start gently palpating the liver of infants low in the abdomen, moving upward with your fingers. This technique helps you avoid missing an extremely enlarged liver that extends down into the pelvis. With a careful examination, you can feel the liver edge in most infants, 1 to 2 cm below the right costal margin.

An enlarged, tender liver may be due to *congestive heart failure* or to *storage diseases*. Among newborns, causes of hepatomegaly include *hepatitis, storage diseases, vascular congestion,* and *biliary obstruction.*

One technique for assessing liver size in infants is simultaneous percussion and auscultation.[14] Percuss and simultaneously auscultate, noting a change in sound as you percuss over the liver or beyond it.

The *spleen*, like the liver, is felt easily in most infants. It too is soft with a sharp edge, and it projects downward like a tongue from under the left costal margin. The spleen is moveable and rarely extends more than 1 cm to 2 cm below the left costal margin.

Several diseases can cause splenomegaly, including *infections, hemolytic anemias, infiltrative disorders, inflammatory* or *autoimmune diseases,* and *portal hypertension.*

Palpate the *other abdominal structures.* You will commonly note pulsations in the epigastrium caused by the aorta. This is felt on deep palpation to the left of the midline.

In fact, the kidneys of infants may be palpated by carefully placing the fingers of one hand in front of and those of the other behind each kidney. The descending colon is a sausage-like mass in the left lower quadrant.

Abnormal abdominal masses in infants can be associated with the kidney (e.g., *hydronephrosis*), bladder (e.g., *urethral obstruction*), bowel (e.g., *Hirschsprung disease* or *intussusception*), and tumors.

Once the normal structures in the infant's abdomen have been identified, use palpation to identify abnormal masses.

In *pyloric stenosis,* deep palpation in the right upper quadrant or midline can reveal an "olive," or a 2-cm firm pyloric mass. While feeding, some infants with this condition will have visible peristaltic waves pass across their abdomen, followed by projectile vomiting.

Male Genitalia

Inspect the male genitalia with the infant supine, noting the appearance of the penis, testes, and scrotum. The *foreskin* completely covers the *glans penis.* It is nonretractable at birth, though you may be able to retract it enough to visualize the external urethral meatus. Retraction of the foreskin in the uncircumcised male occurs months to years later. The rate of circumcision has declined recently in North America and varies worldwide, depending on cultural practices.

A *hypospadias* is present when the urethral orifice appears at some point along the ventral surface of the glans or shaft of the penis (see Table 23-12, The Male Genitourinary System, p. 836). The foreskin is incompletely formed ventrally.

Inspect the *shaft of the penis,* noting any abnormalities on the ventral surface. Make sure the penis appears straight.

A fixed, downward bowing of the penis is a *chordee;* this may accompany a hypospadias.

Inspect the *scrotum,* noting rugae, which should be present by 40 weeks' gestation. Palpate the testes in the scrotal sacs, proceeding downward from the external inguinal ring to the scrotum. If you feel a testis up in the inguinal canal, gently milk it downward into the scrotum. The newborn's testes should be about 10 mm in width and 15 mm in length and should lie in the scrotal sacs most of the time.

In newborns with an *undescended testicle* (*cryptorchidism*), the scrotum often appears underdeveloped and tight, and palpation reveals an absence of scrotal contents (see Table 23-12, The Male Genitourinary System, p. 836).

Examine the testes for swelling within the scrotal sac and over the inguinal ring. If you detect swelling in the scrotal sac, try to differentiate it from the testis. Note whether the size changes when the infant increases abdominal pressure by crying.

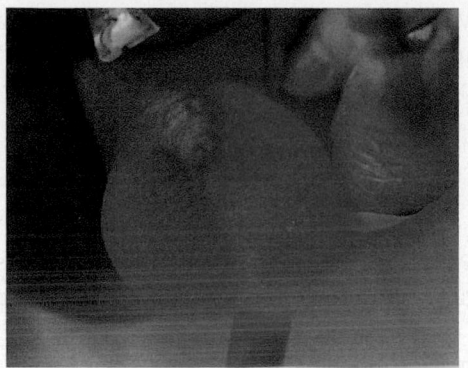

TRANSILLUMINATION OF A HYDROCELE
From Fletcher M, Physical Diagnosis in Neonatology. Philadelphia: Lippincott-Raven, 1998.

Two common scrotal masses in newborns are *hydroceles* and *inguinal hernias;* frequently both coexist, and both are more common on the right side. Hydroceles overlie the testes and the spermatic cord, are not reducible, and can be transilluminated (see photo at left). Most resolve by 18 months. Hernias are separate from the testes, are usually reducible, and often do not transilluminate. They do not resolve

Female Genitalia

In the infant female, the labia majora and minora have a dull pink color in light-skinned infants and may be hyperpigmented in dark-skinned infants.

Ambiguous genitalia, involving masculinization of the female external genitalia, is a rare condition caused by endocrine disorders such as *congenital adrenal hyperplasia.*

Examine the female genitalia with the infant supine.

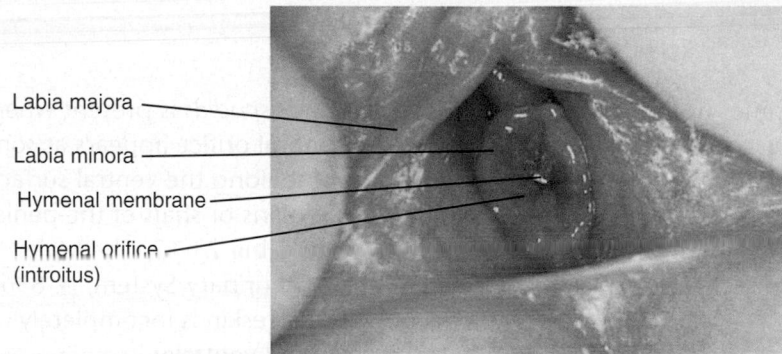

Labia majora
Labia minora
Hymenal membrane
Hymenal orifice (introitus)

Examine the different structures systematically, including the size of the clitoris, the color and size of the labia majora, and any rashes, bruises, or external lesions. Next, separate the labia majora at their midpoint with the thumb of each hand for young infants. Infants will not mind the examination because they are used to having their diapers changed and their bodies washed.

Labial adhesions occur not infrequently, tend to be paper thin, and often disappear without treatment.

Inspect the urethral orifice and the labia minora. Inspect the hymen, which in infants is a thickened, avascular structure with a central orifice, covering the vaginal opening. You should note a vaginal opening, although the hymen will be thickened. Note any discharge.

An imperforate hymen may be noted at birth.

Rectal Examination

The rectal examination generally is not performed for infants or children.

The Musculoskeletal System

Enormous changes in the musculoskeletal system occur during infancy. Much of the examination focuses on detection of congenital abnormalities, particularly in the hands, spine, hips, legs, and feet. With a little practice, you will be able to combine the musculoskeletal examination with the neurologic and developmental examination.

Palpate along the *clavicle*, noting any lumps, tenderness, or crepitus; these may indicate a fracture.

Inspect the *spine* carefully. Subtle abnormalities such as pigmented spots, hairy patches, or deep pits within 1 cm or so of the midline may overlie external openings of sinus tracts that extend to the spinal canal. Palpate the spine in the lumbosacral region, noting any deformities of the vertebrae.

Examine the infant's *hips* carefully at each examination for signs of dislocation.[16] The photos to the right and below and text demonstrate the technique to test for the presence of a posteriorly dislocated hip (*Ortolani test*).[15]

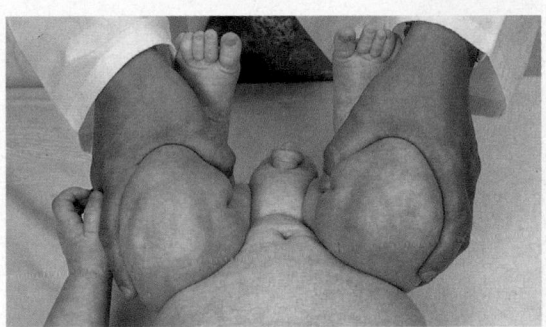

ORTOLANI TEST

Make sure the baby is relaxed. For the *Ortolani test*, place the baby supine with the legs pointing toward you. Flex the legs to form right angles at the hips and knees, placing your index fingers over the greater trochanter of each femur and your thumbs over the lesser trochanters. Abduct both hips simultaneously until the lateral aspect of each knee touches the examining table.

Careful inspection can reveal gross deformities such as dwarfism, congenital abnormalities of the extremities or digits, and annular bands that constrict an extremity.

Spina bifida occulta (a defect of the vertebral bodies) may be associated with defects of the spinal cord, which can cause severe neurologic dysfunction.

A soft audible "click" heard with these maneuvers does not prove a dislocated hip, but should prompt a careful examination.

With a *hip dysplasia,* you feel a "clunk" as the femoral head, which lies posterior to the acetabulum, enters the acetabulum. A palpable movement of the femoral head back into place constitutes a *positive Ortolani sign.*

Congenital hip dysplasia is important to detect: Early appropriate treatment has excellent outcomes.

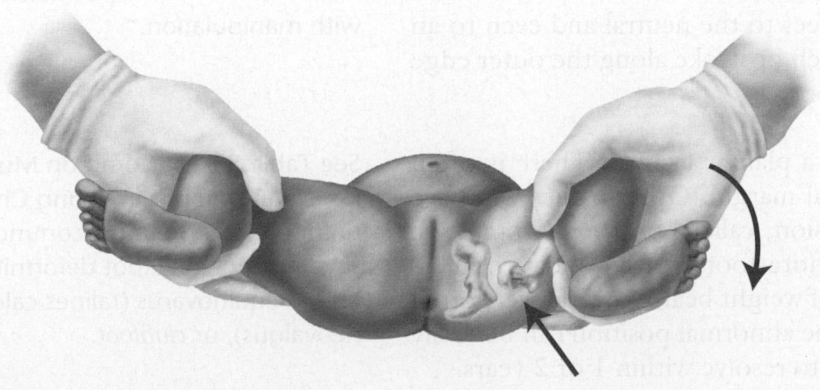

In addition to examining the hips, it is important to examine an infant's *legs and feet* to detect developmental abnormalities. Assess symmetry, bowing, and torsion of the legs. There should be no discrepancy in leg length. It is common for normal infants to have asymmetric thigh skin folds, but if you do detect asymmetry, make sure you perform the instability tests because dislocated hips are commonly associated with this finding.

Most infants are *bowlegged,* reflecting their curled-up intrauterine position.

Another finding after 3 months of age is apparent femoral shortening (*positive Galeazzi* or *Allis test*). This picture demonstrates the technique. Place the feet together and note any difference in knee heights.

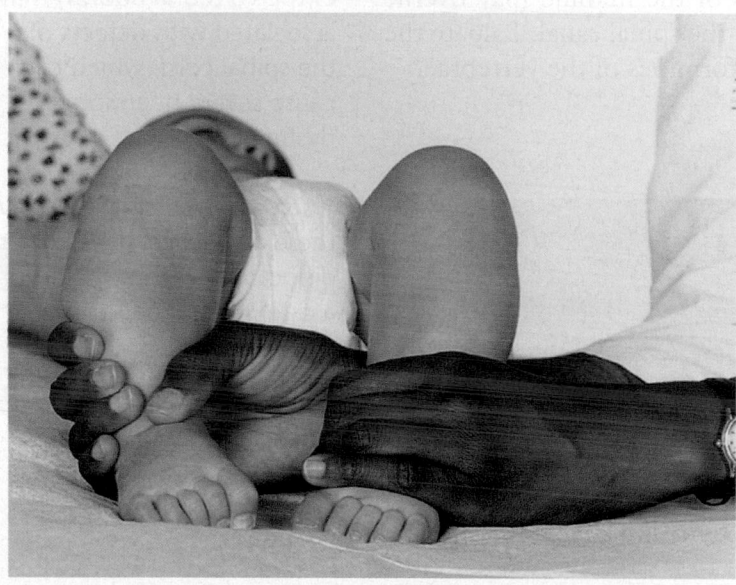

Some normal infants exhibit twisting or *torsion of the tibia* inwardly or outwardly on its longitudinal axis. Parents may be concerned about a toeing in or toeing out of the foot and an awkward gait, all of which are usually normal. Tibial torsion corrects itself during the second year of life after months of weight bearing.

Pathologic tibial torsion occurs only in association with *deformities of the feet or hips*

Now examine the feet. At birth, the feet may appear deformed from retaining their intrauterine positioning, often turned inward as shown on the next page. You should be able to correct the feet to the neutral and even to an overcorrected position. You can also scratch or stroke along the outer edge to see if the foot assumes a normal position.

True *deformities of the feet do not* return to the neutral position even with manipulation.

The infant's foot appears flat because of a plantar fat pad. There is often inversion of the foot, elevating the medial margin. Other babies will have adduction of the forefoot without inversion, called *metatarsus adductus.* Still others will have adduction of the entire foot. Finally, most toddlers have some pronation during early stages of weight bearing, with eversion of the foot. In all of these normal variants, the abnormal position can be easily overcorrected past midline. They all tend to resolve within 1 or 2 years.

See Table 23-13, Common Musculoskeletal Findings in Young Children, p. 836. The most common severe congenital foot deformity is talipes equinovarus (talipes calcaneovalgus), or *clubfoot.*

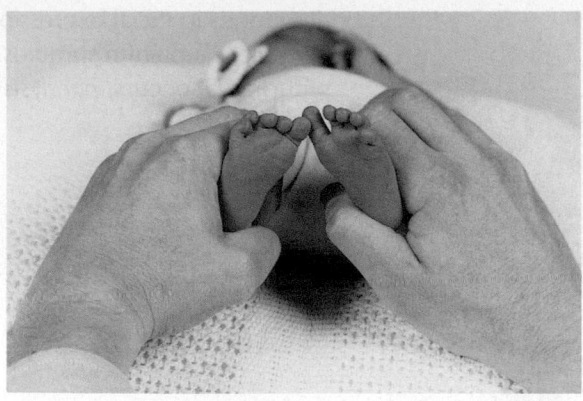
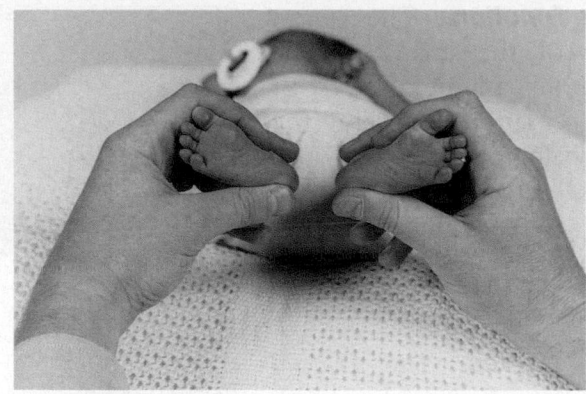

The Nervous System

The examination of the nervous system in infants includes techniques that are highly specific to this particular age. Further, unlike many neurologic abnormalities in adults that produce asymmetric localized findings, neurologic abnormalities in infants often present as developmental abnormalities such as failure to do age-appropriate tasks. Therefore, the neurologic and developmental examinations need to proceed hand in hand. Finding a developmental abnormality should prompt you to pay particular attention to the neurologic examination.

The neurologic screening examination of all infants should include assessment of mental status, gross and fine motor function, tone, cry, deep tendon reflexes, and primitive reflexes. More detailed examination of cranial nerve function, sensory function, and less common primitive reflexes are indicated if you suspect any abnormalities from the history or screening.[16]

The neurologic examination can reveal extensive disease but will not pinpoint specific functional deficits or minute lesions.

Mental Status. Infants should appear alert when awake, regard faces, and attend to their parents' voices. The infant should display mental activity appropriate for his or her age.

Motor Function and Tone. Assess the *motor tone* of infants, first by carefully watching their position at rest and testing their resistance to passive movement.

Then assess *tone* as you move each major joint through its range of motion, noting any spasticity or flaccidity. Hold the baby in your hands, as shown in the figure, to determine whether the tone is normal, increased, or decreased. Either increased or decreased tone may indicate intracranial disease, although such disease is usually accompanied by a number of other signs.

Signs of severe neurologic disease include extreme irritability; persistent asymmetry of posture; persistent extension of extremities; constant turning of the head to one side; marked extension of the head, neck, and extremities (opisthotonus); severe flaccidity; and limited response to pain.

Persistent irritability in the newborn may be a sign of *neurologic insult* or may reflect a variety of *metabolic, infectious,* or other *constitutional abnormalities,* or environmental conditions such as *drug withdrawal.*

Infants with *hypotonia* often lie in a frog-leg position, with arms flexed and hands near the ears. Hypotonia can be caused by a variety of *central nervous system abnormalities* and *disorders of the motor unit.*

Sensory Function. The *sensory function* of the infant can be tested in only a limited way. Test for pain sensation by flicking the infant's palm or sole with your finger. Observe for withdrawal, arousal, and change in facial expression. Do not use a pin to test for pain.

Cranial Nerves. The *cranial nerves* of the infant can be tested, but requires methods that differ from those used for the older child or adult. The following table provides useful strategies.

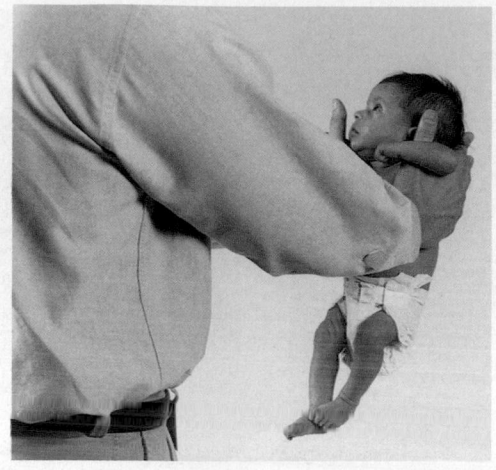

If changes in facial expression or cry follow a painful stimulus but no withdrawal occurs, *paralysis* may be present.

Abnormalities in the cranial nerves suggest an intracranial lesion such as hemorrhage or a congenital malformation.

● **Strategies to Assess Cranial Nerves in Newborns and Infants**

Cranial Nerve		Strategy
I	Olfactory	Difficult to test
II	Visual acuity	Have baby regard your face and look for facial response and tracking.
II, III	Response to light	Darken room; raise baby to sitting position to open eyes. Use light and test for *optic blink reflex* (blinking in response to light). Use the otoscope (no speculum) to assess papillary responses.
III, IV, VI	Extraocular movements	Observe how well the baby tracks your smiling face. Use light if needed.
V	Motor	Test rooting reflex. Test sucking reflex (watch baby suck breast, bottle, or pacifier).
VII	Facial	Observe baby crying and smiling; note symmetry of face and forehead.
VIII	Acoustic	Test acoustic blink reflex (blinking of both eyes in response to loud noise). Observe tracking in response to sound.

(continued)

● Strategies to Assess Cranial Nerves in Newborns and Infants (continued)

Cranial Nerve		Strategy
IX, X	Swallow	Observe coordination during swallowing.
	Gag	Test for gag reflex.
XI	Spinal accessory	Observe symmetry of shoulders.
XII	Hypoglossal	Observe coordination of sucking, swallowing, and tongue thrusting. Pinch nostrils; observe reflex opening of mouth with tip of tongue to midline.

Deep Tendon Reflexes.   The *deep tendon reflexes* are variable in infants because the corticospinal pathways are not fully developed. Thus, their exaggerated presence or their absence has little diagnostic significance, unless this response is different from results of previous testing or extreme responses are observed.

Use the same techniques to elicit deep tendon reflexes as you would for an adult. You can substitute your index or middle finger for the neurologic hammer, as shown below.

A progressive increase in deep tendon reflexes during the first year of life may indicate central nervous system disease such as *cerebral palsy*, especially if it is coupled with increased tone.

As in adults, asymmetric reflexes suggest a lesion of the peripheral nerves or spinal segment.

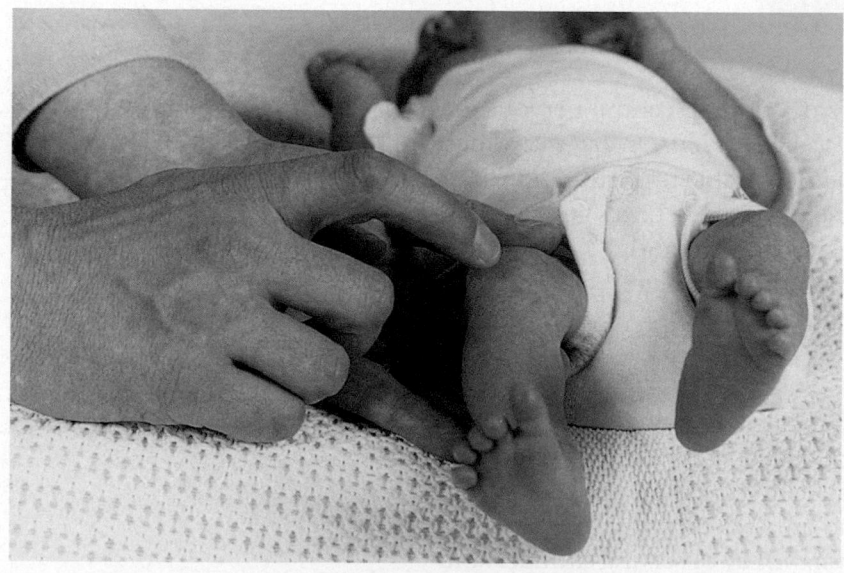

The triceps, brachioradialis, and abdominal reflexes are difficult to elicit before 6 months of age. The *anal reflex* is present at birth and important to elicit if a spinal cord lesion is suspected.

An absent anal reflex suggests loss of innervation of the external sphincter muscle caused by a spinal cord abnormality such as a congenital anomaly (e.g., *spina bifida*), *tumor*, or *injury*.

Although a normal flexion plantar response is obtained in 90% of infants, a *Babinski response* to plantar stimulation (dorsiflexion of big toe and fanning of other toes) can be elicited in some normal babies until 2 years of age.

Try to elicit the ankle reflex as for adults by tapping on the Achilles tendon but often there will not be a response. Another method, shown next, is to grasp the infant's malleolus with one hand and abruptly dorsiflex the ankle. Don't be surprised if you note rapid, rhythmic plantar flexion of the newborn's foot (*ankle clonus*) in response to this maneuver. Up to 10 beats are normal in newborns and young infants; this is *unsustained ankle clonus*.

When the contractions are continuous (*sustained ankle clonus*), *central nervous system disease* should be suspected.

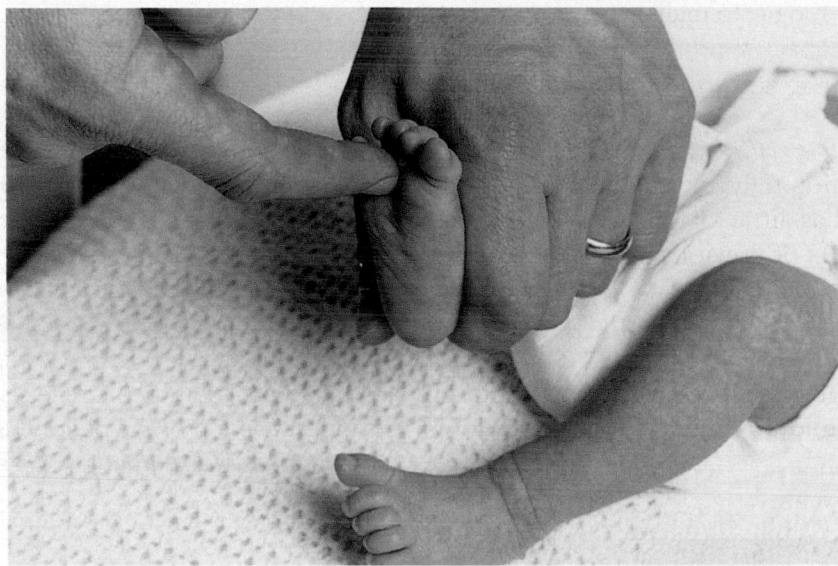

Primitive Reflexes. Evaluate the infant's developing central nervous system by assessing *infantile automatisms*, called *primitive reflexes*. These develop during gestation, are generally demonstrable at birth, and disappear at defined ages. Abnormalities in these primitive reflexes suggest neurologic disease and merit more intensive investigation.[17] The most important primitive reflexes are illustrated on the next page.

A *neurologic* or *developmental abnormality* is suspected if primitive reflexes are

● Absent at appropriate age
● Present longer than normal
● Asymmetric
● Associated with posturing or twitching

Development. Refer to the developmental milestones on p. 737, or utilize the DENVER II on page 742–743 to learn which age-specific developmental tasks to evaluate. By observation and play with the infant, you can do both a developmental screening examination and an assessment for gross and fine motor achievement. Specifically, look for *weakness* by observing sitting, standing, and transitions. Note *station*, or the posture of sitting or standing. Carefully observe the *gait* of the toddler, including balance and fluidity of movements. Fine motor development can be assessed in a similar way, combining the neurologic and developmental exam. Key milestones include the development of the pincer grasp, ability to manipulate objects with the hands, and more precise tasks, such as building a tower of cubes or scribbling, as fine motor development progresses in a proximal to distal direction.

Assess the infant's cognitive and social–emotional development as you proceed with the comprehensive neurologic and developmental examination. Some neurologic abnormalities produce deficits or slowing in cognitive and social development. As stated, infants who have developmental delay may have abnormalities found on the neurologic examination because much of the examination is based on age-specific norms.

● Primitive Reflex

Primitive Reflex		Maneuver	Ages	
Palmar Grasp Reflex		Place your fingers into the baby's hands and press against the palmar surfaces. The baby will flex all fingers to grasp your fingers.	Birth to 3–4 months	Persistence beyond 4 months suggests pyramidal tract dysfunction. Persistence of clenched hand beyond 2 months suggests central nervous system damage, especially if fingers overlap thumb.
Plantar Grasp Reflex		Touch the sole at the base of the toes. The toes curl.	Birth to 6–8 months	Persistence beyond 8 months suggests pyramidal tract dysfunction.
Moro Reflex (Startle Reflex)		Hold the baby supine, supporting the head, back, and legs. Abruptly lower the entire body about 2 feet. The arms abduct and extend, hands open, and legs flex. Baby may cry.	Birth to 4 months	Persistence beyond 4 months suggests neurologic disease (e.g., cerebral palsy); beyond 6 months strongly suggests it. Asymmetric response suggests fracture of clavicle or humerus or brachial plexus injury.
Asymmetric Tonic Neck Reflex		With baby supine, turn head to one side, holding jaw over shoulder. The arms/legs on side to which head is turned extend while the opposite arm/leg flex. Repeat on other side.	Birth to 2 months	Persistence beyond 2 months suggests asymmetric central nervous system development and sometimes predicts the development of cerebral palsy.
Positive Support Reflex		Hold the baby around the trunk and lower until the feet touch a flat surface. The hips, knees, and ankles extend; the baby stands up, partially bearing weight, and sags after 20–30 seconds.	Birth or 2 months until 6 months	Lack of reflex suggests hypotonia or flaccidity. Fixed extension and adduction of legs (scissoring) suggests spasticity from neurologic disease, such as cerebral palsy.

(continued)

● Primitive Reflex (continued)

Primitive Reflex		Maneuver	Ages	
Rooting Reflex		Stroke the perioral skin at the corners of the mouth. The mouth will open and baby will turn the head toward the stimulated side and suck.	Birth to 3–4 months	Absence of rooting indicates severe generalized or central nervous system disease.
Trunk Incurvation (Galant) Reflex		Support the baby prone with one hand, and stroke one side of the back 1 cm from midline, from shoulder to buttocks. The spine will curve toward the stimulated side.	Birth to 2 months	Absence suggests a transverse spinal cord lesion or injury. Persistence may indicate delayed development.
Placing and Stepping Reflexes		Hold baby upright from behind as in positive support reflex. Have one sole touch the tabletop. The hip and knee of that foot will flex and the other foot will step forward. Alternate stepping will occur.	Birth (best after 4 days). Variable age to disappear	Absence of placing may indicate paralysis. Babies born by breech delivery may not have placing reflex.
Landau Reflex		Suspend the baby prone with one hand. The head will lift up, and the spine will straighten.	Birth to 6 months	Persistence may indicate delayed development.
Parachute Reflex		Suspend the baby prone and slowly lower the head toward a surface. The arms and legs will extend in a protective fashion.	4–6 months and does not disappear	Delay in appearance may predict future delays in voluntary motor development.

HEALTH PROMOTION AND COUNSELING

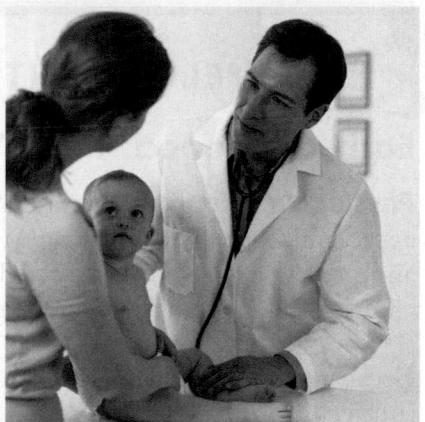

The AAP and an expert group, Bright Futures, recommend health supervision visits for infants and their parents when infants are the following ages: birth, within the first week, and 1, 2, 4, 6, 9, and 12 months. This is called the *Infant Periodicity Schedule*. Health supervision visits provide opportunities to answer questions for parents, assess the infant's growth and development, perform a comprehensive physical examination, and provide anticipatory guidance. Age-appropriate anticipatory guidance includes healthy habits and behaviors, social competence of caregivers, family relationships, and community interactions.

Parents usually are receptive to suggestions about health promotion, which can have major, long-term influences on the child and family.

Review the critical components of a health supervision visit for a 6-month-old. Adjust the content to the appropriate developmental level of the infant.

COMPONENTS OF A HEALTH SUPERVISION VISIT FOR A 6-MONTH-OLD

Discussions With Parents
- Address parents' concerns/questions
- Provide advice
- Perform social history
- Assess development, nutrition, safety, oral health, family relationships, community

Developmental Assessment
- Assess milestones by history (may use DENVER II)
- Measure milestones by examination (may use DENVER II)

Physical Examination
- Perform a careful examination, including growth parameters with percentiles for age

Screening Tests
- Vision and hearing (by exam), possibly hematocrit and lead (if high risk), screen for social risk factors

Immunizations
- See schedule on website http://www.cdc.gov/vaccines/recs/schedules/child-schedule.htm

Anticipatory Guidance
Healthy Habits and Behaviors
- Injury and illness prevention
  Infant seat, rolling walker, poisons, tobacco exposure, "back to sleep" position
- Nutrition
  Breast-feeding or bottle, solids, limit juice, prevent choking, overfeeding
- Oral health
  No bottle in bed, fluoride, brushing teeth

Parent–Infant Interaction
- Promoting development

Family Relationships
- Time for self; babysitters

Community Interaction
- Child care, resources

ASSESSING YOUNG AND SCHOOL-AGED CHILDREN

DEVELOPMENT

Early Childhood: 1 to 4 Years

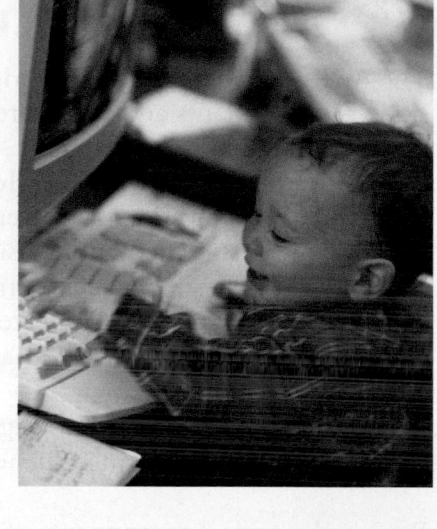

Physical Development. After infancy, the rate of physical growth slows by approximately half. After 2 years, toddlers gain about 2 to 3 kg (4.5–6.5 lbs) and grow 5 cm (2 in) per year. Physical changes are impressive. Chubby, clumsy toddlers transform into leaner, more muscular preschoolers.

Gross motor skills also develop quickly. Most children walk by 15 months, run well by 2 years, and pedal a tricycle and jump by 4 years. Fine motor skills develop through neurologic maturation and environmental manipulation. The 18-month-old who scribbles becomes a 2-year-old who draws lines and then a 4-year-old who makes circles.

Cognitive and Language Development. Toddlers move from sensorimotor learning (through touching and looking) to symbolic thinking, solving simple problems, remembering songs, and engaging in imitative play. Language develops with extraordinary speed. An 18-month-old with 10 to 20 words becomes a 2-year-old with three-word sentences, and then a 3-year-old who converses well. By 4 years, preschoolers form complex sentences. They remain preoperational, however, without sustained logical thought processes.

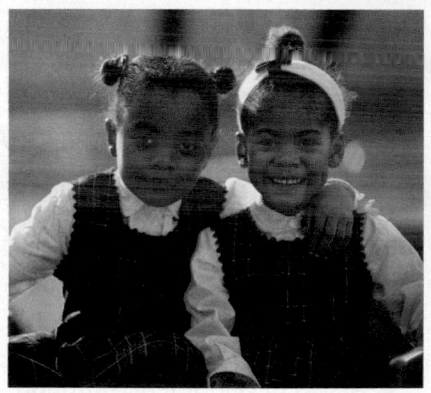

Social and Emotional Development. New intellectual pursuits are surpassed only by an emerging drive for independence. Because toddlers are impulsive, temper tantrums are common.

Developmental Milestones During Early Childhood

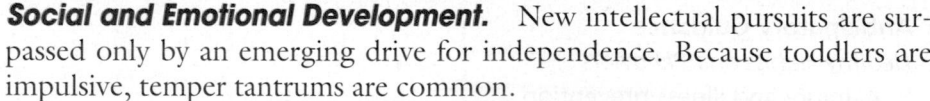

	1 yr	2 yr	3 yr	4 yr	5 yr
Physical/ Motor	Walks	Throws	Jumps in place Balances on 1 foot	Hops Pedals tricycle	Skips Balances well
Cognitive/ Language	2-3 words	2-3 word phrases	Sentences	Speech all understandable	Copies figures Defines words
Social/ Emotional	Plays games (peek-a-boo)	Imitates activities	Feeds self	Imaginative Sings	Dresses self Plays games

Middle Childhood: 5 to 10 Years

Despite Freud's view, middle childhood certainly is not a latent period. Goal-directed exploration, increased physical and cognitive abilities, and achievements by trial and error mark this stage. Physical examination is more straightforward, but always consider the developmental stages and tasks that school-age children are facing.

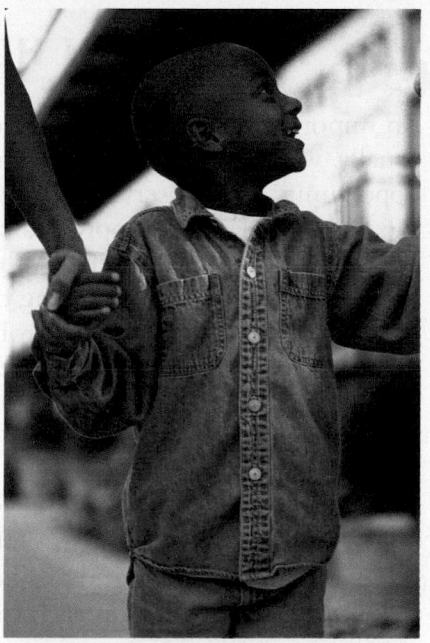

Physical Development. Children grow steadily but more slowly. Nevertheless, strength and coordination improve dramatically, with more participation in activities. This is also when children with physical disabilities or chronic illnesses become more aware of their limitations.

Cognitive and Language Development. Children become "concrete operational"—capable of limited logic and more complex learning. They remain rooted in the present, with little ability to understand consequences or abstractions. School, family, and environment greatly influence learning. A major developmental task is self-efficacy, or the ability to thrive in different situations. Language becomes increasingly complex.

Social and Emotional Development. Children become progressively more independent, initiating activities and enjoying accomplishments. Achievements are critical for self-esteem and developing a "fit" within major social structures—family, school, and peer activity groups. Guilt and poor self-esteem also may emerge. Family and environment contribute enormously to the child's self-image. Moral development remains simple and concrete, with a clear sense of "right and wrong."

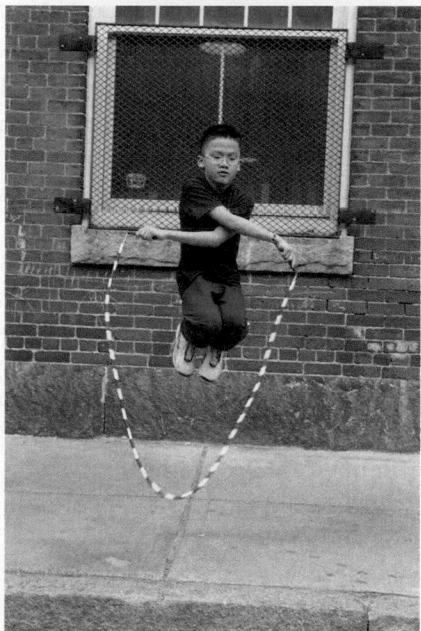

● Developmental Tasks During Middle Childhood

Task	Characteristic	Health Care Needs
Physical	Enhanced strength and coordination	Screening for strengths, assessing problems
	Competence in various tasks and activities	Involving parents
		Support for disabilities
		Anticipatory guidance: safety
Cognitive	"Concrete operational": focus on the present	Emphasis on short-term consequences
	Achievement of knowledge and skills, self-efficacy	Support; screening about skills and school performance
Social	Achieving good "fit" with family, friends, school	Assessment, support, advice about interactions
	Sustained self-esteem	Support, emphasis on strengths
	Evolving self-identity	Understanding, advice, support

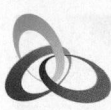 **THE HEALTH HISTORY**

An important and unique aspect of examining children is that parents are usually watching and taking part in the interaction, providing you the opportunity to observe the parent–child interaction. Note whether the child displays age-appropriate behaviors. Assess the "goodness of fit" between parents and child. Although some abnormal interactions may result from the unnatural setting of the examination room, others may be a consequence of interactional problems. Careful *observation* of the child's interactions with parents and the child's unstructured play in the examination room can reveal *abnormalities in physical, cognitive, and social development.*

The health history of the child is similar to the infant health history on pp. 737–739, updated for the child's developmental level. A complete history would be obtained if the child is a new patient. Otherwise, the history is continuously updated at each visit.

Normal toddlers are occasionally terrified or angry at the examiner. Often, they are completely uncooperative. Most eventually warm up to you. If this behavior continues or is not developmentally appropriate, there may be an *underlying behavioral or developmental abnormality.* Older, school-aged children have more self-control and prior experience with nurses and are generally cooperative with the examination. You can detect a surprising amount by using observation.

ABNORMALITIES DETECTED WHILE OBSERVING PLAY

Behavioral Problems*
Poor parent–child interactions
Sibling rivalry
Inappropriate parental discipline
"Difficult temperament"

Developmental Delay
Gross motor delay
Fine motor delay
Language delay (expressive, receptive)
Delay in social or emotional tasks (may use Denver II)

Social or Environmental Problems
Parental problem (e.g., stress, depression)
Risk for abuse or neglect

Neurologic Problems
Weakness
Abnormal posture
Spasticity
Clumsiness
Attentional problems and hyperactivity
Autistic features
Musculoskeletal abnormalities
Foot deformities
Gait problems

*Note: The child's behavior during the visit may not represent typical behavior, but your observations may serve as a springboard for discussion with parents.

Assessing Younger Children

One of the most difficult challenges one faces in examining children in this age group is avoiding a physical struggle, a crying child, or a distraught parent.

Let the child remain dressed during the interview to minimize the child's apprehension. It also allows you to interact more naturally and observe the child playing, interacting with the parents, and undressing and dressing.

Toddlers who are 9 to 15 months may have *stranger anxiety,* a fear of strangers that is developmentally normal. It signals the toddler's growing awareness that the stranger is "new." You should not approach these toddlers quickly. Make sure they remain solidly in their parent's lap throughout much of the examination.

The following are useful tips in examining young children.

● Some Tips for Examining Young Children (1–4-Year-Olds)

Useful Strategies for Examination	Useful Toys and Aids
Examine a child sitting on parent's lap. Try to be at the child's eye level.	"Blow out" the otoscope light.
First examine the child's toy or teddy bear, then the child.	"Beep" the stethoscope on your nose.
Let the child do some of the exam (e.g., move the stethoscope). Then go back and "get the places we missed."	Make tongue-depressor puppets.
Ask the toddler who keeps pushing you away to "hold your hand." Then have the toddler "help you" with the exam.	Use the child's own toys for play.
Some toddlers believe that if they cannot see you, then you are not there. Perform the exam while the child stands on the parent's lap, facing the parent.	Jingle your keys to test for hearing.
If 2-year-olds are holding something in each hand (such as tongue depressors), they cannot fight or resist!	Shine the otoscope through the tip of your finger, "lighting it up," and then examine the child's ears with it.

Engage children in age-appropriate conversation. Ask simple questions about their illness or toys. Compliment their appearance or behavior, tell a story, or play a simple game to "break the ice." If a child is shy, turn your attention to the parent to allow the child to warm up gradually.

With certain exceptions, physical examination does not require use of the examining table—it can be done on the floor or with the child in a parent's lap. The key is to engage the child's cooperation. For young children who resist undressing, expose only the body part being examined. When examining siblings, begin with the oldest child, who is more likely to cooperate and set a good example. Approach the child pleasantly. Explain each step as you perform it. Continue conversing with the family to provide distraction.

Plan the examination to start with the least distressing procedures and end with the most distressing (usually involving the throat and ears). Begin with parts that can be done with the child sitting, such as examining the eyes or palpating the neck. Lying down may make a child feel vulnerable, so change positions with care. Once a child is supine, start with the abdomen, saving the throat and ears or genitalia for last. A parent's help may be needed to hold the child for examination of the ears or throat; however, use of formal restraints is inappropriate. Patience, distraction, play, flexibility in the order of the examination, and a caring but firm and gentle approach are all key to successfully examining the young child.

MORE TIPS FOR EXAMINING THE YOUNG CHILD

Use a reassuring voice throughout the examination.
Let the child see and touch the examination tools you will be using.
Avoid asking permission to examine a body part because you will do the examination anyway. Instead, ask the child which ear or which part of the body he or she would like you to examine "first."
Examine the child in the parent's lap. Let the parent undress the child.
If unable to console the child, give the child a short break.
Make a game out of the examination! For example, "Let's see how big your tongue is!" or, for lung examination, "Blow out the light" using a penlight.

Reassure parents that resistance to examination is developmentally appropriate. Some embarrassed parents scold the child, compounding the problem. Involve parents in the examination. Learn which techniques and approaches work best and are most comfortable for you.

Assessing Older Children

Many children at this age are modest. Providing gowns and leaving underwear in place as long as possible are wise approaches. Suggest that children disrobe behind a curtain. Consider leaving the room while they change with parents' help. Some children may prefer opposite-sex siblings to leave, but most prefer a parent of either sex to remain in the room. Parents of children younger than 11 years should stay with them.

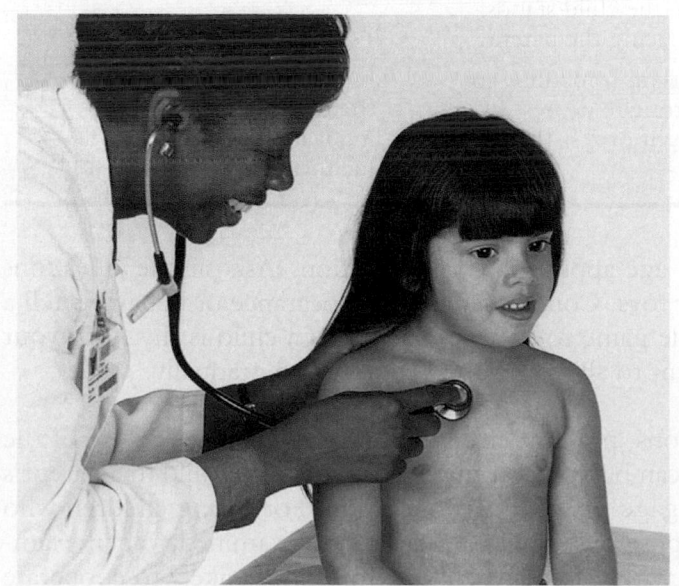

Children usually are accompanied by a parent or caregiver. Even when alone, they are often seeking health care at the request of their parents—indeed, the parent is usually sitting in the waiting room. When interviewing a child, you need to consider the needs and perspectives of both the child and the caregivers.

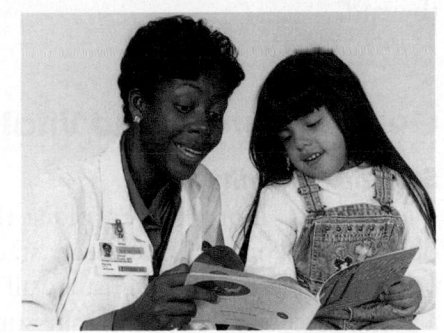

Establishing Rapport.   Begin the interview by greeting and establishing rapport with each person present. Refer to the child by name rather than by "him" or "her." Clarify the role or relationship of all of the adults and children. "Now, are you Jimmy's grandmother?" "Please help me by telling me Jimmy's relationship to everyone here." Address the parents as "Mr. Smith" and "Ms. Smith" rather than by their first names or "Mom" or "Dad." When the family structure is not immediately clear, you may avoid embarrassment by asking directly about other members. "Who else lives in the home?" "Who is Jimmy's father?" "Do you live together?" Do not assume that just because parents are separated, only one parent is actively involved in the child's life.

To establish rapport, meet children on their own level. Use your personal experiences with children to guide how you interact in a health care setting. Eye contact on their level, participating in playful engagement, and talking about what interests them are always good strategies. Ask children about their clothes, one of their toys, what book or TV show they like, or their adult companion in an enthusiastic but gentle style. Spending time at the beginning of the interview to calm down and connect with an anxious child can put both the child and the caregiver at ease.

Working With Families.   One challenge when several people are present is deciding to whom to direct your questions. While eventually you need to get information from both the child and the parent, it is useful to start with the child. Asking simple open-ended questions like "Are you sick? . . . Tell me about it," followed by more specific questions, often provides much of the clinical data. The parents can then verify the information, add details that give you the larger context, and identify other issues you need to address. Characterize symptom attributes the same way you do with adults. Sometimes children are embarrassed to begin, but once the parent has started the conversation, direct questions back to the child:

> Your mom tells me that you get stomachaches. Tell me about them.
> Show me where you get the pain. What does it feel like?
> Is it sharp like a pin prick, or does it ache?
> Does it stay in the same spot, or does it move around?
> What helps make it go away? What makes it worse?
> What do you think causes it?

The presence of family members allows you to observe how they interact with the child. A child may be able to sit still or may get restless and start fidgeting. Watch how the parents set limits or fail to set limits when needed.

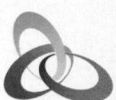

PHYSICAL EXAMINATION OF YOUNG AND SCHOOL-AGED CHILDREN

The order of the examination now begins to follow that used for adults. Examine painful areas last, and forewarn children about areas you are going to examine. If a child resists part of the examination, you can return to it at the end.

General Survey and Vital Signs

Somatic Growth

Height.   For children older than 2 years, measure standing height, optimally using wall-mounted stadiometers. Have the child stand with heels, back, and head against a wall or the back of the stadiometer. If using a wall with a marked ruler, make sure to place a flat board or surface against the top of the child's head and at right angles to the ruler. Stand-up weight scales with a height attachment are not very accurate.

Rule of thumb on height: After age 2 years, children should grow at least 5 cm (2.5 in) per year.

Short stature, defined as subnormal height for age, can be a normal variant or caused by endocrine or other diseases. Normal variants include *familial short stature* and *constitutional delay.* Chronic diseases include *growth hormone deficiency,* other endocrine diseases, *gastrointestinal disease, renal* or *metabolic disease,* and *genetic syndromes.*

Weight.   Young children who can stand and school-age children should be weighed in their underpants or in a gown on a stand-up scale. Although initially nervous, most young children can be coaxed onto such scales. Use the same scales if possible for each visit.

Young children can have inadequate weight and height gain if caloric intake is insufficient. Etiologies of failure to thrive include *psychosocial, interactional, gastrointestinal, and endocrine disorders.*

Head Circumference.   In general, head circumference is measured until the child reaches 24 months. Afterward, head circumference measurement may be helpful if you suspect a genetic or central nervous system disorder.

Most children with exogenous obesity are also tall for their age. Children with endocrine causes of obesity tend to be short.

Body Mass Index for Age.   Age- and sex-specific charts are now available to assess BMI in children (see the following table for interpreting a child's BMI.). BMI in children is associated with body fat, related to subsequent health risks for obesity. BMI measurements are helpful for early detection of obesity in children older than 2 years. Obesity is now a major childhood epidemic, and it often begins before 6 to 8 years. Consequences of childhood obesity include hypertension, diabetes, metabolic syndrome, and poor self-esteem. Childhood obesity often leads to adult obesity and shortened lifespan.

Childhood obesity is a major epidemic: 36% of U.S. children have a BMI >85th percentile, and 16% have a BMI ≥95th percentile.[18] Long-term morbidity from childhood obesity spans many organ systems, including cardiovascular, endocrine, renal, musculoskeletal, gastrointestinal, and psychological. Prevention, early detection, and aggressive management are needed.

● Interpreting BMI in Children	
Group	**BMI-for-Age**
Underweight	<5th percentile
At risk of overweight	≥85th percentile
Overweight	≥95th percentile

Vital Signs

Blood Pressure.   Hypertension during childhood is more common than previously thought, and it is important to recognize, confirm, and appropriately manage it. Thus, you must learn to accurately measure blood pressure in children.

Children have elevated blood pressure during exercise, crying, and anxiety. Although young children may be anxious at first, when the procedure is explained and demonstrated beforehand, most children are cooperative. If the blood pressure is initially elevated, you can perform blood pressure readings again at the end of the examination; one trick is to leave the cuff on the arm (deflated) and repeat the reading later. Elevated readings must always be confirmed by subsequent measurements.

The most frequent "cause" of an elevated blood pressure in children is an *improperly performed examination,* often due to an incorrect cuff size.

Select the blood pressure cuff as you would for adults. It should be wide enough to cover two thirds of the upper arm or leg. A cuff that is too narrow falsely elevates the blood pressure reading, whereas a wider cuff lowers it and may interfere with proper placement of the stethoscope diaphragm over the artery. *Thus, a proper cuff size is essential for accurate determinations of blood pressure in children.*

In children, as in adults, systolic blood pressure readings from the thigh are approximately 10 mm Hg higher than those from the upper arm. If they are the same or lower, *coarctation of the aorta* should be suspected.

With children, as with adults, the point at which the Korotkoff sounds disappear constitutes the diastolic pressure. At times, especially among chubby young children, the Korotkoff sounds are not easily heard. In such instances, use palpation to determine the systolic blood pressure, remembering that the systolic pressure is approximately 10 mm Hg lower by palpation than by auscultation.

An electronic sphygmomanometer can be used if the Korotkoff sounds are inaudible. The child's limb must be still during the measurement. Gentle restraint may be necessary to prevent movement.

Transient hypertension in children can be caused by some common childhood medications, including those to treat asthma (e.g., prednisone) and attention deficit hyperactivity disorder (ADHD; e.g., Ritalin).

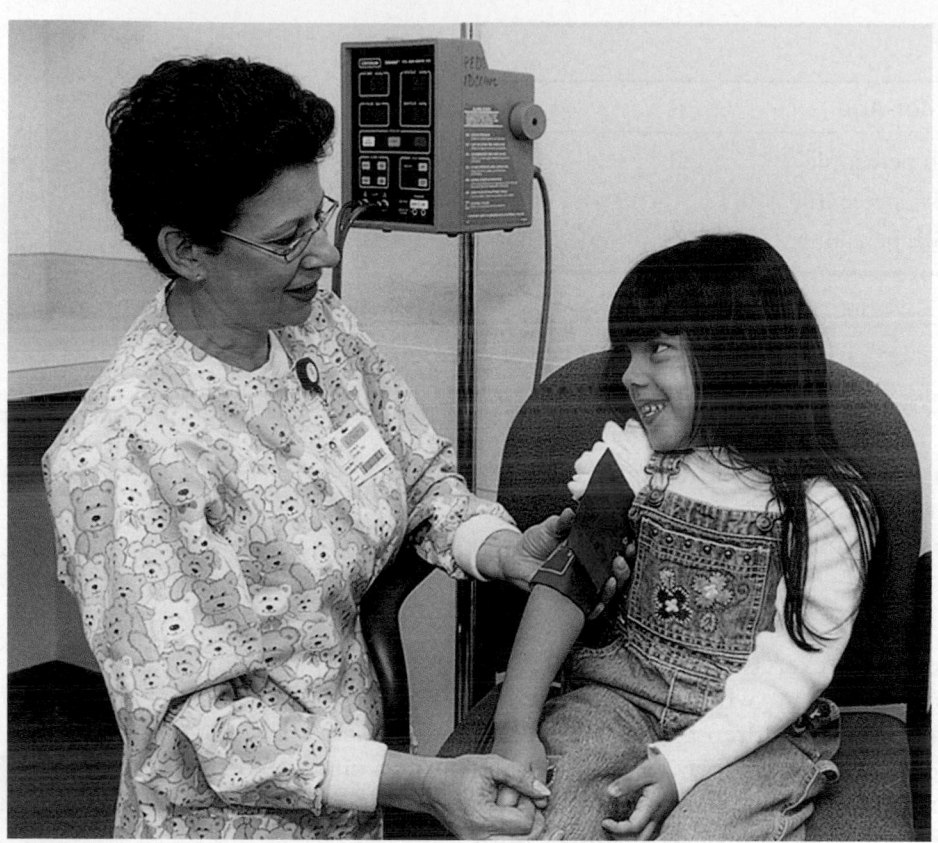

In 2004, the National Heart, Lung, and Blood Institute's National High Blood Pressure Working Group on Hypertension Control in Children and Adolescents defined normal, high-normal, and high blood pressure as follows, with measurements on at least three separate occasions:[19]

Causes of *sustained hypertension* in childhood include renal parenchymal or artery disease, coarctation of the aorta, and primary hypertension.

● Blood Pressure

Blood Pressure Category	Average Systolic and/or Diastolic Blood Pressure for Age, Sex, and Height
Normal	<90th percentile
Prehypertensive	90th–95th percentile
Hypertensive	≥95th percentile

See Table 23-1, Abnormalities in Heart Rhythm and Blood Pressure, p. 824.

Children who have hypertension should be evaluated extensively to determine the cause. For infants and young children, a specific cause can usually be found. An increasing proportion of older children and adolescents, however, have essential or primary hypertension. In all cases, it is important to repeat measurements to reduce the possibility that the elevation reflects anxiety. Sometimes repeating measurements in school is a way to obtain readings in a more relaxed environment. Hypertension and obesity often coexist in children.

It is also important not to *falsely label* a child or adolescent as having hypertension, because of the stigma of labeling, potential limitations to activities, and possible side effects of treatment.

Pulse.   Average heart rates and ranges of normal are shown in the table below. Measure the heart rate over a 60-second interval.

● **Average Heart Rate of Children at Rest**		
Age	Average Rate	Range (Two Standard Deviations)
1–2 years	110	70–150
2–6 years	103	68–138
6–10 years	95	65–125

Sinus bradycardia is a heart rate <100 beats per minute in children younger than 3 years, and <60 beats per minute in children 3 to 9 years.

Respiratory Rate. The rate of respirations per minute ranges from 20 to 40 during early childhood, and 15 to 25 during late childhood, reaching adult levels at around 15 years of age.

For young children, observe the movements of the chest wall for two 30-second intervals or over 1 minute, preferably before stimulating them. Direct auscultation of the chest or placing the stethoscope in front of the mouth is also useful for counting respirations, but the measurement may be falsely elevated if the child becomes agitated. For older children, use the same technique as that used for adults.

The commonly accepted cutoff for tachypnea in children older than 1 year is a respiratory rate greater than 40 breaths per minute.

Children with respiratory diseases such as *bronchiolitis* or *pneumonia* have rapid respirations (up to 80 to 90/min) but *also* increased work of breathing such as grunting, nasal flaring, or use of accessory muscles.

The best single physical finding for ruling out *pneumonia* is an absence of tachypnea.

Temperature. In children, auditory canal or temporal artery temperature recordings are preferable because they can be obtained quickly with essentially no discomfort.

Young children with infections can have extremely high fevers (up to 104°F or 40°C). Children younger than 3 years, who appear very ill with a fever, should be evaluated for possible sepsis, urinary tract infection, pneumonia, or other infectious etiology.

The Skin

After a child's first year of life, the techniques of examination are the same as those for the adult (see Chapter 9, The Integumentary System.)

See Table 23-3, Warts, Lesions that Resemble Warts, and Other Raised Lesions and Table 23-4, Common Skin Lesions During Childhood, p. 826.

The Head

In examining the head and neck, tailor your examination to the child's stage of growth and development.

Even before touching the child, carefully observe the shape of the head, its symmetry, and the presence of abnormal facies. Abnormal facies may not be apparent until later in childhood; therefore, carefully examine the face as well as the head of all children.

See Table 23-6, Diagnostic Facies in Infancy and Childhood, pp. 828–829.

The Eyes

The two most important components of the eye examination for young children are to determine whether the gaze is conjugate or symmetric and to test visual acuity in each eye.

Conjugate Gaze. Use the methods described in Chapter 11, The Eyes, for adults to assess *conjugate gaze,* or the *position and alignment of the eyes,* and the function of the extraocular muscles. The corneal light reflex test and the cover–uncover test are particularly useful in young children.

Perform the cover–uncover test as a game by having the young child watch your nose or tell you if you are smiling or not while you cover one of the child's eyes.

Visual Acuity. It may not be possible to measure the visual acuity of children younger than 3 years who cannot identify pictures on an eye chart. For these children, the simplest examination is to assess for fixation preference by alternately covering one eye; the child with normal vision will not object, but a child with poor vision in one eye will object to having the good eye covered. In all tests of visual acuity, it is important that both eyes show the same result.

Strabismus in children requires treatment by an ophthalmologist.

Both *ocular strabismus* and *anisometropia* (eyes with significantly different refractive errors) can result in *amblyopia,* or reduced vision in an otherwise normal eye. *Amblyopia* can lead to a "lazy eye," with permanently reduced visual acuity if not corrected early (generally by 6 years).

Reduced visual acuity is more likely among children who were born prematurely, and among those with other neurologic or developmental disorders.

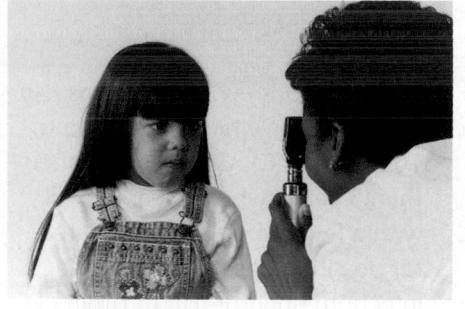
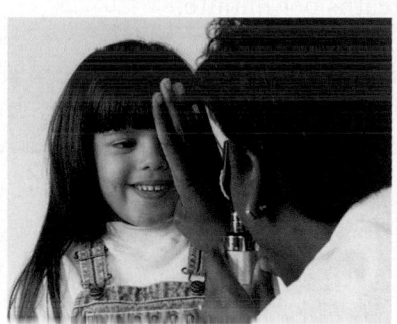

● Visual Acuity	
Age	Acuity
3 months	Eyes converge, baby reaches
12 months	~20/200
Less than 4 years	20/40
4 years and older	20/30

Any difference in visual acuity between the eyes (e.g., 20/20 on the left and 20/30 on the right) is abnormal, and the patient should be referred to an ophthalmologist.

As shown on the next page, visual acuity in children 3 years and older can usually be formally tested using an eye chart with one of a variety of optotypes (characters or symbols).[20] A child who does not know letters or numbers reliably can be tested using pictures, symbols, or the "E" chart. Using the "E" chart, most children will cooperate by telling you in which direction the "E" is pointing.

The most common visual disorder of childhood is *myopia,* which can be easily detected using this examination technique.

Visual Fields. The *visual fields* can be examined in infants and young children with the child sitting on the parent's lap. One eye should be tested at a time with the other eye covered. Hold the child's head in the midline while bringing an object such as a toy into the field of vision from behind the child. The overall method is the same as that for adults, except that you will have to make this into a game for your patient.

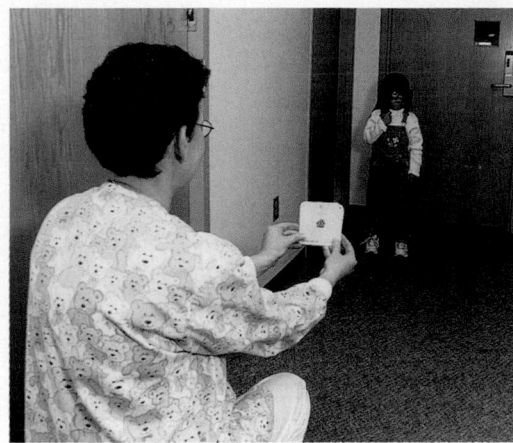
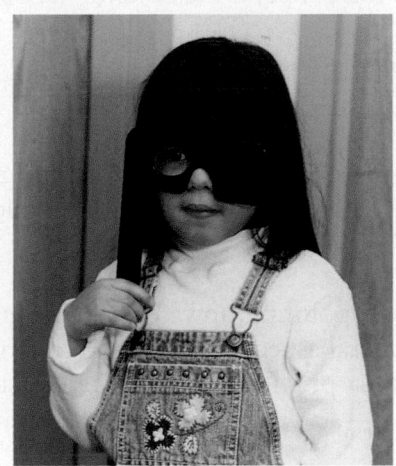

The Ears

If the child is not too fearful, examine the ears with the child sitting on a parent's lap. It is helpful to make a game out of the otoscopic examination or talking playfully to allay fears. It may help to place the otoscopic speculum gently into the external auditory canal of one ear and then withdraw it so the child gets used to the procedure, before the actual examination.

Ask the parent for a preference regarding the positioning of the child for the examination. There are two common positions—the child lying down and restrained, and the child sitting in the parent's lap. If the child is held supine, have the parent hold the arms either extended or close to the sides to limit motions. Hold the head and retract the tragus with one hand while you hold the otoscope with your other hand. If the child is on the parent's lap, the child's legs should be between the parent's legs. The parent could help by placing one arm around the child's body and using the second arm to steady the head.

Tympanic Membranes. Until approximately 3 years the external auditory canal is directed downward similar to infants and the auricle must be pulled downward and backward to afford the best view. After about 3 years the ear canal assumes an adult like slope and the auricle is pulled upward and backward. Hold the child's head with one hand (your left hand if you are right-handed), and with that same hand pull on the auricle. With your other hand, position the otoscope.

TIPS FOR CONDUCTING THE OTOSCOPIC EXAMINATION

Use the best angle of the otoscope.
Use the largest possible speculum.
   A larger speculum allows you to better visualize the tympanic membrane.
Don't apply too much pressure, which will cause the child to cry.
Insert the speculum ¼ to ½ inch into the canal.
First find the landmarks.
   Sometimes the ear canal resembles the tympanic membrane—do not be fooled!
Note whether the tympanic membrane is abnormal.

Not only are there two positions for the child (lying down or sitting), but also there are two ways to hold the otoscope, as illustrated by the following photos:

● The first is with the otoscope handle pointing upward or laterally while you pull on the auricle. Hold the lateral aspect of your hand that has the otoscope against the child's head to provide a buffer against sudden movements by the patient.

● The second technique is used by many nurses because of the different angle of the auditory canal in children. Hold the otoscope with the handle pointing down toward the child's feet while you pull on the auricle. Hold the head and pull up on the auricle with one hand while you hold the otoscope with the other hand.

Acute otitis media is a common condition of childhood. A symptomatic child typically has a red, bulging tympanic membrane, with a dull or absent light reflex. Purulent material may also be seen behind the tympanic membrane. See Table 23-7, Abnormalities of the Eyes, Ears, and Mouth, p. 830. The most useful symptom in making the diagnosis is ear pain, if combined with the above signs.[21,22]

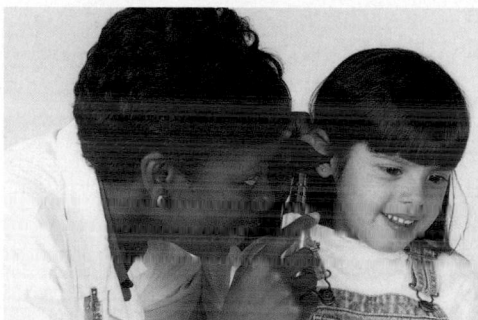

Gently move and pull on the *pinna* before or during your otoscopic examination. Carefully inspect the area behind the pinna, over the mastoid bone.

With acute *mastoiditis,* the auricle may protrude forward, and the area over the mastoid bone is red, swollen, and tender.

Formal Hearing Testing. Although formal hearing testing is necessary for accurate detection of hearing deficits in young children, you can grossly test for hearing by using the whispered voice test. To do this, stand behind the child (so that the child cannot read your lips), cover one of the child's ear canals, and rub the tragus, using a circular motion. Whisper letters,

Younger children who fail these screening maneuvers or who have speech delay should have audiometric testing. These children may have *hearing deficits.*

numbers, or a word and have the child repeat it; then test the other ear. This technique has relatively high sensitivity and specificity compared with formal testing.[23]

Up to 15% of school-aged children have at least mild hearing loss, emphasizing the importance of screening for hearing prior to school age.[23]

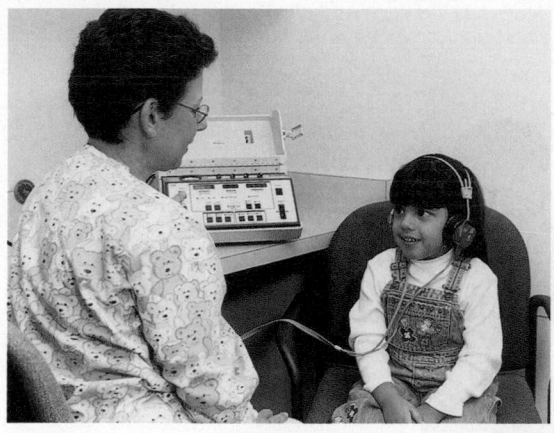

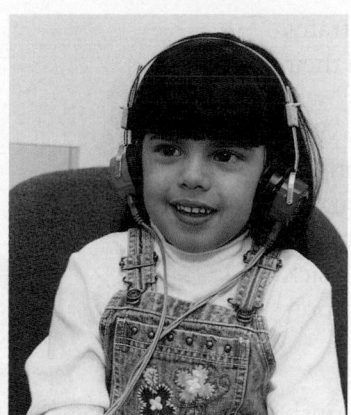

The Nose and Sinuses

Inspect the anterior portion of the nose by using a large speculum on your otoscope. Inspect the nasal mucous membranes, noting their color and condition. Look for nasal septal deviation and the presence of polyps.

Pale, boggy nasal mucous membranes are found in children with *chronic (perennial) allergic rhinitis*.

Purulent rhinitis is common in viral infections but may be part of the constellation of symptoms of *sinusitis*.

Foul-smelling, purulent, unilateral discharge from the nose may be due to a *foreign body* in the nose. This is particularly common among young preschool children, who tend to stick objects into any body orifice.

Nasal polyps are flesh-colored growths inside the nares. They are generally isolated findings but in some cases are present as part of a syndrome.

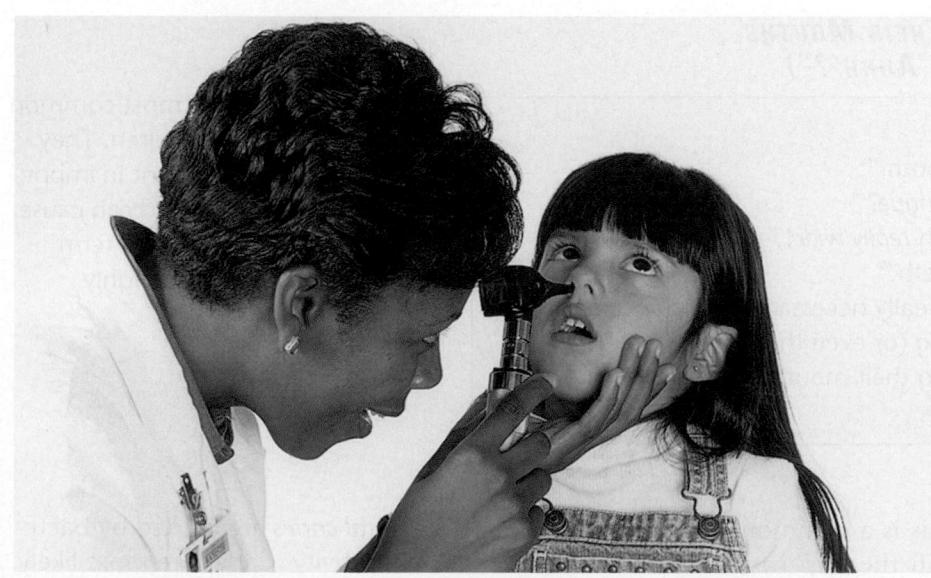

Maxillary sinuses are noted on x-rays by age 4 years, sphenoid sinuses by age 6, and frontal sinuses by age 6 to 7. The sinuses of older children can be palpated as in adults, looking for tenderness.[24]

Children with purulent rhinorrhea (generally unilateral) and also headache, sore throat, and tenderness over the sinuses may have *sinusitis*.

The Mouth and Pharynx

For anxious or young children, perform this part of the examination toward the end, because it may require parental assistance. The young, cooperative child may be more comfortable sitting in the parent's lap.

The accompanying figure demonstrates some tricks to getting children to open their mouths. The child who can say "ahhh" will usually offer a sufficient (albeit brief) view of the posterior pharynx so that a tongue blade is unnecessary. Healthy children are more likely to cooperate with this examination than sick children, especially if the sick child sees the tongue blade or has had previous experience with throat cultures.

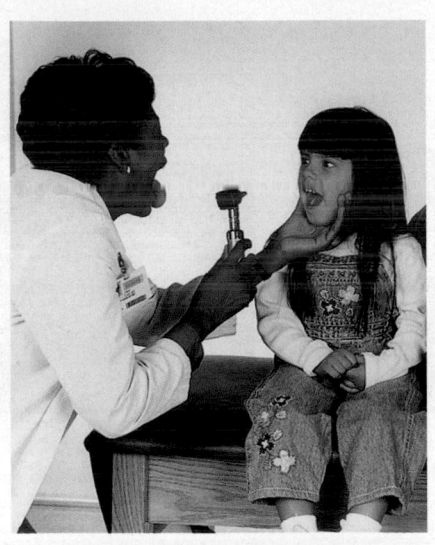

If you need to use the tongue blade, push down and pull slightly forward toward yourself while the child says "ahhh," being careful not to place the blade too far posteriorly, eliciting a gag reflex.

Examine the *teeth* for the timing and sequence of eruption, number, character, condition, and position. Abnormalities of the enamel may reflect local or general disease.

HOW TO GET CHILDREN TO OPEN THEIR MOUTHS (AKA, "WOULD YOU PLEASE SAY 'AHHH'?")

- Turn it into a game.
  - "Now let's see what's in your mouth."
  - "Can you stick out your *whole tongue*?"
  - "I bet you can't open your mouth really wide!"
  - "Let me see the inside of your teeth."
- Don't show a tongue blade unless really necessary.
- Demonstrate first on an older sibling (or even the parent).
- Offer enthusiastic praise for opening their mouths a little, and encourage them to open even wider!

Dental caries are the most common health problem in children. They are particularly prevalent in impoverished populations and can cause both short-term and long-term problems.[25] Caries are highly treatable.

Carefully inspect the upper teeth. This is a common location for *nursing-bottle caries*. The technique, called "lift the lip," can facilitate visualization of dental caries. Gently raise the child's upper lip with your gloved thumb to visualize the outside of the upper teeth. Visualize the inside of the upper teeth by having the child look up at the ceiling with the mouth wide open.

Dental caries are caused by bacterial activity. Caries are more likely among young children who are put to bed nursing from a bottle, allowing formula to pool around the teeth ("nursing-bottle caries"). See Table 23-8, Abnormalities of the Teeth, Pharynx and Neck, p. 831.

The table below displays a common pattern of teeth eruption. In general, lower teeth erupt a bit earlier than upper teeth.

Staining of the teeth may be intrinsic or extrinsic. Intrinsic stains may be from tetracycline use before 8 years (yellow, gray, or brown stain). Iron preparation (black stain) is an example of extrinsic stain. Extrinsic stains can be polished off; intrinsic stains cannot. See Table 23-8, Abnormalities of the Teeth, Pharynx and Neck, p. 831.

● Tooth Types and Age of Eruption[26]

Tooth Type	Approximate Age of Eruption	
	Primary (months)	Permanent (years)
Central incisor	5–8	6–8
Lateral incisor	5–11	7–9
Cuspids	24–30	11–12
First bicuspids	—	10–12
Second bicuspids	—	10–12
First molars	16–20	6–7
Second molars	24–30	11–13
Third molars	—	17–23

Look for abnormalities of the position of the teeth. These include malocclusion, maxillary protrusion (*overbite*), and mandibular protrusion (*underbite*). You can demonstrate the latter two by asking the child to bite down hard while either you or the child parts the lips. Observe the true bite. In normal children, the lower teeth are contained within the arch formed by the upper teeth.

Malocclusion and misalignment of teeth are often from excessive thumb sucking and are reversible if the habit is arrested by 6 or 7 years. Malocclusion can also be a hereditary condition or from premature loss of primary teeth.

Carefully inspect the *tongue*, including the underside. Most children will happily stick their tongue out at you, move it from side to side, and demonstrate its color (the blue tongue below is from eating candy!).

Common abnormalities include *coated tongue* in viral infections, *congenital geographic tongue,* and *strawberry tongue,* found in scarlet fever.

Some young children have a tight frenulum. Children who are severely "tongue-tied" might have a speech impediment. Have the child touch the tongue to the roof of the mouth to diagnose this condition, which is easily treated.

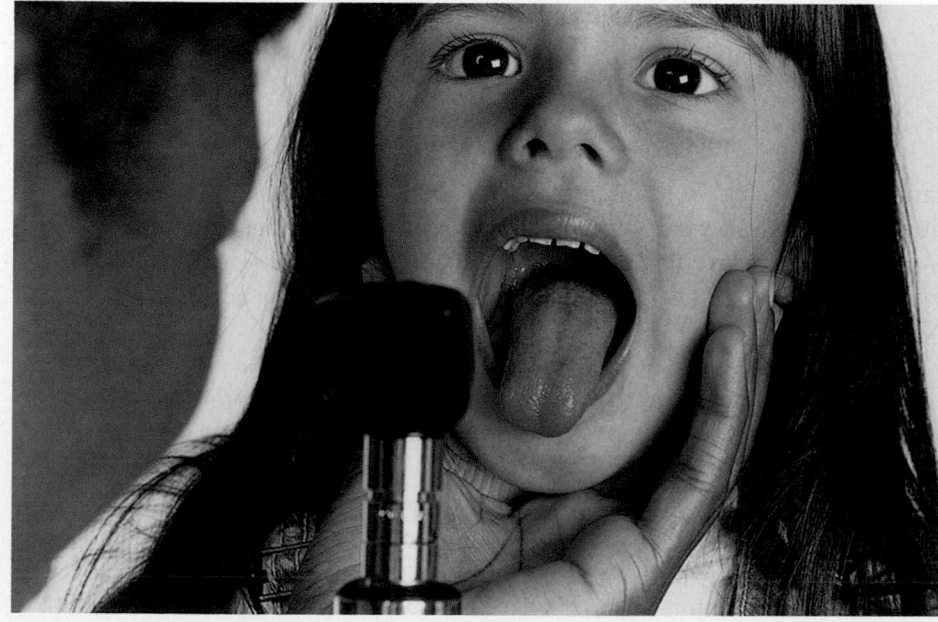

Note the size, position, symmetry, and appearance of the *tonsils*. The peak growth of tonsillar tissue is between 8 and 16 years (see figure in Table 23-8, p. 831). The size of the tonsils varies considerably in children and is often categorized on a scale of 1+ to 4+, with 1+ being easy visibility of the gap between the tonsils, and 4+ being tonsils that touch in the midline with the mouth wide open. The tonsils in children often appear more obstructive than they really are.

Streptococcal pharyngitis typically produces a strawberry tongue, white or yellow exudates on the tonsils or posterior pharynx, a beefy-red uvula, and palatal petechiae. See Table 23-8, Abnormalities of the Teeth, Pharynx and Neck, p. 831. Together with these signs, the most helpful historical information is exposure to strep throat infection within 2 weeks.[27]

Tonsils in children usually have deep crypts on their surfaces, which often have white concretions or food particles protruding from their depths. This does not indicate disease.

A *peritonsillar abscess* is suggested by asymmetric enlargement of the tonsils and lateral displacement of the uvula.

Look for clues of a submucosal cleft palate, such as notching of the posterior margin of the hard palate or a bifid *uvula*. Because the mucosa is intact, the underlying defect is easily missed.

Rarely, you may encounter a child who has a sore throat and has difficulty swallowing saliva, who is sitting up stiffly in a "tripod" position because of throat obstruction. Do not open this child's mouth because he or she may have acute epiglottitis.

Acute epiglottitis is now rare in the United States because of immunization against *Haemophilus influenzae* type B. This is a contraindication to examination of the throat because of potential gagging and laryngeal obstruction.

You may note an abnormal breath odor, which may help lead to a specific diagnosis.

Halitosis in a child can be caused by upper respiratory, pharyngeal, or mouth infection; foreign body in the nose; dental disease; and gastroesophageal reflux.

The Neck

Beyond infancy, the techniques for examining the neck are the same as for adults. Lymphadenopathy is unusual during infancy but very common during childhood. The child's lymphatic system reaches its zenith of growth at 12 years, and cervical or tonsillar lymph nodes reach their peak size between 8 and 16 years.

Lymphadenopathy is usually from viral or bacterial infections. See Table 23-8, Abnormalities of the Teeth, Pharynx and Neck, p. 831.

The vast majority of enlarged lymph nodes in children are due to infections (mostly viral but also bacterial) and not to malignant disease, even though the latter is a concern for many parents. It is important to differentiate normal lymph nodes from abnormal ones or from congenital cysts of the neck.

The figure on p. 756 demonstrates the typical anatomic locations of lymph nodes.

Malignancy is more likely if the node is greater than 2 cm, is hard, is fixed to the skin or underlying tissues (i.e., not mobile), or is accompanied by serious systemic signs such as weight loss, and, in the case of cervical lymph nodes, if the chest x-ray findings are abnormal.

Check for *neck mobility*. It is important to ensure that the neck of all children is supple and easily mobile in all directions. This is particularly important when the patient is holding the head in an asymmetric manner, and when central nervous system disease such as meningitis is suspected.

In young children with small necks, it may be difficult to differentiate low posterior cervical lymph nodes from *supraclavicular lymph nodes* (which are always abnormal and raise suspicion for malignancy).

In children, the presence of nuchal rigidity is a more reliable indicator of meningeal irritation than the *Brudzinski sign* or *Kernig sign*. To detect nuchal rigidity in older children, ask the child to sit with legs extended on the examining table. Normally, children should be able to sit upright and touch their chins to their chests. Younger children can be persuaded to flex their necks by having them follow a small toy or light beam. You also can test for nuchal rigidity with the child lying on the examining table, as shown. Nearly all children with nuchal rigidity will be extremely sick, irritable, and difficult to examine.

Nuchal rigidity is marked resistance to movement of the head in any direction. It suggests meningeal irritation due to *meningitis, bleeding, tumor,* or *other causes.* These children are extremely irritable and difficult to console and may have "paradoxical irritability"—increased irritability when being held.

When meningeal irritation is present, the child assumes the *tripod position* and is unable to assume a full upright position to perform the chin-to-chest maneuver.

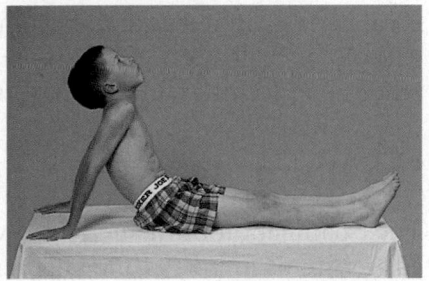

The Thorax and Lungs

As children age, lung examination becomes similar to that for adults. Cooperation is critical. Auscultation usually is easiest when a child barely notices (as when in a parent's lap). Let a toddler who seems fearful of the stethoscope play with it before touching the child's chest.

With upper airway obstruction such as croup, inspiration is prolonged and accompanied by other signs such as stridor, cough, or rhonchi. With lower airway obstruction such as asthma, expiration is prolonged and often accompanied by wheezing.

Assess the relative proportion of time spent on inspiration versus expiration. The normal ratio is about 1:1. Prolonged inspirations or expirations are a clue to disease location. Degree of prolongation and effort, or "work of breathing," are related to disease severity.

Young children asked to "take deep breaths" often hold their breath, further complicating auscultation. It is easier to let preschoolers breathe normally. Demonstrate to older children how to take nice, quiet, deep breaths. Make it a game. To accomplish a forced expiratory maneuver, ask the child to blow out candles on an imaginary birthday cake.

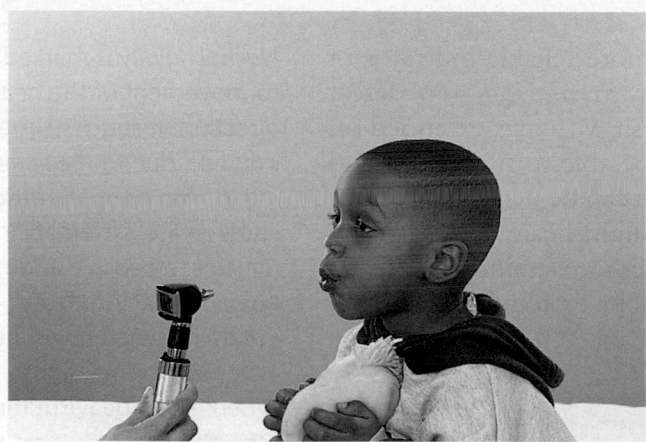

Older children will be cooperative for the respiratory examination and can even go through the maneuvers of assessing fremitus or listening to "E to A" changes (see p. 315). As children grow, the evaluation by observation discussed on the previous page, such as assessing the work of breathing, nasal flaring, and grunting, becomes less helpful in assessing for respiratory pathology. Palpation, percussion, and auscultation achieve greater importance in a careful examination of the thorax and lungs.

Pneumonia in young children generally is manifested by fever, tachypnea, dyspnea, and increased work of breathing.

While *upper respiratory infections* due to viruses can cause young infants to appear quite ill, upper respiratory infections in children present with the same signs as in adults, and children can appear well, without lower respiratory signs.

Childhood asthma is an extremely common condition throughout the world. Children with acute asthma present with varying severity and often have increased work of breathing. Expiratory wheezing and a prolonged expiratory phase, caused by reversible bronchospasm, can be heard without the stethoscope and are apparent on auscultation. Wheezes are often accompanied by inspiratory rhonchi caused by viruses that triggered the asthma.[28]

The Heart

The examination of the heart and vascular systems in infants and children is similar to that in adults, but recognition of their fear, their inability to cooperate, and in many instances, their desire to play will make the examination easier and more productive. Use your knowledge of the developmental stage of each child. A 2-year-old may be easiest to examine while standing or sitting on the mother's lap, facing her shoulder, or being held, as shown. Give young children something to hold in each hand. They cannot figure out how to drop the object and therefore have no hand free to push you away. Endless chatter to small children will hold their attention and they will forget you are examining them. Let children move the stethoscope themselves, going back to listen properly. Use your imagination to make the examination work!

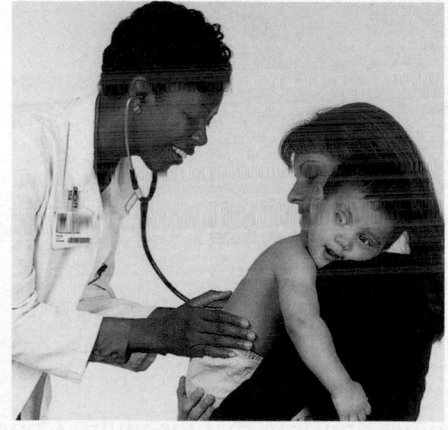

Benign Murmurs. Preschool and school-aged children often have benign murmurs (see figure on next page). The most common (*Still murmur*) is a grade I–II/VI, musical, vibratory, early and midsystolic murmur with multiple overtones, located over the mid- or lower left sternal border, but also frequently heard over the carotid arteries. Carotid artery compression will usually cause the precordial murmur to disappear. This murmur may be extremely variable and may be accentuated when cardiac output is increased, as occurs with fever or exercise.

Also in preschool or school-age children, you may detect a *venous hum*. This is a soft, hollow, continuous sound, louder in diastole, heard just below the right clavicle. It can be completely eliminated by maneuvers that affect venous return, such as lying supine, changing head position, or jugular venous compression. It has the same quality as breath sounds and therefore is frequently overlooked.

Among young children, murmurs without the recognizable features of the two common benign sounds below may signify underlying heart disease and should be evaluated thoroughly by a pediatric cardiologist.

Pathologic murmurs that signify cardiac disease can first appear after infancy and during childhood. Examples include aortic stenosis and mitral valve disease. See Table 23-10, Congenital Heart Murmurs, pp. 833–834.

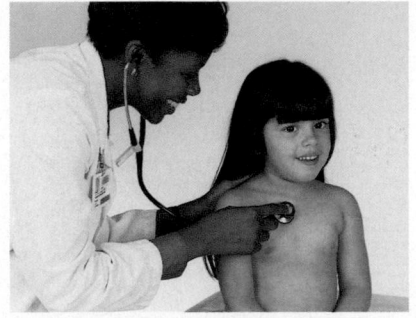
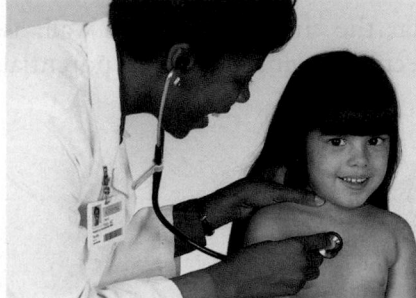

● Location and Characteristics of Benign Heart Murmurs in Children

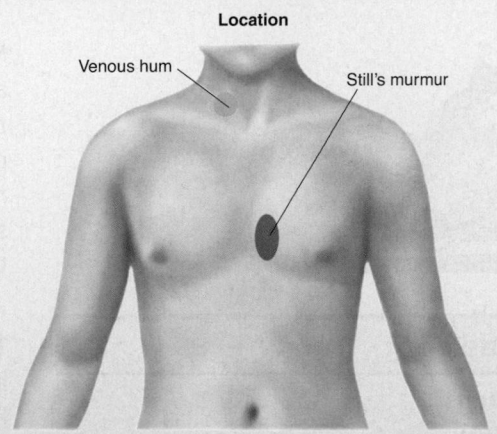

Location

Typical Age	Name	Characteristics	Description and Location
Preschool or early school age	*Still murmur*	I 〜 II	Grade I–II/VI, musical, vibratory Multiple overtones Early and midsystolic Mid-/lower left sternal border Frequently also a carotid bruit
Preschool or early school age	*Venous hum*	I 〜 II I	Soft, hollow, continuous Louder in diastole Under clavicle Can be eliminated by maneuvers

The Abdomen

Toddlers and young children commonly have protuberant abdomens, most apparent when they are upright. The examination can follow the same order as for adults, except the child may need to be distracted during the examination.

Most children are ticklish when a hand is first placed on their abdomens for *palpation*. This reaction tends to disappear, particularly if the child is distracted with conversation and the whole hand is placed flush on the abdominal surface for a few moments without probing. For children who are particularly sensitive and who tighten their abdominal muscles, start by placing the child's hand under yours. Eventually the child's hand can be removed and the abdomen freely palpated.

Also try flexing the knees and hips to relax the child's abdominal wall, as shown. Palpate lightly in all areas, then deeply, leaving the site of potential pathology to the end.

An exaggerated "pot-belly appearance" may indicate malabsorption from *celiac disease, cystic fibrosis,* or *constipation* or *aerophagia.*

A common condition of childhood that can occasionally cause a protuberant abdomen is constipation. The abdomen is often tympanic on percussion, and stool is often felt on palpation.

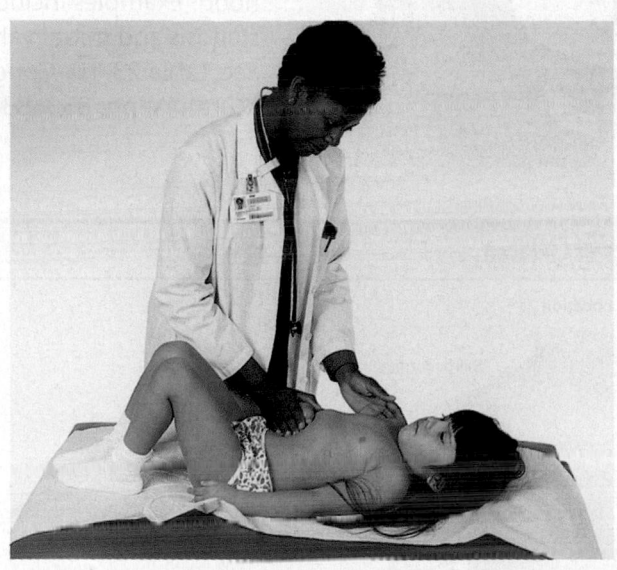

Many children present with abdominal pain from *acute gastroenteritis.* Despite pain, their physical examination is relatively normal except for increased bowel sounds on auscultation and mild tenderness on palpation.

The childhood obesity epidemic has resulted in many children who have extremely *obese abdomens.* While it is difficult to accurately examine these children, the steps to the examination are the same as for normal children.

⬤ Expected Liver Span of Children by Percussion

Age in Years	Mean Estimated Liver Span (cm)	
	Males	Females
2	3.5	3.6
3	4.0	4.0
4	4.4	4.3
5	4.8	4.5
6	5.1	4.8
8	5.6	5.1
10	6.1	5.4

One method to determine the lower border of the liver involves the *scratch test,* shown below. Place the diaphragm of your stethoscope just above the right costal margin at the midclavicular line. With your fingernail, lightly scratch the skin of the abdomen along the midclavicular line, moving from below the umbilicus toward the costal margin. When your scratching finger reaches the liver's edge, you will hear a change in the scratching sound as it passes through the liver to your stethoscope.[29]

Hepatomegaly in young children is unusual. It can be caused by cystic fibrosis, protein malabsorption, parasites, and tumors.

Various diseases can cause splenomegaly, including *infections, hematologic disorders* such as *hemolytic anemias, infiltrative disorders,* and *inflammatory* or *autoimmune diseases,* as well as congestion from *portal hypertension.*

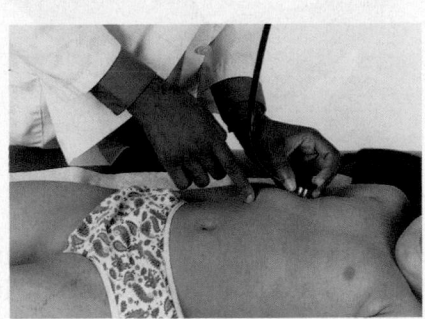

The *spleen,* like the liver, is felt easily in most children. It too is soft with a sharp edge, and it projects downward like a tongue from under the left costal margin. The spleen is moveable and rarely extends more than 1 cm to 2 cm below the costal margin.

Palpate the *other abdominal structures.* You will commonly note pulsations in the epigastrium caused by the aorta. This is felt most easily to the left of the midline, on deep palpation.

Palpating for abdominal tenderness in an older child is the same as for the adult; localization of tenderness may help you pinpoint the abdominal structures most likely to be causing the abdominal pain.

In a child with an acute abdomen, as in *acute appendicitis,* special techniques are helpful, such as checking for involuntary rigidity, rebound tenderness, a Rovsing sign, or a positive psoas or obturator sign (see p. 465).[30] *Gastroenteritis, constipation,* and *gastrointestinal obstruction* may be the causes.

Male Genitalia

Inspect the penis. The size in prepubertal children has little significance unless it is abnormally large. In obese boys, the fat pad over the symphysis pubis may obscure the penis.

In *precocious puberty,* the penis and testes are enlarged, with signs of pubertal changes. This is caused by a variety of conditions associated with excess androgens, including *adrenal or pituitary tumors.* Other pubertal changes also occur.

There is an art to *palpation* of the young boy's scrotum and testes because many have an extremely active cremasteric reflex that may cause the testis to retract upward into the inguinal canal and thereby appear to be undescended. Examine the child when he is relaxed because anxiety stimulates the cremasteric reflex. With warm hands, palpate the lower abdomen, working your way downward toward the scrotum along the inguinal canal. This will minimize retraction of the testes into the canal.

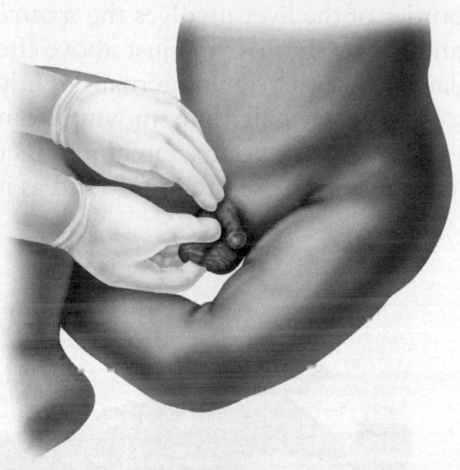

A useful technique is to have the boy sit cross-legged on the examining table, as shown here. You can also give him a balloon to inflate or an object to lift to increase intra-abdominal pressure. If you can detect the testis in the scrotum, it is descended even if it spends much time in the inguinal canal.

The cremasteric reflex can be tested by scratching the medial aspect of the thigh. The testis on the side being scratched will move upward.

Cryptorchidism may be noted at this age. It requires surgical correction. It should be differentiated from a retractible testis.

A painful testicle requires rapid treatment; common causes include Infection such as *epididymitis* or *orchitis, torsion of the testicle,* or *torsion of the appendix testis.*

Female Genitalia

The genital examination can be anxiety provoking for the older child and adolescent (especially if you are of the opposite sex), for parents, and for you; however, if not performed, a significant finding may be missed. Depending on the child's developmental stage, explain what parts of the body you will check, and that this is part of the routine examination.

After infancy, the labia majora and minora flatten out, and the hymenal membrane becomes thin, translucent, and vascular, with the edges easily identified.

The appearance of pubic hair before 7 years should be considered *precocious puberty* and required evaluation to determine the cause.

The genital examination is the same for all ages of children, from late infancy until adolescence. Use a calm, gentle approach, including a developmentally appropriate explanation as you do the examination. A bright light source is essential. Most children can be examined in the supine, frog-leg position.

Rashes on the external genitals can be from various causes such as physical irritation, sweating, and candidal or bacterial infections.

If the child seems reluctant, it may be helpful to have the parent sit on the examination table with the child; alternatively, the examination may be performed while the child sits in the parent's lap. Do not use stirrups, as these may frighten the child. The following diagram demonstrates a 5-year-old child sitting on her parent's lap with the parent holding her knees outstretched.

Examine the genitalia in an efficient and systematic manner. Inspect the external genitalia for pubic hair, the size of the clitoris, the color and size of the labia majora, and the presence of rashes, bruises, or other lesions.

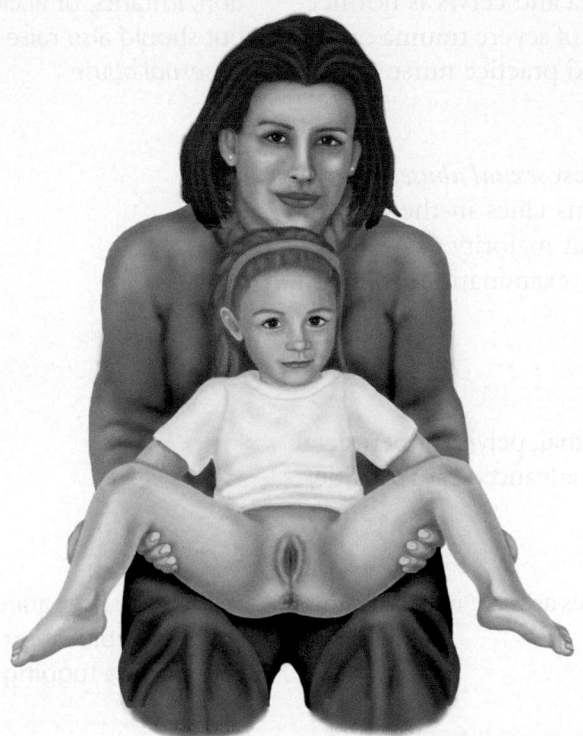

Next, visualize the structures by separating the labia with your fingers as shown below. *Labial adhesions*, or fusion of the labia minora, may be noted in prepubertal children and can obscure the vaginal and urethral orifices. They may be a normal variant.

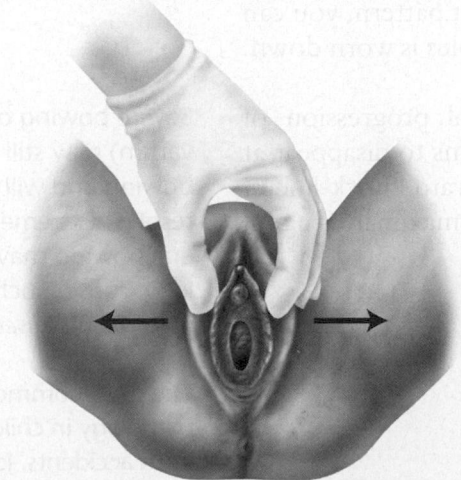

A *vaginal discharge* in early childhood can be from *perineal irritation* (e.g., bubble baths or soaps), *foreign body*, *vaginitis*, or a *sexually transmitted disease* from sexual abuse.

Vaginal bleeding is always concerning. Etiologies include *vaginal irritation*, *accidental trauma*, *sexual abuse*, *foreign body*, and *tumors*. *Precocious puberty* from many causes can induce menses in a young girl.

Purulent, profuse, malodorous, and blood-tinged discharge should be evaluated for the presence of *infiltration*, *foreign body*, or *trauma*.

Sexual abuse is unfortunately far too common throughout the world. Up to 25% of women report some history of sexual abuse; while many of these do not involve severe physical trauma, some do. See Table 23-11, Physical Signs of Sexual Abuse, p. 835.

Avoid touching the hymenal edges because the hymen is exquisitely tender without the protective effects of hormones. Examine for discharge, labial adhesions, lesions, and hygiene. A thin, white discharge (leukorrhea) is often present. A speculum examination of the vagina and cervix is not necessary in a prepubertal child unless there is suspicion of severe trauma or foreign body. An experienced gynecologist or advanced practice nurse should perform the speculum examination.

Abrasions or signs of trauma of the external genitalia can be from benign causes such as masturbation, irritants, or accidental trauma, but should also raise the possibility of *sexual abuse.*

The physical examination may reveal signs that suggest *sexual abuse,* and the exam is particularly important if there are suspicious clues in the history. Bear in mind that, even with known abuse, the great majority of examinations will be unremarkable; thus, a normal genital examination does not rule out sexual abuse.

The Rectal Examination

The rectal examination is not routine. If intra-abdominal, pelvic, or perirectal disease is suspected, the child should be referred to an advanced care provider.

The Musculoskeletal System

In older children, abnormalities of the upper extremities are rare in the absence of injury.

Toddlers may acquire *nursemaid's elbow* or subluxation of the radial head from a tugging injury.

The normal young child has increased lumbar concavity and decreased thoracic convexity compared with the adult, and often a protuberant abdomen.

Observe the child standing and walking barefoot. You can also ask the child to touch the toes, rise from sitting, run a short distance, and pick up objects. You will detect most abnormalities by watching carefully from both front and behind. To indirectly assess the child's gait pattern, you can also note the soles of the shoes to see which side of the soles is worn down.

During early infancy, there is a common and normal progression of increased bowlegged growth (see below left), which begins to disappear at about 18 months of age, often followed by transition toward knock-knees. The *knock-knee pattern* (as shown below right) is usually maximal by age 3 to 4 years and gradually corrects by age 9 or 10 years.

Severe bowing of the legs (genu varum) may still be physiologic bowing and will spontaneously resolve. Extreme bowing or unilateral bowing may be from pathologic causes such as *rickets* or *tibia vara (Blount disease).*

The most common lower extremity pathology in childhood is injury from accidents. Joint injuries, fractures, sprains, strains, and serious ligament injuries such as anterior cruciate ligament (ACL) tears of the knee are all too common in children.

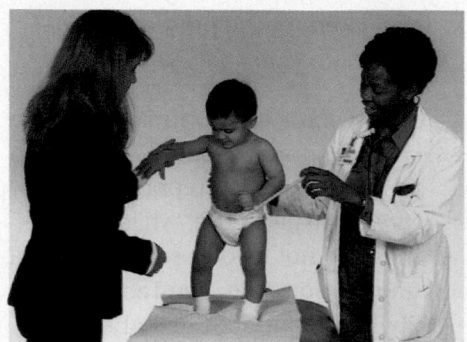
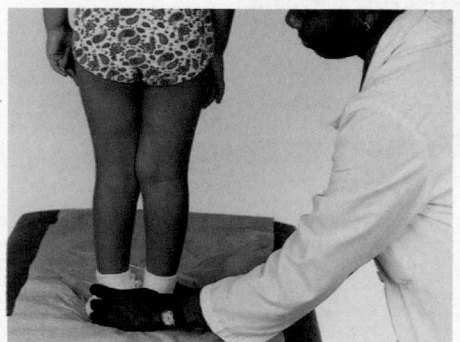

Children may *toe in* when they begin to walk. This may increase up to 4 years of age and then gradually disappear by about 10 years of age.

Inspect any child who can stand for *scoliosis,* using techniques described under "Adolescents."

Also, have the child stand straight and place your hands horizontally over the iliac crests from behind. Small discrepancies can be appreciated. If such a discrepancy is noted and you suspect leg length discrepancy, with one iliac crest higher than the other, a clever trick is to place a book under the shorter leg; this should eliminate the discrepancy.

Test for severe hip disease, with its associated weakness of the gluteus medius muscle. Observe from behind as the child shifts weight from one leg to the other. A pelvis that remains level when weight is borne on the unaffected side is a *negative Trendelenburg sign.*[31] With an abnormal positive sign in *severe hip disease,* the pelvis tilts toward the unaffected hip during weight bearing on the affected side (positive Trendelenburg sign).

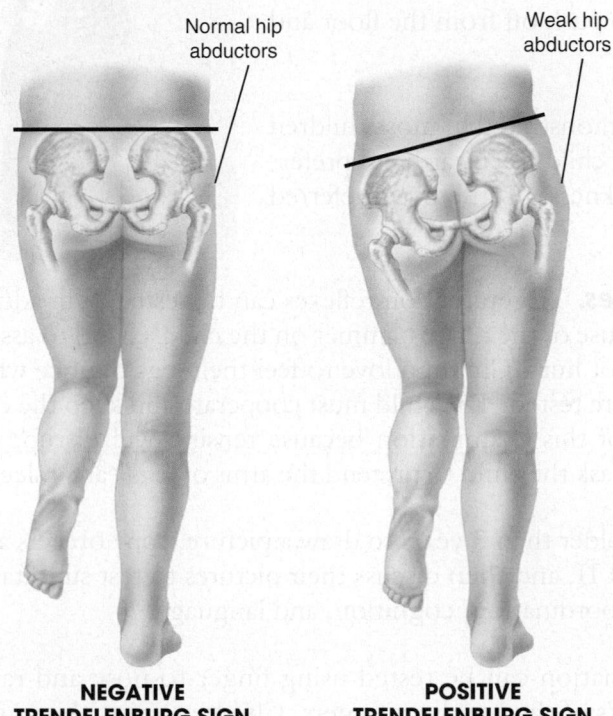

Normal hip abductors

Weak hip abductors

NEGATIVE TRENDELENBURG SIGN

POSITIVE TRENDELENBURG SIGN

The Nervous System

Beyond infancy, the neurologic examination includes the components evaluated in adults. Again, you should combine the neurologic and developmental assessment and will need to turn this into a game with the child to assess optimal development and neurologic performance.

Perform the DENVER II, up to 6 years, as shown on pp. 742–743. Children usually enjoy this component, and you can too. Remember that the DENVER II is better at detecting delays in motor skills than in language or cognitive milestones. Many practitioners now use other standardized developmental instruments.

Sensation. The sensory examination can be performed by using a cotton ball or cotton swab. This is best performed with the child's eyes closed. Do not use pin pricks, which may scare the child.

Children with *spastic diplegias* will often have hypotonia as infants and then excessive tone with spasticity, scissoring, and perhaps clenched fists as toddlers and young children.

Gait, Strength, and Coordination. Observe the child's gait while the child is walking and, optimally, running. Note any asymmetries, weakness, undue tripping, or clumsiness. You can follow the DENVER II examination milestones to test for appropriate maneuvers such as heel-to-toe walking (photo below), hopping, and jumping. Use a toy to test for coordination and strength of the upper extremities.

In children with uncoordinated gait, be sure to distinguish *orthopedic causes* such as positional deformities of the hip, knee, or foot from *neurologic abnormalities* such as *cerebral palsy, ataxia,* or *neuromuscular conditions.*

If you are concerned about the child's strength, have the child lie on the floor and then stand up, and closely observe the stages. Most normal children will first sit up, then flex the knees and extend the arms to the side to push off from the floor and stand up.

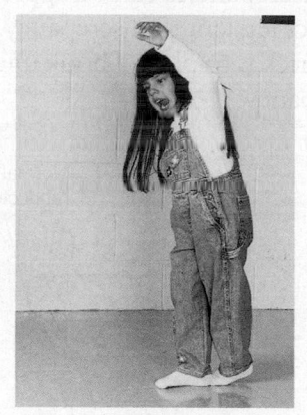

In certain forms of *muscular dystrophy* with weakness of the pelvic girdle muscles, children will rise to standing by rolling over prone and pushing off the floor with the arms while the legs remain extended (*Gower sign*).

Hand preference is demonstrated in most children by age 2. If a younger child has clear hand preference, check for weakness in the nonpreferred upper extremity.

Deep Tendon Reflexes. Deep tendon reflexes can be tested as in adults. First demonstrate the use of the reflex hammer on the child's hand to assure the child that it will not hurt. Children love to feel their legs bounce when their patellar reflexes are tested. The child must cooperate and keep the eyes closed during some of this examination because tensing will disrupt the results. One trick is to ask the child to pretend the arms or legs "are asleep."

Children with mild cerebral palsy may have both slightly increased tone and hyperreflexia.

You can ask children older than 3 years to draw a picture, copy objects as is done in the DENVER II, and then discuss their pictures to test simultaneously for fine motor coordination, cognition, and language.

The cerebellar examination can be tested using finger-to-nose and rapid alternating movements of the hands or fingers. Children enjoy this game. Children older than 5 years should be able to tell right from left, so you can assign them right–left discrimination tasks, as is done in the adult patient.

Distinguish between isolated delays in one aspect of development (e.g., coordination or language) and more generalized delays that occur in several components. The latter is more likely to reflect global neurologic disorders such as *cognitive disabilities* that can be caused by many etiologies.

Some children with *ADHD* will have great difficulty cooperating with your neurologic and developmental examination because of problems focusing. These children often have high energy levels, cannot stay still for extended periods, and have a history of difficulty in school or structured situations.

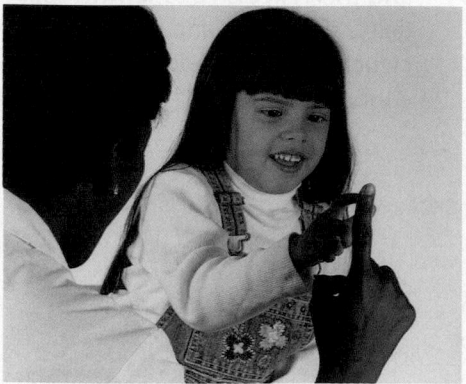

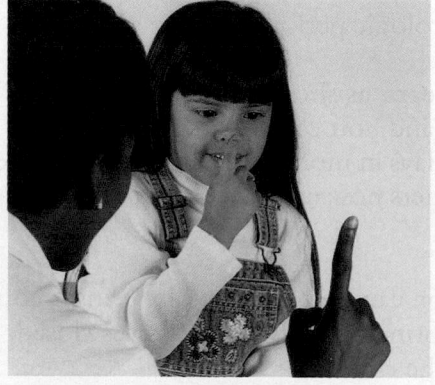

Cranial Nerves.   The cranial nerves can be assessed quite well using developmentally appropriate strategies, as shown in the following table:

● Strategies to Assess Cranial Nerves in Young Children		
Cranial Nerve		**Strategy**
I	Olfactory	Testable in older children.
II	Visual acuity	Use Snellen chart after age 3 years. Test visual fields as for an adult. A parent may need to hold the child's head.
III, IV, VI	Extraocular movements	Have the child track a light or an object (a toy is preferable). A parent may need to hold the child's head.
V	Motor	Play a game with a soft cotton ball to test sensation. Have the child clench the teeth and chew or swallow some food.
VII	Facial	Have the child "make faces" or imitate you as you make faces (including moving your eyebrows), and observe symmetry and facial movements.
VII	Acoustic	Perform auditory testing after age 4 years. Whisper a word or command behind the child's back and have the child repeat it.
IX, X	Swallow and gag	Have the child stick the "whole tongue out" or "say 'ah'." Observe movement of the uvula and soft palate. Test the gag reflex.
XI	Spinal accessory	Have the child push your hand away with his or her head. Have the child shrug his or her shoulders while you push down with your hands to "see how strong you are."
XII	Hypoglossal	Ask the child to "stick out your tongue all the way."

Localizing neurologic signs are rare in children but can be caused by trauma, brain tumor, intracranial bleed, or infection.

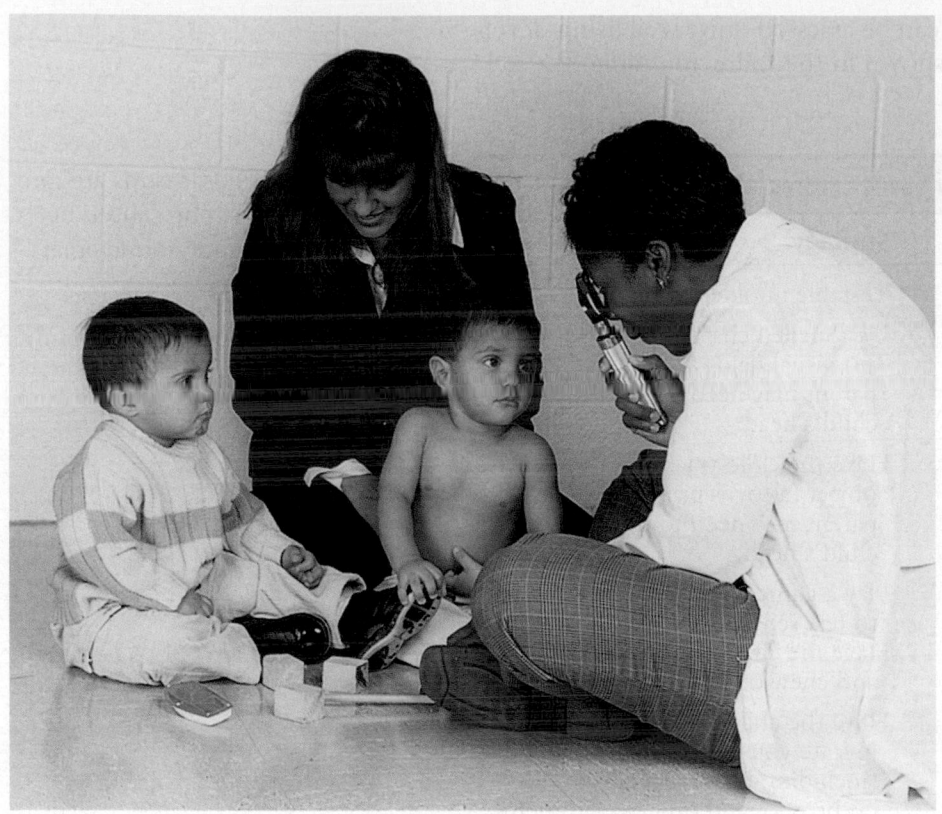

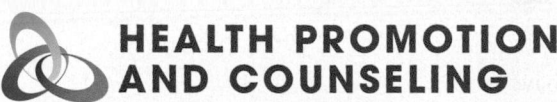

HEALTH PROMOTION AND COUNSELING
Children 1 to 4 Years

The AAP and Bright Futures periodicity schedules for children include health supervision visits at 12, 15, 18, and 24 months, followed by annual visits when the child is 3 and 4 years old.[2] An additional visit at 30 months is also recommended to assess the child's development.

During these health supervision visits, nurses address concerns and questions from parents, evaluate the child's growth and development, perform a comprehensive physical examination, and provide anticipatory guidance about healthy habits and behaviors, social competence of caregivers, family relationships, and community interactions.

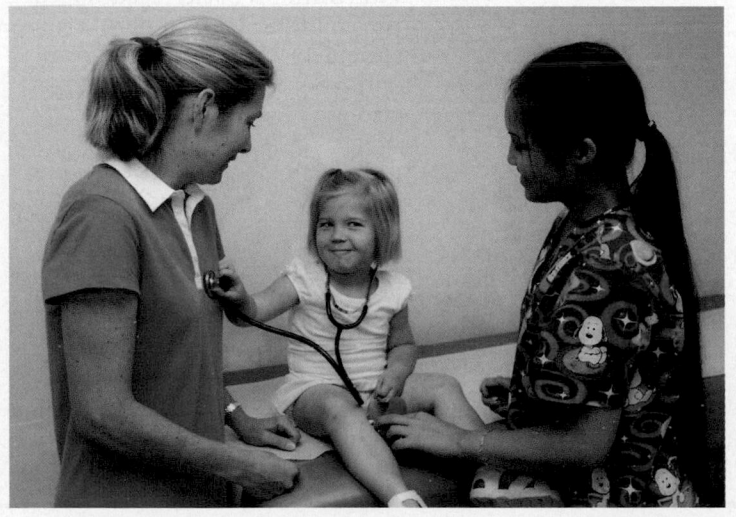

This is a critical age for preventing childhood obesity: many children begin their trajectory toward obesity between ages 3 and 4. It is also important to adequately assess the child's development. Standardized developmental screening instruments are increasingly being recommended to measure the different dimensions of a child's development. Similarly, it is important to differentiate normal (but potentially challenging) childhood behavior from abnormal behavioral or mental health problems.

The following box demonstrates the major components of a health supervision visit for a 3-year-old, stressing health promotion. You do not have to wait for a health supervision visit to address many of these health promotion issues—they can be addressed during other types of visits, even when the child is mildly ill.

COMPONENTS OF A HEALTH SUPERVISION VISIT FOR A 3-YEAR-OLD

Discussions With Parents
- Address parent concerns
- Provide advice
- Assess childcare, school, social environments
- Assess major topic areas: development, nutrition, safety, oral health, family relationships, community

Developmental Assessment
- Assess milestones may use (DENVER II): gross and fine motor, social–personal, language

Physical Examination
- Perform a careful examination, including growth parameters with percentiles for age.

Screening Tests
- Vision and hearing (formal testing at age 4), hematocrit and lead (if high risk or at ages 1–3), screen for social risk factors

Immunizations
- See schedule on the CDC website: http://www.cdc.gov/vaccines/recs/schedules/child-schedule.htm

Anticipatory Guidance
Healthy Habits and Behaviors
- Injury and illness prevention
  Car seat, poisons, tobacco exposure, supervision of activities
- Nutrition
  Obesity assessment; healthy meals and snacks
- Oral health
  Brushing teeth; dentist visits
Parent–Infant Interaction
- Reading and fun times, TV, computer usage
Family Relationships
- Activities, babysitters
Community Interaction
- Childcare, family resources

See Table 23-14, The Power of Prevention: Vaccine-Preventable Diseases, p. 837.

Children 5 to 10 Years

The AAP and Bright Futures periodicity schedules for children recommend annual health supervision visits during this period.[32] As for prior ages, these visits present wonderful opportunities to assess the child's physical, mental, and developmental health and the parent–child relationship. Once again, health promotion should be incorporated into all interactions with children and families—take advantage of any opportunity to promote optimal health and development!

One of the most satisfying components of health promotion for the older child involves talking directly with the child. In addition to discussing issues of health, safety, development, and anticipatory guidance with parents, you should be including the child in these conversations, using age-appropriate language and concepts. For example, the child's major environment beyond the family involves school. Discuss the child's experience and perceptions of school, as well as other cognitive and social activities. During these discussions, focus on healthy habits such as good nutrition, exercise, reading, stimulating activities, and safety.

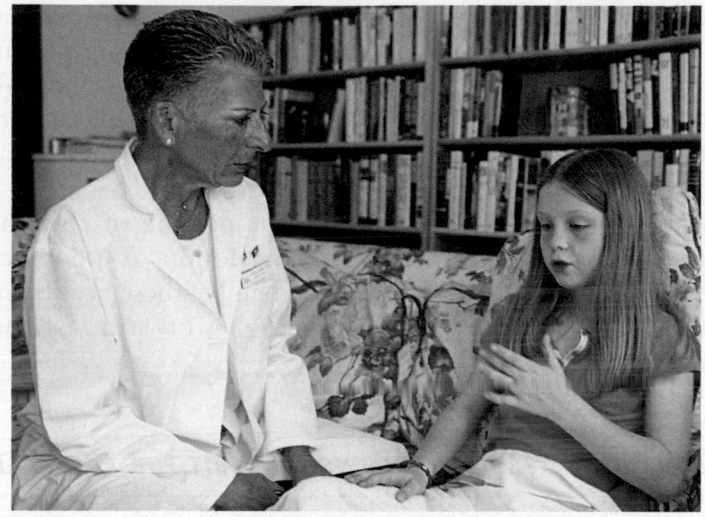

About 12% to 20% of children have some type of chronic physical, developmental, or mental condition.[33] Also, some behaviors that become established at this age can lead to or exacerbate chronic conditions such as obesity or eating disorders. Therefore, health promotion is critical to optimize healthy habits and minimize unhealthy ones. Further, helping families and children with chronic diseases deal most effectively with these disorders is a key part of health promotion. For all children, the well-being of the family is critical to the child's health; thus, health promotion involves assessing and promoting the family's overall health.

The specific components of the health supervision visit for older children are the same as the components for younger children, shown in the box on page 805. "Components of a Health Supervision Visit for a 3-Year-Old." Emphasize school performance and experiences, as well as appropriate and safe sports and activities.

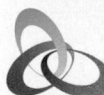 ## ASSESSING ADOLESCENTS

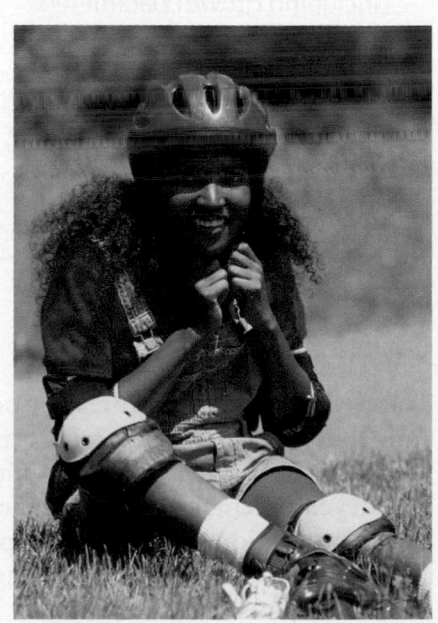

DEVELOPMENT: 11 TO 20 YEARS

Adolescence can be divided into three stages: early, middle, and late, as shown in the table on the next page. Your interview and examination techniques will vary widely depending on the adolescent's physical, cognitive, and social–emotional levels of development.

Physical Development. Adolescence is the period of transition from childhood to adulthood. The physical transformation generally occurs over a period of years, beginning at an average age of 10 in girls and 11 in boys.

On average, girls end pubertal development with a growth spurt by age 14 and boys by age 16. The age of onset and duration of puberty vary widely, although the stages follow the same sequence in all adolescents. Early adolescents are preoccupied with these physical changes.

Cognitive Development. Although less obvious, cognitive changes during adolescence are as dramatic as changes in physique. Most adolescents progress from concrete to formal operational thinking, acquiring an ability to reason logically and abstractly and to consider future implications of current actions. Although the interview and examination resemble those of adults, keep in mind the wide variability in cognitive development of adolescents and their often erratic and still limited ability to see beyond simple solutions. Moral thinking becomes sophisticated, with lots of time spent debating issues.

Social and Emotional Development. Adolescence is a tumultuous time, marked by the transition from family-dominated influences to increasing autonomy and peer influence. The struggle for identity, independence, and eventually intimacy leads to much stress, many health-related problems, and, often, high-risk behaviors. This struggle also provides you with an important opportunity for health promotion.

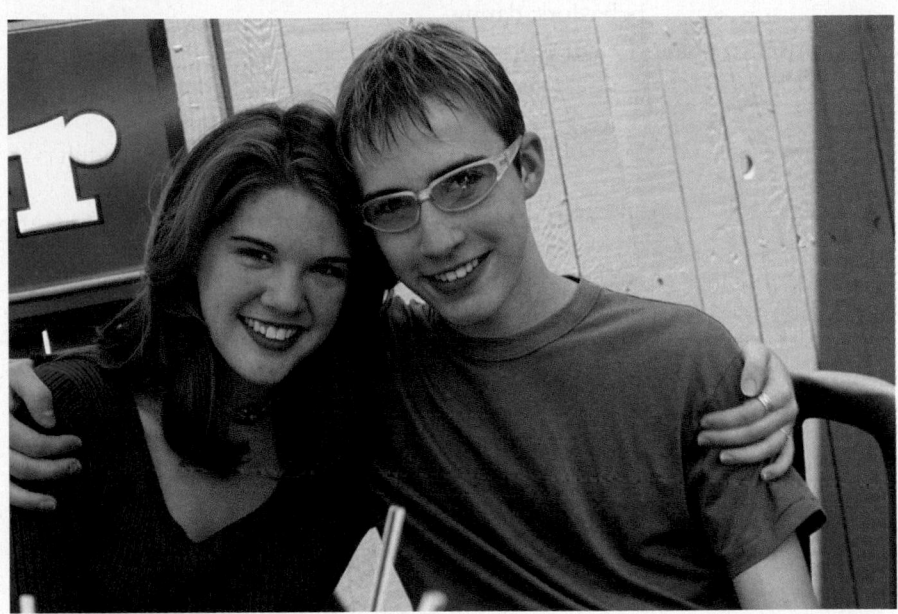

● Developmental Tasks of Adolescence		
Task	**Characteristic**	**Health Care Approaches**
Early Adolescence (10–14-year-olds)		
Physical	Puberty (F: 10–14; M: 11–16) variable	Confidentiality; privacy
Cognitive	"Concrete operational"	Emphasis on short term
Social	Am I normal? Peers increasingly important	Reassurance and positive attitude
Identity		
Independence	Ambivalence (family, self, peers)	Support for growing autonomy

(continued)

● Developmental Tasks of Adolescence (continued)

Task	Characteristic	Health Care Approaches
Middle Adolescence (15–16-year-olds)		
Physical	Females more comfortable, males awkward	Support if patient varies from "normal"
Cognitive	Transition; many ideas	Problem solving; decision making
Social		
Identity	Who am I? Much introspection; global issues	Nonjudgmental acceptance
Independence	Limit testing; "experimental" behaviors; dating	Consistency; limit setting
Late Adolescence (17–20-year-olds)		
Physical	Adult appearance	Minimal unless chronic illness
Cognitive	"Formal operational"	Approach as an adult
Social		
Identity	Role with respect to others; sexuality; future	Encouragement of identity to allow growth
Independence	Separation from family; toward real independence	Support, anticipatory guidance

THE HEALTH HISTORY

The key to successfully examining adolescents is a comfortable, confidential environment. This makes the examination more relaxed and informative. Consider the teen's cognitive and social development when deciding issues of privacy, parental involvement, and confidentiality.

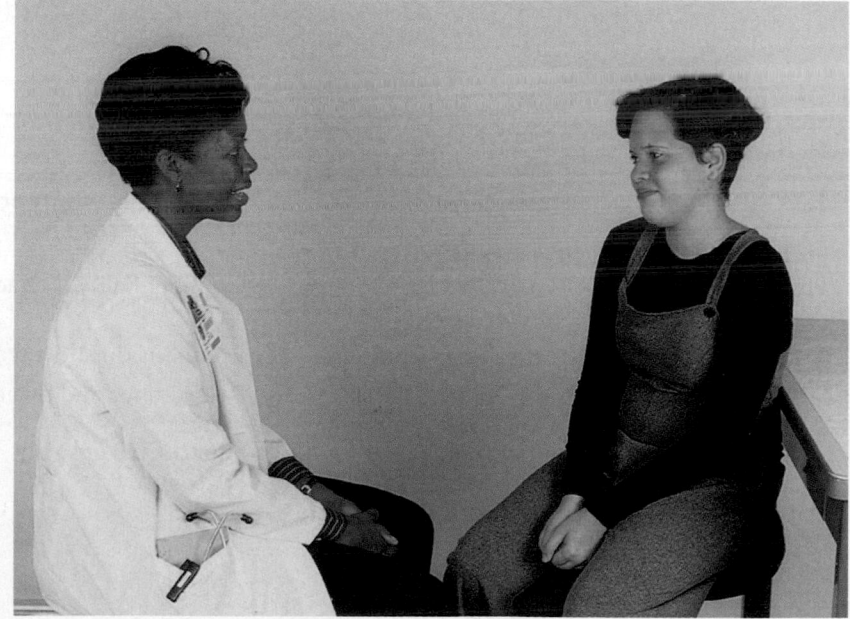

Like most people, adolescents usually respond positively to anyone demonstrating a genuine interest in them. Show such interest early and then sustain the connection for effective communication.

Adolescents are more likely to open up when the interview focuses on them rather than on their problems. In contrast to most other interviews, *start with specific questions* to build trust and rapport and get the conversation going. The nurse has to do more talking than usual, at the beginning. A good way to start is to chat informally about friends, school, hobbies, and family. Using silence in an attempt to get adolescents to talk or asking about feelings directly is usually not a good idea.

It is particularly important to use summarization and transitional statements and to explain what will happen during the physical examination. The physical examination can also be an opportunity to engage young persons. Once rapport is established, return to more open-ended questions. At that point, make sure to ask what concerns or questions the adolescent may have. Because adolescents are often reluctant to ask their most important questions (which are sometimes about sensitive topics), ask if the adolescent has anything else to discuss. A useful phrase to use is "tell me what other questions you have."

Remember also that adolescents' behavior is related to their developmental stage, and not necessarily to chronologic age or physical maturation. Their age and appearance may fool you into assuming that they are functioning on a more future-oriented and realistic level. This is particularly true regarding "early bloomers," who look older than their age. The reverse can also be true, especially in teens with delayed puberty or chronic illness.

Issues of *confidentiality* are important in adolescence. Explain to both parents and adolescents that the best health care allows adolescents some degree of independence and confidentiality. It helps if the nurse starts asking the parent to leave the room for part of the interview when the child is age 10 or 11 years. This prepares both parents and teens for future visits when the patient spends time alone with the nurse.

Before the parent leaves, obtain relevant medical history, such as certain elements of past history, and clarify the parent's agenda for the visit. Also discuss the need for confidentiality. Explain that the purpose of confidentiality is to improve health care, not to keep secrets. Adolescents need to know that you will hold in confidence what they discuss. However, never make confidentiality unlimited. Always state explicitly that you will act on information if concerned about safety: "I will not tell your parents what we talk about unless you give me permission or I am concerned about your safety—for example, if you were to talk to me about killing yourself and I thought that you really were at risk to follow through, I would need to discuss it with others in order to help you."

The goal is to help adolescents bring their concerns or questions to their parents. Encourage adolescents to discuss sensitive issues with their parents and offer to be present or help. Although young people may believe that their parents would "kill them if they only knew," you may be able to promote more open dialogue. This entails a careful assessment of the parents' perspective and the full and explicit consent of the young person.

As in middle childhood, modesty is important. The patient should remain dressed until the examination begins, and should have privacy while putting on a gown. Most adolescents older than 13 years prefer to be examined without a parent in the room, but this depends on the patient's developmental level, familiarity with the examiner, relationship with the parent, and cultural medical issues. For younger adolescents, ask the adolescent and parent their preferences.

The sequence and content of the physical examination of the adolescent are similar to those in the adult. Keep in mind, however, particular issues unique to adolescents, such as puberty, growth, development, family and peer relationships, sexuality, decision making, and high-risk behaviors.

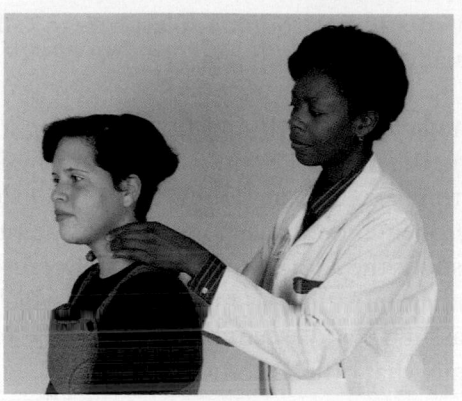

 ## PHYSICAL EXAMINATION OF THE ADOLESCENT

General Survey and Vital Signs

Somatic Growth. Adolescents should wear gowns to be weighed. This is particularly important for adolescent girls being evaluated for underweight problems. Ideally, serial weights (and heights) should use the same scales.

Both obesity and eating disorders among adolescent girls are major public health problems, requiring frequent assessments of weight.

Vital Signs. Ongoing evaluations of blood pressure are important for adolescents.[20] The average heart rate from age 10 to 14 years is 85 beats per minute, with a range of 55 to 115 beats per minute considered normal. Average heart rate for those 15 years and older is 60 to 100 beats per minute.

Causes of sustained hypertension for this age group include *primary hypertension, renal parenchymal disease,* and *drug use.*

The Skin

Examine the adolescent's skin carefully. Many teens will have concerns about various skin lesions, such as acne, dimples, blemishes, and moles.

Adolescent acne, a very common skin condition, tends to resolve eventually but often benefits from proper treatment. It tends to begin during middle to late puberty.

Many adolescents spend considerable time in the sun and at tanning salons. You may detect this during a comprehensive health history or by noticing signs of tanning during the physical examination. This is a good opportunity to counsel adolescents about the dangers of excessive ultraviolet exposure, the need for sunscreen, and the risks of tanning salons.

Moles or benign nevi may appear during adolescence. Their characteristics differentiate them from atypical nevi, discussed in the Integumentary System chapter.

Counsel adolescents to begin performing a regular self-examination of the skin, as shown on pp. 166–167.

Head, Ears, Eyes, Throat, and Neck

The examination of these body parts is the same as for adults.

Refractive errors become common and it is important to test visual acuity during the annual health supervision visit.

The Heart

The technique and sequence of examination are the same as those for adults. Murmurs are a continued cardiovascular issue for evaluation.

● **Location and Characteristics of Benign Heart Murmurs in Adolescents**

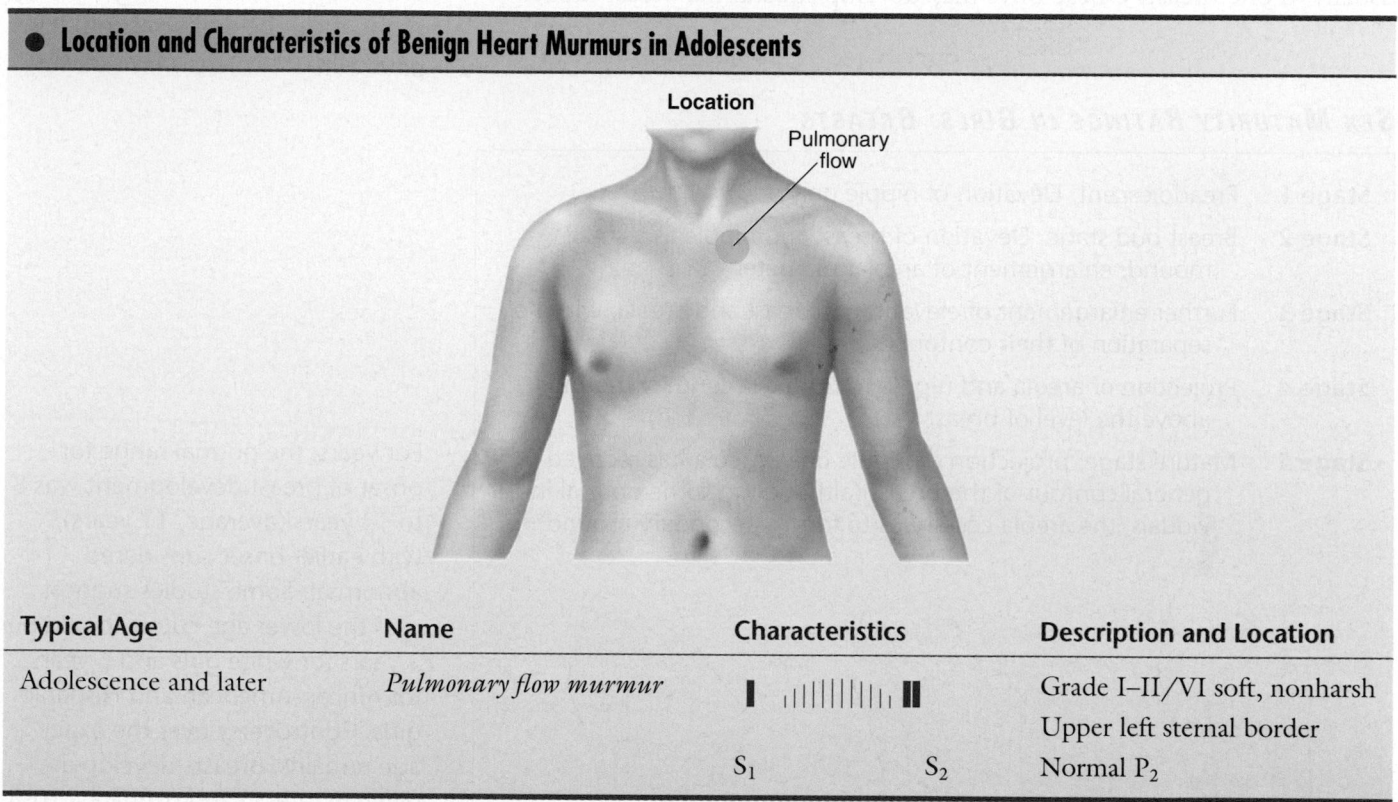

Location

Pulmonary flow

Typical Age	Name	Characteristics	Description and Location
Adolescence and later	*Pulmonary flow murmur*	S_1 S_2	Grade I–II/VI soft, nonharsh Upper left sternal border Normal P_2

The *benign pulmonary flow murmur* is a grade I–II/VI soft, nonharsh murmur, beginning after the first sound and ending before the second sound.

A pulmonary flow murmur accompanied by a fixed split-second heart sound suggests right-heart volume load such as an *atrial septal defect*. See Table 23-10, Congenital Heart Murmurs, pp. 833–834.

The Breasts

Physical changes in a young girl's breasts are one of the first signs of puberty. As in most developmental changes, there is a systematic progression. Generally, over a 4-year period, the breasts progress through five stages, called Tanner stages or Tanner sex maturity rating (SMR) stages, as shown on the next page. Breast buds in the preadolescent stage progress to subsequent enlargement and change in the contour of the

Masses or nodules in the breasts of adolescent girls should be examined carefully. They are usually *benign fibroadenomas* or *cysts;* less likely etiologies include *abscesses* or *lipomas*. Breast carcinoma is

breasts and areola. These stages are accompanied by the development of pubic hair and other secondary sexual characteristics, as shown on p. 816. Menarche usually occurs when a girl is in breast stage 3 or 4, and by then she has passed her peak growth spurt (see the figure on p. 817).

Older adolescent girls should undergo a comprehensive breast examination with instructions for self-examination (see pp. 505–506). A second person (parent or health care provider) should be present during the exam.

Breasts in boys consist of a small nipple and areola. During puberty about one third of boys develop a firm button of tissue 2 cm or more in diameter, usually in one breast. Obese boys may develop substantial breast tissue.

extremely rare in adolescence and nearly always occurs in families with a strong history of the disease.[34]

Many adolescent boys develop *gynecomastia* (enlarged breasts) on one or both sides. Although usually slight, it can be embarrassing. It generally resolves in a few years.

SEX MATURITY RATINGS IN GIRLS: BREASTS

Stage 1   Preadolescent. Elevation of nipple only

Stage 2   Breast bud stage. Elevation of breast and nipple as a small mound; enlargement of areolar diameter

Stage 3   Further enlargement of elevation of breast and areola, with no separation of their contours

Stage 4   Projection of areola and nipple to form a secondary mound above the level of breast

Stage 5   Mature stage; projection of nipple only. Areola has receded to general contour of the breast (although in some normal individuals, the areola continues to form a secondary mound).

For years, the normal range for onset of breast development was 8 to 13 years (average, 11 years), with earlier onset considered abnormal. Some studies suggest that the lower age cutoff should be 7 years for white girls and 6 years for African-American and Hispanic girls. Controversy over the exact age remains. Breasts develop at different rates in approximately 10% of girls, with resultant asymmetry of size or Tanner stage. Reassurance that this generally resolves is helpful to the patient.

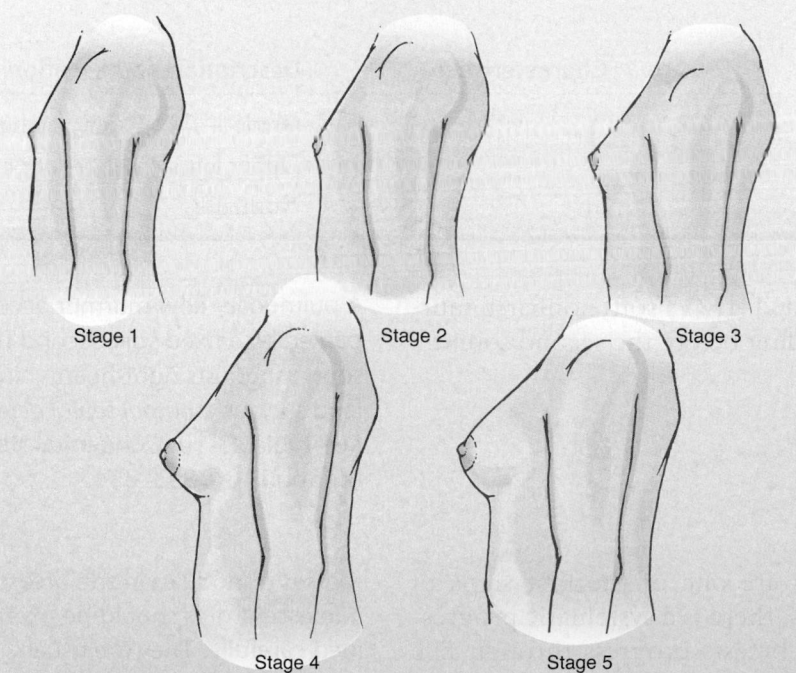

Stage 1   Stage 2   Stage 3

Stage 4   Stage 5

Tanner, J.M. (1962). Growth at adolescence (2nd ed.). Oxford: Blackwell Scientific Publications.

The Abdomen

Techniques of abdominal examination are the same as for adults. The size of the liver approaches the adult size as the teen progresses through puberty, and is related to the adolescent's overall height.

Hepatomegaly in teens may be from infections such as hepatitis or infectious mononucleosis, inflammatory bowel disease, or tumors.

Male Genitalia

The genital examination of the adolescent boy proceeds like the examination of the adult male. Be particularly aware of the embarrassment of many boys regarding this aspect of the examination.

Important anatomic changes in the male genitalia accompany puberty and help to define its progress. The first reliable sign of puberty, starting between ages 9 and 13.5 years, is an increase in the size of the testes. Next, pubic hair appears, along with progressive enlargement of the penis. The complete change from preadolescent to adult anatomy requires about 3 years, with a range of 1.8 to 5 years.

Delayed puberty is suspected in boys who have no signs of pubertal development by 14 years of age.

When examining the adolescent male, assign a sexual maturity rating. The five stages of sexual development, first described by Tanner, are outlined and illustrated below. These involve changes in the penis, testes, and scrotum. In addition, in about 80% of men, pubic hair spreads farther up the abdomen in a triangular pattern pointing toward the umbilicus; this phase is not completed until the 20s.

The most common cause of delayed puberty in males is constitutional delay, frequently a familial condition involving delayed bone and physical maturation but normal hormonal levels.

● **Sex Maturity Ratings in Boys**

In assigning SMRs in boys, observe each of the three characteristics separately because they may develop at different rates. Record two separate ratings: pubic hair and genital. If the penis and testes differ in their stages, average the two into a single figure for the genital rating.

	Pubic Hair	**Penis**	**Testes and Scrotum**
Stage 1 Stage 1	Preadolescent—no pubic hair except for the fine body hair (vellus hair) similar to that on the abdomen	Preadolescent—same size and proportions as in childhood	Preadolescent—same size and proportions as in childhood

(continued)

● Sex Maturity Ratings in Boys (continued)

	Pubic Hair	Penis	Testes and Scrotum
Stage 2 Stage 2	Sparse growth of long, slightly pigmented, downy hair, straight or only slightly curled, chiefly at the base of the penis	Slight or no enlargement	Testes larger; scrotum larger, somewhat reddened, and altered in texture
Stage 3 Stage 3	Darker, coarser, curlier hair spreading sparsely over the pubic symphysis	Larger, especially in length	Further enlarged
Stage 4 Stage 4	Coarse and curly hair, as in the adult; area covered greater than in stage 3 but not as great as in the adult and not yet including the thighs	Further enlarged in length and breadth, with development of the glans	Further enlarged; scrotal skin darkened
Stage 5 Stage 5	Hair adult in quantity and quality, spread to the medial surfaces of the thighs but not up over the abdomen	Adult in size and shape	Adult in size and shape

Tanner, J.M. (1962). Growth at adolescence (2nd ed.). Oxford: Blackwell Scientific Publications.

An important developmental principle is that physical pubertal changes progress along a well-established sequence (below). Although age ranges for start and completion are wide, the sequence for each boy is nevertheless the same. This is helpful in counseling an anxious adolescent regarding his current and future maturation, and regarding the normality of pubertal changes along a wide age range. It is also helpful for detecting abnormal physical changes.

Although nocturnal or daytime ejaculation tends to begin around sexual maturity rating 3, a finding on either history or physical examination of penile discharge may indicate a *sexually transmitted disease.*

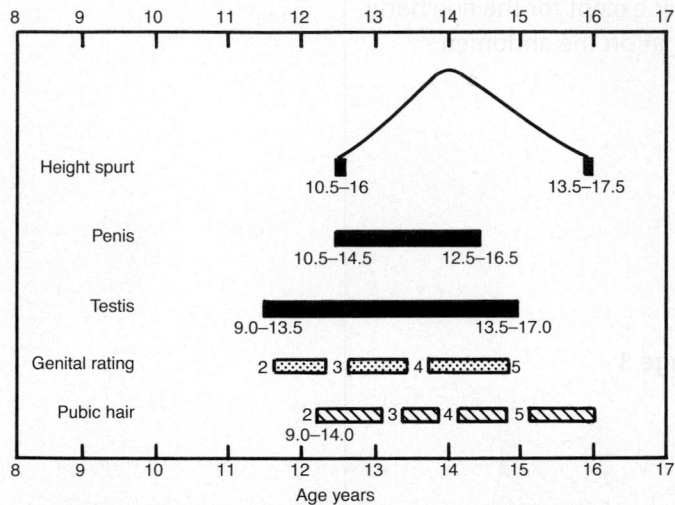

Numbers below the bars indicate the ranges in age within which certain changes occur. (Redrawn from Marshall WA, Tanner JM. Variations in the patterns of pubertal changes in boys. Arch Dis Child 45:22, 1970.)

Female Genitalia

The external examination of adolescent female genitalia proceeds in the same manner as for school-age children. An adolescent's first pelvic examination should be performed by an experienced health care provider. If it is necessary to complete a full pelvic examination on an adolescent, the actual technique is the same as that used for an adult, including the rectal examination. A full explanation of the steps of the examination, demonstration of the instruments, and a gentle, reassuring approach are necessary because the adolescent is usually quite anxious. A parent or another health care provider must be present.

Vaginal discharge in a young adolescent should be treated as in the adult. Causes include *physiologic leukorrhea, sexually transmitted diseases* from consensual sexual activity or *sexual abuse, bacterial vaginosis, foreign body,* and *external irritants.*

A girl's initial signs of puberty are hymenal changes secondary to estrogen, widening of the hips, and beginning of a height spurt, although these changes are difficult to detect. The first easily detectable sign of puberty is usually the appearance of breast buds, although pubic hair sometimes appears earlier. The average age of the appearance of pubic hair has decreased in recent years, and current consensus is that the appearance of pubic hair as early as 7 years can be normal, particularly in dark-skinned girls who develop secondary sexual characteristics at an earlier age.

Pubertal development prior to the normal age ranges may signify *precocious puberty,* which has a variety of endocrine and central nervous system causes.

Assign a sexual maturity rating to every female, irrespective of chronologic age. The assessment of sexual maturity in girls is based on both growth of pubic hair and the development of breasts. The assessment (Tanner staging) of pubic hair growth is shown in the figure below. See p. 812 for breast development assessment. Counsel girls about this sequence and their current stage.

SEX MATURITY RATINGS IN GIRLS: PUBIC HAIR

Stage 1

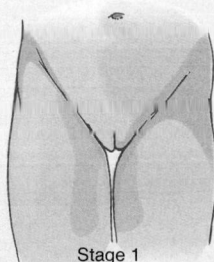

Stage 1

Preadolescent—no pubic hair except for the fine body hair (vellus hair) similar to that on the abdomen

Stage 2

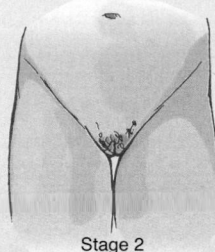

Stage 2

Sparse growth of long, slightly pigmented, downy hair, straight or only slightly curled, chiefly along the labia

Stage 3

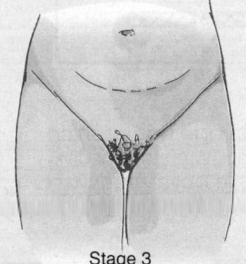

Stage 3

Darker, coarser, curlier hair, spreading sparsely over the pubic symphysis

Stage 4

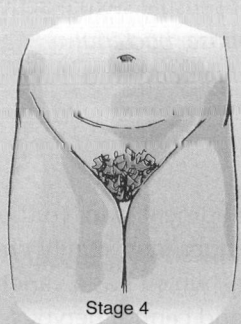

Stage 4

Coarse and curly hair as in adults; area covered greater than in stage 3 but not as great as in the adult and not yet including the thighs

Stage 5

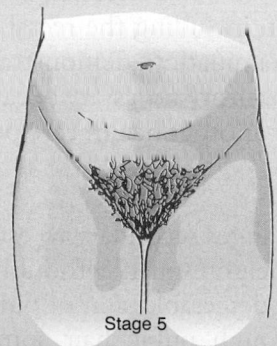

Stage 5

Hair adult in quantity and quality, spread on the medial surfaces of the thighs but not up over the abdomen

Tanner, J.M. (1962). Growth at adolescence (2nd ed.). Oxford: Blackwell Scientific Publications.

Although there is a wide variation in the age of onset and completion of puberty, remember that the stages occur in a predictable sequence, as shown next.

Delayed puberty in an adolescent female below the 3rd percentile in height may be from Turner syndrome or chronic disease. The two most common causes of delayed sexual development in an extremely thin adolescent girl are anorexia nervosa and chronic disease.

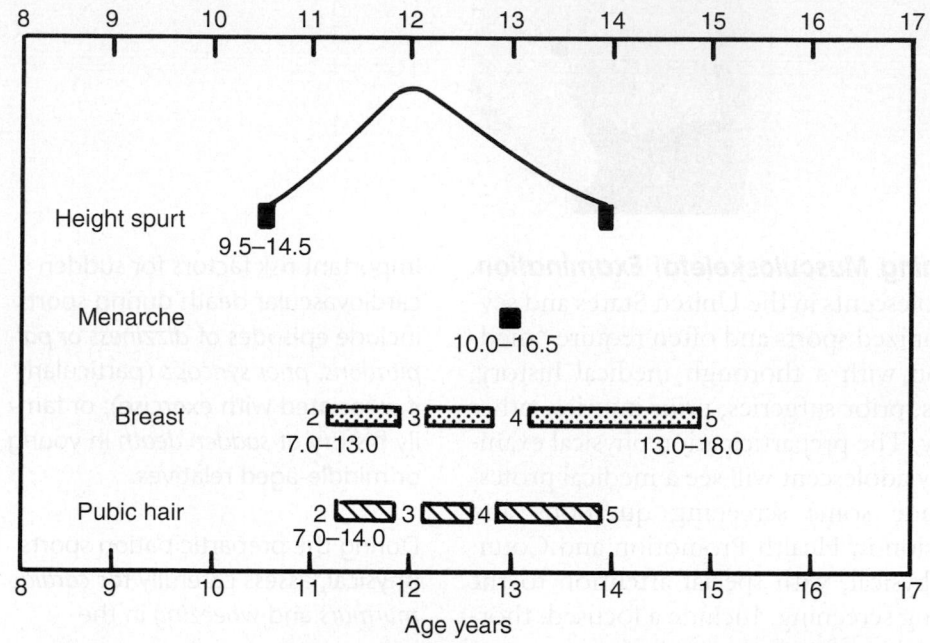

Numbers below the bars indicate the ranges in age within which certain changes occur.
(Redrawn from Marshall WA, Tanner JM. Variations in the pattern of pubertal changes in girls. Arch Dis Child 45:22, 1970.)

The Musculoskeletal System

Evaluations for scoliosis and screening for participation in sports remain common components of examination in adolescents. Other segments of the musculoskeletal examination are the same as for adults.

Assessing for Scoliosis. Make sure the child bends forward with the knees straight (Adams bend test). Evaluate any asymmetry in positioning or gait. Scoliosis in a young child is unusual and abnormal; mild scoliosis in an older child is not uncommon.

If scoliosis is detected, use a scoliometer to test for the degree of scoliosis. With the patient standing, look for asymmetry of the shoulder blades or gluteal folds. Have the teen bend forward as described. Look for prominence of the posterior ribs. Place the scoliometer over the spine at a point of maximum prominence, making sure that the spine is parallel to the floor at that point, as shown above. Have the teen bend fully forward to assess lumbar scoliosis, and less so to assess thoracic scoliosis.

Several types of *scoliosis* may present during childhood. Idiopathic scoliosis (75% of cases), seen mostly in girls, is usually detected in early adolescence.

A *plumb line,* a string with a weight attached, can also be used to assess symmetry of the back. Place the top of the plumb line at C-7 and have the child stand straight. The plumb line should extend to the gluteal crease (not shown here).

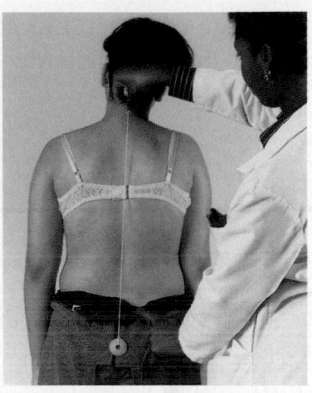

Apparent scoliosis, including an abnormal plumb line test, can be caused by a *leg-length discrepancy.*

The Sports Preparticipation Screening Musculoskeletal Examination.

More than 25 million children and adolescents in the United States and several other countries participate in organized sports and often require "medical clearance." Start the examination with a thorough medical history, focusing on cardiovascular risk factors, prior surgeries, prior injuries, other medical problems, and a family history. The preparticipation physical examination is often the only time a healthy adolescent will see a medical professional, so it is important to include some screening questions and anticipatory guidance (see the discussion in Health Promotion and Counseling). Finally, perform a general physical, with special attention to the heart and lungs and a vision and hearing screening. Include a focused, thorough musculoskeletal examination, looking for weakness, limited range of motion, and evidence of previous injury.

Important risk factors for sudden cardiovascular death during sports include episodes of *dizziness or palpitations, prior syncope* (particularly if associated with exercise), or family history of *sudden death* in young or middle-aged relatives.

During the preparticipation sports physical, assess carefully for *cardiac murmurs* and *wheezing* in the lungs.

The Nervous System

The neurologic examination of the adolescent and the adult is the same. Still, assess the adolescent's developmental achievement according to age-specific milestones, as described on pp. 806–808.

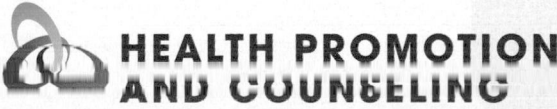

HEALTH PROMOTION AND COUNSELING

The AAP recommends annual health supervision visits for adolescents.[2] Because adolescents tend to be seen less frequently than do younger children for any health care visit, be sure to include health promotion during all health encounters with youth. In addition, adolescents with chronic problems or high-risk behaviors may require additional visits for health promotion and anticipatory guidance.

Most chronic diseases of adults have their antecedents in childhood or adolescence. For example, obesity, cardiovascular disease, addiction (to drugs, tobacco, or alcohol), and depression are all influenced by childhood and teen experiences and by behaviors established during adolescence. More specifically, most obese adults were obese as adolescents or had abnormal indicators such as elevated BMI scores. Almost all adults who are addicted to tobacco began their tobacco habits before 18 years. Therefore, a major component of health promotion for adolescents includes discussions about health behaviors or habits. Effective health promotion can help patients develop healthy habits and lifestyles and avoid several chronic health problems.

Because some health promotion topics involve confidential issues such as mental health, addiction, sexual behavior, and eating disorders, speak to adolescents (particularly older youth) privately during part of a visit that involves health supervision.

COMPONENTS OF A HEALTH SUPERVISION VISIT FOR ADOLESCENTS 11–18 YEARS

Discussions With Parents
- Address parent concerns
- Provide advice
- Discuss school, activities, social interactions
- Discuss youth's behaviors and habits, mental health

Discussions With Adolescent
- *Social and Emotional Development:* mental health, friends, family
- *Physical Development:* puberty, self-concept
- *Behaviors and Habits:* nutrition, exercise, TV, video games or computer screen time, drug/alcohol
- *Relationships and Sexuality:* dating, sexual activity, forced sex
- *Family Functioning:* relations with parents and siblings
- *School Performance:* activities, strengths

Physical Examination
- Perform a careful examination; note growth parameters, sexual maturity ratings

Screening Tests
- Vision and hearing, blood pressure; consider hematocrit; assess emotional health and risk factors

Immunizations
- See schedule on the CDC website: http://www.cdc.gov/vaccines/recs/schedules/child-schedule.htm

Anticipatory Guidance—Teen
Promote Healthy Habits and Behaviors:
- Injury and illness prevention
  Seat belts, drunk driving, helmets, sun, weapons
- Nutrition
  Healthy meals/snacks, obesity prevention
- Oral health: dentist, brushing and flossing

Sexuality:
- Confidentiality, sexual behaviors, safer sex, contraception if needed

Substance Abuse:
- Prevention strategies; treatment if appropriate
- Parent–teen interaction
- Communication, rules

Social Achievement:
- Activities, school, future

Community Interaction
- Resources, involvement

Anticipatory Guidance—Parent
Positive interactions, support, safety, limit setting, family values, modeling behaviors

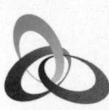

RECORDING YOUR FINDINGS

Note the modifications necessary to accommodate reports from the small child's parent, rather than from the child.

RECORDING THE EXAMINATION: THE PEDIATRIC PATIENT

3/11/11

Brian is an active, 26-month-old boy accompanied by his mother for concern about his development and behavior.

Referral. None.

Source and Reliability. Mother (Mom).

Chief Complaint. Slow development and difficult behavior.

Present Illness. Brian appears to be developing more slowly than his older sister did. He uses only single words and simple phrases, rarely combines words, and appears frustrated with not being able to communicate. People understand approximately 25% of his speech. Physical development seems appropriate for his age; he can throw a ball, kick, scribble, and dress himself well. He has had no head trauma, chronic illnesses, seizures, or regression in his milestones.

Mom also is concerned about his behavior. Brian is extremely stubborn, frequently has tantrums, gets angry easily (especially with his older sister), throws objects, bites, and physically strikes others when he doesn't get his way. His behavior seems worse around Mom, who reports that he is "fine" at his childcare center. He moves from one activity to another with an inability to sit still to read or play a game.

Brian is an extremely picky eater who eats a large quantity of junk food and little else. He will not eat fruits or vegetables and drinks enormous quantities of juice and soda. His mother has tried everything to get him to eat healthy food, to no avail.

The family has been under substantial stress during the past year from Brian's father being unemployed. Although Brian now has Medicaid insurance, the parents are uninsured.

Medications. One multivitamin daily.

Past History

Pregnancy. Uneventful. Mom reduced tobacco intake to a half-pack a day and drank a glass of wine once a month. She denies use of other drugs or having infections.

Newborn Period. Born vaginally at 40 weeks; left the hospital in 2 days. Birth weight 2.5 kg (5 lbs, 8 oz). Mom does not know why Brian was small at birth.

Illnesses. Only minor illnesses; no hospitalizations.

Accidents. Required sutures last year for a facial laceration secondary to a fall on the road.

(continued)

RECORDING THE EXAMINATION: THE PEDIATRIC PATIENT (continued)

Preventive Care.   Regular preventive check-ups. 6 months ago, his regular physician said that Brian was a bit behind on some developmental milestones and suggested a childcare center and increased parental attention to reading, speaking, playing, and stimulation. Immunizations up-to-date. Lead level was elevated mildly last year, and Mom reports he had "low blood." Physician recommended iron supplements and foods high in iron, but Brian won't eat these foods.

Family History

Strong family history of diabetes (two grandparents, none with diabetes as children) and hypertension. No family history of childhood developmental, psychiatric, or chronic illnesses.

Developmental History.   Sat up at 6 months, crawled at 9 months, and walked at 13 months. First words ("mama" and "car") said at approximately 1 year.

Personal and Social History.   Parents are married and live with the two children in a rented apartment. Dad has not had a steady job for 1 year but has worked intermittently in construction. Mom works as a waitress part-time while Brian is in childcare.

Mom had depression during Brian's first year and attended some counseling sessions, but stopped because she could not pay for them or medications. She gets support from her mother who lives 30 minutes away, and many friends, some of whom babysit occasionally.

Despite substantial family stress, Mom describes a loving and intact family. They try to eat dinner together daily, limit television, read to both children (although Brian won't sit still), and go to the nearby park regularly to play.
Environmental Exposures. Both parents smoke, although generally outside the house.
Safety.   Mom reports this as a major concern: she can barely leave Brian out of her sight without him getting into something. She fears he will run in front of a car; the family is thinking of fencing in their small yard. Brian sits in his car seat most of the time; smoke detectors work in the home. Guns are locked; medications are in a cabinet in the parents' bedroom.

Review of Systems
General.   Denies major illnesses.

Skin.   Dry and itchy. Last year hydrocortisone prescribed, which relieved the itching.

Head, Eyes, Ears, Nose, and Throat (HEENT).   *Head*: Denies trauma. *Eyes*: Vision fine. *Ears*: Multiple infections in the past year. Frequently ignores parents' requests; they can't tell if this is purposeful or if he can't hear well. *Nose*: Often runny; Mom wonders about allergies. *Mouth*: No dentist visit yet. Brushes teeth sometimes (a frequent source of dispute).

Neck.   Denies lumps but glands in neck seem "large."

(continued)

RECORDING THE EXAMINATION: THE PEDIATRIC PATIENT (continued)

Respiratory. Frequent cough and whistle in chest. Mom cannot identify trigger; it tends to go away. He can run around all day without seeming to get tired.

Cardiovascular. No known heart disease. Murmur when younger, but went away.

Gastrointestinal. Appetite and eating habits described above. Daily bowel movements. In the process of toilet training and wears pull-ups at night and underwear during day.

Urinary. Good stream. Denies prior urinary tract infections.

Genital. Appropriate for age.

Musculoskeletal. He is "all boy" and never gets tired. Minor bumps and bruises occasionally; denies fractures and pain.

Neurologic. Walks and runs well; seems coordinated for age. Denies stiffness, seizures, or fainting. Mom says his memory seems great, but his attention span is "poor."

Psychiatric. Generally seems happy. Cries easily; bounces back and forth from trying to be independent to needing cuddling and comforting.

Physical Examination

Active and energetic toddler. Plays with reflex hammer, pretending it is a truck. Appears closely bonded with his mother, looking at her occasionally for comfort. She seems concerned that Brian will break something. His face and clothes are clean.

Vital Signs. Ht 90 cm (90th percentile). Wt 16 kg (>95th percentile). BMI 19.8 (>95th percentile). Head circumference 50 cm (75th percentile). Blood pressure (BP) 108/58. Heart rate 90 and regular. Respiratory rate 30; varies with activity. Temperature (ear) 37.5°C. No obvious pain.

Skin. Olive, visible bruises on legs; patchy, dry skin over external surface of elbows; elastic, turgor <2 seconds.

HEENT *Head:* Normocephalic, no lesions. *Eyes:* Difficult to examine due to movement. Symmetric with equal extraocular movements bilaterally. Pupils 4 to 5 mm constricting. Discs difficult to visualize, no hemorrhages noted. *Ears:* Pinna, no external lesions. External canals and tympanic membranes (TMs) without exudate, cerumen, or foreign objects bilaterally. *Nose:* Nares equal; septum midline. *Mouth:* Several darkened teeth (inside surface of upper incisors). One clear cavity on upper right incisor. Tongue pink, midline, full range of motion. Cobblestoning of posterior pharynx; no exudates. Tonsils +3/4, pink.

Neck. Supple, midline trachea, thyroid not palpable.

Lymph Nodes. 0.5 cm tonsillar lymph nodes bilaterally. 0.5 cm inguinal nodes bilaterally. Palpable lymph nodes round, mobile, and nontender.

(continued)

RECORDING THE EXAMINATION: THE PEDIATRIC PATIENT (continued)

Lungs.   Equal expansion. No tachypnea or dyspnea. Congestion audible, but seems to be upper airway (louder near mouth, symmetric). No rhonchi, rales, or wheezes. Clear to auscultation.

Cardiovascular.   Apical impulse in 4th intercostal space medial to the MCL. Positive S_1 and S_2, regular rhythm. No murmurs or abnormal heart sounds. Femoral pulses and dorsalis pedis pulses 2+ bilaterally.

Breasts.   Minimal fat bilaterally.

Abdomen.   Protuberant, soft; no masses or tenderness. Liver span 2 cm below right costal margin (RCM) and not tender. Spleen and kidneys not palpable.

Genitalia.   Tanner I circumcised penis; no pubic hair, lesions, or discharge. Testes descended, difficult to palpate because of active cremasteric reflex. Scrotum equal bilaterally.

Musculoskeletal.   FROM of upper and lower extremities and all joints BL. Spine straight. Gait coordinated, wide-based.

Neurologic.   *Mental Status:* Happy, cooperative child. *Developmental (DENVER II):* Gross motor—Jumps and throws objects. Fine motor—Imitates vertical line. Language—Does not combine words; single words only, three to four noted during examination. Personal-social—Washes face, brushes teeth, and puts on shirt. Overall—At level, except for language, which appears delayed. *Cranial Nerves:* Intact, although several difficult to elicit. *Cerebellar:* Gait age appropriate with steady balance and opposite arm swing. *Deep tendon reflexes (DTRs):* 2+ and symmetric throughout with plantar response BL. *Sensory:* Deferred.

TABLE 23-1

Abnormalities in Heart Rhythm and Blood Pressure

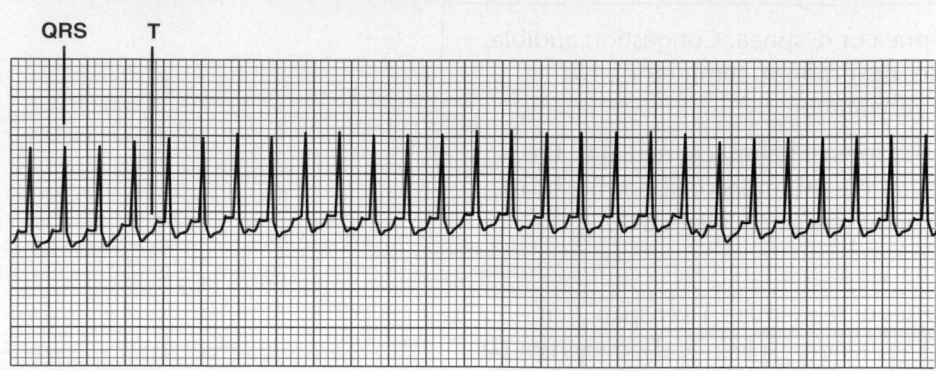

Supraventricular Tachycardia

Paroxysmal supraventricular tachycardia (SVT) is the most common dysrhythmia in children. Some infants with SVT look well or may be somewhat pale with tachypnea, but have a heart rate of 240 beats per minute or greater. Others are ill and in cardiovascular collapse.

SVT in infants is usually sustained, requiring medical therapy for conversion to a normal rate and rhythm. In older children, it is more likely to be truly paroxysmal, with episodes of varying duration and frequency.

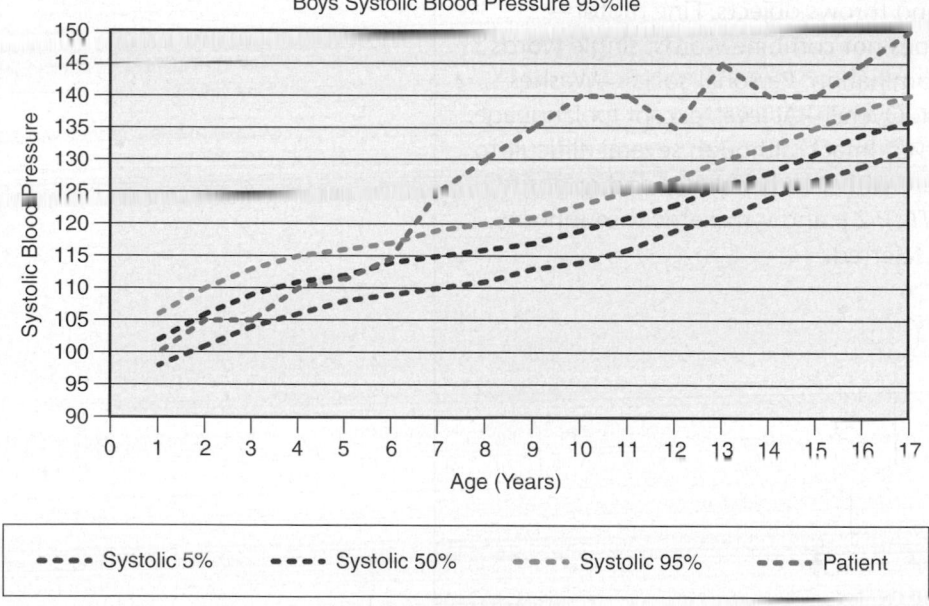

Hypertension in Childhood—A Typical Example[19]

Hypertension can start in childhood. While elevated blood pressure in young children is more likely to have a renal, cardiac, or endocrine cause, adolescents with hypertension are most likely to have primary or essential hypertension.

This child developed hypertension and it "tracked" into adulthood. Children tend to remain in the same percentile for blood pressure as they grow. This tracking of blood pressure continues into adulthood, supporting the concept that adult essential hypertension often begins during childhood.

The consequences of untreated hypertension can be severe.

TABLE
23-2

Common Skin Rashes and Skin Findings in Newborns and Infants

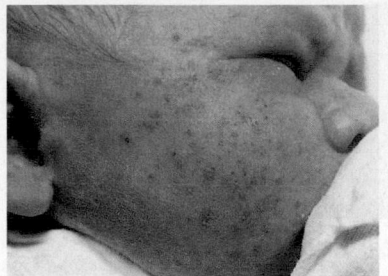

Erythema Toxicum
These common yellow or white pustules are surrounded by a red base.

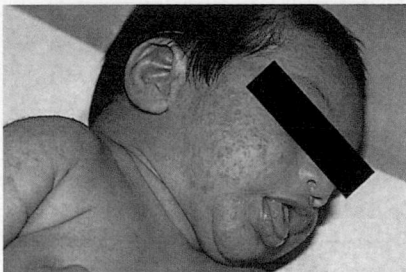

Neonatal Acne
Red pustules and papules are most prominent over the cheeks and nose of some normal newborns.

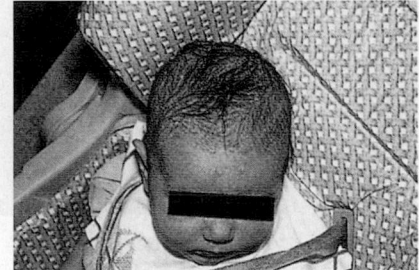

Seborrhea
The salmon red, scaly eruption often involves the face, neck, axilla, diaper area, and behind the ears.

Body and Extremities

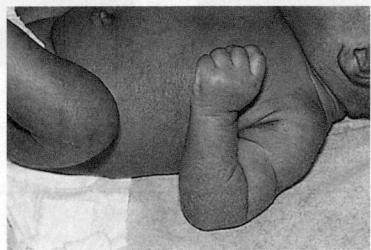
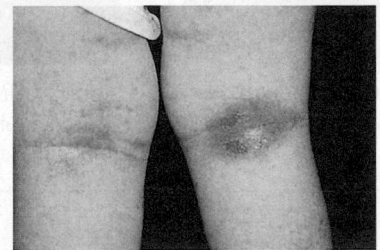

Atopic Dermatitis (Eczema)
Erythema, scaling, dry skin, and intense itching characterize this condition.

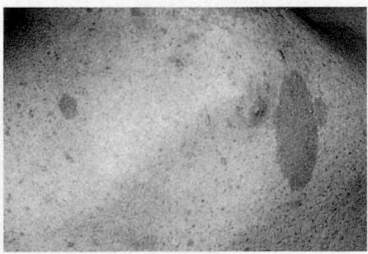

Neurofibromatosis
Characteristic features include more than 5 café-au-lait spots and axillary freckling, both shown above. Later findings include neurofibromas and Lish nodules (not shown).

Diaper Region

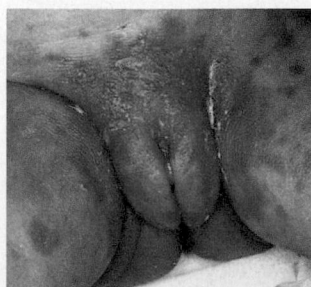

Candidal Diaper Dermatitis
This bright red rash involves the intertriginous folds, with small "satellite lesions" along the edges.

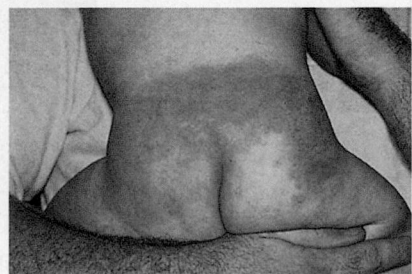

Contact Diaper Dermatitis
This irritant rash is secondary to diarrhea or irritation and is noted along contact areas (here, the area touching the diaper).

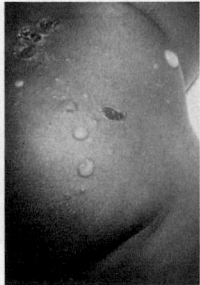

Impetigo
This infection is due to bacteria and can appear bullous or crusty and yellowed with some pus.

TABLE 23-3

Warts, Lesions That Resemble Warts, and Other Raised Lesions

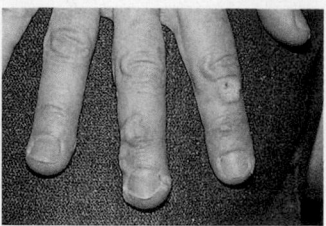

Verruca Vulqaris
Dry, rough warts on hands

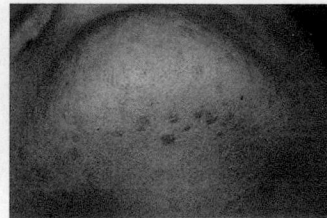

Verruca Plana
Small, flat warts

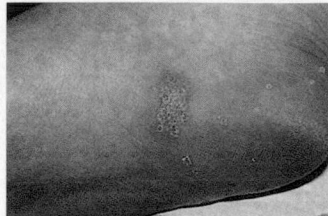

Plantar Warts
Tender warts on feet

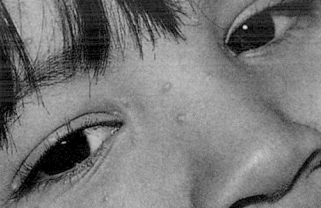

Molluscum Contagiosum
Dome-shaped, fleshy lesions

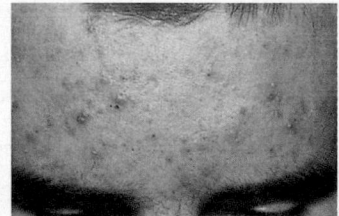
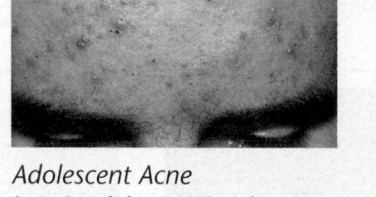

Adolescent Acne
Acne in adolescents involves open comedones (blackheads) and closed comedones (whiteheads) shown at the left, and inflamed pustules (right).

TABLE 23-4

Common Skin Lesions During Childhood

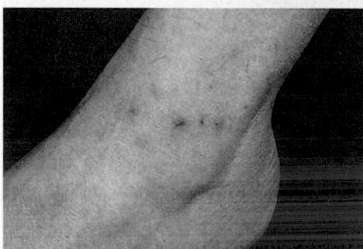

Insect Bites
Intensely pruritic, red, distinct papules characterize these lesions.

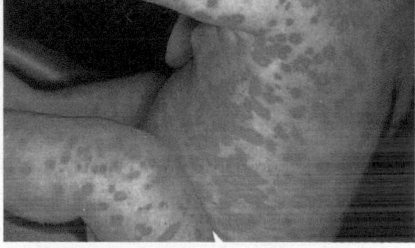

Urticaria (Hives)
This pruritic, allergic sensitivity reaction changes shape quickly.

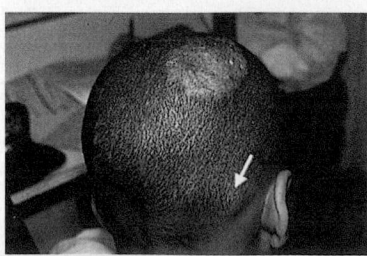

Tinea Capitis
Scaling, crusting, and hair loss are seen in the scalp, along with a painful plaque (kerion) and occipital lymph node (*arrow*).

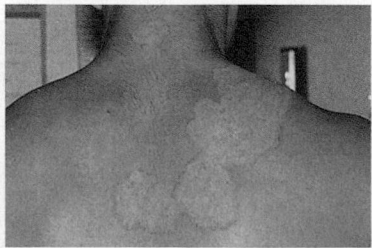

Tinea Corporis
This annular lesion has central clearing and papules along the border.

(Source of all photos except *Urticaria*—Goodheart H. A Photoguide of Common Skin Disorders. Baltimore: Williams & Wilkins, 1999.)

TABLE
23-5

Abnormalities of the Head

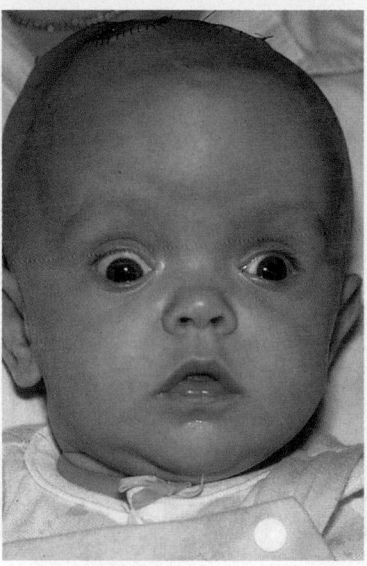

Hydrocephalus

In hydrocephaly, the anterior fontanelle is bulging, and the eyes may be deviated downward, revealing the upper scleras and creating the *setting sun* sign, as shown here. The setting sun sign is also seen briefly in some normal newborns. (From Zitelli BJ, Davis HW. Atlas of Pediatric Physical Diagnosis, 3rd ed. St. Louis, Mosby–Year Book, 1997. Courtesy of Dr. Albert Briglan, Children's Hospital of Pittsburgh.)

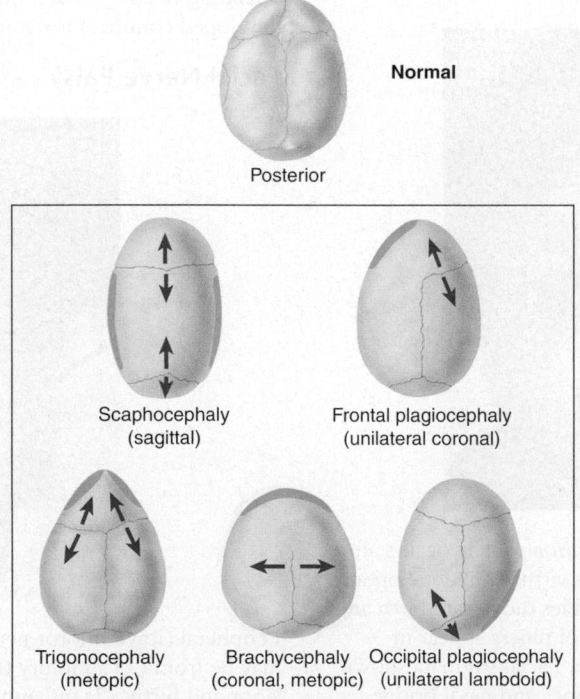

Craniosynostosis

Craniosynostosis is a condition of premature closure of one or more sutures of the skull. This results in an abnormal growth and shape of the skull because growth will occur across sutures that are not affected but not across sutures that are affected. The figures demonstrate different skull shapes associated with the various types of craniosynostosis. The prematurely closed suture line is noted by the absence of a suture line in each figure. Scaphocephaly and frontal plagiocephaly are most common. The *blue shading* shows areas of maximal flattening. The *red arrows* show the direction of continued growth across the sutures, which is normal.

Fetal Alcohol Syndrome

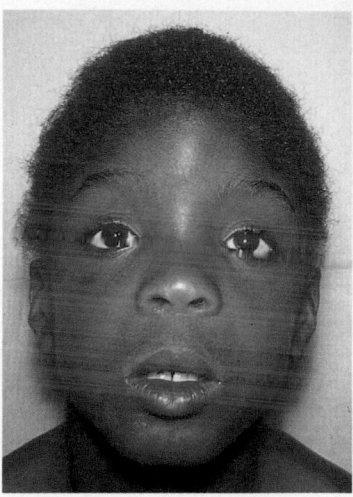

Babies born to women with chronic alcoholism are at increased risk for growth deficiency, microcephaly, and mental retardation. Facial characteristics include short palpebral fissures, a wide and flattened philtrum (the vertical groove in the midline of the upper lip), and thin lips.

Congenital Syphilis

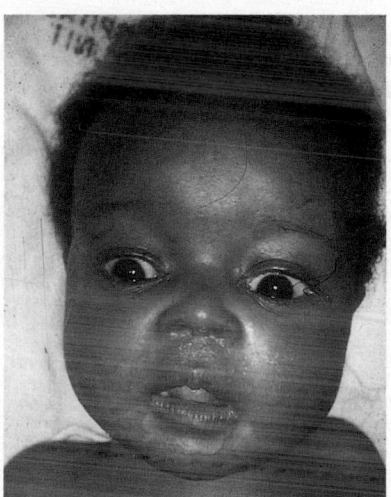

In utero infection by *Treponema pallidum* usually occurs after the 16th week of gestation and affects virtually all fetal organs. If it is not treated, 25% of infected babies die before birth and another 30% shortly thereafter. Signs of illness appear in survivors within the first month of life. Facial stigmata shown here include bulging of the frontal bones and nasal bridge depression (*saddle nose*), both from periostitis; rhinitis from weeping nasal mucosal lesions (*snuffles*); and a circumoral rash. Mucocutaneous inflammation and fissuring of the mouth and lips (*rhagades*), not shown here, may also occur as stigmata of congenital syphilis, as may craniotabes tibial periostitis (*saber shins*) and dental dysplasia (*Hutchinson's teeth*—see p. 288).

Congenital Hypothyroidism

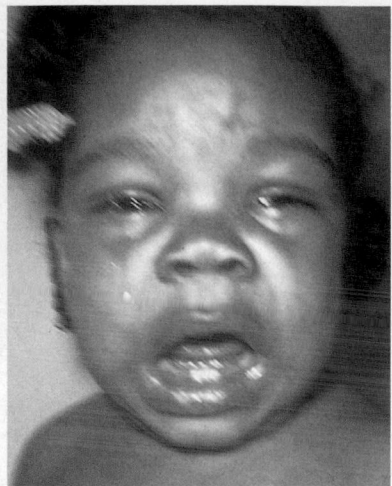

The child with congenital hypothyroidism (*cretinism*) has coarse facial features, a low-set hair line, sparse eyebrows, and an enlarged tongue. Associated features include a hoarse cry, umbilical hernia, dry and cold extremities, myxedema, mottled skin, and mental retardation. Most infants with congenital hypothyroidism have no physical stigmata; this has led to screening of all newborns in the United States and most other developed countries for congenital hypothyroidism.

Facial Nerve Palsy

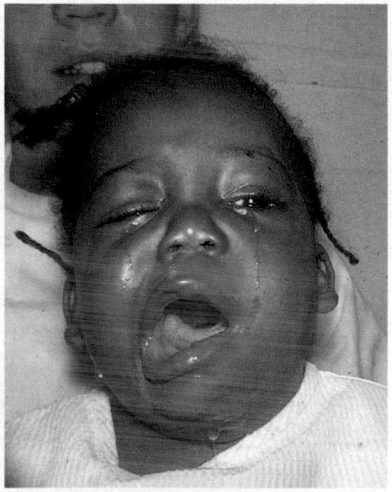

Peripheral (lower motor neuron) paralysis of the facial nerve may be from (1) an injury to the nerve from pressure during labor and birth, (2) inflammation of the middle ear branch of the nerve during episodes of acute or chronic otitis media, or (3) unknown causes (Bell's palsy). The nasolabial fold on the affected left side is flattened, and the eye does not close. This is accentuated during crying, as shown here. Full recovery occurs in ≥ 90% of those affected.

(table continues on page 829)

Down Syndrome

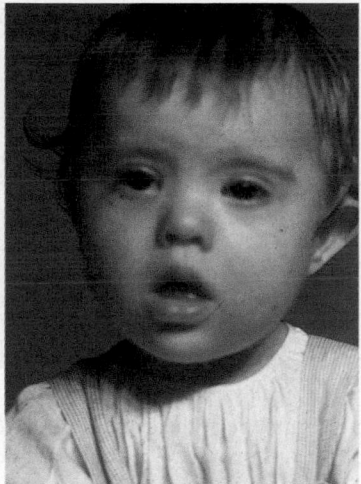

The child with Down syndrome (trisomy 21) usually has a small, rounded head, a flattened nasal bridge, oblique palpebral fissures, prominent epicanthal folds, small, low-set, shell-like ears, and a relatively large tongue. Associated features include generalized hypotonia, transverse palmar creases (*simian lines*), shortening and incurving of the 5th fingers (*clinodactyly*), Brushfield's spots (see p. 830), and mental retardation.

Battered Child Syndrome

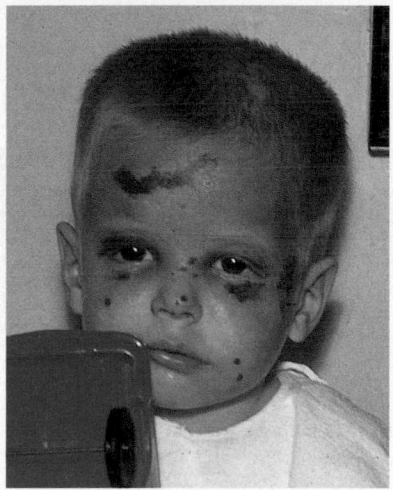

The child who has been physically abused (battered) may have old *and* fresh bruises on the head and face and may either look sad and forlorn or be actively seeking to please, sometimes even particularly involved with and attentive to the abusing parent. Other stigmata include bruises in areas (axilla and groin) not usually subject to injury rather than the bony prominences; x-ray evidence of fractures of the skull, ribs, and long bones in various stages of healing; and skin lesions that are morphologically similar to implements used to inflict trauma (hand, belt buckle, strap, rope, coat hanger, or lighted cigarette).

Perennial Allergic Rhinitis

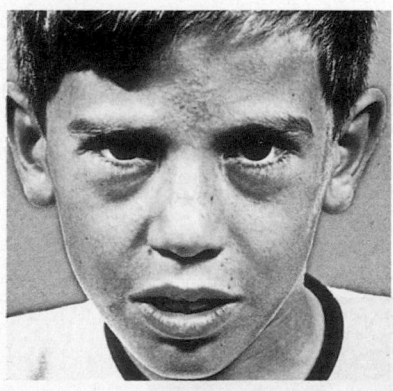

The child suffering from perennial allergic rhinitis has an open mouth (cannot breathe through the nose) and edema and discoloration of the lower orbitopalpebral grooves ("allergic shiners"). Such a child is often seen to push the nose upward and backward with a hand ("allergic salute") and to grimace (wrinkle the nose and mouth) to relieve nasal itching and obstruction. (Photograph reproduced with permission from Marks MB. Allergic shiners: dark circles under the eyes in children. Clin Pediatr 5:656, 1966.)

Hyperthyroidism

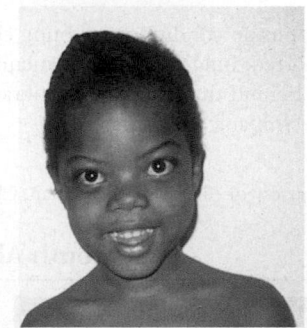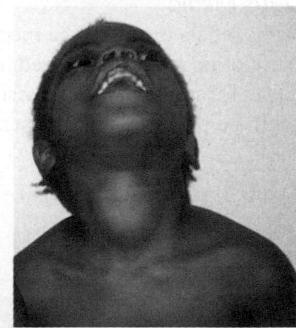

Thyrotoxicosis (*Graves' disease*) occurs in approximately 2 per 1,000 children younger than 10 years. Affected children exhibit hypermetabolism and accelerated linear growth. Facial characteristics shown in this 6-year-old girl are "staring" eyes (not true exophthalmos, which is rare in children) and an enlarged thyroid gland (*goiter*). See p. 209.

TABLE
23-7

Abnormalities of the Eyes, Ears, and Mouth

Eye Abnormalities

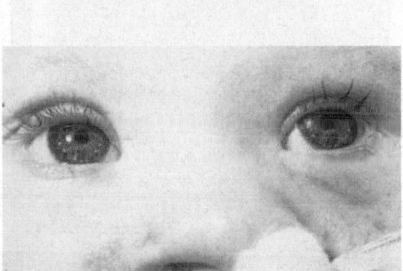

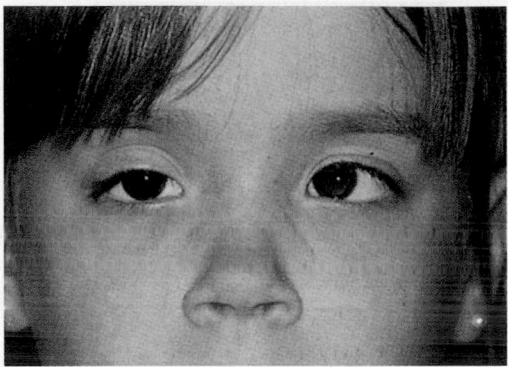

Brushfield's Spots
These abnormal speckling spots on the iris suggest Down syndrome.

Strabismus
Strabismus, or misalignment of the eyes, can lead to visual impairment. Esotropia, shown here, is an inward deviation.

Ear Abnormalities

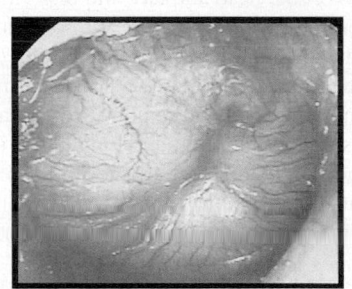

A

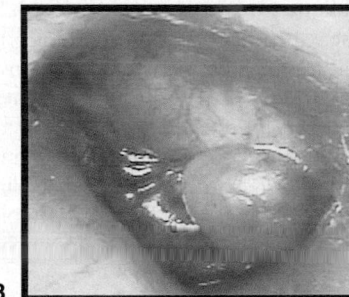

B

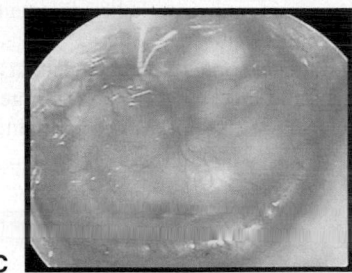

C

Otitis Media
Otitis media is one of the most common conditions in young children. The spectrum of otitis media is shown here. (**A**) Typical acute otitis media with a red, distorted, bulging tympanic membrane in a highly symptomatic child. (**B**) Acute otitis media with bullae formation and fluid visible behind the tympanic membrane. (**C**) Otitis media with effusion, showing a yellowish fluid behind a retracted and thickened tympanic membrane.

(Source of photos: *Otitis Media*—Courtesy of Alejandro Hoberman, Children's Hospital of Pittsburgh, University of Pittsburgh.)

Mouth Abnormalities

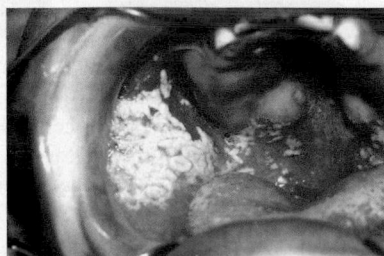

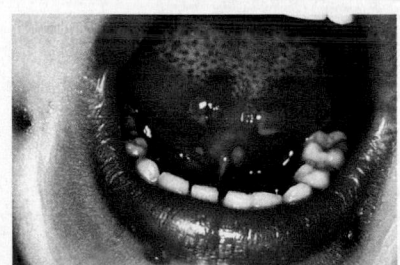

Oral Candidiasis ("thrush")
This infection is common in infants. The white plaques do not rub off.

Herpetic Stomatitis
Tender ulcerations on the oral mucosa are surrounded by erythema.

TABLE 23-8

Abnormalities of the Teeth, Pharynx, and Neck

Dental Abnormalities

Dental Caries

Dental caries is a major global health and pediatric problem. The photographs below show different characteristics of caries.

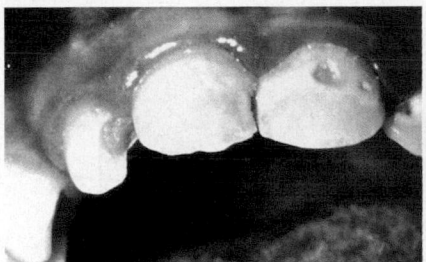

Nursing-bottle caries

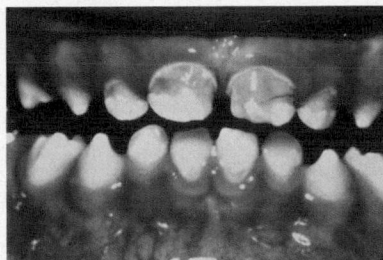

Erosion of teeth

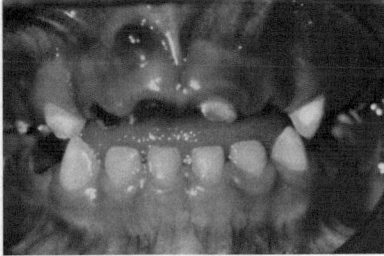

Severe erosion

Staining of the Teeth

Various causes can lead to staining of the teeth of children, including intrinsic stains such as tetracycline (right) or extrinsic stains such as poor oral hygiene (not shown). Extrinsic stains can be removed.

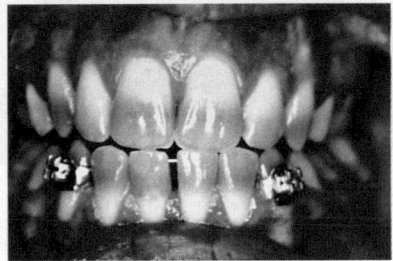

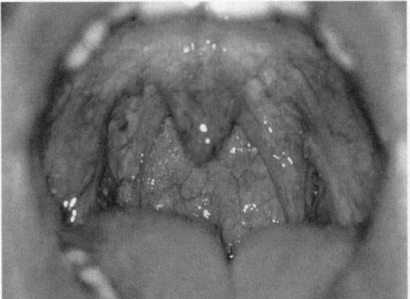

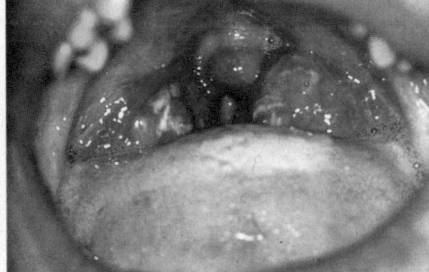

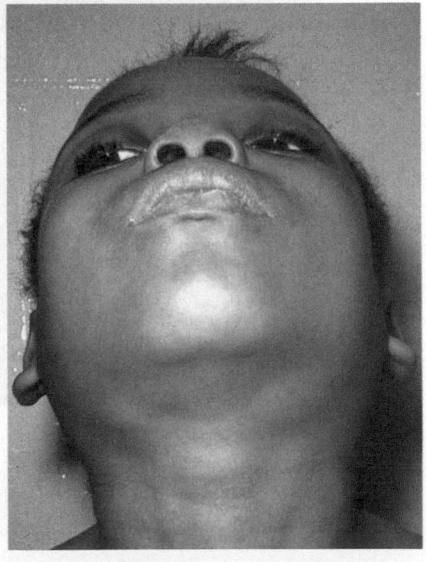

Streptococcal Pharyngitis ("strep throat")

This common childhood infection has a classic presentation of erythema of the posterior pharynx and palatal petechiae (*left*). A foul-smelling exudate (*right*) is also commonly noted.

Lymphadenopathy

Enlarged and tender cervical lymph nodes are common in children. The most likely causes are viral and bacterial infections. Lymph node enlargement can be bilateral, as shown above.

(Sources of photos: *Dental Caries* and *Staining of the Teeth*—Courtesy of American Academy of Pediatrics; *Streptococcal Pharyngitis* and *Lymphadenopathy*—Fleisher G, Ludwig S. Textbook of Pediatric Emergency Medicine, 4th ed. Philadelphia, Lippincott Williams & Wilkins, 2000.)

TABLE
23-9

Cyanosis in Children

It is important to recognize cyanosis. The best location to examine is the mucous membranes. Cyanosis is a "raspberry" color, whereas normal mucous membranes should have a "strawberry" color. Try to identify the cyanosis in these photographs before reading the captions.

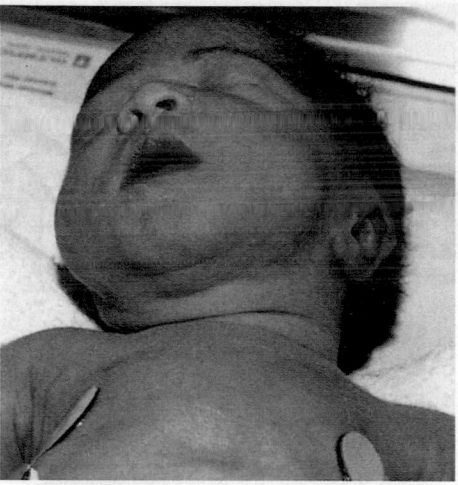

Generalized Cyanosis
This baby has total anomalous pulmonary venous return and an oxygen saturation level of 80%.

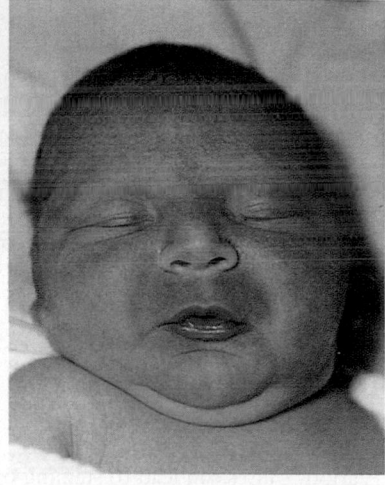

Perioral Cyanosis
This baby has mild cyanosis above the lips, but the mucous membranes remain pink.

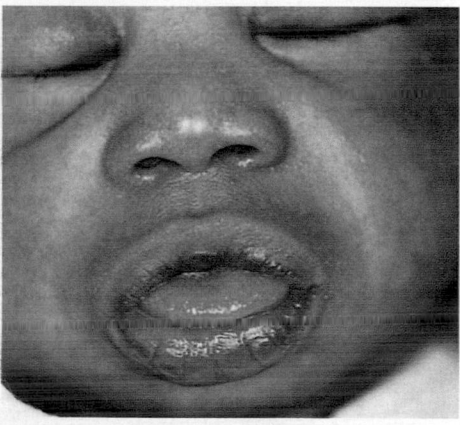

Bluish Lips, Giving Appearance of Cyanosis
Normal pigment deposition in the vermilion border of the lips gives them a bluish hue, but the mucous membranes are pink.

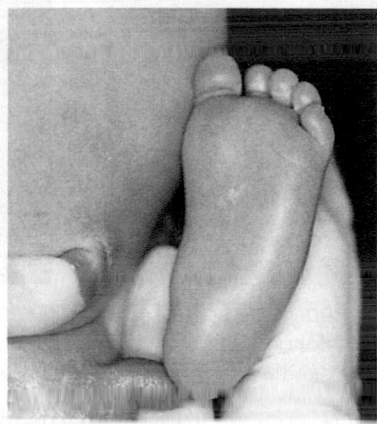

Acrocyanosis
This commonly appears on the feet and hands of babies shortly after birth. This infant is a 32-week newborn.

(Source of photos: Fletcher M. Physical Diagnosis in Neonatology. Philadelphia, Lippincott-Raven, 1998.)

TABLE
23-10
Congenital Heart Murmurs

Some heart murmurs reflect underlying heart disease. If you understand their physiologic causes, you will more readily be able to identify and distinguish them from innocent heart murmurs. Obstructive lesions result when blood flows through valves that are too small. Because this problem does not depend on the drop in pulmonary vascular resistance following birth, these murmurs are audible at birth. Defects with left-to-right shunts, on the other hand, depend on the drop in pulmonary vascular resistance. High-pressured shunts such as ventricular septal defect, patent ductus arteriosus, and persistent truncus arteriosus are not heard until 1 week or more after birth. Low-pressured left-to-right shunts, such as in atrial septal defects, may not be heard for considerably longer, usually first being noted at 1 year or more. Many children with congenital cardiac defects have combinations of defects or variations of abnormalities, so findings on cardiac examination may not follow these classic patterns. This table shows a limited selection of the more common defects.

Congenital Defect and Mechanism	Characteristics of the Murmur	Associated Findings
Pulmonary Valve Stenosis Usually a normal valve anulus with fusion of some or most of the valve leaflets, restricting flow across the valve *Mild* 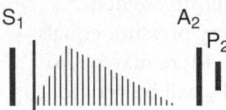 *Severe* 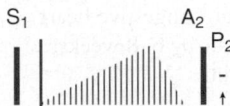	*Location.* Upper left sternal border *Radiation.* In mild degrees of stenosis, the murmur may be heard over the course of the pulmonary arteries in the lung fields. *Intensity.* Increases in intensity and duration as the degree of obstruction increases *Quality.* Ejection, peaking later in systole as the obstruction increases	Usually a prominent ejection click in early systole Pulmonary component of the second sounds at the base (P₂) becomes delayed and softer, disappearing as obstruction increases. Inspiration may increase murmur; expiration may increase click. Growth is usually normal. Newborns with severe stenosis may be cyanotic from right-to-left atrial shunting and rapidly develop congestive heart failure.
Aortic Valve Stenosis Usually a bicuspid valve with progressive obstruction, but there may be a dysplastic valve or damage from rheumatic fever or degenerative disease 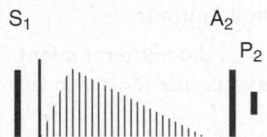	*Location.* Midsternum, upper right sternal border *Radiation.* To the carotid arteries and suprasternal notch; may also be a thrill *Intensity.* Varies, louder with increasingly severe obstruction *Quality.* An ejection, often harsh, systolic murmur	May be an associated ejection click The aortic closure sound may be increased in intensity. There may be a diastolic murmur of aortic valve regurgitation. Newborns with severe stenosis may have weak or absent pulses and severe congestive heart failure. May not be audible until adulthood even though the valve is congenitally abnormal
Tetralogy of Fallot Complex defect with ventricular septal defect, infundibular and usually valvular right ventricular outflow obstruction, malrotation of the aorta, and right-to-left shunting at ventricular septal level *With Pulmonic Stenosis* 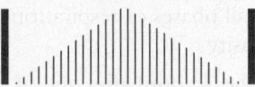 *With Pulmonic Atresia* 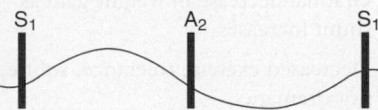	*General.* Variable cyanosis, increasing with activity *Location.* Mid-to-upper left sternal border. If pulmonary atresia, there is no systolic murmur but the continuous murmur of ductus arteriosus flow at upper left sternal border or in the back. *Radiation.* Little, to upper left sternal border, occasionally to lung fields *Intensity.* Usually grade III–IV *Quality.* Midpeaking, systolic ejection murmur	Normal pulses The pulmonary closure sound is usually not heard. May have abrupt hypercyanotic spells with sudden increase in cyanosis, air hunger, altered level of awareness Failure to gain weight with persistent and increasingly severe cyanosis Long-term persistence of cyanosis accompanied by clubbing of fingers and toes Persistent hypoxemia leads to polycythemia, which will accentuate the cyanosis.

(*table continues on page 834*)

TABLE
23-10   Congenital Heart Murmurs (continued)

Congenital Defect and Mechanism	Characteristics of the Murmur	Associated Findings
Transposition of the Great Arteries A severe defect with failure of rotation of the great vessels, leaving the aorta to arise from the right ventricle and the pulmonary artery from the left ventricle	*General.* Intense generalized cyanosis *Location.* No characteristic murmur. If present, it may reflect an associated defect such as VSD. *Radiation and Quality.* Depends on associated abnormalities	Single loud second sound of the anterior aortic valve Frequent rapid development of congestive heart failure Frequent associated defects as described at the left
Ventricular Septal Defect Blood going from a high-pressured left ventricle through a defect in the septum to the lower-pressured right ventricle creates turbulence, usually throughout systole. *Small to Moderate* 	*Location.* Lower left sternal border *Radiation.* Little *Intensity.* Variable, only partially determined by the size of the shunt. Small shunts with a high pressure gradient may have very loud murmurs. Large defects with elevated pulmonary vascular resistance may have no murmur. Grade II–IV/VI with a thrill if grade IV/VI or higher. *Quality.* Pansystolic, usually harsh, may obscure S_1 and S_2 if loud enough	With large shunts, there may be a low-pitched middiastolic murmur of relative mitral stenosis at the apex. As pulmonary artery pressure increases, the pulmonic component of the second sounds at the base increases in intensity. When pulmonary artery pressure equals aortic pressure, there may be no murmur, and P_2 will be very loud. In low-volume shunts, growth is normal. In larger shunts, congestive heart failure may occur by 6–8 weeks; poor weight gain. Associated defects are frequent.
Patent Ductus Arteriosus Continuous flow from aorta to pulmonary artery throughout the cardiac cycle when ductus arteriosus does not close after birth *Small to Moderate* 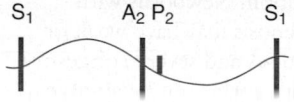	*Location.* Upper left sternal border and to left *Radiation.* Sometimes to the back *Intensity.* Varies depending on size of the shunt, usually grade II–III/VI. *Quality.* A rather hollow, sometimes machinery-like murmur that is continuous throughout the cardiac cycle, although occasionally almost inaudible in late diastole, uninterrupted by the heart sounds, louder in systole	Full to bounding pulses Noticed at birth in the premature infant who may have bounding pulses, a hyperdynamic precordium, and an atypical murmur Noticed later in the full-term infant as pulmonary vascular resistance falls May develop congestive heart failure at 4–6 weeks if large shunt Poor weight gain related to size of shunt Pulmonary hypertension affects murmur as above.
Atrial Septal Defect Left-to-right shunt through an opening in the atrial septum, possible at various levels 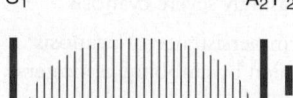	*Location.* Upper left sternal border *Radiation.* To the back *Intensity.* Variable, usually grade II–III/VI *Quality.* Ejection but without the harsh quality	Widely split second sounds throughout all phases of respiration, normal intensity Usually not heard until after age of 1 year Gradual decrease in weight gain as shunt increases Decreased exercise tolerance, subtle, not dramatic Congestive heart failure is rare.

TABLE
23-11

Physical Signs of Sexual Abuse

Possible Indications

1. Marked and immediate dilatation of the anus in knee–chest position, with no constipation, stool in the vault, or neurologic disorders
2. Hymenal notch or cleft that extends greater than 50% of the inferior hymenal rim (confirmed in knee–chest position)
3. Condyloma acuminata in a child older than 3 years
4. Bruising, abrasions, lacerations, or bite marks of labia or perihymenal tissue
5. Herpes of the anogenital area beyond the neonatal period
6. Purulent or malodorous vaginal discharge in a young girl (culture and view all discharges under a microscope for evidence of a sexually transmitted disease)

Strong Indications

1. Lacerations, ecchymoses, and newly healed scars of the hymen or the posterior fourchette
2. No hymenal tissue from 3 to 9 o'clock (confirmed in various positions)
3. Healed hymenal transections, especially between 3 and 9 o'clock (complete cleft)
4. Perianal lacerations extending to external sphincter

A child with concerning physical signs must be evaluated by a sexual abuse expert for a complete history and sexual abuse examination.

Any physical sign must be evaluated in light of the entire history, other parts of the physical examination, and laboratory data.

Key to Photos

(**A**) Acute hemorrhage and ecchymoses of tissues (10-mo-old)

(**B**) Erythema and superficial abrasions to the labia minora (5-yr-old)

(**C**) Healed interruption of hymenal membrane at 9 o'clock (4-yr-old)

(**D**) Narrowed posterior ring continuous with floor of vagina (12-yr-old)

(**E**) Copious vaginal discharge and erythema (9-yr-old)

(**F**) Extensive condylomata around the anus (2-yr-old)

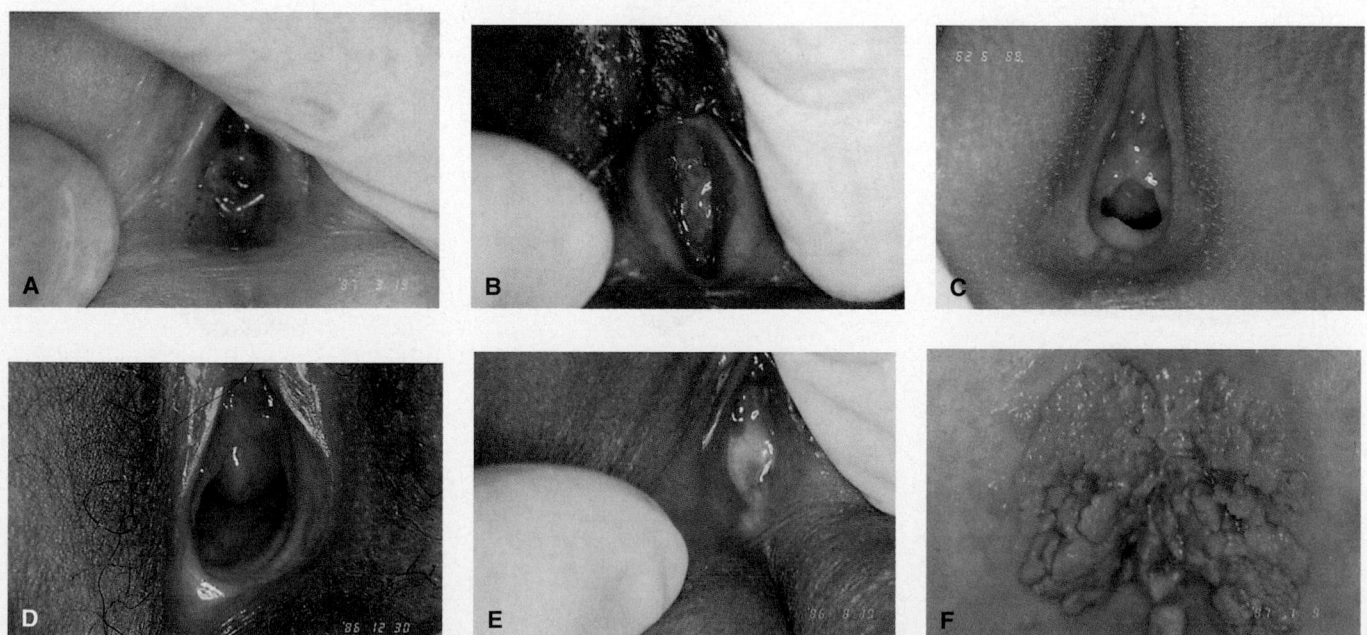

(Source: Reece R, Ludwig S, eds. Child Abuse Medical Diagnosis and Management, 2nd ed. Philadelphia, Lippincott Williams & Wilkins, 2001.)

TABLE
23-12

The Male Genitourinary System

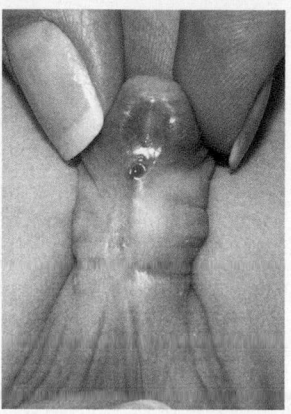

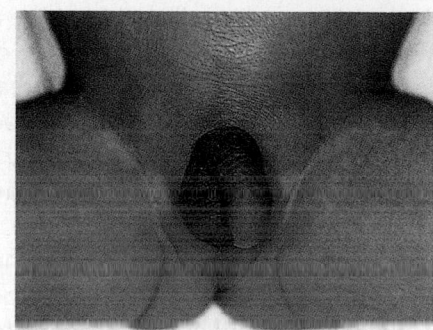

Hypospadias

Hypospadias is the most common congenital penile abnormality. The urethral meatus opens abnormally on the ventral surface of the penis. One form is shown above; more severe forms involve openings on the lower shaft or scrotum.

Undescended Testicle

You should distinguish between undescended testes, shown above (with testes in the inguinal canals), from highly retractile testes from an active cremasteric reflex.

(Sources of photos: *Hypospadias*—Courtesy of Warren Snodgrass, MD, UT–Southwestern Medical Center at Dallas; *Undescended Testicle*—Fletcher M. Physical Diagnosis in Neonatology. Philadelphia: Lippincott-Raven, 1998.)

TABLE
23-13

Common Musculoskeletal Findings in Young Children

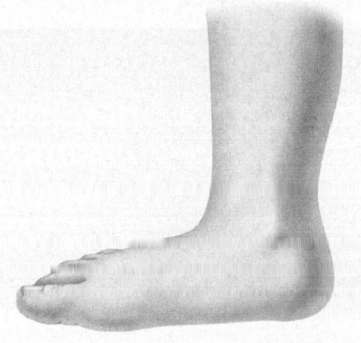

Flat feet or *pes planus* from laxity of the soft-tissue structures of the foot

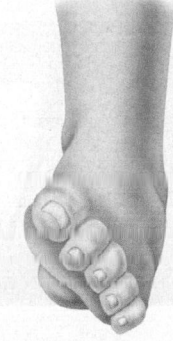

Inversion of the foot (*varus*)

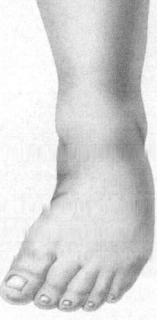

Metatarsus adductus in a child. The forefoot is adducted and not inverted.

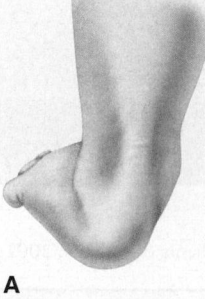

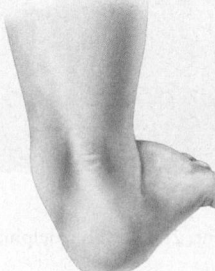

A

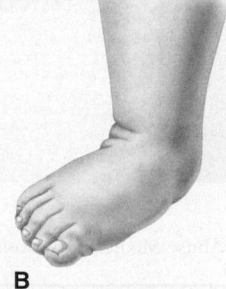

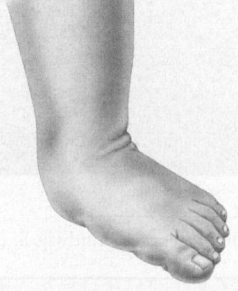

B

Pronation in a toddler. (**A**) When viewed from behind, the hindfoot is everted. (**B**) When viewed from the front, the forefoot is everted and abducted.

TABLE
23-14

The Power of Prevention: Vaccine-Preventable Diseases

This table shows photographs of children with vaccine-preventable diseases. Childhood vaccines have been named the single most important medical intervention in the world in terms of influence on public health. Because of vaccinations, we hope you will never see many of these conditions, but you should be able to identify them. Try to identify the diseases before reading the captions.

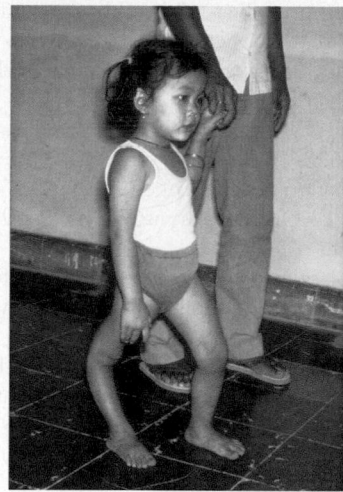

Polio
The deformed leg of this child is from polio.

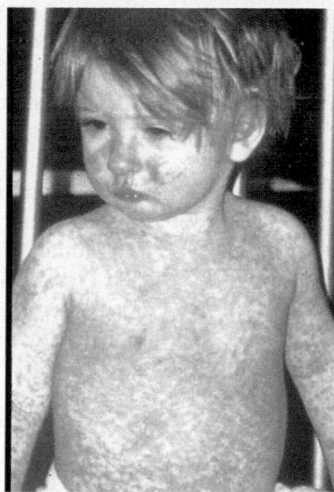

Measles
Characteristic rash of measles

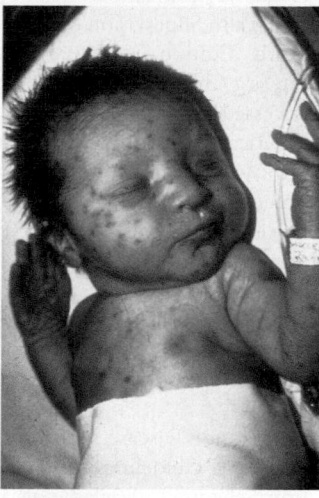

Rubella
Infant born with congenital rubella syndrome

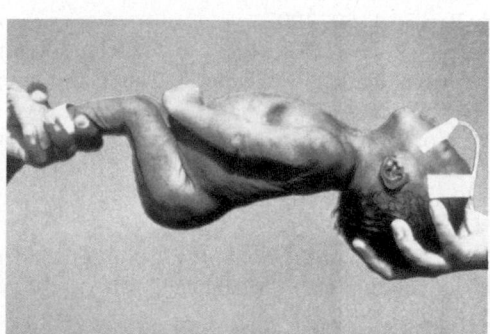

Tetanus
Rigid newborn with neonatal tetanus

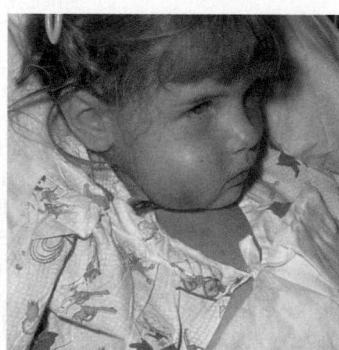

Haemophilus influenzae Type b
Periorbital cellulitis from this invasive bacterial disease

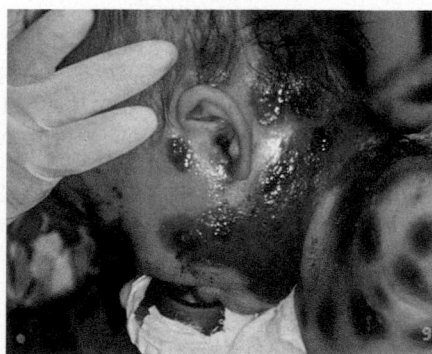

Varicella
An infant with a severe form of varicella

(Sources of photos: _Polio_—Courtesy of World Health Organization; _Haemophilus influenzae_—Courtesy of American Academy of Pediatrics; _Varicella_—Courtesy of Barbara Watson, MD, Albert Einstein Medical Center and Division of Disease Control, Philadelphia Department of Health; all others courtesy of Centers for Disease Control and Prevention.)

BIBLIOGRAPHY

CITATIONS

1. Levine MD, Carey WB, Crocker AC. Developmental–Behavioral Pediatrics, 3rd ed. Philadelphia: WB Saunders, 2002.

2. Hagan JF, Shaw JS, Duncan P, eds. Bright Futures Guidelines for Health Supervision of Infants, Children, and Adolescents—Third Edition, 2008. Available at: http://brightfutures.aap.org/3rd_Edition_Guidelines_and_Pocket_Guide.html. Accessed May 26, 2011.

3. American Academy of Pediatrics. Bright Futures. Available at: http://brightfutures.aap.org/. Accessed May 26, 2011.

4. American Medical Association. Guidelines for Adolescent Preventive Services (GAPS). Available at: http://www.ama-assn.org/ama/upload/mm/39/gapsmono.pdf. Accessed May 26, 2011.

5. U.S. Preventive Services Task Force (USPSTF). Focus on Children and Adolescents. Available at: http://www.uspreventiveservicestaskforce.org/tfchfocus.htm. Accessed May 26, 2011.

6. Centers for Disease Control and Prevention. Recommendations and Guidelines: 2008 Child & Adolescent Immunization Schedules. Available at: http://www.cdc.gov/vaccines/recs/schedules/child-schedule.htm. Accessed May 26, 2011. American Academy of Pediatrics, Immunization Schedules 2011. Available at: http://www.aap.org/immunization/IZSchedule.html. Accessed May 26, 2011. Johnson CP, Blasco PA. Infant growth and development. Pediatr Rev 18(7):224–242, 1997.

7. American Academy of Pediatrics. Immunization Schedules 2011. Available at: http://www.aap.org/immunization/IZSchedule.html. Accessed May 26, 2011.

8. Johnson CP, Blasco PA. Infant growth and development. Pediatr Rev 18(7):224–242,1997.

9. Colson ER, Dworkin PH. Toddler development. Pediatr Rev 18(8):255–259, 1997.

10. Conelan T. Normal speech and development. Pediatr Rev 18:91–100, 1998.

11. Fong CT. Clinical diagnosis of genetic diseases. Pediatr Ann 22(5):277–281, 1993.

12. Hyvarinen L. Assessment of visually impaired infants. Ophthalm Clin North Am 7:219, 1994.

13. Gessner IH. What makes a heart murmur innocent? Pediatr Ann 26(2):82–84, 87–88, 90–91, 1997.

14. Callahan CW Jr, Alpert B. Simultaneous percussion auscultation technique for the determination of liver span. Arch Pediatr Adolesc Med 148(8):873–875, 1994.

15. Burger BJ, Burger JD, Bos CF, et al. Neonatal screening and staggered early treatment for congenital dislocation or dysplasia of the hip. Lancet 336(8730):1549–1553, 1990.

16. Zafeiriou DI. Primitive reflexes and postural reactions in the neurodevelopmental examination. Pediatr Neurol 31(1):1–8, 2004.

17. Schott JM, Rossor MN. The grasp and other primitive reflexes. J Neurol Neurosurg Psychiatry 74(5):558–560, 2003.

18. Ogden CL, Carroll MD, Curtin LR, et al. Prevalence of overweight and obesity in the United States, 1999–2004. JAMA 295:1549–1555, 2006.

19. National High Blood Pressure Education Program Working Group on High Blood Pressure in Children and Adolescents. The Fourth Report on the Diagnosis, Evaluation, and Treatment of High Blood Pressure in Children and Adolescents. Pediatrics 114:555–576, 2004. Also available at: http://www.nhlbi.nih.gov/health/prof/heart/hbp/hbp_ped.pdf. Accessed May 26, 2011.

20. Shamis, DI. Collecting the "facts": vision assessment techniques: perils and pitfalls. Am Orthop J 46:7, 1996.

21. Rothman R, Owens T, Simel DL. Does this child have acute otitis media? JAMA 290:1633–1640, 2003.

22. Blomgren K, Pitkaranta A. Current challenges in diagnosis of acute otitis media. Intl J Ped Otorhinolaryn 69(3):295–299, 2005.

23. Pirozzo S, Papinczak T, Glasziou P. Whispered voice test for screening for hearing impairment in adults and children: systematic review. BMJ 327(7421):967, 2003.

24. Wolf G, Anderhuber W, Kuhn F. Development of the paranasal sinuses in children: implications for paranasal sinus surgery. Ann Otol Rhinol Laryngol 102(9):705–711, 1993.

25. Selwitz RH, Ismail AI, Pitts NB. Dental caries. Lancet 369 (9555):51–59, 2007.

26. Lunt RC, Law DB. A review of the chronology of eruption of deciduous teeth. J Am Dent Assoc 89:872, 1974.

27. Ebell MH, Smith MA, Barry HC, et al. Does this patient have strep throat? JAMA 284:2912–2918, 2000.

28. Centers for Disease Control and Prevention. National Surveillance for Asthma—United States, 1980–2004. MMWR Morb Mortal Wkly Rep 56:1–60, 2007.

29. Tucker WN, Saab S, Leland SR, et al. The scratch test is unreliable for determining the liver edge. J Clin Gastroenterol 25:410–414, 1997.

30. Ashcraft KW. Consultation with the specialist: acute abdominal pain. Pediatr Rev 21:363–367, 2000.

31. Bruce RW. Torsional and angular deformities. Pediatr Clin North Am 43:867–881, 1996.

32. Newacheck PW, Strickland B, Shonkoff JP, et al. An epidemiologic profile of children with special health care needs. Pediatrics 102:117–123, 1998.

33. ACOG Committee. Opinion no. 350, November 2006: Breast concerns in the adolescent. Obstet Gynecol 108(5): 1329–1336, 2006.

34. Herman-Giddens ME, Slora EJ, Wasserman RC, et al. Secondary sexual characteristics and menses in young girls seen in office practice: a study from the Pediatric Research in Office Settings Network. Pediatrics 99(4):505–512, 1997.

ADDITIONAL REFERENCES

AHRQ-Agency for Healthcare Research and Quality. Guide to Clinical Preventive Services, 2010–2011, Recommendations of the U.S. Preventive Services Task Force: Section 3. Recommendations for Children and Adolescents. Available at: http://www.ahrq.gov/clinic/pocketgd1011/gcp10s3.htm. Accessed June 10, 2011.

Bergen D. Human Development: Traditional and Contemporary Theories. Upper Saddle River, NJ: Pearson/Prentice Hall, 2008.

Burns CE, Dunn AM, Brady MA, et al. Pediatric Primary Care: A Handbook for Nurse Practitioners, 3rd ed. St. Louis: Saunders, 2004.

Chiocca EM. Advanced Pediatric Assessment. Philadelphia: Lippincott, Williams and Wilkins, 2010.

Colyar MR. Well-child Assessment for Primary Care Providers. Philadelphia: FA Davis, 2003.

Cote P, Kreitz BG, Cassidy JD, et al. A study of the diagnostic accuracy and reliability of the scoliometer and Adam's forward bend test. Spine 23:796–802; discussion, 803, 1998.

Dixon SD, Stein MT. Encounters with Children: Pediatric Behavior and Development, 4th ed. Philadelphia: Mosby, 2006.

Emans SJ, Laufer MR, Goldstein DP. Pediatric and Adolescent Gynecology, 5th ed. Philadelphia: Lippincott Williams & Wilkins, 2004.

Fenichel G. Clinical Pediatric Neurology: A Signs and Symptoms Approach, 5th ed. Philadelphia: Saunders, 2005.

Hockenberry MJ, Wilson, D. Wong's Nursing Care of Infants and Children, 9th ed. St. Louis: Mosby, 2010.

Korovessis PG, Stamatakis MV. Prediction of scoliotic Cobb angle with the use of the scoliometer. Spine 21:1661–1666, 1996.

Neinstein LS. Adolescent Health Care: A Practical Guide, 4th ed. Philadelphia: Lippincott Williams & Wilkins, 2002.

Sass P, Hassan G. Lower extremity abnormalities in children. Am Fam Phys 68:661–668, 2003.

Viviani GR, Budgell L, Dok C, et al. Assessment of accuracy of the scoliosis school screening examination. Am J Public Health 74:497–498, 1984.

Wallace GB, Newton RW. Gowers' sign revisited. Arch Dis Child 64:1317–1319, 1989.

Zitelli BJ, Davis HW. Atlas of Pediatric Physical Diagnosis, 4th ed. St. Louis: Mosby, 2002.

Assessing Older Adults

LEARNING OBJECTIVES

The student will:

1. Utilize the techniques that best facilitate the health history and physical examination of the older adult.

2. Identify focus areas during the health history specific to the older adult.

3. Recognize normal physiologic changes in the older adult.

4. Utilize screening tools in the assessment of older adults.

5. Perform a health history on an older adult.

6. Perform a physical examination on an older adult.

7. Document the older adult assessment findings.

8. Address areas of health promotion and counseling specific to the older adult.

Older adults now number more than 39 million in the United States and are expected to reach 72 million by 2030.[1] These seniors will live longer than previous generations: life span at birth is currently 80 years for women and 75 years for men. Those older than 85 years are projected to increase to 5% of the U.S. population within 20 years. Hence, the "demographic imperative" is to maximize not only the life span but also the "health span" of our older population, so that seniors maintain full function for as long as possible, enjoying rich and active lives in their homes and communities.

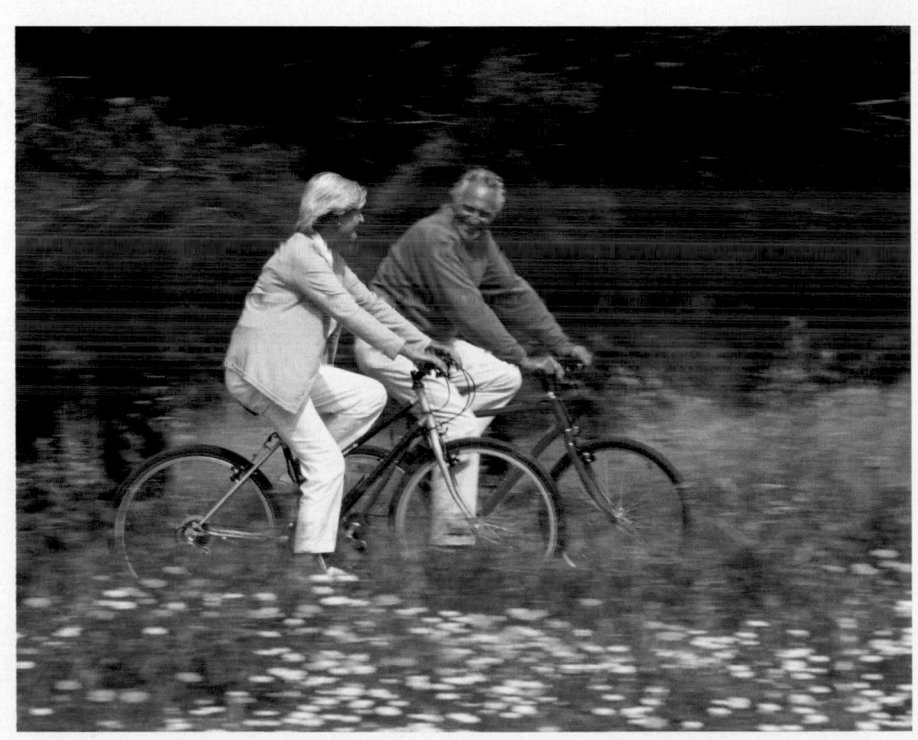

Clinicians now recognize frailty as one of society's common myths about aging—more than 95% of Americans older than 65 years live in the community, and only 5% reside in long-term care facilities.[1,2] Over the past 20 years, seniors actually have become more active and less disabled. These changes call for new goals for nursing care—"an informed, active patient interacting with a prepared proactive team, resulting in high quality satisfying encounters and improved outcomes"—and a distinct set of clinical attitudes and skills.[3,4]

Assessing the older adult presents special opportunities and special challenges. Many of these are quite different from the disease-oriented approach of history taking and physical examination for younger patients: the focus on healthy or "successful" aging; the need to understand and mobilize family, social, and community supports; the importance of functional assessment skills; and the opportunities for promoting the older adult's long-term health and safety. It is important to distinguish between normal aging changes and abnormalities commonly found in an elderly person.

See Table 24-1, Minimum Geriatrics Competencies, p. 875.

Chapter Overview: The Aging Adult

- Anatomy and Physiology: Changes of Aging
- The Health History
  - Approach to the Patient: adjusting the environment; shaping the content and pace of the visit; eliciting symptoms; responsiveness to the cultural dimensions of aging
  - Focus Areas: functional assessment; activities of daily living; instrumental activities of daily living; medications; nutrition; acute and chronic pain; sexuality; urinary incontinence; smoking and alcohol
- Physical Examination of the Older Adult
- Recording Your Findings
- Health Promotion and Counseling
  - Includes screening, cancer screening, immunizations, household safety, falls, driving safety, exercise, depression, dementia, elder mistreatment, advance directives, and palliative care

 ## ANATOMY AND PHYSIOLOGY

Primary aging reflects changes in physiologic reserves over time that are independent of and not induced by any disease. These changes are likely to appear during periods of stress, such as exposure to fluctuating temperatures, dehydration, or even shock. Decreased cutaneous vasoconstriction and sweat production can impair responses to heat; declines in thirst may delay recovery from dehydration; and the physiologic drops in maximum cardiac output, left ventricular filling, and maximum heart rate present with aging may impair the response to shock.

At the same time, the aging population displays marked heterogeneity. Researchers have identified vast differences in how people age and have distinguished "usual" aging, with its complexity of diseases and impairments, from "optimal" aging. Optimal aging occurs in those people who escape debilitating disease entirely and maintain healthy lives late into their 80s and 90s. Studies of centenarians show that genes account for approximately 20% probability of living to 100, with healthy lifestyles accounting for approximately 20% to 30%.[5-7]

These findings provide compelling evidence for promoting optimal nutrition, strength training and exercise, and daily function for older adults to delay unnecessary depletion of physiologic reserves.

Vital Signs

Blood Pressure. In Western societies, systolic blood pressure tends to rise from childhood through old age. The aorta and large arteries stiffen and become atherosclerotic. As the aorta becomes less distensible, a given stroke volume causes a greater rise in systolic blood pressure; *systolic hypertension* with a *widened pulse pressure* often ensues. Diastolic blood pressure stops rising at approximately the sixth decade. At the other extreme, some elderly people develop a tendency toward *postural (orthostatic) hypotension*—a sudden drop in blood pressure when they rise to standing.

Heart Rate and Rhythm. In older adults, resting heart rate remains unchanged, but pacemaker cells decline in the sinoatrial node, as does maximal heart rate, affecting response to physiologic stress.[8]

Elderly people are more likely to have abnormal heart rhythms such as atrial or ventricular ectopy. Asymptomatic rhythm changes are generally benign. Like postural hypotension, however, they may cause *syncope,* or temporary loss of consciousness.

Respiratory Rate and Temperature. Respiratory rate is unchanged, but changes in temperature regulation lead to a susceptibility to *hypothermia*.

Skin, Nails, and Hair.

With age, the skin wrinkles, becomes lax, and loses turgor. The vascularity of the dermis decreases, causing lighter skin to look paler and more opaque. Skin on the backs of the hands and forearms appears thin, fragile, loose, and transparent. There may be purple patches or macules, termed actinic purpura, that fade over time. These spots and patches come from blood that has leaked through poorly supported capillaries and spread within the dermis.

Nails lose luster with age and may yellow and thicken, especially on the toes.

Hair undergoes a series of changes. Scalp hair loses its pigment, producing the well-known graying. Hair loss on the scalp is genetically determined. As early as 20 years, a man's hairline may start to recede at the temples; hair loss at the vertex follows. In women, hair loss follows a similar but less severe pattern. In both sexes, the number of scalp hairs decreases in a generalized pattern, and the diameter of each hair gets smaller. Less familiar, but probably more important clinically, is normal hair loss elsewhere on the body: the trunk, pubic areas, axillae, and limbs. As women reach age 55 years, coarse facial hairs appear on the chin and upper lip but do not increase further thereafter.

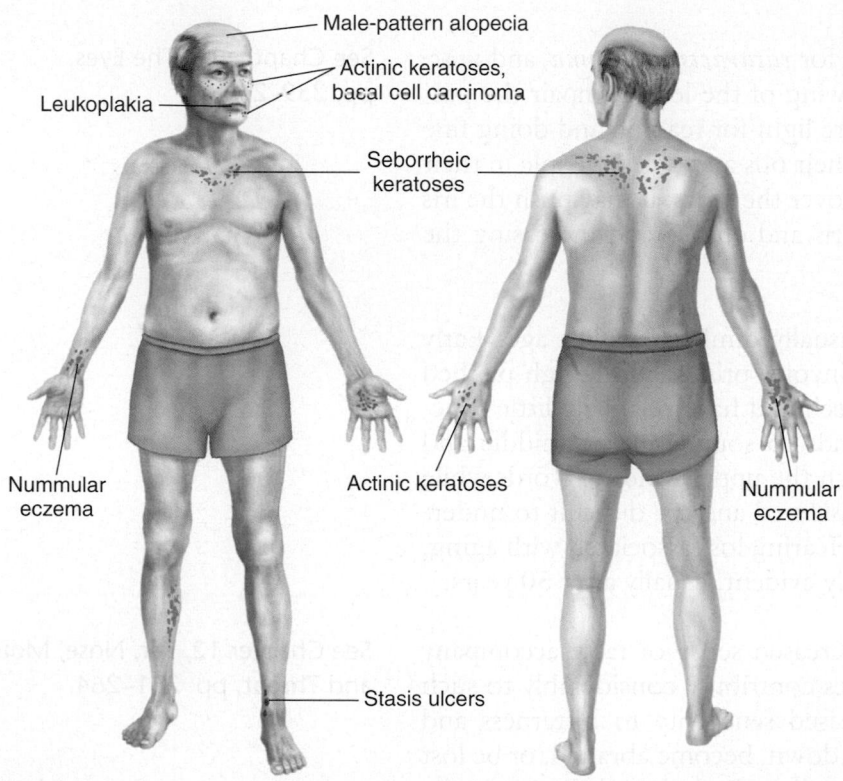

Many of the changes described here pertain to lighter-skinned people and do not necessarily apply to those with darker skin tones. For example, Native American men have relatively little facial and body hair compared with lighter-skinned men and should be evaluated according to their own norms.

Head and Neck.   The eyes, ears, and mouth bear the brunt of old age. The fat that surrounds and cushions the eye within the bony orbit may atrophy, allowing the eyeball to recede somewhat. The skin of the eyelids becomes wrinkled, occasionally hanging in loose folds. Fat may push the fascia of the eyelids forward, creating soft bulges, especially in the lower lids and the inner third of the upper lids. Because their eyes produce fewer lacrimal secretions, aging patients may complain of dry eyes. The corneas lose some of their luster.

The pupils become smaller, which makes it more difficult to examine the ocular fundi. The pupils may also become slightly irregular but should continue to respond to light and accommodate with near vision.

Visual acuity remains fairly constant between 20 and 50 years. It diminishes gradually until approximately 70 years and then more rapidly. Nevertheless, most elderly people retain good to adequate vision (20/20 to 20/70 corrected vision as measured by standard charts). Near vision, however, begins to blur noticeably for virtually everyone. From childhood on, the lens gradually loses its elasticity, and the eye grows progressively less able to accommodate and focus on nearby objects. Ensuing *presbyopia* usually becomes noticeable during the fifth decade.

Aging affects the lenses and increases risk for *cataracts, glaucoma,* and *macular degeneration.* Thickening and yellowing of the lenses impair the passage of light to the retinas, requiring more light for reading and doing fine work. Cataracts affect 1 in 10 people in their 60s and 1 in 3 people in their 80s. Because the lens continues to grow over the years, it may push the iris forward, narrowing the angle between iris and cornea and increasing the risk of *narrow-angle glaucoma.*

See Chapter 11, The Eyes, pp. 239–240.

Acuity of hearing, like that of vision, usually diminishes with age. Early losses, which start in young adulthood, involve primarily the high-pitched sounds beyond the range of human speech and have relatively little functional significance. Gradually, loss extends to sounds in the middle and lower ranges. When a person fails to catch the upper tones of words while hearing the lower tones, words sound distorted and are difficult to understand, especially in noisy environments. Hearing loss associated with aging, known as *presbycusis,* becomes increasingly evident, usually after 50 years.

Diminished salivary secretions and a decreased sense of taste accompany aging, but medications or various diseases contribute considerably to such changes. Decreased olfaction and increased sensitivity to bitterness and saltiness also affect taste. Teeth may wear down, become abraded, or be lost to dental caries or other conditions over time. Periodontal disease is the chief cause of tooth loss in most adults. If a person has no teeth, the lower portion of the face looks small and sunken, with accentuated "purse string" wrinkles radiating from the mouth. Overclosure of the mouth may lead to maceration of the skin at the corners, a condition known as *angular cheilitis.* The bony ridges of the jaws that once surrounded the tooth sockets are gradually resorbed, especially in the lower jaw.

See Chapter 12, Ear, Nose, Mouth and Throat, pp. 261–264.

The frequency of palpable cervical nodes gradually diminishes with age and, according to one study, falls below 50% between 50 and 60 years. In contrast to the lymph nodes, the submandibular glands become easier to feel.

Thorax and Lungs.
As people age, their capacity for exercise decreases. The chest wall becomes stiffer and harder to move, respiratory muscles may weaken, and the lungs lose some of their elastic recoil. Lung mass declines, and residual volume increases. The speed of breathing out with maximal effort gradually diminishes, and the cough becomes less effective.

Skeletal changes associated with aging may accentuate the dorsal curve of the thoracic spine, producing kyphosis from osteoporotic vertebral collapse and increasing the anteroposterior diameter of the chest. The resulting "barrel chest," however, has little effect on function.

Cardiovascular System.   Cardiovascular findings vary significantly with age. Aging also affects vascular sounds in the neck and adds to the significance of extra heart sounds like S_3 and S_4 and of selected systolic murmurs.

Neck Vessels.

Lengthening and tortuosity of the aorta and its branches occasionally result in kinking or buckling of the carotid artery low in the neck, especially on the right. The resulting pulsatile mass, occurring chiefly in women with hypertension, may be mistaken for a carotid aneurysm—a true dilation of the artery. A tortuous aorta occasionally raises the pressure in the jugular veins on the left side of the neck by impairing their drainage within the thorax.

In older adults, systolic bruits heard in the middle or upper portions of the carotid arteries suggest, but do not prove, partial arterial obstruction from atherosclerosis. In contrast, cervical bruits in younger people are usually innocent.

Extra Heart Sounds—S_3 and S_4.

A physiologic *third heart sound,* commonly heard in children and young adults, may persist as late as age 40, especially in women. After age 40, however, an S_3 strongly suggests congestive heart failure from volume overload of the left ventricle, as in coronary artery disease or valvular heart disease (e.g., mitral regurgitation). In contrast, a *fourth heart sound* is seldom heard in young adults other than well-conditioned athletes. An S_4 can be heard in otherwise healthy older people, but often suggests decreased ventricular compliance and impaired ventricular filling.

See Table 14-7, p. 390, Extra Heart Sounds in Diastole.

Cardiac Murmurs.

Middle-aged and older adults commonly have a *systolic aortic murmur.* This murmur is detected in approximately one third of people close to 60 years, and in more than half of those reaching 85 years. Aging thickens the bases of the aortic cusps with fibrous tissue. Calcification follows, resulting in audible vibrations. Turbulence produced by blood flow into a dilated aorta may further augment this murmur. In most people, the process of fibrosis and calcification—known as *aortic sclerosis*—does not impede blood flow. In some, the aortic valve leaflets become calcified and immobile, resulting in *aortic stenosis* and outflow obstruction. Both carry increased risk for cardiovascular morbidity and mortality.

Similar changes alter the mitral valve, approximately one decade later than aortic sclerosis. Calcification of the mitral valve annulus, or valve ring, impedes normal valve closure during systole, causing the systolic murmur of *mitral regurgitation.* This murmur may become pathologic as volume overload increases in the left ventricle.

Peripheral Vascular System.   Aging itself confers relatively few clinically important changes for the peripheral vascular system. Although arterial and venous disorders, especially atherosclerosis, do affect older people more frequently, they probably cannot be considered part of normal aging. Peripheral arteries tend to lengthen, become tortuous, and feel harder and less resilient. These changes do not necessarily indicate atherosclerosis, however, or pathologic changes in the coronary or cerebral vessels.

The common changes in skin, nails, and hair discussed earlier are not specific for arterial insufficiency, even though they are classically associated with it. Loss of arterial pulsations is not typical, however, and demands careful evaluation. Rarely, in those older than 50 years, the temporal arteries may become subject to giant cell, or temporal arteritis, leading to loss of vision in 15% of those affected, and to complaints of headache and jaw claudication in others. Mean age of onset is 72 years. An important concern is a possible aneurysm in the abdominal aorta in older adults with abdominal or back pain, especially those who are male, smoke, and have coronary disease.

Breasts and Axillae.   The normal adult breast may be soft, but also granular, nodular, or lumpy. This uneven texture represents physiologic nodularity. It may be bilateral and palpable throughout or only in parts of the breast. With aging, the female breasts tend to diminish as glandular tissue atrophies and is replaced by fat. Although the proportion of fat increases, its total amount may decrease. The breasts often become flaccid and more pendulous. The ducts surrounding the nipple may become more easily palpable as firm, stringy strands. Axillary hair diminishes.

Abdomen.   During the middle and later years, fat tends to accumulate in the lower abdomen and near the hips, even when total body weight is stable. This accumulation, together with weakening of the abdominal muscles, often produces a soft, more protruding abdomen. Occasionally a person notes this change with alarm and interprets it as fluid or evidence of disease.

Aging may blunt the manifestations of acute abdominal disease. Pain may be less severe, fever is often less pronounced, and signs of peritoneal inflammation, such as muscular guarding and rebound tenderness, may be diminished or even absent.

See Chapter 16, Gastrointestinal and Renal Systems)

Male and Female Genitalia, Anus, Rectum, and Prostate.   As men age, sexual interest appears to remain intact, although frequency of intercourse declines. Several physiologic changes accompany decreasing testosterone levels. Erections become more dependent on tactile stimulation and less responsive to erotic cues. The penis decreases in size, and the testicles drop lower in the scrotum. Protracted illnesses, more than aging, lead to decreased testicular size. Pubic hair may decrease and become gray. Erectile dysfunction, or the inability to have an erection, affects approximately 50% of older men. Usual causes include: hypogastric cavernous arterial insufficiency or venous leakage through the subtunical venules.[9]

In men, proliferation of prostate epithelial and stromal tissue, termed benign prostatic hyperplasia (BPH), begins in the third decade, yet prostate enlargement results in only about half, and symptoms occur in only about half of men with enlargement.[10] Symptoms of urinary hesitancy, dribbling, and incomplete emptying can often be traced to causes other than BPH, such as: coexisting disease, use of medication, lower urinary tract abnormalities. Hyperplasia continues to increase prostate volume until the seventh decade, then appears to plateau. These changes are androgen dependent.

In women, ovarian function usually starts to diminish during the fifth decade; on average, menstrual periods cease between 45 and 52 years. As estrogen stimulation falls, many women experience hot flashes, sometimes for up to 5 years. Symptoms range from: flushing, sweating, and palpitations to chills and anxiety. Sleep disruption and mood changes are common. Women may report vaginal dryness, urge incontinence, or dyspareunia. Several vulvovaginal changes occur: pubic hair becomes sparse as well as gray, the labia and clitoris become smaller, the vagina narrows and shortens, and the vaginal mucosa becomes thin, pale, and dry, with loss of lubrication. The uterus and ovaries diminish in size. Within 10 years after menopause, the ovaries are usually no longer palpable. The suspensory ligaments of the adnexa, uterus, and bladder may also relax. Sexuality and sexual interest are often unchanged.[11]

Musculoskeletal System. Musculoskeletal changes continue throughout the adult years. Soon after maturity, subtle losses in height begin; significant shortening is obvious by old age. Most loss of height occurs in the trunk as intervertebral discs become thinner and the vertebral bodies shorten or even collapse from osteoporosis. Flexion at the knees and hips may also contribute to shortened stature. Alterations in the discs and vertebrae also contribute to the kyphosis of aging and increase the anteroposterior diameter of the chest, especially in women. For these reasons, the limbs of an elderly person tend to look long in proportion to the trunk.

With aging, skeletal muscles decrease in bulk and power, and ligaments lose some of their tensile strength. Range of motion diminishes, partly because of osteoarthritis.

Nervous System and Mental Status Assessment. Aging may affect all aspects of the nervous system, from mental status to motor and sensory function and reflexes. Age related losses can exact a heavy toll. Older adults experience the death of loved ones and friends, retirement from valued employment, diminution in income, decreased physical capacities including impairments in vision and hearing, and often growing social isolation. Moreover, the aging brain experiences biologic changes. Brain volume and the number of cortical brain cells decrease, and both microanatomic and biochemical changes have been identified. Nevertheless, most adults adapt well to getting older. They maintain self-esteem, adapt to their changing capacities and circumstances, and eventually prepare themselves for death.

Most elderly people do well on the mental status examination, but selected impairments may become evident, especially at advanced ages. Many older people complain about their memories. "benign forgetfulness" is the usual explanation and may occur at any age. This term refers to difficulty recalling the names of people or objects or certain details of specific events. Identifying this common phenomenon, when appropriate, may assuage worries about Alzheimer disease. In addition to this circumscribed forgetfulness, elderly people retrieve and process data more slowly, and take more time to learn new material. Their motor responses may slow, and their ability to perform complex tasks may become impaired.

Frequently, the nurse distinguishes these age-related changes in the nervous system from manifestations of specific mental disorders whose prevalence increases with aging, such as depression and dementia. Sorting out these ailments may be difficult, because both mood disturbances and cognitive changes can alter the patient's ability to recognize or report symptoms. Older patients are also more susceptible to delirium, a temporary state of confusion that may be the first clue to infection, problems with medications, or changes in the environment such as hospitalization. The nurse must learn to recognize these conditions promptly and to protect the patient from harm. Some findings that would be abnormal in younger people, however, occur so often in the elderly that they can be attributed to aging alone, such as the changes in hearing, vision, extraocular movements, and pupillary size, shape, and reactivity described earlier.

Review Chapter 19 Mental Status, pp. 595–612 and Table 24-2, p. 876, Delirium and Dementia.

Changes in the motor system are common. Older adults move and react with less speed and agility than younger ones, and skeletal muscles decrease in bulk. The hands of an aged person often look thin and bony as a result of atrophy of the interosseous muscles, causing muscle wasting in the backs of the hands that leaves concavities or grooves. As illustrated on p. 525, this change may first appear between the thumb and the hand (1st and 2nd metacarpals) but may also be seen between the other metacarpals. Small muscle wasting may also flatten the thenar and hypothenar eminences of the palms. Arm and leg muscles can also show signs of atrophy, exaggerating the apparent size of adjacent joints. Muscle strength, though diminished, is relatively well maintained.

Occasionally, an older person develops a benign essential tremor in the head, jaw, lips, or hands that may be confused with parkinsonism (pp. 670–671). Unlike parkinsonian tremors, however, benign tremors are slightly faster and disappear at rest, and there is no associated muscle rigidity.

See Chapter 20 The Nervous System, Table 20-1, pp. 670–671, Tremors and Involuntary Movement.

Aging may also affect vibratory sense and reflexes. Older adults frequently lose some or all vibration sense in the feet and ankles (but not in the fingers or over the shins). Less commonly, position sense may diminish or disappear. The gag reflex may be diminished or absent. Abdominal reflexes may diminish or disappear. Ankle reflexes may be symmetrically decreased or absent, even when reinforced. Less commonly, knee reflexes are similarly affected. Partly because of musculoskeletal changes in the feet, the plantar responses become less obvious and more difficult to interpret. If other neurologic abnormalities accompany these changes, or if atrophy and reflex changes are asymmetric, search for an explanation other than age alone.

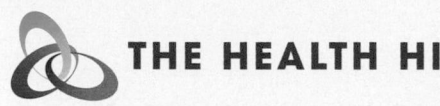

THE HEALTH HISTORY

APPROACH TO THE PATIENT

Refine your interviewing techniques when talking with older adults and obtaining the Health History. The nurses demeanor should convey respect, patience, and cultural awareness. Be sure to address patients by an appropriate title and their last name (e.g., Mr. Jones or Mrs./Ms. Thomas).

Approach to the Older Adult Patient

- Adjust the environment
- Shape the content and pace of the visit
- Elicit symptoms
- Address the cultural dimensions of aging

Adjust the Environment. First, take the time to adapt the environment of the office, hospital, or nursing home to put the patient at ease. Recall the physiologic changes in temperature regulation, and make sure the office is neither too cool nor too warm. Brighter lighting helps compensate for changes in lens proteins—a well-lit room allows the older adult to see your facial expressions and gestures, ensure the patient's back is to the window rather than facing the window as the glare may impair the ability to see well. The nurse should face the patient directly, sitting at eye level.

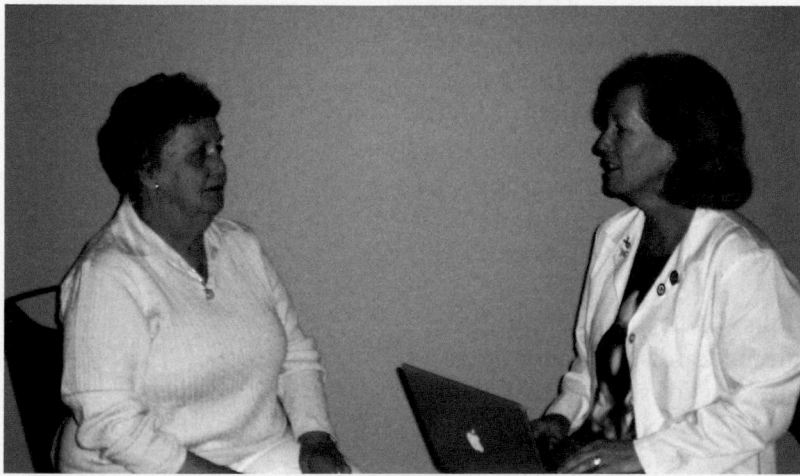

More than 50% of older adults have hearing deficits, especially loss of high-tone discrimination, so a quiet room, free of distractions or noise, is most conducive to good communication. In the hospital setting, turn off the radio or television before starting a discussion. If appropriate, consider using a "pocket talker," a microphone that amplifies your voice and connects to an earpiece inserted by the patient. Adopt low speaking tones, and make sure the patient is using glasses, hearing aids, and dentures when needed to assist with communication. Patients with quadriceps weakness benefit from chairs with higher seating and a wide stool with a handrail leading up to the examining table.[12]

Shape the Content and Pace of the Visit. With older adults, plan to alter the traditional format of the initial or follow-up visit. From middle age on, people begin to measure their lives in terms of years left rather than years lived. Older people often reminisce about the past and reflect on previous experiences. Listening to this process of life review provides important insights and helps support patients as they work through painful feelings or recapture joys and accomplishments.

At the same time, it is important to balance the need to assess complex problems with the patient's endurance and possible fatigue. To provide enough time to fully listen to the patient but prevent exhaustion, make ample use of brief screening tools, information from home visits and the medical record, and reports from family members, caregivers, and allied health disciplines. Consider dividing the initial assessment into two visits. Two or more shorter visits may be less fatiguing and more productive because older patients frequently need more time to respond to questions, and their explanations may be slow and lengthy.

See brief screening tools, p. 853.

Elicit Symptoms in the Older Adult. Eliciting the history from older adults calls for an astute nurse: patients may accidentally or purposefully underreport symptoms; the presentation of acute illnesses may be different; common symptoms may mask a geriatric syndrome; or patients may have cognitive impairment.

Older patients tend to overestimate their health when affected by increasing disease and disability.[12] It is best to start the visit with open-ended questions like "How can I help you today?" Older patients may be reluctant to report their symptoms. Some are afraid or embarrassed; others try to avoid medical unpleasantries or the discomforts of diagnosis and treatment. Still others overlook their symptoms (e.g., pain), thinking them to be merely part of aging, and simply forget about them. To reduce the risk for late recognition and delayed intervention, you may need to adopt more directed questions or health screening tools, as well as consult with family members and caregivers.

Acute illnesses present differently in older adults. Older patients with infections are less likely to have a fever. In those with myocardial infarction, reports of chest pain fall with increasing age, and complaints of shortness of breath, syncope, stroke, and acute confusion become more common.[13] Older patients with hyperthyroidism and hypothyroidism present with fewer symptoms and signs. In hyperthyroidism, fatigue, weight loss, and tachycardia comprise the most common symptom triad in patients age 50 or older.[14] Older patients are more likely to have anorexia and atrial fibrillation; heat intolerance, increased sweating, and hyperreflexia are more rare. In hypothyroidism, fatigue and weakness are common but notably nonspecific; the usual chills, paresthesias, weight gain, and cramps found in younger patients are uncommon.[15]

Managing an increasing number of interrelated conditions calls for recognizing the symptom clusters typical of different *geriatric syndromes*. These are understood to have the following features: multifactorial origin; typically in older, often frail adults; often precipitated by an acute event; episodic; and often followed by functional decline. Because consensus on the definition is still in flux, some prefer the term *geriatric conditions,* or "a collection of symptoms and signs common in older adults not necessarily related to a specific disease."[16] Examples of geriatric syndromes or conditions include: delirium, cognitive impairment, falls, dizziness, depression, urinary incontinence, and functional impairment.[16,17] Student nurses need to learn about these syndromes because one symptom may relate to several others in a pattern unfamiliar to the patient. Searching for the usual "unifying diagnosis" may pertain to fewer than 50% of older adults.[18] It is important for nurses to obtain an accurate assessment utilizing both subjective and objective information.

Finally, the student must be knowledgeable about how cognitive impairment affects the patient's history. Evidence suggests that when older patients do report symptoms, their reports are reliable and contain more symptoms than reports from family or collateral sources.[19–21] When compared with unimpaired counterparts, even elders with mild cognitive impairment provide sufficient history to reveal concurrent disorders.[9] Use simple sentences with prompts about necessary information. For patients with more severe impairments, confirm key symptoms with family members or caregivers with the patients consent and in their presence.

Learn to recognize and avoid stereotypes that distort your appreciation of each patient as unique, with a treasure of life experiences. Discover how older patients see themselves and their situations. Listen for their priorities, goals, and coping skills. Such knowledge strengthens your alliance with older patients as you plan for their care.

TIPS FOR COMMUNICATING EFFECTIVELY WITH OLDER ADULTS

- Provide a well-lit, moderately warm setting with minimal background noise, a safe chair, and access to the examining table.
- Face the patient and speak in low tones; make sure the patient is using glasses, hearing devices, and dentures if needed.
- Adjust the pace and content of the interview to the stamina of the patient; consider two visits for initial evaluations when indicated.
- Allow time for open-ended questions and reminiscing; include family and caregivers when needed, especially if the patient has a cognitive impairment.
- Make use of brief screening instruments, the medical record, and reports from allied disciplines.
- Carefully assess symptoms, especially fatigue, loss of appetite, dizziness, and pain, for clues to underlying disorders.
- Make sure written instructions are in large print and easy to read.

Addressing Cultural Dimensions of Aging. Nurses must acquire new knowledge and awareness about the health beliefs and culture that shape the older adult's response to illness and the health care system.[23] Ethnic groups in the U.S. continue to change and nurses need to be aware of the the changing population. Between 1990 and 2000, Hispanics, African Americans, Native Americans, and other ethnic groups accounted for approximately 43% of the total growth of the population.[24] By 2050, the overall older adult population will increase by 230%, with the minority older adult population growing by 510%.[25] The broad categories used for federal reporting no longer capture the wide array of cultural differences that affect how older adults understand suffering, illness, and decisions about care, ranging from use of alternative therapies to timing of health care visits. Immigrant and refugee groups in the United States with particular health care needs include: Vietnamese, Laotians, Haitians, Somalis, Russians and Eastern Europeans, Afghans, and Bosnians.

Cultural differences affect the epidemiology of illness and mental health, the process of acculturation, the specific concerns of the elderly, and disparities in health outcomes.[25-28] Learn culturally specific ways to show respect to elders and use appropriate nonverbal communication styles. Direct eye contact or handshaking, for example, may not be culturally appropriate. Identify critical experiences that affect the patient's outlook and psyche arising from the country of origin or migration history. Ask about spiritual advisors and native healers.

Cultural values particularly affect decisions about the end of life. Elders, family, and even an extended community group may make these decisions with or for the older patient. Such group decision making is in contrast to the patient autonomy and informed consent that many contemporary health care providers value, expect, and automatically assume to be desired by all.[24] Being sensitive to the stresses of migration and acculturation, using translators effectively, enlisting "patient navigators" from the family and community, and accessing culturally validated assessment tools like the Geriatric Depression Scale are important for empathic care of older adults.[26]

See Chapter 3, Interviewing and Communication, on working with translators, p. 55.

FOCUS AREAS WHEN ASSESSING OLDER ADULTS

Common Concerns

- Functional assessment
- Activities of daily living
- Instrumental activities of daily living
- Medications
- Nutrition
- Acute and persistent pain
- Sexuality
- Urinary incontinence
- Smoking and alcohol

Symptoms in the older adult can have many meanings and interconnections, as seen in the geriatric syndromes. Explore the meaning of these symptoms with all patients, and review the Common or Concerning Symptoms sections in previous chapters. For older adults, be sure to place these symptoms in the context of the overall functional assessment. Several areas warrant special attention as the health history is gathered. Approach the following areas with extra thoroughness and sensitivity, always focusing on helping the older adult to maintain optimal well-being and level of function.

Functional Assessment. The 10-Minute Geriatric Screener evaluates for age-related changes that help older adults maintain optimal function. It covers the three important domains of geriatric assessment: physical, cognitive, and psychosocial function. Note that it addresses vision and hearing, key sensory modalities that can be followed with additional objective testing such as using an eye chart for vision, asking the patient about hearing, followed by the whisper test and more formal testing if indicated. It also includes questions about mobility, urinary incontinence (an often unreported problem), nutrition, memory, depression, and physical disabilities. All these components can affect social interaction and self-esteem in the elderly.

● 10-Minute Geriatric Screener

Problem	Screening Measure	Positive Screen
Vision	2 Parts: Ask: "Do you have difficulty driving, or watching television, or reading, or doing any of your daily activities because of your eyesight?" If yes, then: Test each eye with the Snellen chart while the patient wears corrective lenses (if applicable).	Yes to question and inability to read greater than 20/40 on Snellen chart
Hearing	Use audioscope set at 40 dB. Test hearing using 1,000 and 2,000 Hz.	Inability to hear 1,000 or 2,000 Hz in both ears or either of these frequencies in one ear
Leg mobility	Time the patient after asking: "Rise from the chair. Walk 20 feet briskly, turn, walk back to the chair, and sit down."	Unable to complete task in 15 seconds
Urinary incontinence	2 Parts: Ask: "In the last year, have you ever lost your urine and gotten wet?" If yes, then ask: "Have you lost urine on at least 6 separate dates?"	Yes to both questions

(continued)

● **10-Minute Geriatric Screener** (continued)

Problem	Screening Measure	Positive Screen

Nutrition/weight loss	2 Parts:
	  Ask: "Have you lost 10 lbs over the past 6 months
	    without trying to do so?"
	Weigh the patient.
		Yes to the question or weight
		<100 lbs

Memory	Three-item recall	Unable to remember all three items after 1 minute
Depression	Ask: "Do you often feel sad or depressed?"	Yes to the question

Physical disability	Six questions: "Are you able to. . . :
	  "Do strenuous activities like fast walking or
	    bicycling?"
	  "Do heavy work around the house like washing
	    windows, walls, or floors?"
	  "Go shopping for groceries or clothes?"
	  "Get to places out of walking distance?"
	  "Bathe, either a sponge bath, tub bath, or shower?"
	  "Dress, like putting on a shirt, buttoning and zipping,
	    or putting on shoes?"
		Yes to any of the questions

(Source: Moore AA, Siu AL. Screening for common problems in ambulatory elderly: clinical confirmation of a screening instrument. Am J Med 100:438–440, 1996.)

Activities of Daily Living. Learning how older adults, especially those with chronic illness, function in terms of daily activities is essential and provides an important baseline for the future. First, ask about the capacity to perform the *Activities of Daily Living (ADLs)*—these consist of basic self-care abilities—and then move on to inquiries about capacity for higher level functions, the *Instrumental Activities of Daily Living (IADLs)* as listed on the next page. Can the patient perform these activities independently, need some help, or is the patient entirely dependent on others?

Start with an open-ended request such as: "Tell me about your typical day" or "Tell me about your day yesterday." Then move to a greater level of detail . . . "You got up at 8 AM?" "How is it getting out of bed?" . . . "What did you do next?" Ask how things have changed, who is available for help, and what helpers actually do. Remember that assessing the patient's safety is one of your priorities.

Medications. Prescription drug statistics expose the dramatic rationale for obtaining a complete drug history.[3] Approximately 80% of older adults have at least one chronic disease and take at least one prescription drug each day. Those older than 65 years receive approximately 30% of all prescriptions. Roughly 30% take more than eight prescribed drugs each day! Older adults have more than 50% of all reported adverse drug reactions causing hospital admission, reflecting pharmacodynamic changes in the distribution, metabolism, and elimination of drugs that place them at increased risk.

● Activities of Daily Living and Instrumental Activities of Daily Living	
Physical Activities of Daily Living (ADLs)	**Instrumental Activities of Daily Living (IADLs)**
Bathing	Using the telephone
Dressing	Shopping
Toileting	Preparing food
Transferring	Housekeeping
Continence	Doing laundry
Feeding	Transportation, including driving
	Taking medicine
	Managing money

Take a thorough medication history, including name, dose, frequency, and indication for each drug. Be sure to explore all components of polypharmacy, including suboptimal prescribing, concurrent use of multiple drugs, underuse, inappropriate use, and nonadherence. Ask about use of over-the-counter medications, vitamin and nutritional supplements, and mood-altering drugs such as narcotics, benzodiazepines, and recreational substances. Assess medications for drug interactions. Be particularly careful with patients being treated for insomnia, as it is estimated to occur in approximately 40% of older adults. Increased exercise may be the best remedy. Recall that medications are the most common modifiable risk factor associated with falls. Review strategies for avoiding polypharmacy and collaborate with the patient's physician or nurse practitioner. It is wise to keep the number of drugs prescribed to a minimum. Learn about drug–drug interactions and drugs contraindicated in older adults.[29,30]

Nutrition.   Taking a diet history and Mini Nutritional Assessment (MNA) are especially important in older adults. Prevalence of malnutrition increases with age, affecting 22.6% of the elderly; with 40% of those being hospitalized elders and 50% in rehabilitation facilities.[31] Those with chronic disease are particularly at risk, especially those with poor dentition, oral or gastrointestinal disorders, depression or other psychiatric illness, and drug regimens that affect appetite and oral secretions. For underweight elders, the serum albumin is an independent risk factor for all-cause mortality.[32]

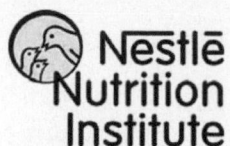

Mini Nutritional Assessment
MNA®

Last name:		First name:		
Sex:	Age:	Weight, kg:	Height, cm:	Date:

Complete the screen by filling in the boxes with the appropriate numbers. Total the numbers for the final screening score.

Screening

A Has food intake declined over the past 3 months due to loss of appetite, digestive problems, chewing or swallowing difficulties?
0 = severe decrease in food intake
1 = moderate decrease in food intake

B Weight loss during the last 3 months
0 = weight loss greater than 3 kg (6.6 lbs)
1 = does not know
2 = weight loss between 1 and 3 kg (2.2 and 6.6 lbs)

C Mobility
0 = bed or chair bound
1 = able to get out of bed / chair but does not go out
2 = goes out

D Has suffered psychological stress or acute disease in the past 3 months?

E Neuropsychological problems
0 = severe dementia or depression
1 = mild dementia

F1 Body Mass Index (BMI) (weight in kg) / (height in m²)
0 = BMI less than 19
1 = BMI 19 to less than 21
2 = BMI 21 to less than 23

IF BMI IS NOT AVAILABLE, REPLACE QUESTION F1 WITH QUESTION F2.
DO NOT ANSWER QUESTION F2 IF QUESTION F1 IS ALREADY COMPLETED.

F2 Calf circumference (CC) in cm
0 = CC less than 31

(max. 14 points)

12-14 points: Normal nutritional status
8-11 points: At risk of malnutrition
0-7 points: Malnourished

Ref.   Vellas B, Villars H, Abellan G, et al. *Overview of the MNA® - Its History and Challenges.* J Nutr Health Aging 2006;10:456-465.

Rubenstein LZ, Harker JO, Salva A, Guigoz Y, Vellas B. *Screening for Undernutrition in Geriatric Practice: Developing the Short-Form Mini Nutritional Assessment (MNA-SF).* J. Geront 2001;56A: M366-377.

Guigoz Y. *The Mini-Nutritional Assessment (MNA®) Review of the Literature - What does it tell us?* J Nutr Health Aging 2006; 10:466-487.

Kaiser MJ, Bauer JM, Ramsch C, et al. *Validation of the Mini Nutritional Assessment Short-Form (MNA®-SF): A practical tool for identification of nutritional status.* J Nutr Health Aging 2009; 13:782-788.

® Société des Produits Nestlé, S.A., Vevey, Switzerland, Trademark Owners

© Nestlé, 1994, Revision 2009. N67200 12/99 10M

For more information: www.mna-elderly.com

Acute and Persistent Pain. Pain and associated complaints account for 80% of clinician visits. Prevalence of pain may reach 25% to 50% in community-dwelling adults and 40% to 80% in nursing home residents. Pain usually arises from musculoskeletal complaints like back and joint pain.[33] Headache, neuralgias from diabetes and herpes zoster, nighttime leg pain, and cancer pain are also common. Older patients are less likely to report pain, leading to undue suffering, depression, social isolation, physical disability, and loss of function. The American Geriatrics Society favors the term *persistent pain,* because chronic pain is associated with negative stereotypes.[34]

● **Characteristics of Acute and Persistent Pain**	
Acute Pain	**Persistent Pain**
Distinct onset	Lasts more than 3 months
Obvious pathology	Often associated with psychological or functional impairment
Short duration	Can fluctuate in character and intensity over time
Common causes: postsurgical, trauma, headache	Common causes: arthritis, cancer, claudication, leg cramps, neuropathy, radiculopathy

(Source: Reuben DB, Herr KA, Pacala JT, et al. Geriatrics at Your Fingertips: 2004, 6th ed., p. 119. Malden, MA: Blackwell Publishing, Inc., for the American Geriatrics Society, 2004.)

Inquire about pain *each time* you meet with an older patient. Assessing pain in older adults is challenging. Patients may not want to report symptoms because of fears of additional testing, costs, or progression of disease.[35] There may be cognitive or verbal impairments or barriers of trust, language, or cultural understanding. Or the patient may report multiple conditions that complicate assessment. Nonetheless, evidence shows that pain reporting by patients with even mild to moderate cognitive impairment is reliable. Ask specifically, "Are you having any pain right now? How about during the past week?" Be alert for red flags of untreated pain, such as use of the terms "burning," "discomfort," or "soreness"; depressed affect; and nonverbal change in posture or gait. Many multidimensional and unidimensional pain scales are available. Unidimensional scales such as the Visual Analog Scale, graphic pictures, and the Verbal 0–10 Scale have all been validated and are easiest to use.[33,36] Recruit caregivers or family members for relevant history in patients with severe cognitive deficits.

Refer to the pain scale in Chapter 7, General Survey, Vital Signs, and Pain, p. 123.

Learn to distinguish acute pain from persistent pain and thoroughly investigate its cause. In older adults, confusion, restlessness, fatigue, or irritability may all arise from conditions causing pain. Assessing pain includes comprehensive evaluation of its effects on quality of life, social interactions, and functional level. Multidisciplinary assessment is warranted if the cause cannot be identified and risks of disability and comorbidity are high. Study

See the *10-Minute Geriatric Screener* for functional assessment on pp. 853–854.

the many modalities of pain relief, ranging from analgesics to the full range of nonpharmacologic therapies, especially those that engage patients directly and actively in their treatment plan and build self-reliance. Patient education alone has been shown effective.[34] Relaxation techniques, tai chi, acupuncture, massage, and biofeedback can avert adding more medications.

Sex.   Sex continues throughout a person's life. Use open-ended questions, such as "Tell me about your sex life," which may bring up some valid concerns requiring attention. The physical assessment section will address changes that occur with aging, including pain. Suggestions to alleviate pain might be changes in positions, use of lubrication, heat application, and warm baths.

Often older adults do not want to ask and nurses may not want to "pry" into the sexual history, especially after the loss of a lifetime partner; however, sex education and the use of condoms should be taught to older adults. During the review of systems, it is important for nurses to address the risks and the symptoms of sexually transmitted diseases as older adults are also at risk for diseases.

Urinary Incontinence.   Urinary incontinence is often not mentioned by patients as they may be embarrassed or may believe it is a normal part of aging. During the health history, questions should address:

Onset: When did the incontinence/leaking begin? Has it occurred before? How often does it occur? Does it occur when something else happens (sneezing, laughing, jumping)?
Location: Where are you when this occurs?
Duration: Does it last all day? Occasionally? Is there a pattern?
Characteristic Symptoms: Describe the urine (color, odor, amount, and times per day).
Associated Manifestations: What else is occurring? (Use the mnemonic DIAPERS or DDRRIIPP below.) How is this affecting the quality of life?
Relieving Factors: Does changing the amount, type, or timing of fluid intake influence the incontinence?
Treatment: Have you seen anyone for this? What have you done? Bladder training? Kegel exercises?

These mnemonics help students assess incontinence:

DIAPERS
Delirium
Infection
Atrophic urethritis/vaginitis
Pharmaceuticals
Excess urine output from conditions like hyperglycemia or congestive heart failure
Restricted mobility
Stool impaction

DDRRIIPP

Delirium

Drug side effects

Retention of feces

Restricted mobility

Infection of urine

Inflammation

Polyuria

Psychogenic[37,38]

Smoking and Alcohol. Smoking is harmful at all ages. At each visit, advise elderly smokers to quit. The commitment to stop smoking may take time, but quitting is an important step in reducing risk for heart disease, pulmonary disease, malignancy, and loss of daily function.

An estimated 5% to 10% of adults older than 65 years have alcohol-related problems.[39] Lifelong prevalence of alcohol abuse or dependency among community residents older than 65 years ranges from 4% to 8%.[40] Rates of alcoholism in older patients in hospital, emergency room, and clinic settings have been reported to reach 21%, 24%, and 36%, respectively, and account for approximately 1% of hospital admissions for this age group.[40] The number of older people with problem drinking is expected to rise as the population ages over the coming decades.

Despite the prevalence of alcohol problems among the elderly, rates of detection and treatment are low. Detection is especially important, because as many as 100 medications have adverse interactions with alcohol, and up to 30% of older adult drinkers exacerbate chronic ailments like cirrhosis, gastrointestinal bleeding, reflux disease, gout, hypertension, diabetes, insomnia, gait disorders, or depression.[41] Look for the clues shown in the accompanying box, especially in elders with recent bereavement or losses, pain, disability or depression, or a family history of alcohol disorders.

DETECTING ALCOHOL USE DISORDERS IN OLDER ADULTS: CLINICAL CLUES

- Memory loss,
- Cognitive impairment
- Depression, anxiety
- Change in hygiene or appearance
- Poor appetite, malnutrition
- Sleep difficulties
- Hypertension refractory to therapy
- Labile blood glucose
- Seizures
- Impaired balance and gait, and increased falls
- Frequent complaints of gastritis or esophagitis

Use the CAGE questions to uncover problem drinking. Although symptoms and signs are subtler in older adults, making early detection more difficult, the four CAGE questions remain sensitive and specific in this age group, using the conventional cutoff score of 2 or more.[40,41]

See Chapter 4, Health History, Alcohol and Illicit Drugs, pp. 67–68.

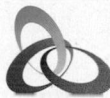

PHYSICAL EXAMINATION OF THE OLDER ADULT

General Survey. Deepen the observations about the patient that you have been compiling since the visit began.

What is the patient's apparent state of health and degree of vitality?
What about mood and affect?
Is screening for cognitive changes needed?
Note the patient's hygiene and how the patient is dressed.
How does the patient walk into the room? Move onto the examining table?
Are there changes in posture or involuntary movements?

Impoverished affect in *depression, Parkinson disease,* or *Alzheimer disease.*

See Table 24-3, p. 877, Screening for Dementia: The Mini-Cog, for a brief and well-validated screening tool for dementia.[42,43]

Undernutrition, slowed motor performance, loss of muscle mass, or weakness suggests frailty.

Kyphosis or abnormal gait can impair balance and increase risk of falls.

Vital Signs. Measure blood pressure using recommended techniques, checking for increased systolic blood pressure (SBP) and widened pulse pressure (PP), defined as systolic blood pressure minus diastolic blood pressure. With aging, systolic blood pressure and peripheral vascular resistance increase, whereas diastolic blood pressure decreases.

Isolated systolic hypertension (SBP ≥140) after age 50 triples the risk for coronary heart disease in men and increases risk of stroke; however, caution is advised when lowering BP in the "oldest old" older than 80 years.[44–46] PP ≥60 is a risk factor for cardiovascular and renal disease and stroke.[47–50]

Assess the patient for orthostatic hypotension, defined as a drop in systolic blood pressure of ≥20 mm Hg or diastolic blood pressure of ≥10 mm Hg within 3 minutes of standing.[51,52] Measure blood pressure and heart rate in two positions: supine after the patient rests for up to 10 minutes, then within 3 minutes of standing.

Review the Joint National Committee 7th Report categories of prehypertension to help you with early detection and treatment of hypertension (p. 116).

Orthostatic hypotension occurs in 10% to 20% of older adults and in up to 30% of frail nursing home residents, especially when they first arise in the morning. Presentation may include: light-headedness, weakness, unsteadiness, visual blurring, and, in 20% to 30% of patients, syncope. Causes include: medications, autonomic disorders, diabetes, prolonged bed rest, blood loss, and cardiovascular disorders.[47,53–55]

Measure heart rate, respiratory rate, and temperature. The apical heart rate may yield more information about arrhythmias in older patients. Use thermometers accurate for lower temperatures.

Respiratory rate ≥25 breaths per minute indicates lower respiratory infection; also congestive heart failure (CHF) and chronic obstructive pulmonary disease (COPD) exacerbation.

Hypothermia is more common in elderly patients.[12]

Weight and height are especially important in the elderly and needed for calculation of the body mass index. Weight should be measured at every visit.

Low weight is a key indicator of poor nutrition.

Undernutrition is seen with depression, alcoholism, cognitive impairment, malignancy, chronic organ failure (cardiac, renal, pulmonary), medication use, social isolation, and poverty.

Skin. Note physiologic changes of aging, such as thinning, loss of elastic tissue and turgor, and wrinkling. Skin may be dry, flaky, rough, and often itchy (*asteatosis*), with a latticework of shallow fissures that creates a mosaic of small polygons, especially on the legs.

Observe any patchy changes in color. Check the extensor surface of the hands and forearms for white depigmented patches, or *pseudoscars,* and for well-demarcated vividly purple macules or patches that may fade after several weeks (*actinic purpura*).

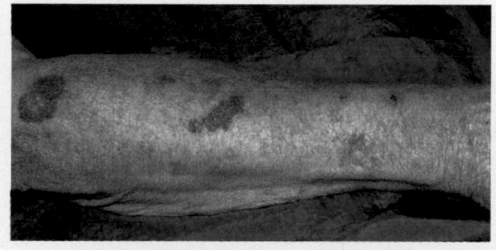

ACTINIC PURPURA—FOREARM

Look for changes from sun exposure. Areas of skin may appear weather beaten, thickened, yellowed, and deeply furrowed; there may be *solar lentigines*, or "liver spots," and *actinic keratoses*, superficial flattened papules covered by a dry scale.

Inspect for the benign lesions of aging, namely, *comedones*, or blackheads, on the cheeks or around the eyes; *cherry angiomas*, which often appear early in adulthood; and *seborrheic keratoses*, raised yellowish lesions that feel greasy and velvety or warty.

Distinguish such lesions from a *basal cell carcinoma*, initially a translucent nodule that spreads and leaves a depressed center with a firm elevated border, and from a *squamous cell carcinoma*, a firm reddish-appearing lesion often emerging in a sun-exposed area. A dark raised asymmetric lesion with irregular borders may be a *melanoma*. See Table 9-9, p. 180, Skin Tumors, and Table 9-10, p. 181, Benign and Malignant Nevi.

Watch for any painful vesicular lesions in a dermatomal distribution.

Suspect *herpes zoster* from reactivation of latent varicella-zoster virus in the dorsal root ganglia. Risk increases with age and impaired cell-mediated immunity.[56]

In older bed-bound patients, especially when emaciated or neurologically impaired, inspect the skin thoroughly for damage or ulceration.

Pressure sores may develop from obliteration of arteriolar and capillary blood flow to the skin or from shear forces during movement across sheets or when lifted upright incorrectly. See Table 9-12, p. 183, Pressure Ulcers.

Head and Neck.   Conduct a careful and thorough evaluation of the head and neck.

See Chapter 10, The Head and Neck.

Inspect the eyelids, the bony orbit, and the eye. The eye may appear recessed from atrophy of fat in the surrounding tissues. Observe any *senile ptosis* arising from weakening of the levator palpebrae, relaxation of the skin, and increased weight of the upper eyelid. Check the lower lids for *ectropion* or *entropion*. Note yellowing of the sclera, and *arcus senilis*, a benign whitish ring around the limbus.

See Table 11-2, p. 237, Variations and Abnormalities of the Eyelids and Table 11-4, p. 239, Opacities of the Cornea and Lens.

Test visual acuity, using a pocket Snellen chart or wall-mounted chart. Note any *presbyopia*, the loss of near vision arising from decreased elasticity of the lens related to aging.

More than 40 million Americans have refractive errors.

The pupils should respond to light and near effort. Except for possible impairment in upward gaze, extraocular movements should remain intact.

Using your ophthalmoscope, carefully examine the lens and fundi.

Cataracts, glaucoma, and macular degeneration all increase with aging.[57]

Inspect each lens carefully for any opacities. Do not depend on the flash-light alone because the lens may look clear superficially.

Cataracts are the world's leading cause of blindness. Risk factors include cigarette smoking, exposure to UV-B light, high alcohol intake, diabetes, medications (including steroids), and trauma. See Table 11-4, p. 239.

In older adults, the fundi lose their youthful shine and light reflections, and the arteries look narrowed, paler, straighter, and less brilliant. Assess the cup-to-disc ratio, usually 1:2 or less.

Inspect the fundi for colloid bodies causing alterations in pigmentation, called *drusen*.

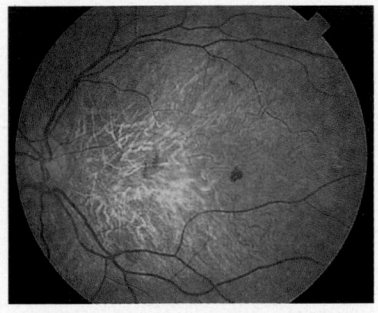

An increased cup-to-disc ratio suggests open angle *glaucoma*, caused by irreversible optic neuropathy and leading to loss of peripheral and central vision and blindness. Prevalence is three to four times higher in African Americans than in the general population.[58]

Test hearing by occluding one ear and using the techniques for whispered voice or an audioscope. Be sure to inspect the ear canals for cerumen, because removal can quickly improve hearing.

See techniques for testing hearing, pp. 269–270. Screening by asking if hearing loss is present is effective.

Examine the oral cavity for odor, appearance of the gingival mucosa, any caries, mobility of the teeth, and quantity of saliva; if the patient has dentures, check the fit as they should not wobble or fall out. Inspect closely for lesions on any of the mucosal surfaces. Ask the patient to remove the dentures to check the gums for sores.

Continue your usual examination of the thyroid gland and lymph nodes.

Malodor may occur with poor oral hygiene, periodontitis or caries. *Gingivitis* may arise from periodontal disease. Dental plaque and cavitation may cause caries. Increased tooth mobility from abscesses or advanced caries warrants removal to prevent aspiration. Decreased salivation may develop from medications, radiation, Sjögren syndrome, or dehydration. Lesions may arise from *oral tumors*, usually on the lateral borders of the tongue and floor of the mouth.[59]

Thorax and Lungs. Complete the usual examination, making note of subtle signs of changes in pulmonary function.

Increased anteroposterior diameter, purse-lipped breathing, and dyspnea with talking or minimal exertion suggest *chronic obstructive pulmonary disease.*

Cardiovascular System. Review the findings from blood pressure and heart rate measurements.

As with younger adults, begin by inspecting the jugular venous pressure (JVP), palpating the carotid upstrokes, and listening for any overlying carotid bruits.

Assess the point of maximum impulse (PMI) or apical impulse and auscultate for S_1 and S_2. Listen also for the extra sounds of S_3 and S_4.

Beginning in the second right interspace, listen for cardiac murmurs in all areas of auscultation (see pp. 373–375). Describe the timing, shape, location of maximal intensity, radiation, intensity, pitch, and quality of each murmur you detect.

For systolic murmurs over the clavicle, check for delay between the brachial and radial pulses.

Peripheral Vascular System. Auscultate the abdomen for aortic, renal, or femoral artery bruits.

Isolated systolic hypertension and a widened pulse pressure are cardiac risk factors, prompting a search for *left ventricular hypertrophy (LVH)*.

A *tortuous atherosclerotic aorta* can raise pressure in the left jugular veins by impairing drainage into the right atrium. It may also cause kinking of the carotid artery low in the neck on the right, chiefly in women with hypertension, which can be mistaken for a carotid aneurysm.

Carotid bruits in the elderly warrant further investigation for possible carotid stenosis due to risk for ipsilateral stroke.

Sustained PMI in LVH; diffuse PMI in congestive heart failure (see pp. 363–366.)

In older adults an S_3 suggests dilatation of the left ventricle from congestive heart failure or cardiomyopathy; an S_4 often accompanies hypertension.

Delay during simultaneous palpation (but not compression) of the brachial and radial pulses denotes aortic stenosis.[60]

A harsh holosystolic murmur at the apex suggests mitral regurgitation, also common in the elderly.

Bruits over these vessels are found in *atherosclerotic disease*.

Assess the width of the abdominal aorta in the epigastric area and examine for a pulsatile mass.

Consider *abdominal aortic aneurysm* if aortic width is ≥3 cm or with a pulsatile mass, especially in older male smokers with coronary disease.

Palpate pulses carefully.

Diminished or absent pulses may indicate *arterial occlusion*. Consider confirmation with an ankle–brachial index. Note that ≤33% of patients with peripheral vascular disease have symptoms of claudication.[61]

Breasts and Axillae.   Palpate the breasts carefully for lumps or masses. Include palpation of the tail of Spence that extends into the axilla. Examine the axillae for lymphadenopathy.

Lumps or masses in older women, and rarely in older men, mandate further investigation for possible malignancy.

Abdomen.   Continue your usual examination of the abdomen. Check for any bruits over the aorta, renal arteries, and femoral arteries. Inspect the upper abdomen; palpate to the left of the midline for any aortic pulsations. Try to assess the width of the aorta by pressing more deeply with one hand on each of its lateral margins (see pp. 459–460).

Bruits are found in atherosclerotic vascular disease

Widened aorta and pulsatile mass are found in *abdominal aortic aneurysm*

Female Genitalia.[62-64]   Inspect for changes related to menopause such as thinning of the skin or loss of pubic hair. Note redness, discharge, lesions, prolapsed uterus, or mutilation.

Male Genitalia and Prostate.   Examine the penis, retracting the foreskin if present. Examine the scrotum, testes, and epididymis. Note redness, lesions, discharge, or lumps.

Findings include smegma, penile cancer, and scrotal hydroceles.

Musculoskeletal System.   Begin your evaluation with the 10-Minute Geriatric Screener (pp. 853–854). If you find joint deformity, deficits in mobility, or pain with movement, conduct a more thorough examination. Review the techniques for examining individual joints in Chapter 18, The Musculoskeletal System.

Degenerative joint changes are found in *osteoarthritis;* joint inflammation in *rheumatoid* or *gouty arthritis*

See Chapter 18, The Musculoskeletal System; see Tables 18-1 to 18-8, pp. 584–592.

Nervous System and Mental Status.   As with the musculoskeletal examination, begin your evaluation of the nervous system with the 10-Minute Geriatric Screener (pp. 853–854).

Pursue further examination if you note any deficits. Focus especially on memory and affect. Screen for depression using the Geriatric Depression Scale and utilize the Mini-Cog (Table 24-3, p. 877) when screening for dementia.

Learn to distinguish delirium from depression and dementia (see Table 24-2, p. 876). Careful search for underlying causes is warranted.[65]

Also pay close attention to gait and balance, particularly standing balance; timed 8-foot walk; stride characteristics including: width, pace, and length of stride, and ease of turning.

Note that standard neuromuscular tests have not been shown to predict impairments in mobility.[69] Further, although neurologic abnormalities are common in the older population, their prevalence without identifiable disease increases with age, ranging from 30% to 50%.[70] Examples of age related abnormalities include: unequal pupil size, decreased arm swing and spontaneous movements, increased leg rigidity and abnormal gait, presence of the snout and grasp reflexes, and decreased toe vibratory sense.

Search for evidence of tremor, rigidity, bradykinesia, micrographia, shuffling gait, difficulty turning in bed, opening jars, or rising from a chair.

In summary, the assessment of the older adult does not follow the traditional format of the history and physical examination. It calls for enhanced techniques of interviewing, special emphasis on daily function and key topics related to elder health, and a focus on functional assessment during the physical examination.

Abnormalities of gait and balance, especially widening of the base, slowing and lengthening of stride, and difficulty turning, are correlated with risk for falls.[66–68]

The snout reflex is a pursing of the lips or pouting after tapping of the closed lips near the midline. If present, then involvement of the frontal lobe, such as dementia, or closed head injury is suspected.

These findings are seen in *Parkinson disease,* found in 1% of adults 65 years or older and 2% of those 85 years or older.[71,72] Tremor is of slow frequency and occurs at rest, with a "pill-rolling" quality. It is aggravated by stress and inhibited during sleep or movement. *Essential tremor* if bilateral and symmetric, with positive family history, and if diminished by alcohol.

Persistent blinking after tap on forehead and difficulty walking heel-to-toe in *Parkinson disease* are also more common.

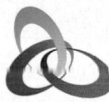

RECORDING YOUR FINDINGS

As you read through this physical examination, notice some atypical findings. Interpret these findings in the context of all you have learned about the examination of the older adult.

RECORDING THE PHYSICAL EXAMINATION— THE OLDER ADULT

> Mr. J, 82 year old appears healthy but overweight, with positive muscle bulk. He is alert and interactive, with recall of his life history. Accompanied by his son.
>
> **Vital Signs**
> Ht 5'10" (178 cm). Wt (dressed) 208 lbs (92 kg). Body mass index (BMI) 31. BP 145/88 right arm, supine; 154/94 left arm, supine. Orthostatic BP without changes. Heart rate (HR) 98 and regular. Respiratory rate (RR) 18, regular. Temperature (oral) 98.6°F.
>
> *(continued)*

RECORDING THE PHYSICAL EXAMINATION—
THE OLDER ADULT (continued)

10-Minute Geriatric Screener
(See pp. 853–854)

Vision. Patient reports difficulty reading. Visual acuity 20/40 on Snellen chart with glasses.

Needs further evaluation for glasses and possibly hearing aid

Hearing. Whisper test R intact, L on 3rd attempt. Cannot hear 1,000 or 2,000 Hz with audioscope in either ear.

Leg Mobility. Can walk 20 feet briskly, turn, walk back to chair, and sit down in 14 seconds.

Urinary Incontinence. Has lost urine and gotten wet on 20 separate days in the past 2 months.

Needs further evaluation for incontinence, including "DIAPERS" assessment (see p. 858), referral for prostate examination, and postvoid residual, which is normally ≤50 mL (requires bladder catheterization)

Nutrition. Has lost 15 lbs over the past 6 months without trying.

Needs nutritional screen, p. 855

Memory. Can remember three items after 1 minute.

Depression. Does not often feel sad or depressed.

Physical Disability. Walks fast but cannot ride a bicycle (never learned). Does moderate but not heavy work around the house. Shops for groceries or clothes. Goes to places out of walking distance (son drives). Bathes each day without difficulty. Dresses independently, including buttons, zippers, and ties shoes.

Consider exercise regimen with strength training

Physical Examination
Skin, Hair, Nails. Tan, warm and moist. 1.5 cm solar lentigo above R eyebrow. Gray hair thinning at crown, dry with moderate amount of flakes, gray hairs evenly distributed over body. Nails without clubbing or cyanosis, slightly yellow and thick.

Head, Eyes, Ears, Nose, Throat (HEENT). Scalp without lesions. Skull normocephalic/atraumatic. Eyes-symmetrical, lids- close BL, no ptosis or edema, conjunctiva pink, sclera muddy, iris brown. Lacrimal apparatus moist without additional drainage PERRLA 2 mm constricting to 1 mm BL. EOMs intact. Disc margins sharp, without hemorrhages or exudates. Mild arteriolar narrowing. Snellen with corrective glasses on 20/40 OD, OS, OU and 20/70 without correction. Ears- auricles and pinna without lumps, lesions or tenderness, (TMs) with cone of light, minimal tan, sticky cerumen BL. Weber midline, AC ≥ BC, whisper test R intact, L on 3rd attempt. Nose- patent BL, mucosa and turbinates pink. No odor or fronal or maxillary sinus tenderness, exudates, polyps or bleeding. Septum midline. Lips- pink, moist, without lesions or ulcerations. Mouth- mucosa pink, moist, without lesions or bleeding. Dentition fair, some loose teeth. Caries present. Tongue midline, slight beefy redness, no lesions. Uvula midline. Pharynx without exudates.

(continued)

RECORDING THE PHYSICAL EXAMINATION—THE OLDER ADULT (continued)

Neck. Supple. Trachea midline. Thyroid lobes slightly enlarged, no nodules.

Lymph Nodes. No preauricular, postauricular, occipital, tonsillar, sub-mandibular, submental, superficial, posterior cervical, deep cervical chain, supraclavicular, cervical, axillary, epitrochlear, or inguinal lymph nodes.

Thorax and Lungs. Mild kyphosis A&P thorax symmetric without retractions or bulging. No tenderness, crepitus or lesions. Positive tactile fremitus. Lungs resonant throughout. Equal expansion. Diaphragmatic excursion descends 4 cm BL. Vesicular breath sounds in all fields. No adventitious sounds.

Cardiovascular. No visible pulsations. Carotid upstrokes brisk, without bruits. PMI 2 cm in diameter, tapping, in the 5th ICS L MCL. II/VI harsh holosystolic murmur at the apex, radiating to the axilla. No S_3, S_4, or other murmurs.

Abdomen. Protuberant, symmetric without lesions, peristalsis, pulsations or increased vasculature, Soft, nontender. No masses or hepatosplenomegaly. Liver span 7 cm in R MCL; edge smooth and palpable. No CVAT. Active bowel sounds, no aortic, renal or iliac bruits.

Genitourinary. Circumcised male. No penile lesions, lumps, tenderness or redness. Testes descended BL, smooth.

Extremities. Upper and lower - warm, without edema, bruising, pain, or increased vascularity.

Peripheral Vascular. Bilateral (BL) radial, brachial, femoral, popliteal, dorsalis pedis, and posterior tibial pulses 2+ and symmetric.

Musculoskeletal. Mild degenerative changes in spine and at the knees, with quadriceps wasting. FROM in all joints. Motor: Decreased quadriceps bulk. Tone intact. Strength 4/5 throughout.

Neurologic. Ox3, dressed appropriately for the weather, good spirits. Mini-Mental Status exam: score 29. Cranial Nerves II–XII intact. BL RAMs, finger-to-nose sequence intact. Gait with widened base. Sensation intact to pinprick, light touch, position, and vibration (upper/lower extremities intact). Romberg negative. BL biceps, triceps, brachioradialis, knee, and ankle reflexes 2+ and symmetric, with plantar response.

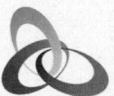

HEALTH PROMOTION AND COUNSELING

Important Topics for Health Promotion and Counseling in the Older Adult

- Screening
- Cancer screening
- Immunizations
- Household safety
- Fall assessment
- Driving safety
- Exercise
- Depression
- Dementia
- Elder mistreatment
- Advanced directive and palliative care

Screening. As the life span for older adults extends into the 80s and beyond, new issues for screening emerge. Given the heterogeneity of the aging population, guiding principles for deciding who might benefit from screening and when screening might be stopped are helpful, especially because evidence for screening decisions is not always available. In general, base screening decisions on each older person's particular circumstances, rather than age alone. Three factors should be considered: life expectancy, time interval until benefit from screening accrues, and patient preference.[73] The American Geriatrics Society recommends that if life expectancy is short, give priority to treatment that will benefit the patient in the time that remains. Consider deferring screening if it places added burdens on the older adult with multiple medical problems, a shortened life expectancy, or dementia. Tests that help with prognosis and planning, however, are still warranted even if the patient would not pursue treatment.[74]

Vision and Hearing. Screening for age-related changes in *vision* and *hearing* is important in helping older adults maintain optimal function, and is included in the 10-Minute Geriatric Screener.[75] Test *vision* objectively using an eye chart. Asking the patient about any *hearing* loss may be adequate, followed by the whisper test and more formal testing if indicated.

See 10-Minute Geriatric Screener, pp. 853–854.

See Chapter 10, The Head and Neck, techniques for assessing hearing, pp. 225–227.

Cancer Screening. Cancer screening for selected conditions can be controversial because of limited evidence supporting its use for adults older than 70 to 80 years. The American Geriatrics Society recommends annual or biennial mammography for breast cancer screening up to age 75 years, then every 2 to 3 years if life expectancy remains more than 4 years. Although the prevalence of cervical cancer has declined in the United States, 40% to 50% of deaths from cervical cancer are in women older than 65 years. Provide Pap smears every 1 to 3 years until age 65 to 70 years when there is no history of cervical pathology. Colonoscopy is recommended for colon cancer screening every 10 years beginning at 50 years. This examination is difficult for many older patients, who may decline despite encouragement.

Immunizations. Advise your patients to have the pneumococcal vaccine, the influenza vaccine, and the zoster vaccine.[76,77]

See also Chapter 13, Respiratory System, p. 323.

- *Influenza vaccine.* The following groups should receive the *influenza vaccine* each year: people 50 years or older; any older adult with chronic disorders of the cardiovascular or pulmonary systems, diabetes, renal or hepatic dysfunction, immunosuppression, or HIV/AIDS; residents and health care personnel of nursing homes and long-term care facilities; caregivers of children; or anyone requesting the vaccination.[78]

- *Pneumococcal vaccine.* The *pneumococcal vaccine* should be given every 5 years to adults 65 years or older with chronic disorders of the cardiovascular or pulmonary systems, diabetes, renal or hepatic dysfunction, asplenia, chronic alcoholism, immunosuppression, cerebrospinal fluid leak, or HIV/AIDS; residents of nursing homes or long-term care facilities; and Alaska Natives and selected American Indian populations, such as the Navajo and Apache.

● *Zoster vaccine. Zoster vaccine* is recommended at age 60 years, regardless of whether the patient reports a prior episode of herpes zoster. Studies show that vaccination reduces incidence of herpes zoster by approximately 50% and incidence of postherpetic neuralgia by more than 65%.[79]

Household Safety. Emergency room visits for household injuries are increasing at a rapid rate, particularly for adults older than 75 years. In a special report in 2002, the U.S. Consumer Product Safety Commission estimated that almost 1.5 million adults older than 65 years were treated for injuries related to household products, including more than 60% of those with falls.[80] ER visits and deaths were most likely to involve yard and garden equipment, ladders and stepstools, personal use items like hair dryers and flammable clothing, and bathroom and sports injuries. Encourage older adults to adopt corrective measures for poor lighting, chairs at awkward heights, slippery or irregular surfaces, and environmental hazards.

See also Fall Assessment, below.

HOME SAFETY TIPS FOR OLDER ADULTS

- Handrails on both sides of any stairway
- Well-lit stairways, paths, and walkways
- Rugs secured by nonslip backing or adhesive tape
- Removal of clutter or electric cords
- Grab bars and nonslip mat or safety strips in the bath or shower
- Carbon monoxide and smoke alarms with a plan for escaping

Fall Assessment. A veritable avalanche of evidence links falls to morbidity and mortality in our older population. Each year approximately 35% to 40% of healthy community-dwelling older adults experience falls. Incidence rates in nursing homes and hospitals are almost three times higher, with related injuries in approximately 25%. Loss of confidence from fear of falling and postfall anxiety further impair full recovery.[37,38]

Fall-related assessments should include details about the how the fall occurred, especially from witnesses, and identification of risk factors, medical comorbidities, functional status, and environmental risks—coupled with interventions for prevention.[81] Gait velocity is also emerging as a significant predictor of falls and related adverse events.[82] The Heinrich II Fall Risk Model tool is able to screen for those at risk of falling. Effective single interventions include gait and balance training and exercise to strengthen muscles, reduction of home hazards, discontinuation of psychotropic medication, and multifactorial assessment with targeted interventions. Additional useful strategies include addressing change in postural blood pressure, attention to concurrent acute illness, reduction in medications to fewer than four, detection of sensory neuropathy and impairment of proprioception, investigation of any episodes of syncope, patient and family education, treatment of osteoporosis, and possible use of hip protectors.[83]

Hendrich II Fall Risk Model®

Confusion Disorientation Impulsivity	4	
Symptomatic Depression	2	
Altered Elimination	1	
Dizziness Vertigo	1	
Male Gender	1	
Any Administered Antiepileptics	2	
Any Administered Benzodiazepines	1	
Get Up & Go Test		
Ability to rise in a single movement- No Loss of Balance with Steps	0	
Pushes up, successful in one attempt	1	
Multiple attempts, but successful	3	
Unable to rise without assistance during test (OR if a medical order states the same and/or complete bed rest is ordered) *If unable to assess, document this on the patient chart with the date and time	4	

A Score of 5 or Greater = High Risk   Total Score

Driving Safety. Driving symbolizes independence, and losing this is difficult. It is not a subject easily broached by the health care provider or the family, and determining when someone should stop driving is not based on age but on one's ability. As people age, their vision, hearing, strength, and cognitive skills may diminish, and it is important to evaluate each person individually. Observation of the person's driving while noting deficiencies is important. The family may report unexplained vehicle damage, and suggesting a driving evaluation from a driving specialist is warranted. Ensure there is an alternative manner of transportation available if the person gives up driving so as not to isolate him or her.

Exercise. Recommend regular aerobic exercise to improve strength and aerobic capacity, increase physiologic reserve, improve energy level for doing ADLs, and slow onset of disability.

The American College of Sports Medicine and the American Heart Association Recommendations on Physical Activity and Public Health for Older Adults advocate a physically active lifestyle and target intensity of aerobic activity based on the older adult's degree of aerobic fitness, activities that increase muscle strength and flexibility, balance exercises for those at risk of falls, and therapeutic plans that integrate both treatment and prevention, including at the community level. Older adults are advised to perform moderate-intensity aerobic activities for at least 30 minutes 5 days each week, or vigorous-intensity activity for at least 20 minutes 3 days each week.[84]

Depression. *Depression* affects 10% of older adults but is both underdiagnosed and undertreated.[85] A positive response to asking "Do you often feel sad or depressed?" is approximately 80% sensitive and specific and should prompt further investigation, possibly with the Geriatric Depression Scale. Depressed men older than 65 years have the highest incidence of suicide and require careful assessment and evaluation.

See Chapter 19, Mental Status, Depression, p. 610.

Dementia and Mild Cognitive Impairment. *Dementia*, "an acquired syndrome of decline in memory and at least one other cognitive domain such as language, visuospatial, or executive function sufficient to interfere with social or occupational functioning in an alert person," affects 11% of Americans older than 65 years, or roughly 4.5 million people.[86,87] Prominent features include short- and long-term memory deficits and impaired judgment. Thought processes are impoverished; speech may be hesitant as a result of difficulty in finding words. Loss of orientation to place may make navigating by foot or car problematic or even dangerous. Most dementias represent Alzheimer disease (50% to 85%) or vascular multi-infarct dementia (10% to 20%). Watch for Alzheimer disease in patients with a positive family history, because their risk is three times higher than the risk in the general population.

See Table 24-2, Delirium and Dementia, p. 876, and Table 24-3, Screening for Dementia: The Mini-Cog, p. 877.

Dementia often has a slow, insidious onset and may escape detection by both families and clinicians, especially in the early stages of *mild cognitive impairment (MCI)*. MCI refers to a milder syndrome of cognitive loss compared with dementia; specifically, the impairment is not of such magnitude as to interfere with social or vocational function. The person may or may not complain of cognitive deterioration, but standardized cognitive testing reveals reasonable evidence of significant decline in at least one cognitive domain. When the domain affected is memory, the disorder is called *amnestic MCI;* when the domain affected is not memory but language or visuospatial function, for example, the disorder is called *nonamnestic MCI.* A significant percentage, but not all, of these people progress to a clinical diagnosis of Alzheimer disease. There are syndromes of even milder cognitive change later in the life cycle, such as *age-associated cognitive impairment (AACI).* The clinical significance of AACI and related mild cognitive loss syndromes is not yet known. Current research seeks to identify the clinical features of these various syndromes.[88–93]

In Alzheimer dementia, look for amnestic memory impairment, deterioration of language, and visuospatial deficits. Initial loss of independent activities of daily living (IADLs) such as check writing and use of public transportation progresses to eventual loss of basic activities like eating and grooming. Mood change and apathy often appear early; psychosis and agitation emerge in the later stages.[87] Watch for family complaints of new or unusual behaviors. Testing with the Mini-Mental State Examination may be helpful, although level of education and cultural variables such as language may affect scores. If you identify cognitive changes, investigate contributing factors such as medications, depression, metabolic abnormalities, or other medical and psychiatric conditions. In patients with dementia, counsel families about the potential for disruptive behavior, accidents, falls, and termination of driving privileges. Foster discussion of legal arrangements such as power of attorney and advance directives while the patient can still contribute to decision making.

Elder Mistreatment.   Finally, consider screening all older patients for possible *elder mistreatment,* which includes abuse, neglect, exploitation, and abandonment. Depression, dementia, and malnutrition are independent risk factors. Prevalence of elder mistreatment is approximately 1% to 5% of the older population; however, that statistic is based solely on self-reported cases of elder mistreatment, and many more cases may remain undetected. Self-neglect is a growing national concern and represents more than 50% of adult protective service referrals.[94] Although several screening instruments are available, no single instrument has emerged for rapid yet accurate assessment and diagnosis of these important problems.[94–96]

Advance Directives and Palliative Care.   Many older patients are interested in expressing their wishes about end-of-life decisions and would like providers to initiate these discussions before any serious illness develops.[97] Advance care planning involves several tasks—providing information, invoking the patient's preferences, identifying proxy decision makers, and conveying empathy and support. Use clear and simple language. Often begin the discussion by relating these decisions to a current illness or experiences with relatives or friends. Ask about preferences relating to written "Do Not Resuscitate" orders specifying life support measures "if the heart

See also Chapter 3, The Patient With Altered Capacity, pp. 52–53, and Death and the Dying Patient, pp. 87–88.

or lungs were to stop or give out." Second, encourage the patient to establish in writing a health care proxy or durable power of attorney for health care, "someone who can make decisions reflecting your wishes in case of confusion or emergency." These conversations, although difficult at first, convey your respect and concern for patients and help them and their families prepare openly and in advance for a peaceful death.[98] It is preferable to hold these discussions outside a stressful environment if possible.

For patients with advanced or terminal illnesses, include these discussions in an overall plan for palliative care. The goal of palliative care is "to relieve suffering and improve the quality of life for patients with advanced illnesses and their families through specific knowledge and skills, including communication with patients and family members; management of pain and other symptoms; psychosocial, spiritual, and bereavement support; and coordination of an array of medical and social services."[99] To ease patient and family distress, accent your communication skills: make good eye contact; ask open-ended questions; respond to anxiety, depression, or changes in the patient's affect; and show empathy.

TABLE
24-1

Minimum Geriatric Competencies*

Medication Management

1 Explain impact of age-related changes on drug selection and dose based on knowledge of age-related changes in renal and hepatic function, body composition, and central nervous system sensitivity.
2 Identify medications, including: anticholinergic, psychoactive, anticoagulant, analgesic, hypoglycemic, and cardiovascular drugs, that should be avoided or used with caution in older adults and explain the potential problems associated with each.
3 Document a patient's complete medication list, including prescribed, herbal, and over-the-counter medications, and for each medication provide the dose, frequency, indication, benefit, side effects, and an assessment of adherence.

Cognitive and Behavioral Disorders

4 Define and distinguish among the clinical presentations of delirium, dementia, and depression.
5 Formulate a differential diagnosis and implement initial evaluation in a patient who exhibits cognitive impairment.
6 Urgently initiate a diagnostic workup to determine the root cause (etiology) of delirium in an older patient.
7 Perform and interpret a cognitive assessment in older patients for whom there are concerns regarding memory or function.
8 Develop an evaluation and nonpharmacologic management plan for agitated, demented, or delirious patients.

Self-Care Capacity

9 Assess and describe baseline and current functional abilities (instrumental activities of daily living, activities of daily living, and special senses) in an older patient by collecting historical data from multiple sources and performing a confirmatory physical examination.
10 Develop a preliminary management plan for patients presenting with functional deficits, including adaptive interventions and involvement of interdisciplinary team members from appropriate disciplines, such as: social work, nursing, rehabilitation, nutrition, and pharmacy.
11 Identify and assess safety risks in the home environment, and make recommendations to mitigate these.

Falls, Balance, Gait Disorders

12 Ask all patients older than 65 years of age, or their caregivers, about falls in the last year; watch the patient rise from a chair and walk (or transfer); and then record and interpret the findings.
13 For a patient who has fallen, construct a differential diagnosis and evaluation plan that addresses the multiple etiologies identified by history, physical examination, and functional assessment.

Health Care Planning and Promotion

14 Define and differentiate among types of code status, health care proxies, and advanced directives in the site where one is training.
15 Accurately identify clinical situations where life expectancy, functional status, patient preference, or goals of care should override standard recommendations for screening tests in older adults.
16 Accurately identify clinical situations where life expectancy, functional status, patient preference, or goals of care should override standard recommendations for treatment in older adults.

Atypical Presentation of Disease

17 Identify at least three physiologic changes of aging for each organ system and their impact on the patient, including their contribution to homeostenosis (the age-related narrowing or homeostatic reserve mechanisms).
18 Generate a differential diagnosis based on recognition of the unique presentations of common conditions in older adults, including acute coronary syndrome, dehydration, urinary tract infection, acute abdomen, and pneumonia.

Palliative Care

19 Assess and provide initial management of pain and key nonpain symptoms based on the patient's goals of care.
20 Identify the psychological, social, and spiritual needs of patients with advanced illness and their family members, and link these identified needs with the appropriate interdisciplinary team members.
21 Present palliative care (including hospice) as a positive, active treatment option for a patient with advanced disease.

Hospital Care for Elders

22 Identify potential hazards of hospitalization for all older adult patients (including immobility, delirium, medication side effects, malnutrition, pressure ulcers, procedures, peri- and postoperative periods, and hospital-acquired infections) and identify potential prevention strategies.
23 Explain the risks, indications, alternatives, and contraindications for indwelling (Foley) catheter use in the older adult patient.
24 Explain the risks, indications, alternatives, and contraindications for physical and pharmacologic restraint use.
25 Communicate the key components of a safe discharge plan (e.g., accurate medication list, plan for follow-up), including comparing/contrasting potential sites for discharge.
26 Conduct a surveillance examination of areas of the skin at high risk for pressure ulcers and describe existing ulcers.

(Source: Association of American Medical Colleges/John A. Hartford Foundation, Inc. A Consensus Conference on Competencies in Geriatrics Education, October 5, 2007.)

Delirium and Dementia

Delirium and dementia are common. They each affect multiple aspects of mental status and have many possible causes. Some clinical features and their effects on mental status are compared below. Note: A delirium may be superimposed on dementia.

	Delirium	**Dementia**
Clinical Features		
Onset	Acute	Insidious
Course	Fluctuating, with lucid intervals; worse at night	Slowly progressive
Duration	Hours to weeks	Months to years
Sleep/Wake Cycle	Always disrupted	Sleep fragmented
General Medical Illness or Drug Toxicity	Either or both present	Often absent, especially in Alzheimer disease
Mental Status		
Level of Consciousness	Disturbed. Person less clearly aware of the environment and less able to focus, sustain, or shift attention	Usually normal until late in the course of the illness
Behavior	Activity often abnormally decreased (somnolence) or increased (agitation, hypervigilance)	Normal to slow; may become inappropriate
Speech	May be hesitant, slow or rapid, incoherent	Difficulty in finding words, aphasia
Mood	Fluctuating, labile, from fearful or irritable to normal or depressed	Often flat, depressed
Thought Processes	Disorganized, may be incoherent	Impoverished. Speech gives little information.
Thought Content	Delusions common, often transient	Delusions may occur.
Perceptions	Illusions, hallucinations, most often visual	Hallucinations may occur.
Judgment	Impaired, often to a varying degree	Increasingly impaired over the course of the illness
Orientation	Usually disoriented, especially for time. A known place may seem unfamiliar.	Fairly well maintained, but becomes impaired in the later stages of illness
Attention	Fluctuates. Person easily distracted, unable to concentrate on selected tasks	Usually unaffected until late in the illness
Memory	Immediate and recent memory impaired	Recent memory and new learning especially impaired
Examples of Cause	Infection (lungs, urine, skin) Medications (anticholinergics, CNS depressants) Environment (hospital)	*Reversible:* Vitamin B$_{12}$ and folate deficiency Thyroid disorders Substance abuse *Irreversible:* Alzheimer, Parkinson and Huntington disease, vascular dementia (from multiple infarcts), dementia due to head trauma

TABLE
24-3

Screening for Dementia: The Mini-Cog

Administration

The test is administered as follows:

1. Instruct the patient to listen carefully to and remember 3 unrelated words and then to repeat the words.

2. Instruct the patient to draw the face of a clock, either on a blank sheet of paper or on a sheet with the clock circle already drawn on the page. After the patient puts the numbers on the clock face, ask him or her to draw the hands of the clock to read a specific time.

3. Ask the patient to repeat the 3 previously stated words.

Scoring

Give 1 point for each recalled word after the clock drawing test (CDT) distractor.
Patients recalling none of the three words are classified as demented (Score = 0).
Patients recalling all three words are classified as nondemented (Score = 3).
Patients with intermediate word recall of 1–2 words are classified based on the CDT (Abnormal = demented; Normal = nondemented).

Note: The CDT is considered normal if all numbers are present in the correct sequence and position, and the hands readably display the requested time.

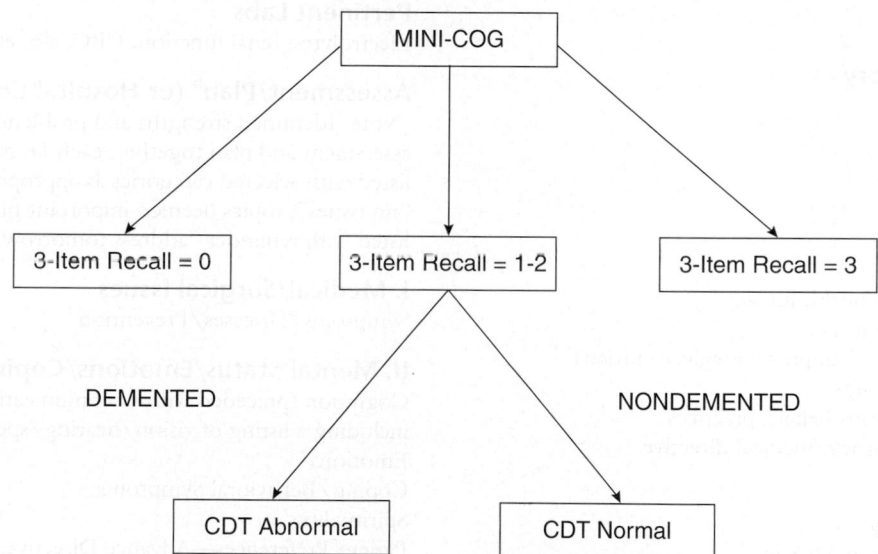

(From Borson S, Scanlan J, Brush M, et al. The Mini-Cog: a cognitive 'vital signs' measure for dementia screening in multi-lingual elderly. Int J Geriatr Psychiatry 15(11):1021–1027, 2000. Copyright John Wiley & Sons Limited. Reproduced with permission.)

TABLE
24-4

Caring for Older Adults: The Siebens Domain Management Model

One framework to guide care of older adults is the Siebens Domain Management Model.[a,b] With practicality as a goal, the model organizes a patient's health-related problems and strengths into four domains: I. Medical/Surgical Issues; II. Mental Status/Emotions/Coping; III. Physical Function; and IV. Living Environment. Using these domain headings helps make care planning and documentation efficient and comprehensive and promotes interdisciplinary teamwork.

Format for Provider History & Physical Reports
(Modify as needed for Follow-Up Visits)
Revised with Siebens Domain Management Model (SDMM)[a]

Subjective[b]

Chief Concern or Reason for Visit (follow-up)

History of Present Illness
Symptoms/Workups to date/Patient's Perspective/Worries

Medications

Allergies

Past Medical History
Health maintenance

Family History

Social History
Education/functional health literacy
Marital status, Children, Pets
Nature of relationships (support/caregiver burden)
Alcohol/Tobacco/Drugs
Spirituality and Religious beliefs, practices
Health Power of Attorney/medical directive

Functional History
Prior level of function in Mobility,
Self-care,
Medication mgmt, paying bills
Work/Leisure/Fun activities

Review of Systems
Inclusive of sexuality

Objective[b]

Pertinent Physical Exam
Vital Signs and pertinent organ systems

Cognition, Affect
Mobility—moving in bed, getting out of bed or a chair, walking, etc.

Pertinent Labs
Electrolytes, renal function, CBC, alb, etc.

Assessment/Plan[b] (or Hospital Course)
(Note: Identified strengths and problems are best listed with assessment and plan together; each Domain must, ideally, be listed with selected categories as appropriate or else described as "no issues"; topics deemed important but not assessed can be listed with reminder "address tomorrow/next visit.")

I. Medical/Surgical Issues
Symptoms/Diseases/Prevention

II. Mental Status/Emotions/Coping
Cognition (preceded with Communication if any issues including a listing of vision/hearing/speech/language issues)
Emotions
Coping/Behavioral Symptoms
Spirituality
Patient Preferences—Advance Directives

III. Physical Function
Basic ADLs (self care—dressing, bathing, home mobility, etc.)
Instrumental ADLs (meals, medication and money management, etc.)
Advanced ADLs—(sexuality, work, parenting, leisure/fun, driving, general physical activity/exercise, etc.)

IV. Living Environment
A. Physical (home, adaptations, community)
B. Social (family supports/coping, social interactions, etc.)
C. Financial (health insurance, personal income, etc.) & Community Resources

---

[a]Siebens H. Applying the Domain Management Model in Treating Patients with Chronic Diseases Jt. Comm J Qual Improvement 2001;27:302–314.
Siebens H. Proposing a Practical Clinical Model. Top Stroke Rehabil 2011;18:60–65.
[b]Note that information is also organized in the familiar SOAP format—Subjective, Objective, Assessment, Plan.
© Hilary C. Siebens, MD, 2005.
Also available at: www.siebenspcc.com as SDMM CCard

BIBLIOGRAPHY

CITATIONS

1. Administration on Aging, Department of Health and Human Services. Statistics: A Profile on Older Americans.http://www.aoa.gov/AoARoot/Aging_Statistics/index.aspx. Accessed May 21, 2011.

2. Fries JF. Measuring and monitoring success in compressing morbidity. Ann Intern Med Suppl 139(5):455, 2003.

3. Bodenheimer T, Wagner EH, Grumbach K. Improving primary care for patients with chronic illness. JAMA 288(14):1775–1779, 2002.

4. Geriatrics Interdisciplinary Advisory Group, American Geriatrics Society. Interdisciplinary care for older adults with complex needs: American Geriatrics Society Position Statement. J Am Geriatr Soc 54(5):849–852, 2006.

5. Perls TT. Understanding the determinants of exceptional longevity. Ann Intern Med Suppl 139(5):445, 2003.

6. Perls TT, Kunkel LM, Puca AA. The genetics of exceptional human longevity. J Am Geriatr Soc 50:359–368, 2002.

7. Rowe JW, Kahn RL. Human aging: usual and successful. Science 237:143–149, 1987.

8. Taffet GE. Physiology of aging. In: Cassel CK, Leipzig RM, Cohen HJ, et al, eds. Geriatric Medicine, 4th ed. New York: Springer, 2003:27–36.

9. Mulligan T, Saddiqi W. Changes in male sexuality. In: Cassel CK, Leipzig RM, Cohen HJ, et al, eds. Geriatric Medicine, 4th ed. New York: Springer, 2003:719–726.

10. DuBeau CE. Benign prostatic hyperplasia. In: Cassel CK, Leipzig RM, Cohen HJ, et al, eds. Geriatric Medicine, 4th ed. New York: Springer, 2003:755–768.

11. Kaiser FE. Sexual function and the older woman. In: Cassel CK, Leipzig RM, Cohen HJ, et al, eds. Geriatric Medicine, 4th ed. New York: Springer, 2003:727–736.

12. Tangarorang GL, Kerins GJ, Besdine RW. Clinical approach to the older patient: an overview. In: Cassel CK, Leipzig RM, Cohen HJ, et al, eds. Geriatric Medicine, 4th ed. New York: Springer, 2003:149–162.

13. Bayer AJ, Chadna JS, Farag RR, et al. Changing presentation of myocardial infarction with increasing old age. J Am Geriatr Soc 34:263–266, 1986.

14. Trivalle C, Doucet J, Chassagrie P, et al. Differences in the signs and symptoms of hyperthyroidism in older and younger patients. J Am Geriatr Soc 44:50–53, 1996.

15. Doucet J, Trivalle C, Chassagrie P, et al. Does age play a role in clinical presentation of hypothyroidism? J Am Geriatr Soc 42:984–986, 1994.

16. Cigolle CT, Langa KM, Kabeto MU, et al. Geriatric conditions and disability: the health and retirement study. Ann Intern Med 147(3):156–164, 2007.

17. Tinetti ME, Williams CS, Gill TM. Dizziness among older adults: a possible geriatric syndrome. Ann Intern Med 132(5):337–344, 2000.

18. Fried LP, Sotrer DJ, King DE, et al. Diagnosis of illness presentation in the elderly. J Am Geriatr Soc 39:117–123, 1991.

19. Davis PB, Robins LN. History-taking in the elderly with and without cognitive impairment. J Am Geriatr Soc 37:249–255, 1989.

20. Ferraro KF, Su YP. Physician-evaluated and self-reported morbidity for predicting disability. Am J Public Health 90(1):103–108, 2000.

21. Kuczmarski MF, Kuczmarski RJ, Najjar M. Effects of age on validity of self-reported height, weight and body mass index: findings from the third National Health and Nutrition Examination Survey, 1988–1994. J Am Diet Assoc 101(1):28–34, 2001.

22. Lagaay AM, van der Meij JC, Hijmans W. Validation of medical history taking as part of a population based survey in subjects aged 85 and over. BMJ 304:1091–1092, 1992.

23. Kobylarz FA, Heath JM, Lide RC. The ETHNIC(S) mnemonic: a clinical tool for ethnogeriatric education. J Am Geriatr Soc 50(9):1582–1589, 2002.

24. United States Census 2010: 2010 Census Demographic Profiles. Washington D.C. Available at: http://2010.census.gov/2010census/data/index.php. Accessed May 22, 2011.

25. Xakellis G, Brangman SA, Ladson H, et al. Curricular framework: core competencies in multicultural geriatric care. J Am Geriatr Soc 52(1):137–142, 2004.

26. Goldstein MZ, Griswold K. Practical geriatrics: cultural sensitivity and aging. Psychiatric Serv 49:769–771, 1998.

27. Lee SJ, Moody-Ayers SY, Landfeld CS, et al. The relationship between self-rated health and mortality in older black and white Americans. J Am Geriatr Soc 55(10):1624–1629, 2007.

28. Sudore RL, Mehta KM, Simonsick EM, et al. Limited literacy in older people and disparities in health and healthcare access. J Am Geriatr Soc 54(5):770–776, 2006.

29. Fick DM, Cooper JW, Wade WE, et al. Updating the Beers criteria for potentially inappropriate medication use in older adults: results of a US consensus panel of experts. Arch Intern Med 163:2716–2724, 2003.

30. Reuben DB, Herr KA, Pacala JT, et al. Geriatrics at Your Fingertips, 6th ed. Malden, MA: Blackwell Science, Inc., for the American Geriatrics Society, 2004:9–12.

31. The Mini Nutritional Assessment (MNA): The Profile. Nestlé Research Center, Lausanne, Switzerland. Available at: http://www.mna-elderly.com/the_problem_malnutrition.html Accessed May 22, 2011.

32. Corti MC, Guralnik JM, Salive ME, et al. Serum albumin level and physical disability as predictors of mortality in older persons. JAMA 272(13):1036–1042, 1994.

33. Ferrell BA. Acute and chronic pain. In: Cassel CK, Leipzig RM, Cohen HJ, et al, eds. Geriatric Medicine, 4th ed. New York: Springer, 2003:323–342.

34. American Geriatrics Society Panel on Persistent Pain in Older Persons. Pharmacological Management of Persistent Pain in Older Persons. American Geriatrics Society. J Am Geriatr Soc 2009 (in press). Available at: http://www.americangeriatrics.org/health_care_professionals/clinical_practice/clinical_guidelines_recommendations/persistent_pain_executive_summary Accessed May 23, 2011.

35. Charlton JE, ed. Core Curriculum for Professional Education in Pain, 3rd ed. Seattle: International Association for the Study of Pain, 2005. Available at: http//www.iasp-pain.org/. Accessed May 23, 2011.

36. American Medical Association. Pain Management Module 5: Assessing and Treating Pain in Older Adults. Available at: http://www.ama-cmeonline.com/pain_mgmt/module05/index.htm. Accessed May 23, 2011.

37. Resnick NM. Urinary incontinence. In: Cassel CK, Leipzig RM, Cohen HJ, et al, eds. Geriatric Medicine, 4th ed. New York: Springer, 2003:931–956.

38. Dowling-Castronovo A, Bradway C. Nursing standard of practice protocol: urinary incontinence (UI) in older adults admitted to acute care. Updated January 2008 Available at: http://consultgerirn.org/topics/urinary_incontinence/want_to_know_more. Accessed May 23, 2011.

39. Jones TV, Lindsey BA, Yount P, et al. Alcoholism screening questionnaires: are they valid in elderly medical outpatients? J Gen Intern Med 8(12):674–678, 1993.

40. Callahan CM, Tierney WM. Health services use and mortality among older primary care patients with alcoholism. J Am Geriatr Soc 43(12):1378–1383, 1995.

41. Naegle M. Alcohol use screening and assessment for older adults best practices in care to the older adult from the Hartford Institute for Geriatric Nursing. Available at: http://consultgerirn.org/topics/urinary_incontinence/want_to_know_more. Accessed May 23, 2011.

42. Borson S, Scanlan J, Brush M, et al. The Mini-Cog: a cognitive "vital signs" measure for dementia screening in multi-lingual elderly. Int J Geriatric Psychiatry 15(11):1021–1027, 2000.

43. Borson S, Scanlan JM, Chen P, et al. The Mini-Cog as a screen for dementia: validation in a population-based sample. J Am Geriatr Soc 51(10):1451–1454, 2003.

44. Bulpitt CJ, Beckett NS, Cooke J, et al. Results of the pilot study for the hypertension in the very elderly trial. J Hypertens 21(12):2409–2417, 2003.

45. Oates DJ, Berlowitz DR, Glickman ME, et al. Blood pressure and survival in the oldest old. J Am Geriatr Soc 55(3):383–388, 2007

46. Lloyd-Jones DM, Evans JC, Levy D. Hypertension in adults across the age spectrum: current outcomes and control in the community. JAMA 294(4):466–472, 2005.

47. Bobrie G, Genes N, Vaur L, et al. Is "isolated home" hypertension as opposed to "isolated office" hypertension a sign of greater cardiovascular risk? Arch Intern Med 161(18):2205–2211, 2001.

48. Chaudhry SI, Krumholz HM, Foody JM. Systolic hypertension in older persons. JAMA 292(9):1074–1080, 2004.

49. Papademetriou V. Comparative prognostic value of systolic, diastolic, and pulse pressure. Am J Cardiol 91(4):433–435, 2003.

50. Vaccarino V, Bergue H J, Krumholz J, et al. Pulse pressure and risk of cardiovascular events in the systolic hypertension in the elderly program. Am J Cardiol 88(9):980–986, 2001.

51. Carlson JE. Assessment of orthostatic blood pressure: measurement technique and clinical applications. South Med J 92(2):167–173, 1999.

52. Consensus Committee of the American Autonomic Society and the American Academy of Neurology. Consensus statement on the definition of orthostatic hypotension, pure autonomic failure, and multiple system atrophy. Neurology 46(5):1470, 1996.

53. McGee S, Abernethy WB, Simel DL. Is this patient hypovolemic? JAMA 281(11):1022–1029, 1999.

54. Ooi WL, Barrett S, Hossain M, et al. Patterns of orthostatic blood pressure change and their clinical correlates in a frail elderly population. JAMA 277(16):1299–1304, 1997.

55. Raiha I, Luntonen S, Piha J, et al. Prevalence, predisposing factors and prognostic importance of postural hypotension. Arch Intern Med 155(9):930–935, 1995.

56. Gnann JW, Whitely RJ. Herpes zoster. N Engl J Med 347(5):340–346, 2002.

57. Congdon NG, Friedman DS, Lietman T. Important causes of visual impairment in the world today. JAMA 290(15):2057–2060, 2003.

58. Freidman DS, Jampel HD, Munoz B, et al. The prevalence of open-angle glaucoma among blacks and whites 73 years and older: the Salisbury Eye Evaluation Glaucoma Study. Arch Ophthalmol 124(11):1625–1630, 2006.

59. Gordon SR, Jahnigen DW. Oral assessment of the dentulous elderly patient. J Am Geriatr Soc 34:276–281, 1986.

60. Leach RM, McBrien DJ. Brachiocardial delay: a new clinical indicator of the severity of aortic stenosis. Lancet 335(8699):1199–1201, 1990.

61. McDermott MM, Greenland P, Liu K, et al. The ankle brachial index is associated with leg function and physical activity: the walking and leg circulation study. Ann Intern Med 136(12):873–883, 2002.

62. Dumesic DA. Pelvic examination: what to focus on in menopausal women. Consultant 36:39–46, 1996.

63. American Geriatrics Society. Screening for cervical carcinoma in older women. J Am Geriatr Soc 49(5):655–657, 2001.

64. Hoffman MS, Cardosi RD, Roberts WS, et al. Accuracy of pelvic examination in the assessment of patients with operable cervical cancer. Am J Obstet Gynecol 190(4):986–993, 2004.

65. Holsinger T, Deveau J, Boustani M, et al. Does this patient have dementia? JAMA 297(21):2391–2404, 2007.

66. Baloh RW, Ying SH, Jacobson KM. A longitudinal study of gait and balance dysfunction in normal older people. Arch Neurol 60:835–839, 2003.

67. Guralnik JM, Ferrucci L, Simonsek E et al. Lower extremity function in persons over the age of 70 years as a predictor of subsequent disability. N Engl J Med 332(9):556–561, 1995.

68. Tinetti ME, Williams TF, Mayewski R. Fall risk index for elderly patients based on number of chronic disabilities. Am J Med 80(3):429–434, 1986.

69. Tinetti ME, Ginter SF. Identifying mobility dysfunctions in elderly patients. JAMA 259(8):1190–1193, 1988.

70. Odenheimer G, Funkenstein HH, Beckett L, et al. Comparison of neurologic changes in 'successfully aging' persons vs. the total aging population. Arch Neurol 51(6):573–580, 1994.

71. Rao G, Fisch L, Srinivasan S, et al. Does this patient have Parkinson disease? JAMA 289(3):347–353, 2003.

72. Nutt JG, Wooten GF. Diagnosis and initial management of Parkinson's disease. N Engl J Med 353(10):1021–1027, 2005.

73. Beck LH. Periodic health examination and screening tests in adults. Hosp Pract 15:121–126, 1999.

74. Hall K, Chyun D. General screening recommendations for chronic disease and risk factors in older adults. Available at: http://consultgerirn.org/uploads/File/trythis/try_this_27.pdf. Access May 23, 2011.

75. Bogardus ST, Yueh B, Shekelle PG. Screening and management of adult hearing loss in primary care: clinical applications. JAMA 289(15):1986–1990, 2003.

76. Centers for Disease Control and Prevention (CDC). Recommended Adult Immunization Schedule 2010. Available at: http://www.cdc.gov/mmwr/preview/mmwrhtml/mm5901 a5.htm?s_cid=mm5901a5_w. Accessed May 23, 2011.

77. Centers for Disease Control and Prevention (CDC). Vaccines and Immunizations. Recommendations and Guidelines. Adult Immunization Schedule. Updated February 2011. Available at: http://www.cdc.gov/vaccines/recs/schedules/adult-schedule. htm#chgs. Accessed May 23, 2011.

78. Nichol KL, Nordin JD, Nelson DB, et al. Effectiveness of influenza vaccine in the community-dwelling elderly. N Engl J Med 357(14):1373–1381, 2007.

79. Oxman MN, Levin MJ, Johnson GR, et al. A vaccine to prevent herpes zoster and postherpetic neuralgia in older adults. N Engl J Med 352(22):2271–2284, 2005.

80. U.S. Consumer Product Safety Commission. Special Report: Emergency Room Injuries—Adults 65 and Older. 2002. Available at: http://www.cpsc.gov/LIBRARY/FOIA/ FOIA05/os/older.pdf. Accessed May 23, 2011.

81. Ganz DA, Bao Y, Shekelle PG, et al. Will my patient fall? JAMA 297(1):77–86, 2007.

82. Montero-Odasso M, Schapira M, Soriano ER, et al. Simple gait velocity assessment predicts adverse events in healthy seniors aged 75 years and older. J Gerontol A Biol Sci Med Sci 60(10):1304–1309, 2005.

83. Tinetti ME. Preventing falls in elderly persons. N Engl J Med 348(1):42–48, 2003.

84. Nelson ME, Rejeski WJ, Blair SN, et al, American College of Sports Medicine, American Heart Association. Physical activity and public health in older adults: recommendation from the American College of Sports Medicine and the American Heart Association. Circulation 116(9): 1094–1105, 2007.

85. Unutzer J. Late-life depression. N Engl J Med 357(22): 2269–2276, 2007.

86. U.S. Preventive Services Task Force. Screening for Dementia: Recommendations and Rationale. June 2003. Rockville, MD: Agency for Healthcare Research and Quality. Available at: http://www.ahrq.gov/clinic/3rduspstf/dementia/dementrr. htm. Accessed February 23, 2008.

87. Cummings JL. Alzheimer's disease. N Engl J Med 351(1): 56–67, 2004.

88. Small BJ, Gagnon E, Robinson B. Early identification of cognitive deficits: preclinical Alzheimer's disease and mild cognitive impairment. Geriatrics 62(4):19–23, 2007.

89. Karlawish JHT, Clark CM. Diagnostic evaluation of elderly patients with mild memory problems. Ann Intern Med 138(5):411–419, 2003.

90. Budson AE, Price BH. Memory dysfunction. N Engl J Med 352(7):692–699, 2005.

91. Tschanz JT, Weklsg-Bohmer KA, Lyketsos CG, et al. Conversion to dementia from mild cognitive disorder: the Cache County Study. Neurology 67(2):229–234, 2006.

92. Boyle PA, Wilson RS, Aggarwal NT, et al. Mild cognitive impairment: risk of Alzheimer's disease and rate of cognitive decline. Neurology 67(3):441–445, 2006.

93. Busse A, Hensel A, Guhne U, et al. Mild cognitive impairment: long-term course of four clinical subtypes. Neurology 67(12):2176–2185, 2006.

94. Dyer CB, Pickens S, Burnett J. Vulnerable elders: when it is no longer safe to live alone. JAMA 298(12):1448–1450, 2007.

95. Fulmer T, Guadagno L, Dyer CB, et al. Progress in elder abuse screening and assessment instruments. J Am Geriatr Soc 52:297–304, 2004.

96. Fulmer T, Hernandez M. Elder mistreatment. In: Cassel CK, Leipzig RM, Cohen HJ, et al, eds. Geriatric Medicine, 4th ed. New York: Springer, 2003:1057–1066.

97. Tulsky JA. Doctor-patient communication issues. In: Cassel CK, Leipzig RM, Cohen HJ, et al, eds. Geriatric Medicine, 4th ed. New York: Springer, 2003:287–298.

98. Callahan D. The value of achieving a peaceful death. In: Cassel CK, Leipzig RM, Cohen HJ, et al, eds. Geriatric Medicine, 4th ed. New York: Springer, 2003:351–360.

99. Morrison RS, Meier DE. Clinical practice: palliative care. N Engl J Med 350(25):2582–2590, 2004.

ADDITIONAL REFERENCES

Ahmed A. Clinical manifestations, diagnostic assessment, and etiology of heart failure in older adults. Clin Geriatr Med 23: 11–30, 2007.

American Geriatrics Society, Ethnogeriatrics Steering Committee. Doorway Thoughts: Cross-Cultural Health Care for Older Adults. Sudbury, MA: Jones and Bartlett, 2004.

Amin SH, Kuhle CL, Fitzpatrick LA. Comprehensive evaluation of the older woman. Mayo Clin Proc 78(9):1157–1185, 2003.

Beckett NS, Peters R, Fletcher AE, et al, for the HYVET Study Group. Treatment of hypertension in patients 80 years of age or older. N Engl J Med 78(9):1887–1898, 2008.

Burks K. Osteoarthritis in older adults: current treatments. J Gerontol Nurs 31(5):11–19, 2005.

Cassel CK. Geriatric Medicine: An Evidence-based Approach, 4th ed. New York: Springer, 2003.

Carolan Doerflinger DM. How to try this: the mini-cog. Am J Nurs 107(12):62–71, 2007.

Chobanion AV. Isolated systolic hypertension in the elderly. N Engl J Med 357(80):789–796, 2007.

Clark CM, Karlawish JHT. Alzheimer disease: current concepts and emerging diagnostic and therapeutic strategies. Ann Intern Med 138(5):400–410, 2003.

Donowitz GR, Cox HL. Bacterial community-acquired pneumonia in older patients. Clin Geriatr Med 23(5):515–534, 2007.

Ene-Stroescu D, Gorbien MJ. Gouty arthritis: a primer on late-onset gout. Geriatrics 60(7):24–31, 2005.

Fantl, A., Newman, D. K., Colling, J., DeLancey, J. O. L., Keeys, C., & Loughery, R. Urinary incontinence in adults: acute and chronic management. Agency for Health Care Policy and Research, Publication No. 92-0047: Rockville, MD. Evidence Level I: CPCG Based on Systematic Review, 1996.

Gupta V, Lipsitz LA. Orthostatic hypotension in the elderly: diagnosis and treatment. Am J Med 120(10):841–847, 2007.

Hazzard WR. Principles of Geriatric Medicine and Gerontology, 5th ed. New York: McGraw-Hill/Professional, 2003.

Hartford Institute for Geriatric Nursing. Available at: www. ConsultGeriRN.org. Accessd May 24, 2011.

Inouye SK. Delirium in older persons. N Engl J Med 354(11): 1157–1165, 2006.

Kales HC, Mellow AM. Race and depression: does race affect the diagnosis and treatment of late-life depression? Geriatrics 61(5):18–21, 2006.

Karlawish JHT, Clark CM. Diagnostic evaluation of elderly patients with mild memory problems. Ann Intern Med 138(5):411–419, 2003.

Kennedy-Malone L, Fletcher KR, Plank LR. Management Guidelines for Nurse Practitioners Working With Older Adults, 2nd ed. Philadelphia: FA Davis, 2004.

Khan AA, Hodsman AB, Papaioannou A, et al. Management of osteoporosis in men: an update and case example. CMAJ 176(3):345–348, 2007.

Kobylarz FA, Pomidor A, Heath JM. SPEAK: a mnemonic tool for addressing health literacy concerns in geriatric clinical encounters. Geriatrics 61(7):20–26, 2006.

Landefeld CS. Current Geriatric Diagnosis & Treatment. New York: Lange Medical Books–McGraw-Hill, 2004.

Meldon SW, Ma OJ, Woolard R, for American College of Emergency Physicians. Geriatric Emergency Medicine. New York: McGraw-Hill, 2004.

Moylan KC, Binder EF. Falls in older adults: risk assessment, management and prevention. Am J Med 120(6):493–497, 2007.

Morrison LJ, Morrison RS. Palliative care and pain management. Med Clin North Am 90(5):983–1004, 2006.

Nakasato YR, Carnes BA. Health promotion in older adults: promoting successful aging in primary care settings. Geriatrics 61(4):27–31, 2006.

Norton P, Brubaker L. Urinary incontinence in women. Lancet 367(9504):57–67, 2006.

Nusbaum MR, Lenahan P, Sadovsky R. Sexual health in aging men and women: addressing the physiologic and psychological sexual changes that occur with age. Geriatrics 60(9):18–23, 2005.

Scalf LA, Shenefelt PD. Contact dermatitis: diagnosing and treating skin conditions in the elderly. Geriatrics 62(6):14–19, 2007.

Small BJ, Gagnon E, Robinson B. Early identification of cognitive deficits: preclinical Alzheimer's disease and mild cognitive impairment. Geriatrics 62(4):19–23, 2007.

Springhouse Corporation, ed. Handbook of Geriatric Nursing Care, 2nd ed. Philadelphia: Lippincott Williams & Wilkins, 2002.

Staats DO. Preventing injury in older adults. Geriatrics 63(4): 12–17, 2008.

Villareal DT, Apovian CM, Kushner RF, et al. Obesity in older adults: technical review and position statement of the American Society for Nutrition and NAASO, The Obesity Society. Am J Clin Nutr 82(5):923–934, 2005.

Vistamehr S, Shelsta HN, Pammisano PC, et al. Glaucoma screening in a high-risk population. J Glaucoma 15(6):534–540, 2006.

Walter LC, Lewis CL, Barton MB. Screening for colorectal, breast, and cervical cancer in the elderly: a review of the evidence. Am J Med 118(10):1078–1086, 2005.

Weiner DK. Office management of chronic pain in the elderly. Am J Med 120(4):306–315, 2007.

Wolkove N, Elkholy O, Baltzan M, et al. Sleep and aging: sleep disorders commonly found in older people. CMAJ 176(9): 1299–1304, 2007.

GLOSSARY

accommodation   change in size to adjust for seeing objects at various distances.

achalasia   failure to relax smooth muscles of the gastrointestinal tract.

acral   pertaining to extremities.

actinic keratosis   localized thickening of outer layers of the skin from prolonged sun exposure, precursor to skin cancer.

afterload   resistance to left ventricular ejection; the forces that impede the flow of blood out of the heart, i.e. the compliance of the aorta and the volume of blood in the left ventricle.

alopecia   hair loss.

anhedonia   inability to enjoy what is usually likable.

aperture   opening for the light.

arciform   arcurate, bowed; shaped like an arc.

arcus lipoides   a white ring around the limbus of the eye, due to lipid deposition in the peripheral cornea.

articular   pertaining to joints.

atelectasis   a collapsed or airless condition of the lung.

atherosclerosis   the formation of fibrofatty deposits in the intimal lining of large and medium arteries, which leads to hardening and narrowing of the arteries.

atraumatic   without injury.

atrophy   a wasting or decrease in size or physiologic activity of a part of the body.

bipolar disorder   affective disorder in which the person has both manic and depressive episodes.

bradycardia   slow heart beat, usually less than 60 beats per minute.

bradykinesia   extreme slowness of movement.

bronchitis   inflammation of the mucous membrane of the bronchial airways, caused by irritation or infection.

bulbar conjunctiva   thin and transparent covering of the sclera on the anterior of the eye.

canthi   corners of the eyes; singular is canthus.

cerumen (earwax)   a yellowish or brownish waxy substance secreted in the ear canal; helps to clean, lubricate, and protect from infections or insects.

claudication   pain with walking.

coitus   sexual intercourse.

contractility   the ability of the heart muscle fiber to stretch during ventricular filling; in the healthy heart the stretch is proportional to the force of the contraction; the intrinsic ability of cardiac muscle to develop force for a given muscle length.

convergence   movement of two objects toward a common point.

crude touch   sensation perceived as light touch but without accurate localization.

cryptorchidism   undescended testicle.

dermatome   area of the body innervated by the sensory root of a single spinal nerve.

diaphoresis   profuse sweating.

diopters   measurement of the optical powers of a lens.

diplopia   double vision.

dyslipidemia   An abnormal concentration of lipids or lipoproteins in the blood.

dyspareunia   abnormal pain during sexual intercourse.

dyspepsia   chronic or recurrent discomfort or pain centered in the upper abdomen.

dysphagia   difficulty swallowing.

dysplasia   abnormal development of tissue.

dyspnea   labored or difficult breathing, shortness of breath.

dysthymia   loss of interest or pleasure in all usual activities or pastimes but not severe enough to meet major depressive episode criteria.

dysuria   pain or difficulty voiding.

ectasia   a dilated milk duct.

ectopy   displacement.

ectropion   eversion, usually of the eyelid.

edema   abnormal accumulation of fluid in the intercellular spaces of the body.

edentulous   without teeth.

embolus   undissolved matter in the blood, such as a blood clot.

entropion   turning inward, usually eyelid turns in toward the eye.

equilibrium   state of balance.

erythema   reddening of the skin; a non-specific sign of skin inflammation, injury or irritation; caused by dilation of the skin capillaries.

euphoria   a state of happiness.

evert   turning outward of the foot.

facies   the appearance of the face.

fascia   fibrous connective tissue.

fever   abnormal elevation in body temperature.

fibrillation   uncoordinated electrical activity of the heart; quivering or spontaneous contraction of individual muscle fibers, which can be atrial or ventricular.

fibroadenoma   small, solid, noncancerous lump composed of glandular and fibrous tissues.

flank pain   pain in one side of the body between the upper abdomen and the back.

fossa   a furrow or shallow depression.

fundus   back portion of the interior of the eye, visible through the pupil using the ophthalmoscope.

gait   the manner or style of walking.

granuloma   small nodule, inflammation.

hematuria   blood in the urine.

hemianopsia   inability to see half of the visual field, generally on one side.

hemolysis   the destruction of red blood cells.

hemoptysis   expectoration of blood that arises from the larynx, trachea, bronchi or lungs.

Hertz   a unit of frequency equal to one cycle per second.

hydrocele   accumulation of serous fluid in a saclike cavity in the scrotum.

hyperopia   farsighted or inability of the eye to focus on objects close by.

hyperplasia   abnormal proliferation of cells.

hyperresonance   an increased resonance during percussion, caused by over inflation of the lungs as in emphysema or asthma.

hypertrophy   increase in the size of an organ or body part, such as a muscle.

hypothermia   decrease in temperature.

icterus (icteric)   jaundice, a generalized yellowing of the skin, often secondary to liver disease. (icteric is adjective).

insomnia   inability to sleep or remain asleep.

inspissated   thickened by dehydration, evaporation or absorption.

intertriginous   an area where two skin areas may touch or rub together.

kyphosis   exaggerated outward or convex curvature of the thoracic spine.

lateral decubitus position   the patient lies on his side.

leukoplakia   precancerous change in mucous membrane (usually thick and white lesions).

lordosis   exaggerated inward or concave curvature of the lumbar spine.

lymphedema   swelling of a body part that is due to pooling of interstitial fluid caused by the blockage of a lymph node or vessel.

maceration   the process of softening a solid by steeping in a fluid. Maceration of the skin occurs when it is consistently wet. The skin softens, turns white, and can easily get infected with bacteria or fungi.

malaise   feeling of sickness or indisposition.

malignant   progressive or deadly.

mastitis   infection of the breast resulting in pain, redness, swelling and warmth.

mastoid   hard, bony structure behind the ear.

microglossia   abnormally small tongue.

myopia   nearsighted or inability of the eye to focus on objects at a distance.

neoplasm   a new and abnormal formation of tissue, as a tumor or growth, which serves no useful function. It may be benign or malignant.

nocturia   urinary frequency at night.

normocephalic   a person whose head and all major organs of the head are in a normal condition and without significant abnormalities.

nummular   coin shaped.

odynophagia   pain with swallowing.

orchitis   inflammation of a testis.

orthopnea   labored breathing that occurs when lying flat and is relieved by sitting up.

otitis externa   inflammation of the skin of the ear canal.

otoscope   a medical instrument consisting of a magnifying lens and light and used for examining the ear.

palpebral conjunctiva thick, opaque, vascular lining of the inner surface of the eyelids.

palpebral fissures opening between the upper and lower eyelids.

palpitations a sensation of rapid or irregular beating of the heart. The patient may describe the sensation as thudding, fluttering or throbbing under the sternum.

palsy paralysis.

parenchyma the essential elements of an organ essential to its functioning, as distinct from the capsule that encompasses it and other supporting structures.

parethesia sensation of numbness, prickling or tingling.

paroxysmal nocturnal dyspnea (PND) sudden attacks of dyspnea that occur when patients are asleep in bed.

pedunculated attached to a base by means of a *peduncle*, or slender stalk, e.g., a skin tag or polyp.

percutaneous through the skin.

phobia irrational fear of an object, activity, or situation.

photophobia light sensitivity from excess light entering the eye, which may overstimulate the photoreceptors in the retina, which then stimulates the optic nerve.

pleximeter finger finger that receives the percussion strike from the opposite hand, usually the third finger of the non-dominant hand.

plexor finger finger that strikes the finger pressing on the patient's body during percussion, usually the third finger of the dominant hand.

pneumothorax a collection of air in the pleural cavity, "collapsed lung."

polyuria significant increase in 24-hour urine.

precordium the area on the anterior chest that overlies the heart and great vessels.

preload the end-diastolic stretch of a heart muscle fiber; end diastolic volume.

presbyopia changes with age, farsightedness due to decreased elasticity in the lens.

prodrome early symptom(s) before the onset of a disease.

proliferative grow or produce by multiplication of parts.

protuberant rounded.

ptosis drooping of the upper eyelid.

radicular pertaining to a spinal nerve root.

regurgitation a backward flowing, as in the return of solids or fluids to the mouth from the stomach or the back flow of blood through a defective heart valve.

resonance quality of the sound heard during percussion of the normal lung.

scaling removal of the surface.

scaphoid concave or hollowed.

scoliosis lateral curvature of the spine.

sebum a fatty secretion of the sebaceous glands of the skin.

serpiginous a term used to describe the shape or arrangement of lesions that have a wavy or serpent-like patter.

shotty hard and round, resembling shotgun pellets.

somatoform has psychological symptoms that are similar to those of a physical disease.

speculum instrument for inserting into and holding open a cavity of the body, e.g., the vagina.

strabismus eyes are not directed at the same point; crossed eyes.

stadiometer instrument to measure height, attach to the wall to insure accuracy.

stasis slowed or stopped flow, e.g., blood flow in veins.

stenosis the constriction or narrowing of a passage or orifice, e.g., a heart valve or blood vessel.

stroke volume the amount of blood ejected by the left ventricle with each contraction.

syncope the transient and usually sudden loss of consciousness, accompanied by an inability to remain standing; fainting.

tachycardia an abnormally fast heartbeat, usually over 100 beats per minute.

tangential lighting lighting from the side to be able to better see small movements or pulsations of the body and decrease shadows.

teres round and smooth; cylindrical; used to describe certain muscles and ligaments.

thelarche the beginning of breast development.

thrill a palpable vibration felt over the precordium or an artery due to blood turbulence, associated with grade 4 to 6 heart murmurs.

thrombophlebitis   inflammation of a vein in conjunction with the formation of a thrombus.

thrombosis   a blood clot that adheres to the wall of a blood vessel, usually a vein.

tinnitus   a ringing or buzzing sound that is heard by the patient.

torticollis   contraction of the muscles of the neck, which draw the head to one side.

traumatic brain injury (TBI)   occurs when an outside force traumatically injures the brain.

tympany   a clear hollow drum-like note heard during percussion over gas filled organs, such as the stomach and bowels.

valgus   bent; turned outward; the distal part of leg is deviated outward, i.e., knock-kneed.

varus   a term for the inward angulation of the distal segment of a bone or joint, i.e., bowleg.

vertigo   patients feel they or their surroundings are in a state of constant movement; usually due to a problem with the inner ear, but can also be caused by visual problems.

viscera   internal organs enclosed within a cavity.

xanthelasma   yellow, lipid rich plaque present on the eyelids, associated with hyperlipidemia.

INDEX

Page numbers followed by b indicate in-chapter boxed material, those followed by t indicate end-of-chapter tables, and those followed by f indicate figures.

A

ABCDE method, for moles, 166–168
Abdomen
  in adults
    health assessment of, 727
    physical examination of, 103
    protuberant, 449, 451, 463, 483t
    tender, 453, 485t–486t
  in children
    adolescents, 813
    infants, 763–765
    obese, 796
    school-aged, 796–797, 796f, 796t, 797f
  in elderly, 846, 865
Abdominal aorta, 433, 433f
Abdominal aortic aneurysm
  in elderly, 865
  palpation for, 459, 460f
  prevention and early identification of, 422
Abdominal cavity, 433
Abdominal discomfort. See Abdominal pain
Abdominal distention, protein deficiency, 133
Abdominal examination, 448–459
  aorta in, 459, 460f
  auscultation in, 450–451
    abdominal sounds, 450, 484t
    bruits and friction rub, 450–451, 484t
  inspection in, 448–450
    abdominal wall bulges, localized, 449, 482t
    protuberant abdomen, 449, 483t
  kidneys in, 457–459
    left kidney palpation in, 457–458
    percussion tenderness in, 458–459, 459f
    right kidney palpation in, 458, 458f
  liver in, 454–457
    enlarged, 456–457, 456f, 487t
    palpation of, 455–457, 455f–457f
    percussion of, 454–455, 454f, 455f
  palpation in, 452–453
    deep, 453, 453f
    light, 452, 452f
    peritoneal inflammation assessment, 453
    rebound tenderness in, 453, 453f
    tender abdomen, 453, 485t–486t
  percussion in, 451–452
    protuberant abdomen, 451, 483t
    tympany and dullness, 451
Abdominal fullness, 441
Abdominal masses, 453, 466
Abdominal pain, 435–436, 436f, 472t–473t
  in appendicitis, 439, 465–466, 472t–473t,
      486t (See also Appendicitis)
  GI symptoms with, 440–441
  lower
    acute, 439
    chronic, 440
    parietal, 436
    referred, 436

upper
  acute, 437–438
  chronic, 438–439
  visceral, 435–436, 436f, 485t
Abdominal quadrants, 432,
    432f
Abdominal reflexes
  in adults, 650, 650f
  in elderly, 848
Abdominal wall
  lipomas in, 482t
  localized bulges in, 449, 482t
  mass in, 466
  tenderness of, 485t
Abduction
  fingers, 549, 550f
  hands, 549, 549f
  hip, 563t, 565, 565f
  shoulder, 534f, 536f
  thumbs, 549, 549f
  wrist, 546f, 546t
Abductor group, hip, 560, 560f
Abnormal uterine bleeding,
    687, 689
Absence seizure, 669t
Absent reflexes, 645
Abstract thinking, 608
Abuse
  alcohol, 611
    in elderly, 859–860
    screening for, 467–468
    stroke risk from, 660t
  child, 76
  elder, 873
  physical, 75–76
  sexual
    in children, 799, 800, 835t
    in female adults, 694
  substance, 611
Acanthosis nigricans, 170t, 503
Accommodation, 216, 631
Acetabulum, 559, 559f
Achilles reflex, 649, 649f
Achilles tendinitis, 570
Achilles tendon, 570
  palpation of, 574
  rupture of, 570
Acid reflux, 438
Acne (vulgaris)
  in adolescents, 810, 826t
  in adults, 159, 160, 197
  lesions of, 178t
  neonatal, 825t
  pustule in, 175t
Acoustic neuroma, 632
Acquired immunodeficiency syndrome
    (AIDS), 698
Acrocyanosis, in infant, 832t

Acromioclavicular joint
  anatomy and physiology of, 530, 530f
  examination maneuvers for, 536, 536f
Acromion, 530, 530f
Acronyms. See Mnemonics and acronyms;
    specific acronyms
Actinic cheilitis, 282t
Actinic keratosis
  in adults, 180t
  in elderly, 862
Actinic purpura, 861, 861f
Action tremors, 670t
Active listening, 47
Active range of motion, 523
Activities of daily living (ADL), in elderly,
    854, 855t
Activity, motor, 107
Activity-exercise, 72t
Acute coronary syndrome, 351
Acute myocardial infarction. See Myocardial
    infarction
Acute otitis externa, 268, 268f
Acute otitis media, 254
  auricle in, 266
  in children, 788, 830t
  ear canal and drum in, 268, 830t
  with purulent effusion, 280t
Adam's bend test, 555, 817, 817f
Added breath sounds, 314–315, 314t, 331t
Addiction, 122. See also specific substances
Addison disease, skin in, 182t
Adduction
  hands, 549, 549f
  hip, 563t, 565, 565f
  shoulder, 535f, 536, 536f
  thumbs, 549, 549f
  wrist, 546f, 546t
Adductor group, hip, 560, 560f
ADHD, in children, 802
Adipose tissue
  breast, female, 491, 491f
  skin, 154f, 155
Adnexa, 685
Adolescents, 806–819. See also Children
  confidentiality issues with, 809
  development of
    cognitive, 807, 807t–808t
    physical, 806–807, 807t–808t
    social and emotional, 807, 807t–808t
  health history in, 808–810, 810f
  health promotion and counseling in, 818–819
  physical examination of, 810–818
    abdomen, 813
    breasts, female, 811–812, 812f
    genitalia, female, 815–817, 816t, 817f
    genitalia, male, 813–815, 813t–814t, 815f
    head, ears, eyes, throat, and neck, 811
    heart, 811

Adolescents *(continued)*
  musculoskeletal system, 817–818, 817f, 818f, 836t
  nervous system, 818
  skin, 810
  somatic growth, 810
  vital signs, 810
  recording findings on, 820–823
ADPIE, 14–15
Adult illnesses, 66
Advance directives, in elderly, 873–874
Adventitia, 399f, 400
Adventitious (extra) breath sounds, 314t, 331t, 332t–333t
  anterior auscultation for, 320
  posterior auscultation for, 314–315, 314t
Aerophagia, 438
Affect, 599t, 602, 860
Afterload, 347
Age. *See also* Older adults
  in organizing clinical data, 24–25
Age-associated cognitive impairment (AACI), 873
Agenda for interview, establishing, 41
Agitated depression, 601
Agitated patients, 601
Air and bone conduction, 633
Air conduction
  anatomy and physiology of, 252, 252f
  physical examination of, 269, 269f
Air hunger, 300
"Alarm symptoms," 439
Alcohol
  odor of, 107
  in past history, 67–68
Alcohol abuse, 611
  in elderly, 859–860
  screening for, 467–468
  stroke risk from, 660t
Alcoholic hepatitis, visceral pain in, 435
Alertness, 598, 652t
Alignment, eye, 223
Allen test, 117 118, 117f 418f
Allergic rhinitis, 258
  chronic (perennial), 789
  nose in, 271
  perennial, 789, 829t
Allergies, 66. *See also specific types*
  circles under eyes from, 133
Allis test, 768
Alopecia, 164
Alopecia areata, 184t
Altered capacity, interviewing patient with, 52–53
Alveolar mucosa, 261, 261f
Alveoli, 298
Alzheimer dementia, 873
Ambiguous genitalia, 766
Amblyopia, in children, 786
Amenorrhea, 687, 689, 690
American Sign Language, 56
Amnestic mild cognitive impairment, 873
Amylase, in pancreatitis, 31
Anabolic agents, 582
Analgesia, 640
Analgesic rebound, 206t–207t
Anatomic snuffbox, 544, 544f

Anemia
  pallor in, 158
  skin color in, 133
Anesthesia, 640
Aneurysm
  femoral, 413, 414
  popliteal, 414
Aneurysmal artery, 410
"Angel kisses," 748, 749t
Angina pectoris, 351
  chest pain in, 327t
  epidemiology of, 351
  exertional, 351
  as heartburn, 438
  as "indigestion," 438
Angioedema, on mouth, 282t
Angle of Louis, 293, 293t
Angry patient, interviewing, 54–55
Angular cheilitis
  in adults, 282t
  in elderly, 844
Anhedonia, 610
Anisocoria, 225, 240t, 631
Anisometropia, in children, 786
Ankle, 572–576
  bony structures and joints of, 572–573, 573f
  function of, 572
  muscle groups and ligaments of, 573, 573f
  physical examination of
    inspection in, 574
    palpation in, 574, 574f
    range of motion and maneuvers in, 575–576, 575f, 575t, 576f
Ankle–brachial index (ABI), 419–420, 419f
Ankle clonus, 650, 772
Ankle reflex
  in adults, 649, 649f
  in elderly, 848
  in infants, 772, 772f
Ankyloglossia, 755
Ankylosing spondylitis, 557, 584t
Ankylosis, 524
Annular skin lesions, 172t
Annulus fibrosis, 552, 552f
Anorexia (nervosa), 440, 441
  clinical features of, 442t
  dress in, 108
Anserine bursa, 569, 569f
Anterior axillary line, 295, 295f, 296, 296f
Anterior cerebral artery (ACA) stroke, 664t–665t
Anterior chamber, eye, 213, 213f
Anterior chest examination, 316–320
  auscultation in
    for adventitious (extra) sounds, 320, 331t, 372t
    for breath sounds, 319–320
  inspection in, 316, 329t
  palpation in, 316–317, 317f
  percussion in, 318–319, 318f, 319f
Anterior cruciate ligament (ACL), 568, 568f
Anterior fontanelle, 750, 750f
Anterior horn cell lesion, 678t
Anterior naris, 256, 256f
Anterior pillar, 263, 263f
Anterior talofibular ligament, 573, 573f

Anterior triangle, 193, 194f
Anticipatory guidance, for children, 735
Antiresorptive agents, 582
Anxiety
  breathing difficulties in, 301
  chest pain in, 328t
  dyspnea with, 300
  with hyperventilation, 324t–325t
Aorta, 338–339, 338f, 400
  abdominal, anatomy of, 433, 433f
  coarctation of, 114, 746, 760, 783, 784
  in elderly, 845
  tortuous atherosclerotic, 864
Aortic aneurysm, dissecting, chest pain in, 328t
Aortic area, 363f, 367, 370f
Aortic dissection
  blood pressure in, 112
  chest pain in, 328t, 351
Aortic ejection sound, 389t
Aortic insufficiency, 344
  arm pulses in, 410, 410f
  heart sounds in, 362
Aortic pressure, 341, 341f
Aortic regurgitation, 343–344
  general findings in, 375
  heart murmurs in, 375, 394t
Aortic sclerosis
  in elderly, 845
  general findings in, 375
Aortic stenosis, 343, 344f
  in elderly, 845, 864
  general findings in, 375
  heart murmurs in, 374, 375, 393t
  heart sounds in, 362
  in infants, 763
  syncope from, 666t–667t
Aortic valve, 339, 339f
Aortic valve murmur, 357, 833t
Aortic valve stenosis, congenital, 833t
AP diameter, in chronic obstructive pulmonary disease, 306
Aphasia, 602–603, 603t, 674t
  Broca, 674t
  from stroke, 659
  Wernicke, 674t
Aphonia, 671t
Aphthous stomatitis, 177t
Aphthous ulcer, 272, 272f, 290t
Apical impulse
  definition and representation of, 363
  palpation of, 338
  physical examination of, 363–366, 364f–366f
    diameter and amplitude in, 365, 365f
    duration in, 366
    identification in, 364, 364f
    location of, 364, 365, 365f
  variations and abnormalities of, 386t
Apical pulse, 112, 115, 116
Apley scratch test, 536f
Apnea, 756
Apparent state of health, 106
Appearance
  clinical, 38–39
  general, 106–109 (*See also* General appearance)
  in mental status, 601–602

Appendicitis
  in adults
    abdominal pain in, 439, 465–466,
        472t–473t
    abdominal tenderness in, 486t
    visceral periumbilical pain in, 436
  in children, 797
Appendix, 433f, 434
Apprehension sign, positive, 588t
Approach, patient. *See also specific systems*
  reflecting on, 91–92
Aqueous humor, 213
Arch, of foot, 573, 573f
Arciform skin lesions, 172t
Arcus senilis, 862
Areola
  female, 491–492, 491f, 492f
  male, 492
Argyll Robertson pupils, 226, 240t
Arms
  flaccid, 655, 655f
  physical examination of, 409–410, 409t
    equipment list for, 408
    inspection in, 409
    palpation in, 409–410, 409f
Arousal (consciousness), 702
  level of, 106
    in comatose patient, 652–653
    in mental health assessment, 598, 598t, 601
Arousal system, 615
Arrhythmias. *See also specific types*
  blood pressure measurement with, 115
  syncope from, 666t–667t
Arterial bruit, 483t
Arterial insufficiency
  in elderly, 846
  of legs
    advanced, 426t
    characteristics of, 426t
    evaluation of, 418–419, 418f–419f
    leg temperature in, 411
    symptoms of, 406
    ulcers in, 427t
Arterial intima, 399, 399f
Arterial occlusion
  acute peripheral vascular, 424t–425t
  arm pulses in, 410, 410f
  in arms, 417, 417f–418f
Arterial pulses, 347–348, 348f, 429t
  blood pressure and, 347–348, 348f, 429t
  grading amplitude of, 410
Arteries, 399–401, 399f–401f
Arterioles, 400
Arteriosclerosis obliterans, of thigh, 414, 414f
Arthritis. *See also* Osteoarthritis
  acute gouty
    of foot, 591t
    joint pain in, 586t–587t
  ankle and foot, 555
  carpometacarpal, 545
  gonococcal, 521
  hands, 589t
  post-traumatic, 545
  rheumatoid, 521
    ankle and foot, 574

  hands and wrist, 543, 544, 589t
  intervertebral joints, 556
  joint pain in, 586t–587t
  joints in, 523, 524
  metacarpophalangeal joints, 545
  muscle atrophy/weakness in, 524
  signs of, 524
  of spine, 554
Articular capsule, shoulder, 532, 532f
Articular cartilage, 519, 519f
Articular disease, 518
Articular facets, 551, 551f
Articular processes, 551, 551f
Articular structures, 518
A's, four, 121
Asbestosis, dyspnea in, 324t–325t
Ascites
  assessing, 465–466
  examination for, 463–464
    abdomen and flanks in, 449, 451, 463,
        463f, 483t
    fluid wave in, 464, 464f
    shifting dullness in, 463, 464f
  from protein deficiency, 133
Ascitic fluid, 483t
Assessment. *See also specific systems*
  comprehensive health (*See* Health assessment,
      comprehensive)
  cultural, 78–84
    collaborative partnerships in, 82, 83
    cultural competence in, 79, 80f
    cultural humility in, 80–83
    culture defined in, 78–79
    health history in, 83–84
    overview of, 78–79
    respectful communication in, 82–83
    self-awareness in, 82
  focused, 61, 62t
  health, 3–10 (*See also* Health assessment;
      specific systems)
  integration of, 31–32
  nursing process, 14, 15–19
    steps in
      cluster findings, 16
      develop plan, 19
      identify abnormal or positive findings, 16
      interpret findings as probable process,
          16–17
      making diagnosis, 18
      making hypotheses, 17
      types of reasoning in, 15–16
  problem-oriented, 61
  spiritual, 85–86, 85–87
    approach to, 85–86
    listening in, 86
    presence in, 85–86
    spiritual distress in, 85–86
    spirituality in, 85
    Stoll's guidelines for, 86–87
Associated manifestations, 12, 65
Asteatosis, 861
Astereognosis, 642
Asthma
  childhood, 794
  cough in, 326t

  dyspnea in, 324t–325t
  physical findings in, 333t
Astigmatism, headache from, 206t–207t
Asymmetric tonic neck reflex, 773t
Ataxia, 637, 638
  cerebellar, 638, 675t
  sensory, 675t
Ataxic breathing, 124t
Atelectasis, 332t
Atheroma, 399, 399f
Atherosclerosis
  on arterial circulation of thigh, 414, 414f
  in elderly, 864
  insufficient arterial supply to legs in
      evaluation of, 418–419, 418f–419f
    of legs, 426t
    leg ulcers in, 427t
    symptoms of, 406
  of mesenteric or celiac arteries, 407
  peripheral vascular, 424t–425t
  of renal artery, 423
Athetosis, 671t
Athlete's foot, 177t
Atonic seizure, 669t
Atopic dermatitis, in infants, 825t
Atopic eczema, 171t
Atrial fibrillation, 385t, 660t–661t
Atrial flutter, 385t
Atrial gallop, 390t
Atrial premature contractions, 385t
Atrial septal defect, in children
  adolescents, 811, 811t
  infants, 763
  murmurs in, 834t
Atrial sound, 390t
Atrioventricular (AV) block, 385t
Atrioventricular (AV) node, 345f
Atrioventricular valve, 339, 339f
Atrioventricular valve regurgitation, in infants,
    763
Atrophic glossitis, 289t
Atrophy, muscular, 524–525
Attention, 598, 598t
Attention deficit hyperactivity disorder
    (ADHD), in children, 802
Attention tests, 606
Atypical absences, 669t
Atypical nevus, 181t
Auditory acuity, 268
Aura, with seizures, 668t
Auricle, 250, 250f, 266
Auscultation, 98, 99. *See also specific systems*
  in anterior chest examination
    for adventitious (extra) sounds, 320, 331t
    for breath sounds, 319–320
  of heart, 368–375
    for heart murmurs, 372–375 (*See also*
        Heart murmurs)
    for heart sounds, 372, 372t
    overview of, 368
    S_1 and S_2 timing in, 370–371, 371f
    stethoscope components and use in, 368,
        368f, 369f
    stethoscope "inching" in, 369, 370f
  in posterior chest examination, 312–315

Auscultation *(continued)*
  for adventitious (extra) sounds, 314–315, 314t, 331t
  for breath (lung) sounds, 312–314, 313t, 330t
  for transmitted voice sounds, 315, 330t, 332t–333t
  use of, 312
Auscultatory gap, 111–112
Automatisms, 668t, 772
Autonomic nerve supply, to eyes, 216, 216f
Axillae examination, 102, 503–504. *See also* Breasts and axillae
Axillary lumps, 494
Axillary lymph nodes
  anatomy and physiology of, 102, 402f, 493, 493f
  in health assessment, 726
  physical examination of, 503
Axillary temperature, 116, 118
Axiohumeral group, 531, 531f
Axioscapular group, 531, 531f
Axons, 614

B

Babinski response
  in adults, 651, 651f, 772
  in infants, 772
Babinski sign, 645
Back
  chronic stiffness of, 584t
  physical examination of, 102
Back pain
  low, 522, 579, 584t
    idiopathic, 522
    radicular, 584t
    midline, 522
    off the midline, 522
Bacteremia, shaking chills in, 118
Bacterial meningitis, stiff neck in, 656
Bacterial vaginosis, 712t
Balance, in elderly, 866
Balance beam scale, 132, 132f
Balanitis, 705
Balanoposthitis, 705
Ball and socket joints, 520, 520f
Barrel chest, 329t
Bartholin's glands
  anatomy and physiology of, 684, 684f
  infection of, 711t
Basal cell carcinoma
  of ear, 278t
  in elderly, 862
  of skin, 165, 180t
Basal ganglia
  anatomy and physiology of, 614, 614f
  diseases of, 620
  function of, 619
  lesions of, 676t–677t
Basal ganglia system, 619
Basilar artery occlusion, 664t
Battered child syndrome, facies in, 829t
Beau lines, 186t
Beckwith-Wiedemann syndrome, 755

Behavior. *See also* Mental status; *specific types*
  clinical, 38–39
  health and, 595
  in mental status, 596–597, 601–602
  motor, 601
Bell, of stethoscope, 368
Bell palsy, 633
Belt, 108
"Benign forgetfulness," 847–848
Benign prostatic hyperplasia (BPH), 704–705, 846–847
Beverage intake record, 131
Bias, 81, 82
Bias, unconscious, 81
Biceps muscle, 538, 538f
Biceps reflex, 646–647, 646f
Biceps tendon, 532, 532f
Bicipital tendinitis, 537f
Bigeminal pulse, 429t
Biliary colic, abdominal pain in, 472t–473t
Binocular diplopia, 631
Binocular vision, 214, 214f
Biot breathing, 124t
Birthmarks, infant, 748, 749t
Bisferiens pulse, 429t
Bite, insect
  in adults, 175t
  in children, 826t
Bitemporal hemianopsia, 222f, 236t
Bladder
  anatomy of, 433f, 434
  control of functions of, 434
  distention of, 434, 459
  infection of, suprapubic pain in, 445
  physical examination of, 459
Blepharitis, 224
Blind patient, interviewing of, 57
Blind right eye, 236t
Bloating, 438
Blood loss, symptoms of, 440
Blood pressure, 109–115. *See also* Hypertension; Hypotension, orthostatic (postural)
  arterial pulses and, 347–348, 348f, 429t
  in children
    infants, 746
    school-aged, 783–784, 784t
  classification of, 113–114, 113t, 377t
  diet on, 139, 148t
  in elderly, 842, 860
  monitoring of, home, 109, 123
  orthostatic (postural), 114
  physical examination of, 355
  self-monitoring of, 109, 123
Blood pressure cuff
  in adults, 109–110, 110f
  in children, 783
Blood pressure measurement
  after lymph node dissection, 115
  with arrhythmias, 115
  auscultatory gap in, 111–112
  in dialysis patients, 115
  false readings in, 111, 113
  in leg, 114
  in obese or very thin patient, 115

  self-monitoring in, 109
  technique for, 110–113
  weak/inaudible Korotkoff sounds in, 115
  with weak pulse, 114–115
Blount's disease, 800
Blurred vision, 218
Body fat
  central, 133, 744, 745f
  female breast, 491, 491f
  under skin, 154f, 155
Body frame, 131
Body mass index (BMI). *See also* Obesity; Weight
  calculation of, 131, 134, 134t–135t
  classification of, 137, 137t
  excessive low, 142t
  in health assessment, 723
  high, 127
  low, 127, 138
  risk factors and, 137
  in school-aged children, 782, 783t
  table of, 135t
Body odors, 107
Body systems. *See also specific systems*
  in organizing clinical data, 25
Bone conduction
  anatomy and physiology of, 252, 252f
  physical examination of, 269, 269f
Bone density, 580
Bone pain, from vitamin D deficiency, 134
Bone quality, 580
Bone strength, 580
Bony landmarks, 293–295, 293t–295t
Borborygmi, 450
Bouchard nodes, 543, 545, 589t
Bounding pulse, 410, 429t
Boutonnière deformity, 589t
Bowel function change, 441
Bowel habits change, 440
Bowel sounds, 450, 484t
Bowing, leg (bowlegged), 134, 768, 800
Brachial artery, 357, 357f, 400, 400f
  in blood pressure measurement, 111
  physical examination of, 357, 357f
Brachial pulse palpation, 410, 410f
Brachioradialis muscle, 538, 538f
Brachioradialis reflex, 647, 647f
Braden scale, for pressure sore risk, 161, 162t–163t
Bradycardia, in infants, 717
Bradykinesia, 620
Bradypnea, 124t
Brain, 613–615, 613f, 614f
Brain injury, 193
Brainstem, 615
Brainstem lesions, 676t–677t
Brain tumor, headache from, 206t–207t
BRCA1/2 mutations, 509
BRCA 1/2 mutation screening, 510
Breast augmentation patient, 505
Breast awareness, 505–506
Breast cancer
  breast masses in, 514t
  counseling on, 512–513
  male, 503
  risk assessment for, 507

risk factors for, 497, 507–510, 508t
  benign breast disorders, 509, 510t
  BRCA1/2 mutations, 509
  breast density, 510
visible signs of, 495, 515t
Breast cancer screening, 510–512
  BRCA 1/2, 510
  breast self-examination in, 505–506, 511
  chemoprevention in, 512
  clinical breast examination in, 497–502, 511
    (*See also* Clinical breast examination
    (CBE), female)
  individualized screening in, 510
  mammography in, 510–511
  MRI in, 511–512, 512t
Breast changes, 507
Breast cysts, 501, 514t
Breast density, 510
Breast dimpling, 495, 515t
Breast disorders, benign, breast cancer and, 509,
    510t
Breast edema, 495, 515t
Breast examination
  clinical, 497–502, 511 (*See also* Clinical breast
    examination (CBE), female)
  self-examination, 505–506, 511
Breast lumps
  history of, 494, 514t, 515t
  palpation of, 502f, 503
Breast masses
  in adolescents, 811–812
  in adults, 501, 507, 514t
  palpable, 507
Breast nodules, 500, 501
Breasts and axillae, 490–515
  in adults
    in health assessment, 726
    physical examination of, 102, 103
    in review of systems, 70
  anatomy and physiology of, 490–493
    in female breast, 490–492
    lymphatics in, 493, 493f
    in male breast, 492
  breast masses
    in adolescents, 811–812
    in adults, 501, 514t
  in children
    adolescent breast development in,
        811–812, 812f
    infants, 763
  in elderly, 846, 865
  health history in, 493–496
    change in shape, 494
    common and concerning symptoms, 493
    dimpling, 495
    discharge or edema, 495
    family history, 496–497
    general, 495–496
    lifestyle habits, 497
    lumps and masses, 494, 514t, 515t
    pain or discomfort, 494
    rashes or scaling, 495
    retraction, 495
  health promotion and counseling on, 507–513
    benign breast disorders, 509, 510t

BRCA1/2 mutations, 509
breast cancer counseling, 512–513
breast cancer risk assessment, 507
breast cancer risk factors, 497, 507–510, 508t
  (*See also* Breast cancer, risk factors for)
breast cancer screening, 510–512
breast density, 510
chemoprevention, 512
female breast changes, 507
female breast symptoms, 507
palpable masses, 507
physical examination in, 497–506
  axillae, 102, 503–504
  breast augmentation patient, 505
  breast awareness and self-examination,
      505–506, 511
  female, 497–502 (*See also* Clinical breast
      examination (CBE), female)
  male breast, 503
  mastectomy patient, 505
  nipple discharge, 504
  recording findings on, 506
Breast self-examination, 505–506, 511
Breast shape change, 494, 514t, 515t
Breath, shortness of, 352. *See also* Dyspnea
Breathing. *See also* Respiration
  abnormalities in, 124t
  anatomy and physiology of, 298–299, 299f
  difficulties with, 300–301
  in exercise, 299, 299f
  lungs in, 298–299, 299f
  normal, 299, 299f
Breath odors, 107
Breath (lung) sounds, 312–314, 313t, 330t
  added, 314–315, 314t, 331t
  adventitious (extra), 314t, 331t, 332t–333t
    anterior auscultation for, 319–320
    posterior auscultation for, 314–315, 314t
  auscultation for
    anterior chest, 319–320
    posterior chest, 312–315, 313t, 330t
  in infants, 759, 759t
Bridging veins, 402, 402f
Broca aphasia, 603, 674t
Bronchi, major, 297, 298f
Bronchiectasis
  cough in, 326t
  hemoptysis in, 326t
Bronchitis, chronic
  cough in, 326t
  dyspnea in, 324t–325t
  hemoptysis in, 326t
  physical findings in, 332t
Bronchophony, 315, 330t
Brudzinski sign
  in adults, 656
  in children, 793
Bruits
  abdominal
    in adults, 450–451, 483t
    in elderly, 865
  arterial, 483t
  carotid, 357, 864
Brushfield spots, 753, 830t
Buccal mucosa, 263, 263f

Buerger disease
  pain in, 424t–425t
  wrist pulses in, 416f, 417
Bulbar conjunctiva, 211
Bulimia nervosa, 142t, 440
Bulla, 175t
Bullous myringitis, 280t
Bundle of His, 345, 345f
Bundling, excessive, 747
Bursae, 519, 520
  anserine, 569, 569f
  hip, 561
  iliopectineal, 561
  iliopsoas, 561
  ischial (ischiogluteal), 559f, 560f, 561
  olecranon, 539, 539f
  prepatellar, 569, 569f
  psoas, 559f, 561
  shoulder, 532, 532f
  subacromial, 532, 532f
  subscapular, 532
  trochanteric, 559f, 560f, 561
Bursitis, 521
  olecranon, 539
  trochanteric, 521

C

Café-au-lait spots
  in adults, 170t, 173t
  in infants, 748, 749t
CAGE questionnaire, 67–68, 467
Calcaneofibular ligament, 573, 573f
Calcaneus, 573, 573f
Calcium intake, 581–582, 582t
Calculating ability, 607
Callus, 592t
Campinha-Bacote model, 79
Canal of Schlemm, 213, 213f
Cancer. *See also specific types*
  in children, 792
  night sweats in, 118
  protuberant abdomens in, 483t
Cancer screening
  BRCA 1/2 mutation, 510
  breast, 510–512
    BRCA 1/2, 510
    breast self-examination in, 505–506, 511
    chemoprevention in, 512
    clinical breast examination in, 497–502,
        511 (*See also* Clinical breast
        examination (CBE))
    individualized screening in, 510
    mammography in, 510–511
    MRI in, 511–512, 512t
  cervical, 696
  colorectal, 469–471
  in elderly, 869
  prostate, 708–710
Candidal diaper dermatitis, 825t
Candidal vaginitis, 712t
Candidiasis, oral
  in children, 830t
  in infants, 755
  on palate, 285t
  on tongue, 289t

Canine teeth, 262f
Canker sore, 272, 272f, 290t
Capacity, patient, 52–53
Capillaries, 400
Capillary bed, in fluid exchange, 404–405, 404f
Capillary hemangioma, 748, 749t
Capillary leak syndrome, 428t
Caput medusa, 467
Carcinoma. *See also* Cancer screening; *specific types*
    of floor of mouth, 290t
    of lip, 283t
Cardiac apex, 337, 337f
Cardiac chambers, 339, 339f
Cardiac circulation, 339, 339f
Cardiac cycle, 340–342
    valve openings and closings in, 340–341, 341f, 342f
    ventricular pressures in, 340, 340f
Cardiac murmurs. *See* Heart murmurs, in adults
Cardiac output, 347
Cardiac syncope, 626
Cardinal directions, of extraocular movements, 217, 217f
Cardinal fields, 226–227, 227f, 242t
Cardiomegaly, in infants, 760
Cardiomyopathy, hypertrophic
    heart murmurs in, 393t
    syncope from, 666t–667t
Cardiopulmonary resuscitation (CPR), 88
Cardiovascular disease. *See also specific types*
    incidence of, 377
    lifestyle modifications for prevention of, 382
    risk assessment tools for, 380–381
    risk factor screening for, 381
Cardiovascular system, 336–395
    anatomy and physiology of, 337–350
        arterial pulses and blood pressure, 347–348, 348f, 429t
        auscultatory findings and chest wall, 344, 345f
        cardiac chambers, valves, and circulation, 339, 339f
        cardiac cycle, 340–342
            valve openings and closings, 340–341, 341f, 342f
            ventricular pressures, 340, 340f
        conduction system, 345–346, 345f, 346f
        heart and great vessel location, 337–339, 337f, 338f
        heart as pump, 347
        heart murmurs, 343–344, 344f
        heart sound splitting
            split S₁, 343
            split S₂, 342–343, 343f, 372t
        heart wall, 339
        jugular venous pressure, 348–350, 349f, 350f
        jugular venous undulations, 348, 348f
            vs. carotid pulsations, 359t
            highest point of, estimating, 349–350, 350f, 360, 360f
            measurement of, 359–360
    documenting findings in, 376
    ECG components and, normal, 346, 346f
    in elderly, 845, 864
    functions of, 336

in health assessment, 726
health history in, 350–354
    cardiac history, 354
    chest pain, 351
    cough, 353
    cyanosis and pallor, 353
    edema, 353
    family history, 354
    fatigue, 353
    lifestyle habits, 354
    nocturia, 353, 479t
    palpitations, 352
    shortness of breath, 352
health promotion in
    cholesterol, high, 378
    diabetes and metabolic syndrome, 378
    healthy lifestyles, 381–383
    hypertension, 377–378, 377t (*See also* Hypertension)
    incidence of cardiovascular disease, 377
    risk reduction, 379–381
    heart rates in, 384t
    heart rhythms in
        irregular, 384t, 385t
        normal, 384t
    heart sound variations in
        both systolic and diastolic components, 395t
        extra
            in diastole, 372t, 390t
            in systole, 372t, 389t
        first heart sound (S₁), 387t
        second heart sound (S₂), 388t
    integrating assessment in, 376
    physical examination of, 102, 354–376
        auscultation, heart murmurs in, 391t–394t
        blood pressure and heart rate review, 355
        face, 355
        great vessels of neck, 355–360
            brachial artery, 357, 357f
            carotid artery pulse, 355–357, 356f
            carotid thrills and bruits, 357
            jugular venous pressure, 259t, 357–360, 360f
        heart, 361–375 (*See also* Heart, physical examination of)
        hepatojugular reflux, 360
        patient preparation, 354–355
    in review of systems, 70
Caries, dental
    in children, 790, 831t
    nursing bottle, 790, 831t
Carotene, 155
Carotenemia, 159, 169t
Carotid arteries
    anatomy and physiology of, 194, 194f
    in elderly, 845
    physical examination of, 202
Carotid artery disease, stroke risk from, 661t
Carotid artery pulse, 355–357, 356f
    amplitude and contour of, 355–356, 356f
    thrill and bruits in, 357
Carotid bruits
    in adults, 357
    in elderly, 864

Carotid pulsations, *vs.* jugular venous undulations, 359
Carotid sinus, 356, 356f
Carpal bones, 541, 541f
Carpal tunnel, 543, 543f
Carpal tunnel syndrome, 544, 547, 547f
    causes of, 548
    maneuvers to test for, 547–548, 547f, 548f
Carpometacarpal arthritis, 545
Cartilage, 518
Cartilage, articular, 519, 519f
Cartilaginous joints, 519, 519f, 519t
Cataracts, 239t, 844, 863
Cat scratches, 177t
Cauda equina, 615
Cauda equina syndrome, 522
Cellulitis, pain in, 424t–425t
Central cyanosis
    in adults, 159
    in infants, 748, 759, 763, 832t
Central lymph nodes, 493, 493f
Central nervous system, 613–616. *See also specific structures*
    brain, 613–615, 613f, 614f
    spinal cord, 615, 615f
Central nervous system disorders, 676t–677t
Central venous pressure (CVP), 348
Cerebellar ataxia, 638, 675t
Cerebellar incoordination, 638
Cerebellar system, 619
Cerebellum, 613, 613f, 615
    damage to, 620
    diseases of, 635–636
    lesions of, 677t
Cerebral accidents, sudden, hemiplegia of, 655, 655f
Cerebral cortex lesions, 676t–677t
Cerebral palsy, mild, in children, 802
Cerebrum, 613, 613f
Cerumen, 250, 268
Cervical cancer screening, 696
Cervical cord compression, 585t
Cervical lymph nodes, in children, 793, 831t
Cervical myelopathy, 585t
Cervical radiculopathy, 585t
Cervical spondylosis, 585t
Cervix (uterine), 685, 685f
Chalazion, 241t
Chancre, syphilitic, 177t
    in female, 711t
    in male, 714t
    on mouth, 283t
Chancroid, in male, 714t
Characteristic symptom, 12, 65
Charting. *See* Documentation; *specific systems*
Cheilitis
    actinic, 282t
    angular, 282t
Chemical irritation, 326t
Chemoprevention, for breast cancer, 512
Cherry angioma
    in adults, 179t
    in elderly, 862
Chest examination, anterior, 316–320
    for adventitious (extra) sounds, 320, 331t

auscultation in, 319–320, 331t
inspection in, 316, 329t
palpation in, 316–317, 317f
percussion in, 318–319, 318f, 319f
Chest examination, posterior, 306–315, 307f
auscultation in, 312–315
for adventitious (extra) sounds, 314–315, 314t, 331t
for breath (lung) sounds, 312–314, 313t, 330t
for transmitted voice sounds, 315, 330t, 332t–333t
use of, 312
inspection in, 306–307, 329t
palpation in, 307–308, 307f, 308f
percussion in
diaphragmatic excursion in, 311–312, 311f
notes in, 310–312, 310t, 311f
technique in, 308–309, 309f
Chest expansion, 307
Chest findings, 293–296
around circumference of chest, 295–296, 295f, 296f
locating posterior, 294, 294t
locating vertical, 293–294, 293t
Chest indrawing, 758
Chest pain, 302–303, 327t–328t
anterior, 351
in cardiovascular health history, 351
exertional, 351
Chest wall
anatomy and physiology of, 292
auscultatory findings and, 344, 345f
in elderly, 844
pain in, 328t
Cheyne-Stokes breathing, 124t
"Chicken breast deformity," 756
Chicken pox, skin in, 182t
Chief complaint, 19, 41, 63t, 64. See also specific systems
Child abuse, 76
Child development. See Development
Childhood illnesses, 66
Children, 731–837. See also specific topics
adolescents, 806–819 (See also Adolescents)
development in, 733–734
health promotion and counseling in, 734–736
infants, 736–775 (See also Infants)
medical record for, 732
recording findings on, 820–823
school-aged, 776–806 (See also School-aged children)
sequence of examination in, 732
vaccine-preventable diseases in, 837t
Chilliness, 118
Chills, 118
Chlamydia, 698
Choanal atresia, 754
Cholecystitis
abdominal pain in, 437, 472t–473t
abdominal tenderness in, 486t
acute, 466
Chondrodermatitis helicis, of ear, 278t
Chondromalacia, of knee, 570
ChooseMyPlate, 128, 147t

Chordee, 765
Chorea, 671t
Chronic arterial insufficiency, of legs
advanced, 426t
evaluation of, 418–419, 418f–419f
leg temperature in, 411
leg ulcers in, 427t
symptoms of, 406
Chronic obstructive pulmonary disease (COPD)
AP diameter in, 306
dyspnea in, 324t–325t
in elderly, 863
hepatomegaly in, 487t
liver position in, 319, 319f
physical findings in, 333t
posture in, 107
Chronic otitis externa, 268, 268f
Chronic otitis media, 254
Chronic renal disease, skin in, 182t
Chronic venous insufficiency, 399
advanced, 426t
deep, pain in, 424t–425t
edema in, 428t
of leg
characteristics of, 426t
physical examination of, 411, 424t–427t
stasis ulcers in, 177t, 427t
Ciliary body, 212, 213, 213f
Circulation, cardiac, 339, 339f
Circumduction, 675t
Circumlocutions, 603
Cirrhosis, hepatomegaly in, 487t
Clarifying, in interview questioning, 48
Claudication, intermittent, 413
Clavicles, in children, 756, 767
Cleft palate, 792
Clinical breast examination (CBE), female, 497–502, 511
inspection in
arms at sides, 498, 498f
arms over heads, 499, 499f
general, 497
hands pressed against hips, 499, 499f
leaning forward, 499, 499f
overview of, 497
palpation in
breast, 500–502, 500f–502f
lump, 502f, 503
nipple, 502, 502f
Clinical breast examination (CBE), male, 503
Clinical data organization
age in, 24–25
body systems in, 25
challenges in, 24–26
data quality in, 26
multisystem conditions in, 25
sifting through data in, 25
single vs. multiple problems in, 24–25
symptom timing in, 25
Clinical findings. See also specific disorders and systems
clustering of, 16
evaluation of, 30–31
identify abnormal or positive, 16
as probable process, 16–17

recording of, 19–30 (See also Recording findings)
reliability of, 30
sensitivity of, 31–32
specificity of, 31
validity of, 30
Clinical reasoning, 15–19
hypothesis creation in, 17–18
integration of, 31–32
Clitoris, 684, 684f
Clonus, 650, 650f
Clubbing, of fingers and nails, 185t, 306
Clubfoot, 768
Clustered skin lesions, 172t
Cluster headache, 205t
CN VII facial paralysis, 673t
Coarctation of aorta, 114, 746, 760, 783, 784
Cochlea, 251
Cognitive development
in adolescents, 807, 807t–808t
in early childhood, 776, 776f
in infants, 737, 737f
in middle childhood, 777, 777t
Cognitive disabilities
in children, 802
interviewing patient with, 57
Cognitive functions
higher, 599t, 607–608
physical examination for, 605–607
Cold sore, 282t
Colic
biliary, abdominal pain in, 472t–473t
renal, 447
ureteral, 447
Collaborative partnerships, 82, 83
Colles fracture, 544, 544f
Colloid oncotic pressure, plasma protein, 404–405, 404f, 428t
Colon, 433–434, 433f
Colorectal cancer
bowel habits change in, 440
screening and risk factors for, 469–471
Coma (comatose patient), 601
abbreviated assessment of, 651–657
don'ts, 652
further examination, 656–657
general, 651–652, 662t, 663t
Glasgow Coma Scale, 653, 653t
level of consciousness, 652–653
meningeal signs, 656, 656f
neurologic evaluation, 544f, 654–656, 654f, 663t, 679t
abnormal postures in, 654, 662t
pupils in, 654, 679t
structural, 663t
toxic-metabolic, 663t
Comfort, patient, 93
Communicating veins, 402, 402f
Communication. See also Interviewing
about end-of-life treatment, 88
with dying patient, 87–88
effective, 88
experience of illness, patient, 36
nonverbal, 49
patient, in physical examination, 93

Communication *(continued)*
purpose of conversation in, 35
respectful, 82–83
supportive interaction in, 35
trust in, 35
Compartment syndrome, pain in, 424t–425t
Competence
cultural, 79, 80f
patient, 53
Complaint, chief, 63t, 64. *See also specific systems*
Complex atheromas, 399, 399f
Complex partial seizures, 668t
Compliance, heart, 342
Comprehensive health assessment. *See*
Health assessment, comprehensive;
specific systems
Comprehensive physical examination. *See*
Physical examination, comprehensive
Concave curves, spine, 550, 552f, 554f
Conduction system, 345–346, 345f, 346f
Conductive hearing loss
anatomy and physiology of, 251, 253
cranial nerves and, 633
physical examination for, 269, 269f, 281t
Conductive phase, 251
Condylar joints, 520, 520f
Condylar synovial joint, 528, 528f
Condyle
lateral, of femur, 566f, 567
medial, of tibia, 566, 566f, 569f
Condyloma acuminatum
in female
adults, 711t
children, 835t
in male, 714t
Cone, symptom, 44
Cone of light, 251, 251f, 268, 268f
Confabulation, 604
Confidentiality, patient
adolescent issues with, 809
in interview, 40, 58
Confusing patient, interviewing of, 52
Congenital cysts, of neck, 755
Congenital dermal melanocytosis, 748, 749t
Congenital heart disease, central cyanosis in,
748, 750, 822t
Congenital hypothyroidism, facies in, 828t
Congestive heart failure. *See* Heart failure
Conjugate gaze, in children, 786
Conjugate movements, 226
Conjunctiva
anatomy and physiology of, 211
physical examination of, 224, 224f, 238t
upper palpebral, 233, 233f
Conjunctivitis, 238t
Consciousness. *See also* Mental status
level of, 106
in comatose patient, 652–653
in mental health assessment, 598, 598t,
601
loss of, 626, 666t–667t
Consensual reaction, 215, 215f, 226
Consolidation, 330t
physical findings in, 332t
pneumonic, 758

Constipation
in adults, 442–443, 475t
in children, 795
Constitutional delay, in adolescent males, 813
Constrictive pericarditis, paradoxical pulse in,
421, 429t
Constructional ability, 608
Contact diaper dermatitis, 825t
Contact lens care, 235
Continuers, 48
Contraception, 690
Contractility, myocardial, 347
Convergence (eyes), 216, 228, 228f, 631
Conversation, purpose of, 35
Conversion reaction, 666t–667t
Convex curves, of spine, 550, 552t, 554f
Coordination
cerebellum in, 638
in children, 802, 802f
gait (*See also* Gait)
abnormalities of, 675t
in adults, 637–638, 637f
in children, 802, 802f
general, 635
point-to-point movements in, 636, 636f, 637f
rapid alternating movements in, 635–636,
635f, 636f
stance in, 638, 638f
Coping–stress-tolerance, 72t
Coracoid process, 530, 530f, 532f
Corn, 592t
Cornea, 225, 239t
Corneal arcus, 239t
Corneal infection, 238t
Corneal injury, 238t
Corneal light reflex, 228, 228f, 242t
Corneal opacities, 225, 239t
Corneal reflex, 632
Corneal scar, 239t
Corona, 699, 699f
Coronary heart disease
epidemiology of, 351
risk assessment for, 380
risk reduction for, 379
Corpis, 685, 685f
Corpora cavernosa, 699, 699f
Corpora spongiosum, 699, 699f
Cortical lesion, unilateral, 634–635
Corticobulbar tracts, 619, 620f
Corticospinal tract, 619, 620f
Corticospinal tract injury, 619
Costochondritis, chest pain in, 328t
Costovertebral angle, 434, 434f
Costovertebral angle tenderness, 458–459,
459f, 556
Cough, 301–302, 326t, 353
Cough syncope, 666t–667t
Cover–uncover test, 228, 242t
Coxsackie A virus, skin in, 182t
"Crabs," 694, 705
Crackles
in adults, 314–315, 314t, 331t
in infants, 759
Cranial nerve(s)
in adults, 616

anatomy and physiology of, 616,
616f–618f, 617t–618t
physical examination of, 630–635, 630t
in children
newborns and infants, 770, 770t–771t
school-aged, 803, 803t
disorders of, 206t–207t, 242t
Cranial nerve I (olfactory)
function of, 617t
physical examination of, 630
Cranial nerve II (optic)
function of, 617t
physical examination of, 630–631
Cranial nerve III (oculomotor)
disorders of, 631
function of, 617f, 617t
palsy of, 631
paralysis of, 242t
physical examination of, 631
Cranial nerve IV (trochlear)
function of, 617f, 617t
paralysis of, 242t
physical examination of, 631
Cranial nerve V (trigeminal)
function of, 617f, 617t
physical examination of, 631–632, 632f
Cranial nerve VI (abducens)
function of, 617f, 617t
paralysis of, 242t
physical examination of, 631
Cranial nerve VII (facial)
function of, 617t
physical examination of, 633, 633f
Cranial nerve VIII (acoustic)
function of, 617t
physical examination of, 633
Cranial nerve IX (glossopharyngeal)
function of, 618t
physical examination of, 633–634
Cranial nerve X (vagus)
function of, 618t
physical examination of, 633–634
Cranial nerve XI (spinal accessory)
function of, 618f, 618t
physical examination of, 634
Cranial nerve XII (hypoglossal)
function of, 618t
physical examination of, 634–635
Craniosynostosis, 751, 827t
Craniotabes, 751
Cranium, 616
Cremasteric reflex, in children, 797–798, 798f
Crepitus
definition of, 524
knee, 569, 570
Crescendo-decrescendo murmur, 374, 374f
Crescendo murmur, 374, 374f
Crescents, in optic disc, 243t
Cretinism, facies in, 828t
Cricoid cartilage, 195, 195f
Cries, abnormal infant, 755, 755t
Critical thinking, 11–33
data collection in, 32, 32f
objective, 13
subjective, 12

definition and overview of, 11–12
evaluating clinical findings in, 30–31
hypothesis creation in, 17–18, 32, 32f
hypothesis testing in, 32, 32f
integrating reasoning, assessment, and
    evidence analysis in, 31–32
nursing process in, 14–15 (*See also* Nursing
    process)
OLD CART in, 12
recording findings on, 19–30
    (*See also* Recording findings)
sample scenarios for, 13
signs in, 13
steps in, 13
symptoms in, 12
Crossed eyes
    in infants, 753
    in school-aged children, 786
Crossover test, shoulder, 535f, 536f
Croup, 757, 793
Crude touch, 621, 621f
Crust, 176t
Crying patient, interviewing of, 54
Cryptorchidism
    in adults, 706, 715t
    in children
        infants, 765
        school-aged, 798
Cultural assessment, 78–84
    collaborative partnerships in, 83
    cultural competence in, 79, 80f
    cultural humility in, 80–83
    culture defined in, 78–79
    health history and, 83–84
    overview of, 78–79
    respectful communication in, 82–83
    self-awareness in, 82
Cultural background, 81
Cultural competence, 79, 80f
Cultural desire, 79, 80f
Cultural humility, 80–83
Cultural identity, 82
Culture
    definition of, 78–79
    in health assessment, 79
Cushing disease, skin in, 182t
Cutaneous cyst, ear, 278t
Cutaneous hyperesthesia, 465–466
Cutaneous stimulation reflexes, 623, 623t,
    650–651
    abdominal, 650, 650f
    plantar response, 651, 651f
Cuticle, 156, 156f
Cyanosis, 155, 159, 169t, 306
    in cardiovascular health history, 353
    central
        in adults, 159
        in infants, 748, 759, 763, 832t
    in children, 832t
Cyanotic cardiac disease, 747
Cyst, 174t
    breast, 501, 514t
    congenital, of neck, 755
    cutaneous, of ear, 278t
    epidermal inclusion, 174t

epidermoid
    of ear, 278t
    female, 711t
    male, 706
epididymis, 716t
pilar, 197
thyroglossal duct, 754

D

Dacryocystitis, 241t, 753
Data. *See also specific types*
    clinical (*See* Clinical data)
    identifying, 63t, 64
    integration of, 31–32
    objective, 13
    subjective, 12
Data collection
    objective, 13
    sequence of, 32, 32f
    subjective, 12
Date, of history, 64
Deaf, interviewing of, 56–57
Deafness, 275
Death and dying patient, 87–88
Decerebrate rigidity, 662t
Decision maker, surrogate, 53
Decision making, evidence-based, 17
Decision-making capacity, patient, 53
Decorticate rigidity, 662t
Decrescendo murmur, 374, 374f, 375
Decubitus ulcers, 161, 162t–163t, 183t, 427t
Deep cervical chains, 198, 199
Deep tendon reflexes, in adults, 645–650
    ankle (Achilles), 649, 649f
    biceps, 646–647, 646f
    clonus, 650, 650f
    grading scale, 645, 645t
    knee, 648, 648f
    reinforcement, 646, 646f
    supinator or brachioradialis, 647, 647f
    technique, 645, 645f
    triceps, 647, 647f
Deep tendon reflexes, in children
    infants, 771–772, 771f, 772f
    school-aged, 802, 802f
Deep tendon response, 622, 622t
Deep veins, of legs, 401
Deep venous thrombosis (DVT), 398–399,
    424t–425t
    Homan sign in, 31
    prevention and early identification of, 423
    venous tenderness in, 413
Degenerative joint disease
    on hands, 589t
    joint pain in, 586t–587t
Dehydration
    in infants
        fontanelles in, 750, 750f
        skin in, 748
    membranes in, 133
    prevention of, 140–141
    skin in, 159
    tachycardia from, 133
    turgor recoil in, 133

Delayed puberty
    in adolescent males, 813
    in females, 694
    in males, 813
Delirium, 599, 876t
Deltoid ligament, 573, 573f
Dementia, 599
    Alzheimer, 873
    appearance in, 109
    in elderly, 872
Dental caries
    in children, 790, 831t
    nursing bottle, 790, 831t
Dental screening, 275–276
Dentin, 262, 262f
Dentures, 863
DENVER II, 741, 742f–743f,
    801
Deoxyhemoglobin, 155
Dependence, physical, 122
Dependent edema, 353
Depression, 601, 610
    affect in, 106
    agitated, 601
    appearance in, 109
    in elderly, 872
    major, 610
de Quervain tenosynovitis, 547, 547f
Dermatitis
    atopic, in infants, 825t
    diaper
        candidal, 825t
        contact, 825t
    neurodermatitis, 176t
    seborrheic, 197
Dermatofibroma, 174t
Dermatomes, 622, 642–644, 643f, 644f
Dermatomyositis, 170t
Dermis, 154f, 155
Detrusor muscle, 434
Development, child
    early childhood, 776, 776f
    infant, 736–737
        cognitive and language, 737, 737f
        physical, 736–737, 737f
        social and emotional, 737, 737f
    middle childhood, 777, 777t
    principles of, 733–734
Developmental delay, 741, 742f–743f
Developmental milestone testing, 741,
    742f–743f
Deviation
    of eye, 223, 224, 226
    of trachea, 200
Dextrocardia, 363
Diabetes mellitus
    breath odor in, 107
    neuropathic ulcer in, 427t
    pedal pulses in, 415, 415f
    risks with, 378
    skin in, 182t
    stroke risk from, 660t
Diabetic amyotrophy, 661
Diabetic retinopathy, ocular fundi in,
    247t

Diagnosis, nursing process, 14, 17. *See also specific systems*
basis of, 18
clinical reasoning in, 17–18
Diagnostic hypotheses, in interview, 44
Dialysis patients, blood pressure measurement in, 115
Diaper dermatitis, 825t
DIAPERS assessment, 858–859, 867
Diaphoresis, 159
Diaphragm (body), 298
Diaphragm (stethoscope), 368
Diaphragmatic excursion, percussion of, 311–312, 311f
Diarrhea, 442, 476t–477t
Diastasis recti, 482t, 764
Diastole
extra heart sounds in, 372t, 390t
jugular venous undulations in, 348, 348f, 349
pressures and heart sounds in, 340–342, 340f–342f
Diastole murmurs, 391t–394t
Diastolic blood pressure, in elderly, 860
Diastolic heart sounds, 395t
Diastolic hypertension, in elderly, 842
Diastolic murmurs, 373
Diastolic pressure, 348, 348f
Diet (dietary intake), 138–139
on blood pressure, 139, 148t
cardiovascular disease and, 382–383
counseling on, 136–137
in elderly, 860, 861
for health promotion, 138, 147t
rapid screen for, 143t
Diffuse esophageal spasm, chest pain in, 328t
Diffuse interstitial lung diseases, dyspnea in, 324t–325t
Digital rectal examination (DRE), 710
Digital scale, 132
Dimpling, skin, in breast cancer, 495, 515t
Diphtheria, on mouth, 285t
Diplegias, spastic, in children, 801
Diplopia, 219, 631
Direct reaction, 215, 215f, 226, 240t
Disc herniation, 555, 556, 584t
Discomfort, upper abdominal, 438
Discriminative sensations, 641–642, 642f
Discs, intervertebral, 552, 552f
Disease, 44
Disease/illness distinction model, 44
Disorientation, 605
Disruptive patient, interviewing of, 54–55
Dissecting aortic aneurysm, chest pain in, 328t
Disseminated intravascular coagulation, skin in, 182t
Distal air sacs, 298
Distal interphalangeal (DIP) joints, 541f, 542, 545, 545f
Distraction, in infant approach, 739
Distress
signs of, 108
spiritual, 85–86
Diverticulitis
abdominal pain in, 472t–473t
abdominal tenderness in, 486t

Dizziness
ear and, 254–255, 277t
neurological, 623–624, 664t–665t
(*See also* Stroke)
Documentation
of cardiovascular system findings, 376
in health assessment, 4
of health history, 76
of peripheral vascular system findings, 416–417
Doll's eye movements, 654, 679t
Do Not Resuscitate (DNR) status, 88
Doppler ultrasound stethoscope, 114
Dorsalis pedis artery
in adults, 401, 401f
in infants, 760
Dorsalis pedis pulse palpation, 415, 415f
Dorsiflexors, 573
Double vision, 219
Down syndrome
eyes in, 753
facies in, 829t
palpebral fissure in, 223
Draping, of patient, 93
Dress, 108, 602
Driving safety, in elderly, 872
Drop-arm test, 536, 537f, 588t
Drop attack, 669t
Drugs, illicit, in past history, 67–68
Drusen, 232, 863
Dry skin, 159, 176t
Dub. *See* Second heart sound (S₂)
Dullness. *See also specific systems*
in chest percussion, 310, 318, 332t–333t
diaphragmatic, in chest percussion, 311
liver, 454–455, 454f, 455f
Duodenum, 433, 433f
Dupuytren contracture, 523, 544, 590t
Durable power of attorney, 53
Duration, 12, 65
Dysarthria, 602, 634, 674t
Dysconjugate gaze, 226, 228, 228f, 242t
Dysdiadochokinesia, 635
Dysequilibrium, 277t
Dysesthesias, 625
Dyskinesia, tardive, 670t
Dyslipidemia, skin in, 182t
Dysmenorrhea, 687, 688
Dyspareunia, 689, 692
Dyspepsia, 438, 472t–473t
Dysphagia, 265, 441, 474t
Dysphonia, 674t
Dysplastic nevus, 181t
Dyspnea, 300–301, 324t–325t
in cardiovascular health history, 352
paroxysmal nocturnal, 352
Dysrhythmia, in infants, 761
Dystonia, 671t
Dysuria, 445, 479t

E

Earache, 253–254
Ear canal
anatomy and physiology of, 250, 250f
physical examination of, 267–268, 267f, 268f

Ear discharge, 254, 280t
Eardrum
abnormalities of, 279t–280t
normal, 279t
perforation of, 279t
physical examination of, 267–268, 267f, 268f
Earlobe, 250, 250f
Early childhood development, 776, 776f. *See also* Children; School-aged children
Early satiety, 441
Early systolic ejection sounds, 341, 389t
Ears, in adults, 249
anatomy and physiology of
equilibrium in, 252
pathways of hearing in, 251–252, 252f
structures in, 250 251, 250f
eardrum in
abnormalities of, 279t–280t
normal, 279t
in health assessment, 724
health history for, 252–256
common or concerning symptoms in, 252
dizziness and vertigo in, 254–255, 277t
earache in, 253–254
ear discharge in, 254, 280t
family history in, 255
hearing loss in, 252–253
lifestyle habits in, 255–256
past history in, 255
purpose and opening questions in, 252
tinnitus in, 254
health promotion for
hearing loss in, 275
hearing screening in, 275
physical examination of, 266–269
air and bone conduction in, 269, 269f
auditory acuity in, 268
auricle in, 266
ear canal and drum in, 267–268, 267f, 268f, 279t–280t
lumps in, 278t
recording findings on, 274
Ears, in children
abnormalities of, 830t
adolescents, 811
infants, 754, 754f
school-aged, 788–789, 788f
general examination, 706
hearing test, formal, 788–789, 789f
otoscopic examination, 788
tympanic membranes, 787–788, 788f
Ears, nose, mouth, and throat, in adults. *See specific organs*
Eating, healthy, 382–383
Eating disorders
in adolescents, 810
in adults, 127, 142t
Ecchymosis, 133, 179t
Ectocervix, 685
Ectropion, 226, 237t, 862
Eczema, atopic
in adults, 171t
in newborns and infants, 825t
Edema, 160
angioedema, on mouth, 282t

breast, 495, 515t
cardiovascular, 353
in chronic venous insufficiency, 428t
dependent, 353
in health history, 353
in left-sided heart failure, 353
of legs, palpation for, 411–412, 411f, 412f
leg swelling in, 411
from lymphatic dysfunction, 405
lymphedema
of arm and hand, 409
causes of, 428t
mechanisms of, 405
nonpitting, 428t
from overhydration, 133
peripheral, 376, 405, 412, 412f, 428t
of arm and hand, 409
causes of, 412, 428t
in heart examination, 376
of legs, 411–412, 411f, 412f, 428t
pitting
of legs, 412, 412f, 428t
vs. nonpitting, 160, 405
skin signs of, 160
from protein deficiency, 133
scrotal, 713t
skin
in breast cancer, 495, 515t
examination for, 160
Education, health, 3, 9. *See also specific systems*
Egophony, 315, 330t
Ejaculation, 703
Ejaculatory duct, 699f, 700
Ejection sounds
aortic, 389t
early systolic, 341, 389t
pulmonic, 389t, 393t
systolic, 372t
Elastic laminae, 400
Elastin, 400
Elbow, 538–541
bony structures and joints in, 538–539, 538f, 539f
muscle groups in, 538, 538f
olecranon bursae in, 539, 539f
physical examination of, 539–541
inspection in, 539, 539f
palpation in, 539, 539f
range of motion and maneuvers in, 540, 540f, 540t, 541f
posterior dislocation of, 539, 539f
supracondylar fracture of, 539, 539f
Elderly. *See* Older adults
Elder mistreatment, 873
Electrical vectors, 346, 346f
Electrocardiogram (ECG)
components of, normal, 346, 346f
electrical vectors in, 346, 346f
limb and chest leads in, 346, 346f
patterns of heart rhythms on, 384t, 385t
11th rib, 294, 294f
Embolism
acute peripheral vascular, 424t–425t
sudden arterial occlusion from, on limbs, 415
Emergency history, 62

Emotional cues, 42
Emotional development
in adolescents, 807, 807t–808t
in early childhood, 776, 776f
in infants, 737, 737f
in middle childhood, 777, 777t
Empathic responses, 49
Empowerment, patient, 51
Empty can test, 537f
Endocardium, 339
Endocrine system, in review of systems, 71
End-of-life decisions, 88
Entropion, 237t, 862
Environment
for interview, preparing, 39
for physical examination, 92–93, 92f, 93f
Epicondyle
lateral, of tibia, 567
medial, of femur, 566, 566f, 569f
Epicondylitis
lateral, 539
medial, 539
Epidermal inclusion cyst, 174t
Epidermis, 154–155, 154f
Epidermoid cysts
of ear, 278t
female, 711t
male, 706
Epididymis, 699f, 700
Epididymis abnormalities, 716t
Epididymis cyst, 716t
Epididymitis, acute, 716t
Epigastric hernia, 482t
Epigastric pain, 437
Epiglottitis, in children, 792
Episcleritis, 241t
Episcleritis, nodular, 224, 224f
Epispadias, 713t
Epistaxis, 259–260, 271
Epitrochlear lymph nodes
anatomy and physiology of, 402, 402f
physical examination of, 102, 410, 410f
Epstein pearls, 754
Epulis, 287t
Equilibrium, 252
Erb's point, 363f
Erectile dysfunction
in adults, 702–703
in elderly, 846
Erections, in elderly, 846
Erosion, 177t
Errors of refraction, 206t–207t
Erythema, 164, 169t
Erythema infectiosum, 169t, 182t
Erythema toxicum, 825t
Esophageal dysphagia, 441, 474t
Esophageal spasm, diffuse, 328t
Esophagitis, reflux, 303, 328t
Esotropia, 242t, 753
Essential tremors, in elderly, 848, 866
Estrogen replacement, 689
Ethics, of interviewing, 58–59
Ethnicity, 79
Eustachian tube, 250f, 253

Evaluation, nursing process, 15, 18
Eversion, ankle, 575t, 576f
Evidence-based decision making, 17
Exacerbating factors, 65
Examination, physical. *See* Physical examination
Excoriation, 177t
Exercise
on bone density, 583
breathing in, 299, 299f
cardiovascular disease and, 383
in elderly, 872
moderate and vigorous, 140t
on musculoskeletal system, 578–579
nutrition and, 139–140, 140t
stroke risk reduction in, 660t
Exertional angina, 351
Exertional pain, 351
Exophthalmos, 237t
Exostoses, 267, 267f
Exotropia, 242t, 753
Expectation, patient, 45
Experience of illness, for patient, 36
Expiration, 299, 299f
Expression, facial, 106, 602
Extension
ankle, 575t
elbow, 540, 540t, 541f
hand, 548
hip, 563t, 565, 565f
knee, 571f, 571t
neck, 557t
shoulder, 534f
spinal column, 558
thumb, 549, 549f
wrist, 546f, 546t
Extensor group, hip, 560, 560f
Extensor response, abnormal, 662t
External ear, 250, 250f
External elastic lamina, 400
External inguinal ring, 701, 701f
External jugular vein, 194, 194f
External pterygoids, 528, 528f
External rotation
hip, 563t, 566, 566f
knee, 571t
shoulder, 535f, 536f
Extinction, 642
Extra-articular disease, 518
Extra-articular joint pain, 521
Extra-articular structures, 518
Extra breath sounds, 314–315, 314t
Extraocular movements, 242t
anatomy and physiology of, 226–227, 227f
cardinal directions of, 217, 217f
cranial nerves in, 631
Extraocular muscles, 226–228, 242t
cardinal fields and extraocular movements, 226–227, 227f, 242t
convergence, 228, 228f
corneal light reflex, 228, 228f, 242t
cover–uncover test, 228, 242t
Extremities, lower, 103
Eyebrows, 223
Eye chart, Snellen, 221, 221f

Eye disorders, 236t–247t
  dysconjugate gaze, 226, 228, 228f, 242t
  eyelid variations and abnormalities, 223–224, 237t
  headache from, 206t–207t
  lumps and swellings, 226, 241t
  ocular fundi
    in diabetic retinopathy, 247t
    normal and hypertensive, 246t
  opacities of cornea and lens, 225, 239t
  optic disc abnormalities, 229–231, 230f, 244t
  optic disc variations, normal, 229–231, 230f, 243t
  pupillary abnormalities, 225–226, 240t
  red eyes, 224, 224f, 238t
  retinal arteries and arteriovenous crossings, 231, 245t
  visual field defects, 222–223, 222f, 223f, 236t
Eyelid patch, 749t
Eyelids
  examination of, 223–224
  variations and abnormalities of, 223–224, 237t
Eye movements
  adult (See Extraocular movements; Extraocular muscles)
  infant, 752–753
Eye protection, 235
Eyes, in adult, 211–247, 724
  anatomy and physiology of, 211–217
    autonomic nerve supply, 216, 216f
    extraocular movements, 217, 217f
    eye structures, 211–213, 211f–213f
    pupillary reactions in
      consensual reaction, 226
      direct reaction, 215, 215f, 226, 240t
      light reaction, 215, 215f, 225–226
      near reaction, 216, 216f, 226
    visual fields, 214, 214f
    visual pathway, 214–215, 215f
  health history for, 217–220
    common or concerning symptoms in, 217
    eye history in, 219–220
    family history in, 220
    general questions in, 218–219
    lifestyle habits in, 220
    purpose of, 218
  health promotion in
    contact lens care in, 235
    eye protection in, 235
    vision screening in, 234–235
  physical examination of, 220–233
    components, 220–221
    equipment, 221
    external eye, 223–226
      conjunctiva and sclera, 224, 224f, 238t
      cornea and lens, 225, 239t
      deviation, 223, 224, 226
      eyebrows, 223
      eyelids, 223–224, 237t
      iris, 225
      lacrimal apparatus, 226, 241t
      lumps and swellings, 226, 241t
      position and alignment, 223
      pupils, 225–226, 240t
    extraocular muscles, 226–228, 242t

cardinal fields and extraocular movements, 226–227, 227f, 242t
      convergence, 228, 228f
      corneal light reflex, 228, 228f, 242t
      cover–uncover test, 228, 242t
    nasolacrimal duct obstruction, 232, 232f
    ophthalmoscopic examination, 228–232
      mydriatic drop contraindications in, 228
      ophthalmoscope and its use in, 94, 94f, 228f, 229
      optic disc examination, steps for, 229–231, 230f, 243t–244t
        (See also Optic disc examination)
      retina examination, 231–232, 231f, 232f, 245t–247t
    patient preparation, 220
    upper palpebral conjunctiva, 233, 233f
    vision tests, 221–223
      peripheral vision, 222–223, 222f, 223f
      visual acuity, distal, 221, 221f
      visual acuity, near vision, 222
  recording findings on, 234
Eyes, in children
  abnormalities of, 830t
  adolescents, 811
  infants, 752–753, 752f
  school-aged, 785–787
    visual acuity, 786, 786f, 786t
    visual fields, 787, 787f

F

Face
  in cardiovascular assessment, 355
  in health assessment, 724
  myxedema, 208t
  physical examination of, 197
Faces Pain Scale, 119, 120f
Facets
  asymmetric, 106
  six, 3, 6, 9
Facial expression, 106, 602
Facial nerve palsy, in children, 828t
Facial nerve paralysis, 673t
Facial paralysis, 633, 673t
Facial symmetry, in infants, 752
Facies
  in adult
    acromegaly, 208t
    Cushing syndrome, 208t
    facial swelling, 208t
    myxedema, 208t
    nephrotic syndrome, 208t
    Parkinson disease, 208t
    parotid gland enlargement, 208t
  in children
    diagnostic, 752, 828t–829t
    infants, 752
Failure to thrive, 745
Faint, 666t–667t
Fainting, hysterical, 666t–667t
Fallopian tube, 685, 685f
Falls
  assessment of, in elderly, 870, 871f
  prevention of, 203, 579

False negative, 31
False positive, 31
Familial megalocephaly, 745
Familial short stature, 782
Family history, 20–21, 64t, 68
Family planning, 697
Family stress, sample nursing process for, 28
Family violence, 75–76
Farsightedness
  headache from, 206t–207t
  in health history, 218
Fasciculations
  in tongue, 634
  in trapezius muscles, 634
Fat (body)
  central, 133, 744, 745f
  female breast, 491, 491f
  under skin, 154f, 155
Fat (dietary), healthy vs. unhealthy, 382–383
Fatigue, 107–108, 353
Fecal impaction, 475t
Feelings, patient, 45, 49
Female breast. See Breasts and axillae
Female reproductive system. See Reproductive system, female
Femoral aneurysm, 413, 414
Femoral artery, 401, 401f
Femoral canal, 701
Femoral hernias, 717t
Femoral pulse palpation
  in adults, 413, 413f
  in infants, 760
Festination, 675t
Fetal alcohol syndrome, facies in, 828t
Fever, 116, 118
  causes of, 117
  in infants, 747
  on respiratory rate, 747
  rheumatic, 521
Fever blister, 282t
Fibroadenoma, 514t
Fibrocystic breast, 492
Fibromyalgia, neck pain from, 585t
Fibromyalgia syndrome, joint pain in, 586t–587t
Fibrous connective tissues, female breast, 491, 491f
Fibrous joints, 519t, 520, 520f. See also specific joints
Fibula, 572
FIFE, 45
Fifth disease, 169t, 182t
Findings, clinical. See Clinical findings; specific systems
Fine touch, 621, 621f
Fingernails. See Nails
Fingers. See also Hands
  muscle strength tests of, 549, 550f
  pleximeter, 99
  plexor, 99
  range of motion of, 548–549, 549f
Finger-to-nose test, 636
First branchial cleft, 754
First-degree heart block, 362

First heart sound (S$_1$)
  auscultation of, 370–372, 370f, 371f, 372t
  production of, 341, 341f
  splitting of, 343
  timing of, 370–371, 371f
  variations in, 372t, 387t
Fissure
  lung, 296–297, 296f, 297f
  skin, 177t
  tongue, 289t
Fitness
  exercise for (*See* Exercise)
  nutrition and, 139–140, 140t
Flaccidity, muscle, 526, 680t
Flail chest, traumatic, 329t
Flank pain, 447, 447f
Flash, across field of vision, 219
Flat feet
  in adults, 591t
  in children, 836t
Flatus
  passing excess, 441
  protuberant abdomens in, 483t
Flexion
  ankle, 575t
  elbow, 540, 540f, 540t
  hand, 548
  hip, 563–564, 563t, 564f
  knee, 571t, 572f
  neck, 557t
  plantar, 573
  shoulder, 534f
  spinal column, 557
  thumb, 549, 549f
  wrist, 546f, 546t
Flexor group, hip, 560, 560f
Flexor response, abnormal, 662t
Flexor retinaculum, 543, 543f
Flight of ideas, 604
Floaters, 219
Floaters, vitreous, 232
Floating ribs, 294, 294f
Floor of mouth, 273
Fluid exchange, capillary bed in, 404–405, 404f
Focused assessment, 61, 62t
Focused questions, 47–48
Focusing approach, 42
Follice-stimulating hormone (FSH), 689
Follow-up history, 61
Fontanelles, 750, 750f
Food intake record, 131
Foot, 572–576
  abnormalities of
    general, 591t
    toes and soles, 592t
  bony structures and joints of, 572–573, 573f
  deformities of, in infants, 768
  function of, 572
  in infants, 768–769
  muscle groups and ligaments of, 573, 573f
  physical examination of
    inspection in, 574
    palpation in, 574, 574f
    range of motion and maneuvers in, 575–576, 575f, 575t, 576f

Foot inversion, 836t
Forced expiratory time, 321
Fordyce spots (granules), 286t
Forearm supination, testing, 538f
Foreign body, nose, 789
Foreskin
  in adults, 699, 699f
  in infants, 765
Forgetfulness, "benign," 847–848
Fornices, 685, 685f
Four As, 121
Fourth heart sound (S$_4$)
  in elderly, 845, 864
  in infants, 762
Fovea
  anatomy and physiology of, 213, 213f
  examination of, 232
Fractured rib, 321
Fremitus (tactile)
  in anterior chest examination, 317, 317f
  chest disorders with, 332t–333t
  in infants, 758
  in posterior chest examination, 307–308, 308f
Frenulum, in children, 791
Friction rub
  abdominal, 450–451, 484t
  pericardial, 395t
  pleural, 331t
Frontal sinus
  anatomy and physiology of, 257, 257f
  physical examination of, 271, 271f
Function, patient, 45
Functional incontinence, 446, 480t–481t
Functional murmurs, 375
Functional syndromes, 596
Fundus, ocular
  anatomy and physiology of, 213, 213f
  in diabetic retinopathy, 247t
  in elderly, 863
  normal and hypertensive, 246t
Fundus, uterine, 685, 685f
Funnel chest, 329t, 756

G

Gag reflex
  in adults, 634
  in elderly, 848
Gait
  abnormalities of, 675t
  in adults, 107
    coordination of, 637–638, 637f
    hips and, 561, 561f
  in children
    infants, 772
    school-aged, 801, 802, 802f
    toe-in, 801
  in elderly, 860, 866
  velocity of, in elderly, 870
Galactorrhea, 494–495
Galant reflex, 774t
Galeazzi test, 768
Gallbladder, 433, 433f
Gallop, atrial, 390t
Gallstone pancreatitis, 437

Ganglion, wrist, 590t
Gas
  passing excess, 441
  protuberant abdomens in, 483t
Gas irritation, 326t
Gastric cancer, abdominal pain in, 472t–473t
Gastric emptying, delayed, 438
Gastritis, epigastric pain in, 437
Gastrocnemius muscle, 570
Gastroenteritis, in children
  infants, 764
  school-aged, 796
Gastroesophageal reflux, 326t
Gastrointestinal reflux disease (GERD)
  "alarm symptoms" in, 439
  endoscopy for, 439
  epigastric pain in, 437
  pharyngeal symptoms in, 438
  respiratory symptoms in, 438
Gastrointestinal system, 431–487
  anatomy and physiology of, 431–434
    abdominal cavity, 433
    landmarks, 431, 432f
    left lower quadrant, 432, 432f, 433–434, 433f
    left upper quadrant, 432, 432f, 433, 433f
    right lower quadrant, 432, 432f, 433f, 434
    right upper quadrant, 432, 432f, 433, 433f
  health history in, 435–444
    abdominal pain, 435–436, 436f, 472t–473t
    bowel function change, 441
    common or concerning symptoms, 435
    constipation, 442–443, 475t
    diarrhea, 442, 476t–477t
    dysphagia, 441, 474t
    gastrointestinal complaints, 435
    genitourinary tract symptoms, 435
    GI symptoms with abdominal pain, 440–441
    jaundice, 443–444
    lower abdominal pain or discomfort
      acute, 439
      chronic, 440
    odynophagia, 441
    upper abdominal pain or discomfort
      acute, 437–438
      chronic, 438–439
  health promotion in, 467–471
    alcohol abuse screening, 467–468, 611
    colorectal cancer screening and risk factors, 469–471
    hepatitis A risk factors, 468
    hepatitis B risk factors, 468–469
    hepatitis C risk factors, 469
  physical examination of, 447–460
    abdomen, 448–459 (*See also* Abdominal examination)
    equipment, 447–448
    tips, 448
  recording findings on, 466
  in review of systems, 70
  special techniques in, 460–465
    for abdominal wall mass, 466
    for ascites, 449, 451, 463–464, 463f, 464f, 483t (*See also* Ascites)

Gastrointestinal system *(continued)*
　for cholecystitis, 466
　for spleen, 460–463, 461f–463f
　　(See also Spleen)
　for ventral hernias, 466
　stools, black and bloody, 443, 478t
Gaze preference, 654
General appearance, 106–109
　apparent state of health in, 106
　dress, grooming, and personal hygiene in,
　　108, 602
　facial expression in, 106, 602
　fatigue in, 107–108
　level of consciousness in, 106
　motor activity and speech in, 107
　odors in, body and breath, 107
　posture and gait in, 107
　signs of distress in, 107
　vital signs in *(See* Vital signs)
　weakness in, 108
Generalized seizures, 626, 669t
General points, 70
General survey, 105–106, 131. *See also specific*
　　systems
　in comprehensive physical examination, 101
　in elderly, 860
　in head-to-toe sequence sample, 723–726
　in infants, 744
Genital herpes simplex
　in female, 711t
　in male, 714t
Genitalia
　in adults *(See* Reproductive system)
　ambiguous, 766
Genitalia, female
　in adults, external, 694
　in children
　　adolescents, 815–817, 816t, 817f
　　infants, 766
　　school-aged, 798–800, 799f
　in elderly, 847, 865
Genitalia, male
　in children
　　adolescents, 813–815, 813t–814t, 815f
　　infants, 765–766
　　school-aged children, 797–798, 798f
　　in elderly, 846–847, 865
Genital warts
　in men, 714t
　in women, 711t
Genitourinary tract symptoms, 435. *See also*
　　Renal system
Genogram, 69f, 72t
Geographic skin lesions, 172t
Geographic tongue, 289t
Geriatric screener, 10-minute, 853, 853t–854t,
　　865
German measles, skin in, 182t
Giant cell arteritis
　in elderly, 846
　headache from, 206t–207t
Gingiva, 261, 261f, 262f
Gingival hyperplasia, 287t
Gingival margins, 261, 261f, 262f
Gingival sulcus, 261, 262f

Gingivitis, 265, 266, 272
　acute necrotizing ulcerative, 287t
　in elderly, 863
　marginal, 287t
Glandular tissue, female breast, 491, 491f
Glans penis
　in adults, 699, 699f, 705
　in infants, 765
Glasgow Coma Scale, 653, 653t
Glaucoma
　cupping in, 244t
　in elderly, 844, 863
　headache from, 206t–207t
　narrow-angle, 225
　open-angle, 225, 863
　red eyes in, 238t
Glenohumeral joint, 530, 530f
Glossitis, atrophic, 289t
Gluteus maximus muscle, 560, 560f
Gluteus minimus muscle, 560
Goals
　for interview, 38
　provider- *vs.* patient-centered, 38
Goiter, 200
　multinodular, 209t
　neck symptoms in, 196
Golfer's elbow, 539
Gonococcal arthritis, 521
Gonococcal urethritis, 706
Gonorrhea, 698
Gout, chronic tophaceous, 589t
Gouty arthritis, acute
　on foot, 591t
　joint pain in, 586t–587t
Gower sign, 802
Graded response, questioning for, 48
Grand mal seizure, 669t
Granuloma, pyogenic, 287t
Graphesthesia, 642, 642f
Graves disease. *See* Hyperthyroidism
Gravida-para notation, 690
Gray matter, 614, 614f
Gray matter lesions, subcortical, 676t–677t
Greater trochanter, 559f, 560f, 561
Greater tubercle of humerus, 530, 530f
Great saphenous vein, 402, 402f
Great vessels, location of, 337f, 338–339, 339f
Great vessels of neck, 355–360
　brachial artery, 357, 357f
　carotid artery pulse, 355–357, 356f
　carotid thrills and bruits, 357
　jugular venous pressure, 259t, 357–360, 360f
Greeting, of patient, 39–41
Grip strength, 547, 547f
Groin anatomy, male, 700
Groin hernias, 717t
　femoral, 717t
　inguinal, 562, 717t
　　anatomy and physiology of, 701
　　direct, 717t
　　indirect, 713t, 717t
　　inspection of, 706–707
　　pain and swelling in, 704
　inspection of, 717t
Grooming, 108, 602

Growth charts, 744
Growth in children, somatic
　adolescents, 810
　infants, 744–745
　　head circumference, 745, 745f
　　length, 744, 745f
　　weight, 745
　school-aged
　　head circumference, 782
　　height, 782
　　weight, 782, 783t
Growth velocity, reduced, 744
Guidance, anticipatory, for children, 735
Guided questioning, 47–49
Gums
　anatomy and physiology of, 261, 261f, 262f
　bleeding of, 265
　findings in, 272
　　gingival hyperplasia, 287t
　　gingivitis
　　　acute necrotizing ulcerative, 287t
　　　marginal, 287t
　　　pregnancy tumor, 287t
　　recession, 288t
　physical examination of, 272
　vitamin deficiencies on, 133
Gynecomastia
　in adolescents, 812
　in adults, 503

H

Haemophilus influenzae type B, 837t
Hair
　anatomy and physiology of, 154f, 155
　in elderly, 842–843, 843f
　"grown-out," 109
　physical examination of, 164, 197
　vitamin deficiencies on, 133
Hair loss, 184t
Hairy leukoplakia, 289t
Hairy tongue, 289t
Halitosis, in children, 792
Hallux valgus, 591t
Hammer, reflex, 95, 95f
Hammer grip, 267
Hammer toe, 592t
Hamstring muscle, 560f, 561f
Handle of malleus, 251, 251f, 268, 268f
Hands, 541–550
　arterial supply to, 416f–417f, 417–418
　arthritis of, 589t
　bony structures of, 541, 541f
　carpal tunnel of, 543, 543f
　joints of, 541f, 542, 542f
　muscle groups of, 542
　physical examination of, 543–545, 548–550
　　inspection in, 543–544
　　palpation in, 544–545, 544f
　　range of motion in
　　　fingers, 548–549, 549f, 550f
　　　thumbs, 549, 549f, 550f
　rheumatoid arthritis on, 589t
　swellings and deformities of, 589t, 590t
　tendons and tendon sheaths of, 543

Hard of hearing, 56–57
Hashimoto thyroiditis, 202
Hay fever, 258
Head, in adults, 189–196
    anatomy and physiology of, 189, 190f
    eyes, ears, nose, throat (HEENT), 70, 101–102
    in health assessment, 724
    health history for, 194–196
        headache, 190–192
        head trauma or brain injury, 193
        traumatic brain injury, 193
    physical examination of, 197–202 (*See also
        under* Head and neck)
    preventing injury to, 203–204
    recording findings on, 202
Head, in children
    adolescents, 811
    craniosynostosis, 751, 827t
    diagnostic facies in, 828t–829t
    infants, 750–752, 750f
        facial symmetry of, 752
        hydrocephalus, 827t
        skull symmetry and head circumference in,
            751, 751f
        sutures and fontanelles in, 750, 750f
    school-aged, 785
Headache, 205t–207t, 623
    from eye disorders, 206t–207t
    health history in, 190–192
    migraine, 205t
        health history in, 190–192
        prodrome of, 192
        progress note on, sample, 33t
        sample nursing process for, 19–23, 26–27
    posttraumatic, 206t–207t
    primary, 190, 205t
    secondary, 190, 206t–207t
    from subarachnoid hemorrhage, 206t–207t,
        623
Head and neck. *See also* Head; Neck
    in elderly, 843–844, 862–863, 863f
    physical examination of, 197–202
        carotid arteries and jugular veins, 202
        equipment for, 197
        face, 197
        hair, 197
        lymph nodes, 198–199, 198f, 199f
        neck, 198
        scalp, 197
        skin, 197
        skull, 197
        thyroid gland, 200f–201f, 201–202
        trachea, 199–200
    recording findings on, 202
    traumatic brain injury prevention in, 203–204
Head and neck disorders. *See also* Headache;
    specific disorders
    facies in
        acromegaly, 208t
        Cushing syndrome, 208t
        facial swelling, 208t
        myxedema, 208t
        nephrotic syndrome, 208t
        Parkinson disease, 208t
        parotid gland enlargement, 208t

thyroid dysfunction (*See also*
        Hyperthyroidism; Hypothyroidism)
    enlargement, 209t
    multinodular goiter, 209t
    signs and symptoms of, 209t
    singular nodule, 209t
Head circumference
    in infants, 745, 745f
    physical examination of, 751, 751f
    in school-aged children, 782
Head-to-toe health assessment, 721, 722–728
    patient lying down, 726–727
    patient seated
        general survey, 723–726
        specific systems, 727–728
    patient standing, 728
    visual acuity, 728
Head trauma, 193
Healed perforation, of eardrum, 279t
Health
    apparent state of, 106
    definition of, 3
    patient view of, 7
    six facets of, 3, 6, 9
Health assessment, 3–10, 720–728.
        See also specific systems
    on admission, extent of, 5–6
    asking questions in, 9–10
    comprehensive, 62t
        chief complaint in, 63t, 64
        date and time of history in, 64
        family history in, 20–21, 64t, 68
        health patterns in, 64t, 72
        history of present illness in, 63t–64t, 64–66
        identifying data in, 63t, 64
        past history in, 64t, 66–68
        reliability in, 63t, 64
        review of systems in, 64t, 69–71
        seven components of, 63, 63t–64t
        source of history in, 63t, 64
        source of referral in, 63t, 64
    definition of, 720
    detecting patient changes in, 9–10
    documentation in, 4
    equipment for, 721t–722t
    focused, 720
    gaining confidence in, 720–721
    head-to-toe sequence of, 721
    head-to-toe sequence sample for, 722–728
        patient lying down, 726–727
        patient seated
            general survey, 723–726
            specific systems, 727–728
        patient standing, 728
        visual acuity, 728
    health care team and, 6
    health education in, 3, 9
    health history in, 4, 5
    health promotion in, 7–8
    listening and understanding in, 5, 9
    vs. medical health assessment, 6
    nurse role in, 8–10
    nursing care plan development in, 6, 9
    nursing process in, 4
    patient view of health in, 7

physical examination in, 4
preventive care and, 6, 7
purpose of, 4–5
sample case on, 8–9
scope of, 4
six facets in, 3, 6, 9
use of, 720
vital role of, 9
Health care delivery, scope of, 6–7
Health care proxy, 53
Health care team, 6
Health events, major, 69
Health history, 4, 5, 61–76. *See also*
        Communication; Interviewing; *specific
        disorders and topics*
    comprehensive assessment in (*See* Health
        assessment, comprehensive)
    cultural assessment in, 83–84
    documentation of, 76
    emergency history in, 62
    fluidity of, 63
    focused assessment in, 61, 62t
    follow-up history in, 61
    format of, 36
    interviewing process in, 36
    nutrition in, 128–131 (*See also* Nutrition)
    problem-oriented assessment in, 61
    purpose and use of, 61
    sensitive topics in, 72–76
        guidelines for, 73
        mental health history in, 75
        overview of, 72–73
        sexual history in, 73–75
    source of, 63t, 64
    transcultural perspectives on, 83–84
        (*See also* Cultural assessment)
Health indicators, 4
Health maintenance, 18, 29, 67. *See also specific
        systems*
Health patterns, 64t, 72
Health promotion, 7–8, 122–123
Health supervision visits, 735
Healthy People 2020
    health indicators in, 4
    purpose and scope of, 3–4
Hearing
    air conduction in, 252, 252f
    bone conduction in, 252, 252f
    in elderly, 863
    hard of, 56–57
    pathways of, 251–252, 252f, 253
    screening of, 274
Hearing deficits
    in adults, 56–57
    in children
        infants, 754
        school-aged, 788–789, 789f
    in elderly, 863
Hearing loss, 252–253, 275
    conductive, 251, 253, 281t, 633
    congenital, 253
    cranial nerves and, 633
    in elderly, 844
    interviewing patient with, 56–57
    from medications, 253

Hearing loss (continued)
  physical examination for, 269, 269f
  prevention of, 275
  screening for, 275
  sensorineural, 251, 253, 281t, 633
  vertigo with, 633
Hearing screening
  in adults, 275
  in elderly, 869
Hearing test, in children, 788–789, 789f
Heart
  in adults
    functions of, 336
    location of, 337–339, 337f, 338f
    as pump, 347
  in children
    adolescents, 811
    infants, 759–763
      auscultation of, 761–762, 762f
      heart murmurs in, 762–763, 833t–834t
      inspection of, 759–760
      palpation of, 760–761, 761f
    school-aged, 794–795, 794f, 795f
Heart, physical examination of, 361–375
  anatomic location in, 361
  aortic area in, 363f, 367, 370f
  apical impulse in, 363–366, 364f–366f, 386t
  auscultation of, 368–375
    heart murmurs, 372–375 (See also Heart
      murmurs)
    heart sounds, 372, 372t
    overview, 368
    S1 and S2 timing, 370–371, 371f
    stethoscope components and use, 368,
      368f, 369f
    stethoscope "inching," 369, 370f
  inspection in, 362
  integrating cardiovascular assessment in, 376
  palpation in, 363, 363f
  patient position in, 361, 361f
  percussion in, 367–368
  peripheral edema and, 376
  pulmonic area in, 363f, 367, 370f
  right ventricular area in, 366–367, 366f, 367f
  sequence of, 362, 362t
  timing and intensity of impulses/sounds in,
    361–362, 361f
Heart block
  atrioventricular (AV), 385t
  first-degree, 362
Heartburn, 438
Heart chambers, 339, 339f
Heart disease risk score, 380
Heart failure, 347
  cyanosis in, 159
  general findings in, 375
  in infants, 760, 762
  left-sided
    dyspnea in, 324t–325t
    edema in, 353
    physical findings in, 332t
    posture in, 107
Heart murmurs, in adults, 343–344, 344f,
    372–375
  aortic regurgitation, 375, 394t

aortic stenosis, 374, 375, 393t
aortic stenosis or aortic insufficiency, 344,
    344f
aortic valve, 357
auscultation of, 372–375, 391t–394t
    (See also Heart murmurs)
  diastolic, 373, 394t
  elderly, 845, 864
  grades of, 375t
  holosystolic, 373, 391t
  in hypertrophic cardiomyopathy, 393t
  innocent, 392t
  late systolic, 373
  locations of, 344, 345f
  midsystolic, 373, 392t, 393t
  mitral regurgitation, 374, 391t
  mitral stenosis, 374, 394t
  overview, 372, 372t
  pansystolic, 373, 391t
  pulmonic stenosis, 393t
  regurgitant, 344
  stenotic valve, 343
  timing, 373
  tricuspid regurgitation, 391t
  ventricular septal defect, 391t
Heart murmurs, in children
  adolescents, 811, 811t
  congenital, 833t–834t
  infants, 762–763
  school-aged, benign, 794–795, 795t
Heart rate, 384t, 385t. See also Pulse;
    specific disorders
  in elderly, 842, 860, 861
  in infants, 746–747, 746t
  physical examination of, 355
  from pulse, 116, 116f
  in school-aged children, 785, 785t
Heart rhythm, 116, 116f. See also specific
    disorders
  classification of, 384t
  in elderly, 842
  in infants, 761
  irregular, 385t
  regular, 384t
Heart sounds
  auscultation of, 370–372, 370f, 371f, 372t
    in diastole, 340–342, 340t–342t
    in elderly, 845, 864
  extra
    in diastole, 372t, 390t
    in systole, 372t, 389t
  first (S1)
    production of, 341, 341f
    splitting of, 343
    timing of, 370–372, 371f
    variations in, 387t
  fourth (S4), physiologic, 390t
  from heart valve closing, 339
  in infants, 761–762
  locations of, 344, 345f
  second (S2)
    production of, 341, 341f
    splitting of, 342–343, 343f, 372t
    timing of, 370–371, 371f
    variations in, 388t

  splitting of, 372, 372t
    split S1, 343
    split S2, 342–343, 343f
  third (S3), physiologic vs. pathologic, 390t
Heart valves, 339, 339f. See also specific valves
Heart wall, 339
Heatstroke, educating patients on, 122
Heaves, palpation for, 363
Heberden nodes, 543, 545, 545f, 589t
Heel, 573, 573f
Heel pain, 574
Heel-to-shin test, 636, 637f
Heel-walk, 637
Height
  in adults, 128
  in children
    infants, 744, 745f
    school-aged, 782
  in elderly, 847, 861
  measurement of, 131–132
Heinrich II Fall Risk Model, 870, 871f
Helix, 250, 250f
Hemangioma, 173t
Hematemesis, 440
Hematochezia, 443, 478t
Hematologic system, in review of systems, 71
Hematuria, 446
Hemianopsia, 223
  bitemporal, 222f, 236t
  homonymous, 222f, 223, 223f
  left homonymous, 236t
  temporal, 223, 223f
Hemiparesis, 526
Hemiparesis, spastic, 675t
Hemiplegia, 526, 662t
  acute
    arms in, 655, 655f
    legs in, 655–656, 655f
    of sudden cerebral accidents, 655, 655f
Hemisensory loss, 639
Hemoglobin, 155
Hemoptysis, 302, 326t
Hepatic bruit, 483t
Hepatitis
  alcoholic, visceral pain in, 435
  risk factors for, 444
  hepatitis A, 468
  hepatitis B, 468–469
  hepatitis C, 469
Hepatojugular reflux, 360
Hepatomegaly
  in adults, 456–457, 456f, 487t
  in children
    adolescents, 813
    school-aged, 797
Herald lesion, 171t
Hereditary hemorrhagic telangiectasia, 283t
Hernia
  epigastric, 482t
  groin
    femoral, 717t
    inguinal, 562
      anatomy and physiology of, 701
      direct, 717t
      indirect, 713t, 717t

in infant, 766, 766f
  inspection of, 706–707, 717t
  pain and swelling in, 704
  inspection of, 717t
  incisional, 482t
  scrotal, 713t
  umbilical, 482t, 764
  ventral, 466
Herniated disc, 555, 556, 584t
Herpes (simplex)
  genital, 172t, 174t
    in female, 711t
    in male, 714t
  mouth, 282t
Herpes simplex virus 6 (HSV 6), skin in, 182t
Herpes zoster
  in adults, 160, 174t, 182t
  in elderly, 862
  immunization for, in elderly, 870
Herpetic stomatitis, 830t
Heterochromia, 240t
Hidradenitis suppurativa, 503
Higher cognitive functions, 599t, 607–608
Hinge joints, 520, 520f
Hip disease, in children, 801
Hip dysplasia, 767, 767f
Hips, 559–566
  bony structures and joints of, 559–560, 559f, 560f
  bursae of, 561
  in children, 767, 767f
  flexion deformity of, 562, 563–564, 564f
  muscle groups of, 560, 560f
  physical examination of, 561–566
    inspection in, 561–562, 561f
    maneuvers in, 563–566, 564f–566f
    palpation in
      bony landmarks, 562
      inguinal structures, 562, 562f
      range of motion in, 563, 563t, 564f
  stability of, 559
Hirsutism, 197
History. *See also specific systems*
  emergency, 62
  family, 20–21, 64t, 68
  follow-up, 61
  health (*See* Communication; Health history; Interviewing)
  mental health, 75
  past, 20, 64t, 66–68
  personal and social, 21
  recording of, 20–21
  sexual, 73–75
History of present illness (HPI), 63t–64t, 64–66. *See also specific systems*
  key elements of, 65
  past occurrences of symptom in, 66
  pertinent positives and negatives in, 66
  risk factors or other pertinent information in, 66
  self-treatment in, 65
  seven attributes of symptom in, 65
  symptom cone in, 44
Hives
  in adults, 174t
  in children, 826t

Hoarseness, 196, 264–265, 633
Holosystolic murmurs
  in adults, 373, 391t
  in elderly, 864
Homan sign, in deep venous thrombosis, 31
Homonymous hemianopsia, 222f, 223, 223f, 630
Homonymous hemianopsia, left, 236t
Homonymous left superior quadrantic defects, 236t
Hoover sign, 758
Hop in place, 637
Hordeolum, 241t
Horizontal defect, 236t
Horizontal fissures, 296f, 297, 297f
Horizontal group, 404, 404f
Horner syndrome, pupils in, 225, 240t, 631
Hospice care, 88
"Hot flashes," 696
Household safety, for elderly, 870
HPV. *See* Human papillomavirus (HPV)
Human behavior, health and. *See* Behavior; Mental status; *specific disorders*
Human immunodeficiency virus (HIV)
  infection with, 692
  prevention of infection with
    in females, 697–698
    in males, 707–708
Human papillomavirus (HPV)
  infection with, 696
    condyloma acuminatum from
      in female, 711t
      in male, 714t
    vaccine for, 696–697
Humeroulnar joint, 538, 538f
Humerus dislocation, anterior, 588t
Humility, cultural, 80–83
Hydration, 140–141
Hydration status, 128, 140–141
Hydrocele, 713t, 766, 766f
Hydrocephalus, 827t
Hydrostatic pressure, 404, 404f, 428t
Hygiene, personal, 108, 602
Hymen, 684, 684f
  in children
    imperforate, 766
    school-aged, 798, 800
  sexual abuse on, 835t
Hyoid bone, 195, 195f
Hypalgesia, 640
Hyperactive reflexes, 645
Hyperalgesia, 640
Hypercholesterolemia risks, 378, 379
Hyperesthesia, 640
Hyperesthesia, cutaneous, 465–466
Hyperextension, hip, 563t, 565, 565f
Hyperlipidemia, stroke risk with, 660t
Hyperopia, 218
  headache from, 206t–207t
  optic disc examination in, 230
Hyperpnea, 124t
Hyperpyrexia, 116
Hyperreflexia, 645
Hyperresonance, in chest percussion, 311, 318, 333t

Hypertension
  in adults, 113–114, 113t
    classification of, 113–114, 113t, 377t
    diet recommendations for, 139, 148t
    eyes in, 223, 227f
    facts on, 378
    incidence of, 377
    lifestyle modifications for, 382
    ocular fundi in, 246t
    retinal arteries and arteriovenous crossings in, 231, 245t
    risk factors in, 379
    risk reduction for, 379
    risks with, 378
    stroke risk from, 660t
    unequal arm/leg blood pressures in, 114
    white coat, 115
  in children, 824t
    adolescents, 810
    infants, pulmonary hypertension, 761
    newborns, sustained, 746
    transient, 783
  in elderly, 842
  health promotion for, 377–378, 377t
  isolated systolic
    in adults, 114
    in elderly, 860, 864
  sample nursing process for, 27–28
Hypertensive retinopathy, ocular fundi in, 246t
Hyperthyroidism
  in children, facies in, 829t
  exophthalmos in, 237t
  eye convergence in, 228
  eyes in, 223, 227f
  hair in, 164, 197
  lid lag in, 226, 227
  motor activity in, 107
  signs and symptoms of, 209t
  skin in, 159, 182t
  stare of, 106
  symptoms of, 196
  thyroid gland in, 202
Hypertrophic cardiomyopathy
  heart murmurs in, 393t
  syncope from, 666t–667t
Hypertrophic scar, 176t
Hypertrophy, muscular, 524
Hyperventilation, 124t, 666t–667t
Hypervolemia, jugular venous pressure in, 358
Hypesthesia, 640
Hypoactive reflexes, 645
Hypocapnia, from hyperventilation, 666t–667t
Hypopnea, 124t
Hyporeflexia, 645
Hypospadias
  in general, 705, 713t, 765
  in infants, 765, 836t
Hypotension, orthostatic (postural)
  in adults, 114, 666t–667t
  in elderly, 842, 860–861
Hypothalamus, 614, 614f
Hypothenar atrophy, 590t
Hypothermia, 116
  educating patients on, 123
  in elderly, 842, 861

Hypothesis testing, 32, 32f
Hypothyroidism
  congenital, facies in, 828t
  dress in, 108
  hair in, 164, 197
  hoarseness in, 196
  motor activity in, 107
  myxedema face in, 208t
  signs and symptoms of, 196, 209t
  skin in, 159, 182t
  weight gain in, 127
Hypotonia, muscle
  in adults, 526
  in infants, 769
Hypoventilation, 124t
Hypovolemia
  jugular venous pressure in, 358
  syncope with, 666t
Hysterical fainting, 666t–667t

I

Ichthyosis vulgaris, 176t
Ideas, patient, 45
Identifying data, 63t, 64
Idiopathic low back pain, 522
Idiopathic pain, 121
Idiopathic pulmonary fibrosis, 324t–325t
Iliofemoral thrombosis, 413
Iliopectineal bursa, 561
Iliopsoas bursa, 561
Iliopsoas muscle, 560, 560f
Ilium, 559, 559f
Illness, 44
Immunization, 67. *See also specific
        immunizations*
  childhood, 735
  in elderly, 869
  for influenza, 323
  pneumococcal vaccine, 323
  for *S. pneumoniae* pneumonia, 323
Imperforate hymen, 766
Impetigo, 176t, 825t
Implementation, nursing process, 15, 18
Impoverished affect, 860
Incisional hernia, 482t
Incisors, 262f
Incoherence, 604
Incontinence, urinary, 446, 480t–481t
  in elderly, 858–859
  functional, 446, 480t–481t
  overflow, 446, 480t–481t
  prevention of, 471
  stress, 29–30, 445, 446, 480t–481t
  urge, 446, 480t–481t
Incoordination, cerebellar, 638
Incus, 250f, 251, 251f, 268, 268f
Indigestion, 440
Indirect inguinal hernia, 713t
Infant cries, abnormal, 755, 755t
Infantile automatisms, 772
Infant Periodicity Schedule, 775
Infants, 736–775. *See also* Children
  development of, 736–737
    cognitive and language, 737, 737f

    physical, 736–737, 737f
    social and emotional, 737, 737f
  health history in, 737–743
    approach in, 739
    birth history in, 738
    developmental milestone testing in, 741,
        742f–743f
    family history in, 738
    general guidelines on, 740
    health maintenance in, 738–739
    health patterns in, 739
    past history in, 738
  health promotion and counseling in, 775
  physical examination of, 743–774
    abdomen, 763–765
    birthmarks, 748, 749t
    breasts, 763
    ears, 754, 754f, 830t
    eyes, 752–753, 752f, 830t
    facies, 828t–829t
    general survey and vital signs, 744
    genitalia
      female, 766, 766f
      male, 765–766, 836t
    head, 750–752, 750f, 751f, 827t
    heart, 759–763, 833t–834t (*See also* Heart,
        in infants)
    mouth and pharynx, 754–759 (*See also*
        Mouth and pharynx, in children)
    musculoskeletal system, 767–768, 767f,
        768f, 836t
    neck, 755–756, 756f
    nervous system, 768–774 (*See also* Nervous
        system, in children)
    nose and sinuses, 754
    rectum, 766
    skin, 748, 749t, 825t, 826t
    somatic growth, 744–745
      head circumference, 745, 745f
      length, 744, 745f
      weight, 745
    thorax and lungs, 756–759
    vital signs, 746–747
      blood pressure, 746
      pulse, 746–747, 746t
      respiratory rate, 747
      temperature, 747
  recording findings on, 820–823
Infarct
  lacunar, 664t
  myocardial (*See* Myocardial infarction)
Inferior vena cava, 338f, 339, 401
Inflammation, signs of, 524
Influenza immunization
  in adult, 323
  in elderly, 869
Informant, surrogate, 53
Information, 607
Infraclavicular, 297
Infraclavicular lymph nodes, 493, 493f
Infrascapular, 297
Infraspinatus muscle, 531, 531f, 537f
Ingrown toenail, 592t
Inguinal canal, 701, 701f
Inguinal hernia, 562

  anatomy and physiology of, 701
  direct, 717t
  indirect, 713t, 717t
  in infant, 766, 766f
  inspection of, 562, 706–707, 717t
  pain and swelling in, 704
Inguinal ligament
  anatomy and physiology of, 701, 701f
  physical examination of, 562, 562f
Inguinal (lymph) nodes, 404
  male, 700
  superficial, palpation of, 415
Inguinal pain, 704
Inguinal ring, 701, 701f
Inguinal swelling, 704
Insect bite
  in adults, 175t
  in children, 826t
Insight, 598, 598t–599t, 605
Inspection, 98, 99
Inspiration, 298, 299f
Instrumental activities of daily living (IADL), in
        elderly, 854, 855t
Integumentary system, 153–186
  anatomy and physiology of, 154–156
    functions in, 154
    hair in, 154f, 155
    nails in, 156, 156f
    sebaceous glands in, 154f, 156
    skin in, 154–155, 154f
    sweat glands in, 154f, 156
  diseases and skin conditions in, 182t
  hair loss in, 181t
  in health assessment, 723–724
  health history in, 156–158
    common or concerning symptoms in, 156
    family history in, 157
    lifestyle and personal habits in, 157–158
    past history in, 157
    purpose of, 156
  health promotion and counseling on, 165–168
  physical examination of, 101, 158–162
    hair, 164
    nails, 164, 164f
    pressure ulcers, 161, 162t–163t, 183t,
        427t
    skin, 158–163
    skin lesions, 160–161, 162t–163t,
        171t–181t (*See also* Skin lesions)
  recording findings on, 165
  in review of systems, 70
  skin cancer in, 165–168 (*See also* Skin cancer)
  vitamin deficiencies on, 133
Intelligence limitations, interviewing patient
        with, 57
Intention tremors, 636, 670t
Intercarpal joint, 542, 542f
Intercostal spaces, 292, 293, 293t
Interdental papillae, 261, 261f
Intermittent claudication, 413
Internal capsule, of brain, 615
Internal elastic lamina, 400
Internal inguinal ring, 701, 701f
Internal jugular vein, 194, 194f
Internal pterygoids, 528, 528f

Internal rotation
  hip, 563t, 566, 566f
  knee, 571t
  shoulder, 535f, 536f
Interobserver reliability, 30
Interpersonal space, 41
Interphalangeal joints, 541f, 542
Interpreter, working with, 55–56
Interscapular, 297
Interstitial colloid oncotic pressure, 404, 404f
Interstitial lung diseases, diffuse, 324t–325t
Interventions, nursing, 18
Intervertebral discs, 552, 552f
Intervertebral foramen, 551, 551f
Interviewing, 35–59. *See also* Communication;
      specific systems
  adaptation of
    for silent patient, 51–52
  ethics and professionalism in, 58–59
  experience of illness in, patient, 36
  health history format in, 36
  phases of, 36–46 (*See also specific phases*)
    introduction, 36, 39–41
    pre-interview, 36, 37–39
    termination, 37, 46
    working, 37, 41–46
  process of, 36
  purpose of conversation in, 35
  setting goals in, 38
  sexuality and nurse–patient relationship in,
      58
  for special patients, adapting, 51–58
    angry or disruptive patient, 54–55
    confusing patient, 52
    crying patient, 54
    hearing impairment, 56–57
    intelligence limitations, 57
    language barrier, 55–56
    low literacy, 56
    patient with altered capacity, 52–53
    personal problems, 57–58
    talkative patient, 53–54
    vision impairment, 57
  supportive interaction in, 35
  therapeutic communication techniques in,
      46–51 (*See also* Therapeutic
      communication techniques)
  trust in, 35
Interviewing process, 36
Intestinal ischemia, 407
Intestinal obstruction, abdominal pain in,
      472t–473t
Intima
  arterial, 399, 399f
  venous, 401
Intracranial pressure, in infants, 750
Intraobserver reliability, 30
Intraurethral pressure, 434
Introduction phase, of interview, 36, 39–41. *See
      also specific systems*
  arranging room in, 40–41
  confidentiality in, 40
  greeting patient and establishing rapport in,
      39–41
Introitus, 684, 684f, 685f

Inversion
  ankle, 575t, 576f
  foot, 836t
Involuntary movements, 627, 670t–672t
Iris, 225
Iritis, 238t
Irritability, in newborn
  extreme, 769
  persistent, 769
Irritable bowel syndrome
  bowel habits change in, 440
  constipation in, 475t
Ischemia
  intestinal, 407
  mesenteric, abdominal pain in, 472t–473t
  myocardial (*See* Myocardial infarction)
  stroke (*See* Stroke; Transient ischemic attack)
Ischial (ischiogluteal) bursa, 559f, 560f, 561
Ischial tuberosity, 555f, 556f, 561
Ischium, 559, 559f
Isolated systolic hypertension
  in adults, 114
  in elderly, 860, 864

J

Jacksonian seizure, 668t
Jaundice
  artificial light on, 158
  in health history, 443–444
  in infants, 748, 748f
  sclera in, 224, 224f
  skin in, 155, 159, 169t
Joint anatomy and physiology, 519–520. *See also*
      Musculoskeletal system; *specific joints*
  acromioclavicular, 530, 530f
  bursae in, 520
  cartilaginous, 519, 519f, 519t
  condylar, 520, 520f
  fibrous, 519t, 520, 520f
  glenohumeral, 530, 530f
  hinge, 520, 520f
  intercarpal, 542, 542f
  knee, 567
  metacarpophalangeal, 542, 542f
  pain in, 521
  patellofemoral, 567
  radiocarpal, 542, 542f
  radioulnar, distal, 542, 542f
  spheroidal (ball and socket), 520, 520f
  sternoclavicular, 530, 530f
  synovial, 519–520, 519f, 519t, 520f
  tibiofemoral, 567
Joint capsule, 519, 519f
Joint examination, 523–577. *See also specific joints*
  acromioclavicular, 536, 536f
  ankle and foot, 572–576
  elbow, 538–541
  general points on, 523
  hips, 559–566
  inflammation and arthritis signs in, 524
  knee, 566–572
  leg length in
    changes in, 562
    measurement of, 576–577, 577f
    unequal, 555

  limited motion description in, 577, 577f
  muscle bulk in, 524–525, 525f
  muscle strength in, 526–527
  muscle tone in, 525–526
  pain patterns in, 586t–587t
  recording findings on, 578
  shoulder, 529–538, 588t
  spine, 550–559
  temporomandibular, 527–529
  terminology in, 518–519
  tips for, 523–524
  wrist and hands, 541–550
Joint pain, 521. *See also specific joints*
  extra-articular, 521
  patterns of, 586t–587t
Judgment, patient, 598, 599t, 605
Jugular veins
  anatomy and physiology of, 194, 194f,
      348–349, 349f
  in children, 357
  physical examination of, 202
Jugular venous pressure (JVP), 348–349
  anatomy and physiology of, 348–350, 349f
  in hypervolemia, 358
  in hypovolemia, 358
  physical examination of, 259t, 357–360, 360f
  steps for assessment of, 358–360, 360f
Jugular venous undulations, 348, 348f, 349, 359
  vs. carotid pulsations, 359t
  highest point of, estimating, 349–350, 350f,
      360, 360f
  measurement of, 359–360

K

Kaposi sarcoma, in AIDS, 285t
Kawasaki disease, skin in, 182t
Keloids, 176t, 278t
Kernig sign
  in adults, 656, 656f
  in children, 793
Kidneys. *See also* Renal system
  anatomy of, 434, 434f
  enlargement of, 458
  pain in, 447, 447f, 458
  physical examination of, 457–459
    left kidney palpation in, 457–458
    percussion tenderness in, 458–459, 459f
    right kidney palpation in, 458, 458f
  right, lower pole of, 433, 433f
Kidney stone, 437, 439
Klebsiella pneumonia, 326t
Klinefelter syndrome, small testis in, 715t
Knee, 566–572
  bony structures of, 566–567, 566f
  joints of, 567
  ligaments in, 566, 566f
  mechanisms of, 566
  menisci and ligaments of, 567–568, 568f
  muscle groups of, 567, 567f
  physical examination of, 568–572
    inspection in, 568
    maneuvers in, 571–572
    palpation in, 569–570, 569f–570f
    range of motion in, 571, 571f, 571t, 572f

Knee bend, shallow, 637
Knee reflex, 648, 648f
  in elderly, 848
  reinforcement of, 646, 646f
Knock-knee pattern, 800
Koplik spots, 286t
Korotkoff sounds, 111
  in paradoxical pulse, 421, 429t
  weak/inaudible, 115
Kubler-Ross, 87
Kussmaul breathing, 124t
Kyphoscoliosis, thoracic, 329t
Kyphosis, 554f
  in elderly, 844–845, 847, 860
  thoracic, 554, 554f

L

Labia, genital, in children
  infants, 766
  school-aged, 798
Labial adhesions, in children
  infant, 766
  school-aged, 799
Labial frenulum, 261, 261f
Labial mucosa, 261, 261f
Labia majora, 684, 684f
Labia minora, 684, 684f
Lacrimal apparatus, 226, 241t
Lacrimal gland, 212, 212f
Lacrimal puncta, 212, 212f
Lacrimal sac, 212, 212f
Lacunar infarcts, 664t
Lamina, 551, 551f
Landau reflex, 774t
Landmarks, bony, 293–295, 293t–295t
Language, in mental status, 599t, 602–603, 603t
Language barrier, interviewing patient with, 55–56
Language development
  in early childhood, 776, 776f
  in infants, 737, 737f
  in middle childhood, 777, 777t
Laryngitis, 326t
Lateral bending
  neck, 557t
  spinal column, 558
Lateral collateral ligament (LCL), 568, 568f
Lateral condyle of femur, 566f, 567
Lateral epicondyle of tibia, 567
Lateral epicondylitis, 539
Lateral joint, 573, 573f
Lateral lymph nodes, 493, 493f, 504
Lateral menisci, 568, 568f
Lateral nail folds, 156, 156f
Latissimus dorsi muscle, 553, 553f
Leading questions, 48
Lead poisoning, oral mucosa in, 272
Learning ability, new, 607
Left atrial pressure, 340–341, 341f
Left-beating nystagmus, 672t
Left homonymous hemianopsia, 236t
Left lower quadrant, 432, 432f, 433–434, 433f
Left lower quadrant pain, 439

Left-sided heart failure
  dyspnea in, 324t–325t
  edema in, 353
  physical findings in, 332t
  posture in, 107
Left upper quadrant, 432, 432f, 433, 433f
Left ventricle, 338, 338f
Left ventricular failure
  cough in, 326t
  hemoptysis in, 326t
Left ventricular pressure, 340–341, 340f, 341f
Leg bowing, 134, 768, 800
Leg length
  changes in, 562
  measuring, 576–577, 577f
  unequal, 555
Legs
  arterial supply to, 418–419, 418f–419f
  blood pressure in, 114
  flaccid, 655–656, 655f
  in infants, 768
  physical examination of, 409t, 410–416
    inspection in, 410–411
    palpation in, 411–416
      for DVT, 413
      for edema, 411–412, 411f, 412f
      pulses in, 413–415, 413f–415f, 429t
      for temperature, 411
Length, in infants, 744, 745f
Lens, eye
  in adults, 225, 239t
  in elderly, 863
  opacities of, 225, 239t
Lethargy, 601, 652t
Leukokoria, 753
Leukonychia, 186t
Leukoplakia
  hairy, 289t
  mouth findings in, 286t
  on tongue, 290t
Leukorrhea, 686, 800
Levator palpebrae, 212, 212f
Level of arousal, in comatose, 652–653
Level of consciousness, 106
  in comatose, 652–653
  in mental health assessment, 598, 599t, 601
Lhermitte's sign, 585t
Libido, male, 702
Lice, 694, 705
Lichenification, 176t
Lid lag, 226, 227
Lid retraction, 237t
Lifting, low back and, 579
Ligamentous laxity, 524
Ligaments, 518
Light-headedness, 623
Lighting, 92–93, 92f, 93f
Light reaction, 215, 215f
Light sensitivity, 217
Light touch, 640
Linear epidermal nevus, 172t
Linear skin lesions, 172t
Lingual frenulum, 262, 263f

Lipid disorders
  risk reduction in, 379
  risks with, 378
Lipomas, abdominal wall, 482t
Lips. *See also* Mouth and pharynx
  abnormalities of, 282t–283t
  anatomy and physiology of, 261, 261f
  carcinoma of, 283t
  physical examination of, 272
Listening
  active, 47
  to dying patient, 87–88
  in health assessment, 5, 9
  in interview, 51
  in spiritual assessment, 86
Literacy, low, interviewing patient with, 56
Liver, in adults
  anatomy of, 433, 433f
  in COPD, position of, 319, 319f
  physical examination of, 454–457
    enlarged, 456–457, 456f, 487t
    palpation in, 455–457, 455f–457f
    percussion in, 454–455, 454f, 455f
Liver, in children
  infants, 764
  school-aged, 796t, 797, 797f
Liver disease, skin in, 182t
Liver span
  in adults, 454–455, 454f, 455f
  in children, 796t
"Liver spots," 862
Lobar pneumonia, 330t
Lobes
  of brain, 613, 614f
  of ear, 250, 250f
  of lung, 296–297, 296f, 297f
  Riedel, 487t
Lobule, of ear, 250, 250f
Location, 12, 65
Longitudinal arch, 573, 573f
Lordosis, 554f
  lumbar, 564, 564f
  problems with, 562
Loss of consciousness, 626, 666t–667t
Loss of sensation, 625–626
Low back pain, 522, 579, 584t
  idiopathic, 522
  radicular, 584t
  sample nursing process for, 29
Lower extremities, 103
Lower motor neuron injury, 619
Lower motor neurons, 618
Lower respiratory infection, nasal flaring in, 757
Low literacy, interviewing patient with, 56
Lub. *See* First heart sound (S_1)
Lumbar curvature, 550, 552f, 554f
Lumbar lordosis, 564, 564f
Lumbosacral junction, 552, 552f
Lumps
  breast or axillary
    history of, 494, 514t, 515t
    palpation of, 502f, 503.
  ear, 278t
  eye, 226, 241t

Lung abscess
  cough in, 326t
  hemoptysis in, 326t
Lung cancer
  cough in, 326t
  hemoptysis in, 326t
Lungs
  air-filled, 330t
  airless, 330t
  in children, 793–794, 794f
  in elderly, 844
  physical examination of, 102
Lung sounds. *See* Breath (lung) sounds
Lunula, 156, 156f
Luteinizing hormone (LH), 689
Lymphadenopathy, 196, 198, 199
  in adults, 196, 198, 199, 415, 503
  in children, 792, 831t
Lymphangitis, acute, 424t–425t
Lymphatic system and lymph nodes, 195–196, 195f
  anatomy and physiology of, 403–404, 403f, 404f
  breast, 493, 493f
  fluid exchange and capillary bed in, 404–405, 404f
  health history in, 405–408
  peripheral disorders of, painful, 424t–425t
  physical examination of, 410, 410f, 415–416
  reproductive system
    female, 686
    male, 700
Lymphedema
  of arm and hand, 409
  causes of, 428t
Lymph nodes, 493, 493f. *See also* Lymphatic system and lymph nodes
  anatomy and physiology of, 195–196, 195f, 402–403, 402f
  axillary
    anatomy and physiology of, 402, 402f, 493, 493f
    in health assessment, 726
    physical examination of, 503
  central, 493, 493f
  cervical, in children, 793, 831t
  dissection of, blood pressure after, 115
  epitrochlear, 402, 402f
  infraclavicular, 493, 493f
  lateral, 493, 493f, 504
  of neck, in infants, 755, 756f
  pectoral, 493, 493f, 504
  physical examination of, 198–199, 198f, 199f
  subscapular, 493, 493f, 504
  supraclavicular
    in adults, 198, 199, 493, 493f
    in children, school-aged, 793
  tonsillar, 198

M

Macrocephaly, 197, 745, 751
Macroglossia, 755
Macula, 213, 213f
Macula examination, 232, 232f

Macular degeneration
  in adults, 232, 232f
  in elderly, 844
Macular star, 246t
Macule, 173t
Major fissures, 296f, 297, 297f
Major health events, 69
Malabsorption, in children, 795
Male breast, 492, 503
Male reproductive system. *See* Reproductive system, male
Malignancy. *See* Cancer
Malignant melanoma, 165–168. *See also* Skin cancer
  in adults, 165–168, 181t
  in elderly, 862
Malleus, 250f, 251, 251f
Malocclusion, in children, 791
Malodor, 863
Mammary duct ectasia, 501
Mammography, 509, 510–511
Manic episode, 601
Manner, 602
Manubrium, 530, 530f
Masseter muscles, 528, 528f, 529
Mastectomy
  patient examination after, 505
  prophylactic bilateral, 512
Mastoiditis, in children, 788
Mastoid process, 250f, 251
Maxillary sinus
  anatomy and physiology of, 257, 257f
  physical examination of, 271, 271f
Measles, 182t, 837t
Measurement error, 744
Media
  arterial, 399f, 400
  venous, 401
Medial collateral ligament (MCL), 568, 568f, 569f
Medial condyle, of tibia, 566, 566f, 569f
Medial epicondyle, of femur, 566, 566f, 569f
Medial epicondylitis, 539
Medial malleolus, 573, 573f
Medial menisci, 568, 568f
Median nerve
  in carpal tunnel, 543, 543f
  on forearm, 539
Medically unexplained symptom, 596
Medical records, review of, 38
Medications, in past history, 66
Medullated nerve fibers, in optic disc, 243t
Mees lines, 186t
Megalocephaly, 745
Meibomian glands, 212, 212f
Melanin, 155
Melanoma, malignant, 165–168
  in adults, 165–168, 181t (*See also* Skin cancer)
  in elderly, 862
Melena, 443, 478t
Memory, 598, 598t
  recent, 607
  remote, 607
Menarche, 687, 688, 812
Ménière disease, 254, 633

Meningeal irritation, in children, 793
Meningeal signs, in comatose, 656, 656f
Meningitis, headache in, 206t–207t, 623
Meningococcemia, skin in, 182t
Menisci, 568, 568f
Menopause, 687, 689, 696
Menorrhagia, 689
Menstrual history, 687–689
Mental health history, 75
Mental health screening
  high-yield questions for, 597
  mental status examination in, 52, 598t–599t, 600–601
  mini-mental status examination in, 609, 873
  patient identifiers for, 597
Mental status, 595–611
  in elderly, 847–848, 865–866
  in health assessment, 723
  health history in, 597–599
    attention, mood, and speech in, 598, 598t–599t
    delirium or dementia in, 599
    insight, orientation, and memory in, 598, 598t–599t, 605–606
    mental status examination in, 598t–599t
    overview of, 598
  health promotion and counseling on
    for alcohol and substance abuse, 467–468, 611
    for depression, 610
    for suicide, 611
  in infants, 769
  physical examination in, 599–609
    appearance and behavior, 601–602
    cognitive functions, 605–607
    equipment, 599
    higher cognitive functions, 599t, 607–608
    mental status examination, 600–601
    mini-mental status examination, 609
    mood, 603–604
    speech and language, 602–603, 603t
    thought and perceptions, 604–605
  recording findings on, 609
  symptoms and behavior in, 596–597
    patient identifiers for selective screening, 597
    patient symptoms, 596
    unexplained symptoms, 596
Mental status examination (MSE), 52, 598t–599t, 600–601
Mesenteric ischemia, abdominal pain in, 472t–473t
Metabolic coma, 663t
Metabolic syndrome
  definition of, 378
  risks with, 378
  weight and, 137
Metabolic syndrome tool, 380
Metacarpal bones, 541, 541f
Metacarpophalangeal joints (MCPs), 541f, 542, 542f
  inspection of, 544–545, 544f
  in rheumatoid arthritis, 545
  synovitis in, 544, 544f
Metatarsalgia, 574
Metatarsals, 573

Metatarsophalangeal joint, 573, 573f, 574
Metatarsophalangeal joint range of motion, 575t, 576, 576f
Metatarsus adductor, 768, 836t
Metrorrhagia, 689
Microcephaly, 745, 751
Micrognathia, 752
Micturition syncope, 666t–667t
Midaxillary line, 296, 296f
Midclavicular line, 295, 295f, 365, 365f
Middle cerebral artery (MCA) stroke, 659, 664t–665t
Middle childhood development, 777, 777t
Middle ear, 250f, 251
Midline back pain, 522
Midline structures, 195, 195f
Midsternal line, 295, 295f, 365f
Midsystolic murmurs, 373, 392t–393t
Migraine headache, 205t
    health history in, 190–192
    prodrome of, 192
    progress note on, sample, 33t
    sample nursing process for, 19–23, 26–27
Mild cognitive impairment (MCI), 872–873
"Milk letdown," 492
"Milk line," 492, 492f
Milky discharge, 504
Mini-Cog, 865, 877t
Mini-Mental Status Examination (MMSE), 609, 873
Minimum geriatric competencies, 875t
Mini Nutritional Assessment (MNA), 855, 856f
Minor fissures, 296f, 297, 297f
Miosis, 225
Mitral area, 370f
Mitral regurgitation
    in elderly, 845
    heart murmurs in, 374, 391t
Mitral stenosis
    cough in, 326t, 344f
    heart murmurs in, 374, 394t
    heart sounds in, 362
    hemoptysis in, 326t
Mitral valve, 339, 339f
Mitral valve prolapse, 389t
Mitral valve stenosis, 342, 390t
Mnemonics and acronyms
    ADPIE, 14–15
    FIFE, 45
    NURS, 42
    OLD CART, 12, 43, 65
    OPQRST, 43
    SnNout, 31
    SpPin, 31
Mobility, skin, 159
Molars, 262f
Moles. See Nevus (nevi)
Molluscum contagiosum, 826t
Mongolian spots, 748, 749t
Monocular vision, 214, 214f
Mononeuritis multiplex, 661
Mood
    health history for, 598, 598t–599t
    physical examination for, 603–604
Morton neuroma, 591t

Motor activity, 107
Motor behavior, 601
Motor function, in infants, 769
Motor nerves, 616
Motor pathways, 618–620, 618f, 620f
Motor system, 635–638
    coordination
        gait, 637–638, 637f
        general, 635
        point-to-point movements, 636, 636f, 637f
        rapid alternating movements, 635–636, 635f, 636f
        stance, 638, 638f
Motor tone, in infants, 769
Motor vehicle accidents, preventing head injuries in, 203–204
Mouth, 249
Mouth and pharynx, in adults, 261–266
    anatomy and physiology of, 261–263, 261f–263f
        gums, 261, 261f, 262f
        lips, 261, 261f
        teeth, 262, 262f
        tongue, 262–263, 263f
    floor of mouth, 273
    in health assessment, 725
    health history for, 264–266
        dysphagia in, 265
        family history in, 266
        gum bleeding in, 265
        hoarseness in, 264–265
        lifestyle habits in, 266
        past history in, 266
        sore throat in, 264
        sore tongue in, 265
        toothache in, 265
    health promotion in
        oral and dental screening in, 275–276
        salivary flow in, 276
    lip abnormalities in, 282t–283t
    pharynx, palate, and oral mucosa findings, 284t–286t
        diphtheria, 285t
        Fordyce spots (granules), 286t
        Kaposi sarcoma, 285t
        Koplik spots, 286t
        leukoplakia, 286t
        petechiae, 286t
        pharyngitis, 284t
        thrush, 285t
        tonsils
            exudative, 284t
            large normal, 284t
        torus palatinus, 273, 285t
    physical examination of, 272–274, 285t
        gums and teeth, 272
        lips, 272
        oral mucosa, 272, 272f
        pharynx, 274
        roof of mouth, 273, 285t
        tongue and floor of mouth, 273, 273f
    recording findings on, 274
Mouth and pharynx, in children
    abnormalities of, 830t

infants, 754–759
    auscultation in, 758–759, 759t
    inspection in, 754–758, 757t
    palpation in, 758
    school-aged, 790–792, 791f, 791t
MRSA precautions, 100–101
Mucoid sputum, 301
Mucous patch, of syphilis, 290t
Multinodular goiter, 209t
Multiple-choice answers, in interview questioning, 48
Multisystem conditions, in organizing clinical data, 25
Murmurs, heart. See Heart murmurs
Murphy sign, 466
Muscle bulk, 524–525
Muscle flaccidity, 134, 526
Muscle hypotonia, 526
Muscle strength, 526–527
    in children, 802, 802f
    fingers, 549, 550f
    neck, 556
    spinal column, 559
    supraspinatus muscle, 537f
    wrist
        extension, 546, 546f
        grip, 547, 547f
Muscle tone, 525–526
    with basal ganglia lesions, 620
    basal ganglia system on, 619
    with cerebellar lesions, 620
    in coma, 654–655, 655f, 662t
    corticospinal tract on, 619
    disorders of, 680t
    with lower motor neuron lesions, 619
    motor pathways for, 619
    with upper motor neuron lesions, 619
Muscle wasting, protein deficiency, 134
Muscular atrophy, 524–525, 525f
Muscular dystrophy, 802
Muscular hypertrophy, 524
Muscular pseudohypertrophy, 525
Musculoskeletal pain, sample nursing process for, 29
Musculoskeletal system, in adults, 517–592
    in elderly, 847, 865
    feet abnormalities in, 591t
    hands in
        arthritis in, 589t
        swellings and deformities of, 590t
    in health assessment, 727, 728
    health history in, 521–522
        joint pain, 521
        low back pain, 522, 584t
        midline back pain, 522
        neck pain, 522–523, 585t
        off the midline back pain, 522
        questioning, 521–522
    health promotion in, 578–583
        fall prevention, 579
        low back, 579
        nutrition, exercise, and weight, 578–579
        osteoporosis, 579–583
    joint examination in, 523–577 (See also Joint examination)

joint pain patterns, 586t–587t
joints in (*See also* Joint; *specific joints*)
  bursae in, 520
  types of, 519–520, 519f–520, 519t
physical examination of, 102, 103, 104
recording findings on, 578
in review of systems, 71
terminology for, 518–519
toe and sole abnormalities of, 592t
Musculoskeletal system, in children
  adolescents, 817–818, 817f, 818f, 836t
  infants, 767–768, 767f, 768f, 836t
  school-aged, 800–801, 800f, 836t
Mycoplasma pneumonia, 326t
Mycosis fungoides, 172t
Mydriasis, 225
Mydriatic drops, contraindications to, 228
Myocardial contractility, 347
Myocardial dysfunction, in infants, 760
Myocardial infarction
  chest pain in, 327t
  epidemiology of, 351
  epigastric pain in, 436
  syncope from, 666t–667t
Myocardium, 339
Myoclonus, 669t
Myopathy, 108, 566
Myopia, 218, 221
  headache from, 206t–207t
  optic disc examination in, 230
MyPlate, 128, 147t
Myringitis, bullous, 280t

N

Nail bed, 156, 156f
Nail folds, 156, 156f
Nail pitting, 186t
Nail plate, 156, 156f
Nail polish
  "grown out," 109
  vitamin deficiencies on, 133
Nail root, 156, 156f
Nails
  anatomy and physiology of, 156, 156f
  in elderly, 842
  findings in, 185t–186t
  fingernails, 109
  nutrition and, 133
  physical examination of, 109, 164, 164f
Narrow-angle glaucoma, 225, 844
Nasal breathers, obligate, 754
Nasal cavity
  cross section of, 257, 257f
  lateral wall of, 256–257, 257f
  medial wall of, 256, 256f
  physical examination of, 270–271
Nasal congestion, 258
Nasal flaring, in infants, 757
Nasal mucosa, 270f, 271
Nasal obstruction, 270
Nasal passage, 270, 270f
Nasal polyps
  in adults, 271
  in children, 789

Nasal septum, 256, 256f, 270f, 271
Nasolacrimal duct, 212, 212f, 256–257
Nasolacrimal duct obstruction, 232, 232f
Nausea, 440
Near reaction, 216, 216f
Near response, 631
Nearsightedness, 206t–207t, 218
Near syncope, 626
Near vision, 222
Neck, in adults, 193–196. *See also* Spine
  anatomy and physiology of, 193–196
    anterior triangle in, 193, 194f
    great vessels in, 194, 194f
    lymph nodes in, 195–196, 195f
    midline structures in, 195, 195f
    posterior triangle in, 193, 194f
    thyroid gland in, 195, 195f
  in health assessment, 725
  muscle strength of, 556
  physical examination of, 102, 198
    (*See also under* Head and neck)
  range of motion of, 556–557
  recording findings on, 202
  in review of systems, 70
  symptoms of, 196
Neck, in children
  adolescents, 811
  infants, 755–756, 756f
  school-aged, 792–793, 793f
Neck mobility
  in children, 793
  in coma, 656
Neck pain, 522–523, 585t
Neck stiffness
  in bacterial meningitis, 656
  in subarachnoid hemorrhage, 656
Neck vessels, 355–360
  brachial artery, 357, 357f
  carotid artery pulse, 355–357, 356f
  carotid thrills and bruits, 357
  in elderly, 845
  jugular venous pressure, 259t, 357–360, 360f
Negative
  false, 31
  true, 31
Neonatal acne, 825t
Nerve cells, 614
Nerve root compression
  low back, 584t
  neck, 585t
Nervous system, in adults, 613–680
  abbreviated assessment of comatose patient
    in, 651–657
    don'ts, 652
    further examination, 656–657
    general, 651–652, 662t, 663t
    Glasgow Coma Scale, 653, 653t
    level of consciousness, 652–653
    meningeal signs, 656, 656f
    muscle tone, 680t
    neurologic evaluation, 544f, 654–656, 654f, 663t, 679t
    pupils, 679t
  anatomy and physiology of, 613–623
    central nervous system, 613–616

    brain, 613–615, 613f, 614f
    spinal cord, 615, 615f
    peripheral nervous system, 616–623
      cranial nerves, 616, 616f–618f, 617t–618t
      dermatomes, 622
      motor pathways, 618–620, 618f, 620f
      peripheral nerves, 616–618
      sensory pathways, 620–622, 621f
      spinal reflex, cutaneous stimulation, 623, 623t
      spinal reflex, deep tendon, 622, 622t
  coma, 663t
  elderly, 847–848, 865–866
  in health assessment, 727–728
  health history in, 623–627
    dizziness or vertigo, 277t, 623–624, 664t–665t (*See also* Stroke)
    headache, 623
    loss of consciousness, 626, 666t–667t
    loss of sensation, 625–626
    seizures, 626–627, 668t–669t
    tremors and involuntary movements, 627, 670t–672t
    weakness, 624–625
  health promotion and counseling on, 657–661
    peripheral neuropathy risk reduction in, 661
    stroke at a glance in, 658–659
    stroke prevention in, 657–658
    stroke risk factors in
      primary prevention, 659, 659t–660t
      secondary prevention, 659
    stroke warning signs in, 658
    transient ischemic attack prevention in, 657–658
  physical examination of, 103–104, 627–651
    appropriate detail of, 629
    categories of, 630
    coordination, 635–638
      gait, 637–638, 637f, 675t
      general, 635
      point-to-point movements, 636, 636f, 637f
      rapid alternating movements, 635–636, 635f, 636f
      stance, 638, 638f
    cranial nerves, 630–635
      cranial nerve I, 630
      cranial nerve II, 630–631
      cranial nerve III, 631
      cranial nerve IV, 631
      cranial nerve V, 631–632, 632f
      cranial nerve VI, 631
      cranial nerve VII, 633, 633f, 673t
      cranial nerve VIII, 633
      cranial nerve IX, 633–634
      cranial nerve X, 633–634, 674t
      cranial nerve XI, 634
      cranial nerve XII, 634–635
      summary, 630t
    cutaneous stimulation reflexes, 650–651
      abdominal, 650, 650f
      plantar, 651, 651f
    deep tendon reflexes, 645–650
      ankle (Achilles), 649, 649f

Nervous system *(continued)*
    biceps, 646–647, 646f
    clonus, 650, 650f
    grading scale, 645, 645t
    knee, 648, 648f
    reinforcement, 646, 646f
    supinator or brachioradialis, 647, 647f
    technique, 645, 645f
    triceps, 647, 647f
  disorders of
    central, 676t–677t
    peripheral, 678t
  equipment for, 628
  guidelines for, 627–628
  screening examination in, 629
  sensory system, 639–644
    dermatomes, 642–644, 643f, 644f
    discriminative sensations, 641–642, 642f
    general, 639
    light touch, 640
    pain, 640
    patterns of testing of, 639–640, 640f
    proprioception, 641, 641f
    temperature, 640
    vibration, 640–641, 641f
  speech disorders, 675t
  postural hypotension, 114, 666t–667t
  recording findings on, 657
  syncope, 666t–667t
Nervous system, in children
  adolescents, 818
  infants, 768–774
    age-specific techniques for, 769
    cranial nerves in, 770, 770t–771t
    development of, 772–773
    mental status in, 769
    motor function and tone in, 769
    neurologic screening in, 769
    reflexes in, deep tendon, 771–772, 771f, 772f
    reflexes in, primitive, 772, 773t–774t
    sensory function in, 770
  school-aged, 801–803, 802f, 803t
    cranial nerves, 803, 803t
    DENVER II, 801
    gait, strength, and coordination, 802, 802f
    reflexes, deep-tendon, 802, 802f
    sensation, 801
Neuralgias, cranial, 206t–207t
Neurodermatitis, 176t
Neurofibromatosis, 555
  in infants, 748, 749t, 825t
  in newborns, 825t
Neurologic screening, in infants, 769
Neurologic system, in review of systems, 71
Neuromuscular junction disorder, 678t
Neurons, 614
Neuropathic pain, 121
Neuropathic ulcer, 427t, 592t
Neuropathy, weakness in, 108
Nevus (nevi)
  in adolescents, 810
  in adults
    atypical (dysplastic), 181t
    benign, 181t

    linear epidermal, 172t
    malignant, 181t
Nevus simplex, 748, 749t
New learning ability, 607
Night sweats, 118
Nipple
  female, 491–492, 491f, 492f
  male, 492
  Paget disease of, 515t
  supernumerary, 492, 492f
Nipple discharge, 494–495, 504, 504f
Nipple retraction, 495, 515t
Nociceptive pain, 121
Nocturia, 353, 445–446, 479t
Nodal premature contractions, 385t
Nodule
  breast, 500, 501
  skin, 174t
  subcutaneous, 524
Nonamnestic mild cognitive impairment, 873
Nonfocusing approach, 42
Nongonococcal urethritis, 706
Nonpitting edema, 160, 405, 428t
Nonverbal communication, 49
Normal sinus rhythm (NSR), 346, 346f
Nose and paranasal sinuses, in adults, 249
  anatomy and physiology of, 256–257
  functions of, 256
  in health assessment, 725
  health history for, 258–261
    change in smell in, 260
    congestion in, 259
    epistaxis in, 259–260
    lifestyle habits in, 260
    opening questions in, 258
    past and family histories in, 260
    rhinorrhea in, 258–259
  physical examination of, 270–271
    equipment for, 270
    inside of nose, 270, 270f
    nasal cavity, 271
    nasal obstruction, 270
    sinus tenderness, 271, 271f
    recording findings on, 274
Nose and paranasal sinuses, in children
  infants, 754
  school-aged, 788, 788f
Notetaking, pre-interview, 39
Nuchal rigidity, in children, 793
Nuclear cataract, 239t
Nucleus pulposus, 519, 519f, 552, 552f
Number identification, 642, 642f
Number list, 606
Numbness, 625
NURS, 42
Nursemaid's elbow, 800
Nurse–patient relationship, sexuality and, 58
Nursing care plan
  development of
    critical thinking in, 19
    in health assessment, 6, 9
    negotiation of, 46
Nursing presence, 85–86

Nursing process
  ADPIE in, 14–15
  assessment in, 15–19, 17 (*See also* Assessment, nursing process)
  in critical thinking, 14–15
  definition of, 4, 14
  diagnosis in, 17
  elements of, 14–15 (*See also specific elements*)
  evaluation in, 18
  in health assessment, 4
  implementation/interventions in, 18
  for migraine headache case, sample, 19–23, 33t
  planning in, 17–18
  sample cases on
    family stress, 28
    health maintenance, 29
    hypertension, 27–28
    low back pain, musculoskeletal, 29
    migraine headache case, 26–27
    overweight, 28
    stress incontinence, 29–30
    tobacco use (smoking), 28–29
Nursing records, review of, 38
Nutrients, sources of, 148t
Nutrition, 72t, 127–148
  cardiovascular disease and, 382–383
  counseling on, 136–137
  in elderly, 855, 856f, 860
  health history in, 128–131
    common or concerning symptoms in, 128
    sample questions in, 129–130
    weight changes in, 129–131
  health promotion and counseling on, 136–141
    blood pressure and diet, 139, 148t
    BMI and risk factors, 137
    BMI calculation, 131, 134, 134t–135t
    BMI classification, 137, 137t
    dietary intake, 138–139, 147t
    exercise, 139–140, 140t
    hydration, 140–141
    hypertension, dietary changes for, 139, 148t
    nine key messages, 138–139, 147t
    nutrient sources, 148t
    obesity, 136, 136t, 145t
    optimal weight, nutrition, and diet, 136, 136t
    risk factors, 136, 145t
    tips, 137
  hydration status in, 128, 140–141
  on musculoskeletal system, 578–579
  nutritional disorder evaluation in, 131, 144
  nutritional status in, 127–128
  physical examination in, 131–135
    BMI calculation, 134, 134t–135t
    BMI table, 135t
    cardiovascular and peripheral vascular, 133
    gastrointestinal, 133
    HEENT, 133
    height measurement, 131–132
    musculoskeletal, 134
    neurologic, 134
    overview, 131
    skin, hair, and nails, 133
    weight measurement, 132, 132f

screening on, 143t
vitamin and mineral deficiencies in, 128
Nutritional status, 127–128
Nystagmus
  in adults, 226, 227, 631, 672t
  in children, 830t
  in infants, 752–753

O

Obesity, 136, 136t. *See also* Body mass index (BMI)
  childhood
    adolescent, 810
    school-aged, 782, 783t
  classification of, 137, 137t
  overview of, 136–137
  protuberant abdomens in, 483t
  responding to, 137–138, 146t
  risk factors and diseases in, 136, 145t
  stages of change model and readiness assessment in, 146t
  stroke risk from, 660t
Objective data, 13
Objective information, 13
Obligate nasal breathers, 754
Oblique fissures, 296f, 297, 297f
Obstetric history, 690–692
Obstipation, 443
Obstructive airway disease, paradoxical pulse in, 421, 429t
Obstructive breathing, 124t
Obtundation, 601, 652t
Obturator sign, 465
Occipital nodes, 198, 199
Occlusive aortic disease, 114
Ocular fundi
  anatomy and physiology of, 213, 213f
  in diabetic retinopathy, 247t
  normal and hypertensive, 246t
Ocular motor weakness, 753
Ocular strabismus, in children, 753, 786, 830t
Oculocephalic reflex, 654
Oculomotor nerve, 215f, 216, 216f
Oculomotor nerve paralysis, 240t
Odors, body and breath, 107
Odynophagia, 441
Off the midline back pain, 522
OLD CART, 12, 43, 65
Older adults, 840–878
  anatomy and physiology of, 841–848
    abdomen, 846
    breasts and axillae, 846
    cardiovascular system, 845
    delirium, 876t
    dementia, 876t, 877t
    genitalia, 846–847
    head and neck, 843–844
    heterogeneity in, 842
    mental status, 847–848, 876t, 877t
    motor system, 848
    musculoskeletal system, 847
    nervous system, 847–848
    peripheral vascular system, 845–846
    primary changes, 841

skin, nails, and hair, 842–843, 843f
thorax and lungs, 844–845
vital signs, 842
dementia screening in: Mini-Cog, 865, 876t, 877t
demographics of, 840
examination techniques for, 874
frailty myths and, 841
health history in, 849–860
  approach to patient in, 849–852
    content and pace, 850
    cultural dimensions, 852
    effective communication, 851
    eliciting symptoms, 850–851
    environment, 849–850
  focus areas in, 852–860
    10-minute geriatric screener, 853, 853t–854t, 865
    activities of daily living, 854, 855t
    common concerns, 852
    functional assessment, 853, 853t–854t
    medications, 854–855
    nutrition, 855, 856f
    pain, 857–858, 857t
    sex, 858
    smoking and alcohol, 859–860
    symptoms, 853
    urinary incontinence, 858–859
health promotion and counseling in, 868–874
  advance directives and palliative care, 873–874
  cancer screening, 869
  dementia, 872
  depression, 872
  driving safety, 872
  elder mistreatment, 873
  exercise, 872
  fall assessment, 870, 871f
  household safety, 870
  immunizations
    influenza, 869
    pneumococcal, 869
    zoster, 870
  mild cognitive impairment, 872–873
  screening, 869
  vision and hearing, 869
minimum geriatric competencies in, 875t
physical examination of, 860–866
  abdomen, 865
  breasts and axillae, 865
  cardiovascular system, 864
  genitalia, 865
  head and neck, 862–863, 863f
  musculoskeletal system, 865
  nervous system and mental status, 865–866
  overview, 860
  peripheral vascular system, 864–865
  skin, 861–862, 861f
  thorax and lungs, 863
  vital signs, 860–861
recording findings in, 866–868
Siebens domain management model for, 878t
Olecranon bursae, 539, 539f
Olecranon bursitis, 539
Oligomenorrhea, 689

Onset, 12, 65
Onycholysis, 185t
Open-angle glaucoma
  in adults, 225
  in elderly, 863
Open-ended questions, to focused questions, 47–48
Opening snap (OS), 342, 390t
Ophthalmoscope, 94, 94f, 228f, 229
Ophthalmoscopic examination
  of adults, 228–232
    mydriatic drop contraindications in, 228
    ophthalmoscope and its use in, 94, 94f, 228f, 229
    optic disc examination steps in, 229–231, 230f, 243t–244t (*See also* Optic disc examination)
    retina examination in, 231–232, 231f, 232f, 245t–247t
  of infants, 753
Opisthotonos, 769
Opposition, thumbs, 549, 549f, 550
OPQRST, 43
Optic atrophy, 244t
Optic blink reflex, 753
Optic disc, 213, 213f
  abnormalities of, 229–231, 230f, 244t
  normal variations of, 229–231, 230f, 243t
Optic disc examination, 229–231, 230f
  abnormalities in, 244t
  in myopia and hyperopia, 230f
  papilledema in, 231, 231f, 244t
  positioning in, 229
  in refractive error, 230f
  steps in, 230–231, 231f
  technique in, 230
  variations in, normal, 243t
Optic fundi, 630
Optic nerve, 213, 213f, 215f
Optic radiation, 215, 216f, 236t
Oral candidiasis
  in children, 830t
  in infants, 755
  on palate, 285t
  on tongue, 289t
Oral-facial dyskinesias, 670t
Oral mucosa
  anatomy and physiology of, 261, 261f, 262f
  physical examination of, 272, 272f
Oral screening, 275–276
Oral temperature, 116–117
Oral thermometers, 117
Oral tumors, in elderly, 863
Orange peel sign, 515t
Orchitis, 715t
Orgasm, male, 703
Orientation, 598, 598t, 605–606
Oropharyngeal dysphagia, 441, 474t
Orthopnea, 352
Orthostatic blood pressure, 114
Orthostatic hypotension
  in adults, 114, 666t–667t
  in elderly, 842, 860–861
Ortolani test, 767, 767f
Ossicles, 250f, 251

Osteoarthritis
  in elderly, 865
  hands and wrists, 543, 589t
  hip, 565, 566
  joint pain in, 586t–587t
  knee, 569, 570
Osteomyelitis, 524
Osteopenia, 580
Osteoporosis, 579–583
Otitis externa, 253
  auricle in, 266
  chronic, 268, 268f
  ear canal and drum in, 268, 268f
Otitis media, 253, 254
  acute, 254
    auricle in, 266
    in children, 788, 830t
    ear canal and drum in, 268, 830t
    with purulent effusion, 280t
  chronic, 254
Otoscope, 94, 94f
  examination with, in children, 788
  grips for, 267
Ovaries
  in adults, 685–686, 685f
  in elderly, 847
Overbite, 791
Overflow incontinence, 446, 480t–481t
Overhydration
  edema from, 133
  pulse in, 133
Overload
  pressure, 347
  volume, 347
Overweight, 28, 137, 137t. See also Body mass
    index (BMI); Obesity
Oximetry, pulse, 320, 320f
Oxyhemoglobin, 155, 158

P

Paget disease of breast, 504
Paget disease of nipple, 515t
Pain, 106, 118–122. See also specific systems
  chronic, 119
  definition of, 119
  in elderly, 857–858, 857t
  epidemiology of, 118–119
  health disparities and, 120
  idiopathic, 121
  management of, 121
  neurologic, 625
  neuropathic, 121
  nociceptive (somatic), 121
  nonverbal cues to, 120
  patient history in, 119–120, 120f
  psychogenic, 121
  scales of, 119, 120f
  sensation of, 621, 621f, 640
  types of, 120–121
Palate movements, 633
Palliative care, in elderly, 873–874
Pallor, 158, 159, 353
Palmar grasp reflex, 773t
Palpation, 98, 99. See also specific systems

Palpebral conjunctiva, 211
Palpebral fissure, 211, 223
Palpitations, cardiovascular, 352
Pancreas, 433, 433f
Pancreatic cancer, 472t–473t
Pancreatitis
  abdominal pain in, 472t–473t
  abdominal tenderness in, 486t
  amylase in, 31
  gallstone, 437
Pansystolic murmurs
  in adults, 373, 391t
  in elderly, 864
Papilledema, 231, 231f, 244t
Papilloma, breast, 504, 504f
Pap smear, 696
Papule, 174t
Parachute reflex, 774t
Paradoxical pulse, 421, 429t
Paralanguage, 49
Paralysis
  facial, 633, 673t
  facial nerve, 673t
  in infants, 770
  vocal cord, 633
Paranasal sinuses, 257, 257f
Paraphasias, 603
Paraphimosis, 705
Paraplegia, 526
Parasternal muscles, 298
Paratonia, 680t
Paraurethral glands, 684, 684f
Paravertebral muscles, 555, 556f
Paresis, 526
Paresthesias, 625
Parietal pain, 436
Parietal pleura, 298
Parkinson disease, 106, 866
Parkinsonian gait, 675t
Parkinsonism, 106
Paronychia, 185t
Parotid duct, 263, 263f
Parotid gland, 189, 190t
Paroxysmal nocturnal dyspnea (PND), 352
Paroxysmal supraventricular tachycardia, in
    infants, 746, 824t
Pars flaccida, 251, 251f, 266, 268f, 279t
Pars tensa, 251, 251f, 268, 268f, 279t
Partial seizures, 668t
Partial seizures that have become generalized, 668t
Particulate irritation, 326t
Partnerships, collaborative, culture and, 82, 83
Passive range of motion, 523
Past history, 20, 64t, 66–68
Past pointing, 636
Patch, 173t
Patella, 569
Patellar tendon, 567, 569, 569f
Patellofemoral grinding test, 570
Patellofemoral joint, 567
Patellofemoral syndrome, 570
Patent ductus arteriosus, heart sounds in
  in adults, 395t
  in children, 834t
  in infants, 763

Patient. See also specific topics
  empowerment of, 51
  on health, 7
  perspective on illness of, 42, 45–46
  reflecting on approach to, 91–92
  story of
    expanding and clarifying, 43–44
    inviting, 41–42
Patient-centered goals, 38
Patient identifiers, for mental health screening,
    597
Peau d'orange sign, 515t
Pectoral lymph nodes, 493, 493f, 504
Pectoris muscle, whipcord, 315, 330t
Pectus carinatum, 329t, 756
Pectus excavatum, 329t, 756
Pedal pulses, 415, 415f
Pediatrics. See Adolescents; Children; Infants;
    School-aged children
Pedicle, 551, 551f
Pediculosis pubis, 694
Pelvic examination, 693–694
Pencil grip, 267
Penile discharge
  in adults, 703–704, 713t–715t
  in male adolescents, 815
  in STDs, 815
Penile lesions, 703–704, 713t–715t
Penis
  in adults
    abnormalities of, 705–706, 713t
    physical examination of, 705–706, 713t
    shaft of, 699, 699f
  in children
    infants, 765
    school-aged, 797, 798f
  in elderly, 846
Penis carcinoma, 713t
Peptic ulcer, abdominal pain in, 472t–473t
Perceptions, 598, 598t, 605
Percussion, 98, 99
  in anterior chest examination, 318–319, 318f,
    319f
  in posterior chest examination
    diaphragmatic excursion in, 311–312, 311f
    notes in, 310–312, 310t, 311f
    technique in, 308–309, 309f
Perennial allergic rhinitis, 789, 829t
Pericardial friction rub, heart sounds in, 395t
Pericardial tamponade, paradoxical pulse in,
    421, 429t
Pericarditis
  chest pain in, 327t
  constrictive, paradoxical pulse in, 421, 429t
Pericardium, 339
Perimenopause, 687, 689
Perineum, 684, 684f, 685f
Periodontal disease, in elderly, 844
Peripheral arterial disease (PAD), 398, 422
Peripheral arteries, in elderly, 846
Peripheral cataract, 239t
Peripheral edema, 376, 405, 428t
  of arm and hand, 409
  causes of, 412, 428t
  of legs, 412, 412f, 428t

Peripheral nerve disorders, 678t. *See also specific disorders*
  mononeuropathy, 678t
  neuropathy, reducing risk for, 661
  polyneuropathy, 678t
Peripheral nerves, 616–618
Peripheral nervous system, 616–623. *See also specific parts*
  cranial nerves, 616, 616f–618f, 617t–618t
  dermatomes, 622
  motor pathways, 618–620, 618f, 620f
  peripheral nerves, 616–618
  sensory pathways, 620–622, 621f
  spinal reflex
    cutaneous stimulation reflexes, 623, 623t
    deep tendon response, 622, 622t
Peripheral pulses, in infants, 760
Peripheral vascular system, 398–429
  anatomy and physiology of, 398–402
    arteries in, 399–401, 399f–401f
    veins in, 401–402, 402f
  disorders of, 421
    arterial pulse and pressure wave abnormalities, 429t
    chronic insufficiency of arteries and veins, 399, 424t–427t
    edema, 428t
    painful, and their mimics, 424t–425t
    prevention and early identification of, 422–423
    skin, 182t
    ulcers, ankle and foot, 427t
  in elderly, 845–846, 864–865
  fluid exchange and capillary bed in, 404–405, 404f
  in health assessment, 727
  health history in, 405–408
    family history in, 408
    lifestyle and health patterns in, 408
    past history in, 407–408
    questioning in, 406–407
  health promotion and counseling on, 422–423
  physical examination of, 103, 104, 408–421
    ankle–brachial index, 419–420, 419f
    arms, 409–410, 409t (*See also* Arms, physical examination of)
    equipment list for, 408
    hand arterial supply, 416f–417f, 417–418
    leg arterial supply, 418–419, 418f–419f
    legs, 409t, 410–416 (*See also* Legs, physical examination of)
    paradoxical pulse, 421, 429t
    pulsus alternans, 356, 421, 429t
    saphenous vein, 416, 416f
    ulnar pulse, 417, 417f–418f
    venous valve competency, 421
  recording findings on, 416–417, 423
  in review of systems, 70
Peripheral vision, 222–223, 222f, 223f
Peripheral visual fields by confrontation, 222–223, 222f, 223f
Peritoneal inflammation
  abdominal tenderness in, 486t
  palpation for, 453

Peritonitis, in infants, 764
Peritonsillar abscess, in children, 792
Perpendicular lighting, 92, 93f
Persistent pain, in elderly, 857–858, 857t
Personal and social history, 21
Personal hygiene, 108, 602
Personal problems, response to, in interview, 57–58
Pertinent positives and negatives, 63t, 66
Pes planus
  in adults, 591t
  in children, 836t
Petechiae, 179t
  in mouth, 286t
  from vitamin A deficiency, 133
Petit mal absences, 669t
Peutz-Jeghers syndrome, 283t
Phalanges, 541, 541f
Phalen's sign (test), 549, 549f
Pharyngitis, 284t
  lymph nodes in, 196
  streptococcal
    in adults, 264
    in children, 792, 831t
Pharynx, 249. *See also* Mouth and pharynx
  anatomy of, 263, 263f
  findings in, 284t–286t
  in health assessment, 725
  physical examination of, 274
Phimosis, 705
Photophobia, 217, 219
Physical abuse, 75–76
Physical dependence, 122
Physical development
  in adolescents, 806–807, 807t–808t
  in early childhood, 776, 776f
  in infants, 736–737, 737f
  in middle childhood, 777, 777t
Physical examination, 4
  complete, 91
  focused, 91
  head-to-toe sequence sample, 721, 722–728
    patient lying down, 726–727
    patient seated
      general survey, 723–726
      specific systems, 727–728
    patient standing, 728
    visual acuity, 728
  purpose of, 90
  recording findings in, 22–23
Physical examination, comprehensive, 90–104
  equipment for, 94–96
    ophthalmoscope, 94, 94f, 228f, 229
    other, 94
    otoscope, 94, 94f
    reflex hammer, 95, 95f
    stadiometer, 94
    stethoscope, 95, 95f
    tuning forks, 96, 96f
  overview of, 101–104
    abdomen, 103
    breasts, axillae, and epitrochlear nodes, 102, 103
    cardiovascular system, 102
    conclusion of, 104

  general survey, 101
  HEENT, 101–102
  lower extremities, 103
  musculoskeletal system, 102, 104
  neck and back, 102
  nervous system, 103–104
    with patient sitting, 103–104
    with patient standing, 104
    with patient supine, 102–103
  peripheral vascular system, 103, 104
  precordium, 102–103
  skin, 101
  thorax and lungs, 102
  vital signs, 101
  patient communication in, 93
  preparing for, 91–97
    equipment check, 94–96
    lighting and environment, 92–93, 92f, 93f
    patient approach, reflecting on, 91–92
    patient comfort, 93
    sequence
      choosing, 96–97
      patient lying down, 98
      patient seated, 98
      patient seated-anterior, 97
      patient seated-posterior, 98
      patient standing, 98
    sequence of, suggested, 97–98
    techniques of, 98–101
      cardinal, 98, 99
      sequence and positioning, 100
      standard and MRSA precautions, 100–101
      universal precautions, 101
Physical symptom, 596
Physiologic cupping, optic disc, 243t
Physiologic nodularity, 492
Pierre Robin syndrome, 752
Pigeon chest, 329t
Pilar cysts, 197, 278t
Pillars, tongue, 263, 263f
Pinguecula, 241t
Pinpoint pupils, 679t
Pitcher's elbow, 539
Pitting, nail, 186t
Pitting edema
  of legs, 412, 412f, 428t
  vs. nonpitting, 160, 405
  skin signs of, 160
Pityriasis rosea, 171t
Placing and stepping reflexes, 774t
Plagiocephaly, 751
Plan, nursing care
  development of
    critical thinking in, 19
    in health assessment, 6, 9
  negotiation of, 46
Planning, nursing process, 14, 17–18
Plantar flexion, 573
Plantar grasp reflex, 773t
Plantar response
  in adults, 651, 651f
  in elderly, 848
Plantar warts
  in adults, 592t
  in children, 826t

Plaque, 173t
Plateau murmur, 374, 374f
Play, in infant approach, 739
Pleurae, 298
Pleural effusion, 333t
Pleural (friction) rub, 331t
Pleural space, 298
Pleurisy
  epigastric pain in, 436
  tender abdomen in, 485t
Pleuritic pain, 327t
Pleximeter finger, 99
Plexor finger, 99
Plumb line, in scoliosis, 818, 818f
Pneumococcal pneumonia, 326t
Pneumococcal vaccine
  in adult, 323
  in elderly, 869
Pneumonia
  in adults
    dyspnea in, 324t–325t
    Klebsiella, cough in, 326t
    lobar, 330t
    Mycoplasma, cough in, 326t
    pneumococcal, cough in, 326t
    viral, cough in, 326t
  in children
    infants, ruling out, 757
    school-aged, 794
Pneumonic consolidation, 758
Pneumothorax, 333t
Point localization, 642
Point of maximal impulse (PMI)
  anatomy and physiology of, 338, 338f
  in elderly, 864
  physical examination of, 363–366,
    364f–366f, 386t
  variations/abnormalities in, 386t
Point-to-point movements, 636, 636f, 637f
Polio, 837t
Polycystic ovary syndrome, 197
Polymenorrhea, 689
Polyneuropathy, 566, 639
Polyps, nasal
  in adults, 271
  in children, 799
Polyuria, 445–446, 479t
Popliteal aneurysm, 414
Popliteal artery, 401, 401f
Popliteal pulse palpation, 414, 414f
Position
  of eye, 223
  matching, 49
  patient, 100
Positioning, 100
Position sense
  in adults, 621, 621f, 641, 641f
  in elderly, 848
  loss of, 638, 641
Positive
  false, 31
  true, 31
Positive support reflex, 773t
Postcoital bleeding, 689
Posterior auricular nodes, 198, 199

Posterior axillary line, 296, 296f
Posterior cerebral artery (PCA) stroke,
    664t–665t
Posterior cervical chain, 198, 199
Posterior chamber, of eye, 213, 213f
Posterior chest examination, 306–315, 307f. See
    also Chest examination, posterior
Posterior circulation stroke, 664t–665t
Posterior column disease, 641
Posterior columns, 621, 621f
Posterior cruciate ligament (PCL), 568, 568f
Posterior fontanelle, 750, 750f
Posterior pillar, 263, 263f
Posterior talofibular ligament, 573, 573f
Posterior tibial artery, 401, 401f
Posterior tibial pulse palpation, 415, 415f
Posterior triangle, 193, 194f
Postictal state, 626
Postmenopausal bleeding, 687
Postnasal drip, 326t
Post-traumatic arthritis, 545
Posttraumatic headache, 206t–207t
Postural blood pressure, 114
Postural hypotension
  in adults, 114, 666t–667t
  in elderly, 842, 860–861
Postural tremors, 670t
Posture
  abnormalities of, 675t
  in adults, 107
  in infants, 772
  in mental status, 601
"Pot-belly" appearance, 795
Power of attorney, durable, 53
Preauricular nodes, 198, 199
Precocious puberty
  in females, 798, 815
  in males, 797
Precordial impulse, 338
Precordium, 102–103, 337
Pregnancy
  protuberant abdomens in, 483t
  skin in, 182t
Pregnancy tumor, 287t
Prehypertension
  in adults, 113–114, 113t
  in elderly, 861
Pre-interview, 36, 37–39
Preload, 347
Premature ejaculation, 703
Premature thelarche, 763
Premenstrual syndrome (PMS), 687, 688–689
Premolars, 262f
Prenatal care, early, 697
Prepatellar bursa, 569, 569f
Prepuce, 684, 684f, 699, 699f
Presbycusis
  in adults, 633
  in elderly, 844
Presbyopia
  in adults, 218, 222
  in elderly, 844, 862
Presence, nursing, 85–86
Present illness, 19–20
Presenting problem, 41

Pressure
  aortic, 341, 341f
  left atrial, 340–341, 341f
  left ventricular, 340–341, 340f, 341f
Pressure overload, 347
Pressure sores (ulcers)
  in adults, 161, 162t–163t, 183t, 427t
  in elderly, 862
Presyncope, 277t, 626
Preventive care. See also specific systems
  examples of, 6, 7
  in health assessment, 6, 7
  levels of, 6
Primary prevention, 6, 7
Primitive reflexes, in infants, 772,
    773t–774t
PR interval, 346, 346f
Problem list, 14
  assessment for, 17
  generation of, 24
  health maintenance in, 18
  prioritizing of, 14
  sample, 24
Problem-oriented assessment, 61
Prodrome, migraine, 192
Professionalism, 58–59
Progress note, sample, 33t
Pronation, elbow, 540, 540f, 540t
Pronation, toddler, 836t
Pronator drift, 638
Pronator teres muscle, 538, 538f
Proprioception, 641, 641f
Proptosis, 227
Prostate, in elderly, 865
Prostate cancer, 708–710
Prostate cancer screening, 710
Prostate-specific antigen (PSA), 710
Prostatic pain, 445
Prostatitis, 704
Protein deficiency
  abdominal distention from, 133
  ascites from, 133
  edema from, 133
  muscle wasting and flaccidity from, 134
Protuberant abdomen, 119, 151, 153, 483t
Proverbs, 608
Provider-centered goals, 38
Proximal interphalangeal (PIP) joints, 545
Proxy, health care, 53
Pseudohypertrophy, muscular, 525
Pseudoscars, 861, 861f
Pseudoseizures, 669t
Psoas bursa, 559f, 561
Psoas muscle, 553
Psoas sign, 465
Psoriasis, 160, 171t, 173t–174t, 197
Psychiatric sytem, in review of systems, 71
Psychogenic pain, 121
Pterygium, 239t
Pterygoids, 528, 528f
Ptosis, 237t, 240t, 242t, 631
Puberty
  delayed
    in females, 694
    in males, 813

precocious
  in females, 798, 815
  in males, 797
Pubic hair
  female
    in elderly, 847
    Tanner staging of, 816t, 817f
  male, in elderly, 846
Pulmonary artery, 337f, 338, 338f, 400
Pulmonary embolism
  cough in, 326t
  dyspnea in, 324t–325t
  hemoptysis in, 326t
  syncope from, 666t–667t
Pulmonary flow murmur, in adolescents, 811, 811t
Pulmonary function assessment, clinical, 320
Pulmonary hypertension, in infants, 761
Pulmonary tuberculosis
  cough in, 326t
  hemoptysis in, 326t
Pulmonary valve stenosis, congenital, 833t
Pulmonic area, 363f, 367, 370f
Pulmonic ejection sound, 389t, 393t
Pulmonic stenosis, heart murmurs in
  in adults, 393t
  in infants, 763
Pulmonic valve, 339, 339f
Pulse, in adults
  apical, 112, 115, 116
  arm, 410, 410f
  arterial, 347–348, 348f, 410, 429t
    blood pressure and, 347–348, 348f, 429t
    grading amplitude of, 410
  bigeminal, 429t
  bounding
    in overhydration, 133
    in peripheral vascular disorders, 429t
  brachial, 410, 410f
  carotid artery, 355–357, 356f
    amplitude and contour of, 355–356, 356f
    thrill and bruits in, 357
  dorsalis pedis, 415, 415f
  educating patients on, 123
  in elderly, 865
  femoral, 413, 413f
  grading of, 410t
  in legs, 413–415, 413f–415f, 429t
  in overhydration, 133
  paradoxical, 421, 429t
  pedal, 415, 415f
  popliteal, 414, 414f
  posterior tibial, 415, 415f
  radial
    heart rate and rhythm from, 116, 116f
    palpation of, 409
  ulnar, 417, 417f–418f
  weak
    blood pressure measurement with, 114–115
    grading of, 410
    palpation of, 415
    in peripheral vascular disorders, 429t
Pulse, in children
  infants, 746–747, 746t
    femoral pulse, 760

  peripheral, 760
  tibial, 760
  school-aged, 785, 785t
Pulse oximetry, 320, 320f
Pulse pressure, 347, 348f
  abnormalities of, 429t
  in elderly, 842, 860
Pulsus alternans, 356, 421, 429t
Pupillary constriction, 216
Pupillary reactions
  consensual reaction, 226
  direct reaction, 215, 215f, 226, 240t
  to light, 631
  light reaction, 215, 215f, 225–226
  near reaction, 216, 216f, 226
Pupils, 225–226, 240t
  abnormalities of, 225–226, 240t
  in comatose patients, 654, 679t
  in elderly, 862
  pinpoint, 679t
Purpura, 179t
Purpuric lesions, of skin, 179t
Purulent rhinitis, 789
Purulent rhinorrhea, 789
Purulent sputum, 301
Pustule, 175t
P wave, 346, 346f
Pyloric stenosis, in infants, 765
Pyogenic granuloma, 287t
Pyramidal tract, 619

Q

QRS complex, 346, 346f
Quadrantanopia, 630
Quadrantic defects, 222f, 236t
Quadrants, abdominal, 432, 432f
  left lower, 432, 432f, 433–434, 433f
  left upper, 432, 432f, 433, 433f
  right lower, 432, 432f, 433f, 434
  right upper, 432, 432f, 433, 433f
Quadriceps femoris, 567, 567f
Quadriplegia, 526
Questioning. See also specific systems
  asking questions in, 9–10
  eliciting graded response via, 48
  focused, 47–48
  guided, 47–49
  leading, 48
  open-ended
    in interviewing, 41
    moving to focused questions from, 47–48
Q wave, 346, 346f

R

Radial artery, 400, 400f
Radial deviation, wrist, 546f, 546t
Radial pulse
  heart rate and rhythm from, 116, 116f
  palpation of, 409
Radicular pain, 522
  cervical, 585t
  low back, 584t
Radiocarpal joint, 542, 542f

Radiohumeral joint, 538, 538f
Radioulnar joint, 538, 538f
Radioulnar joint, distal, 542, 542f
Rales
  in adults, 314–315, 314t, 331t
  in infants, 759
Range of motion, 523. See also specific joints
  active vs. passive, 523
  describing limited, 577, 577f
  limitations for, 524
Rape victims, 694
Rapid alternating movements, 635–636, 635f, 636f
Rapport
  in interview, 39–41
  matching position for, 49
Raynaud disease, 407, 409, 424t–425t
Reasoning, clinical, 15–19, 17–18. See also Assessment, nursing process
Reassurance, 50
Rebound tenderness, 453, 465
Recent memory, 607
Recession of gums, 288t
Recording findings, 19–30. See also specific systems
  case study on, 19–23
  chief complaint in, 19
  clinical data challenges in, 24–26
  family history in, 20–21
  nursing process in, sample case, 19–23, 33t
  nursing process in, sample cases, 26–30
  past history in, 20
  personal and social history in, 21
  physical examination in, 22–23
  present illness in, 19–20
  problem list generation in, 24
  progress note in, sample, 33t
  on reflexes, 23
  review of systems in, 21–22
Rectal examination
  in children
    infants, 766
    school-aged, 800
  digital, 710
Rectal temperature
  in adults, 116, 117
  in infants, 747
Red eyes, 224, 224f, 238t
Red reflex, 230
Reduced growth velocity, 744
Referral, source of, 63t, 64
Referred pain
  abdominal, 436
  to back, 584t
Reflection, in interview questioning, 48–49
Reflexes. See also specific reflexes
  abdominal, 650, 650f
  absent, 645
  deep tendon, 645–650
    ankle (Achilles), 649, 649f
    biceps, 646–647, 646f
  in children
    infants, 771–772, 771f, 772f
    school-aged, 802, 802f
  clonus, 650, 650f

Reflexes (continued)
  grading scale, 645, 645t
  knee, 648, 648f
  reinforcement, 646, 646f
  supinator or brachioradialis, 647, 647f
  technique, 645, 645f
  triceps, 647, 647f
  definition of, 622
  in elderly, 848
  hyperactive, 645
  hypoactive, 645
  primitive, 772, 773t–774t
  recording findings on, 23
  spinal
    cutaneous stimulation, 623, 623t
    deep tendon, 622, 622t
Reflex hammer, 95, 95f
Reflux esophagitis, 303, 328t
Refraction, errors of, 206t–207t, 230
Regurgitant murmur, 344
Regurgitation, 438, 440
Reinforcement, 646, 646f
Relationships, 602
Reliability, 30, 63t, 64
Relieving factors, 12, 65
Religion, 85. See also Spiritual assessment
Remote memory, 607
Renal arterial disease, atherosclerotic, 123
Renal artery stenosis, 450
Renal colic, 447
Renal disease, skin in, 182t
Renal stone, 437, 439
Renal system
  anatomy and physiology of, 431–432,
    432f–434f, 434
  health history in, 444–447
    common or concerning symptoms in, 435
    dysuria, urgency, or frequency, 445, 479t
    general questions, 444–445
    hematuria, 446
    kidney or flank pain, 447
    polyuria or nocturia, 445–446, 479t
    suprapubic pain, 445
    ureteral colic, 447
    urinary incontinence, 446, 480t–481t
  physical examination of
    bladder, 459
    kidneys, 457–459
      left kidney palpation in, 457–458
      percussion tenderness in, 458–459, 459f
      right kidney palpation in, 458, 458f
    urinary incontinence prevention in, 471
Reproductive system, female, 684–698
  anatomy and physiology of, 684–686, 694f,
    695f
  health history in, 686–692
    menstrual history, 687–689
    obstetric history, 690–692
    phases, 687
    vaginal discharge, 690, 712t
    vulvar lesions, 690, 711t
  health promotion and counseling on, 695–698
    cervical cancer screening, 696
    family planning, 697
    HPV infection, 696

    HPV vaccine, 696–697
    menopause changes, 696
    reproductive system education, 696
    STDs and HIV prevention, 697–698
  physical examination of, 692–695
    approach to pelvic examination, 693–694
    equipment, 694
    external, 694
    internal, 695
    patient positioning, 694
    patient preparation, 692
    for rape victims, 694
  recording findings on, 695
  in review of systems, 71
Reproductive system, male, 699–710
  anatomy and physiology of, 699–701, 699f,
    701f
  health history in, 701–705
    benign prostate hyperplasia, 704
    inguinal pain or swelling, 704
    penile discharge or lesions, 703–704, 714t
    scrotal pain or swelling, 704
    sexual preference and sexual response,
      702–703
  health promotion and counseling on, 707–710
    prostate cancer, 708–710
    STD and HIV prevention, 707–708
    testicular self-examination, 708–709, 709f
  hernias, groin, 701, 704, 706–707, 713t,
    717t (See also Hernia, groin)
  physical examination of, 705–707
    epididymis and spermatic cord
      abnormalities, 716t
    penis, 705–706, 713t
    scrotum and its contents, 704, 706, 713t
    sexually transmitted diseases, 714t
    testis abnormalities, 715t
  recording findings on, 707
  in review of systems, 71
Resonant chest percussion, 310, 311f, 330t
Respectful communication, 82–83
Respiration. See also Breathing
  educating patients on, 123
  in infants, 756–757, 757t
  sighing, 124t
Respiratory infection
  lower, nasal flaring in, 757
  upper, in children
    infants, nasal flaring in, 757
    school-aged, 794
Respiratory rate
  in adults, 116, 124t
  in elderly, 842, 861
  in infants, 747
  in school-aged children, 785, 795
Respiratory rhythm, 116, 124t
Respiratory system, 292–333
  anatomy and physiology of, 292–299
    bony landmarks, 293–295, 293t–295t
    breathing, 298–299, 299f
    chest findings, 293–296
      circumference of chest, 295–296, 295f,
        296f
      posterior, 294, 294t
      vertical, 293–294, 293t

    chest locations in, 297
    chest wall, 292
    lung, fissures, and lobes, 296–297, 296f,
      297f
    pleurae, 298
    spinous processes, 295, 295t
    trachea and major bronchi, 297, 298f
  health history in, 299–304
    anxious patients, 300
    breathing difficulty, 300–301
    chest pain, 302–303, 327t–328t
    cough, 301–302, 326t
    dyspnea, 300–301, 324t–325t
    family history, 304
    hemoptysis, 302, 326t
    lifestyle and personal habits, 304
    overview, 299–300
    past history, 303–304
    wheezing, 30
  health promotion and counseling on, 321–323
    immunizations, 323
    tobacco cessation, 321–322
  physical examination of, 305–321
    anterior chest, 316–320 (See also Chest
      examination, anterior)
    chest disorder findings, 332t–333t (See also
      specific disorders)
    forced expiratory time, 321
    fractured rib in, 321
    with patient sitting, 305
    with patient supine, 305
    with patients who cannot sit up without
      aid, 305
    posterior chest, 306–315 (See also Chest
      examination, posterior)
    pulmonary function assessment, clinical,
      320
    pulse oximetry, 320, 320f
    respiration and thorax, 124t, 305–306
    thorax deformities, 306–307, 316, 329t
  recording findings on, 321
  in review of systems, 70
Response
  empathic, 49
  graded, questioning for, 48
  to personal problems, 57–58
Resting tremors, 670t
Restless legs syndrome, 627
Retching, 440
Reticular activating system, 615
Retina examination, 231–232, 231f, 232f
  ocular fundi in, 246t–247t
  retinal arteries and arteriovenous crossings,
    231, 245t
Retinal arteries and arteriovenous crossings,
    231, 245t
Retinopathy
  diabetic, 247t
  hypertensive, 246t
Retracted drum, 279t
Retraction, 306
  lid, 237t
  nipple, 495, 515t
Retractions, 758
Retrograde filling test, 421

Retropulsion, 675t
Review of systems, 64t, 69–71. *See also specific systems*
Reynolds Risk Score, 380–381
Rheumatic fever, 521
Rheumatoid arthritis, 521
 ankle and foot, 574
 hands and wrists, 543, 544, 589t
 intervertebral joints, 556
 joint pain in, 586t–587t
 joints in, 523, 524
 metacarpophalangeal joints, 545
 muscle atrophy/weakness in, 524
 proximal interphalangeal joints, 545
Rheumatoid nodules
 of ear, 278t
 of feet, 574
Rhinitis
 allergic, 258
 chronic (perennial) allergic, 789, 829t
 nose in, 271
Rhinitis medicamentosa, 258
Rhinorrhea
 in adults, 258–259
 purulent, in children, 789
Rhonchi
 in adults, 314–315, 314t, 331t
 in infants, 759
Rib
 2nd, 293, 293f, 294f
 11th, 294, 294f
 12th, 294, 294f
 floating, 294, 294f
 fractured, 321
Rickets
 in infants, 751
 in school-aged children, 800
Riedel lobe, 487t
Right lower quadrant, 432, 432f, 433f, 434
Right lower quadrant pain, acute, 439
Right upper quadrant, 432, 432f, 433, 433f
Right ventricle
 anatomy and physiology of, 337, 337f
 palpation of, 363
Right ventricular area, 366–367, 366f, 367f
Rigidity, 526, 680t
 decerebrate, 662t
 decorticate, 662t
Rings, optic disc, 243t
Ringworm, hair loss in, 184t
Rinne test, 269, 269f, 633
Risk factors. *See also specific disorders and systems*
 in history of present illness, 67
 in past history, 67
Role-relationship, 72t
Romberg sign, 638, 675t
Romberg test, 638
Room, interview, arranging, 40–41
Rooting reflex, 774
Roseola infantum, skin in, 182t
Rotation
 external
  hip, 563t, 566, 566f
  knee, 571t
  shoulder, 535f, 536f

hip, 563t, 566, 566f
internal
 hip, 563t, 566, 566f
 knee, 571t
 shoulder, 535f, 536f
knee, 571t
neck, 557t
spinal column, 558
Rotator cuff muscles, 531, 531f
 pain in, 588, 588t
 physical examination maneuvers for, 536, 536f–537f
Rotator cuff tear, 533, 537f–538f, 588t
Rotator cuff tendinitis, 588t
Rovsing sign, 465
Rubella, 182t, 837t
Rubeola, 182t
Rubor, 419
R wave, 346, 346f

S

S_1 heart sounds
 production of, 341, 341f
 splitting of, 343
 timing of, 370–372, 371f
 variations in, 387t
S_2 heart sounds
 production of, 341, 341f
 splitting of, 342–343, 343f, 372t
 timing of, 370–371, 371f
 variations in, 388t
S_3 heart sound, 390t
S_4 heart sound, 390t
Sacral curvature, 550, 552f, 554f
Sacroiliac joint, 554, 556f
Sacroiliitis, 554
Sacrospinalis muscle, 553
Safety measures, 67
Sagittal suture synostosis, 751
Salivary flow
 in adults, 276
 in elderly, 844
Salivary glands, 189, 190f
"Salmon patch," 748, 749t
Salpingitis, tender abdomen in, 485t
Saphenous veins
 anatomy and physiology of, 402, 402f
 physical examination of, 416, 416f
Sarcoidosis, dyspnea in, 324t–325t
Satiety, early, 441
Scabies, 175t
Scale
 balance beam, 132, 132f
 digital, 132
 on skin, 176t
Scalene muscles, 298, 299
Scaling, breast, 495
Scalp, 197
Scaphoid fracture, 544, 544f
Scapula, inferior tip of, 294, 294f
Scapular line, 296, 296f
Scapulohumeral group, 531, 531f, 533
Scapulothoracic articulation, 529
Scars, 176t

School-aged children, 776–806. *See also* Children
development of
 in early childhood, 776, 776f
 in middle childhood, 777, 777t
health history in, 778–781
 abnormalities while observing play in, 778, 778t
 general points on, 778
 in older children, 780–781
 in younger children, 779–780, 779t
health promotion and counseling in, 804–806
 early childhood, 804–805
 middle childhood, 805–806
physical examination in, 781
 abdomen, 796–797, 796f, 796t, 797f
 ears, 786–789, 788f, 830t (*See also* Ears, in children)
 eyes, 785–786, 786f, 786t, 830t
 facies, 828t–829t
 genitalia
  female, 798–800, 799f, 835t
  male, 797–798, 798f, 836t
 head, 785, 828t–829t
 heart, 794–795, 794f, 795f, 833t–834t
 mouth and pharynx, 790–792, 791f, 791t, 830t (*See also* Mouth and pharynx, in children)
 musculoskeletal system, 800–801, 800f, 836t
 neck, 792–793, 793f
 nervous system, 801–803, 802f, 803t (*See also* Nervous system, in children)
 nose and sinuses, 789, 789f
 rectum, 800
 skin, 785, 826t
 somatic growth, 782
 thorax and lungs, 793–794, 794f
 vital signs, 783–785
  blood pressure, 783–784, 784t
  pulse, 785, 785t
  respiratory rate, 785
  temperature, 785
 recording findings on, 820–823
 vaccine-preventable diseases in, 837t
Sciatica, 522, 584t
Sciatic nerve, 553f
 course of, 555f, 556f
 inspection of, 555–556, 555f
 tenderness of, 555
Scissors gait, 675t
Sclera, 224, 224f, 238t
Scleroderma, 160
Scoliosis, 555, 555f, 557
 adolescent assessment for, 817–818, 817f, 818f
 in children, 801
 on shoulder, 533
Scotoma, 217, 219
Screening. *See also specific systems; specific tests*
 10-minute geriatric, 853, 853t–854t, 865
 alcohol abuse, 467–468, 611
 cancer (*See* Cancer screening)
 cardiovascular risk factor, 381
 children, 735

Screening *(continued)*
  dental, 275–276
  dietary intake, rapid, 143t
  elderly, 869
  hearing, 275, 869
  mental health
    dementia: Mini-Cog, 865, 876t, 877t
    high-yield questions for, 597
    mental status examination in, 52,
      598t–599t, 600–601
    mini-mental status examination,
      609, 873
    patient identifiers for, 597
  nervous system
    adult, 629
    infant, 769
  nutrition, 143t
  oral, 275–276
  osteoporosis, 579–583
  in past history, 67
  sports preparticipation, adolescent, 818
  vision, 234–235
    in adults, 234–235
    in elderly, 869
Scrotal edema, 713t
Scrotal hernia, 713t
Scrotal pain, 704, 706, 713t
Scrotal swelling, 704, 706, 713t
Scrotum, 704, 706, 713t
  abnormalities of, 704, 706, 713t
  in children
    infants, 765
    school-aged, 797–798
  physical examination of, 705, 706, 713t
Sebaceous cyst, ear, 278t
Sebaceous glands, 154f, 156
Seborrhea, in newborns and infants, 825t
Seborrheic dermatitis, 197
Seborrheic keratosis
  in adults, 180t
  in elderly, 862
2nd rib, 293, 293f, 294f
Secondary prevention, 6, 7
Second heart sound (S₂)
  auscultation of, 370–372, 370f, 371f, 372t
  production of, 341, 341f
  splitting of, 342–343, 343f, 372t
  variations in, 570–571, 571t
  variations in, 388t
Seizures and seizure disorders, 668t–669t
  absence, 669t
  atonic, 669t
  complex partial seizures, 668t
  definition of, 626–627
  generalized, 626, 669t
  grand mal, 669t
  history of, 626–627
  Jacksonian, 668t
  partial, 668t
  partial that have become generalized, 668t
  pseudoseizures *vs.*, 669t
  simple partial, 668t
  tonic-clonic, 669t
  types of, 668t–669t
Self-awareness, of personal bias, 82

Self-examination
  breast, 505–506, 511
  skin, 166–168, 181t
  testicular, 708–709, 709f
Self-perception–self-concept, 72t
Self-reflection, 37–38
Self-treatment, 65
Seminal vesicle, 699f, 700
Senile ptosis, 862
Sensation, loss of, 625–626
Sensitive topics, 72–76
  guidelines for, 73
  mental health history in, 75
  overview of, 72–73
  sexual history in, 73–75
Sensitivity
  definition and example of, 31
  use of, 31–32
Sensorineural hearing loss
  anatomy and physiology of, 251, 253
  physical examination for, 269, 269f, 281t
Sensorineural phase, 251
Sensory ataxia, 675t
Sensory cortex lesions, 642
Sensory function, in infants, 770
Sensory loss, hemisensory, 639
Sensory mapping, 639
Sensory nerves, 616
Sensory pathways
  anatomy and physiology of, 620–622, 621f
  lesions of, 621–622
Sensory system, 639–644
  dermatomes, 642–644, 643f, 644f
  discriminative sensations, 641–642, 642f
  general, 639
  in health assessment, 728
  light touch, 640
  pain, 640
  patterns of testing, 639–640, 640f
  proprioception (position), 641, 641f
  temperature, 640
  vibration, 640–641, 641f
Sequence
  of data collection, 32, 32f
  of hypothesis testing, 32, 32f
  of symptoms, 13
Sequence, of physical examination, 100
  flowshop, 96–97
  patient lying down, 96
  patient seated, 98
  patient seated-anterior, 97
  patient seated-posterior, 98
  patient standing, 98
  positioning and, 100
Serial 7s, 606
Serous effusion, of ear, 280t
Serpiginous skin lesions, 172t
Setting sun sign, 827t
Seven attributes, of symptom, 65
Sevens, serial, 606
Sex, in elderly, 858
Sex maturity ratings
  in females, 816t
  in girls, 812t
  in males, 813t–814t

Sexual abuse, signs of
  in children, 799, 800, 835t
  in female adults, 694
Sexual advances, by patient, 58
Sexual function, male, 700
Sexual history, 73–75
Sexuality, nurse–patient relationship and, 58
Sexually transmitted diseases (STDs), 692
  in females, 697–698
  in males, 703–704, 714t
  penile discharge in, 815
  prevention of
    in females, 697–698
    in males, 707–708
Sexual maturity, 694
Sexual preference
  in females, 690–691
  in males, 702
Sexual response
  in females, 690–691
  in males, 702–703
Shaft, of penis
  in adults, 699, 699f
  in infants, 765
Shaking chill, 118
Shared understanding, of problem, 44–46
Shingles (herpes zoster)
  in adults, 160, 174t, 182t
  in elderly, 870
Shoes, 108
Shortness of breath, 352. *See also* Dyspnea
Short process of malleus, 251, 251f, 268, 268f
Short stature, 782
Shoulder, 529–538
  additional structures of, 532, 532f
  anterior dislocation of, 533, 588t
  anterior view of, 532f
  articular capsule and bursae in, 532, 532f
  bony structures in, 529–530, 530f
  joints in, 530, 530f
  muscle groups in, 531, 531f
  overview of, 529
  pain in, 533, 588t
  physical examination of
    inspection in, 533
    maneuvers in, 536, 536f, 538f
    palpation in, 533, 533f
    ranges of motion in, 533, 561f, 562f
    rotation in, 536, 536f, 588, 588t
  in scoliosis, 555
Siebens domain management model, 878t
Sighing respiration, 124t
Signposting, 50
Signs. *See also specific systems and disorders*
  definition of, 13
  identifying, 16
Silence, 51
Silent patient, interviewing, 51–52
Similarities, 608
Simple partial seizures, 668t
Sinoatrial (SA) node, 345f
Sinus arrhythmia, 385t
Sinuses
  in health assessment, 725
  physical examination of, 271, 271f

Sinusitis
  acute bacterial, 259
  in children, 789
  headache from, 206t–207t
  physical examination for, 271, 271f
Sinus node, 345, 345f
SITS muscles, 531, 531f, 533
Sitting position, rising from, 638
Situs inversus, 363, 452
Six facets, 3, 6, 9
Skene glands, 684, 684f
Skin, in adults. *See also* Integumentary system
  anatomy and physiology of, 154–155, 154f
  in anemia, 133
  color of, 133, 155
  dry, 159, 176t
  elderly
    anatomy and physiology of, 842–843, 843f
    physical examination of, 861–862, 861f
  layers of, 154–155, 154f
  oily, 159
  physical examination of, 101, 158–163, 197
    color, 158–159, 169t–170t
    edema, 160
    lesions, 160–161
    mobility and turgor, 159
    moisture, 159
    recording findings on, 165
    self-, 181t
    self-examination in, 166–168
    temperature, 159
    texture, 159
    total-body, 166
  in review of systems, 70
  sebaceous glands in, 154f, 156
  sweat glands in, 154f, 156
  temperature of, 118
  vitamin deficiencies on, 133
Skin, in children
  adolescents, 810, 825t
  infants, 748, 749t, 825t
  newborn and infant rashes and findings, 825t
  school-aged, 785, 825t
Skin cancer, 165–168
  prevention of, 168
  risk factors for, 166
  skin examination in
    instructions for self-examination in, 166–168, 181t
    mole detection in, 168
    recording findings on, 165
    total-body, 166
  types of, 165–166
Skin dimpling, in breast cancer, 495, 515t
Skin lesions, 160–161, 162t–163t, 171t–181t
  acne vulgaris, 178t
  anatomic location and distribution of, 160, 171t
  nevi, benign and malignant, 181t
  patterns and shapes of, 160, 172t
  physical examination of, 160–163
  pressure ulcers as, 161, 162t–163t, 183t
  primary
    burrow, 175t
    elevations

  palpable fluid-filled, 174t–175t
  palpable solid masses, 173t–174t
  flat, nonpalpable, 173t
  initial presentation of, 173t–175t
  purpuric, 179t
  secondary
    crust, 176t
    depressed, 177t
    erosion, 177t
    excoriation, 177t
    fissure, 177t
    keloids, 176t
    lichenification, 176t
    scale, 176t
    scars, 176t
    ulcer, 177t
    tumors, 180t
    vascular, 179t
Skin self-examination, 166–168, 181t
Skin tumors, 180t
Skull, 197
Skull symmetry, infant, 751, 751f
Sleep-rest, 72t
Small arteries, 400
Small bowel obstruction, 440
Small pox, 175t
Small saphenous vein, 402, 402f
Smegma, 699
Smell. *See also* Nose and paranasal sinuses
  change in, 260
  loss of, 630
  sense of, 630
Smoking
  cessation of, 321–322
  in elderly, 859
  sample nursing process for, 28–29
  stroke risk from, 660t
Smooth tongue, 289t
Snellen eye chart, 221, 221f
SnNout, 31
Snout reflex, 866
Snuffbox, anatomic, 544, 544f
SOAP format, 33
Social development
  in adolescents, 807, 807t–808t
  in early childhood, 776, 776f
  in infants, 737, 737f
  in middle childhood, 777, 777t
Social history, 21
Sodium, on blood pressure, 139, 148t
Solar lentigines, 862
Soles of feet, abnormalities of, 592t
Soleus muscle, 570
Somatic growth, in children
  adolescents, 810
  infants, 744–745
    head circumference, 745, 745f
    length, 744, 745f
    weight, 745
  school-aged
    head circumference in, 782
    height, 782
    weight, 782, 783t
Somatic pain, 121
Somatic symptom, 596

Somatization disorder, 52
Somatoform symptom, 596
Sore throat, 264
Source
  of history, 63t, 64
  of referral, 63t, 64
Space, interpersonal, 41
Spastic diplegias, 801
Spastic hemiparesis, 675t
Spasticity, 526, 680t
Specificity, 31
Specks, visual, 219
Speculum, 267, 267f, 268f
Speech
  disorders of, 674t
  in general appearance, 107
  in mental status, 598, 602–603, 603t
Spelling backward, 606
Spermatic cord, 699f, 700, 701f
  abnormalities of, 716t
  torsion of, 716t
  varicocele of, 716t
Spermatocele, 716t
Spheroidal joints, 520, 520f
Sphygmomanometer, 109–110, 110f
Spider angioma, 179t
Spider vein, 179t
Spina bifida, 555
Spina bifida occulta, 767
Spinal column. *See also* Spine
  muscle strength of, 559
  range of motion of, 557, 557f–558f
Spinal cord, 615, 615f
  anatomy of, 618f
  lesions of, 676t–677t
Spinal cord defect, in infants, 748
Spinal cord syndromes, 639
Spinal nerve, 616
Spinal nerve lesion, 678t
Spinal reflexes
  cutaneous stimulation, 623, 623t
  deep tendon, 622, 622t
Spinal root lesion, 678t
Spinal stenosis, 522
Spine, 550–559
  bony structures of, 551–552, 551f
  in children, 767
  curves of, 550, 552f
  in elderly, 844–845
  in health assessment, 728
  joints of, 552, 552f
  muscle groups of, 553, 553f
  muscles in mechanics of, 551
  physical examination of, 553–559
    inspection in, 553–554, 553f–555f
    muscle strength in
      neck, 556
      spinal column, 559
    palpation in, 554–556
    range of motion in
      neck, 556–557
      spinal column, 557, 557f–558f
Spinothalamic tract, 621, 621f
Spinous processes, 295, 295t, 551, 551f

Spiritual assessment, 85–86, 85–87
  approach to, 85–86
  listening in, 86
  presence in, 85–86
  spiritual distress in, 85–86
  spirituality defined in, 85
  Stoll's guidelines for, 86–87
Spiritual distress, 85–86
Spirituality, 85
Spleen, in adults
  anatomy of, 433, 433f
  examination of, 460–463
    palpation in, 462, 462f, 463f
    percussion in, 461–462, 461f
Spleen, in children
  infants, 765
  school-aged, 797
Splenic percussion sign, 461–462, 461f
Splenius capitis muscle, 553, 553f
Splenius cervicis muscle, 553
Splenomegaly
  in adults, 457, 460–462, 461f–463f
  in children
    infants, 765
    school-aged, 797
Split S2, in infants, 761
Spondylosis, cervical, 585t
Spontaneous pneumothorax, 324t–325t
Sports preparticipation screening, adolescent, 818
SpPin, 31
Sputum
  mucoid, 301
  purulent, 301
Squamous cell carcinoma
  in adults, 165, 180t
  in elderly, 862
Stadiometer, 94
Staining of teeth, in children, 791, 831t
Stance, 561, 561f, 638, 638f
Standard precautions, 100–101
Stapes, 250f, 251
Stasis ulcer, 177t, 427t
Static tremors, 670t
Station, in infants, 770
Stature, short, 782
Stenotic valve, 343
Stensen duct, 263, 263f
Steppage gait, 675t
Stepping reflex, 774t
Stereognosis, 611, 642
Stereotyping, cultural, 81
Sternal angle, 293, 293t, 294t
Sternoclavicular joint, 530, 530f
Sternomastoid muscles, in breathing during
    exercise, 299, 299f
Steroid injection, hypertrophic scar from, 176t
Stethoscope, 95, 95f
  auscultation with, 99
  bell of, 368
  diaphragm of, 368
  Doppler ultrasound, 114
  heads for, 368, 368f, 369f
  "inching" of, 369, 370f
  use of, 368
Stiffness, chronic back, 584t

Still murmur, 794–795, 795f, 795t
Stimulation reflexes. See also specific reflexes
  cutaneous, 623, 623t
  deep tendon response, 622, 622t
Stoll's guidelines for spiritual assessment, 86–87
Stomach cancer, abdominal pain in, 472t–473t
Stomatitis
  aphthous, 177t
  herpetic, 830t
Stone, renal, 437, 439
Stools
  black and bloody, 443, 478t
  color of, 444
"Stork bite," 748, 749t
Story, patient's
  expanding and clarifying, 43–44
  inviting, 41–42
Strabismus
  in infants, 753
  in school-aged children, 786, 830t
Strawberry tongue, 791
Strength, bone, 580
Strength, muscle, 526–527
  in children, 802, 802f
  fingers, 549, 550f
  neck, 556
  spinal column, 559
  supraspinatus muscle, 537f
  wrist
    extension, 546, 546f
    grip, 547, 547f
Strep throat
  in adults, 264
  in children, 792, 831t
Streptococcal pharyngitis
  in adults, 264
  in children, 792, 831t
Streptococcus pneumoniae pneumonia
    immunization, 323
Stress, family, 28
Stress incontinence, 445, 446, 480t–481t
  nursing process for, 29–30
  sample nursing process for, 29–30
Stridor, 331t
  audible, 306
  in infants, 757
Stroke
  anterior cerebral artery, 664t–665t
  definition of, 658
  dizziness or vertigo in, 624
  at a glance, 658–659
  middle cerebral artery, 659, 664t–665t
  posterior cerebral artery, 664t–665t
  posterior circulation, 664t–665t
  prevention of, 382, 657–658
  risk factors in
    primary prevention, 659, 659t–660t
    secondary prevention, 659
  types of, 664t–665t
  warning signs of, 658
  weakness in, 624
Stroke volume, 343
Structural coma, 663t
Stupor, 601, 653t
Sty, 241t

Subacromial bursa, 532, 532f
Subarachnoid hemorrhage
  headache from, 206t–207t, 623
  neck stiffness in, 656
Subclavian steal syndrome, blood pressure in, 112
Subconjunctival hemorrhage, 238t
Subcutaneous nodules, 524
Subcutaneous tissue, 154f, 155
Subjective data, 12
Subjective information, 13
Submandibular gland, 189, 190f
Submandibular gland ducts, 262, 263f
Submandibular nodes, 198, 199
Submental nodes, 198, 199
Subscapular bursa, 532
Subscapularis muscle, 531, 531t
Subscapular lymph nodes, 493, 493f, 504
Substance abuse, 611
Subtalar joint, 572, 573f
Subtalar joint range of motion, 575t, 576, 576f
Sudden infant death syndrome (SIDS), 756
Suicide, 611
Summarization, in interviewing, 50
Superficial cervical chain, 198, 199
Superficial inguinal nodes, 404, 415
Superficial reflexes, 623, 623t, 650–651
  abdominal, 650, 650f
  plantar response, 651, 651f
Superficial temporal artery, 189, 190f
Superficial thrombophlebitis, 413, 424t–425t
Superficial veins, of legs, 402, 402f
Superior vena cava, 338f, 339, 401
Supernumerary nipples, 492, 492f
Supernumerary teeth, 754
Supination
  elbow, 540, 540f, 540t
  forearm, 538f
Supinator muscle, 538, 538f
Supinator reflex, 647, 647f
Supraclavicular, 297
Supraclavicular lymph nodes
  in adults, 198, 199
    anatomy and physiology of, 190, 190f
  in children, 793
Suprapatellar pouch, 569, 569f
Suprapubic pain, 445
Supraspinatus muscle, 531, 531f, 532f
Supraspinatus muscle strength testing, 537f
Supraspinatus tendon, 532, 532f
Supraventricular premature contractions, 385t
Surrogate decision maker, 53
Surrogate informant, 53
Survey, general, 105–106, 131. See also specific
    systems
  in comprehensive physical examination, 101
  in elderly, 860
  in head-to-toe sequence sample, 723–726
  in infants, 744
Sutures, 750, 750f
Swallowing, thyroid in, 200–201, 200f–201f
Swan neck deformities, 589t
S wave, 346, 346f
Sweat glands, 154f, 156
Sweats, night, 118
Swing, 561, 561f

Symptom cone, 44
Symptoms. *See also specific symptoms and systems*
    characteristic, 12
    definition of, 12
    identifying, 16
    multiple, in confusing patient, 52
    past occurrences of, 66
    patient, meaning of, 596
    sequence and time course of, 43
    seven attributes of, 43, 65
    timing of, 245
Syncope, 626, 666t–667t
    cardiac, 626
    disorders resembling, 666t–667t
    in elderly, 842
    micturition, 666t–667t
    near syncope, 626
    presyncope, 277t, 626
    vasodepressor, 626, 666t–667t
    vasovagal, 626, 666t–667t
Synostosis, sagittal suture, 751
Synovial fluid, 519, 519f
Synovial joints
    anatomy and articulation in, 519, 519f, 519t
    condylar, 528, 528f
    structure of, 520, 520f
Synovial membrane, 519, 519f
Synovitis, 524
    knee, 570
    metacarpophalangeal joint, 544, 544f
Syphilis, 698
    congenital, on facies, 828t
    primary, in male, 714t
Syphilitic chancre, 177t
    in female, 711t
    in male, 714t
    on mouth, 283t
Systemic lupus erythematosus (SLE), skin in, 182t
Systems review, 64t, 69–71. *See also specific systems*
Systole
    extra heart sounds in, 372t, 389t
    jugular venous undulations in, 348, 348f, 349
    pressures and heart sounds in, 340–341, 340f, 341f
Systolic aortic murmur, in elderly, 845
Systolic blood pressure, in elderly, 860
Systolic clicks, 389t
Systolic ejection sound, early, 341, 389t
Systolic heart sounds, 395t
Systolic hypertension
    in elderly, 842
    isolated
        in adults, 114
        in elderly, 860, 864
Systolic murmurs
    in adults, 373
    in elderly, 845, 864
Systolic pressure, 348, 348f

T

Tachycardia
    from dehydration, 133
    paroxysmal supraventricular, in infants, 746, 824t

Tachypnea
    in adults, 124t
    in infants, 747
Tactile fremitus
    in anterior chest examination, 317, 317f
    chest disorders with, 332t–333t
    in infants, 758
    in posterior chest examination, 307–308, 308f
Talipes calcaneovalgus, 768
Talipes equinovarus, 768
Talkative patient, 53–54
Talocalcaneal joint, 572, 573f
Talocalcaneal joint range of motion, 575t, 576, 576f
Talofibular ligament
    anterior, 573, 573f
    posterior, 573, 573f
Talus, 572, 573f
Tandem walking, 637, 637f
Tangential lighting, 92–93, 92f
Tanner stages
    for females, 686, 694, 812t, 816t, 817f
    for males, 813t–814t
Tardive dyskinesia, 670t
Tarsal plates, 212, 212f
Tear fluid, 212
Tearing, excessive, 226
Teeth, in adults
    anatomy and physiology of, 262, 262f
    in elderly, 844
    findings in, 287t–288t
        abrasion with notching, 288t
        attrition, 288t
        erosion, 288t
        Hutchinson teeth, 288t
    physical examination of, 272
Teeth, in children
    abnormalities of, 831t
    eruption of, 755, 791, 791t
    school-aged, 790
    staining of, 791, 831t
    supernumerary, 754
Telangiectatic nevus, 748, 749t
Temperature, 116–118
    axillary, 116, 118
    in children
        infants, 747
        school-aged, 116–118, 785
    chills, 118
    educating patients on, 122–123
    in elderly, 842, 861
    fever, 118
    hypothermia, 116
        educating patients on, 123
        in elderly, 842, 861
    leg, in arterial insufficiency, 411
    night sweats, 118
    oral, 116–117
    oral thermometers for, 117
    rectal
        in adults, 116, 117
        in infants, 747
    sensation of, 621, 621f, 640
    skin, 118, 159

temporal artery, 117–118
    tympanic membrane, 117
Temperature instability, in newborn, 747
Temporal arteritis
    in elderly, 846
    headache from, 206t–207t
Temporal artery, superficial, 189, 190f
Temporal artery temperature, 117–118
Temporal hemianopsia, 223, 223f
Temporalis (temporal) muscles, 528, 528f, 529
Temporomandibular joint, 527–529
    anatomy of, 527–528, 527f
    muscle groups and nerves in, 528, 528f, 529
    physical examination of, 528–529, 528f
    10-minute geriatric screener, 853, 853t–854t, 865
Tender abdomen, 453, 485t–486t
Tendinitis, 521, 524. *See also specific types*
Tendons, 518
Tennis elbow, 539
Tenosynovitis, 521
Tension headaches, 205t
Teres minor muscle, 531, 531f
Terminal hair, 155
Termination phase, of interview, 37, 46
Terry nails, 185t
Tertiary prevention, 6, 7
Testes (testicles)
    abnormalities of, 715t
    in adults, 699–700, 699f
    in elderly, 846
    small, 715t
    undescended
        in adults, 836t
        in infants, 765, 836t
Testicular self-examination, 708–709, 709f
Testicular tumor, 715t
Testosterone, 700
Test selection and use, 30–31. *See also specific systems*
Tetanus, 837t
Tetralogy of Fallot, murmurs in, 833t
Thalamus, 613f, 614, 614f
Thelarche, premature, 763
Thenar atrophy, 544, 548–549, 590t
Therapeutic communication techniques, 46–51. *See also* Interviewing
    active listening in, 47
    empathic responses in, 49
    guided questioning in, 47–49
    nonverbal communication in, 49
    patient empowerment in, 51
    reassurance in, 50
    summarization in, 50
    transitions in, 50–51
    validation in, 49–50
Thermometers, oral, 117
Thinking
    abstract, 608
    critical (*See* Critical thinking)
Third heart sound (S₃)
    in elderly, 845, 864
    in infants, 762
Thoracic curvature, 550, 552f, 554f
Thoracic kyphoscoliosis, 329t

Thoracic kyphosis, 554
Thorax
    deformities of, 306–307, 316, 329t
    in health assessment
        anterior, 726
        posterior, 725
    normal adult, 306–307, 316, 329t
    physical examination of, 102
    in school-aged children, 793–794, 794f
Thorax and lungs
    in adults, 102
    in children
        infants, 756–759
        school aged, 793–794, 794f
    in elderly, 844–845, 863
Thought, 604–605
Thought content, 599t, 604–605
Thought processes, 599t, 604–605. *See also*
        Mental status
Thrills
    carotid, 357
    in infants, 760–761, 761f
    palpation for, 363
Throat, 249, 274. *See also* Mouth and pharynx
Thromboangiitis obliterans
    pain in, 424t–425t
    wrist pulses in, 416f, 417
Thrombocytopenic purpura, skin in, 182t
Thrombophlebitis, 398
Thrombophlebitis, superficial, 413, 424t–425t
Thrombosis. *See also* Myocardial infarction
    acute peripheral vascular, 424t–425t
    deep venous, 398–399, 424t–425t
        Homan sign in, 31
        prevention and early identification of,
            422–423
        venous tenderness in, 413
    venous, 398
Thrush
    in children, 830t
    in infants, 755
    on palate, 285t
    on tongue, 289t
Thumb. *See also* Hands
    adduction of, 549, 549f
    range of motion of, 549, 549f
Thyroglossal duct cysts, 754
Thyroid cartilage, 195, 195f
Thyroid dysfunction. *See also* Hyperthyroidism;
        Hypothyroidism
    enlargement, 209t
    multinodular goiter, 209t
    signs and symptoms of, 209t
    singular nodule, 209t
Thyroid gland
    anatomy and physiology of, 195, 195f
    enlargement of, 209t
    inspection of, 200–201
    location of, 199
    palpation of, 201–202, 201f
    physical examination of, 200f–201f, 201–202
    swallowing on, 200–201, 200f–201f
Thyroid isthmus, 195, 195f, 201, 202
Thyrotoxicosis, children's facies in, 829t
Tibia, 572, 573f

Tibial artery, posterior, 401, 401f
Tibial pulse, in infants, 760
Tibial tuberosity, 566f, 567, 569, 569f
Tibia torsion, in infants, 768
Tibia vara, 800
Tibiofemoral joint, 567, 568–569, 568f, 569f
Tibiotalar joint, 572, 573f
Tibiotalar joint range of motion, 575, 575t, 576f
Tics, 671t
Time, of history, 64
Time course, of symptoms, 43
Tinea capitis
    in adults, 184t
    in children, 816t
Tinea corporis, 172t
Tinea faciale, 172t
Tinea tonsurans, 184t
Tinea versicolor, 170t, 171t
Tinel's sign (test), 549, 549f
Tinnitus, 254
TMJ syndrome, 528
Tobacco use. *See also* Smoking
    cessation of, 321–322
    sample nursing process for, 28–29
Toe-in walking, in children, 801
Toenail, ingrown, 592t
Toes, abnormalities of, 592t
Tolerance, 121
Tongue, in adults
    anatomy and physiology of, 262–263, 263f
    fasciculations in, 634
    findings in, 289t–290t
        aphthous ulcer (canker sore), 272, 272f,
            290t
        cancer, 273, 273t
        candidiasis, 289t
        carcinoma, floor of mouth, 290t
        fissured tongue, 289t
        geographic tongue, 289t
        hairy leukoplakia, 289t
        hairy tongue, 289t
        leukoplakia, 290t
        mucous patch of syphilis, 290t
        smooth tongue (atrophic glossitis), 289t
        tori mandibulares, 290t
        varicose veins, 290t
    physical examination of, 272, 272f, 273f
    sore, 265
Tongue, in children
    infants, 755
    school-aged, 791
Tongue tie, 755
Tonic-clonic seizure, 669t
Tonic neck reflex, asymmetric, 773t
Tonsillar fossa, 263, 263f
Tonsillar (lymph) nodes, 198, 199
Tonsils
    exudative, 284t
    large normal, 284t
    in school-aged children, 792
Toothache, 265
Tophi, ear, 278t
Tori mandibulares, 290t
Torsion of spermatic cord, 716t
Torsion of tibia, in infants, 768

Torticollis
    in adults, 556, 585t
    in infants, 751
Tortuous atherosclerotic aorta, 864
Torus palatinus, 273, 285t
Total-body skin examination, 166
Touch
    crude, 621, 621f
    fine, 621, 621f
    light, 640
Toxic-metabolic coma, 663t
Trachea, 199–200, 297, 298f
Tracheal deviation, 200
Tracheal rings, 195, 195f
Tracheobronchitis
    chest pain in, 327t
    cough in, 326t
Tragus, 250, 250f
Transcultural perspectives, 83–84
Transient ischemic attack (TIA), 658. *See also*
        Stroke
    dizziness or vertigo in, 624
    prevention of, 657–658
    weakness in, 624
Transitions, in interviewing, 50–51
Transposition of the great arteries, murmurs in,
        834t
Transverse foramen, 551, 551f
Transverse tarsal joint range of motion, 575t,
        576, 576f
Trapezius muscle
    fasciculations of, 634
    physical examination of, 553, 553f
Traube space, 461
Traumatic brain injury (TBI)
    health history in, 193
    prevention of, 203–204
Traumatic flail chest, 329t
Treatments, 65. *See also specific disorders and
        systems*
    definition of, 12
    self-treatment in, 65
Tremors
    in adults, 627, 670t–671t
    in elderly, 848, 866
    intention, 636
Trendelenburg sign, in children, 801, 801f
Trendelenburg test, 421
Triceps muscle, 538, 538t
Triceps reflex, 647, 647f
Trichilemmal cyst, of ear, 278t
Trichomonal vaginitis, 712t
Trichotillomania, 184t
Tricuspid area, 370f
Tricuspid regurgitation, 391t
Tricuspid valve, 339, 339f
Trigeminal neuralgia, 206t–207t, 632
Trigger finger, 590t
Tripod position, in children, 793, 793f
Trochanteric bursa, 559f, 560f, 561
Trochanteric bursitis, 521
Trochlear groove, 567
True negative, 31
True positive, 31
Trunk incurvation reflex, 774t

Tuberculosis, pulmonary
 cough in, 326t
 hemoptysis in, 326t
 night sweats in, 118
Tunica vaginalis, 699f, 700
Tuning forks, 96, 96f
Turbinates, 256–257, 257f, 270, 270f
Turgor, skin
 in adults, 159
 dehydration and, 133
 in infants, 748
Turgor recoil, 133
T wave, 346, 346f
12th rib, 294, 294f
20/200 vision, 221, 222
Two-point discrimination, 642, 642f
Tympanic membranes
 in adults, 250f, 251
 in children, 787–788, 788f
Tympanic membrane temperature, 117
Tympanosclerosis, 279t

U

Ulcer, 177t
 ankles and feet, 427t
 aphthous, 272, 272f, 290t
 in arterial insufficiency of legs, 427t
 decubitus
  in adults, 161, 162t–163t, 183t, 427t
  in elderly, 862
 neuropathic, 427t, 592t
 origin of, 406
 peptic, 472t–473t
 skin, 177t
 stasis, 177t, 427t
 in venous insufficiency, 177t, 427t
Ulnar artery, 400f, 401
Ulnar artery patency, 417–418
Ulnar deviation, wrist, 546f, 546t
Ulnar nerve, in elbow, 539, 539f
Ulnar pulse, 416, 416f
Umbilical hernia, 482t, 764
Umbo, 251, 251f, 268, 268f
Underbite, 791
Undernutrition in elderly, 860, 861
Understanding, in health assessment, 5, 9
Underweight, 137
Undescended testes
 in adults, 836t
 in infants, 766, 836t
Unexplained symptoms, 596
Universal precautions, 101
Upper airway obstruction, in children, 793
Upper motor neuron lesions, 619
Upper motor neurons, 618
Upper palpebral conjunctiva, 233, 233f
Upper respiratory infection
 in children
  infants, nasal flaring in, 757
  school-aged, 794
 cough in, 301
Ureteral colic, 447
Ureteral pain, 447, 447f
Urethra, 685f

Urethral meatus
 female, 684, 684f
 male, 699, 699f
Urethritis
 gonococcal, 706
 nongonococcal, 706
Urge incontinence, 446, 480t–481t
Urinary frequency, 445, 479t
Urinary incontinence, 446, 480t–481t
 in elderly, 858–859
 functional, 446, 480t–481t
 overflow, 446, 480t–481t
 prevention of, 471
 stress, 445, 446, 480t–481t
  nursing process for, 29–30
 urge, 446, 480t–481t
Urinary system, 71
Urinary urgency, 445, 479t
Urination
 pain on, 445, 479t
 problems with, male, 704–705
Urticaria
 in adults, 174t
 in children, 826t
U.S.D.A. MyPlate, 128, 147t
Uterine prolapse, 711t
Uterus
 in adults, 685, 685f
 in elderly, 847
Uvula, 263, 263f

V

Vaccine-preventable diseases, 837t
Vagina
 in adults, 684–685, 684f, 685f
 in elderly, 847
Vaginal bleeding, in children, 799
Vaginal discharge
 in adults, 690, 712t
 in children, 835t
  adolescents, 815
  school-aged, 799
Vaginal itching, 690
Vaginismus, 692
Vaginitis
 candidal, 712t
 trichomonal, 712t
Vaginosis, bacterial, 712t
Validation, in interviewing, 49–50
Validity, 90
Value-belief, 72t
Values, 82
Valves, heart, 339, 339f
Valvular heart disease, 845. See also specific types
Varicella, 182t, 837t
Varicocele of spermatic cord, 716t
Varicose veins, 290t, 416, 416f
Varicosities, saphenous vein, 416, 416f
Varus, in children, 836t
Vasa vasorum, 400
Vascular disease. See Cardiovascular disease;
  Peripheral vascular system; specific types
Vascular lesions, of skin, 179t
Vascular markings, 748, 749t

Vascular system. See Cardiovascular system;
  Peripheral vascular system
Vas deferens, 699f, 700
Vasodepressor syncope, 626, 666t–667t
Vasovagal syncope, 626, 666t–667t
Vectors, electrical, 346, 346f
Veins, 401–402, 402f. See also specific veins
Vein walls, 344
Vellus hair, 155
Venereal wart, 711t
Venous disorders, painful peripheral, 424t–425t
Venous hum
 abdominal, 483t
 in adults, 395t, 483t
 in children, 795, 795f, 795t
Venous insufficiency, chronic, 399
 advanced, 426t
 deep, pain in, 424t–425t
 edema in, 428t
 of leg
  characteristics of, 426t
  physical examination of, 411, 424t–427t
 stasis ulcer of, 177t, 427t
Venous intima, 401
Venous media, 401
Venous obstruction, prominent veins in, 409
Venous stasis, 406
Venous thrombosis, 398
Venous valve competency, 421
Ventral hernias, 466
Ventricle
 left, 338, 338f
 right, 337, 337f
Ventricular failure, left
 cough in, 326t
 hemoptysis in, 326t
Ventricular premature contractions, 385t
Ventricular septal defect, murmurs in
 in adults, 391t
 congenital, 834t
 in infants, 763
Verruca plana, in children, 826t
Verruca vulgaris
 in adults, 592t
 in children, 826t
Vertebrae, 551, 551f
Vertebral arch, 551, 551f
Vertebral body, 551, 551f
Vertebral column, 551, 552f
Vertebral foramen, 551, 551f
Vertebral line, 295, 296, 296f
Vertebral prominens, 295, 295t
Vertical group, 404, 404f
Vertigo
 ear and, 254–255, 277t
 with hearing loss, 633
 neurological, 623–624, 664t–665t (See also
  Stroke)
Vesicles, 160, 174t
Vestibule
 of nose, 256, 256f, 257f
 of vagina, 684, 684f
Vibration sense
 in adults, 621, 621f, 640–641
 in elderly, 848

Violence, family, 75–76
Viral exanthems, 182t
Viral rhinitis, nose in, 271
Visceral pain, 435–436, 436f
Visceral pleura, 298
Visceral tenderness, 485t
Vision impairment, interviewing patient with, 57
Vision screening
    in adults, 234–235
    in elderly, 869
Vision tests, 221–223
    eyelids, 223–224, 237t
    peripheral vision, 222–223, 222f, 223f
Visual acuity
    in adults, 221
        distal, 221, 221f
        elderly, 844
        in health assessment, 728
        near vision, 222
    in children, 786, 786t
Visual fields, 214, 214f
    in children, 787, 787f
    by confrontation, 630
    by confrontation, peripheral, 222–223, 222f, 223f
    defects of, 236t
        cranial nerves in, 630
        physical examination of, 222–223, 222f, 223f
Visual loss, sudden unilateral, 218
Visual milestones of infancy, 753t
Visual pathway, 214–215, 215f
Vital signs, in adults, 101, 106, 109–118. See also specific signs
    blood pressure, 109–115
    elderly, 842, 860–861
    in health assessment, 723
    health promotion and, 122–123
    heart rate and rhythm, 116, 116f, 384t, 385t
    pain, 106, 118–122
    recording findings on, 122
    respiratory rate and rhythm, 116, 124t
Vital signs, in children
    adolescents, 810
    infants, 744, 746–747
        blood pressure, 746
        pulse, 746–747, 746t
        respiratory rate, 747
        temperature, 747
    school-aged, 783–785
        blood pressure, 783–784, 784t
        pulse, 785, 785t
        respiratory rate, 785
        temperature, 116–118, 785
Vitamin A deficiency, 133
Vitamin D deficiency, 134
Vitamin deficiencies, gums in, 133
Vitiligo, 170t, 173t

Vitreous body, 213, 213f
Vitreous floaters, 232
Vitreous humor, 213
Vocabulary, 607
Vocal cord paralysis, 633
Voice sounds, transmitted, 315, 330t, 332t–333t
Voiding, involuntary, 445
Volume overload, 347
Vomiting, 440
Vulva, 684
Vulvar lesions, 690, 711t
Vulvovaginal symptoms, 690

W

Waist circumference, 133, 134
Walking
    tandem, 637, 637f
    toe-in, in children, 801
    on toes and heels, 637
"Walk test," 320
Warts
    in children, 826t
    genital, in men, 714t
    plantar, 592t
    venereal, 711t
Weakness. See also Muscle strength
    in general appearance, 108
    muscular, 526
    neurological, 624–625
Weak pulse
    blood pressure measurement with, 114–115
    grading of, 410
    palpation of, 415
    in peripheral vascular disorders, 429t
Weber test, 269, 269f, 633
Weight. See also Body mass index (BMI); Obesity
    in adults
        cardiovascular disease and, 383
        counseling on, 136–137
        in health assessment, 723
        measurement of, 132, 132f
        on musculoskeletal system, 578–579
        rapid changes in, 129
    in elderly, 861
    exercise for control of, 139–140, 140t
    history taking on changes in, 129–131
    in infants, 745
    in school-aged children, 782, 783t
Weight gain, 127
    causes of, 127, 142t
    nutrition and, 129
    from water retention, 129
Weight loss, 127
    exercise for, 139–140, 140t
    nutrition and, 129
Wernicke aphasia, 603, 674t

Wharton ducts, 262, 263f
Wheal, 174t
Wheezes, 300
    in adults, 314–315, 314t, 331t
    in infants, 759
Wheezing, 300–301, 306, 758
Whiplash, neck pain from, 585t
Whispered pectoriloquy, 315, 330t
Whispered voice test, 633
White bands, nail, 186t
White coat hypertension, 115
White matter, 614, 614f
White spots, in nails, 186t
Wisdom tooth, 262f
Working phase, of interview, 37, 41–46
    diagnostic hypotheses in, 44
    disease/illness distinction model, 44
    emotional cues in, 42
    establishing agenda in, 41
    negotiating a plan in, 46
    patient's perspective on illness in, 42, 45–46
    patient's story in
        expanding and clarifying, 43–44
        inviting, 41–42
    seven attributes of symptoms in, 43
    shared understanding of problem in, 44–46
Wrist, 541–550
    bony structures of, 541, 541f
    carpal tunnel of, 543, 543f
    flexor retinaculum of, 543, 543f
    joints of, 541f, 542, 542f
    muscle groups of, 542
    physical examination of, 543–548
        inspection in, 543–544
        maneuvers in, 547–548, 547f, 548f
        muscle strength tests of
            extension, 546, 546t
            grip, 547, 547f
        palpation in, 544–545, 544f
        range of motion in, 545, 546f, 546t
    tendons and tendon sheaths of, 543
Wrist extension test, 546, 546f

X

Xanthelasma, 241t
Xiphoid process, 432f, 433, 433f

Y

Young children. See School-aged children

Z

Zoster (herpes)
    in adults, 160, 174t, 182t
    in elderly, 862
    immunization for, in elderly, 870
Z scores, 580